Hodgkin's Disease

This volume is published as part of a long-standing cooperative program between the Harvard University Press and the Commonwealth Fund, a philanthropic foundation, to encourage the publication of significant scholarly books in medicine and health.

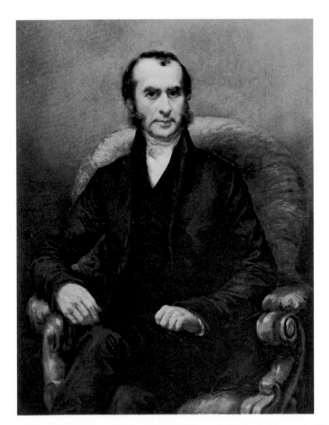

Thomas Hodgkin (1798–1866). The original of this portrait hangs in the Gordon Museum, Guy's Hospital and Medical School, London, and is reproduced here by permission of the Curator.

Henry S. Kaplan

Hodgkin's Disease

SECOND EDITION

Harvard University Press
Cambridge, Massachusetts
London, England
1980

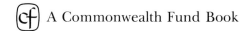 A Commonwealth Fund Book

Library of Congress Cataloging in Publication Data

Kaplan, Henry S   1918–
    Hodgkin's disease.

    "A Commonwealth Fund book."
    Bibliography: p.
    Includes index.
    1. Hodgkin's disease. [DNLM: 1. Hodgkin's
disease. WH500 K17h]
RC644.K35   1980   616.4'2   79-16054
ISBN 0-674-40485-8

Dedicated to the Memory of
David A. Karnofsky, M.D. (1914–1969)
Physician, Scientist, Scholar, Teacher, Friend

Preface to the Second Edition

A torrent of clinical and laboratory research has already rendered obsolete some sections of the first edition of this book, published in 1972. Thus, despite the immensity of the task, the need for this second edition seemed inescapable. The changes have been so extensive that this is in many respects a new book, rather than merely a revision of the first, despite the fact that it has been possible to retain essentially intact sections devoted to historical aspects, sites of presentation of disease, and staging. The literature survey has been carried through 1978, and the bibliography has been greatly expanded. Chapter 2 on etiology and epidemiology has been extensively revised and enlarged to encompass recent developments such as the controversy concerning the transmissibility of Hodgkin's disease. Major new sections in Chapter 3 are devoted to recent advances in cell culture, surface marker characterization, cytogenetics, and other topics bearing on the nature and origin of the Sternberg-Reed cell. Technological advances in diagnostic radiology and nuclear medicine, such as computed tomographic scanning, ultrasonography, and improved radioisotopic scans with some of the newer radionuclides, have been added to Chapter 5. Perhaps the greatest metamorphosis has occurred in Chapter 6, which has more than doubled in size to accommodate the profusion of recent laboratory studies on mechanisms of impairment of cell-mediated immunity in patients with Hodgkin's disease. The three chapters formerly devoted to therapeutics have been extensively revised and are presented in an entirely different sequence. Chapter 9 was formerly devoted to general therapeutic considerations, followed by chapters on radiotherapy and chemotherapy, respectively. For a number of cogent reasons, it has seemed preferable to present the chapters on radiotherapy and chemotherapy first, and then to devote an entirely new Chapter 11 to a detailed analysis of the evidence bearing on selection of optimal treatment and to the presentation of current therapeutic recommendations. Chapter 11 also includes new sections on combined modality therapy and the management of relapsing disease. Although Chapter 12 on prognosis is structurally unchanged, data on survival and freedom from relapse and data on the influence on prognosis of a multiplicity of factors have been updated and made more comprehensive. To conserve space, material that has become obsolete or is no longer relevant has been pruned as thoroughly as possible. For example, the histopathologic classification presented by Cross in 1969, which has clearly not gained widespread acceptance, has been deleted, although some of the original illustrations have been retained and reclassified.

It seems appropriate to comment on the strong emphasis throughout the book on Stanford University Medical Center data. This has been a deliberate policy, which stems not from bias or local chauvinism but rather from the fact that the clinical data which have been collected here at Stanford during the past twenty years are particularly comprehensive, homogeneous, coherent, and reliable. Patients have been examined by the same group of clinicians and subjected to staging laparotomy with splenectomy almost exclusively by a single group of surgeons; biopsies and tissue samples obtained at laparotomy have been examined and classified histopathologically by a single group of pathologists, lymphangiograms evaluated by a single group of diagnostic oncologic radiologists, and radiotherapy and chemotherapy administered by a closely integrated team of radiation oncologists and medical oncologists. There are only a few other institutions in the world in which data of similar quality are available, and these have been cited wherever possible. It is recognized that the picture of Hodgkin's disease that emerges from these data is particularly relevant to North America and Western Europe, and that the disease as it occurs in other parts of the world may well differ with respect to such features as age-specific incidence, relative frequency of histopathologic types, stage distribution at presentation, response to treatment, and prognosis. It is to be hoped that the gaps in our information concerning Hodgkin's disease in Asia, Africa, and Latin America will be filled during the years ahead by systematic, carefully conducted clinical studies from the major medical centers of those continents.

This new edition could not have been written without the help and cooperation of many organizations and individuals. I am deeply grateful to the Rockefeller Foundation for the privilege of having been a visiting scholar at its cultural center, the Villa Serbelloni, at Bellagio, Italy, during the late summer of 1976. The serene, cloistered atmosphere of the villa and the indescribable beauty of its setting on a promontory overlooking Lake Como resulted in a month of extraordinary productivity, during which the first six chapters of this book were extensively rewritten. My grateful acknowledgment is also extended to the Commonwealth Fund, which once again has defrayed a major part of the publication costs of this book. Colleagues at Stanford and elsewhere throughout the world have generously made available material from manuscripts prior to publication or have given approval for the reproduction of selected illustrations from their published papers. Thanks are also extended to the editors of the journals in which those illustrations first appeared. Many colleagues at Stanford have been extremely helpful. The series of randomized clinical trials that are described in detail in Chapter 11, which were supported by research grant CA-05838 from the National Cancer Institute, National Institutes of Health, D.H.E.W., were initiated and have been conducted to the present time in collaboration with Saul A. Rosenberg, M.D., Professor of Medicine and Radiology and Chief of the Division of Medical Oncology. During many of those years, he and I were privileged to have the assistance in the conduct of those trials of Eli Glatstein, M.D., formerly Assistant Professor of Radiology in the Division of Radiation Therapy and now Chief, Radiation Branch, National Cancer Institute, and of Carol S. Portlock, M.D., formerly Assistant Professor of Medicine in the Division of Medical Oncology and now Assistant Professor of Medicine, Yale University School of Medicine.

Other colleagues who have provided invaluable cooperation and assistance include: Richard T. Hoppe, M.D., Assistant Professor of Radiology in the Division of Radiation Therapy; Ronald A. Castellino, M.D., Associate Professor of Radiology in the Division of Diagnostic Radiology; Ronald F. Dorfman, M.D., Professor of Pathology and Co-Director of the Laboratory of Surgical Pathology; and Thomas A. Nelsen, M.D., Professor of Surgery. Anna Varghese, data aide, and Polly Butterfield, programmer, helped with the retrieval and analysis of clinical data from our computerized files. The talented staff of the Medical Illustration unit, and in particular Charlene Levering, Merele Colten, and Deborah Warburg, have applied their skills to the production of the handsome new figures on survival and freedom from relapse and to many other new illustrations in the later chapters of the book. Mrs. Sandra Malko volunteered untold hours in Lane Medical Library to assure that the literature survey would be up to date. The enormous job of typing the new manuscript, of integrating new typescript pages with altered pages of the first edition, of keeping track of correspondence with authors and journals concerning the reproduction of illustrations, and of attending to countless other details has been accomplished by Mrs. Ann Cooney with remarkable skill, speed, and accuracy. The editorial staff of Harvard University Press have once again cooperated fully to expedite the production of a handsome, well-edited volume. Finally, my gratitude goes once again to my family, and particularly to my wife, for the forbearance and understanding that have so vitally assisted me through the arduous effort entailed in this new edition.

Henry S. Kaplan

Stanford, California
May 1979

Preface to the First Edition

There has been no comprehensive book on Hodgkin's disease since the classical work of Jackson and Parker published in 1947. Many significant advances in our understanding of the fundamental nature, epidemiology, histopathologic classification, diagnostic evaluation, clinical staging, radiotherapy, chemotherapy, and prognosis of this fascinating disease have long since rendered their book obsolete for contemporary physicians. It seemed desirable to undertake the formidable task of writing this book, therefore, in an effort to bring together all of the major lines of investigation and the new data derived therefrom between the covers of a single reference source. A second major purpose was to provide an up-to-date compendium on the optimal management of the disease for practicing physicians and students. Although it was my intention initially to approach the task more as editor than as author and to request a number of other colleagues to prepare individual chapters, this approach was superseded by the decision to make this a solo effort, in the hope of gaining from the presentation of a single, cohesive point of view, whatever might be lost in the authoritativeness or comprehensiveness of certain of the chapters of the book. Moreover, I now stand solely responsible for the viewpoints concerning optimal medical management of the disease that appear herein.

An attempt has been made to cover the relevant medical literature assiduously through December 1970. However, there seemed no virtue in attempting an encyclopedic or exhaustive treatment of the vast published literature. In particular, much of the older, richly interesting and varied writing on Hodgkin's disease has been dealt with selectively; the reader interested in pursuing this material in greater detail is referred to the excellent reviews by Hoster et al. (1948) and by Wallhauser (1933). In more recent times, papers that merely added additional confirmatory data to extensively documented topics have been deliberately omitted. Undoubtedly, some inadvertent omissions have also occurred, for which my apologies are due.

This book would not have been published without the cooperation and assistance of a great many individuals. In particular, the contributions of the following persons are acknowledged: Saul A. Rosenberg, M.D., Ronald F. Dorfman, M.D., Malcolm A. Bagshaw, M.D., J. Robert Stewart, M.D., James R. Eltringham, M.D., Eli Glatstein, M.D., Gordon R. Ray, M.D., Paul Wolf, M.D., and other colleagues and fellows at Stanford University Medical Center, for their collaboration in our clinical investigations of Hodgkin's disease and for many helpful suggestions and criticisms; Henry Rappaport, M.D., Robert J. Lukes, M.D., Stephen B. Strum, M.D., Vincent T. DeVita, Jr., M.D., M. Vera Peters, M.D., Professor Sir David W. Smithers, Professor K. Musshoff, and numerous other colleagues elsewhere who have critically reviewed portions of the manuscript, provided helpful suggestions and criticisms, and/or generously permitted the reproduction in this volume of illustrative material from their own published works, as well as the many editors and publishers of those articles, who also gave their permission for the reproduction herein of such illustrative material; the late Professor S. J. De Navasquez, Curator, Gordon Museum, Guy's Hospital, London, and his technical assistant, Mr. J. Dawes, for making available a color photograph of the excellent portrait of Thomas Hodgkin which hangs in the Gordon Museum, photographs of some of Hodgkin's original gross specimens, and histologic sections freshly prepared from them; Mr. W. Hill, Librarian of the Wilks Library, Guy's Hospital, London, for his assistance in providing biographical material concerning Thomas Hodgkin and Sir Samuel Wilks; Peter J. Dawson, M.D.; Morton D. Bogdonoff, M.D., Chief Editor of the *Archives of Internal Medicine;* and B. J. Harries, M.B., B.S., FRCS., Dean of the University College Hospital Medical School, London, for making available the color photograph of the splendid painting by Robert Carswell, and granting permission for its reproduction herein as Figure 1.6; the Commonwealth Fund, New York City; its former Vice President for Medical Affairs, now emeritus, Dr. Colin Mac-Leod; his successor in that position, Dr. Robert J. Glaser; and Mr. Terrence Keenan of its staff, for a special grant which has helped to defray the costs of translations, the reproduction of early historical material, and the generous use of medical illustrations and reproductions of roentgenograms throughout the book; Harvard University Press, its biomedical editor, Mr. Murray Chastain, and the Press staff for their splendid cooperation in expediting the publication of the book, as well as for its handsome format; Miss Jill Leland, for her skillful and resourceful preparation of the many charts, graphs, and medical drawings; Mr. Jules Souté, Photographer of the Department of Radiology, for his expert photographs of the many roentgenograms, charts, and other illustrations; Mrs. Corinne Simonini, chief file room clerk of the Department of Radiology, for making available, and later refiling, the literally dozens of X-ray film folders of patients with Hodgkin's disease from which the roentgenograms reproduced herein were selected; Mrs. Nadine Cline, who skillfully typed portions of the manuscript; my secretary, Miss Ruth McConnell, who typed the remainder of the final manuscript, as well as all of the earlier rough draft versions, and conducted and carefully kept track of the voluminous correspondence with authors, editors, and publishers; Miss Clara Manson, chief librarian, and Mrs. Anna Hoen, reference librarian, of the Lane Library, Stanford University School of Medicine, for their assistance with the bibliographic material; and finally, my wife and family for their patience, tolerance, and understanding during the nearly three years of arduous effort which the writing of this book has entailed. To all of them, and the many others not specifically named here, I extend my warm and grateful appreciation.

Henry S. Kaplan

Stanford, California
February 1971

Contents

Tables

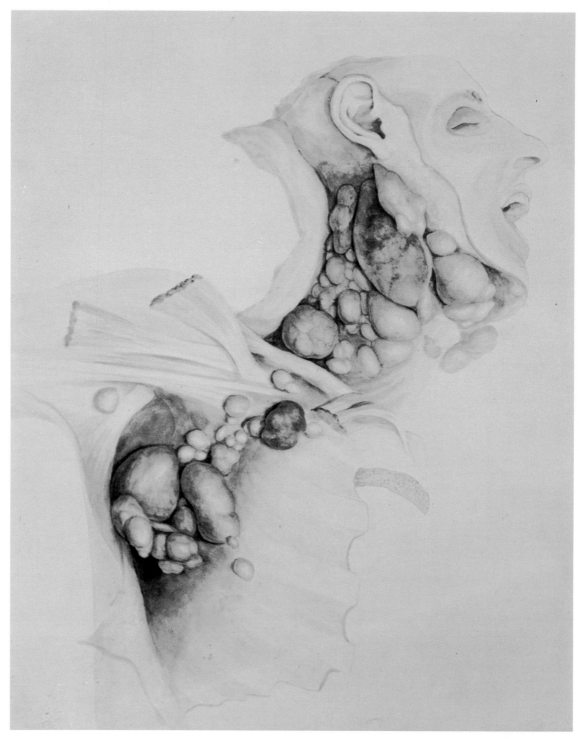

Figure 1.6 Water color painting by Robert Carswell (1793–1857) of a patient seen by him at postmortem examination in 1828; this case was the seventh described in Hodgkin's paper. Carswell's five magnificent water color paintings are the property of University College Medical School, University of London, and were rediscovered by Dr. Peter J. Dawson, who published three of them in an article in the *Archives of Internal Medicine* (121:288–290, 1968). Permission to reproduce Dawson's figure 1 was given by the Dean of University College Hospital Medical School, by Dr. Dawson, and by the Editor of the *Journal of the American Medical Association* and affiliated publications.

Chapter 1

Historical Aspects

The sequential recognition of the various entities of the leukemia-lymphoma family and the intense controversies concerning their nature and etiology constitute one of the most fascinating chapters of medical history. For all practical purposes, the story begins in 1832 with the description by Hodgkin of several cases of a disease which was later to bear his name. The unfolding of the subject may not have ended even at this late date, since a new type of lymphoma was described as recently as 1958 by Burkitt.

Thomas Hodgkin was a scholar dedicated to the careful correlation of clinical medicine and morbid anatomy in the delineation of disease. A perusal of his life history, as recounted by Wilks (1909), Hale White (1924), Cameron (1954), Foxon (1966), Thompson Hancock (1968), and others, is most rewarding. It is not generally recognized, for example, that Hodgkin, in a paper entitled "On the Retroversion of the Valves of the Aorta" (*London Medical Gazette* 3: 433–443, 1829) clearly described aortic insufficiency some five years before Corrigan. He was also a century ahead of his time with respect to his interest in the social aspects of medicine and, in particular, to the medical problems associated with poverty and with underprivileged groups such as the American Indian and the African native. A complete bibliography of Hodgkin's writings, reflecting the eclectic spectrum of his interests, has been assembled by Mr. W. Hill, Librarian of the Wilks Library, Guy's Hospital Medical School (1966).

Hodgkin's historic paper (Fig. 1.1), entitled "On Some Morbid Appearances of the Absorbent Glands and Spleen," was read before the Medical-Chirurgical Society on January 10 and January 24, 1832. Hodgkin's characteristic modesty emerges in the very first paragraph: "The morbid alterations of structure which I am about to describe are probably familiar to many practical morbid anatomists, since they can scarcely have failed to have fallen under their observation in the course of cadaveric inspection. They have not, as far as I am aware,

ON SOME

MORBID APPEARANCES

OF

THE ABSORBENT GLANDS

AND

SPLEEN.

BY DR. HODGKIN.

PRESENTED

BY DR. R. LEE.

READ JANUARY 10TH AND 24TH, 1832.

THE morbid alterations of structure which I am about to describe are probably familiar to many

Figure 1.1 Heading on cover page of Hodgkin's classic article (*Medico-Chirurgical Transactions* 17:68–114, 1832).

been made the subject of special attention, on which account I am induced to bring forward a few cases in which they have occurred to myself, trusting that I shall at least escape severe or general censure, even though a sentence or two should be produced from some existing work, couched in such concise but expressive language, as to render needless the longer details with which I shall trespass on the time of my hearers."

He was probably correct in believing that others had observed the same condition. For example, David Craigie, in his *Elements of General and Pathological Anatomy* (1828, p. 250) in a discussion on the pathology of the lymphatic glands, makes the following statement in a section entitled "Enlargement and Induration (Vascular Sarcoma)": "Either after repeated attacks of inflammation, alternating with resolution, or with a slow and indistinct form of the disease, a gland, or a cluster of glands gradually enlarges, and, resisting all means of resolution, becomes unusually hard . . . The great hardness, and the malignant tendency of this growth, have procured for it from most authors the ominous names of *scirrhus* and *cancer*. Though correct enough for all practical purposes, these epithets are not justified by the anatomical characters."

Craigie mentions a case described by Cruickshank (1786) "in which the tracheobronchial lymphatic glands were affected with this morbid change to such extent as to cause fatal suffocation." However, there is little to indicate that Craigie recognized the distinctive nature of this disease process, whereas Hodgkin's studies had convinced him that he was dealing with a primary disease of the absorbent (lymphatic) glands and not some banal secondary response to an obscure inflammatory condition. He states on pages 85 and 86: "this enlargement of the glands appeared to be a primi-

tive [i.e., primary] affection of those bodies, rather than the result of an irritation propagated to them from some ulcerated surface or other inflamed texture . . . Unless the word inflammation be allowed to have a more indefinite and loose meaning, this affection . . . can hardly be attributed to that cause."

Hodgkin described briefly the clinical histories and gross postmortem findings on six cases (Figs. 1.2, 1.3, 1.4, 1.5) and added a description of a seventh case seen by Carswell (Fig. 1.6). He was aware that the patient in his case 1 had a history of exposure to tuberculosis and had evidence of tuberculosis at autopsy; he was also aware that his patient in case 3 had a history of syphilis treated with mercurials. Yet he included these with the others, suggesting that he believed them to be valid examples of what was later designated as Hodgkin's disease.

In 1838, in a lengthy paper on abdominal tumors, Richard Bright, at that time one of the

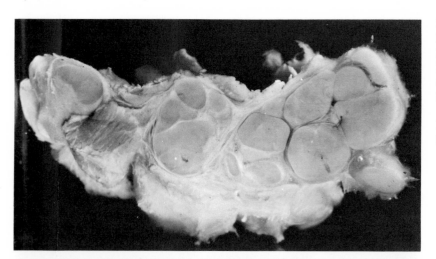

Figure 1.2   Gross specimen of enlarged lymph nodes from Hodgkin's original case 2, Ellenborough King. The photograph of the specimen (Gordon Museum catalog no. 4768) and those of Figures 1.3, 1.4, and 1.5 were provided by Mr. Joseph Daws, assistant to the Curator, Gordon Museum.

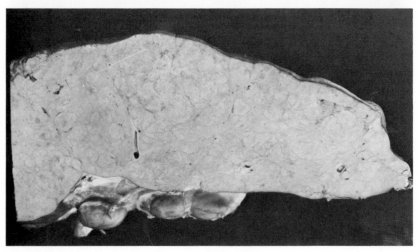

Figure 1.3   Preserved spleen from patient in Hodgkin's original case 2 (Gordon Museum catalog no. 1532).

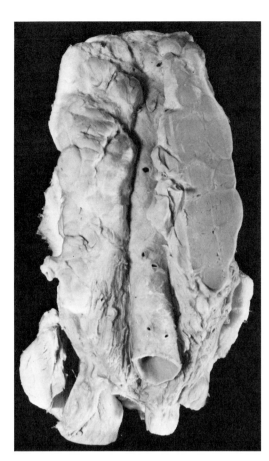

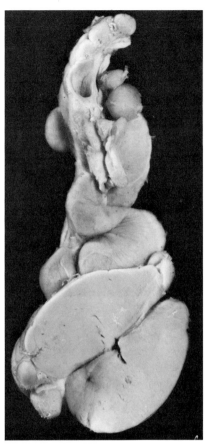

Figure 1.4 Mass of enlarged lymph nodes apparently surrounding a great vessel from Hodgkin's original case 4, Thomas Wescott (Gordon Museum catalog no. 4769).

Figure 1.5 Mass of enlarged lymph nodes from Hodgkin's original case 6, Thomas Black (Gordon Museum catalog no. 4770). After review of microscopic slides prepared many years later from this preserved specimen, Fox (1926) considered it to have been more likely a case of lymphosarcoma than of Hodgkin's disease.

principal consulting physicians at Guy's Hospital, reprinted the history of and postmortem findings on Hodgkin's case 2 (his case 18) and Hodgkin's case 1 (his case 19) and stated: "There is another form of disease, which appears to be of a malignant character, though it varies from the more usual forms of malignant disease; and which has been particularly pointed out by Dr. Hodgkin, as connected with extensive disease of the absorbent glands, more particularly those which accompany the blood vessels."

But for the magnanimous and selfless character of Sir Samuel Wilks, Hodgkin's disease might now be called Wilks' disease, or by some other name, and Hodgkin's contribution would have passed into oblivion. Wilks, who was apparently the first to describe primary and secondary amyloidosis, which he termed "lardaceous disease" (1856),

noted in the course of his delineation of four classes of this disease a fifth variant, of which the principal features were "a peculiar enlargement of the lymphatic glands frequently associated with disease of the spleen" (Fig. 1.7). He described ten such cases, including Hodgkin's original cases 1, 2, 3, and 4 from the Gordon Museum of Guy's Hospital Medical School. In the introduction to his paper, Wilks was clearly under the impression that his observations were original: "The affection of the lymphatic glands, which we shall presently notice, and which appears to bear some close relationship to this form of disease, has not yet (as far as we know) been recognized as a peculiar condition, or deserving of a special name and pathology, although, no doubt, instances of it must be constantly met with." However, by the time he completed writing his paper, Wilks had evidently

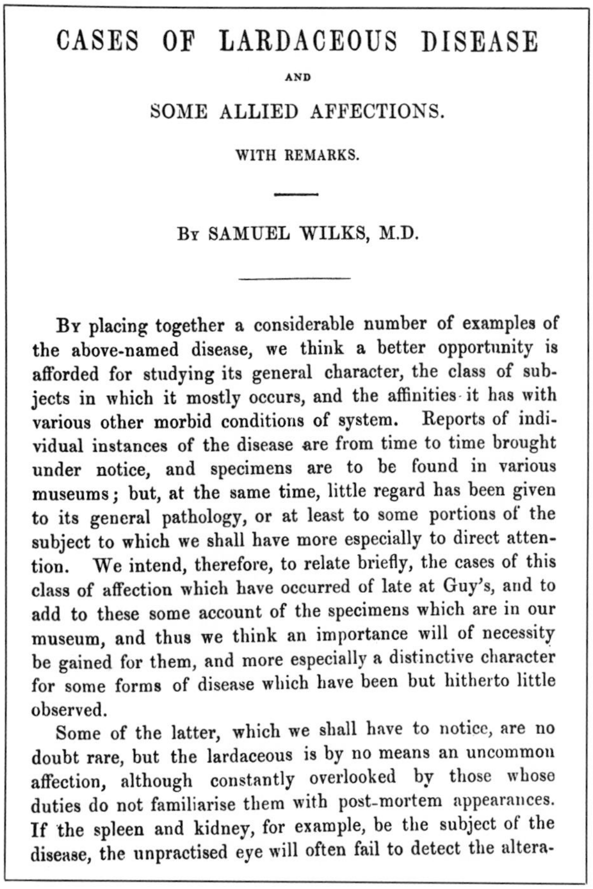

CASES OF LARDACEOUS DISEASE

AND

SOME ALLIED AFFECTIONS.

WITH REMARKS.

———

By SAMUEL WILKS, M.D.

———

By placing together a considerable number of examples of the above-named disease, we think a better opportunity is afforded for studying its general character, the class of subjects in which it mostly occurs, and the affinities it has with various other morbid conditions of system. Reports of individual instances of the disease are from time to time brought under notice, and specimens are to be found in various museums; but, at the same time, little regard has been given to its general pathology, or at least to some portions of the subject to which we shall have more especially to direct attention. We intend, therefore, to relate briefly, the cases of this class of affection which have occurred of late at Guy's, and to add to these some account of the specimens which are in our museum, and thus we think an importance will of necessity be gained for them, and more especially a distinctive character for some forms of disease which have been but hitherto little observed.

Some of the latter, which we shall have to notice, are no doubt rare, but the lardaceous is by no means an uncommon affection, although constantly overlooked by those whose duties do not familiarise them with post-mortem appearances. If the spleen and kidney, for example, be the subject of the disease, the unpractised eye will often fail to detect the altera-

Figure 1.7 Cover page of Wilks' 1856 paper on amyloidosis ("lardaceous disease"), in which some of Hodgkin's original cases were unwittingly redescribed.

encountered Bright's paper (1838), which clearly alludes to Hodgkin's previous observation of similar cases. Wilks was sufficiently diligent to institute a search for Hodgkin's original paper, concerning which he appends the following admirable comment:

While writing this paper, I endeavoured to find the observations of Dr. Hodgkin on a peculiar enlargement of the lymphatic glands, referred to by Dr. Bright, but only now, and on its completion, chanced to meet with them in the seventeenth volume of the "Medico-Chirurgical Transactions."

I there discover that one or two of the cases extracted from our museum have already been published, and Dr. Hodgkin points out the connection of this disease with a peculiar affection of the spleen. Had I known this earlier I should have altered many expressions which I have used with respect to any originality of observation on my part, but otherwise I do not know that I could have done better

than again to refer to these cases, which resemble so exactly those which have come under my own notice. It is only to be lamented that Dr. Hodgkin did not affix a distinct name to the disease, for by so doing I should not have experienced so long an ignorance (which I believe I share with many others) of a very remarkable class of cases, a recognition of which would have guided both myself and others to an explanation of some more recent instances coming under our notice.

Wilks remained interested in this topic and by 1865 had collected a series of fifteen cases in a second paper (Fig. 1.8), the title of which linked Hodgkin's name permanently to this new entity, "Cases of the Enlargement of the Lymphatic Glands and Spleen (or Hodgkin's Disease) with Remarks." In the introduction to this paper, he states: "Having spoken of the lardaceous affection, I must

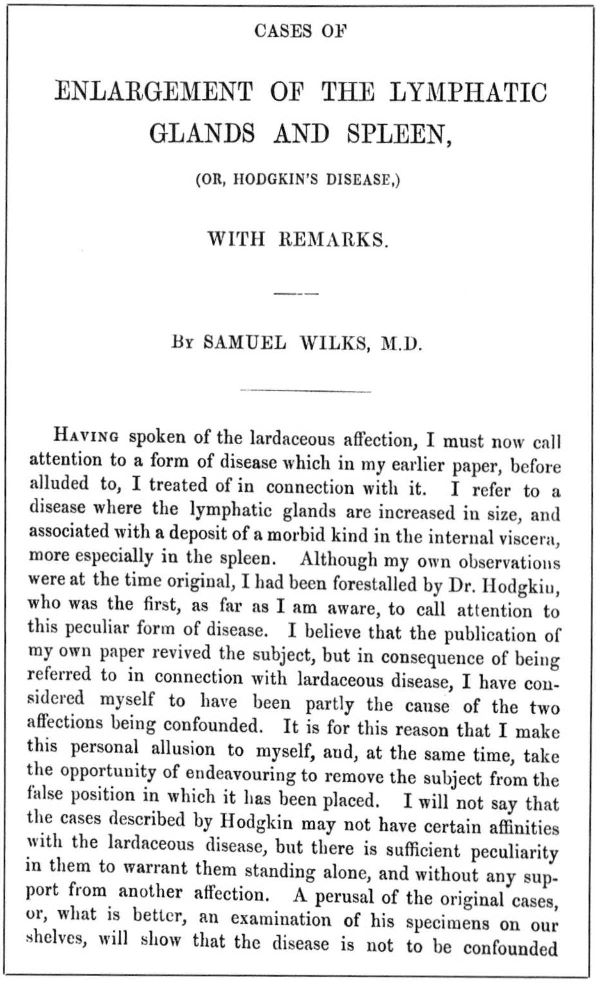

CASES OF

ENLARGEMENT OF THE LYMPHATIC GLANDS AND SPLEEN,

(OR, HODGKIN'S DISEASE,)

WITH REMARKS.

———

By SAMUEL WILKS, M.D.

———

Having spoken of the lardaceous affection, I must now call attention to a form of disease which in my earlier paper, before alluded to, I treated in connection with it. I refer to a disease where the lymphatic glands are increased in size, and associated with a deposit of a morbid kind in the internal viscera, more especially in the spleen. Although my own observations were at the time original, I had been forestalled by Dr. Hodgkin, who was the first, as far as I am aware, to call attention to this peculiar form of disease. I believe that the publication of my own paper revived the subject, but in consequence of being referred to in connection with lardaceous disease, I have considered myself to have been partly the cause of the two affections being confounded. It is for this reason that I make this personal allusion to myself, and, at the same time, take the opportunity of endeavouring to remove the subject from the false position in which it has been placed. I will not say that the cases described by Hodgkin may not have certain affinities with the lardaceous disease, but there is sufficient peculiarity in them to warrant them standing alone, and without any support from another affection. A perusal of the original cases, or, what is better, an examination of his specimens on our shelves, will show that the disease is not to be confounded

Figure 1.8 Cover page of Wilks' 1865 paper, in which the appellation "Hodgkin's disease" is first used.

now call attention to a form of disease which in my earlier paper, before alluded to, I treated of in connection with it. I refer to a disease where the lymphatic glands are increased in size, and associated with a deposit of a morbid kind in the internal viscera, more especially in the spleen. Although my own observations were at the time original, I had been forestalled by Dr. Hodgkin, who was the first, as far as I am aware, to call attention to this peculiar form of disease."

In 1858, apparently unaware of the prior publications of Hodgkin and of Wilks, Wunderlich independently reported two cases of what appears to have been the same entity, for which he suggested the name "progressive multiple lymph gland hypertrophy." Trousseau, in 1865, described several cases of "l'adénie," many of which were undoubtedly instances of Hodgkin's disease, and cited similar earlier case reports by Bonfils (1856) and Cossy (1861). These were but the first of scores of synonyms which were to be applied to the disease by others in ensuing decades. A complete listing of these has been presented by Wallhauser (1933). A few of the more widely used terms include: lymphogranuloma, adénie, granuloma malignum, lymphadenoma, lymphomatosis granulomatosa, and lymphoblastoma.

Meanwhile, thirteen years after Hodgkin's original paper, the first cases of leukemia were reported in 1845 by Craigie, Bennett, and Virchow (Fig. 1.9). Craigie and Bennett were clearly puzzled by the nature of their cases, since they referred to "suppuration of the blood," yet could find no evidence of phlebitis or other inflammatory condition

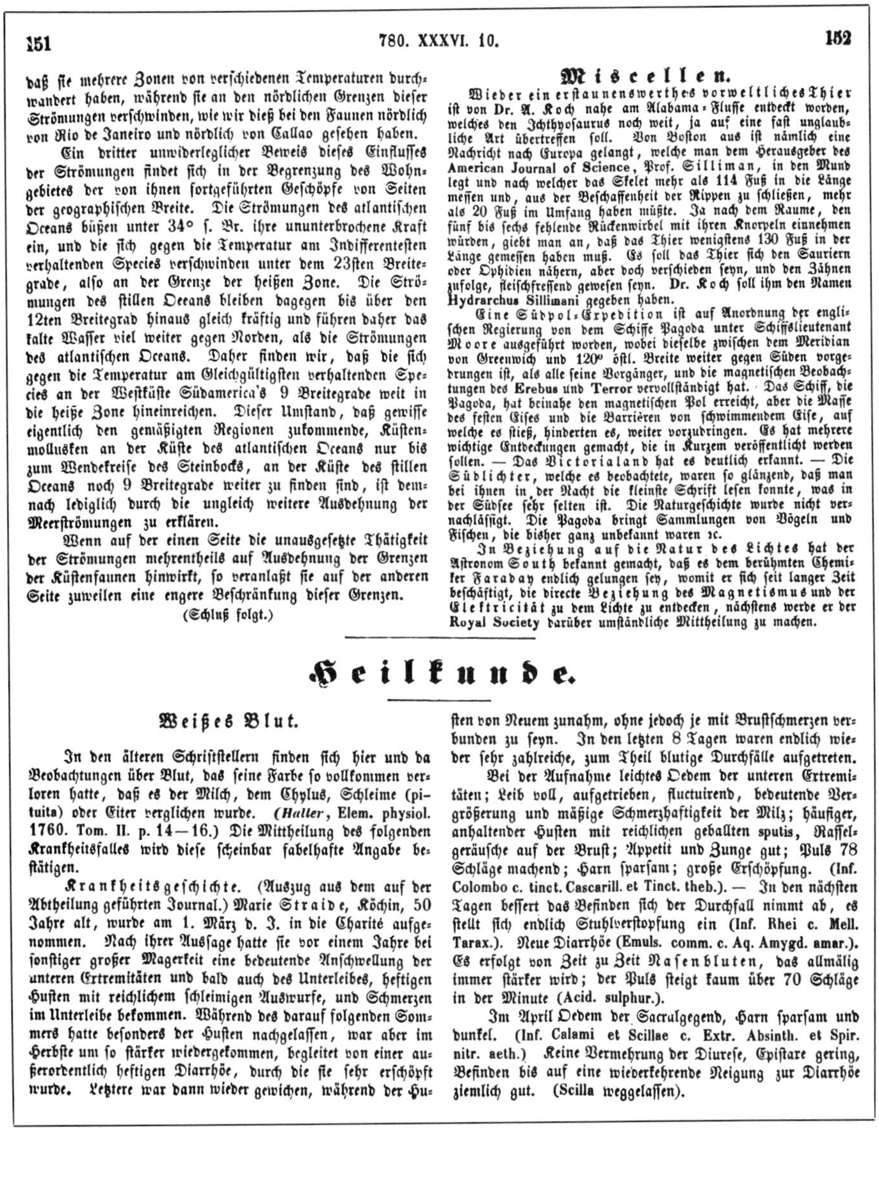

---

151   780. XXXVI. 10.   **152**

daß sie mehrere Zonen von verschiedenen Temperaturen durchwandert haben, während sie an den nördlichen Grenzen dieser Strömungen verschwinden, wie wir dieß bei den Faunen nördlich von Rio de Janeiro und nördlich von Callao gesehen haben.

Ein dritter unwiderleglicher Beweis dieses Einflusses der Strömungen findet sich in der Begrenzung des Wohngebietes der von ihnen fortgeführten Geschöpfe von Seiten der geographischen Breite. Die Strömungen des atlantischen Oceans büßen unter 34° s. Br. ihre ununterbrochene Kraft ein, und die sich gegen die Temperatur an Indifferentes verhaltenden Species verschwinden unter dem 23sten Breitegrade, also an der Grenze der heißen Zone. Die Strömungen des stillen Oceans bleiben dagegen bis über den 12ten Breitegrad hinaus gleich kräftig und führen daher das kalte Wasser viel weiter gegen Norden, als die Strömungen des atlantischen Oceans. Daher finden wir, daß die sich gegen die Temperatur am Gleichgültigsten verhaltenden Species an der Westküste Südamerica's 9 Breitegrade weit in die heiße Zone hineinreichen. Dieser Umstand, daß gewisse eigentlich den gemäßigten Regionen zukommende, Küstenmollusken an der Küste des atlantischen Oceans nur bis zum Wendekreise des Steinbocks, an der Küste des stillen Oceans noch 9 Breitegrade weiter zu finden sind, ist demnach lediglich durch die ungleich weitere Ausdehnung der Meeresströmungen zu erklären.

Wenn auf der einen Seite die unausgesetzte Thätigkeit der Strömungen mehrentheils auf Ausdehnung der Grenzen der Küstenfaunen hinwirkt, so veranlaßt sie auf der anderen Seite zuweilen eine engere Beschränkung dieser Grenzen.

(Schluß folgt.)

Miscellen.

Wieder ein erstaunenswerthes vorweltliches Thier ist von Dr. A. Koch nahe am Alabama-Flusse entdeckt worden, welches den Ichthyosaurus noch weit, ja auf eine fast unglaubliche Art übertreffen soll. Von Boston aus ist nämlich eine Nachricht nach Europa gelangt, welche man dem Herausgeber des American Journal of Science, Prof. Silliman, in den Mund legt und nach welcher das Skelet mehr als 114 Fuß in die Länge messen und, aus der Beschaffenheit der Rippen zu schließen, mehr als 20 Fuß im Umfang haben müßte. Je nach dem Raume, den fünf bis sechs fehlende Rückenwirbel mit ihren Knorpeln einnehmen würden, giebt man an, daß das Thier wenigstens 130 Fuß in der Länge gemessen haben muß. Es soll das Thier sich den Sauriern oder Ophidien nähern, aber doch verschieden seyn, und den Zähnen zufolge, fleischfressend gewesen seyn. Dr. Koch soll ihm den Namen Hydrarchus Sillimani gegeben haben.

Eine Südpol-Expedition ist auf Anordnung der englischen Regierung von dem Schiffe Pagoda unter Schiffslieutenant Moore ausgeführt worden, wobei dieselbe zwischen dem Meridian von Greenwich und 120° östl. Breite weiter gegen Süden vorgedrungen ist, als alle seine Vorgänger, und die magnetischen Beobachtungen der Erebus und Terror vervollständigt hat. Das Schiff, die Pagoda, hat beinahe den magnetischen Pol erreicht, aber die Masse des festen Eises und die Barrieren von schwimmendem Eise, auf welche es stieß, hinderten es, weiter vorzudringen. Es hat mehrere wichtige Entdeckungen gemacht, die in Kurzem veröffentlicht werden sollen. — Das Victorialand hat es deutlich erkannt. — Die Südlichter, welche es beobachtete, waren so glänzend, daß man bei ihnen in der Nacht die kleinste Schrift lesen konnte, was in der Südsee sehr selten ist. Die Naturgeschichte wurde nicht vernachlässigt. Die Pagoda bringt Sammlungen von Vögeln und Fischen, die bisher ganz unbekannt waren 2c.

In Beziehung auf die Natur des Lichtes hat der Astronom South befand gemacht, daß es dem berühmten Chemiker Faraday endlich gelungen sey, womit er sich seit langer Zeit beschäftigt, die directe Beziehung des Magnetismus und der Electricität zu dem Lichte zu entdecken, nächstens werde er der Royal Society darüber umständliche Mittheilung zu machen.

Heilkunde.

Weißes Blut.

In den älteren Schriftstellern finden sich hier und da Beobachtungen über Blut, das seine Farbe so vollkommen verloren hatte, daß es der Milch, dem Chylus, Schleime (pituita) oder Eiter verglichen wurde. (Haller, Elem. physiol. 1760. Tom. II. p. 14—16.) Die Mittheilung des folgenden Krankheitsfalles wird diese scheinbar fabelhafte Angabe bestätigen.

Krankheitsgeschichte. (Auszug aus dem auf der Abtheilung geführten Journal.) Marie Straide, Köchin, 50 Jahre alt, wurde am 1. März d. J. in die Charité aufgenommen. Nach ihrer Aussage hatte sie vor einem Jahre bei sonstiger großer Magerkeit eine bedeutende Anschwellung der unteren Extremitäten und bald auch des Unterleibes, heftigen Husten mit reichlichem schleimigen Auswurfe, und Schmerzen im Unterleibe bekommen. Während des darauf folgenden Sommers hatte besonders der Husten nachgelassen, war aber im Herbste um so stärker wiedergekommen, begleitet von einer außerordentlich heftigen Diarrhöe, durch die sie sehr erschöpft wurde. Letztere war dann wieder gewichen, während der Husten von Neuem zunahm, ohne jedoch je mit Brustschmerzen verbunden zu seyn. In den letzten 8 Tagen waren endlich wieder sehr zahlreiche, zum Theil blutige Durchfälle aufgetreten.

Bei der Aufnahme leichtes Oedem der unteren Extremitäten; Leib voll, aufgetrieben, fluctuirend, bedeutende Vergrößerung und mäßige Schmerzhaftigkeit der Milz; häufiger, anhaltender Husten mit reichlichem geballten sputis, Rasselgeräusche auf der Brust; Appetit und Zunge gut; Puls 78 Schläge machend; Harn sparsam; große Erschöpfung. (Inf. Colombo c. tinct. Cascarill. et Tinct. theb.). — In den nächsten Tagen bessert das Befinden sich die Durchfall nimmt ab, es stellt sich endlich Stuhlverstopfung ein (Inf. Rhei c. Mell. Tarax.). Neue Diarrhöe (Emuls. comm. c. Aq. Amygd. amar.). Es erfolgt von Zeit zu Zeit Nasenbluten, das allmälig immer stärker wird; der Puls steigt kaum über 70 Schläge in der Minute (Acid. sulphur.).

Im April Oedem der Sacralgegend, Harn sparsam und dunkel. (Inf. Calami et Scillae c. Extr. Absinth. et Spir. nitr. aeth.) Keine Vermehrung der Diurese, Epistase gering, Befinden bis auf eine wiederkehrende Neigung zur Diarrhöe ziemlich gut. (Scilla weggelassen).

Figure 1.9 Cover page of Virchow's 1845 paper "Weisses Blut." Craigie and Bennett independently described cases of leukemia in the same year but had a less clear conception of the nature of the disease.

as a possible cause of such a pyogenic response. Virchow, on the other hand, had a much clearer conception of the nature of the disease and even defined two forms, leukemic and aleukemic, the latter of which presumably subsumed many instances of what were later to be defined as lymphosarcoma, Hodgkin's disease, and reticulum cell sarcoma. The term "pseudoleukemia" was introduced in 1865 by Cohnheim to refer to Virchow's aleukemic group. Although Wilks makes no specific mention of the cases described by Craigie, Bennett, and Virchow, he was apparently aware of the existence of "leucocythaemia" and considered Hodgkin's disease to be distinct from it: "It is believed that both spleen and lymphatic glands are involved in the blood-making process, and thus that a leucocythaemia may be produced by disease of these organs; the two conditions of blood being distinguishable by the different sizes of the superabundant white corpuscles. According to my own experience I have never met with well-marked leucocythaemia in Hodgkin's disease, and thus I have always preferred the term anaemia to leucocythaemia lymphatica."

After the delineation of the leukemias, the next nosological advance did not come until almost fifty years later, when Dreschfeld (1892) and Kundrat (1893) independently distinguished from the aleu-

Wiener klinische Wochenschrift

Die »Wiener klinische Wochenschrift« erscheint jeden Donnerstag im Umfange von mindestens zwei Bogen Gross-quart. Zuschriften für die Redaction sind zu richten an Dr. Gustav Riehl, I. Bellariastrasse Nr. 12, Bestellungen und Geldsendungen an die Verlagshandlung.

unter ständiger Mitwirkung der Herren Professoren Drs.

E. Albert, G. Braun, V. R. v. Ebner, S. Exner, M. Gruber, E. R. v. Hofmann, R. Freih. v. Krafft-Ebing, S. Stricker, C. Toldt, A. Vogl, H. Widerhofer, E. Zuckerkandl

begründet von weil. Hofrath Prof. **H. v. Bamberger**

herausgegeben von

Theodor Billroth, Rudolf Chrobak, Ernst Fuchs, Hans Kundrat, Ernst Ludwig und **L. R. v. Schrötter.**

Organ der k. k. Gesellschaft der Aerzte in Wien.

Redigirt von **Dr. Gustav Riehl.** (Telephon Nr. 7260.)

Verlag von Wilhelm Braumüller, k. u. k. Hof- und Universitäts-Buchhändler, I. Graben 21. (Telephon Nr. 6934.)

Abonnementspreis jährlich 10 fl. = 20 Mark. Abonnements und Insertions-Aufträge für das In- und Ausland werden von allen Buchhandlungen u. Postämtern, so wie auch von der Verlagshandlung übernommen. Abonnements, deren Abbestellung nicht erfolgt ist, gelten als erneuert. Inserate werden mit 30 kr. = 50 Pfg. pro 2spaltige Nonpareillezeile berechnet. Grössere Aufträge nach Uebereinkommen.

VI. Jahrgang. Wien, 23. März 1893. Nr. 12.

Inhalt. Ueber Lympho-Sarkomatosis. Von Prof. Kundrat. — Ein Fall von Meningocele spuria traumatica mit osteoplastischem Verschluss des Defectes. Von Primararzt Dr. E. Šlajmer. — Chemische Untersuchung der Neuquelle in Franzensbad. Von Prof. E. Ludwig. — Die Entstehung der Knochendeformitäten. Von Prof. Dr. Adolf Lorenz. (Schluss). — Verhandlungen ärztlicher Gesellschaften und Vereine: Officielles Protokoll der k. k. Gesellschaft der Aerzte in Wien: Bericht des II. Secretärs; Kundrat: Lympho-Sarkomatosis. — Officielles Protokoll der geburtshilflich-gynäkologischen Gesellschaft in Wien. — Société médicale des hôpitaux de Paris. — Referate: v. Rosthorn: Mackenrodt, Dreysel. —.: König. Dittrich: Pohl. Wintersteiner: König. — Klinische und therapeutische Mittheilungen: Kresolsaponat. Glycerin. Bacterienfreies Wasser. Solveol. Krebsbehandlung. Gastroraphie. Trigeminusresection. — Notizen. — Programme.

— Alle Rechte vorbehalten. —

Ueber Lympho-Sarkomatosis.

Von Professor **Kundrat.**

Vortrag, gehalten in der Jahres-Sitzung der k. k. Gesellschaft der Aerzte am 17. März 1893.

Ein alter Brauch in unserer Gesellschaft bringt es mit sich, für diese feierliche Jahres-Sitzung ein Thema von allgemeinem Interesse zu wählen.

Meine Wahl fiel auf das angekündigte Thema: Die Lympho-Sarkomatosis, nicht allein, weil es im Stande ist, dieser Anforderung im weitesten Umfange zu genügen, das Interesse sowohl der Aerzte im Allgemeinen als aller Specialisten zu fesseln, mehr noch deshalb, weil mir nach eigener Erfahrung aus dem Verkehr mit den Praktikern bewusst geworden, dass dieses Thema derzeit dringend einer Besprechung bedarf, einerseits um die erworbene Erkenntniss zum Gemeingut zu machen, anderseits um dadurch eine Anregung für weitere Beobachtung zu geben, für welche die eigene Forschungsrichtung nicht ausreicht, da sie als eine rein anatomische vielfacher Beschränkung unterworfen ist.

Von allgemeinem Interesse ist das Thema wohl schon deshalb, weil weder das Wesen des Lympho-Sarkoms bisher eine genügende Würdigung gefunden, noch die Details der Erkrankung, so vielgestaltig und wichtig sie sind, eine eingehende Erörterung und Zusammenfassung, auch die Stellung desselben zu anderen, namentlich ähnlichen Processen jeder Abgrenzung entbehrt.

Denn soviele einzelne interessante Fälle bekannt und beschrieben sind, die Anschauungen über das Lympho-Sarkom blieben die alten: Es wird noch heute, wie zu jener Zeit, wo man es von anderen lymphatischen Geschwulstbildungen schied, zu den Sarkomen gezählt oder ihnen angereiht, und doch ist es meines Erachtens in jeder Beziehung vollständig von diesen zu trennen.

Ich wage dies zu behaupten, gestützt auf langjährige Erfahrung und eine nun durch 10 Jahre auf diesen Gegenstand gerichtete Beobachtung, die mir ein Material von 50 Fällen von Lympho-Sarkom und der doppelten Anzahl der ähnlichen und verwandten Erkrankungen geliefert.

Gestützt auf dieses Material, von dem ich Ihnen die interessantesten, im Museum aufbewahrten Präparate nebenbei zeigen will, möchte ich Ihnen ein Bild der Erkrankung im Allgemeinen und seiner einzelnen Formen geben — ohne in die Details der einzelnen Fälle einzugehen — damit Sie sich selbst eine eigene Anschauung und ein Urtheil über meine Auffassung bilden können.

Bezüglich der histologischen Beschaffenheit kann ich nichts Neues beibringen. Die Lympho-Sarkome sind charakterisirt durch das reticulirte Grundgewebe mit eingelagerten lymphoïden Zellen; betont muss hier werden, dass dasselbe nie dem normalen reticulirten lymphoïden Gewebe gleicht, indem die typische Ausbildung durch unregelmässige Anordnung des Gerüstes, schwächere oder wieder mehr fibröse Ausbildung desselben, Reichthum und Grösse der Zellen erheblich vom Typus abweicht.

Durch diese wechselnde Ausbildung des Zellreichthums und der Gerüste ist es bedingt, dass wir zwei Formen, medulläre und mehr fibröse, unterscheiden können, die aber nicht scharf geschieden sind, indem erstere aus letzteren hervorgehen können oder vielmehr die anfänglich dichteren Massen durch üppige Zellwucherung in medulläre Formen übergehen, andererseits auch durch partielle Schrumpfungen Verdichtungen sich ausbilden.

Hervorzuheben aber ist, dass das Lympho-Sarkom keine Neigung zu retrograden Metamorphosen besitzt — ebenso wie die leukämischen und pseudoleukämischen Tumoren — Verfettungen sehr selten und nur zellweise getroffen werden — anämische Nekrosen in ihnen Raritäten sind.

Genetisch stehen sie mit dem lymphatischen Apparat in unlöslicher Verbindung. Mir ist kein Fall bekannt, der anderen Ursprung gezeigt — nur sind es nicht, wie die allgemeine Anschauung festhält, die Lymphdrüsen, sondern häufig auch nur Lymphfollikel, und selbst vielleicht das bei einzelnen Individuen in einzelnen Schleimhäuten, vielleicht auch zu gewissen Lebenszeiten und bei manchen eigenthümlichen constitutionellen Zuständen so wechselnd ausgebildete adenoide Gewebe, das ihren Ausgang bildet.

So dürfte es sich erklären, warum wir Lympho-Sarkom primär nur an Lymphdrüsen und manchen Schleimhäuten finden.

Nimmt das Lympho-Sarkom aber auch diesen Ausgang, so bleibt es doch nicht auf diese Gebilde beschränkt und

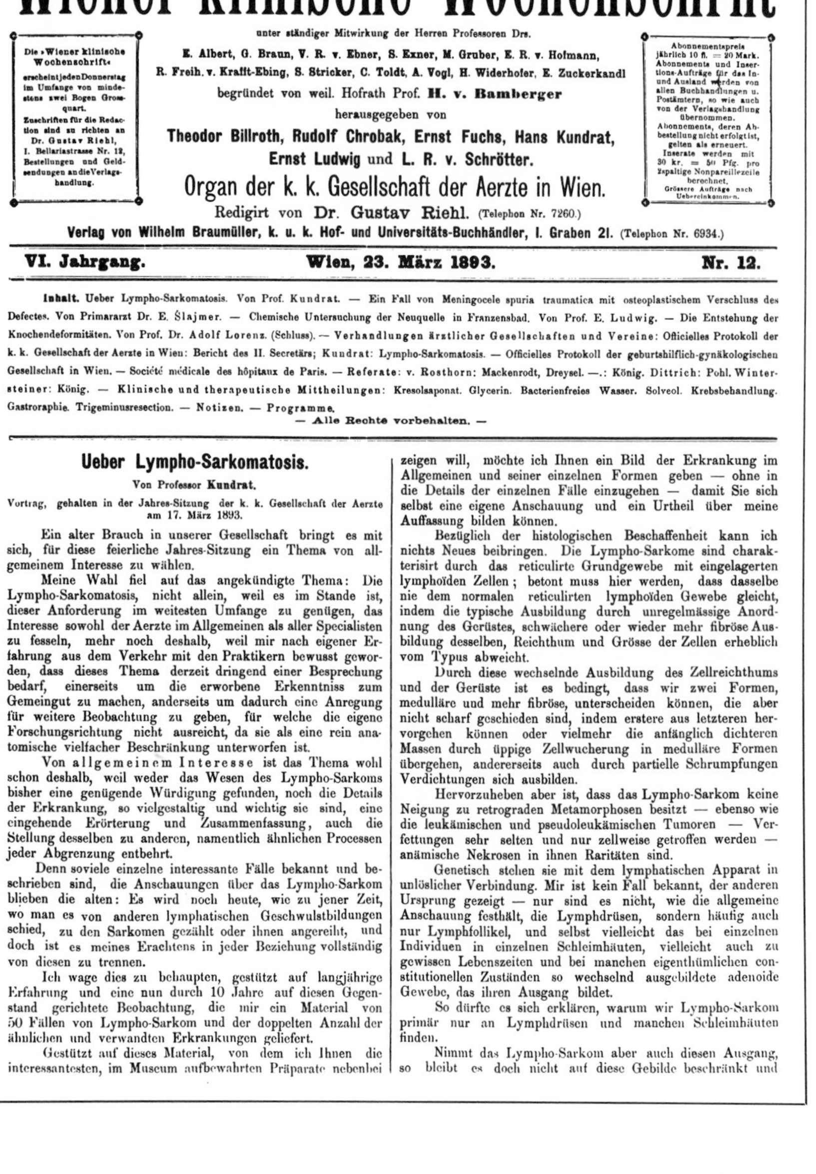

Figure 1.10 Cover page of Kundrat's 1893 article on lymphosarcoma. Another paper independently describing the same entity was published in the preceding year by Dreschfeld.

kemic leukemias a group of cases in which the lymphoid neoplastic cells remained confined for relatively long periods of time to the lymphatic system; to these cases Kundrat gave the name "lymphosarcoma" (Fig. 1.10). Moreover Kundrat specifically pointed out that the differential diagnosis of these cases included not only the pseudoleukemias (Virchow's aleukemic leukemias), but also "granuloma malignum," one the many synonyms for Hodgkin's disease.

The follicular (nodular) lymphomas were not recognized as a separate group until 1925, when

Brill, Baehr, and Rosenthal described the clinical, laboratory, and histopathologic features of two cases (Fig. 1.11), as well as their extraordinary sensitivity to radiation therapy. Two years later, Symmers independently described the same entity — one of the many synonyms for which has therefore been Brill-Symmers disease. Although Brill et al. initially believed that they were dealing with a benign hyperplasia of the lymph nodes, continued observation of the clinical course of their cases led them to revise this opinion and to conclude that they represented malignant neoplasms of rela-

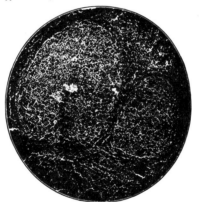

2. LeCount, E. R.: J. Exper. Med. 4: 559, 1899.
3. Ewing, J.: Neoplastic Diseases, Philadelphia, 1919, p. 336.
4. Josselin de Jong, R.: Beitr. z. path. Anat. u. z. allg. Path. (Ziegler's) 69: 185, 1921.
5. Hitzrot, cited by Pool, E. H., and Stillman, R. G.: Surgery of the Spleen, New York, 1923.

Figure 1.11 Cover page of the 1925 paper by Brill, Baehr, and Rosenthal containing the first description of nodular (follicular) lymphoma; Symmers independently reported the same entity in 1927. Reproduction by permission of the Editor of the *Journal of the American Medical Association* and affiliated publications.

tively slow evolution, a conclusion in which they were soon joined by Symmers. In a now classical paper, Rappaport, Winter, and Hicks (1956) pointed out that five types of follicular lymphoma are recognizable, in which the tumor cell type associated with a "giant follicular" pattern might resemble the lymphocyte, lymphoblast, or histiocyte, or mixtures thereof, or exhibit the pleomorphic pattern of Hodgkin's disease.

Reticulum cell sarcoma of bone was first distinguished from the myelomas in 1928 by Oberling, who considered the Ewing sarcoma of bone to be a variant of this group, which he designated as reticuloendothelial sarcoma. Two years later, in 1930, Roulet first separated off the group of primary reticulum cell sarcomas of lymphoid tissue, to which he gave the name *retothele sarcome*. It has been pointed out by some authors that the widely felt need for such a category at that time was reflected in the rapidity with which his terminology, translated into "reticulum cell sarcoma," was generally adopted. A good deal of confusion about the criteria for the histopathologic diagnosis of reticulum cell sarcoma has persisted even to the present time, however, probably due in part to the fact, pointed out by Gall and Mallory (1942), that Roulet "included under the heading of retothele sarcome a group of lesions with a morphologic range which, judging from his descriptions and his illustrations, extends almost from one extreme to the other of the malignant lymphomas." Gall and Mallory suggested that the reticulum cell sarcomas should be further subdivided into two major groups, the stem cell lymphomas and the clasmatocytic lymphomas.

The final entrant to date into the lymphoma family was not reported until as recently as 1958, when Denis Burkitt (Fig. 1.12) described the clinical, roentgenologic, and histologic features in thirty-eight cases of "a sarcoma involving the jaws in African children." Since that time, this tumor, to which the name "Burkitt lymphoma" has generally been given, has become the focus of intense interest on the part of virologists, epidemiologists, pathologists, and clinicians in many parts of the world.

So much for the chronology of the various members of the lymphoma-leukemia complex. Let us now consider the unfolding of concepts concerning their nature, etiology, and pathogenesis. That Hodgkin's disease is an entity was a conviction strongly held by Wilks. He stated: "A perusal of these cases will show that here is an affection presenting as striking peculiarities as any in the noso-

logy, and deserving a distinct appellation." However, such opinions could not possibly rest on solid foundations until the histopathology of Hodgkin's disease had been delineated. Wilks actually used the microscope to study some of his cases, but his descriptions were confined to brief statements, such as "the microscope showed masses of cells and fibres as of new tissue."

The history of the discovery of the pathognomonic giant cells of Hodgkin's disease has been carefully reviewed by Rather (1972) and by Strum (1973). Perhaps the earliest descriptions were those of Ollivier and Ranvier (1867) and Tuckwell (1870). The latter, in an autopsy on a forty-nine-year-old woman with a huge spleen and enlarged abdominal lymph nodes, noted under the microscope "small cells of various shapes" plus "a few larger cells, containing two or three nuclei." Bristowe and Pick (1870), examining cell juice expressed from the involved tissues of Tuckwell's case, noted cells with "a distinct nucleolated nucleus, of large size, which nearly filled the cell . . . In some instances the cells were found to contain two or even, though very rarely, three nuclei." Langhans (1872), Greenfield (1878), and Gowers (1879) also clearly recognized giant, multinucleated cells, and Greenfield (Fig. 1.13) contributed the first drawing of such cells, seen at low magnification in a lymph node. Goldmann (1892), using the staining procedures developed by Ehrlich, was apparently the first to recognize the acidophilia of the nucleolus in these cells. Rather (1972) concludes that "what actually happened in regard to the discovery of the pathognomonic cell of Hodgkin's disease was that many investigators, in Germany, France, and England . . . beginning in the 1860's, recognized and described one, sometimes two, varieties of large cells in a disease characterized especially by enlargement of the lymph nodes and spleen in the absence of a leukemic blood picture." However, Sternberg (1898) and Dorothy Reed (1902) are generally credited with the first definitive and thorough descriptions of the histopathology of Hodgkin's disease, and Reed clearly illustrated the appearance of the multinucleated giant cells with excellent drawings. For these reasons, the names of Sternberg and Reed, rather than those of Ollivier and Ranvier, Tuckwell, Langhans, Greenfield, and Gowers are now associated with these cells. On the basis of her studies, Reed was able to conclude: "We believe then, from the descriptions in the literature and the findings in eight cases examined, that Hodgkin's disease has a peculiar and typical histological picture and could thus rightly be considered a histopathological disease entity."

Using these histologic criteria, Fox (1926) examined microscopic sections which he was able to prepare from gross specimens preserved in the Gordon Museum of Guy's Hospital Medical School of Hodgkin's original cases 2, 4, and 6. Remarkably, Fox found the microanatomy to be perfectly preserved, despite the fact that the tissues had been kept in fixative for ninety-seven years! He was able to confirm the diagnosis of Hodgkin's disease on histopathologic grounds in Hodgkin's cases 2 and 4; a photomicrograph of case 2 reproduced in his article is quite convincing, as are the sections reproduced here (Fig. 1.14). However, Fox considered that case 6 was more likely an example of lymphosarcoma or lymphatic leukemia, though here the tissues were not sufficiently well preserved for him to be entirely certain. He apparently also accepted case 7, which had originally been described to Hodgkin by Carswell, without, however, having examined tissues from it, but rejected case 5 as "systemic lymphomatosis," case 3 as syphilis (a view in which Wilks also concurred), and case 1, which had been accepted by Wilks as exhibiting both tuberculosis and Hodgkin's disease, "as obviously tuberculosis." The last of these conclusions is puz-

---

218   THE BRITISH JOURNAL OF SURGERY

RAPER, F. P. (1956), *Brit. J. Urol.*, **28**, 436.
RAVAULT, P. P., PAPILLAN, J., PINET, F., and JACQUOT, F. J. (1956), *Lyon méd.*, **88**, 453.
ROSS, J. C., and TINCKLER, L. F. (1958), *Brit. J. Surg.*, **46**, 58.
SAMSON, P. (1945), *J. thorac. Surg.*, **14**, 330.
SANTY, P., GALY, P., GONIN, A., MARION, P., PAPILLON, J., and PINET, F. (1957), *Pr. méd.*, **65**, 307.

SCANNELL, J. G., and SHAW, R. S. (1954), *J. thorac. Surg.*, **28**, 163.
TUBBS, O. S. (1946), *Thorax*, **I**, 247.
VAUX, D. M. (1938), *J. Path. Bact.*, **46**, 441.
WALSH, G. C., NORTON, G. I., BAIRD, M. M., and ROBERTSON, R. (1957), *Canad. med. Ass. J.*, **76**, 292.
ZEMAN, F. D. (1945), *J. thorac. Surg.*, **14**, 330.

A SARCOMA INVOLVING THE JAWS IN AFRICAN CHILDREN

By DENIS BURKITT

FROM THE DEPARTMENT OF SURGERY, MAKERERE COLLEGE MEDICAL SCHOOL, AND MULAGO HOSPITAL, KAMPALA, UGANDA

MALIGNANT tumours of the jaws in children, primary or secondary, are generally regarded as rare. A sarcoma involving the jaws in African children has recently come to be recognized at Mulago Hospital as a distinctive clinical condition and certainly the commonest malignancy of childhood.

Thirty-eight patients with this sarcoma in the jaws have been seen during the past 7 years; 32 of them were seen at Mulago Hospital and 6 at district hospitals. The tumour was diagnosed clinically in a further 8 children, but these have not been included in this series owing to lack of histological confirmation.

Records of only 3 cases of this type of jaw sarcoma in children have been traced in the literature (Christiansen, 1938; Salmon and Darlington, 1944; Burford, Ackerman, and Robinson, 1944). Gelfand (1957) published an illustration of a sarcoma of the jaw in an African child without clinical details.

GEOGRAPHICAL DISTRIBUTION

Patients have not been limited to any particular area in Uganda, and have represented 11 different tribes. This sarcoma has also been observed in Kenya (Clifford, 1958), Tanganyika (Morris, 1958; Blackman, 1958), Nigeria (Thomas, 1958), the Belgian Congo (Thijs, 1958), and Southern Rhodesia (Gelfand, 1957). Patients with this syndrome have not yet been recognized in Johannesburg (Oettlé, 1958), Khartoum (Taylor, 1958), Lusaka (Buck, 1958), or Lourenço Marques (Prates, 1958).

CLINICAL FEATURES

These patients were from 2 to 14 years of age, 30 being between the ages of 2 and 7 years (*Fig.* 246).

In most cases the tumour started in the region of the alveolar process of a maxilla (*Fig.* 247) or the mandible (*Fig.* 249). Loosening of the deciduous molars was often the first symptom, the teeth in the involved area soon becoming embedded in tumour tissue only, and losing their insertion in bone. The next stage was irregular displacement of the teeth prior to their falling out. The tumour grew rapidly,

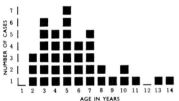

NUMBER OF CASES
AGE IN YEARS
Fig. 246.—Showing age distribution in 38 cases.

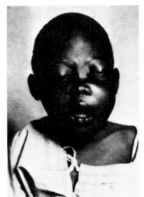

Fig. 247.—Sarcoma involving the left maxilla and arising in relation to the teeth. *Case* 1, taken 2 months after onset of symptoms.

grossly distorting the face. In only one patient (*Case* 20) did it ulcerate through the skin. Œdema of the eyelids and chemosis of the conjunctivæ indicated invasion of the orbit, and if the patient survived the eye became proptosed and finally destroyed. Less commonly the tumour presented as a swelling high in the maxilla with early invasion of the orbit (*Fig.* 248). Pain was not usually as severe as would have been expected from the appearance of the tumour. Within two or three months of onset of symptoms their relatives removed the majority of the children from hospital in a moribund condition.

Unless secondary infection occurred, which was not usual, the regional lymph-nodes were not

---

Figure 1.12 Cover page of Burkitt's original (1958) description of the African lymphoma which now bears his name. This is the most recently recognized of the entities comprising the lymphoma-leukemia complex. Reproduced by permission of the *British Journal of Surgery*.

zling; both Hodgkin and Wilks had clearly stated that the patient in case 1 had tuberculosis, but they were nonetheless impressed with the fact that the abdominal lymphadenopathy and splenomegaly in this instance were not simply additional manifestations of the tuberculous process. Since Fox was unable to obtain any of the tissues from case 1 and thus did not examine them under the microscope, it is difficult to see on what grounds he was able to refute the view that this case was an example of coexistent Hodgkin's disease and tuberculosis. On

---

272   LYMPHATIC SYSTEM.

Jenner, where the presence of a large excess of leucocytes in the blood coincided with the formation of an abscess, the temporary leukæmia disappearing after the abscess was opened. One thing he would urge was that the definition of leukæmia should be restricted to the cases where the white blood-corpuscles abounded in numbers equal to or exceeding the red, and not, as had been loosely stated, when twenty or thirty white corpuscles were visible in the field of the microscope.   *March 19th,* 1878.

---

2. *Specimens illustrative of the pathology of lymphadenoma and leucocythæmia.*

By W. S. GREENFIELD, M.D.

In bringing before the Society specimens illustrative of the pathology of lymphadenoma and leucocythæmia, it will be convenient to give some account of the cases from which most of the specimens are taken, then to describe the histological characters of the morbid changes in different organs, and afterwards to discuss some points in the general pathology and relations of these diseases. But in order to bring more completely into relief the morbid anatomy and histology of lymphadenoma, I have exhibited to the Society a number of specimens from other cases than those now recorded, some of which have already been shown to this and other societies, and have thus endeavoured to illustrate the several stages of the changes in various organs. Briefly to mention these, they are specimens from the liver in two cases, the spleen in three cases, the glands in three cases, and drawings of the naked-eye appearances of the liver and spleen in typical cases. The microscopic specimens were selected from sections of the glands in various parts of the body in seven cases, from the spleen in seven cases, the liver in two, and the skin in two, and also from growths in the omentum, the lungs, &c. Together with these, microscopic drawings illustrative of some of the most important changes are shown.

I have been able only to bring one case of leucocythæmia, of which specimens and drawings from the liver, spleen, and kidney, and microscopic sections and drawings from the same organs, are shown.

Figure 1.13 Cover page of the 1878 paper by Greenfield, which, together with those of Ollivier and Ranvier (1867), Tuckwell (1870), Langhans (1872), and Gowers (1879), contained the first known descriptions of the characteristic binucleate or multinucleate giant cells of Hodgkin's disease, recognition of which is now usually credited to Sternberg (1898) and to Dorothy Reed (1902), and named after them.

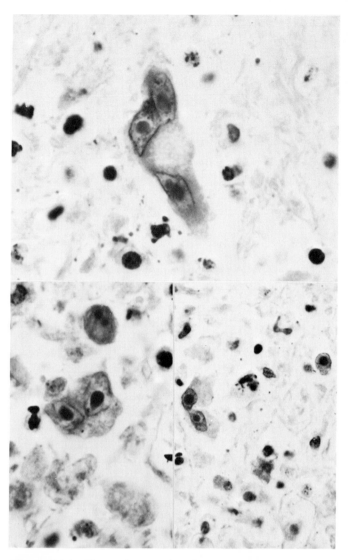

Figure 1.14 Photomicrographs of representative fields from involved lymph nodes in Hodgkin's original case 2, revealing binucleate giant cells with huge nucleoli and other cytologic features readily recognizable, even after fixation for 140 years, as those of Sternberg-Reed cells. The microscopic sections were prepared in 1968 by Mr. Joseph Daws, assistant to the Curator, Gordon Museum.

the evidence currently available, it seems likely that Wilks (1865) was more likely correct in considering that at least four of Hodgkin's cases were, in fact, examples of Hodgkin's disease.

During the first four decades of this century, pathologists began to describe a somewhat broader spectrum of histologic features. However, it was Jackson and Parker, in a classical series of papers (1937, 1939, 1944a,b) and in their book, *Hodgkin's Disease and Allied Disorders* (1947), who presented the first serious effort at a histopathologic classification of different types of Hodgkin's disease. To the main body of typical cases, they assigned the name "Hodgkin's granuloma"; to a much more malignant variant, seen in a relatively small proportion of cases and usually characterized by a great abundance of pleomorphic and anaplastic Sternberg-Reed cells, the name "Hodgkin's sarcoma"; and finally, after Jackson (1939) had first erroneously designated it as "early Hodgkin's disease," they assigned the name "Hodgkin's paragranuloma" to another infrequent variant characterized by extremely slow clinical evolution, a relative paucity of Sternberg-Reed cells, and a great abundance of lymphocytes.

Lukes and his colleagues (1963, 1966) have recognized a rather characteristic subtype within the heterogeneous "granuloma" category, to which they assigned the name "nodular sclerosis." They have proposed a new histopathologic classification, which appears to have appreciably greater prognostic relevance and usefulness than the Jackson-Parker classification (cf. Chapter 3). In historical context, it is of interest that Greenfield (1878) may well have been the first person to describe nodular sclerosing Hodgkin's disease: "the normal structure . . . appears to be entirely lost; it is everywhere traversed by irregular broad bands of fibrous tissue."

Whereas lymphosarcoma, reticulum cell sarcoma, and the Burkitt lymphoma were regarded as malignant neoplasms from the beginning, and the follicular lymphomas came to be so regarded within a few years after their discovery, controversy has raged for over 100 years concerning the nature, etiology, and pathogenesis of Hodgkin's disease. Hodgkin himself considered it to be a kind of "hypertrophy of the lymphatic system," a view on which Wilks (1865) comments: "a most remarkable disorder; in which an interruption to the healthy action of the body is induced by the excessive function of one set of organs." Wilks' own concept of the disease was somewhat closer to the mark: "On the contrary, does the new cell-formation interfere with the function of the gland, and is the latter therefore destroyed instead of being increased? Instead of the life of the patient gradually ceasing from an excess of function from a set of organs, is it not rather through their diminution or cessation of action?" That he believed it to be neoplastic in character is suggested by the statement: "It would appear, then, that this disease represents merely one mode in which an adventitious deposit can affect the organs, and that it must take its place in the rank of malignant diseases, or amongst those

affections which are characterized by the development of new growths in the system."

Of particular interest is the fact that Wilks anticipated the later debates as to whether Hodgkin's disease arises unicentrically or multicentrically; concerning its mode of spread, he states: "The peculiarity of this affection still remains in the fact of the glandular system being especially affected, and which gives rise, therefore, to peculiar symptoms. This may be due to the lymphatic glands being first diseased, for it has not yet been determined, in this class of maladies, how far the constitutional and how far the local causes predominate in causing the propagation of, and in giving the character to, new growth. In the present form of disease, the lymphatic glands appear to be affected for a considerable period, perhaps many years, before the system suffers, and that next the spleen becomes especially involved, and afterwards the other organs; *it is possible, too, that the propagation takes place in the course of the lymphatics, and the reason why the corpuscles of the spleen are thus affected arises from the fact of their being intimately connected with the absorbent system, and in like manner the deposit in Glisson's capsule of the liver may have been transmitted by the same channels.* As regards its degree of malignancy, it appears to take a place between cancer and tubercle" [italics added]. It is also interesting to note the views of Greenfield (1878), who concluded: "that at first it is an essentially local disease, consisting in an irritative overgrowth of some normal lymphatic glandular tissue, which becomes infective, *leading to similar implication of adjacent glands, and thence spreading to more distant areas, usually by contiguity.* Clinically and anatomically, there is little distinction at this stage from cancer, and *it may be regarded as lymphatic cancer*" [italics added].

The view that Hodgkin's disease is a malignant neoplasm was also held and strongly defended by Benda (1904), Mallory (1914), and Warthin (1931). Proponents of its infectious nature were, however, impressed with the frequency of its association with tuberculosis, and Sternberg (1898), finding that the patients in eight of his thirteen cases had coexistent tuberculosis, argued that Hodgkin's disease was a peculiar form of tuberculosis. However, Dorothy Reed (1902), Longcope (1903, 1907), and others refuted this thesis and concluded that Hodgkin's disease was an independent entity, with which tuberculosis might sometimes be associated. Additional details concerning this interesting but now obsolete controversy may be found in the excellent reviews by Wallhauser (1933) and by Hoster et al. (1948). Nonetheless, Reed belonged to the group that considered Hodgkin's disease to be inflammatory in nature. She stated: "Macroscopically, the growth differs from malignant tumor in the absence of capsular infiltration and implication of adjacent tissues. Sarcoma does not confine its growth to gradual extension from gland to gland. We do not know of any malignant neoplasm the metastases of which occur in only one form of tissue. Hodgkin's disease seems not to metastasize by cellular transplantation but by causing a proliferation in pre-existing lymphoid tissue, apparently anywhere in the body . . . Histologically, it might be thought that the changes resemble those of a malignant growth, but we believe that closer study will show a greater similarity to inflammatory processes."

Accordingly, others took up the search for infectious agents other than the tubercle bacillus. In the first two decades of this century, largely as a consequence of the work of Bunting (1914) and Bunting and Yates (1915), great interest was centered on diphtheroid bacteria as possible etiologic agents. Attention was later drawn by Parsons and Poston (1939) and Wise and Poston (1940) to the possible role of *Brucella,* and Jackson and Parker (1947) were for a time interested in an aerobic gas-forming bacillus which they isolated from some of their cases that came to autopsy. It was claimed by L'Esperance (1929, 1931) that she had succeeded in reproducing Hodgkin's disease experimentally with an avian strain of tubercle bacillus, but her claims could not be confirmed by Branch (1931), Van Rooyen (1933), or Jackson and Parker. Various species of fungus were also briefly entertained as possibilities. Finally, Gordon's discovery (1932) that extracts from involved lymph nodes of patients with Hodgkin's disease could induce in rabbits an acute encephalitis, which he erroneously interpreted as being possibly due to virus infection, ushered in a period in which viruses have been strongly suspected of being the etiologic agents of Hodgkin's disease. Views intermediate between the neoplastic and the inflammatory concepts have also been put forward. For example, Chevalier and Bernard (1932) suggested that Hodgkin's disease might arise as an inflammatory reaction secondary to virus infection and later transform into a blastoma. Definitive evidence that Hodgkin's disease is a malignant neoplasm finally emerged during the last decade when cytogenetic studies (detailed in Chapter 3) demonstrated that the giant cells satisfy two of the fundamental attributes of neoplastic cells: aneuploidy and clonal derivation.

Clinical awareness of the existence of autoim-mune disease in man and the growing body of experimental work dealing with immunologic reactions of the graft-versus-host type led Kaplan and Smithers (1959) to suggest that Hodgkin's disease might represent an autoimmune process, involving an interaction between neoplastic and normal lymphoid cells, as a consequence of antigenic abnormalities arising in the neoplastic cells, akin to the graft-versus-host reactions observed in animals. Green and his colleagues (1960) have carried this view further in proposing that Hodgkin's disease might involve a maternal-to-fetal cell chimera, a view for which no firm experimental evidence has since been presented. Order and Hellman (1972) reinterpreted the Kaplan-Smithers hypothesis in the light of modern immunobiology, postulating that "T cells (thymus-derived lymphocytes) are infected by a tumour-inducing virus causing a change in cell-surface antigen. Normal T cells begin to react against the virus-transformed cells. This interaction is protracted in a fashion similar to a chronic graft-versus-host reaction and results in the production of neoplastic reticulum cells." De Vita (1973) characterized this reaction in colorful terms as "a lymphocyte civil war." Similar considerations led Lukes and Collins (1974) to suggest that the giant cells of Hodgkin's disease may be derived from T-lymphocytes which have undergone blastogenic transformation in vivo. However, the recent successful cultivation of Sternberg-Reed and Hodgkin's giant cells in vitro by Kaplan and Gartner (1977) and by Long et al. (1977b) permitted the demonstration that they are aneuploid, heterotransplantable, mitotically active malignant cells with phagocytic and other properties indicative of their origin from macrophages or other closely related cells of the mononuclear phagocyte system, rather than from lymphocytes. Accordingly, the mechanism underlying the lymphocyte depletion and other apparently "autoimmune" phenomena seen in Hodgkin's disease remains unexplained.

Virtually all of the principal clinical features of Hodgkin's disease had been described by the end of the nineteenth century (Fig. 1.15). Only a cursory description of the clinical history and physical findings in his cases was presented by Hodgkin. Wilks (1865) clearly observed the anemia and cachexia of his patients and also called attention to intermittent fever in at least one instance. It was not until 1887, however, that Pel and Ebstein first carefully described the peculiar cyclic bouts of fever which now bear their names. Dorothy Reed (1902) presented a meticulously detailed descrip-

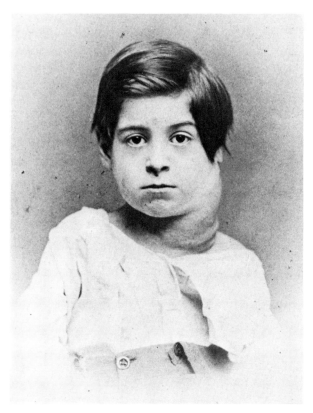

Figure 1.15 This photograph, published by Damon in 1864, is probably the earliest in existence of a patient with a malignant lymphoma. The presence of massive left cervical lymphadenopathy is evident. Although Damon stated that the case was one of "leucocythemia," the differential diagnosis of that condition from Hodgkin's disease was not yet established, and the clinical appearance would be equally consistent with either entity.

tion of the clinical histories and the hematologic findings in her eight cases. Of particular interest is the fact, carefully recorded by her, that "tuberculin was given in five of the cases but without reaction" —probably the earliest observation of the immunologic unresponsiveness so characteristic of the disease. The patient in her first case was tuberculin-negative, despite the fact that he had open and active tuberculosis.

The first systematic investigations of the response to the tuberculin test were made by Parker, Jackson, Fitzhugh, and Spies (1932) and by Steiner (1934a). Both groups of workers found a remarkably high incidence of anergy to tuberculin, and Jackson and Parker, in their book, *Hodgkin's Disease and Allied Disorders* (1947), noted that in some patients the tuberculin test may again become strongly positive after effective roentgen therapy.

Although Dubin (1947) called attention to "the

poverty of the immunological mechanism" in Hodgkin's disease, it was Schier and his associates (1956) who first demonstrated that the relative anergy of patients with Hodgkin's disease is not limited to tuberculin but is also evident with a number of other natural antigens capable of eliciting delayed cutaneous hypersensitivity reactions. Later, after it had been discovered that a number of chemical contact allergens such as dinitrochlorobenzene could also elicit the tuberculin type of reaction, Aisenberg (1962) carried out the first systematic study of a series of patients with Hodgkin's disease, the results of which suggested strongly that the frequency of anergic responses after active sensitization to dinitrochlorobenzene was closely linked to activity of the disease. At low sensitizing concentrations of this agent, Eltringham and Kaplan (1973) found that even patients with stage I disease confined to a single lymph node may have impaired delayed hypersensitivity responses. Levy and Kaplan (1974) developed a sensitive modification of the lymphocyte mitogenic response to phytohemagglutinin (PHA) with which they could detect similar impairment of T-lymphocyte function in vitro. Subsequent studies have revealed that another T-lymphocyte response, the capacity to form spontaneous rosettes with sheep red blood cells, is also frequently decreased (Bobrove et al., 1975); that this response, as well as the response to PHA, may be restored to normal by incubation of peripheral blood lymphocytes in fetal sera (Fuks et al., 1976b); and that a rosette-inhibiting factor can be demonstrated in the sera and in extracts of the involved spleens (Bieber, Fuks, and Kaplan, 1977) of patients with Hodgkin's disease. These and other developments are set forth in greater detail in Chapter 6.

Curiously, few efforts to probe the diagnostic aspects of the disease were made until quite recent years. The introduction by Peters (1950) of a three-stage clinical classification ushered in a new era of increased emphasis on the diagnostic evaluation and systematic analysis of the anatomic extent of involvement. This movement gained great impetus from the development by Kinmonth (1952) of lower extremity lymphangiography, a new technique for the roentgenologic visualization of the pelvic and retroperitoneal lymph nodes which began to be utilized in several major centers after improved oily contrast media became available about 1960. It was soon apparent that lymphangiography was far more sensitive and accurate than clinical palpation, inferior vena cavography, and intravenous urography (the only methods previously available for the detection of para-aortic and pelvic node involvement) and that clinically silent involvement of these nodes could be demonstrated by this new technique in a dismayingly high proportion of cases (Baum et al., 1963; Lee, Nelson, and Schwartz, 1964). In time, other roentgenologic and isotopic procedures, notably pulmonary tomography and skeletal scintigraphy, have further increased the accuracy of the diagnostic evaluation (Davidson and Clarke, 1968).

However, the spleen, splenic hilar nodes, and liver remained silent areas in which foci of disease could lurk undetected by any of these radiologic methods. Laparotomy with splenectomy and biopsy of the splenic hilar, para-aortic, and mesenteric nodes and the liver came into use on a selective basis initially at Stanford University Medical Center. After some years, my colleagues and I (Glatstein et al., 1969) collected a series of sixty-five such cases, in which the frequency of clinically unsuspected splenic involvement was so astonishingly high that we were led to explore the use of laparotomy with splenectomy and biopsy as a *routine* part of the diagnostic evaluation and staging of the disease, again with striking results (Glatstein et al., 1970; Enright, Trueblood, and Nelsen, 1970). Collectively, these diagnostic procedures have provided us for the first time with reliable comprehensive data on the patterns of anatomic distribution of Hodgkin's disease at the time of biopsy diagnosis and have opened the way to refined staging classifications (cf. Chapter 8) which correlate increasingly well with prognosis and to new concepts of the mode of dissemination of the disease which have had important therapeutic implications.

The therapy of Hodgkin's disease and the other lymphomas was essentially symptomatic throughout the nineteenth century. Pusey (1902) was apparently the first to treat the lymphomas with the X rays newly discovered by Roentgen in 1896. Pusey's case 1 involved a twenty-four-year-old male with bilateral cervical lymphadenopathy, biopsy of which revealed "small round cell sarcoma" (presumably some form of lymphosarcoma). This patient was given twenty-one X-ray exposures, from September 2 through September 27, 1901, "with a hard tube and a weak light." Slight erythema appeared on September 17, and by September 27 this had developed into pronounced dermatitis, at which time exposure was stopped. Pusey said: "The effect of the exposures on the tumor was almost magical. Within ten days it had shrunken perceptibly and the motions of the head were freer. On September 17 the circumfer-

ence around the chin was reduced to 17½ inches, a decrease of 3½ inches. On September 25 this was 16¾ inches, and the tumor was reduced to the size of an olive. On October 11 there was no trace of the disease left except a small, freely movable, painless gland not larger than an almond kernel. There was no swelling, no stiffness, and interference with motion had disappeared." No recurrence had developed within the three-month followup period prior to publication of Pusey's paper. Two other cases were apparently osteosarcomas, and the patients had significant relief of pain but little or no tumor regression in response to similar treatments. His fourth and fifth cases, however, were cases of Hodgkin's disease, the first a boy of four, with bilateral cervical involvement, referred for X-ray treatment to the left cervical region after surgical resection of the nodes on the right side by Dr. Ochsner. Pusey reported that under X-ray exposures the swelling rapidly subsided, and in two months the glands were "reduced to the size of an almond." His remaining case, a fifty-year-old man with right axillary and epithrochlear adenopathy, had been under treatment with arsenic without response. Treatment to the epitrochlear nodes elicited a prompt response, and accordingly similar treatment was then initiated to the axillary lymphadenopathy, which had begun to decrease in size and firmness, with improved mobility of the arm, at the time of his epochal publication.

Interestingly enough, the second report on the use of X-ray therapy in the treatment of Hodgkin's disease also emanated from Chicago. In his article in 1903, some fifteen months after Pusey's paper appeared, Nicholas Senn, then professor of surgery at Rush Medical College, described dramatic responses in two patients, both male, one forty-three and the other fifty-three years of age, whom he had referred for roentgen therapy to radiologists at two different hospitals. Senn makes no mention of Pusey's articles, although it is not unreasonable to assume that he was aware of it. (It is perhaps indicative of the low esteem in which the pioneering radiologists of that day were held by a surgeon that Senn did not see fit to invite Dr. W. F. Butterman or Dr. Joseph F. Smith to join him as co-authors on this paper, although they had in fact done all of the work.) Comparison of the pretreatment photograph of the patient in his case 1 with that of the same patient after treatment shows an essentially complete and dramatic regression of the massive lymphadenopathy which was evident initially. These almost complete regressions of disease must have impressed Senn vividly, for he concludes (somewhat prematurely): "The eminent success attained in these two cases by the use of the X-ray can leave no further doubt of the curative effect of the Roentgen ray in the treatment of pseudoleukaemia."

The hopes aroused by such encouraging initial responses were soon dashed by the apparently inevitable appearance of recurrences in the treated area or elsewhere, and the outcome again came to be regarded as inevitably fatal. As is detailed in Chapter 10, the development of megavoltage apparatus during the last thirty years has ushered in a new era in the radiotherapy of Hodgkin's disease and the other malignant lymphomas. Specifically, it has become technically feasible to irradiate to tumoricidal dose levels essentially all of the lymph nodes and other lymphatic tissues in the body ("total lymphoid" radiotherapy) through the development of large fields (the "mantle," "inverted-Y," and variations of these) shaped to the lymphoid tissue distributions in different regions (Kaplan 1962, 1966c; Page, Gardner, and Karzmark, 1970a,b).

During the period from about 1920 to 1950, there was also some interest in the use of radical surgery for the eradication of localized lymphomas. However, in most of the series in which good results were reported, X-ray therapy had been given postoperatively and, therefore, could well have been responsible for the favorable outcome. This consideration and the cosmetically disfiguring end results of such extensive surgery have gradually led most surgeons to consider that radical surgery is not indicated in the primary management of the malignant lymphomas.

In the 1940's, as a byproduct of wartime work on compounds related to the mustard gases, it was discovered that the nitrogen mustards had powerful lymphocytolytic effects, both on normal lymphoid tissues and in preliminary clinical trials in selected cases of Hodgkin's disease and other malignant lymphomas (Goodman et al., 1946). This was the beginning of chemotherapy for the leukemias and lymphomas. Soon the work of organic chemists made available a host of derivatives of the nitrogen mustards, all having in common the great reactivity of their alkylating groups. Some of these agents are still widely utilized in the management of certain leukemias; others are principally effective in Hodgkin's disease and in certain of the malignant lymphomas; and still others have found their way into the treatment of a variety of other types of neoplastic disease. The antimetabolite approach to chemotherapy was introduced by Farber and his associates (1948, 1949), who used aminopterin, an analog of folic acid, for the treatment of childhood leukemia. Since that time, dozens of other antimetabolites have been synthesized and tested both experimentally and clinically, and many of these have now found their way into the clinical armamentarium, as have a number of alkaloids and antibiotics extracted from various plant, fungus, and microbial sources. Experimental studies indicating the desirability of using combinations of agents with nonoverlapping toxicities led to the introduction in 1964 of the highly effective four-drug "MOPP" regimen (De Vita, Serpick, and Carbone, 1970). Some of the patients with advanced disease have now survived relapse-free for ten years or more, indicating that MOPP may have curative potential (De Vita et al., 1976). Moreover, patients with advanced disease have been successfully treated with both total lymphoid radiotherapy and MOPP in various planned sequences (Moore et al., 1972; Kaplan and Rosenberg, 1975; Rosenberg et al., 1978; Hoppe et al., 1979). These developments are detailed in Chapter 11, and their influence on prognosis, especially in stages III and IV, is discussed in Chapter 12. Collectively, these diagnostic and therapeutic advances have brought us close to the total therapeutic conquest of a once inevitably fatal malady (Kaplan, 1976, 1977).

Chapter 2

Etiology and Epidemiology

Although the etiology of Hodgkin's disease is not yet established, the etiology of morphologically similar tumors and of other types of lymphoma has been extensively studied in experimental animals. Epidemiologic studies have also yielded a considerable amount of information concerning age, sex, racial, environmental, and other factors which may significantly modify the susceptibility of human populations to the development of Hodgkin's disease. In this chapter, the discussion of epidemiology has been restricted to Hodgkin's disease, whereas the section on experimental investigations has been deliberately extended to cover certain other lymphomas as well. This approach has been chosen because the existence of a morphologically acceptable equivalent of Hodgkin's disease in experimental animals is still a highly controversial question and the amount of experimental work strictly concerned with Hodgkin's disease is therefore quite limited. Since the insights gained into the problem of etiology of the other lymphomas may well have relevance for Hodgkin's disease as well, the much more voluminous experimental literature pertaining to the other lymphomas seemed appropriate for presentation here.

Experimental Studies

Lymphosarcomas and Lymphatic Leukemias. The availability during the past fifty years of genetically homogenous inbred stains of mice with characteristic patterns of susceptibility or resistance to the development or induction of various types of tumors has made the mouse a particularly useful laboratory animal for such studies. Experimental interest has also been encouraged by the fact that the lymphosarcomas and lymphatic leukemias of the mouse are morphologically indistinguishable from those of man. The spontaneous incidence of leukemias and lymphosarcoma in most inbred strains of mice is quite low, attaining a level of approximately 1 to 2 percent at about two years of age. However, there are certain "high-leukemia" strains (notably strains AKR and C58) in which almost all the untreated animals develop spontaneous lymphosarcoma or lymphatic leukemia during the first year of life. Exposure of "low-leukemia" strains to a variety of physical, chemical, and biological agents has been shown to induce a high incidence of lymphosarcoma and lymphatic leukemia (cf. Kaplan, 1974).

Physical Agents. That exposure to ionizing radiation is leukemogenic for certain strains of mice was first firmly established by the studies of Furth and Furth in 1936. More recently, it has been demonstrated that systemic exposure to the beta rays of radioactive phosphorus or to fission neutrons is also leukemogenic. The induced tumors almost invariably arise in the thymus gland, and their development in irradiated animals may be effectively prevented by prior thymectomy.

Paradoxically, however, local X-irradiation over the thymic region proved to be ineffective; the induction of a high incidence of lymphomas in susceptible strains, such as strain C57BL, required whole-body radiation exposure (Kaplan, 1949; Kaplan and Brown, 1951). It was later shown that the cells of the bone marrow and spleen, by a mechanism which is not yet fully understood, can inhibit or suppress the leukemogenic process initiated in the thymus by X-ray exposure (Kaplan, Brown and Paull, 1953; Lorenz, Congdon and Uphoff, 1953). The capacity of marrow cells to inhibit leukemogenesis is readily inactivated by low doses of X-rays, but the presence of even a small amount of unirradiated bone marrow suffices to confer protection; hence the requirement for whole-body X-ray exposure.

Another curious feature of X-ray leukemogenesis is the relationship between radiation dose and tumor yield. Although tumor incidence decreases as radiation dose is decreased, it does so only over a rather restricted range of doses, and an apparent "threshold" dose is reached at approximately 200 r, below which the associated tumor incidence does not significantly exceed the control level. When the radiation is given in a series of fractionated exposures, separated by intervals of several days, the tumor yield is paradoxically very much greater than when the same total dose is given either as a single massive exposure or in consecutive daily fractions (Kaplan and Brown, 1952).

Further experimentation revealed that radiogenic lymphomas may arise by a completely indirect process, in which nonirradiated cells are induced to become neoplastic by virtue of their residence in an irradiated environment. When young C57BL mice were subjected to thymectomy, exposed to whole-body X-irradiation, and then implanted subcutaneously with a nonirradiated thymus from a baby mouse of the same strain, lymphosarcomas occurred in appreciable yield and could be shown to originate in the thymic implant (Kaplan and Brown, 1954; Kaplan, Carnes, Brown, and Hirsch, 1956). When this experiment was repeated with F_1 hybrid mice from a cross of strains C57BL and C_3H, which were then grafted after thymectomy and irradiation with nonirradiated thymus glands from young C57BL donors, most of the ensuing tumors could be shown to exhibit the transplantation behavior characteristic of the C57BL genotype and thus clearly had been derived from the cells of the thymic implant, which had never been exposed to irradiation (Kaplan, Hirsch, and Brown, 1956). This paradox, which was soon confirmed in other laboratories (Law and Potter, 1956; Barnes et al., 1959) was later explained by the discovery of a leukemogenic viral agent in extracts from such tumors (see under Biologic Agents).

Chemical Agents. It has long been known that the carcinogenic hydrocarbons are leukemogenic in certain strains of mice (Morton and Mider, 1938). Methylcholanthrene and dimethylbenzanthracene have been the two most intensively studied compounds in this category. At almost the same time, the discovery was independently made by investigators in France (Lacassagne, 1937) and in the United States (Gardner, 1937) that the female sex hormone, estrogen, is also a leukemogen in some murine strains, though its activity is less pronounced. In recent years, such compounds as urethane (ethyl carbamate), thiotriethylene phosphoramide and nitroquinoline oxide have swelled the list of chemical leukemogens.

In general, the results of studies on the mechanism of leukemia induction by chemical agents have been consistent with the pattern established by more extensive studies on radiation leukemogenesis. There have now been a series of reports of the successful extraction of cell-free (presumably viral) leukemogenic activity from lymphomas and leukemias induced by the carcinogenic hydrocarbons, urethane, nitroquinoline oxide, and other agents (Irino et al., 1963; Toth, 1963; Kunii et al., 1965; Ribacchi and Giraldo, 1966; Haran-Ghera, 1967; Igel et al., 1969; Ball and McCarter, 1971).

Biologic Agents (Viruses). The knowledge that leukemia may be induced by viruses dates back more than seventy years to the discovery by Ellermann and Bang (1908) that the blood of leukemic chickens contains a subcellular agent capable of transmitting the disease to other chickens. Experimental difficulties made further progress difficult at that time, and this field of investigation languished until the 1940's when Burmester (1952) succeeded in developing better-defined flocks of chickens, with which more reproducible laboratory results could be obtained. It became clear that two major forms of leukemia, each associated with its own viral agent, were involved: a lymphatic (leukosis) form, which is widely endemic and responsible for major economic losses in the poultry industry, and a myeloblastic (occasionally erythromyeloblastic) form. Under certain circumstances, birds infected with the leukosis virus may also develop osteopetrosis, nephroblastic tumors, or other bizarre lesions. The avian leukosis virus was subsequently purified by Beard and his colleagues.

In the four decades that followed the discovery of Ellermann and Bang, many investigators tried unsuccessfully to demonstrate similar viruses in murine leukemias. However, it was not until 1951 that Ludwik Gross succeeded in demonstrating that cell-free filtrates or extracts prepared from spontaneous lymphomas of mice of the high-leukemia AKR strain induce similar lymphatic leukemias *de novo* after inoculation into strain C_3H/Bi test mice. He succeeded where others had failed because he inoculated his filtrates and extracts into newborn rather than adult mice. By serial passage of this subcellular material, Gross was able to increase its leukemogenic potency manyfold.

Particles believed to represent the virus were observed budding from the surfaces of lymphoid tumor cells in electron micrographs of tissues from spontaneous AKR and C58 lymphomas and in those induced in strain C_3H by the Gross virus. These particles, designated as type C, were spherical and had a centrally placed electron-dense nucleoid (Figure 2.1). These observations clearly

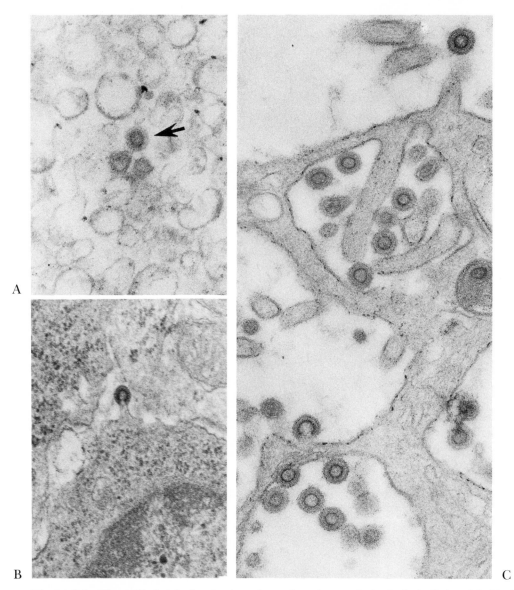

Figure 2.1   The radiation leukemia virus shown here is morphologically indistinguishable from the Gross, Moloney, Friend, Rauscher, and other leukemogenic viruses of the mouse. *A,* solitary virus particle (arrow) in microsomal pellet of cell-free extract from leukemic tissue. *B,* virus particle budding from plasma membrane of lymphocyte in thymus graft inoculated with cell-free extract. *C,* virus particles in cytoplasmic vacuoles of epithelial cell in thymic graft 13 days after inoculation of cell-free extract. Electron micrograph ×60,000, by Mary Lou Hart; glutaraldehyde and osmium tetroxide fixation, uranyl acetate stain. (Reproduced, by permission of *Cancer Research,* from Carnes, Lieberman, Marchildon, and Kaplan, 1968).

identified the etiologic agent of the leukemias induced in strain C₃H/Bi mice as a virus and strongly indicated that the lymphatic leukemias and lymphomas of the high-leukemia AKR and C58 strains, from which the Gross virus had originally been extracted, were also caused by the same agent.

A number of other murine leukemogenic viruses, including the Graffi, Moloney, Friend, and Rauscher viruses, have since been discovered in ex-

tracts prepared, curiously enough, not from lymphomas or leukemias but from long-transplanted epithelial or sarcomatous tumors of mice, in which these viruses appear to be efficiently propagated passengers. All of them have exhibited the type C morphology in electron micrographs. Some of them induce predominantly thymic lymphomas and lymphatic leukemias; others, myeloid leukemias; and still others induce reticulum cell sarcomas and erythroblastic leukemias of splenic

origin (Friend, 1957). On inoculation into thymectomized mice, the Gross and Moloney viruses induce myeloid leukemia; virus recovered from such myeloid leukemias again induces thymic lymphosarcomas and lymphatic leukemias on inoculation into intact animals.

The paradoxical discovery that radiation acts by an indirect mechanism in the induction of thymic lymphomas stimulated a search for the presence of an agent similar to the Gross virus in radiogenic lymphomas. Cell-free extracts prepared from thymic lymphomas induced by X-irradiation in mice of strains C57BL and C_3H were soon shown to contain an agent capable of inducing the same type of neoplasm *de novo* after neonatal injection into non-irradiated mice of the corresponding strains (Kaplan, 1957; Gross, 1958; Lieberman and Kaplan, 1959). Leukemogenic activity of the agent increased and the latent period for tumor induction decreased significantly during serial passage. Subsequent work led to the purification of the radiation leukemia virus (RadLV) which was found to possess the same type C morphology (Fig. 2.1) as the other murine leukemia viruses (Carnes et al., 1968). Thus, a link was established between one of the external leukemogenic agents, radiation, and the leukemia viruses. As mentioned above, similar subcellular leukemogenic agents have also been obtained from lymphomas induced by the chemical leukemogens. Thymic lymphoid cells infected in vitro with RadLV have been demonstrated to undergo neoplastic transformation after return to an in vivo environment (Lieberman and Kaplan, 1966). Moreover, direct neoplastic transformation of lymphoid cells by a murine leukemia virus in vitro has now been achieved (Rosenberg, Baltimore, and Scher, 1975). It may therefore be concluded that viruses are the universal common denominator in the etiology of the murine leukemias and lymphomas (Kaplan, 1967).

Physical and chemical agents appear to act indirectly by altering the host-virus relationship in such a way as to "activate" the latent leukemogenic potentialities of viruses harbored by otherwise low-leukemia strains of mice. Activation of type C viruses from mouse embryo fibroblasts by physical and chemical agents in vitro has also been demonstrated (Lowy et al., 1971; Rowe et al., 1971).

There is evidence that these viruses are transmitted from one generation to the next through the embryo and that they can persist in the tissues of such naturally infected strains throughout life without producing discernible ill effects unless the animals are exposed to such external inducing

s.
m.
infe
polic
vance
herited
vated sta

The ge.
viruses is c
acid (RNA) \
corresponding
mately 10 × 1(
permissive cells,
double-stranded
copy (the proviru
fied enzyme, RNA-
informally known
(Temin and Mizutani,
provirus then undergoe
of the host cell, from wh
ered by the elegantly ser.
nique of molecular hybr.
Kohne, 1968). During activ
quence occurs; the provirus i.
lar DNA and transcribed to vir.
viral proteins are synthesized a
occurs at the cell membrane.

The murine viruses are able to c
riers and induce lymphomas and ly
mias in laboratory rats. This has t
demonstration that a new antigen ap
cells of lymphomas and leukemias induc
the murine leukemia viruses. This antig
same for all tumors induced by a given v
gardless of species. Thus, antisera prepared
rat against lymphomas induced by a given vi
the rat will also react with lymphomas induce
the same virus in the mouse. Such antisera h
been shown to exhibit a number of types of i
munologic reactivity: they prevent the growth o
transplantable lymphomas, produce lethal cytotoxic effects on tumor cells with which they are incubated in vitro, undergo adsorption by lym-
phoma cells, and neutralize viral activity (Geering, Old and Boyse, 1966; Ferrer and Kaplan, 1968).

The Friend, Moloney, and Rauscher (FMR) viruses have been shown to be an immunologically related "family," since antisera prepared against tumors induced by any one of them cross-react extensively against tumors induced by the other two.

The Gross virus a
cally related to ea
group.
Finally, when
avian leukemia
ment with ethe
cific antigen, s
of the murine
spectively, ca
ment-fixation
Huebner,
Huebner, 1
Hilgers et
(competition
gust, 197
Recen
of viruse
has bee
with a
(Opler
chara
electr
leuke
1967
Vir
tro
su
ph
p
s

...d RadLV are also immunologi-
...th other, though not to the FMR
...

...the outer coat of the murine or
...viruses is stripped away by treat-
... and detergent, a new group-spe-
...called because it is common to all
...or the avian leukemia viruses, re-
... be demonstrated by the comple-
...technique (Sarma, Turner, and
...964; Hartley, Rowe, Capps, and
...65), by indirect immunofluorescence
...l., 1972; Declève et al., 1974), and by
... radioimmunoassay (Strand and Au-
...

...vidence extends the leukemogenic role
...to higher mammalian species. Leukemia
...induced in inbred families of guinea pigs
...rus extracted from a guinea pig leukemia
...1967), and virus particles of consistent and
...eristic morphology have been identified in
...n micrographs prepared from the blood of
...nic cats (Jarrett et al., 1964; Kawakami et al.,
...Rickard et al., 1967; Laird et al., 1968).
...s-like particles have also been observed in elec-
...micrographs of the blood and tissues of dogs,
...uman primates, and cattle bearing lym-
...omas and leukemias. Moreover, bovine lym-
...oma may occur in local epidemic outbreaks
...rongly suggestive of an infectious etiology (Ben-
ixen, 1965). The bovine lymphoma virus has
...een isolated and propagated in vitro (Van der
Maaten, Miller, and Boothe, 1974; Graves and Ferrer, 1976), as have simian and gibbon ape leukemia-lymphoma viruses (Kawakami et al., 1972;
Gallo et al., 1978).

Thus, viruses have been proved to be leukemogenic in a broad spectrum of animal species, ranging from chickens to mice, rats, guinea pigs, and
cats, and are strongly implicated in the etiology of
leukemias and lymphomas in primate and bovine
species (Kaplan, 1974, 1978b). Collectively, these
observations render the view increasingly plausible
that the human leukemias and lymphomas will also
ultimately prove due to viruses. Viruses and virus-
like particles have been identified in electron micrographs of blood and tissues from leukemic
human patients, and extracts from such human
leukemias have yielded a variety of infectious and
toxic reactions on inoculation into mice and other
experimental animals. Sophisticated and sensitive
biochemical techniques are now available for the simultaneous detection of viral RNA and reverse
transcriptase in cytoplasmic particles (Schlom and
Spiegelman, 1971), for the detection of the integrated provirus in cellular DNA (Britten and
Kohne, 1968), for the immunologic distinction of
the viral reverse transcriptases of different species
(Parks and Scolnick, 1972; Parks et al., 1972; Sherr
et al., 1975), and for the identification in cells and
viral particles of several virion structural proteins
(Strand and August, 1973; Witte, Weissman, and
Kaplan, 1973). With the aid of these methods, C-
type viruses have now been recovered from human
acute myeloid leukemias (Gallagher and Gallo,
1975; Nooter et al., 1975). More recently, Kaplan
et al. (1977) isolated a C-type RNA virus from a cell
line established in vitro from a human histiocytic
lymphoma (Epstein and Kaplan, 1974); several additional C-type viral isolates were subsequently detected in other permanently established non-
Hodgkin's lymphoma cell lines (Kaplan et al.,
1979). Normal human bone marrow cells have apparently been transformed by cocultivation with a
lethally irradiated human acute monocytic leukemia cell line which, by electron microscopy, contains 50 and 70 nm particles resembling intracellular type A particles (Karpas, Wreghitt, and
Nagington, 1978). However, there is as yet no conclusive proof that such viruses were the etiologic
agents of, rather than merely secondary passengers in, the leukemias and lymphomas in which
they were encountered.

*The Role of Genetic, Constitutional, and Trophic Factors
in Murine Leukemogenesis.* The availability of highly
inbred strains of mice has made it possible to demonstrate convincingly that genetic determinants
exert a powerful control on susceptibility or resistance of various mouse strains to the spontaneous
development or induction of leukemias or lymphomas (Kirschbaum and Mixer, 1947). Genetic
factors have also been shown to control viral
expression and replication in vitro (Lilly and
Pincus, 1973; Rowe, 1973).

Age, sex, nutritional status, and hormonal balance have also been shown to influence susceptibility to leukemia development within a given strain.
Susceptibility to viral induction appears to be maximal at birth and decays rapidly after the first few
weeks of life. The susceptibility of strain C57BL
mice to lymphoma induction by X-rays is also maximal during the first month of life. In several
strains, females are significantly more susceptible
than males. This difference in response can be
eliminated in some strains by orchiectomy, suggesting that it may be due to inhibition by andro-
genic hormones. Simple caloric restriction, which

has long been known to inhibit the development of a variety of other experimental animal neoplasms (Tannenbaum, 1947), has also been shown to inhibit murine leukemia development.

The longstanding controversy concerning the unicentric-vs.-multicentric origin of human lymphomas has been convincingly resolved in the mouse. In most strains, lymphosarcomas exhibit a striking predilection for unifocal origin in one particular lymphoid structure, the thymus; invasion and dissemination to other tissues and organs occur secondarily (Kaplan, 1948, 1957). In this respect, they bear a striking resemblance to the lymphatic leukemias of childhood, which in at least some instances first become clinically manifest as lymphosarcomatous masses replacing the thymus and invading the mediastinum.

Reticulum Cell Sarcoma. In old age, many strains of mice develop a high incidence of tumors which commonly involve the mesenteric lymph nodes initially and then spread to those of the mediastinum and periphery. On histologic examination, these tumors exhibit a pleomorphic cellular pattern dominated by the presence of cells with the morphology of atypical histiocytes (Dunn, 1954). Little information is available concerning the etiology of these reticulum cell neoplasms of the mouse. Their incidence does not appear to be affected significantly by irradiation or some of the chemical leukemogens. A high incidence of reticulum cell tumors has been noted after an appreciably shorter latent period in chimeric F_1 hybrid mice that survive a homologous graft-vs.-host reaction induced by the injection of parental strain spleen cells (Schwartz and Beldotti, 1965). More recently, it has been reported by Cole and Nowell (1970) that some of the lymphomas which developed in their chimeric F_1 hybrid mice injected with parental bone marrow were of donor genotype. Graft-versus-host reactions have been reported to activate latent type C viruses in vivo (Hirsch et al., 1972; Armstrong et al., 1973), suggesting that these reticulum cell neoplasms may also be viral in origin.

A new strain of mouse, the SJL strain, has been developed which characteristically develops this pleomorphic type of neoplasm at a much earlier age (Murphy, 1963; McIntire, 1969). Some of these tumors are known to produce immunoglobulins (McIntire and Law, 1967). The SJL strain is also susceptible to the development of thymic lymphosarcomas induced by irradiation and to the development of lymphosarcomas arising in other lymphoid structures after treatment with dimeth-

ylbenzanthracene. Subcellular, presumably viral, extracts prepared from such tumors have been reported not only to induce lymphosarcomas *de novo* in inoculated mice but also to accelerate the onset of reticulum cell tumors, which would otherwise develop spontaneously in these mice at a much older age (Haran-Ghera, Kotler, and Meshorer, 1967).

Hodgkin's Disease. Experimental work on the etiology of Hodgkin's disease has been seriously hampered by the lack of a morphologically acceptable counterpart of this type of lymphoma in experimental animals (Dunn and Deringer, 1968). Although it has been reported that lymphomas morphologically similar to or identical with Hodgkin's disease occur in dogs (Moulton and Bostick, 1958; Squire, 1969), their incidence is so low and their occurrence so sporadic as to make them of little value for planned experimentation.

Although most of the tumors which arise spontaneously in the SJL/J strain are, as indicated above, more properly classified as reticulum cell sarcomas, some have been interpreted as "Hodgkin's-like" on the basis of their pleomorphic cell pattern and the presence within them of giant cells. Most of these giant cells have proved on careful examination to be of the Langhans type, but in some instances, giant cells said to be consistent with the morphology of Sternberg-Reed cells have been reported. The question remains controversial, however (Dunn and Deringer, 1968). These tumors are seldom transplantable.

Repeated injections of the azo dye trypan blue into adult rats were reported by Gillman et al. (1952) to induce a diffuse proliferative response of endothelial and fixed connective tissue cells, leading to gross enlargement of lymph nodes and progressive distortion of the nodal architecture by infiltrates composed of plasma cells, histiocytes, endothelial cells, "paramonocytes," and hemohistioblasts. These tumor-like processes seldom acquired a histologically malignant appearance, but a few were stated to have been successfully transplanted to other rats. The authors claimed that occasional cells in some of these tumors resembled Sternberg-Reed cells and therefore referred to the corresponding lesions as "Hodgkin's-like sarcomas." However, the tumors observed by Simpson (1952), Marshall (1953), and Brown and Thorson (1956) after prolonged injection of rats with either trypan blue or Evans blue were reticulum cell sarcomas apparently arising in the liver, instead of in the lymph nodes. No mention is made by these investigators of the occurrence of Hodgkin's-like lesions. The controversy grew when Rüttner and Brunner (1959) reported that the lesions they observed were invariably reversible after cessation of dye injection; they concluded that these were dye-induced storage responses of the reticuloendothelial system rather than true neoplasms. Moreover, the claim that such lesions are transplantable could not be confirmed by Brown and Thorson (1956) or Marshall (1956).

However, the subject has been revived by Gillman, Kinns, and Cross (1969) and by Gillman et al. (1973), who claim that batches of trypan blue vary in activity but that "active" batches regularly produce lymphoreticular tumors in Wistar and Babraham rats, and that such tumors are transplantable into syngeneic inbred rats, with an average "take time" of 200 to 400 days. One tumor line was maintained by serial transplantation for more than forty passages. They state that some of the cells of these rat tumors closely resemble the abnormal reticulum cells and occasionally even the classical binucleate Sternberg-Reed cells of Hodgkin's disease. Cells from such lesions are said to reproduce Hodgkin's-like neoplasms regularly on serial passage. Accordingly, the authors suggest that these neoplasms may provide a satisfactory experimental animal model of Hodgkin's disease. In view of the past controversy, however, it would seem wise to regard these views with caution until confirmation is provided by other experimenters and pathologists.

Two other experimental approaches have been utilized by investigators seeking to define the etiology of Hodgkin's disease. In the first, extracts of involved human tissues obtained at biopsy or postmortem examination have been cultured and inoculated into a variety of experimental animals, which have then been observed for the development of characteristic infection or other reproducible disease states. This approach stems from the great emphasis placed by many pathologists and clinicians at the turn of the century on the granulomatous nature of Hodgkin's disease, culminating in the theory, of which Sternberg was the leading proponent, that Hodgkin's disease is an aberrant form of tuberculosis. The historical aspects of this once important but now discredited thesis have been admirably reviewed by Hoster et al. (1948).

For a time, interest also focused on other bacteria as possible etiological factors. At one time or another, the finding of various infections associated with Hodgkin's disease at autopsy has transiently incriminated *Brucella* (Parsons and Poston, 1939;

Wise and Poston, 1940; Forbus, 1942); diphtheroids (Bunting, 1914; Bunting and Yates, 1915); and avian tubercle bacilli (L'Esperance, 1929, 1931; Twort, 1930; Steiner, 1934b; Van Rooyen, 1934; Hoster, Doan, and Schumacher, 1944). Careful investigation has in each instance failed to provide support for the view that these organisms represent anything more than chance secondary invaders.

The incrimination of viruses as etiologic agents in Hodgkin's disease, based on the elicitation of a variety of toxic reactions in experimental animals inoculated with cell-free extracts of involved tissues, has, in at least three instances to date, also failed to withstand the test of careful and sustained investigation.

In the early 1930's, the work of M. H. Gordon and his associates attracted widespread interest. Although Hodgkin's disease lymph node emulsions which they injected into a variety of animal species yielded various responses, attention focused principally on the so-called Gordon test, which involved the production of encephalitis in rabbits. Lymph nodes from patients with Hodgkin's disease were ground and extracted in broth in the cold prior to intracerebral inoculation into rabbits. Within a few days the animals developed a typical syndrome characterized by muscle rigidity, paralysis, spasm, progressive wasting, and death. Smears and cultures failed to reveal the presence of bacterial organisms in the inoculated material, the rabbit brain, or the blood. Histologic sections of the brain revealed loss of Purkinje cells and an intense glial reaction. Almost 75 percent of the nodes from patients with Hodgkin's disease yielded a positive test, compared with about 2 percent of nodes from control patients with various other neoplastic and non-neoplastic conditions.

Special staining techniques for viral elementary bodies revealed large numbers of minute granules of about the same size as the elementary bodies of vaccinia and psittacosis. From this and the consistent failure to demonstrate bacteria in these preparations, it was concluded that the encephalitogenic agent was probably viral (Gordon, 1932, 1936; Gordon et al., 1934). However, all attempts to transmit the encephalitis from affected to normal rabbits were unsuccessful. Rabbits that recovered from the encephalitis exhibited no evidence of immunity, nor did their sera contain complement-fixing antibodies or precipitins.

The most telling evidence against Gordon's hypothesis, however, was that similar encephalitogenic activity was demonstrable in extracts from human bone marrow, spleen, leukocytes, and pus. Several investigators (Turner, Jackson, and Parker, 1938; Edward, 1938; McNaught, 1938) were able to correlate encephalitogenic activity with the relative abundance of eosinophils in diseased human lymph nodes and in normal bone marrow. Leukocyte suspensions containing more than 2,000 eosinophils per cubic millimeter regularly produced the typical pattern of Gordon's encephalitis in rabbits, whereas variations in the numbers of other types of white blood cells were not correlated with a positive response. It is now generally accepted that a positive Gordon test is due to the toxic action of a product extracted from eosinophils, which are characteristically abundant in the lymph nodes of most patients with Hodgkin's disease.

In the next experimental attack on the viral etiology of Hodgkin's disease, Grand (1944, 1949) prepared tissue cultures from fragments of lymph nodes obtained surgically from patients with Hodgkin's disease and from patients with various neoplastic and non-neoplastic diseases who served as controls. These cultures were incubated in a medium consisting of a mixture of chicken plasma, chick embryo extract, and human serum, the latter in some cases from patients with advanced Hodgkin's disease. After forty-eight to seventy-two hours of incubation, large multinucleate giant cells with oval nuclei appeared at the periphery of the cultures. These cells, which he identified as Sternberg-Reed cells, were consistently found in cultures prepared from Hodgkin's disease-involved nodes, but not in those derived from normal lymph nodes and nodes involved by other types of neoplasms. Brilliant cresyl blue, a vital dye with an affinity for viral intracellular inclusion bodies, stained the granular central body in the nucleus of these cells, whereas Janus B green did not. Other types of cells in these cultures showed cytoplasmic inclusions which also stained with brilliant cresyl blue. No such granules or specific staining with brilliant cresyl blue were observed in similar cells in control cultures. A supernatant extract from the Hodgkin's disease cultures, inoculated onto the chorioallantoic membrane of hen's eggs and incubated for six additional days, yielded clusters of white vesicles containing a clear fluid. No such lesions were found in eggs inoculated with control culture fluids. Tissue cultures of portions of the chorioallantoic membrane containing the vesicular lesions were found to stain positively with brilliant cresyl blue for the presence of specific cell inclusions.

However, extensive tissue culture studies by Rottino (1949), Hoster and Reiman (1950), and by Reiman et al. (1950) failed to confirm the findings of Grand. The latter workers found that inclusion bodies identical with those described by Grand may occur in normal explant cells in vitro when the culture medium contains chicken embryo extract or chicken plasma and suggested that this might be due to the fact that the virus of chicken lymphomatosis is a potential contaminant of such materials. An important difference in the techniques employed by the two groups may also have contributed to the discrepancy in their results. Whereas Grand cultured Hodgkin's disease lymph node cells directly, Hoster and his associates worked primarily with cell-free extracts from tissues involved by Hodgkin's disease, which were then added to tissue cultures of normal cells. Siegel and Smith (1961) confirmed the finding of inclusion bodies, similar to those described by Grand, in cultures of normal nodes and in nodes involved by other types of lymphoma, as well as in Hodgkin's disease, suggesting that they are not specific. Stewart et al. (1969) have recently described two types of virus particles in a continuous cell line derived from lymph node biopsy material from a patient with Hodgkin's disease. Further investigations along these lines, aided by the availability of defined tissue culture media and the advanced techniques of modern virology, would seem indicated.

About thirty years ago, it was noted that cell-free extracts prepared from involved lymph nodes of patients with Hodgkin's disease caused an increased mortality after inoculation into embryonated chicken eggs (Bostick, 1948), and the induction of a peculiar edematous state in the eggs (Karnofsky et al., 1948). However, it was not possible to maintain or to concentrate the agent by serial passage. Bostick (1950) also noted that such extracts tended to interfere with the propagation of influenza virus in the amniotic fluid of fertile chicken eggs.

Shifting from chicken eggs to suckling mice, Bostick and Hanna (1955) collected amniotic sac fluids from seven-day embryonated chicken eggs previously inoculated with extracts from lymph nodes involved by Hodgkin's disease, as well as from normal human lymph nodes. These fluids were inoculated intracerebrally by serial blind passage into suckling Princeton strain mice, and, after five to seven passages, material originally derived from three patients with Hodgkin's disease yielded a fatal encephalitis in the recipient animals. Materials from three other patients with Hodgkin's disease and from all of the control tissues were negative. The agent was inactivated at 56C. for thirty minutes, was resistant to ether, and induced no lesions on chicken eggs or in chicken embryo, monkey kidney, or human cell cultures. Complement-fixing antibodies were found in immunized rabbits and in young adult mice, but not in sera from human Hodgkin's disease patients or normal controls.

It seemed clear that the agent was a virus, but initial attempts to identify it with any of the known murine or human viruses were unsuccessful. However, Siegel (1961) later succeeded in identifying the agent as a strain of Theiler's mouse encephalomyelitis virus. This example illustrates very well a major pitfall in this experimental approach: viruses occurring as sporadic "passengers" in the animal species selected for experimentation may be induced to propagate as a consequence either of serial blind passage of animal tissue extracts or, conceivably, of some effect of the Hodgkin's disease tissue extracts. In either case, the result is the production of virus-induced disease in the experimental animals, which, however, is not due to a human virus etiologically related to Hodgkin's disease, but to a quite unrelated virus of the animal host.

More recent investigations, some of which have been reviewed by Sinkovics and Györkey (1973), have employed the techniques of electron microscopy, immunofluorescence, and radioimmunoassay in the search for candidate RNA tumor viruses. Particles bearing a variable degree of resemblance to type C viruses have occasionally been seen by electron microscopy in ultrathin sections of involved lymph nodes (Dmochowski, 1968; Seman and Seman, 1968) and plasma pellets (Hirshaut et al., 1974) from patients with Hodgkin's disease. However, Hirshaut et al. failed to find any such particles in the involved tissues from several patients and, despite a very careful search, were unable to confirm the observation of budding of virus-like particles from cell membranes previously reported by Dmochowski (1968). Moreover, no such particles were seen in the cell cultures studied by Eisinger et al. (1971). Until such particles can be consistently demonstrated in involved tissues or cell cultures and characterized rigorously by virtue of such features as typical morphology, budding, an RNA-containing nucleoid, reverse transcriptase, and/or distinctive virion structural proteins, their significance must remain in doubt. Newell et al. (1968) have pointed out that under certain conditions similar particles may be visualized with al-

most equal frequency in plasma pellets from normal individuals.

The technique of direct immunofluorescence, using an antiserum prepared against a human leukemic plasma pellet containing such virus-like particles, was applied by Hirshaut et al. (1974) to the study of involved tissues from 16 patients with Hodgkin's disease with positive reactions in 4 (25 percent). However, it is very difficult, even after extensive absorption with normal tissues, to render such heterologous antisera monospecific and thus to be certain that the antigens detected are indeed those of the virus-like particles.

Order and his co-workers used heterologous antibody prepared in rabbits to demonstrate the presence of antigens with fast and slow electrophoretic migration patterns in the involved spleens of patients with Hodgkin's disease (Order, Porter, and Hellman, 1971; Katz et al., 1973; Order, Colgan, and Hellman, 1974). The fast antigen was later identified as normal tissue ferritin (Eshhar, Order, and Katz, 1974), a finding presumably relevant to the prior observation of increased ferritin levels in the sera of patients with Hodgkin's disease (Bieber and Bieber, 1973).

Another antigen, unrelated to those studied by Order et al., has been detected in culture supernatants and in cultured cells from the involved spleens of patients with Hodgkin's disease (Long et al., 1973, 1974a, 1974b, 1977a). Heterologous antisera were raised in rabbits to material from the pelleted culture supernatants which sedimented at a specific gravity of $1.15-1.21$ g/ml in sucrose gradients (the density range in which type C viruses, if present, would be expected to occur). These antisera reacted by agar-gel diffusion and immunoelectrophoresis with material from nine of ten cultures derived from positive spleens, two of eight cultures from histologically uninvolved Hodgkin's spleens, three of six cultures from non-Hodgkin's lymphomas, and none of twelve cultures from normal fetal and adult spleen and thymus. Similarly prepared antisera were also used in indirect immunofluorescence studies or were labeled with radioiodine and used in an indirect radioimmunoassay. Fluorescent antibody staining of the cytoplasm was seen in 51 percent of acetone-fixed cells, and surface staining in 48 percent of viable cells from Hodgkin's disease cultures, as compared with 4–8 percent and <5 percent, respectively, of cells from normal cultures. By radioimmunoassay, the anti-Hodgkin's disease sera reacted with an antigen on the surface of cells from the Hodgkin's disease cultures, whereas the same cells did not react with antisera against normal spleen culture supernatants, nor against Hodgkin's disease tissues which had not been cultured. Absorption measurements indicated that the quantity of antigen in cells from Hodgkin's disease cultures was 15- to 30-fold that in cells from normal cultures. No cross-reactivity could be demonstrated against the group-specific antigens or representative feline, murine, or avian RNA tumor viruses, nor against EB or herpes simplex virus-related antigens or antisera derived from them. Long and co-workers (1973) concluded that the antigen is specifically associated with cultivation in vitro of the Hodgkin's disease tissues, but that their evidence does not unambiguously distinguish among three possibilities: that it is a nonviral tumor antigen, that it is a component of a candidate tumor virus, or that it is a differentiation antigen detected by virtue of differences in cellular composition of Hodgkin's disease versus normal lymphoid tissue cultures.

More recently, the same group have used a sensitive radioimmunoassay to quantitate soluble immune complexes (IC) in the sera of patients with Hodgkin's disease and have investigated the binding of IC to their monolayer cultures (Long et al., 1977b). They found that 23 of 90 sera had IC levels >20 μg/ml (normal <10 μg/ml), and that all of these reacted with the cell cultures, as did 5 of 11 borderline sera (10–20 μg/ml), whereas only 4 of 56 sera with normal levels of IC did so. The IC could be removed from the positive sera by absorption with the cultured cells. There was no reaction with IC-containing sera from 19 controls, nor with sera from patients with pericarditis, systemic lupus erythematosus, or on renal dialysis, all of whom had extremely high serum IC levels. Attempts to characterize the IC from Hodgkin's disease sera are in progress.

Spiegelman and his associates used molecular probes to search for nucleic acid sequences homologous to those of Rauscher murine leukemia virus (R-MuLV) in the involved tissues of patients with Hodgkin's disease. In 16 of 24 cases, they reported significant homology between RNA from cytoplasmic fractions of involved tissues and a ^{3}H-labeled DNA probe prepared, with the aid of viral reverse transcriptase, from R-MuLV RNA (Hehlmann, Kufe, and Spiegelman, 1972). Similar observations have been reported by Aulakh and Gallo (1977) in tissues from 3 of 10 patients with Hodgkin's disease. Spiegelman's group also isolated particles at a density of 1.17 g/ml from the postmitochondrial cytoplasmic fraction of disrupted tissues involved by Hodgkin's disease. These particles, which had

previously been found to yield positive simultaneous detection reactions (Schlom and Spiegelman, 1971) indicative of the presence of both 70S RNA and reverse transcriptase, were then used to synthesize ^{3}H-labeled, single-stranded cDNA probes by the endogenous reaction in the presence of actinomycin D. Molecular hybridization was said to reveal homologous sequences in the nuclear DNA of cells from three spleens involved by Hodgkin's disease and not in the DNA of cells from normal spleens (Kufe, Peters, and Spiegelman, 1973). In an extension of these studies, Spiegelman et al. (1973) reported that involved lymph node or spleen tissues from 22 (78 percent) of 28 patients with Hodgkin's disease contained a cytoplasmic particulate fraction with a density of 1.17 g/ml, a positive simultaneous detection reaction, and ^{3}H-cDNA sequences homologous to those of R-MuLV RNA. Chezzi et al. (1976) observed positive simultaneous detection reactions in cytoplasmic particles from 14 (77.8 percent) of 18 spleens from patients with Hodgkin's disease.

Although these observations are undoubtedly intriguing, they are also puzzling, since it is well known that the Sternberg-Reed and Hodgkin's giant cells, which together make up the neoplastic cell population in Hodgkin's disease, seldom constitute more than 1–2 percent, and often less than 0.1 percent of the cells in involved tissues. Accordingly, if sequences homologous to those of R-MuLV RNA or of human virus-like particles are indeed present, they must be derived mainly from the lymphocytes, eosinophils, and other cellular elements of the stromal population, all of which are nonneoplastic. It is also relevant that Long et al. (1973) were unable to detect any reaction by agar-gel diffusion between their anti-Hodgkin's disease sera and intact or disrupted R-MuLV, nor between antisera against the group-specific antigen of R-MuLV and crude supernatant pellets from their Hodgkin's disease spleen cultures.

Thus, several investigative approaches have yielded suggestive indications that tissues involved by Hodgkin's disease, cell cultures prepared from them, or the plasmas of patients with the disease may contain particles with morphologic, immunologic, or biochemical features similar to those of certain RNA tumor viruses. The evidence is still fragmentary, however, and open to alternative interpretations. Intensification of such research efforts is clearly warranted, with due attention to the numerous pitfalls in such a complex system. The successful cultivation of Sternberg-Reed and Hodgkin's giant cells in vitro (Kaplan and Gartner,

1977; Kaplan, unpublished) should facilitate definitive investigations of the possible viral etiology of the disease in pure populations of neoplastic cells.

The Burkitt Lymphoma. A new and unusual lymphoma in central African children was described for the first time by Burkitt in 1958. This tumor is now known to occur endemically in two widely separated parts of the world, central Africa and New Guinea, and has been observed sporadically in North and South America and Europe. Clinically, it exhibits a remarkable tendency to involve the jaws, whereas involvement of the lymph nodes is paradoxically infrequent.

The distinctive epidemiologic features of this tumor (Haddow, 1963; Burkitt and Wright, 1966; Wright, 1967; Burkitt, 1969) strongly suggested the possible involvement of an insect vector and stimulated intense interest in the possibility that it might be of viral etiology. Since systematic laboratory investigation was not feasible in Africa, the first step was to propagate Burkitt lymphoma cells in vitro. This was first accomplished by Epstein and Barr in 1964. Soon thereafter, Epstein, Achong, and Barr (1964) succeeded in demonstrating, in a small but significant number of cells in these cultures, the presence of a virus morphologically similar to those of the herpes group, to which they gave the name EB virus (Fig. 2.2). Since that time, Burkitt lymphoma cells from tumors occurring in other parts of Africa, New Guinea (Pope, et al., 1967) the United States, and the United Kingdom have been successfully cultivated in vitro in a number of laboratories, and, in each instance, a herpes-like virus morphologically indistinguishable from EB virus could be detected by electron microscopy.

EB virus has been shown to differ from all of the known human herpes viruses, both biologically and immunologically. Immunofluorescence tests employing antisera to the EB virus have revealed fluorescence in a small proportion of cells in all African Burkitt lymphoma cultures studied to date (Henle and Henle, 1966b; Klein, Clifford, Klein, and Stjernswärd, 1966). Careful studies by Epstein and Achong (1968) have demonstrated the abundant presence of virus particles in the very same cells that yielded a positive, direct immunofluorescence test and the absence of virus particles in nearby fluorescence-negative cells. Antisera to the known human herpes viruses do not react with virus-bearing cultured Burkitt cells, and conversely, specific antiserum to the EB virus does not react with tissue culture cells infected with herpes

simplex virus, cytomegalovirus, and varicella virus. Thus, it appears that the EB virus is distinct from, though morphologically similar to, the previously known human herpes viruses.

That the virus is probably not present merely as a "passenger" is indicated by the fact that its genome is detectable in the DNA of the Burkitt lymphoma cells, as demonstrated both by molecular hybridization (zur Hausen and Schulte-Holthausen, 1970; Nonoyama and Pagano, 1973) and by positive immunofluorescence reactions for the EB virus genome-associated nuclear antigen, EBNA (Reedman and Klein, 1973). Approximately 97 percent of all African Burkitt lymphoma cell lines studied to date were found to be EBNA-positive (Klein, 1975a). In contrast, tumors morphologically indistinguishable from Burkitt lymphomas which occur sporadically in Europe, North America, and other nonendemic areas have usually lacked EBV genomes (Pagano, Huang, and Levine, 1973), although a small number of cell lines established in vitro from such tumors have been EBNA-positive (Epstein et al., 1976; Gravell et al., 1976).

Henle, Henle, and Diehl (1968), Niederman et al. (1968), and Evans et al. (1968) have demonstrated that a herpes-like virus, morphologically and serologically indistinguishable from the EB virus, is the cause of infectious mononucleosis. Some of the metaphases in cultures of normal leukocytes infected by special techniques with EB virus exhibit chromosomal abnormalities, as do many of the Burkitt culture cell lines. More detailed studies, using the Giemsa banding technique, have revealed a typical chromosome 8q−/14q+ translocation in almost all African Burkitt and other lymphoma cell lines (Manolov and Manolova, 1972; Jarvis et al., 1974; Zech et al., 1976), and in three North American Burkitt lymphoma cell lines (Kaiser-McCaw et al., 1977). This translocation is not present in EB virus-transformed lymphoblastoid cells. The well-known proliferative capacity of the abnormal lymphocytes from infectious mononucleosis and the observed capacity of cultures of Burkitt cell lines, as well as of normal hematopoietic cells infected with the EB virus, to grow unusually well in culture is consistent with the view that this virus may confer an enhanced capacity for proliferation on the lymphoid cells which it infects. A critical review of the evidence bearing on the possible oncogenicity of the EB virus has been presented by Klein (1975b).

Although the EB virus is the agent most consistently demonstrated in Burkitt tumor cells, it is not

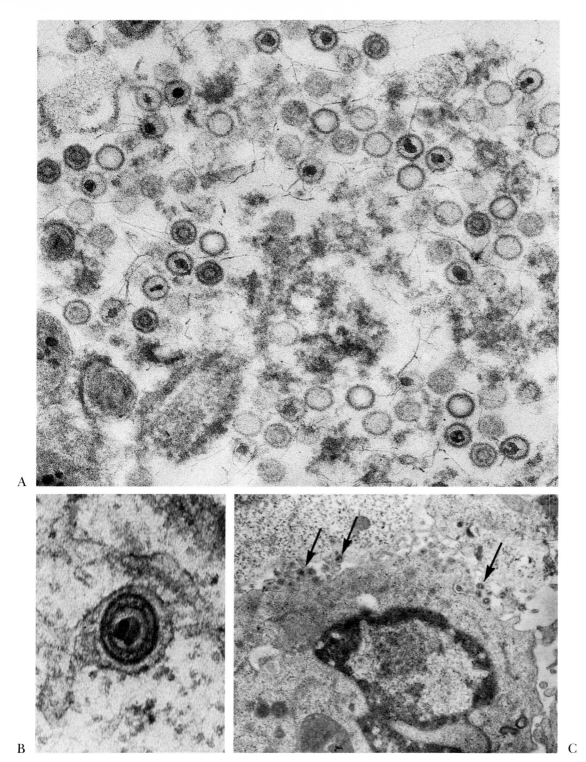

A

B   C

Figure 2.2 *A*, group of immature EB virus particles lying scattered in cellular debris. When favorably oriented to the plane of sectioning, the particles present a hexagonal profile and are either empty or with central ring-shaped or dense nucleoids. Electron micrograph ×72,000. *B*, detail of mature EB virus particle lying within a cytoplasmic membrane-bounded space. The particle has matured by budding through the membrane limiting the space and has become enveloped by an additional outer coat derived from this membrane as the particle has passed through. Electron micrograph ×149,000. *C*, survey picture of portions of three EB virus-producing cells with part of a nucleus below. Mature extracellular EB virus particles lie (arrows) between the cells in intercellular spaces. Electron micrograph ×14,000. (Figure 2.2 was provided by Professor M. A. Epstein, Department of Pathology, University of Bristol, Bristol, England.)

the only such agent. Herpes simplex virus has been isolated from a small number of Burkitt lymphomas (Simons and Ross, 1965; Woodall, et al., 1965). However, these isolations from Burkitt tumors involving the jaw have an incidence which does not significantly exceed that of the usual oral carrier rate for herpes simplex virus. Similarly, the *Mycoplasmas* isolated from some patients with Burkitt's lymphoma (Dalldorf et al., 1966) are generally thought to be commensal "passengers." Finally, the widely prevalent reovirus type III was isolated from some 17 percent of Burkitt lymphomas by Bell et al. (1966). Although it is likely that this represents secondary infection, interest in a possible causal association was for a time stimulated by the report of Stanley et al. (1966) that the serial transplantation of spleen cells from mice with runting syndrome induced by neonatal reovirus III infection in turn elicits a runt disease, the survivors of which developed an unstated, small number of lymphomas. One of these tumors, designated 2731/L, was serially transplanted in mice and was said to exhibit a macroscopic distribution and histologic appearance very similar to that of Burkitt's lymphoma. Smithers (1967, 1969) has commented on the possible relevance of these observations to certain immunologic peculiarities distinctive of Hodgkin's disease. However, the role of reovirus III in the induction of such lymphomas in mice remains improbable.

Epidemiologic Studies

Shimkin (1955) called attention to the progressive increase in mortality from Hodgkin's disease in the United States over the period 1921 to 1951. A similar increase in Hodgkin's disease incidence was noted by Uddströmer (1934) in Sweden in the period 1915 to 1931. However, no significant change in Hodgkin's disease mortality was recorded in Olmsted County, Minnesota, from 1945 through 1969 (Nobrega, Kyle, and Harrison, 1973), in Denmark from 1931 through 1953 (Clemmesen and Sorensen, 1958), or in Australia between 1908 and 1950 (Lancaster, 1955). These and other aspects of the epidemiology of Hodgkin's disease have been reviewed by Correa and O'Conor (1971), Cole (1972), Newell and Rawlings (1972), Abramson (1973), Levine (1974), and Gutensohn and Cole (1977).

Age. MacMahon (1957) noted that the age-specific incidence curve for Hodgkin's disease in the United States is characteristically bimodal (Fig.

2.3). When plotted semilogarithmically, the age-specific incidence curves for reticulum-cell sarcoma and lymphosarcoma exhibit a roughly linear increase in rate from childhood through age seventy-five. In contrast, the curve for Hodgkin's disease, which parallels those of the other two lymphomas at ages over forty-five, exhibits a distinct additional peak in the age range fifteen to forty. The same bimodal character is apparent in age-specific incidence data from the German Federal Republic (Dörken, 1960), Denmark (Clemmesen, 1965), and Israel (Modan et al., 1969). It is also apparent in age-specific mortality rates for both sexes (Fig. 2.4) and in mortality-rate surveys from New York, the United States Army, Saskatchewan, Canada, and Norway. However, several exceptions are known: data from Japan (MacMahon, 1957; Nishiyama and Inoue, 1970; Akazaki and Wakasa, 1974), rural Norway (Stalsberg, 1973), and from the southern United States (Cole, MacMahon, and

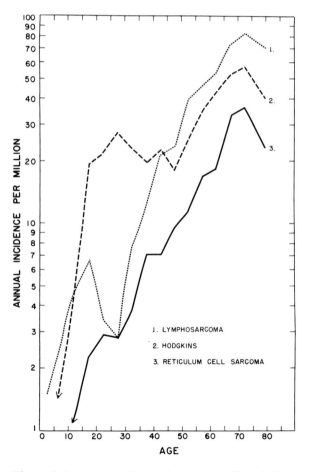

Figure 2.3 Age-specific incidence rates of Hodgkin's disease, lymphosarcoma, and reticulum cell sarcoma, Brooklyn, 1943–52. (Reprinted, by permission of the author and *Cancer Research,* from MacMahon, 1966.)

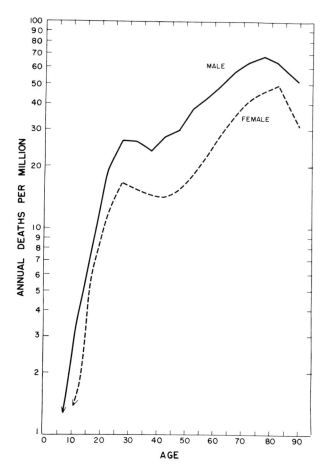

Figure 2.4 Age-specific mortality rates from Hodgkin's disease by sex, United States, 1958–62. (Reprinted, by permission of the author and *Cancer Research,* from MacMahon, 1966.)

the basis of data from ten countries, Correa and O'Conor (1971) noted an apparently inverse relationship between the rates for children and those for young adults, with a rank correlation coefficient of −0.915 (*p* <0.001), as is graphically evident in Figure 2.8.

MacMahon (1966) has suggested that Hodgkin's disease may not be a single entity but a syndrome comprising at least two, and possible three, entities with probably distinct etiologies. Specifically, he postulated that the disease in young adults may be an inflammatory granuloma, whereas that of older individuals is more likely a neoplasm. In a subsequent exchange of published letters, Smithers (1970b) has criticized, and Newell et al. (1970) and MacMahon, Cole, and Newell (1971) have defended, the hypothesis that Hodgkin's disease comprises two distinct entities. Clarke, Anderson, and Davidson (1974) argued that the high frequency of mediastinal involvement in young adult cases constitutes further evidence in support of the MacMahon hypothesis. In the opinion of Smithers, however, Hodgkin's disease is a single progressive neoplastic disorder in which host resistance and clinical manifestations vary as a function of age and sex.

Aisenberg, 1968) reveal an absence of the early peak, but not the peak observed in the later decades of life (Figs. 2.5, 2.6). A quite different pattern has been noted in a number of tropical and subtropical countries, of which Colombia, Peru, El Salvador, and Nigeria are examples: a strikingly high incidence occurs in male children, with a paradoxically low incidence in young adults, followed by the usual second peak of high incidence in older age groups (Correa and O'Conor, 1971; Correa, 1973; Edington, Osunkoya, and Hendrickse, 1973). The difference in age-specific incidence patterns observed in Cali, Colombia, and in rural Norway, as contrasted with those in Connecticut and in urban Norway, respectively, is clearly indicated in Figure 2.7. It will be noted that the curve for males in Colombia is distinctly bimodal, but that the first peak occurs in childhood, rather than in the young-adult range, and the second peak develops some time after 50 years of age. On

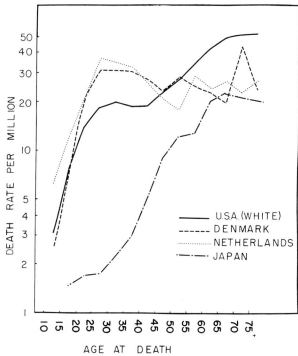

Figure 2.5 Age-specific mortality rates from Hodgkin's disease in four countries, 1950–53. (Reprinted, by permission of the author and *Cancer Research,* from MacMahon, 1966.)

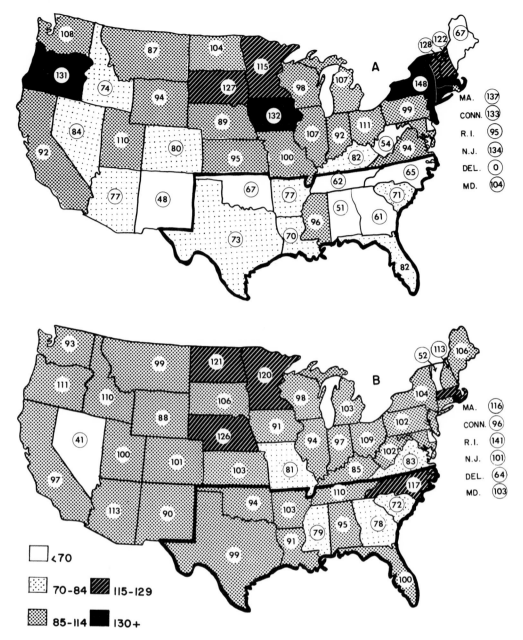

Figure 2.6 Standard mortality ratios for Hodgkin's disease in the white population of the United States, by state and age group, 1959–61; *A* = ages 15–34; *B* = ages ≥ 45. (Reprinted, by permission of the authors and *The Lancet,* from Cole, MacMahon, and Aisenberg, 1968.)

In their assessment of this controversy, Correa and O'Conor (1971) concluded that "the variation in epidemiologic patterns may be the result of the interplay of environmental and host factors influencing the natural history of a single disease . . . In a given population, susceptibility to the agent or agents which cause Hodgkin's disease is related to immunocompetence and host response, the level of which is, in turn, dependent on environmental and socioeconomic factors." Sup-

port for the view that several environmental factors may influence the incidence of Hodgkin's disease has come from studies of the epidemiology of the disease in childhood (Fraumeni and Li, 1969; Dörken, 1975). The influence of environmental factors is also strongly suggested by the fact that a higher incidence of Hodgkin's disease is observed among Japanese in Hawaii (Stemmermann, 1970) and that Hodgkin's disease mortality rates among U.S. Japanese have been shifting toward the

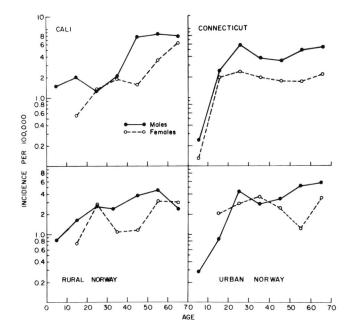

Figure 2.7 Age-specific incidence rates per 100,000 population for each sex in: (a) Cali, Colombia (1962–1966); (b) Connecticut, USA (1960–1962); (c) rural Norway (1964–1966); and (d) urban Norway (1964–1966). (Reprinted, by permission of the authors, and the Editor of the *International Journal of Cancer,* from the paper by Correa and O'Conor, 1971.)

higher rates usually observed in the U.S. white populations (Mason and Fraumeni, 1974). In the context of the one- versus two-entity debate, it is relevant to point out that cultures of Sternberg-Reed and Hodgkin's giant cells from adolescent and young adult as well as older patients have consistently displayed such fundamental attributes of neoplasia as aneuploidy and heterotransplantability (Kaplan and Gartner, 1977). These findings strongly support the view that the disease is neoplastic at all ages.

Sex. It has long been known that Hodgkin's disease is more prevalent in males than in females. Mortality and morbidity data from the United States, United Kingdom, and Denmark reveal a male-female sex ratio ranging from 1.38 to 1.94. Moreover, it appears that the sex ratio for these countries has not changed appreciably over an interval of many years, from data going back to 1911 in the case of England and Wales.

When the age-specific mortality and incidence rates for Hodgkin's disease in the United States are separately considered by sex, the bimodal characteristic described in the previous section is apparent for both sexes (Fig. 2.4). Indeed, bimodality was more striking in females than in males in data from the Greater Boston metropolitan area (Grufferman, Duong, and Cole, 1976). However, this does not appear to be true of the data from Cali, Colombia (Fig. 2.7), nor of that from Connecticut (Greco, Acheson, and Foote, 1974), where the first peak was absent in females. The sex ratio does not remain constant over all age ranges (MacMahon, 1957). In adults, it appears to be appreciably lower (0.91 to 1.20) in the 15- to 34-year-old bracket, increasing sharply and to about an equal extent thereafter in the 35- to 49-year bracket and the 50 or over age group (range 1.44 to 2.35). The sex ratio is particularly high in the 15- to 34-year-old range in the southern United States (Cole, MacMahon, and Aisenberg, 1968), and in childhood cases in Colombia, Peru, and other tropical and subtropical countries of Latin America (Correa, 1973).

Of particular interest are the changing sex ratios during the first fifteen years of life. MacMahon

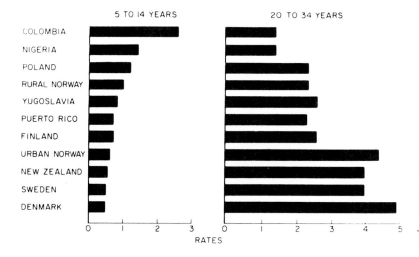

Figure 2.8 Average annual incidence rates per 100,000 population for children (5–14 years) and young adults (20–34 years). Calculated for males in selected countries. (Reprinted by permission of the authors and the Editor of the *International Journal of Cancer,* from the paper by Correa and O'Conor, 1971.)

(1966), in a review of 122 published cases of Hodgkin's disease in children under 10 years of age, found that 85 percent of the patients were male. Miller (1966), in an analysis of computer-tape data by single year of age for all United States cancer deaths occurring in individuals less than 20 years old during the years 1950 to 1959, encountered 1,484 cases of Hodgkin's disease. Males comprised 76 percent of the cases among white children 5 to 11 years of age; this proportion decreased after puberty to 60 percent in the 11 to 19 year age group. There was a gradual increase in mortality rates from Hodgkin's disease for both sexes up to the age of 11, with that for males exceeding the rate of increase in females. After 11 years of age, however, a much steeper rate of increase in incidence was observed, which was particularly marked among females, accounting for the abrupt change in sex ratio relative to puberty. Subtracting the published mean survival time of 2.7 years for Hodgkin's disease in children (Evans and Nyhan, 1964), Miller concluded that the shift in the incidence rates and sex ratios begins at about 9 years of age. Seeking an interpretation of this phenomenon, he raised the question of its possible association with the prepubertal onset of involution of the lymphatic tissues.

Demography. Data published by the World Health Organization (1955) show death rates from Hodgkin's disease in sixteen countries in the years 1950 to 1952 (Table 2.1). It is apparent that only two countries, The Netherlands and Denmark, have overall rates which exceed those in the United States. Particularly noteworthy is the fact that rates in the younger (0 to 39 years) age group are remarkably high, relative to those in the United States, in The Netherlands, Denmark, and Switzerland. MacMahon (1957) called attention to the fact that these three countries are also traditional dairy producers, but Clemmesen (1965) has referred to this suggestion as speculative.

A second noteworthy feature of the table is the remarkably low rate in Japan, and to a lesser extent in Australia, particularly in the younger age group. Incomplete diagnosis may account for part, but is

Table 2.1 Death Rates from Hodgkin's Disease in Selected Countries, 1950 to 1952

Country	Death rate per million[a]			Percentage U.S. rate		
	Age 0–39	Age 40 and more	All ages	Age 0–39	Age 40 and more	All ages
United States (white)	9.9	32.6	18.1	100	100	100
Canada	8.7	29.1	16.0	88	89	88
Denmark	15.0	25.7	18.8	152	79	104
Finland	9.5	21.5	13.8	96	66	76
Norway	11.4	22.8	15.5	115	70	86
Sweden	7.9	22.6	13.2	80	69	73
England and Wales	10.1	25.0	15.4	102	77	85
Ireland	9.5	27.8	16.1	96	85	89
Scotland	10.7	30.2	17.7	108	93	98
France	10.1	20.6	13.9	102	63	77
Germany	9.0	21.7	13.6	91	67	75
Italy	10.7	31.1	18.0	108	95	99
Netherlands	17.6	23.7	19.8	178	73	109
Switzerland	12.9	25.7	17.5	130	79	97
Australia	5.9	21.5	11.5	60	66	64
Japan	1.8	13.3	5.9	18	41	33

Source: Data compiled by the World Health Organization and published in "Mortality from Hodgkin's Disease and from Leukaemia and Aleukaemia," *Epidemiol. and Vital Statist. Rep.,* 8:81–114, 1955.

[a]Within each broad age group all rates have been standardized to the age distribution of the United States white population in five-year groups.

unlikely to account for all, of this remarkable deficit. The very low rates in Japan are consistent with the remarkable paucity of lymphatic leukemia and lymphosarcoma in that country (Wakasa, 1973; Akazaki and Wakasa, 1974).

Wildner and Eckert (1965) have summarized data on Hodgkin's disease incidence rates from the German Democratic Republic and other countries. These are given separately by sexes in Table 2.2. It should be recognized that the accuracy of such statistics may vary widely in different parts of the world. This probably accounts for the fact that the relative incidence rates given by these authors are in several respects at variance with those reported by the World Health Organization (Table 2.1).

A somewhat higher incidence (3.3 in males, 2.5 in females) for Hodgkin's disease in Israel is cited by Robinson (1966), based on data of the Israel Cancer Registry. He noted a higher lymphoma morbidity among Jews of European origin than in those from Asia or Africa, which was statistically significant for lymphosarcoma but not for Hodgkin's disease. It has been stated that a peculiar form of reticulum cell sarcoma, tending to origi-

nate in and involve predominantly the gastrointestinal tract and often associated with preexisting or concurrent malabsorption and steatorrhea, is particularly prevalent in Israel and other countries of the Middle East and North Africa.

It has been reported that Hodgkin's disease is particularly prevalent among children in Peru, Mexico (Solidoro, Guzman, and Chang, 1966), and other Central and South American countries, as well as in Turkey, Lebanon, and other countries of the Middle East (Azzam, 1966; Çavdar et al., 1974) and in central India (Grover and Hardas, 1972). In a review of 660 neoplasms in infants and children under 15 years of age in Ceylon, Cooray and Perera (1966) encountered 164 malignant tumors, of which 23 were Hodgkin's disease. Burn et al. (1971) have reported striking differences in the relative frequencies of four histopathologic types of Hodgkin's disease among East African as compared with English children.

Reports are available on various aspects of the disease as it occurs in Peru (Misad, Brandon, and Albujar, 1973), Argentina (Besuschio and Ghinelli, 1973), Brazil (Marigo, Muller, and Davies, 1969; Carvalho, 1973; Machado et al., 1973), and Costa Rica (Salas, 1973). Similar studies have been presented from several Western European countries, including Norway (Bjelke, 1969) and Finland (Franssila, Heiskala, and Heiskala, 1977). Among the African countries from which such reports have been published are Egypt (Aboul Nasr, Tawfik, and El-Einen, 1973), Nigeria (Edington and Hendrickse, 1973), and Uganda (Olweny et al., 1971; Wright, 1973). Asian countries for which published data are available include Japan (Wakasa, 1973), China (Kaplan, 1978a), Singapore (Tan and Shanmugaratnam, 1973), and Papua New Guinea (Wilkey, 1973). Additional incidence survey data from other countries in which unusual patterns of occurrence of Hodgkin's disease have been reported might furnish important clues to the etiology of the disease.

Extensive reviews of the geographic pathology and demography of Hodgkin's disease have been presented by Lingeman (1969), Correa and O'Conor (1971), Correa (1973), Stalsberg (1973), and Correa (1977). From their analysis of the available world data, Correa and O'Conor (1971) were able to delineate at least three epidemiological patterns of Hodgkin's disease (Figs. 2.7, 2.8). "Type I is characterized by relatively high incidence and mortality rates in male children, low incidence in the third decade, and a second peak of high incidence in the older age groups. A great majority of

Table 2.2 Sex-Specific Incidence Rates for Hodgkin's Disease in Various Countries (Wildner and Eckert, 1965)

Country	Annual incidence per 100,000	
	Male	Female
U.S.S.R.	3.0	1.7
Austria	2.7	2.1
Netherlands	2.5	1.5
Belgium	2.4	1.8
Ireland	2.4	1.6
Italy	2.4	1.5
Sweden	2.4	1.4
Scotland	2.4	1.3
U.S.	2.2	1.4
White	2.3	1.4
Colored	1.3	0.7
West Germany	2.2	1.4
England and Wales	2.2	1.3
East Germany	2.1	1.1
Israel	2.1	0.8
France	1.8	1.3
Canada	1.8	1.2
Australia	1.7	0.6
Norway	1.6	1.8
Hungary	1.5	0.8
Chile	1.0	0.6
Japan	0.6	0.3
Ceylon	0.1	0.1

the cases in populations with this type of curve are classified histologically as mixed cellularity or lymphocyte depletion and thus carry a less favorable prognosis. This pattern seems to prevail in developing countries. Type III is characterized by very low rates in children and a pronounced initial peak in young adults. Nodular sclerosis is the prevalent histological subtype in the wealthy urbanized countries where this type of age incidence curve prevails. An intermediate pattern, which we will designate type II, is found in rural areas of developed countries and apparently in central Europe and the southern part of the United States as well." A shift in pattern from type I to type III apparently occurred in the United States between 1925 and 1950. There may also be a type IV pattern in the Orient, characterized by a relative paucity of cases in all age groups. Correa and O'Conor suggest that susceptibility to the causative agent(s) may be determined by host immunocompetence, which in turn may be linked to nutrition and other environmental and socioeconomic factors.

Ethnic Groups. As in the case of leukemia and lymphosarcoma, both mortality and incidence rates for nonwhites (predominantly Negroes) are appreciably lower than those for whites (MacMahon, 1957). The white-nonwhite ratio fluctuates appreciably with age; from an initial level near 1.0 in the 0–14 year age group it increases sharply to 1.6 for males and 1.7 for females in the 15 to 34 year age group, decreases again at 35 to 49 years (1.1 for males, 1.5 for females), and rises again in the 50 plus age group (1.3 for males, 1.9 for females). Olisa et al. (1976), in an analysis of Hodgkin's disease in American Negroes, concluded that their age distribution pattern is consistent with epidemiologic type II of Correa and O'Conor (1971). In the Brooklyn survey, in which it was noted that leukemia and the lymphomas generally were more common in the Jewish than in the Catholic or Protestant populations, the excess cases of Hodgkin's disease were confined to the Jewish subgroup over 40 years of age (MacMahon and Koller, 1957; MacMahon, 1957). In New York State, deaths due to Hodgkin's disease were noted to be more frequent among males born in Italy than among other white male ethnic groups (Milham and Hesser, 1967).

In Israel, epidemiologists have had an interesting opportunity to compare disease rates in Jews and Arabs, and among Jews who have come from various parts of the world. Meytes and Modan (1969) analyzed data on patients in Israel in whom the diagnosis of Hodgkin's disease was made dur-

ing the years 1960–1964. They noted no statistically significant differences in incidence between Jews and Arabs, nor between Jews born in Europe and those born in America, Africa, Asia, or Israel. Both Jews and Arabs exhibited the bimodal age-specific incidence curve described by MacMahon (1966). Further analysis of their data suggested that bimodality was more distinct among Jews born in Europe, America, and Asia than among those born in Africa. Differences in the relative frequencies of the various histopathologic types of Hodgkin's disease have also been noted in these ethnic subgroups (Sacks, Selzer, and Steinitz, 1973).

Genetic and Familial Factors. It is now well established that the major histocompatibility (H-2) gene locus in mice exerts a strong influence on susceptibility to the development of leukemias and lymphomas (Lilly and Pincus, 1973). Interest was thus stimulated in the possibility that susceptibility to Hodgkin's disease might be similarly correlated with certain antigens of the corresponding HL-A system in man. Beginning with Amiel (1967), several groups have conducted retrospective studies and have observed an apparent association with one or another of the antigens of the HL-A 5/4c complex: W5, HL-A5, W18, and possibly W15 (for references to individual studies, see Forbes and Morris, 1972; Bertrams et al., 1972; Bodmer, 1973; Graff et al., 1974; Hansen et al., 1977). However, other groups have noted an increased frequency of HL-A1 and 8 (Falk and Osoba, 1971; Henderson et al., 1973), as well as a significantly decreased frequency of HL-A3 in newly diagnosed cases (Falk and Osoba, 1971). In an analysis of pooled data from many centers, Svejgaard et al. (1975) found that the three antigens most significantly associated with Hodgkin's disease were A1, B5, and B18.

In some studies, the association with A5 or W5 has been limited to particular histopathologic types, notably mixed cellularity and lymphocyte predominance (Forbes and Morris, 1972; Graff et al., 1974). The fact that such observations must be viewed with caution, however, came to light in an international collaborative study which revealed major discrepancies in the interpretation of histopathologic types of Hodgkin's disease (Chelloul et al., 1972). Moreover, from the data of that international collaborative study, Morris, Lawler, and Oliver (1972) concluded that it was not possible to draw any firm conclusions concerning associations between HL-A antigens and Hodgkin's disease. Although reactions with certain antisera detecting

HL-A1, HL-A8, W18, W27, and W6 were significantly increased, and those of certain antisera detecting HL-A12 and HL-A13 were significantly decreased in the group of Hodgkin's disease patients, relative to controls, there were disturbing inconsistencies in reactions with different antisera defining a given antigen. For example, of four antisera with HL-A1 specificity, only two showed a significant increase in reaction frequency among patients with Hodgkin's disease.

These and other difficulties with the retrospective studies led to a prospective study by Kissmeyer-Nielsen, Kjerbye, and Lamm (1975). In their analysis of data from 201 cases of Hodgkin's disease and 562 normal blood donor controls in Denmark, only one antigen, HL-A1, occurred with a modest increase in frequency, of borderline significance, among the patient group. No evidence was found to support the occurrence of other antigens with significantly increased frequency. They suggested that the earlier retrospective studies may have selected for HL-A antigens associated in some way with improved prognosis, rather than with occurrence, of Hodgkin's disease. In another prospective study involving 65 Swedish cases, Björkholm et al. (1974a) also found that the antigen frequencies in the overall patient group did not deviate from those of normal controls. However, the frequency of HL-A8 was slightly increased in patients over 40 years of age, whereas that of HL-A12 was markedly increased among those under 40 with a favorable histopathology. A significant increase in HL-A28 was noted in patients with advanced disease, particularly those who were anergic to tuberculin.

In addition to a number of individual case reports of Hodgkin's disease occurring in more than one member of the family, there have to date been three systematic studies of familial incidence in larger series. The study of Rigby and associates (1968) refers to leukemia and lymphomas collectively, whereas the other two were specifically oriented toward Hodgkin's disease (DeVore and Doan, 1957; Razis, Diamond, and Craver, 1959a). In all three studies, there was a distinct indication that the close relatives of patients with Hodgkin's disease and perhaps other lymphomas have a significantly, though modestly, increased risk of developing Hodgkin's disease, relative to that in the general population. Razis et al. (1959a) and Fraumeni (1974) have estimated that the risk is increased about threefold, and the data of Rigby et al. (1968) indicated a two-and-one-half-fold increase in frequency.

However, Leighton et al. (1974) have cautioned that the 90 percent confidence limits for the estimates of relative risk in their own and other such studies are so wide as to leave in serious doubt, for the present, whether the relatives of patients with Hodgkin's disease are in fact subject to a significantly increased risk of developing the disease. Most of the reported instances involve Hodgkin's disease in two siblings or in parent and child (Table 2.3). Jackson and Parker (1947) cited a family in which three brothers and one sister all developed Hodgkin's disease. Maldonado, Taswell, and Kiely (1972) and Thorling (1973) have each added instances involving two brothers; Fenelly and McBride (1974) record Hodgkin's disease in three sisters. Additional data on Hodgkin's disease in siblings have been presented by Perlin et al. (1976). Rare instances of concordance in single-ovum twins have been reported (Razis et al., 1959a; Bohunický et al., 1971), although none of the six twin siblings in the study by Johnson and Johnson (1972) had developed a lymphoma or other type of cancer. Smithers (1967) stated that there were six cases involving siblings among the 416 patients with the disease seen at the Royal Marsden Hospital from 1935 to 1964. At Stanford University Medical Center, four pairs of cases involving siblings, three involving parent-child combinations, and four other pairs of cases among close blood relatives have been recorded among some 1,200 patients with Hodgkin's disease admitted during the past twenty years. In several of the multiple-case families, an additional association with immunological deficiency states and autoimmune disease has been noted (Potolsky et al., 1971; Creagan and Fraumeni, 1972; Fenelly and McBride, 1974; Buehler et al., 1975; Lynch et al., 1976). In the Swiss mountain family described by Hardmeier and Rellstab (1975), consanguinity may have been a contributory factor in the occurrence of four cases of Hodgkin's disease, five of myelocytic leukemia, and one each of reticulum cell sarcoma and of melanoma.

In a more recent analysis of 23 cases in which Hodgkin's disease occurred in first-degree blood relatives during a 20-year period, Vianna et al. (1974a) noted 9 sibling pairs, 7 parent-child pairs, 4 pairs of cousins, and 1 pair each of nephew-aunt, nephew-uncle, and grandfather-granddaughter. In a study of 174 patients with Hodgkin's disease with 472 siblings at risk, Johnson and Johnson (1972) noted 2 sibling pairs, both with onsets within a one-year interval. An incidence survey in Greater Boston during 1959–1973 detected 5 sib-

Table 2.3   Some Cases of Familial Hodgkin's Disease Cited in Literature

Reference	Family	Sex and age at onset		Date of onset	
		Proband	Relative	Proband	Relative
Arkin (1926)	1	M. 34	Son 23	1899 (died)	1922
		M. 34	Nephew 20	1899 (died)	1917
Charache (1941)	2	F. 15 (a twin)	Mother	1936	1925 (Twin living and well)
McHeffey and Peterson (1934)	3	M. 11	Brother 13	1931 (Jan.)	1931 (Jan.)
Razis, Diamond, and Craver (1959a)	4	M. 35	Sister (1) 23	1939 (Dec.)	1932 (March)
		M. 35	Sister (2) 34	1939 (Dec.)	1935
	5	F. 38	Son 20	1954 (Aug.)	1954 (Sept.)
	6	M. 30	Brother 37	1951 (Jan.)	1954 (March)
	7	M. 14	Mother 52	1952 (June)	1952 ("End")
	8	F. 38	Father 40	1956 (June)	1934 (Spring)
	9	F. 38	Mother "elderly"	1950 (Aug.)	1948 (Summer)
	10	M. 24	Brother 36	1952 (April)	1951
	11	M. 24	Sister 22	1951 ("End")	1951 ("End")
	12	M. 52	Son 46	1923	1952 (Feb.)
	13	F. 40	Son 13	1950 ("Beginning")	1955 (Summer)
	14	F. 47	Daughter 19	1947 (Dec.)	1948 (Aug.)
	15	M. 50	Sister 40	1953 (Feb.)	1954 (Aug.)
	16	M. 53	Daughter 16	1953 (April)	1955 (Sept.)
Schier (1954)	17	F. 25	Sister 37	1933	1938
		F. 25	Brother 35	1933	1938
	18	M. 35	Brother 35	1943	1952
		M. 35	Nephew 26	1943	1952
Smith (1934)	19	F. 23	Sister 18	1924	1930
Videbaek (1955)	20	M. 26	Brother 27	1945	1950

ling pairs under the age of 45, as compared with an expected number of 0.7, suggesting that siblings of young adults with Hodgkin's disease have about a sevenfold excess risk of the disease (Grufferman et al., 1977). Eight additional sibling pairs were identified in individuals ineligible for the incidence series. Among all 13 pairs, 12 were sex concordant, as compared with an expected number of 6.8 ($p = 0.01$). Grufferman et al. note that of the 46 sibling pairs under the age of 45 recorded in the literature, 30 are sex concordant, versus an expected number of 23.9. Overall, they suggest that siblings of the same sex as an affected person have a risk of developing Hodgkin's disease which is approximately double that of siblings of the opposite sex.

Data from Greater Boston were combined with similar data from a National Cancer Institute series by Gutensohn et al. (1975b) in an analysis of family size, from which they concluded that there is a consistent increase in risk of Hodgkin's disease as sibship size decreases. However, Stoopler et al. (1975)

pointed out that whereas the Boston data were consistent with such an interpretation, those from the National Cancer Institute were not. Moreover, they added data from an Atlanta, Georgia, study which they interpreted as failing to show any consistent relationship between sibship size and the incidence of Hodgkin's disease. In a reply to this criticism, Gutensohn et al. (1975a) argue that the Greater Boston data are more representative than those of the National Cancer Institute series and state that their own statistical analysis of the Atlanta data indicates a significant inverse association between sibship size and the incidence of Hodgkin's disease, thus supporting the Boston data. They conclude that the risk of Hodgkin's disease is low among persons from large families. This question remains controversial, however, since Paffenbarger, Wing, and Hyde (1977) found no evidence of an excess risk associated with sibship size in a retrospective analysis of 50,000 male former college students. Katin (1977) has also presented a brief critique of the Boston study.

Analyzing these instances, MacMahon (1966) has pointed out that most of the sibships involved individuals between 20 and 35 years of age. Razis et al. (1959a) noted that in a number of cases the onset was at similar times in the affected siblings (Table 2.3). A most remarkable pair is that cited by Craver (1968) in which Hodgkin's disease had its onset in the same week in a mother and son who worked in the same room of their home. A pair of sisters and their maternal aunt all developed the disease within an interval of 28 months in the family studied by Creagan and Fraumeni (1972). The mean interval between the times of onset was 2.6 years, and the mean difference between the ages of the siblings was 7.9 years. Similarly, in twelve parent-child pairs the dates of onset in parent and child were relatively close in time in seven of twelve instances. These observations favor an environmental rather than a genetic interpretation.

MacMahon's method of analysis was applied by Vianna et al. (1974a) in a study of 23 familial cases. Intervals of three years or less between times of onset were noted by these investigators in all 7 familial pairs who lived in the same household before and after the time of diagnosis of the first case, and five years or less in 11 of 16 additional pairs who resided in the same county, but not in the same household. Mantel and Blot (1976), in a very penetrating analysis, have pointed out that the restricted nature of the data selected for analysis by Vianna et al. (1974a) renders their use of MacMahon's method a serious misapplication. The fact that only those familial pairs were entered into the analysis in which both diagnoses occurred during a fixed time period (between 1950 and 1970) results in truncation of the age-at-onset distribution, with the extent of truncation increasing for later-born individuals. Another form of truncation stems from the fact that 7 of the pairs were parent-child, and one pair was grandparent-grandchild, because "the earlier born member of the pair is likely precluded from having disease at an early age, since that would be a substantial bar to parenthood." Finally, the fact that several of the pairs resided in the same household can result in a third form of truncation: shared household pairs in a restricted time frame are likely to be parent plus young child, since older children are more likely to leave the household. In such pairs, "The parent must develop the disease at a later age, yet likely close in time." Mantel and Blot cogently add one final caution: "There is a distinct logical difference between the statements: a) if a disease is infec-

tious in origin, then affected family members might be expected to develop the disease at about the same time, and b) if affected family members develop a disease at about the same time, then an infectious agent is involved. Whereas statement a may be generally valid, statement b is not."

Six reports to date describe occurrence of the disease in both husband and wife, the interval between onsets being relatively short in three cases (Mazar and Strauss, 1951; Brennan, 1956; DeVore and Doan, 1957; Berliner and Distenfeld, 1972; Dworsky and Henderson, 1974). Priesel and Winkelbauer (1926) reported an instance of apparently congenital Hodgkin's disease in a girl, four and one-half months old, with lymphadenopathy from the time of her birth, and in her mother, in whom the diagnosis was made by cervical lymph node biopsy during the last month of pregnancy. Querleu et al. (1977), in an exhaustive review of the literature, collected several other such cases, which they interpret as rare examples of transplacental metastasis from the mother.

Environmental and Occupational Factors.
Seasonal Variations. A seasonal trend in the onset of Hodgkin's disease, with a peak in December and January, has been reported by Cridland (1961). However, this peak was observed in a selected sample which included only 106 of a total of 269 cases seen at his institution during the interval concerned. The criteria for selection were limitation of lymphadenopathy to one peripheral site at onset and no deep involvement within six months after onset. Ten percent of the patients had upper respiratory infections at the time of onset, but these were not particularly prevalent in December and January. Two German studies have also indicated the occurrence of an excess of cases with onset in the winter months (Uhl and Hunstein, 1969; Hartwich and Schlabeck, 1970. The determination of the date of onset of Hodgkin's disease is difficult and often erroneous, however. As Innes and Newall (1961) have pointed out, "It must be realized that the results are entirely dependent on the ability of patients to recall the month in which they first noticed enlarged lymph nodes. Unless the nodes had enlarged rapidly, there is no way of being certain that the onset of the disease occurred in this month, and furthermore, it is not an uncommon experience to discover quite large superficial nodes of which the patient is unaware." MacMahon (1966) concluded that such seasonal variation probably "relates to perception and diag-

nosis rather than to etiologic factors." Similar cautions concerning the interpretation of seasonal data have been expressed by Abramson (1973). No seasonal pattern could be detected in American case material analyzed by Newell (1972).

Time-Space Clustering. Gilmore and Zelesnick (1962) reported the occurrence over a thirteen-year interval of three cases of Hodgkin's disease and three of leukemia among four families occupying two adjoining houses in a town in south central Pennsylvania. Evidence of sporadic clustering was noted in two large-scale studies by Ederer et al. (1965) and Lundin et al. (1966). An apparent cluster of three cases (plus a later fourth case) was reported in Utah (Heath et al., 1973), and a small cluster has been described in Great Britain (Evans et al., 1977). Another apparent cluster of three cases in an Amish Kindred has been cited by Halazun, Kerr, and Lukens (1972). In a case-control study of Hodgkin's disease in the New Orleans and Los Angeles areas, clusters involving (a) seven heroin addicts, (b) five students and one teacher from the same junior high school, and (c) a previously cited married couple, were noted in the Los Angeles series (Newell et al., 1973; Dworsky and Henderson, 1974). Ramsey (1975) noted the occurrence of seven cases of Hodgkin's disease or malignant lymphoma during a ten-year period in individuals living within a 200-meter radius.

Klinger and Minton (1973) noted that in Union County, Ohio (1970 population: 23,786), there were 12 recorded cases of Hodgkin's disease in the interval 1960–1971, for an average annual incidence of 4.3/100,000. However, 5 of these cases had occurred in a single community, Darby Township (1970 population: 1,212) for an average annual incidence of 34.4/100,000. They concluded that the difference between these rates was highly significant ($p < 0.0005$). However, a pitfall in methodology casts serious doubt on the significance of their report. The fact is that Union County was *selected* as the study area, rather than chosen at random, due to a report of three cases in Darby Township; thus, the inclusion of those three cases invalidates their analysis. Smith and Pike (1974) have estimated that if the population of the United States were divided into some 8,000 units the same size as Union County, situations more extreme than that reported in Union County would be expected by chance alone in about 160 units (2 percent). Thus, they point out, if each such a posteriori cluster were singled out for publication, reports of this kind could emerge weekly for over

three years and still represent only a chance phenomenon. It is of interest that two conventionally designed studies of time-space clustering, one in the Manchester (U.K.) area, the other in Connecticut, have yielded essentially negative results (Alderson and Nayak, 1971; Kryscio et al., 1973).

Interest in the possibility that Hodgkin's disease might be transmitted like an infectious disease with a long and variable latent period, either directly from case to case or via an intermediate contact, was strongly stimulated by the reports of Vianna et al. (1971a, 1972). The attention of these investigators was drawn to the fact that a number of cases of the disease had occurred in students who had attended a particular high school in Albany, N.Y. They initiated a search for additional cases linked to the initially identified cases either directly, or indirectly through a single contact, and succeeded in identifying 31 such cases among a total of 208 cases diagnosed in Albany County during the interval 1950–1970. Of these, there were 9 instances of case-case, and 25 of case-contact-case linkage, a situation which they termed an "extended epidemic" or "outbreak." Controls for the 31 linked cases (rather than for the total sample population of 208) were burn patients and students at the same high school who were stated to show a significantly lesser degree of linkage. Other linked groups of cases of leukemias and lymphomas, including Hodgkin's disease, have been reported by Wagener and Haanen (1975) and Schimpff et al. (1975). However, the lack of properly matched control groups makes it impossible to assess the statistical significance of such findings (Abramson, 1973; Smith and Pike, 1974; Grufferman, 1977). It has been estimated (Smith and Pike, 1974, 1976) that spurious instances of linkage could occur by chance alone, over a ten-year interval, in about 20 percent of all newly diagnosed cases of Hodgkin's disease among patients 30 years of age. No evidence of clustering was detected by Paffenbarger, Wing, and Hyde (1977) among 45 cases of Hodgkin's disease occurring in a cohort of 50,000 male graduates from two universities.

Another investigation by Vianna and Polan (1973) indicated a significant degree of clustering of cases of Hodgkin's disease among young patients in relation to certain schools in Nassau and Suffolk counties, New York. This report has been challenged (Pike and Smith, 1974; Grufferman, 1977) and defended (Vianna and Polan, 1974) with respect to the possibility that nonascertainment of cases may have occurred which could have introduced serious bias into the analysis. Zack et al.

(1977), in an analysis of high school contacts in Connecticut, concluded that there might be as much as a twofold increase in risk among students enrolled in certain schools.

Studies similar to that of Vianna et al. (1971a, 1972) but employing properly matched controls ("case-control" designs; Mack, 1974) have been conducted in Israel, Oxford, and Boston (Abramson, 1973; Smith and Pike, 1974, 1976; Grufferman, 1977). Data from the Oxford case-control study, recently analyzed by Smith, Pike, Kinlen, Jones, and Harris (1977), provide no support for the hypothesis of transmissibility proposed by Vianna and his colleagues. The Oxford study involved 87 of 97 patients less than 40 years of age who were newly diagnosed during the years 1962–1971 in a defined area around Oxford, England. For each of the 87 cases, a matched control was selected with a diagnosis other than chronic or malignant disease. Both sets of individuals were then interviewed with respect to the schools they had attended, their places of work, and other relevant parameters. In the Hodgkin's disease group, links were established between 40 pairs, as compared with 40.75 expected. When seven postulated "periods of susceptibility" and nine postulated "periods of infectivity" were examined, only one yielded a significant result: 7 pairs of links were found, as against 2.75 expected, among the group "susceptible" ten to five years before diagnosis, and "infective" from the time of diagnosis until two years thereafter. If the parallel studies in Israel and in Boston yield similarly negative results, the controversial issue of the transmissibility of Hodgkin's disease may well be definitively resolved.

Social Class and Occupation. Standardized mortality ratios (SMR's) for Hodgkin's disease, other lymphomas, and leukemias in the five social classes defined by the Registrar General for England and Wales have been summarized by MacMahon (1966). Mortality ratios appeared to be high in the upper social classes for all of the lymphomas and leukemias. However, Abramson (1973) has called attention to a considerable shift in British social class data for Hodgkin's disease during the next ten-year period, which suggests that class differences in the accuracy of ascertainment may have contributed to the association noted in the earlier data. No significant differences in incidence as related to social class were found in the Manchester (U.K.) area among men in whom the disease was diagnosed during 1962–1965 (Alderson and Nayak, 1972).

Gutensohn et al. (1975b) observed a significant inverse relationship between sibship size and the risk of Hodgkin's disease. Their data indicated that an individual who was an only child had an 80 percent greater risk than did a person from a middle-sized family. Gutensohn and Cole (1977), in a review of this and other aspects of the epidemiology of Hodgkin's disease in the young, suggest that it may be "social class in childhood that is pertinent; adult social class may be related . . . only because it reflects childhood social class."

Leshan, Marvin, and Lyerly (1959), in a study of 97 World War II soldiers who developed Hodgkin's disease after military induction, observed that they had significantly higher army general classification test (intelligence) scores than those for the general army population. In a related study of 209 soldiers with Hodgkin's disease according to their prewar occupation, a significantly greater proportion were found to occur in occupational groups having the highest median scores on the same test. Educational level was also found to be relatively high in another study of U.S. military personnel with Hodgkin's disease by Cohen, Smetana, and Miller (1964).

Milham and Hesser (1967), in a review of 1,549 death certificates of white adult males who died of Hodgkin's disease in upstate New York from 1940 to 1953 and from 1957 to 1964, and an equal number of death certificates from a matched control group, noted an apparent preponderance of Hodgkin's disease deaths among men whose occupations involved exposure to wood (carpenters, cabinet makers, lumberjacks, paper mill workers, woodyard foremen, etc). There was also a preponderance of individuals who had been born in Italy, but the two factors were not found to be interdependent. Petersen and Milham (1974) and Grufferman, Duong, and Cole (1976) have also reported an increased relative risk among woodworkers in data from the state of Washington and from the Greater Boston metropolitan area, respectively. Spiers (1969) suggested that the common denominator between woodworking occupations and Hodgkin's disease might be exposure to pine pollen. However, Acheson (1967), reviewing Hodgkin's disease and other lymphoma mortality data from High Wycombe and areas of nearby Buckinghamshire, England, in which the furniture industry is concentrated, found no excess of Hodgkin's disease mortality in these areas, relative to that in the rest of Buckinghamshire, Oxfordshire, or part of Berkshire. Moreover, when deaths were tallied according to occupation, no specific excess of deaths from Hodgkin's disease, relative to that from other lymphomas, was detected among woodworkers or paperworkers as compared with other occupations.

Vianna and his colleagues, in the wake of their studies cited above which indicated the apparent case-case or case-contact-case transmission of Hodgkin's disease, examined the possibility that physicians, as a consequence of their professional exposure to such cases, might be at increased risk of developing the disease. In a survey of teaching hospitals in upstate New York during the thirteen-year period 1960–1972, they encountered 13 cases among an estimated median population of 14,500 male physicians 25 years of age or older (Vianna et al., 1974b). They concluded that the calculated average annual incidence rate of 6.9/100,000 represented a statistically significant 1.8-fold increase in risk relative to other males of corresponding age. A curious feature of their data, however, was the fact that disproportionate numbers of cases failed to occur in the specialties most closely associated with the care of patients with Hodgkin's disease, and none were oncologists. In a similar study in England and Wales during the interval 1951–1966, Smith, Kinlen, and Doll (1974) encountered only 12 cases in physicians, whereas 15.8 would have been expected if physicians were at the same risk as all other males of similar age distribution. Another such study in the Greater Boston metropolitan area (Grufferman, Duong, and Cole, 1976) also failed to confirm the findings of Vianna et al.; no excess relative risk (RR) was encountered among either physicians (RR = 1.2; 95 percent confidence interval 0.4–2.6) or nurses (RR = 0.9; 0.4–1.8). An analysis of causes of death among four groups of specialists (radiologists and radiotherapists, general physicians, ophthalmologists, and otolaryngologists) yielded a total of 13 observed deaths versus 13.17 expected, and no excess of observed deaths among radiologists and radiotherapists (Matanoski, Sartwell, and Elliott, 1975).

The hypothesis of transmissibility was also invoked by Milham (1974) in conjunction with his finding among schoolteachers in Washington State of a twofold to threefold increase in risk of dying of Hodgkin's disease, on the basis that they have above-average contact with young individuals among whom the disease is most prevalent. However, it was pointed out by Hoover (1974) that schoolteachers have a considerably lower mortality from all causes combined than the general population, and that Milham's use of proportionate mortality analysis could explain much of the apparent

excess. A revised analysis based on census data confirmed that the excess death rate from Hodgkin's disease among teachers was much smaller than that reported by Milham. The Boston study (Grufferman, Duong, and Cole, 1976) failed to reveal evidence of a significantly increased risk among teachers (RR = 1.1; 95 percent confidence interval 0.7–1.6).

Associated Medical Conditions.

Epilepsy. There is no evidence that epilepsy per se is related to Hodgkin's disease or the other malignant lymphomas. However, certain of the drugs used to treat the disease have been incriminated as the cause of hypersensitivity reactions associated with lymphadenopathy, biopsy of which may reveal histologic abnormalities essentially indistinguishable from Hodgkin's disease. Meller and Resch (1949) and Saltzstein et al. (1958) were the first to report cases in which pronounced lymphadenopathy, clinically and pathologically mimicking Hodgkin's disease, developed in epileptic patients receiving one of the hydantoin anticonvulsant drugs. In 1959, Saltzstein and Ackerman were able to add seven additional cases. The lymphangiographic appearance of the retroperitoneal lymph nodes also closely resembles that of Hodgkin's disease (Sayoc and Howland, 1974). In these and in a number of similar instances reported by various other authors during the ensuing years (Rosenfeld et al., 1961; LeVan and Bierman, 1962; Doyle and Hellstrom, 1963; Krasznai, 1966; Schreiber and McGregor, 1968), the lymphadenopathy disappeared when use of the drug was stopped. However, cases have been reported in which regression did not occur after cessation of drug administration; these appear to have been true malignant lymphomas (Saltzstein, 1962; Hyman and Sommers, 1966; Gams et al., 1968; Brown, 1971). A review and analysis of all of the cases reported in the literature to 1968 has been presented by Gams et al.; their very convenient tabulations of these cases are reproduced in slightly modified form in Tables 2.4, 2.5, 2.6, and 2.7. Additional reports of such cases have continued to appear (Rausing and Trell, 1971; Li et al., 1975). A history of hydantoin use was noted by Li et al. (1975) in 8 (1.6 percent) of 516 patients with Hodgkin's disease or other lymphomas, as compared with 2 instances among 516 tumor-free control individuals (0.4 percent).

The etiologic role of the hydantoin in such instances remains conjectural. However, depression of immunologic function, invoked as a possible mechanism by Li et al. (1975), has been docu-

Table 2.4 Hydantoin-Induced Lymphoproliferative Reactions   A. Hyperplasia: Architecture Preserved, Pleomorphic Response, Clearly Benign

Reference	Case no.	Age	Sex	Drug	Nodes	Rash	Fever	Eosinophils	Enlarged Liver	Enlarged Spleen	Pathology	Regression after cessation of therapy	Subsequent course
1. Chaiken et al. (1950)	—	29	M	Dilantin	Cervical, axillary, inguinal	+	+	+	+	0	Chronic inflammation; pleomorphic cellular response	Yes	No followup available
2. Olmer et al. (1952)	—	46	M	Mesantoin	Axillary, inguinal	+	+	0	+	0	Pleomorphic hyperplasia; lymphocyte and reticulum	—	Died of dehydration before cessation of drug could be evaluated
3. Lindqvist (1957)	—	18	F	Mesantoin	Generalized	+	+	+	0	0	Pleomorphic hyperplasia; eosinophilia; "non-specific lymphadenitis"	Yes, after steroid therapy	Positive lupus erythematosis preparation; diagnosis: systemic lupus erythematosis; no followup available
4. Saltzstein and Ackerman (1959)	2	6	M	Mesantoin, dilantin	Cervical, axillary, inguinal	+	+	+	0	0	Pleomorphic hyperplasia; lymphocyte and reticulum; eosinophilia; foci of necrosis	Yes	No recurrence after four years
5. Saltzstein and Ackerman (1959)	5	10	M	Mesantoin, dilantin	Cervical	+	+	+	+	0	Pleomorphic hyperplasia; lymphocyte and reticulum; slight fibrosis	Yes	No recurrence after two years
6. Bajoghli (1961)	—	6	F	Dilantin	Generalized	+	+	+	+	+	Pleomorphic hyperplasia; lymphocyte and reticulum; "chronic lymphadenitis"	Yes	No recurrence after 1½ months
7. Griesshaber (1964)	—	14	M	Mesantoin	Axillary, inguinal	+	+	+	0	+	Reticulum cell hyperplasia; "chronic lymphadenitis"	Yes	No followup available

Source: Rearranged and slightly modified from Table IA of Gams, Neal, and Conrad (1968).

Table 2.5 Hydantoin-Induced Lymphoproliferative Reactions   B. Pseudolymphoma: Reticulum Cell Hyperplasia, Suspicious for Malignant Lymphoma

Case	Reference	Case no.	Age	Sex	Drug	Nodes	Rash	Fever	Eosinophils	Enlarged Liver	Enlarged Spleen	Pathology	Regression after cessation of therapy	Subsequent course
1.	Van Wyk and Hoffmann (1948)	—	71	M	Dilantin	Cervical	+	0	0	0	0	Reticulum cell hyperplasia; eosinophila	Died of periarteritis	Diagnosis: reactive lymphadenitis secondary to exfoliative dermatitis
2.	Meller and Resch (1949)	—	—	—	Mesantoin	Not specified	+	+	0	0	0	"Indistinguishable from Hodgkin's disease"	Yes	No followup available
3.	Chiari (1951)	1	21	M	Mesantoin	Cervical	+	0	+	0	0	Reticulum cell hyperplasia; eosinophila; foci of necrosis	Yes	No followup available
4.	Chiari (1951)	2	47	M	Mesantoin	Generalized	+	+	0	0	0	Reticulum cell hyperplasia; mitoses; eosinophilia; foci of necrosis	Yes	No followup available
5.	Olmer et al. (1952)	—	56	M	Mesantoin	Cervical	+	+	+	0	0	Reticulum cell hyperplasia; eosinophilia; foci of necrosis	Yes	No followup available
6.	Olmer et al. (1952)	2	31	F	Mesantoin	Cervical, inguinal	+	0	0	0	0	Reticulum cell hyperplasia; eosinophilia; foci of necrosis	Yes	No followup available
7.	Martin et al. (1954)	—	5	M	Dilantin	Generalized	+	+	0	0	0	Reticulum cell hyperplasia; diffuse sclerosis	Yes	No followup available
8.	Saltzstein and Ackerman (1959)	1	11	M	Milotin	Mesenteric	0	0	0	0	0	Reticulum cell hyperplasia; increased mitoses; eosinophilia; foci of necrosis; "malignant lymphoma"	Yes	No recurrence after five years
9.	Saltzstein and Ackerman (1959)	6	7	M	Peganone	Axillary, cervical	0	+	+	+	+	Pleomorphic hyperplasia; reticulum, lymphocyte, plasma cell, eosinophilia; foci of necrosis; capsular invasion	Yes	No recurrence after four months

Table 2.5 Hydantoin-Induced Lymphoproliferative Reactions   B. Pseudolymphoma: Reticulum Cell Hyperplasia, Suspicious for Malignant Lymphoma (*Cont.*)

Case	Reference	Case no.	Age	Sex	Drug	Nodes	Rash	Fever	Eosinophils	Enlarged Liver	Enlarged Spleen	Pathology	Regression after cessation of therapy	Subsequent course
10.	Saltzstein and Ackerman (1959)	7	45	F	Dilantin	Generalized	+	+	+	0	0	Reticulum cell hyperplasia; increased plasma cells; eosinophilia	Yes	No recurrence after two months
11.	Rosenfeld et al. (1961)	—	31	F	Dilantin	Axillary, cervical	+	+	+	+	+	Lymphatic hyperplasia with mitoses; increased fibrosis; "lymphoblastic lymphosarcoma"	Yes	No followup available
12.	Doyle and Hellstrom (1963)	—	36	M	Mesantoin	Axillary, cervical	+	+	+	0	+	Reticulum cell hyperplasia; increased eosinophils and plasma cells; focal necrosis; "Reed-Sternberg" cells; "Hodgkin's disease"	Yes	No recurrence after seven years
13.	Branco and Gander (1964)	—	30	F	Mesantoin	Supraclavicular	+	+	+	+	0	Reticulum cell hyperplasia with numerous mitoses, capsular and subcapsular sinusoidal invasion; increased eosinophils and plasma cells; "Reed-Sternberg" cells	Yes	No recurrence after three years
14.	Langlands et al. (1967)	—	71	M	Primidone	Cervical	+	+	+	0	0	Reticulum cell hyperplasia; eosinophilia; foci of necrosis (October 1965)	Yes	Died of cancer of stomach, July 1967; no lymphoma

Source: Rearranged and slightly modified from Table IB of Gams, Neal, and Conrad (1968).

Table 2.6 Hydantoin-Induced Lymphoproliferative Reactions   C. Pseudo-Pseudolymphoma: Reticulum Cell Hyperplasia, Suspicious or Frankly Malignant

Case	Reference	Case no.	Age	Sex	Drug	Nodes	Rash	Fever	Eosino-phils	Enlarged Liver	Enlarged Spleen	Pathology	Regression after cessation of therapy	Subsequent course
1.	Saltzstein and Ackerman (1959)	4	26	M	Dilantin Mesantoin Mysoline	Generalized	+	+	+	+	+	September 1956: reticulum cell hyperplasia, mitoses, eosinophilia; January 1960: pleomorphic hyperplasia, eosinophilia; May 1960: reticulum cell hyperplasia, "malignant lymphoma"	Yes, twice / No	Died of lymphoma
2.	Saltzstein and Ackerman (1959)	3	53	F	Dilantin	Cervical, axillary, inguinal	0	0	0	0	0	Reticulum cell hyperplasia; eosinophilia; increased plasma cells; foci of necrosis	Yes, twice	Died of multiple myeloma
3.	Gams et al. (1968)	—	45	M	Dilantin	Generalized	0	0	0	0	0	December 1962: reticulum cell hyperplasia, slight fibrosis; April 1963: reticulum cell hyperplasia, increased mitoses; December 1964: reticulum cell hyperplasia, "malignant lymphoma"	Yes / No	Died of diffuse lymphoma

Source: Rearranged and slightly modified from Table IC of Gams, Neal, and Conrad (1968).

Table 2.7 Hydantoins and Frankly Malignant Lymphomas

Case	Case no.[a]	Age	Sex	Drug	Nodes	Rash	Fever	Eosino-phils	Enlarged		Pathology	Regression after cessation of therapy
									Liver	Spleen		
1.	1	27	F	Dilantin Mysoline Celontin	None	0	0	0	0	0	Anaplastic multinucleated reticulum cells; Reed-Sternberg cells; hyaline nodules; "nodular sclerosing Hodgkin's disease"	No[b]
2.	2	22	F	Dilantin	Cervical	0	+	0	0	0	Lymphocyte hyperplasia; Reed-Sternberg cells; "lymphocyte predominant Hodgkin's disease"	No[b]
3.	3	23	F	Dilantin	Cervical, axillary	0	0	0	0	+	Lymphocyte hyperplasia; Reed-Sternberg cells; capsular invasion; eosinophilia; foci of necrosis; "lymphocyte predominant Hodgkin's disease"	No
4.	4	62	M	Dilantin	Generalized	0	0	0	0	+	Lymphocyte hyperplasia; capsular invasions; "lymphosarcoma"	No[b]
5.	5	68	M	Dilantin	None	0	+	0	0	0	January 1957: lymphocyte hyperplasia; pleomorphic; "consistent with atypical hyperplasia secondary to hydantoins"	No[b]
6.	6	65	M	Dilantin	Abdominal	0	0	0	0	0	No description; "reticulum cell sarcoma"	No[b]
7.	7	30	M	Dilantin	Cervical, axillary	0	0	0	0	0	Reticulum cell hyperplasia; Reed-Sternberg cells; "Hodgkin's disease"	No[b]

Source: Rearranged and slightly modified from Table ID of Gams, Neal, and Conrad (1968).
[a] All cases listed are from Hyman and Sommers (1966).
[b] Administration of Dilantin not stopped.

mented in a series of such patients by Sorrell et al. (1971). Sorrell and Forbes (1975) have also described the occurrence of hypersensitivity reactions to a hydantoin drug in a case of hydantoin-associated Hodgkin's disease.

The Lymphoid Tissue "Barrier." The suggestion by Miller (1966) that the marked upturn of Hodgkin's disease mortality rates at the end of the first decade of life might be related to involution of the tonsils and adenoids has stimulated several investigations of the relationship between tonsillectomy and Hodgkin's disease. Vianna, Greenwald, and Davies (1971b) reviewed hospital records for tonsillectomy histories among 109 patients with Hodgkin's disease and 107 selected controls matched with respect to five-year age group and area of residence (but not socioeconomic status). They observed a 2.9-fold increase in risk of Hodgkin's disease associated with a history of prior tonsillectomy. Johnson and Johnson (1972) obtained a prior history of tonsillectomy in 52 percent of 174 recently treated patients with Hodgkin's disease, as compared with 35 percent among a total of 472 of their siblings. When matched siblings were compared with the patient group, the overall rates were 39 percent vs. 48 percent respectively. When the patients were subdivided according to sex, clinical stage, presence or absence of constitutional symptoms, primary site of involvement, and histopathologic type of Hodgkin's disease, Johnson and Johnson concluded that no statistically significant difference from their matched siblings existed with respect to tonsillectomy history. However, their method of analysis was criticized by three independent groups (Cole et al., 1973; Pike and Smith, 1973; Shimaoka, Bross, and Tidings, 1973), all of whom concluded that their data were consistent with a twofold increase in risk associated with tonsillectomy.

Two case-control studies in which socioeconomic factors were matched revealed no significant excess risk associated with tonsillectomy (Ruuskanen, Vanha-Perttula, and Kouvalainen, 1971; Newell et al., 1973), nor was such an association noted in a retrospective study of Hodgkin's disease in male former college students (Paffenbarger, Wing, and Hyde, 1977). Gutensohn, Cole, and Li (1975a) investigated the tonsillectomy rates in 136 young adults patients with Hodgkin's disease, their 315 siblings, and their 78 spouses. Whereas the case-spouse comparison yielded a risk ratio of Hodgkin's disease among tonsillectomized persons of 3.1, the case-sibling comparison yielded a risk ratio

of only 1.4. Moreover, when the case-sibling data were reanalyzed according to sibship size, an increased risk of Hodgkin's disease was associated with tonsillectomy only within the 37 sibships of size 2. Gutensohn, Cole, and Li concluded that "either the association is non-causal or, if causal, is quite complex and modified by factors related to family size."

Some evidence of an increased risk associated with appendectomy has also been reported (Bierman, 1968; Hyams and Wynder, 1968), but no such finding emerged in three case-control studies in which socioeconomic factors were made comparable (Ruuskanen, Vanha-Perttula, and Kouvalainen, 1971; Newell et al., 1973; Gutensohn, Cole, and Li, 1975a). Data from France (Teillet, Weisgerber, and Feingold, 1973) also failed to reveal an influence of tonsillectomy or appendectomy on the risk of developing Hodgkin's disease.

Congenital and Induced Immunological Disorders. It is now well established that individuals with any of the rare congenital immunodeficiency states, as well as renal transplant recipients and other patients receiving chronic immunosuppressive medication, are highly susceptible to the development of malignant lymphomas (Fraumeni, 1969; Penn, 1976). Histiocytic lymphomas (reticulum cell sarcomas) are by far the most common type of tumor in such instances, accounting for well over half of all cases. However, Hodgkin's disease has developed in children with Chediak-Higashi syndrome (Tan et al., 1971) and ataxia-telangiectasia (Harris and Seeler, 1973), as well as in occasional renal transplant recipients (Sterling et al., 1974; Cerilli et al., 1977). Cases of Hodgkin's disease have also been reported in association with systemic lupus erythematosus (Cammarata, Rodnan, and Jensen, 1963; Nilsen, Missal, and Condemi, 1967) and chronic autoimmune hemolytic anemia (Cazenave et al., 1973). Coexistence of Hodgkin's disease and Down's syndrome has been reported (McCormick, Meyer, and Nesbit, 1971) although the chromosomal abnormality associated with this congenital disorder appears to predispose primarily to the development of leukemia rather than lymphomas.

Moreover, in several of the families in which multiple cases of Hodgkin's disease and other lymphomas have been reported, a variety of immunodeficiency states and other immunologic disorders have also been encountered (Potolsky et al., 1971; Buehler et al., 1975; Lynch et al., 1976). Of particular interest in this context was the finding of a significant defect in cell-mediated immunity in both parents and in all five female siblings of a family in which three of the siblings developed Hodgkin's disease (Fenelly and McBride, 1974).

Only three reports to date have dealt with the possible influence of stimulation of the immune system. In a followup study of 64,126 individuals in the states of Georgia and Alabama who received BCG vaccination over a twenty-one-year period, Comstock, Livesay, and Webster (1971) found 32 cases of leukemia, 15 of Hodgkin's disease, and 13 of lymphosarcoma, none of which significantly exceeded expectation. Skegg (1978) also found no indication that BCG vaccination influenced the incidence of Hodgkin's disease in cohorts of children from the North and South islands of New Zealand. Paffenbarger, Wing, and Hyde (1977), in a study of 50,000 male former college students, noted a consistent inverse relationship between clinically overt contagious diseases of childhood and the risk of later death from Hodgkin's disease. They pointed out that this result could be variously interpreted as indicating: "1) that adult-onset Hodgkin's disease decedents had immune systems inadequately challenged by infectious diseases in early childhood and hence less well conditioned to combat Hodgkin's disease, whether or not it is of infectious origin; 2) they had hyperimmune mechanisms that aborted clinical attacks of common childhood infections and fostered an autoimmune phenomenon, which led to Hodgkin's disease; 3) birth-cohort members of the Hodgkin's disease group failed to survive childhood infections because of inadequate immune systems which predisposed survivors to later fatal Hodgkin's disease."

Infectious Mononucleosis; Epstein-Barr and Other Herpes Viruses. In 1953, Massey, Lane, and Imbriglia reported the case of a 20-year-old female in whom acute infectious mononucleosis and mediastinal Hodgkin's disease existed concurrently. Other instances of the coexistence of these two diseases were reported by Kenis et al. (1958). In his Bradshaw Lecture (1967), Smithers mentions the observation of four cases of prior infectious mononucleosis in a series of 416 cases of Hodgkin's disease. At Stanford University Medical Center, during a period of eight years, inquiries about a history of infectious mononucleosis in patients with Hodgkin's disease and the other malignant lymphomas elicited 37 cases of patients with Hodgkin's disease who had a history of reasonably well-documented or probable prior infectious mononucleosis (Table 2.8). Two of these cases, one of which occurred in a young physician, are of particular interest because

the initial manifestation of Hodgkin's disease presented in a lymph node known to have remained persistently enlarged from the time of its prior involvement by infectious mononucleosis. English (1970) cites the case of a 10-year-old boy who developed well-documented infectious mononucleosis, with splenomegaly, lymphadenopathy, a positive "Monospot" test, and an anti-EBV titer of 1:640 seven months before the diagnosis of Hodgkin's disease. Robinson (1976) has described such a sequence in a 23-year-old man, with onset four years after infectious mononucleosis. Paradoxically, the converse sequence (Hodgkin's disease followed by infectious mononucleosis) has also been noted (Ballas, Saidi, and Coccia 1975). The diagnosis of infectious mononucleosis in such instances should not rest on laboratory evidence alone, however, since false-positive "Monospot" tests have been reported in patients with malignant lymphomas, including Hodgkin's disease (Wolf et al., 1970).

The reported observation of cells morphologically indistinguishable from Sternberg-Reed cells of Hodgkin's disease in lymph node biopsies from patients with infectious mononucleosis (Lukes, Tindle, and Parker, 1969; McMahon, Gordon, and Rosen, 1970; Strum, Park, and Rappaport, 1970; Agliozzo and Reingold, 1971; Salvador, Harrison, and Kyle, 1971; Tindle, Parker, and Lukes, 1972) has sharply increased interest in the possible relationship between this EB virus-induced lymphoproliferative infection and the development of Hodgkin's disease. Indeed, it has been suggested by Lukes, Tindle, and Parker (1969) that "infectious mononucleosis on rare occasions may not be a self-limited lymphoid proliferation, but the initial infectious episode which precedes neoplastic transformation."

However, it is clear that the etiologic link, if any, cannot be elucidated on the basis of such morphologic similarities alone. Several case-control studies have failed to reveal a positive association between prior infectious mononucleosis and lymphoid neoplasms (Fraumeni, 1971; Vianna, Greenwald, and Davies, 1971b; Newell et al., 1973; Miller and Beebe, 1973). The results of the four cohort studies to date have been more intriguing. Miller and Beebe (1973) searched for subsequent deaths due to malignant neoplasms and specifically to lymphomas among a group of 2,437 male veterans with a diagnosis of infectious mononucleosis made during U.S. Army military service in 1944, and among a similar number of controls. They found 23 case deaths and 20 control deaths from all neo-

TABLE 2.8 Hodgkin's Disease (HD) Developing in Patients with a Prior History of Infectious Mononucleosis (IM)[a]

A. Reasonably well-documented cases

Case no.	Initials	Age	Sex	Date of admission	Interval, diagnosis IM to biopsy diagnosis HD	Clinical Features of IM					Laboratory tests[b]			Comment
						Fever	Nodes	Sore throat	Fatigue	Other	H.A.	Spot	Smear	
1	K.A.	21	M	10/17/62	3 yrs.	+	+	?	+	Malaise	+	?	+	Physician states diagnosis definite
2	R.S.	28	M	10/12/64	4 yrs.	?	?	?	?	Malaise	?	?	?	Physician states diagnosis definite
3	S.F.	46	M	9/13/65	8 mos.	?	+	?	+					Daughter had mononucleosis concurrently
4	M.T.	14	M	11/16/65	2 mos.	+	+	+			1:3514			Recovered, then recurrent adenopathy
5	D.S.	21	M	5/23/66	5 yrs.	?	?	?	+	Splenomegaly	1:448			
6	L.S.	28	M	7/ 5/66	7 yrs.	+	+	+	+		−		+	Physician states diagnosis definite
7	C.T.	17	M	9/16/66	4.5 yrs.	?	?	?	?		?	?	?	Physician states diagnosis definite
8	B.D.	29	F	10/31/66	8 yrs.	+	+	+	+	Jaundice	1:448			
9	G.C.L.	18	F	1/19/67	8 mos.	?	+		+		+			Right cervical nodes regressed, then re-enlarged
10	C.E.A.	24	F	2/17/67	20 mos.	?	+				?	?	?	Physician states diagnosis definite
11	C.M.	27	M	3/ 8/67	9.5 yrs.	?	+		+		?	?	?	Adenopathy never fully disappeared
12	D.S.	19	M	4/17/67	4 yrs.	+			+		+?		+	"Blood tests" positive; out of school 2 weeks
13	M.G.	20	F	7/18/67	33 mos.	+	+	+			1:640		+	
14	M.T.	19	M	12/ 7/67	5 yrs.	?	+		+		?	?	?	
15	S.Z.	33	F	4/13/68	12 yrs.	?	?	?			?	?	?	"Definite" diagnosis of IM; no details
16	F.G.	32	M	10/21/68	1 yr.	+	+			Malaise		+	+	
17	R.F.	25	M	11/18/68	3 mos.	+	+		+		+?		+	"Blood tests" positive
18	J.C.	26	M	1/16/69	5 yrs.	+	+			Malaise	+?		?	"Blood tests" positive
19	J.S.	25	M	3/28/69	6 yrs.	+	+				+?		?	"Blood tests" positive
20	E.S.	25	M	4/16/69	4.5 yrs.	?	+				1:7168			Recurrent left cervical adenopathy, 10/68
21	F.B.	23	F	5/29/69	6 yrs.	+	+				?		+	

Table 2.8 Hodgkin's Disease (HD) Developing in Patients with a Prior History of Infectious Mononucleosis (IM)[a] (*Cont.*)

A. Reasonably well-documented cases

Case no.	Initials	Age	Sex	Date of admission	Interval, diagnosis IM to biopsy diagnosis HD	Clinical Features of IM					Laboratory tests[b]			Comment
						Fever	Nodes	Sore throat	Fatigue	Other	H.A.	Spot	Smear	
22	D.R.	19	F	9/ 5/69	2 mos.	+	+				1:450			
23	P.S.	23	F	9/15/69	2 yrs.	?	+		+		+?			"Blood tests" positive
24	W.D.	19	M	4/20/70	4 yrs.	?	?				+?			"Blood tests" positive
25	M.D.	29	M	5/22/70	8 yrs.	+	+			Spleno-megaly	+		+	Persistent right inguinal adenopathy, increasing again 12/69.
26	G.T.	19	M	6/ 4/70	5 mos.	+	+	+				+	+	
27	N.B.	30	F	8/ 3/70	14 yrs.	?	+		+	Bed rest 4 mos.	?		?	M.D. diagnosis definite.
28	A.T.	16	F	10/4/70	7 mos.	+	+					+		
29	L.R.	25	M	10/7/70	9 mos.	+	+		+	Jaundice	+?		+	Persistent left cervical adenopathy, increasing again 9 mos. later.

B. Poorly documented and doubtful cases

Case no.	Initials	Age	Sex	Date of admission	Interval, diagnosis IM to biopsy diagnosis HD	Fever	Nodes	Sore throat	Fatigue	Other	H.A.	Spot	Smear	Comment
1	R.B.	19	F	4/27/64	2 yrs.	?	+		+		None performed			M.D. diagnosis
2	H.A.	25	M	6/17/66	8 yrs.	?	+		?		None performed			"Possible" IM diagnosed in college
3	D.F.	17	M	7/26/66	6 mos.	+	+				None performed			M.D. diagnosis
4	L.J.	23	F	3/29/68	9 mos.	+?	+				None performed			Nodes regressed, enlarged again 9 mos. later
5	D.P.	21	M	11/18/68	?	?	?				1:8 on admission			No definite IM history elicited
6	P.S.	16	F	2/10/69	?	-	-				None performed			No history; sister had definite IM one year earlier
7	F.B.	30	F	2/16/70	10 yrs.	?	+?				None performed			M.D. diagnosis
8	Z.R.	24	F	10/ 4/70	3 mos.	+	+?				None performed			M.D. diagnosis

[a]Stanford University Medical Center cases (H. S. Kaplan, previously unpublished data).
[b]H.A. = heterophile agglutination test (available titer given); Spot = mononucleosis spot test; Smear = increased numbers of atypical lymphocytes in peripheral blood smear.

plasms, of which 6 and 4, respectively, were due to malignant lymphomas, as compared with 2.31 expected. They excluded 1 of 2 cases of Hodgkin's disease from the case group on the ground that the diagnosis of infectious mononucleosis was questionable, leaving a net of 5 cases, an estimated relative risk of 2.2. Connelly and Christine (1974) conducted their investigation in Connecticut, where both cancer and infectious mononucleosis are reportable diseases. They traced 4,529 cases of infectious mononucleosis, representing a total of 36,456 person-years at risk, during the years 1948–1964. These were matched, with the assistance of a computer, against a file of over 230,000 cancer cases diagnosed between 1935 and 1968, inclusive. The observed number of cancers of all kinds in the study cohort was 33, a modest excess over the expected number, 24.4; the relative risk of 1.4 was similar for both sexes. However, among the 33 cancers, the largest single category was the malignant lymphomas, of which there were 7, including 5 cases of Hodgkin's disease (4 females and 1 male). Their average age at occurrence of infectious mononucleosis was 16 years; of Hodgkin's disease, 24 years. The relative risk for all lymphomas was 3.0 for males (not dissimilar from the value of 2.2 found by Miller and Beebe), whereas that for females was 4.4.

A similar study in Denmark by Rosdahl, Larsen, and Clemmesen (1974) was made possible by the fact that comprehensive data on Paul-Bunnell absorbed heterophile agglutination tests had been maintained since 1939 by the Statens Seruminstitut, Copenhagen, and on cases of malignant disease in Denmark since 1943 by the Danish Cancer Registry. In all, 17,073 individuals with titers of 1:32 or higher were identified and again computer-matched against the cancer files to yield a net total of 17 cases (16 male, 1 female) with Hodgkin's disease developing 12 months or more (range 1–7 years) after a positive Paul-Bunnell reaction. Case records, which were available for 12 of these individuals, confirmed that they had had infectious mononucleosis. The observed number of cases in males exceeded the expected number (4) at a high level of significance ($p < 0.00001$). The most recent cohort study by Munoz et al. (1978) involved populations in Aberdeen, Scotland, and in Lund, Malmö, Göteborg, Örebro, and Stockholm, Sweden. Positive titers were taken as $\geq 1:80$ for the Paul-Bunnell and ≥ 1.32 for the Paul-Bunnell-Davidson tests. A total of 1,759 individuals with positive tests during the years 1959–1971 were identified in Aberdeen and 7,695 in the Swedish

populations during the years 1952–1970. When these were matched against lists of patients with malignant lymphomas, nasopharyngeal carcinoma, and cancer of the colon in the respective registries, 7 patients, all of whom had Hodgkin's disease, were disclosed. Of these, 5 were female (4 Swedish, 1 Scottish) and 2 were male (1 in each country). The observed number exceeded the number expected (1.8) significantly for both sexes combined ($p < 0.01$) and for females only ($p < 0.001$). The interval between the positive Paul-Bunnell reaction and the diagnosis of Hodgkin's disease ranged from 3 to 11 years (average 5.6 years); an increased risk of Hodgkin's disease was manifested within 3 years.

Collectively, these cohort studies provide rather strong evidence for an association between Paul-Bunnell-positive infectious mononucleosis and Hodgkin's disease. However, it is obvious that there are disturbing inconsistencies with respect to the observed sex distributions which remain unexplained. Moreover, these findings per se do not establish whether the two diseases are directly linked etiologically or, alternatively, whether an underlying common factor predisposes individuals to develop both of them. Lantorp, Wahren, and Hanngren (1972) demonstrated convincingly that cutaneous delayed hypersensitivity reactions are profoundly suppressed during the course of infectious mononucleosis. They studied a series of 17 patients with infectious mononucleosis, all of whom had been vaccinated with BCG before the age of one year, in 14 of whom the results of earlier tuberculin tests were known. Although 12 of these patients had had prior positive reactions to purified protein derivative (PPD), all 17 patients failed to respond to PPD during the active phase of infectious mononucleosis. In contrast to the profound impairment of cell-mediated immunity revealed by these observations, the function of bone marrow-derived (B) lymphocytes, as judged by immunoglobulin levels, appears to be undisturbed in infectious mononucleosis (Niederman et al., 1968). It is thus possible that the link between infectious mononucleosis and Hodgkin's disease may be selective immunosuppression; susceptibility to the unknown causative agent of Hodgkin's disease may be enhanced during the period of impairment of cell-mediated immunity which accompanies this acute viral disorder.

In many instances, infectious mononucleosis follows an insidious course, and it is widely believed by authorities in this field that a very high proportion of all cases go undiagnosed (Evans,

1960). The *post hoc* ascertainment of the diagnosis has presented a particularly difficult problem, since the heterophile antibody reaction seldom remains positive for as long as one year after the acute phase. The discovery (Henle, Henle, and Diehl, 1968) that the EB virus is the causative agent of Paul-Bunnell-positive, and of many cases of Paul-Bunnell-negative, infectious mononucleosis has opened new avenues of investigation based on serologic reactions to the various antigens associated with the EB virus, since antibodies to these antigens appear and, with rare exceptions (Goldman and Aisenberg, 1970; Hirshaut et al., 1974), persist apparently indefinitely in the blood of such patients.

Several studies have now revealed high antibody titers to EB viral capsid antigen (VCA) (Johansson et al., 1970; Levine et al., 1971; Henle and Henle, 1973; Hesse et al., 1973; Henderson et al., 1973; Langenhuysen et al., 1974; Rocchi et al., 1975); to virus-associated cell membrane antigens (MA) (Johansson et al., 1970); to the early antigen (EA) complex (Henle and Henle, 1973; Hesse et al., 1973; Rocchi et al., 1975); and to the EB nuclear antigen (EBNA) (Rocchi et al., 1975). Elevated levels of EB virus-specific neutralizing antibodies have also been noted (Rocchi, Hewetson, and Henle, 1973). In a series of 44 Brazilian patients with Hodgkin's disease, Carvalho et al. (1973) found antibodies to EB virus in the sera of 43 (97.5 percent), the sole exception being a one-year-old child! Titers of 1:320 or more were found in 18 of these 43 (42 percent), and their geometric mean titer (GMT) was 1:173, as compared with 3.8 percent and a GMT of 1:51 in a group of healthy controls with antibodies to the virus. Analysis of data from Denmark on 185 patients with Hodgkin's disease who were individually matched with healthy controls with respect to age, sex, and social class revealed significantly elevated mean antibody titers to VCA which were most evident among patients with the nodular sclerosis and lymphocyte predominance subtypes of the disease (Hesse et al., 1977).

Similarly elevated titers have not been found for other herpes viruses (Goldman and Aisenberg, 1970; Levine et al., 1971; Henderson et al., 1973)

with the exception of herpes simplex virus, elevated mean antibody titers to which were noted in a Danish case-control study (Hesse et al., 1977), and *herpesvirus hominis* type 2, the incidence of antibody to which was significantly elevated in a series of male patients with Hodgkin's disease (Catalano and Goldman, 1972). Antibody titers to cytomegalovirus (CMV) have been normal in some studies (Henderson et al., 1973) and elevated in others (Langenhuysen et al., 1974; Rocchi et al., 1975). Australia antigen, Au (1), was detected in the sera of 5 (6.3 percent) of 80 patients with Hodgkin's disease, whereas its frequency in the normal U.S. population is only 0.1 percent (Sutnick et al., 1970).

However, EB virus DNA could not be detected by molecular hybridization techniques in the involved spleens of several patients with Hodgkin's disease (Nonoyama et al., 1974), nor have EBV genomes been present, by the EBNA reaction, in any of several cultures of Sternberg-Reed and Hodgkin's giant cells (H.S. Kaplan, W. Henle, and G. Henle, manuscript in preparation). Moreover, serum antibody titers to EB virus-associated antigens were also found to be elevated in a spectrum of other neoplastic and nonneoplastic disorders (see review by Levine, 1974). The obvious improbability of an etiologic role for EB virus in all of these neoplastic states has caused investigators to seek alternative explanations for the abnormal EB virus serology in Hodgkin's disease. Since patients with Hodgkin's disease often exhibit an impairment of cell-mediated immunity (Chapter 6), and susceptibility to herpes virus and CMV infections is known to be increased when cell-mediated immunity is impaired, the hypothesis that impairment of cell-mediated immunity might be the common denominator linking Hodgkin's disease and EB virus serology has seemed attractive. However, careful case-by-case comparisons of humoral vs. cell-mediated immune responses in patients with Hodgkin's disease have failed to provide firm support for this view (Hesse et al., 1973), although the elevated antibody titers to toxoplasma CF antigen observed in another matched-control study (Rocchi et al., 1975) are consistent with such a possibility.

Chapter 3

Pathology

Introduction

The malignant lymphomas comprise a broad spectrum of cell types and histologic patterns, and their accurate diagnosis and classification constitutes one of the more difficult topics in morphologic pathology. At one end of the spectrum, they are difficult to distinguish from benign inflammatory or hyperplastic reactions in lymph nodes; at the other, they may be difficult to differentiate from anaplastic carcinomas; and within the lymphoma category, serious problems of interpretation and classification frequently arise.

Hodgkin's disease undoubtedly stands apart as the most bizarre, the most puzzling, the most diverse of these entities. Although few pathologists today would still argue seriously that Hodgkin's disease is not an entity at all, many would find it difficult, on morphologic grounds alone, to convince themselves that it is indeed a neoplasm rather than an infectious granuloma of unknown etiology or an immunologic aberration associated with secondary lymphoproliferative response. Nonetheless, major advances in our understanding of the histopathology and pathogenesis of Hodgkin's disease have been made during the past three decades, partly as the result of the systematic accumulation and analysis of morphologic evidence and partly, in recent years, through the introduction of more sophisticated investigative methods, such as cell culture, chromosome karyotype analysis, Feulgen microspectrophotometry, the use of tritiated thymidine as a specific label for DNA synthesis, surface marker characterization, electron microscopy, and histochemical procedures. Although these aspects of the subject are still evolving at a rapid pace, an attempt has been made to summarize here the present status of modern developments in the cytology and pathology of Hodgkin's disease, as they appear to a nonpathologist.

Biopsy

An unequivocal diagnosis of Hodgkin's disease can be made only by microscopic examination of one or more tissue specimens. Rarely, such a tissue sample may be obtained initially from such sites as the lung, the liver, the spleen, or the bone marrow. In the vast majority of all cases, however, lymphadenopathy is clinically evident, and removal of one or more of the enlarged lymph nodes provides the tissue sample for the pathologist. It is desirable, whenever possible, to remove entire lymph nodes by excisional biopsy, rather than to resort to wedge biopsy of a portion of an enlarged lymph node.

Biopsy specimens must be processed by conventional permanent fixation, sectioning and staining, rather than as frozen sections. Although metastatic carcinoma in lymph nodes is usually readily detectable in frozen sections, the cytologic characteristics of Sternberg-Reed cells, on which the diagnosis of Hodgkin's disease rests, are not sufficiently well preserved in frozen sections. When mediastinal lymphadenopathy and/or fever of unknown origin cause the diagnosis of Hodgkin's disease to be seriously entertained, and clinically enlarged peripheral lymph nodes suitable for biopsy are not detectable, blind biopsy of the scalene lymph nodes on one or both sides may yield an unequivocal diagnosis (Meyer, 1967).

The sampling problem in the search for a tissue diagnosis should not be underestimated. Slaughter, Economou, and Southwick (1958) mapped the involved and uninvolved nodes in a cervical lymph node dissection and demonstrated convincingly that normal or near-normal nodes were often interspersed among the involved nodes in the surgical specimen. Not infrequently, surgeons may be tempted to remove a small, freely movable superficial lymph node in preference to a more deeply situated, less accessible, often fixed node or mass of nodes. In such instances, failure to find Hodgkin's disease in the node removed for biopsy should not be accepted as a definitive answer by the responsible physician. Instead, an additional lymph node biopsy should be obtained from the same or some other site. Moreover, although very large nodes are usually completely replaced by Hodgkin's disease, small nodes may exhibit virtually normal architecture, except for one or more minute foci of involvement, detection of which might well be missed on single section (Strum and Rappaport, 1970a; Henry, 1971).

Focal involvement in other sites, particularly in the liver and bone marrow, constitutes an even more serious sampling problem. Specimens obtained by needle aspiration from suspect tissues, such as lymph nodes or bone marrow, are particularly unreliable. In the case of the bone marrow, organized tissue specimens obtained with the Jamshidi or other biopsy-type needle may provide diagnostically satisfactory material. However, when such needle biopsies are negative in situations associated with a high clinical index of suspicion, marrow biopsy should be repeated by the open surgical procedure, preferably along the iliac crest.

Some European and South American hematologists and pathologists place great emphasis on the examination of Giemsa-stained imprints and smears of fresh lymph node biopsy material (Lucas, 1955; Pilotti and Rilke, 1972). They argue that in such preparations the finer cytologic details of the lymphoid cell subpopulations are more clearly discernible and differentiable. However, this procedure has not been widely adopted by North American pathologists, primarily owing to their concern about the sampling problems involved and their preference for viewing the topographic relationships of the different cell forms in an organized tissue setting.

Cytologic Features of Hodgkin's Disease

Lymph nodes involved by Hodgkin's disease may exhibit a variety of cell types. On the basis of evidence obtained in recent years, it has become possible with increasing confidence to group these cells into two categories: (1) those cells which are now believed to be the neoplastic cell component, collectively termed "Hodgkin's cells" by Seif and Spriggs (1967), Peckham and Cooper (1969), and others, and (2) those which are believed to represent a reactive, inflammatory, and/or stromal cell component.

The Hodgkin's Cells. The use of this name is justified by Seif and Spriggs (1967) as follows: "As it is cumbersome to speak of Sternberg-Reed cells as if they were different from the mononuclear forms of abnormal reticulum cell with which they are associated, we will call both Hodgkin's cells. This name does not imply that all have specific characteristics by which the disease can be reliably diagnosed. Hodgkin's cells are the large reticulum cells in Hodgkin's disease, with abnormally basophilic nucleoli and a strong tendency to lobe and form butterfly or spectacle shapes and binucleation (Sternberg-Reed cells)."

Morphology. In Giemsa-stained imprints, these cells are described as having an open nuclear chromatin network, large, frequently multiple deep blue-staining nucleoli, and abundant, vacuolated pale blue cytoplasm. An important feature of these cells is their nuclear lobation. Such mononuclear cells are not diagnostic of Hodgkin's disease, since they are known to occur in a number of nonneoplastic inflammatory conditions affecting lymph nodes. Classical Sternberg-Reed cells exhibit the same cytologic staining characteristics, but are binucleate or multinucleate. Hoffmann and Rottino (1950a) described similar morphologic features in unstained Hodgkin's cells examined with phase contrast optics and traced a series of transitional forms of abnormal mononuclear "reticulum cell" precursors of the binucleate Sternberg-Reed cell.

Careful descriptions of the appearance of these cells in fixed hematoxylin- and eosin-stained sections have been presented by Smetana and Cohen (1956), Lukes and Butler (1966), and Rappaport (1966). They are large cells, 15 to 45 μ or more in diameter, with abundant, amphophilic or slightly basophilic cytoplasm, and either multiple or multilobed nuclei (Fig. 3.1). The nuclear membrane is usually intensely stained and not infrequently thickened, and the delicate chromatin network within it typically gives way to a peculiar clear halo-like zone (possibly artifactual) around the nucleolus. The nucleoli are large, sometimes enormous, with smooth margins and a strong affinity for acid dyes, often giving them a striking resemblance to viral inclusion bodies. Mononuclear cells with identical nuclear and nucleolar features are also seen in most sections.

It must be stressed that morphologically similar mononuclear cells are occasionally found in reactive and inflammatory lymphadenopathies, particularly those of viral etiology, and are thus not

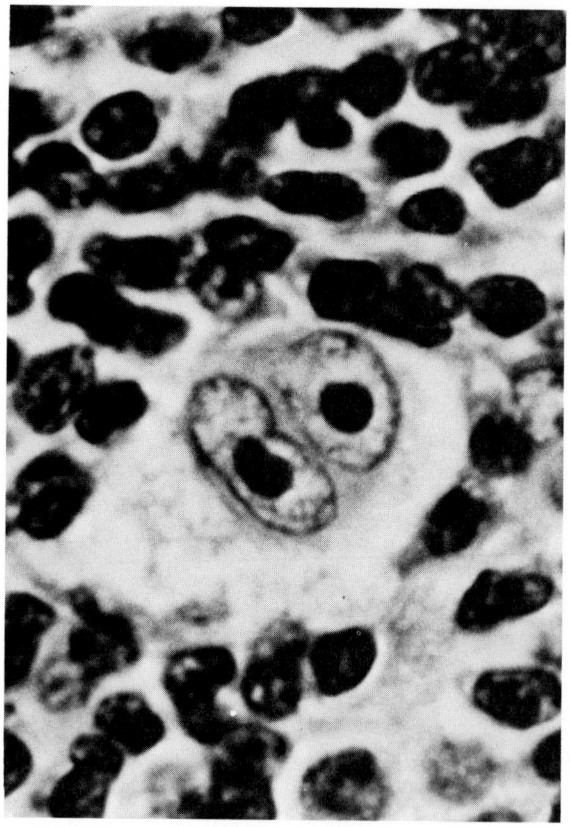

Figure 3.1 Typical large, binucleate Sternberg-Reed cell surrounded by lymphocytes and other stromal cell elements. Note the huge, intensely stained nucleoli, the vacuolated nucleoplasm, the rather coarse nuclear membrane, and the indented, lobated contours of one of the nuclei. Hematoxylin and eosin stain, ×900.

diagnostic of Hodgkin's disease. Accordingly, definitive diagnosis of Hodgkin's disease currently requires the unambiguous identification of one or more Sternberg-Reed cells, the two most distinctive and diagnostically reliable features of which are the huge inclusion-like nucleolus and the multilobate, binucleate or multinucleate nucleus.

However, Lukes et al. (1969) have thrown the subject into turmoil with a brief report stating that they have seen cells indistinguishable from classical Sternberg-Reed cells in lymph node biopsies obtained from patients with infectious mononucleosis. In such instances, however, the surrounding stromal cell population and lymph node architecture are quite different from the appearance ordinarily encountered in Hodgkin's disease. Nonetheless, this report serves a useful purpose in cautioning pathologists that the finding of such a cell per se is not necessarily diagnostic of Hodgkin's disease unless the cell is encountered in an appropriate stroma. Similar observations have been

made by McMahon, Gordon, and Rosen (1970), Agliozzo and Reingold (1971), and Salvador, Harrison, and Kyle (1971). Strum, Park, and Rappaport (1970) reemphasized this point in a report on 13 cases (9 malignant and 4 benign, including 1 of infectious mononucleosis) in which cells closely resembling or indistinguishable from Sternberg-Reed cells were seen. In a later report, Strum (1973) states that such cells can occur not only in infectious mononucleosis but also in a wide range of other conditions, including rubeola, proliferative myositis, thymoma, anticonvulsant-induced lymphadenopathy, epithelial and stromal malignancies such as carcinoma of the lung and breast, myeloproliferative diseases, melanoma, malignant fibroxanthoma, myeloma, mycosis fungoides, Burkitt's lymphoma, and chronic lymphocytic leukemia. Thus, the demonstration of such cells in a tissue section is a necessary but not alone a sufficient condition for the diagnosis of Hodgkin's disease. Criteria for the histopathologic differentiation of infectious mononucleosis from Hodgkin's disease have been detailed by Salvador, Harrison, and Kyle (1971) and by Tindle, Parker, and Lukes (1972).

Special comment is required concerning a variant type of Hodgkin's cell which is typically encountered in the nodular sclerosing type of Hodgkin's disease described by Lukes (1963), Hanson (1964), and Lukes and Butler (1966). This is an unusually large cell, the pale, eosinophilic or clear cytoplasm of which, in formalin-fixed sections, is often retracted, so that the cell appears to rest in a large clear space or lacuna (Fig. 3.2). It has been suggested that cytoplasmic lipid, detected by special staining procedures, may be responsible for the distinctive appearance of these cells (Anagnostou et al., 1977). The nuclei may be mononuclear but have a tendency to be multilobated and to contain nucleoli which, although highly eosinophilic, may be relatively small or variable in size. These bizarre lacunar cells are usually numerous, often clustered in the centers of lymphoid tissue nodules in lymph nodes involved by the nodular sclerosing type of Hodgkin's disease. In contrast, diagnostic Sternberg-Reed cells may be quite sparse and require a careful search.

In the more malignant forms (the Hodgkin's sarcoma and lymphocytic depletion types described below), the Hodgkin's cells are often much more numerous, bizarre, and pleomorphic, with pronounced variations in nuclear size, shape, and staining characteristics. Unless cells that meet the diagnostic criteria for classical Sternberg-Reed

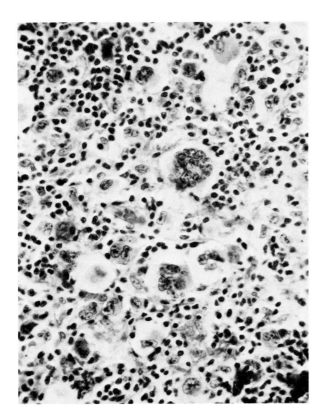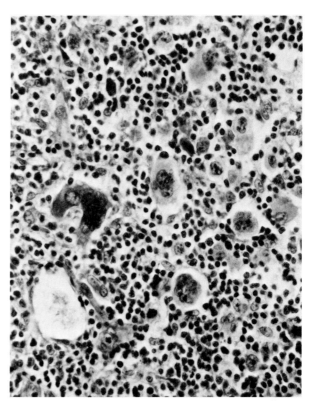

Figure 3.2   Both photomicrographs show "lacunar" Hodgkin's cells characteristically encountered in the nodular sclerosing form of Hodgkin's disease. Note the hyperlobated nuclei and relatively inconspicuous nucleoli. The cytoplasmic retraction which is so prominent in these formalin-fixed preparations, causing the cells to appear to lie in a clear space or lacuna, is in part an artifact of fixation, since it is much less evident in Zenker-fixed sections. (Reprinted, by permission of the authors and the Editor of *Cancer,* from Kadin, Glatstein, and Dorfman, 1971.)

cells can be found, differential diagnosis from diffuse pleomorphic histiocytic lymphomas may not be possible.

Mitotic Figures. Mitotic figures are not ordinarily numerous in Hodgkin's disease, except in some of the more malignant, pleomorphic forms. Since the nucleolus and nuclear membrane disappear during mitosis, the nuclear and nucleolar characteristics on which an unambiguous identification of Sternberg-Reed cells depends are not visible. Nonetheless, when mitoses are seen in extremely large cells with abundant amphophilic cytoplasm, it is generally presumed that they are Sternberg-Reed cells. Thus, it was stated by Dawson, Cooper, and Rambo (1964) that "mitoses were seen in Reed-Sternberg cells in 19 of 21 nodes of Hodgkin's disease."

However, Marmont and Damasio (1967), studying imprints of lymph nodes of patients in whom mitotic arrest had been induced twenty-four hours earlier by treatment with vinblastine, and comparing these with biopsies obtained immediately before treatment, found that most of the arrested mitoses had occurred in large mononuclear cells. They did not observe multipolar or atypical mitoses such as have been observed by others (Rappaport, 1966), nor did they observe mitoses in identifiable Sternberg-Reed cells. Their observations, which were reinforced by the results of tritiated thymidine incorporation studies described below, suggested that the mitotically active component of the Hodgkin's cell population is probably the mononuclear cell form and that the classical binucleate or multinucleate Sternberg-Reed cell is a nonproliferating derivative.

This view, which has been in vogue for several years, has now been refuted by the unambiguous observation of synchronous, apparently aneuploid mitotic figures in both nuclei of binucleate giant cells (Fig. 3.3) in long-term cultures of tissues involved by Hodgkin's disease (Kaplan and Gartner, 1977), indicating that Sternberg-Reed cells are indeed capable of nuclear division, though the rate at which they divide may well be considerably lower than that of mononuclear Hodgkin's cells.

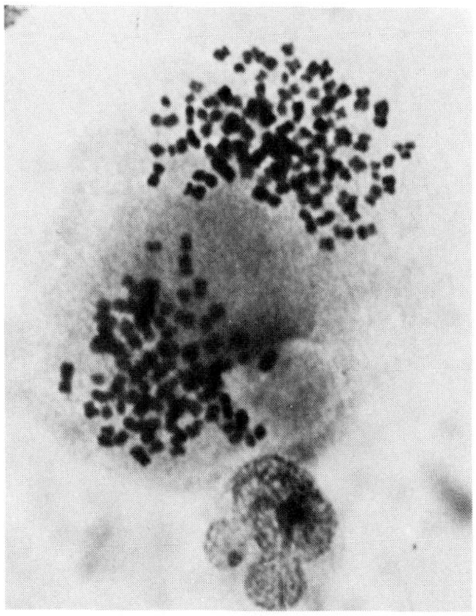

Figure 3.3 Binucleate mitosis in a giant cell from a two-month-old colchicine-treated culture of involved spleen tissue from a patient with stage III$_S$B mixed cellularity Hodgkin's disease. × 850. (Reprinted by permission of the Editor of the *International Journal of Cancer,* from the paper by Kaplan and Gartner, 1977.)

Cell culture studies have also revealed abnormal, multipolar mitoses in mono- and multinucleated cells; in one cell, 45 diplochromosomes were observed, suggesting that Sternberg-Reed cells may arise from mononuclear cells by endoreduplication (Kadin, 1973).

Deoxyribonucleic Acid (DNA) Synthetic Activity. It is now well recognized that the doubling of DNA content, which is a prerequisite for mitosis in all mammalian cells, takes place during a discrete period of DNA synthetic activity, the S period, which occurs during interphase and is separated from the time of actual mitosis, M, by two time intervals, G_1 and G_2, which occur immediately before and immediately after the S period, respectively (Howard and Pelc, 1953). When cells cease to proliferate, either temporarily or permanently, they usually become arrested in G_1 and do not initiate a new round of DNA synthesis.

Thus, evidence that cells are actively synthesizing DNA may be taken as a good indication that they are mitotically active. This approach has other advantages as well. Since the isotopically labeled precursors are incorporated into DNA during interphase, at a time when the nuclear characteristics which permit morphologic identification of the cells are well displayed, it is possible to map and identify individual cells morphologically and then to determine whether they were actively synthesizing DNA. Secondly, since the isotopic labels persist for long periods of time after their incorporation into DNA and since the duration of the S phase is much longer than that of M, it is possible to identify a much larger fraction of the mitotically active population by the labeling technique than by counting cells actually in mitosis at any one point in time.

Peckham and Cooper (1969) prepared cell suspensions from fresh lymph node biopsies of ten patients with Hodgkin's disease. The cell suspensions were incubated at 37C. with tritiated thymidine for thirty minutes, then centrifuged onto slides, fixed, and stained with Giemsa. Representative areas were photographed for morphologic identification and mapping of the cell population. The Giemsa stain was then leached out of some of the preparations, and they were restained by the Feulgen method to permit measurement of DNA content. Autoradiographs were made and the tritiated thymidine-labeled cells identified morphologically by coincidence mapping relative to the original Giemsa-stained preparations.

It was thus possible to demonstrate that cells morphologically identifiable as Hodgkin's cells were consistently labeled with tritiated thymidine, with labeling indices ranging from 8.6 to 34.6 percent in the various specimens studied. No such labeling was observed in a Sternberg-Reed cell, however. Correlation of the number of nucleoli, the Feulgen DNA content, and the frequency of DNA labeling in one case suggested that the labeled cells tended to be those with a single nucleolus and relatively lower DNA content. Accordingly, it was concluded that only a relatively small fraction of Hodgkin's cells are actively proliferating, that the Hodgkin's cells tend to become sterile as they progress to increasing DNA content and aneuploidy, and that the Sternberg-Reed cell is a nonproliferating end stage in this process, perhaps arising from a failure of cytokinesis during mitosis of the mononuclear Hodgkin's cells.

In subsequent reports, however, Peckham and Cooper (1973) and Peckham (1973) were more successful in observing the occurrence of labeling in Sternberg-Reed cells. Although such cells accounted for only 0.7 percent of all labeled cells, as against 29 percent for Hodgkin's cells, their relative abundance in the unlabeled state was about tenfold less than that of Hodgkin's cells, suggesting that the rate at which they enter DNA synthesis may not be very much different from that of their mononuclear variants (Peckham, 1973). Quite convincing illustrations of binucleate giant cells, both nuclei of which were labeled after relatively brief incubation with tritiated thymidine, may be found in the paper by Marinello et al. (1977). Cowley (1978) also observed labeling of some binucleate cells, as well as many more mononuclear Hodgkin cells, in freshly excised lymph nodes injected with tritiated thymidine.

Labeling with tritiated thymidine of all nuclei of binucleate or multinucleate giant cells in long-term cultures from tissues involved by Hodgkin's disease has been unequivocally demonstrated by Kadin and Asbury (1973) and by Kaplan and Gartner (1977). The latter investigators found that binucleate and multinucleate labeled cells constituted 2.2 percent of all labeled cells counted in one of their cases. In a tally of 1,000 cells, 918 were mononuclears, of which 334 (36.5 percent) were labeled, and 82 were binucleate or multinucleate, of which 17 (20.7 percent) were labeled (Fig. 3.4). When labeled cells were incubated overnight with unlabeled cultures, none of the binucleate cells contained a mixture of labeled and unlabeled nuclei, indicating that the binucleate cells arise by nuclear replication rather than by cell fusion. These findings are incompatible with the view that Sternberg-Reed cells are sterile, "end-stage" cells incapable of DNA synthesis.

DNA Content. Under appropriate conditions, the Feulgen reaction is specific for DNA, and the DNA content of individual cells can be measured in stained smears or imprints by Feulgen cytophotometry. If the normal diploid DNA content of human cells is designated 2C, other euploid somatic cells would be expected to exhibit integral multiples of this value (4C, 8C, etc.) for tetraploid, octoploid, and higher ploidy levels. Normal cells may exhibit intermediate values if they are in the process of synthesizing a new round of DNA in preparation for mitosis. Cells with DNA content that is both increased in amount and intermediate between integral higher ploidy levels are usually aneuploid, malignant neoplastic cells.

Petrakis, Bostick, and Siegel (1959) made such measurements on forty-four Sternberg-Reed cells in imprints from the lymph nodes of five patients with Hodgkin's disease. They found that the DNA content of these cells varied widely, from 2C all the way up to 20C. The majority of the cells exhibited diploid or hyperdiploid values, and another large subpopulation were clustered at the hypotetraploid level. Nuclear DNA content per cell tended to increase with increasing nuclear diameter and lobulation and was strikingly increased in the highly multinucleated cells, in which unequal amounts of DNA appeared to be partitioned among the nuclei. These findings have been confirmed and extended by Peckham and Cooper (1969). It is thus clear that aneuploid DNA content, a generally accepted cytologic indicator of

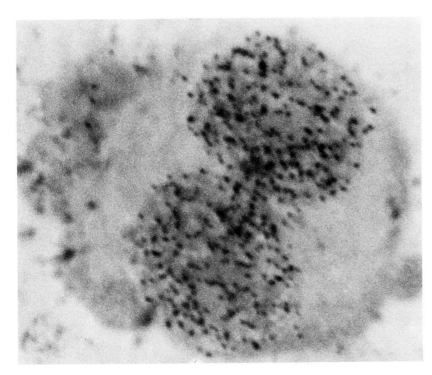

Figure 3.4 Radioautograph after incubation with ³H-thymidine, revealing labeling of both nuclei of a Sternberg-Reed cell in culture. ×2250. (Reprinted by permission of the Editor of the *International Journal of Cancer,* from the paper by Kaplan and Gartner, 1977.)

malignant neoplastic attributes, is frequently observed in Hodgkin's cells, even of the mononuclear type, and is a consistent feature of Sternberg-Reed cells.

Chromosome Number and Morphology. Data concerning chromosome number and morphology in cells obtained from lymph nodes involved by Hodgkin's disease have begun to emerge during the past decade, but our information is still quite limited, in large part because of the great technical difficulty of such cytogenetic studies. Since the mitotic index is usually low, preparations examined promptly after excision often contain too few well-preserved mitotic figures for meaningful analysis. For this reason, investigators have employed the technique of short-term (16- to 72-hour) culture, with or without the addition of phytohemagglutinin. Another serious difficulty is that many of the mitotic figures are small and clearly derived from the lymphoid cells of the reactive stromal population, rather than from the Hodgkin's cells themselves. Thus, failure to find abnormal cells in some studies may merely reflect the sampling problem. Such negative instances cannot be regarded as providing definitive evidence for the normality of chromosome number and/or morphology in Hodgkin's cells.

Data concerning all of the 100 cases of Hodgkin's disease in which chromosome studies were carried out from 1962 through 1978 are summarized in Table 3.1. In 68 of the cases studied to date, two populations of cells in mitosis have been observed, one having a modal chromosome number of 46 and believed to represent normal dividing cells of the lymphoid cell series and the other having pseudodiploid or, more often, distinctly aneuploid chromosome numbers in the hypotetraploid range. In the report by Whitelaw (1969), 31 (16 percent) of 193 scorable mitoses from four cases of Hodgkin's disease were near-tetraploids. It is important to note that aneuploid cells have been observed in three of six cases of paragranuloma or lymphocyte predominance (Table 3.1), as well as in the more aggressive forms of Hodgkin's disease. As is indicated in the table, marker chromosomes have been observed in 40 instances (40 percent of all cases), although no single characteristic type of marker has consistently been noted (Demin et al., 1972). Gastearena et al. (1969) reported a case in which 3 of 20 mitoses contained a giant marker chromosome. Hypodiploid, pseudodiploid, and hypotetraploid cells containing one or two markers have been demonstrated by Castoldi (1973). Miles,

Geller, and O'Neill (1966) described and clearly illustrated one remarkable case in which a near-triploid cell contained two ring chromosomes (Fig. 3.5). The quinacrine fluorescence and Giemsa banding techniques, which permit the detection of subtle structural abnormalities in individually identifiable human chromosomes, have been successfully applied by Fleischmann, Hakanson, and Levan (1971), Reeves (1973), and Fukuhara and Rowley (1978) to the detection of multiple markers in mitotic cells from patients with Hodgkin's disease. Thus, chromosomal studies clearly establish that in many cases of Hodgkin's disease a mitotically active subpopulation of aneuploid, often polyploid cells is present in the lymph nodes and other involved tissues. This evidence alone is strongly indicative of the neoplastic character of the Hodgkin's cells. However, the most compelling evidence is that indicating the clonal derivation of some of the hypotetraploid cells.

It is now generally accepted that perhaps the most fundamental distinction between neoplasia and infection relates to their respective modes of propagation. Infection is usually transmitted *horizontally*, i.e., the infectious agent emerges from affected cells or tissues and spreads through the extracellular fluids, the lymph, and the blood stream to infect other, previously normal cells and tissues. In contrast, the abnormality in neoplastic cells is genetic and is transmitted *vertically* at each mitotic division to the progeny of that division. After several divisions, a clone of neoplastic cells will have been produced which would be expected to exhibit similar or identical abnormalities of chromosome number and morphology.

A most remarkable instance of a clone of aneuploid Hodgkin's cells is that encountered in the seventh of the eight cases studied by Seif and Spriggs (1967). Although most of the metaphases in this case were diploid or near-diploid, 18 of the 63 cells counted had chromosome counts between 77 and 86. Two distinctive, unusually long marker chromosomes were observed (M_1 and M_2); both were present in ten cells, and M_2 alone in an eleventh cell (Figs. 3.6 and 3.7). Detailed karyotype analysis of five of these hypotetraploid cells provided convincing evidence for the comparability of abnormalities within the different subgroups of chromosomes in all five cells, as well as the presence of both markers, thus yielding irrefutable evidence of their clonal derivation.

Similarly, in Case 5 described by Miles et al. (1966), four of five cells with 85 chromosomes were found to have essentially identical karyo-

Table 3.1　Reported Chromosome Studies in Hodgkin's Disease

No.	Ref.[a]	Case	Abnormal mitoses counted[b]				Marker(s) present	Remarks
			~2n	>2n	~3–4n	>4n		
1	1	—			79–90(83)		√	
2	2	—	46[c], 47		92[b]			Prior radiotherapy
3	3	—			79*–83*(83)		√	*Giant marker
4	4	3			70–75			
5	4	4		48, 49				
6	5	—			P[d]		√	
7	6	8		49, 50				
8	6	9	46[e], 47[e], 48[e]					
9	6	10	46[e]	49	69–76			Paragranuloma
10	7	—	43–45, 46[c]	47–51				
11	8	1	46[c], 47		86		√	
12	8	2			~3n			
13	8	3						No aneuploid cells
14	8	4	46		63*–75		√	*2 ring chromosomes
15	8	6			P		√	
16	9	—						Paragranuloma; no aneuploidy
17	10	1			69–70			
18	10	2			71–84(84)			
19	10	3						
20	10	4	46[c]		73, 83			
21	10	5	48					"Unusual variant"
22	10	6	<46, 46					
23	10	7	46		77*–86*(81)		√	*2 giant markers
24	10	8	46[f]		73, 79		√	Paragranuloma
25	11	13						No aneuploid cells
26	11	14	(46)[c]		64–80		√	
27	12	10			~4n			
28	12	11			~4n			
29	12	12			~4n			
30	12	13			~4n			
31	12	14						No aneuploid cells
32	13	—	46[c]				√	Giant marker
33	14	15						LP type; no aneuploidy
34	14	16						LP type; no aneuploidy
35	14	17				115	√	LP type, treated; 2 markers
36	14	18			65*, 75*, 79*, 80*		√	*Same 2 markers
37	14	19			70*, 73*, 74*		√	*Same marker
38	14	20			66*–71*		√	*Same 5 markers
39	14	21		57*	72*		√	*Same marker
40	14	22						Only 1 countable cell (2n)
41	14	23			74*, 76*, 78*–81*		√	*Same 3–4 markers
42	14	24			63*–68*, 73*–81*	152*	√	*Same 2–3 markers
43	14	25						No aneuploid cells
44	14	26						Only 3 countable cells (2n)
45	14	27		51*–54*	65*–72*, 89*–100*		√	*Same and other markers

(*Continued*)

Table 3.1 (*Continued*)

No.	Ref.	Case	Abnormal mitoses counted				Marker(s) present	Remarks
			~2n	>2n	~3–4n	>4n		
46	14	28						Only 2 countable cells (2n)
47	15	—					√	*Clone of 10 cells with same 3 markers
48	16	—	46^c		63*–69*	138*, 140*	√	*One or both of 2 markers
49	17	1	44*,45*,47*	P*			√	*Same giant marker
50	17	2	47*–49*	57*	P*	94*	√	*Same markers
51	17	3	47*, 48*	51*	P*		√	*Same giant marker
52	17	4						No aneuploid cells
53	17	5			P			
54	17	6		55	P			
55	17	7	42*–48*		P*		√	3 aneuploid clones
56	17	8						No aneuploid cells
57	17	9			P			
58	17	10						No aneuploid cells
59	17	11						No aneuploid cells
60	17	12			P			
61	17	13			P			
62	18	1	46^c		74*–83*	160*	√	Multiple markers; see text
63	18	2			85*–90*	102*	√	*Same and other markers; treated
64	18	3			61*–80*		√	*Same and other markers; treated
65	19	1						No aneuploid cells
66	19	2						No aneuploid cells; treated
67	19	3						No aneuploid cells; treated
68	19	4						No aneuploid cells; treated
69	19	5		√*			√	*2 markers; 55% >2n
70	19	6			√			4% < 4n
71	19	7			√*		√	*Same marker; 40% < 3n
72	19	8			√			30% < 3n
73	19	9			√*		√	*2 markers; 30% < 3n
74	19	10				√		10% > 4n
75	19	11				125*, 127*	√	*Same markers, 38% > 5n
76	19	12				102*	√	*Same 4 markers; 46% > 4n
77	19	13				√		4% > 4n
78	19	14			√		√	30% < 4n
79	19	15				√		20% > 4n
80	19	16			√*		√	*50% ~ 3n
81	19	17			√			35% > 3n
82	20	1		√*	√*	√*	√	*Same 2 markers; 14% aneuploid

(*Continued*)

Table 3.1   (*Continued*)

No.	Ref.	Case	~2n	>2n	~3–4n	>4n	Marker(s) present	Remarks
					Abnormal mitoses counted			
83	20	2		√*		√*	√	*Multiple (up to 17) markers
84	21	1						No aneuploid cells
85	21	2						No aneuploid cells
86	21	3	46^c				√	
87	21	4						No aneuploid cells
88	21	5		(52*), 53*		102*	√	*Same 4 markers
89	21	6						No aneuploid cells
90	22	1						No aneuploid cells
91	22	2		(48)				
92	23	1	(45)		90		√	
93	23	2		(48)	88–96	160	√	
94	23	3		(48)		94–98, 130, 170	√	
95	23	4	(46)			93	√	
96	23	5	(46)	56	70–85, 89–93	121–130	√	
97	23	6		<58–66		117–118, 171, 214	√	
98	24	25		(56)			?	
99	24	26	(48)				√	
100	24	27		(66)			√	

a References: 1, Spriggs and Boddington, 1962; 2, Ricci et al., 1962; 3, Galan et al., 1963; 4, Baker and Atkin, 1965; 5, Forteza Bover et al., 1965; 6, Spiers and Baikie, 1966; 7, Sinks and Clein, 1966; 8, Miles et al., 1966; 9, Messinetti et al., 1966; 10, Seif and Spriggs, 1967; 11, Millard, 1968; 12, Whitelaw, 1969; 13, Gastearena et al., 1969; 14, Coutinho et al., 1971; 15, Fleischmann et al., 1971; 16, Olinici, 1972; 17, Demin et al., 1972; 18, Reeves, 1973; 19, Fleischmann et al., 1974; 20, Boecker et al., 1975; 21, Fleischmann and Krizsa, 1976; 22, Abe et al., 1976; 23, Hossfeld and Schmidt, 1978; 24, Fukuhara and Rowley, 1978.

b Modal peaks are noted in parentheses.

c Pseudodiploid or pseudotetraploid.

d Polyploid.

e Deletion of short arm of a 17–18.

f Possible deletion of long arm of a 17–18.

types, including a common marker chromosome. Almost all of the near-tetraploid cells had one or two chromosomes about the size of the 6-12 chromosome group, but with an extremely short short-arm. Moreover, almost all the cells with more than 87 chromosomes had 12 long acrocentrics, and all cells with 85 to 87 chromosomes had 11 long acrocentrics. Thus, it was suggested that all of the aneuploid cells could have arisen from a common progenitor, but that chromosome abnormalities were still in the process of occurring. Another apparent clone manifested by similar homologous abnormalities is that observed in case 2 of Seif and Spriggs (1967).

Clonal distributions of marker chromosomes were also evident in many of the cases more recently reported by Fleischmann, Hakanson, and Levan (1971), Coutinho et al. (1971), Demin et al. (1972), Olinici (1972), Reeves (1973), Fleischman et al. (1974), Fleischmann and Krizsa (1976), and Hossfeld and Schmidt (1978). In the first of the three cases of Hodgkin's disease studied by Reeves (1973), using the Giemsa banding technique, the majority of cells studied were hypotetraploid, with a mode at 81 chromosomes. Six cells were fully and two partially karyotyped. Structural abnormalities common to all of eight cells were a chromosome 14 with extra chromatin on the long (q) arm (14q+) and two small metacentrics, the larger of which was thought to be an isochromosome for the long arms of #18. In addition, deletions of the long arms of a chromosome #6 (6q−) were seen in four of these cells. Other abnormalities included a translocation of much of chromosome #15 onto the long arms of a chromosome 9 and deletion of the short arms of the chromosome 16 (16q−). One cell contained three 9q− chromosomes. Marker chromosomes were also seen in the other two cases studied by Reeves. Case 2 yielded five aneuploid cells, with chromosome numbers of 85, 86, 89, 90, and 102,

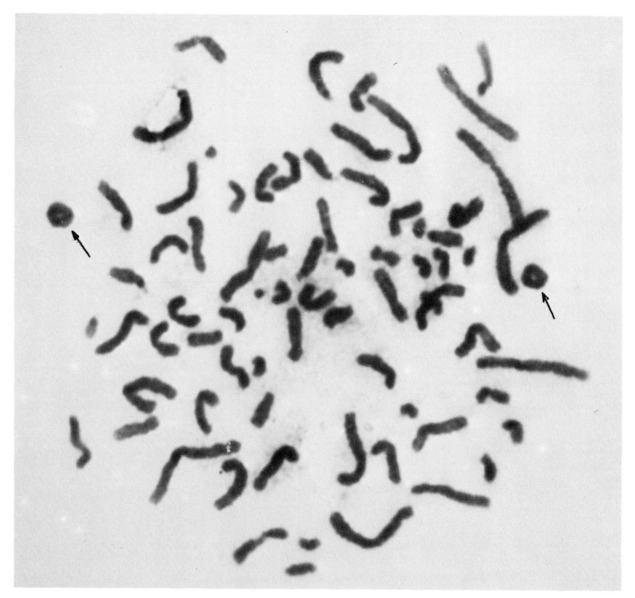

Figure 3.5   Remarkable aneuploid, near-triploid metaphase cell containing two ring chromosomes (arrows) in a direct preparation from freshly biopsied lymph node material in a 29-year-old male with Hodgkin's disease involving the left cervical region. (Reprinted, by permission of the authors and the Editor of *Cancer,* from Miles, Geller, and O'Neill, 1966.)

all of which contained a small ring chromosome, as well as various other markers. In his third case, 18 of 21 mitoses were aneuploid, with chromosome numbers in the range 61–80, all containing extensive karyotypic rearrangements. Karyotypes revealed 6q− deletions in all of the four cells suitable for detailed analysis, as well as a number of other abnormalities. Using the quinacrine fluorescence technique, Fleischmann, Hakanson, and Levan (1971) found three medium-sized markers in each of ten cells studied, two similar in size to a chromo-some #13 and the third similar to a #16. Eight of the ten cells also contained a long telocentric marker, similar in size to a normal #3. Other markers were also observed in three of the ten cells. Fukuhara and Rowley (1978) found the #14q+ marker in all of the karyotypes examined from two of their three patients with Hodgkin's disease. Thus, an impressive number of cytogenetic studies now attest to the fact that Hodgkin's cells are often aneuploid and that in several instances such aneuploid cells are clonally related.

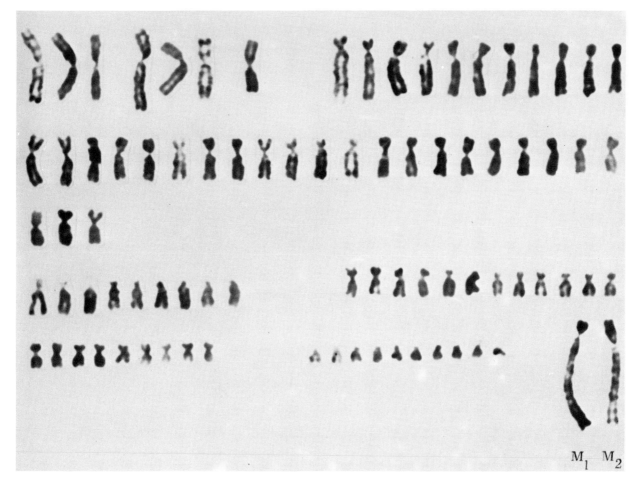

M₁ M₂

Figure 3.6 Karyotype of a cell with 84 chromosomes in a direct preparation from freshly biopsied lymph node material in a 23-year-old male with "sclerocellular" (nodular sclerosing?) Hodgkin's disease (case 7 of Seif and Spriggs, 1967). Note the presence of two distinct marker chromosomes, each longer than chromosome no. 1; the longer of these (M_1) has a nearly terminal centromere, whereas M_2 is submetacentric. (Reprinted from Seif and Spriggs, 1967, by permission of the authors and the *Journal of the National Cancer Institute*.)

Collectively, these observations constitute compelling evidence for the neoplastic nature of Hodgkin's cells and thus of Hodgkin's disease.

Cytochemical Features. There is a remarkable paucity of published information on the cytochemical properties of Sternberg-Reed and other Hodgkin's cells. Certain discrepancies in the literature are no doubt due to the introduction of newer and more specific or more reliable techniques. Thus, whereas Ackerman et al. (1951) reported acid phosphatase activity to be increased in Sternberg-Reed cells in their fixed lymph node biopsy sections, Dorfman (1961, 1964), using newer cryostatic methods, found that Hodgkin's cells, including the Sternberg-Reed cells, were consistently negative for both nonspecific esterase and acid phosphatase.

Since both of these enzymes were regularly present in normal histiocytes, and since the loss of two different enzymes by cells undergoing transition from the normal histiocyte to the Hodgkin's cell seemed highly improbable, he suggested that the Hodgkin's cells may be derived from some other type of cell of primitive mesenchymal origin. Unfortunately, there is still a lack of unanimity on this subject. Yam and Li (1976), Nanba, Itagaki, and Iijima (1975), and Anagnostou et al. (1977) reported that acid phosphatase and nonspecific esterase activity was negative or only very weakly positive in Hodgkin's giant cells, whereas Press and Shvetsova (1975) described distinct, rather granular activity of both enzymes in Hodgkin's giant cells of all types, and Stuart, Williams, and Habeshaw (1977) noted weak nonspecific esterase activity in some of

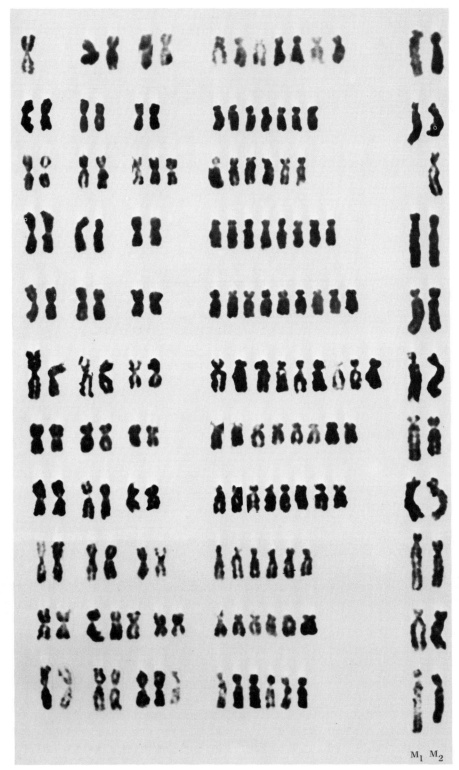

Figure 3.7   Group A and B chromosomes and markers of 11 metaphases in the 16- and 72-hour culture preparations from case 7 of Seif and Spriggs (1967). Ten cells have both the M_1 and M_2 markers; the eleventh has only M_2. (Reprinted by permission of the authors and the *Journal of the National Cancer Institute.*)

M_1 M_2

these cells. Yam and Li (1976), Stuart, Williams, and Habeshaw (1977), and Anagnostou et al. (1977) found such cells to be entirely negative for alkaline phosphatase and peroxidase, and Taylor (1976) was unable to detect the presence of mura-

midase (lysozyme). Dorfman (1964) found both succinic and lactic dehydrogenase activity to be present in Sternberg-Reed cells. Hayhoe et al. (1978) studied a rare case of Sternberg-Reed cell leukemia and observed positive, granular acid phosphatase activity in the giant cells in the peripheral blood. Alkaline phosphatase, peroxidase, Sudan black B, and nonspecific esterase stains were negative.

A high concentration of cytoplasmic RNA is reportedly demonstrable in Hodgkin's and Sternberg-Reed cells stained by the Schiff–methylene blue method (Garvin et al., 1974) or pyronin Y (Rubio and Sorensen, 1972; Anagnostou et al., 1977). Mundkur and his co-workers (1968, 1969) have noted that the azo dyes amido black 10B and palatinechtschwarz selectively bind to and stain the nucleoli of Sternberg-Reed cells. The presence of an abundance of lipid in the cytoplasm of lacunar cells of nodular sclerosing Hodgkin's disease was documented by Anagnostou et al. (1977), who suggested that this feature might explain the characteristic "lacunar" appearance of these cells in formalin-fixed sections. Kass and Schnitzer (1972) observed that the use of an ammoniacal silver stain facilitated the identification of Sternberg-Reed cells in lymph node tissue sections. They appeared as large multinucleated cells with orange-brown nucleoli and bright yellow cytoplasm containing brown-staining granules. The vesicular nuclei were yellow-stained, with brown filamentous strands traversing them. Since the ammoniacal silver stain is said to differentiate between lysine-rich and arginine-rich histones on the basis of color reaction, with lysine-rich histone staining yellow and arginine-rich histone staining brown to black, the observations of Kass and Schnitzer suggest that Sternberg-Reed cells may contain an abundance of lysine-rich histone.

In a most remarkable case of a 78-year-old female patient with a diagnosis of Hodgkin's disease, Sinks and Clein (1966) studied cells interpreted as Sternberg-Reed cells which became apparent in the peripheral blood two months before death. These cells exhibited a mitotic rate of 0.6 percent, and 15 percent of them incorporated tritiated thymidine; by 48 hours after incubation with phytohemagglutinin, the proportion labeled had increased to 42 percent and the mitotic rate to 5 percent. If the responding cells were indeed Sternberg-Reed cells, their capacity to respond to phytohemagglutinin would strongly suggest their derivation from, and residual functional link to, immunocompetent lymphoid cells. Cytochemically, these peripheral blood cells were characterized as yielding negative periodic acid Schiff (PAS), Sudan black B, peroxidase, and acid phosphatase staining reactions; they were moderately reactive for succinic, lactic, and alpha-glycerophosphate dehydrogenases. How-

ever, some pathologists have suggested that the correct diagnosis in this case may well have been histiocytic or undifferentiated lymphoma rather than Hodgkin's disease.

Electron Microscopic Morphology. The ultrastructural morphology of Sternberg-Reed and other Hodgkin's cells has been studied by André et al. (1955), Frajola et al. (1958), Bernhard and Leplus (1964), Forteza Bover et al. (1968), Mori and Lennert (1969), Dorfman et al. (1973), Carr (1975), Glick et al. (1976), Anagnostou et al. (1977), and Hayhoe et al. (1978). Collectively, their descriptions refer to large cells, 15μ or more in diameter, with irregular cytoplasmic outlines and occasionally prominent prolongations and processes. They may have a single nucleus; apparently binucleated cells may be genuinely binucleate in serial section, or they may exhibit slender bridges of nuclear material, indicating that they are actually bilobate. Carr (1975) stated that mitotic figures are found not infrequently in such cells and illustrated an electron micrograph of a mitotic figure in a neoplastic cell from a case of mixed cellularity Hodgkin's disease. Parmley, Spicer, and Garvin (1976) also observed abnormal mitoses in the neoplastic cells of Hodgkin's disease and detected a multilaminar alteration of the endoplasmic reticulum in all such mitotic cells. When multinucleated, their nuclei tend to be more bizarre and irregularly shaped, and their cytoplasm more abundant. The occurrence of a continuous series of transitional forms from the mononuclear to the bi- and multinucleate, all with essentially similar abnormal traits, was emphasized by Frajola, Greider, and Bouroncle (1958).

Within the nucleus, one to three extremely large, electron-dense nucleoli are typically seen, surrounded by nucleoplasm of relatively low and occasionally irregular electron density. The cytoplasmic organelles are less distinctive and may be sparse. Carr (1975) has called attention to the presence of elaborate long fingerlike cytoplasmic processes on the surface of many of the neoplastic cells. Such processes may measure $1–2$ μ in length by 100 nm in diameter, and many contain groups of microfibrils 6 nm in diameter. Carr also noted the presence of small numbers of lysosomes, some having a homogeneously electron-dense interior like that seen in macrophage lysosomes. Microfibrils are numerous in the cytoplasm, especially near the nucleus. The mitochondria, $0.3–0.5$ μ in greatest diameter, are round, ovoid, or elongated and variable in number. The endoplasmic reticulum is predominantly of the smooth type, widely dispersed, and sometimes scanty. Electron-dense lysosomes may be present. Free ribosomes may be uniformly distributed, but some cells exhibit prominent focal collections of polyribosomes. Occasional cells exhibit fine intracytoplasmic filaments in close association with the nucleus, similar to those seen in reticulum cells and monocytes. In the atypical "lacunar" cells of the nodular sclerosing form of Hodgkin's disease, nuclear folding and indentations are more apparent, and multiple nuclei are commonly seen. Such cells may contain swollen mitochondria, numerous cytoplasmic vacuoles, and occasionally prominent Golgi apparatus (Dorfman et al., 1973; Glick et al., 1976; Anagnostou et al., 1977). Small dense granules of unknown origin may be present.

The limitations of purely morphologic methods in the identification of cells of the lymphoid system are well known. It is thus not surprising that pathologists examining electron micrographs of Sternberg-Reed and Hodgkin's giant cells have arrived at widely divergent interpretations of their probable origin. Dorfman et al. (1973) were impressed by the fact that the nuclei of many mononuclear and hyperlobated Hodgkin's cells resembled those of transformed lymphocytes. Glick et al. (1976) concluded that "the ultrastructural similarities between Reed-Sternberg cells and transformed lymphocytes are striking and appear to be indicative of the origin of Reed-Sternberg cells from lymphocytes." This view has also been accepted by Anagnostou et al. (1977). However, Carr (1975) placed greater emphasis on the elaborate cytoplasmic processes, the presence of actin-like cytoplasmic microfibrils, and the presence of moderate numbers of small lysosomes, some closely resembling those present in macrophages, and concluded that "the ultrastructure of the malignant reticulum cell is such as to make it likely that it is of macrophage lineage." As is detailed in the following sections, evidence derived from more dynamic methods of investigation, such as surface marker and cell culture studies, now strongly point to the macrophage, or closely related cells of the mononuclear phagocyte system, as the cell of origin of Sternberg-Reed and Hodgkin's giant cells.

Archibald and Frenster (1973) and Carr (1975) have called attention to the frequency with which lymphocytes are seen completely surrounding Sternberg-Reed cells, and with their cytoplasm in tight apposition to that of the Sternberg-Reed cells in transmission electron micrographs. This observation has now been confirmed by scanning electron microscopy, and the interacting lymphocytes have been shown, by virtue of their capacity for spontaneous rosette formation, to be T-lymphocytes (Braylan, Jaffe, and Berard, 1974; Schnitzer and Mead, 1975; Stuart, Williams, and Habeshaw, 1977). Archibald and Frenster (1973) noted an apparent correlation between the frequency of tight lymphocyte apposition and the presence of cytotoxic changes in neoplastic cells, suggesting that the lymphocytes might be involved in an immunologic attack on these cells. Kay (1976) has described combined phase microscopy and scanning electron microscopy studies of cells teased from involved lymph nodes of patients with Hodgkin's disease in which it was again possible to identify the lymphocytes attacking Sternberg-Reed cells as T-lymphocytes. In short-term culture, contact and attachment of multiple T-lymphocytes to Sternberg-Reed cells were observed, followed by progressive tearing open of gaps in the Sternberg-Reed cell membranes, loss of lamellae, and ultimate disintegration of the membranes with swelling of the cells. He concluded that "killer" T-cells are capable of cytolysis of autologous neoplastic Sternberg-Reed cells. In a subsequent study, Kay and Kadin (1975) concluded that the surface morphology of Sternberg-Reed cells, as seen by scanning electron microscopy, is characteristic of that of normal peritoneal macrophages, suggesting that the Sternberg-Reed cells are of histiocyte-macrophage origin. Curran and Jones (1977) have suggested, in a brief note, that they may be derived from the dendritic histiocyte.

The nuclear body is a distinctive structure which occurs normally in the interphase nucleus of several cell types. In normal human lymph node reticulum cells, Brooks and Siegel (1967) described them as approximately 0.6 μ in diameter, round or elliptical in shape, and containing central electron-dense granules 300–400 Å in diameter embedded in a fine fibrillar matrix. In contrast, those within reticulum cells from lymph nodes involved by Hodgkin's disease were abnormal, frequently multiple, and often fused together. Nuclear bodies were not observed in typical Sternberg-Reed cells.

Surface Markers. It is now well established that each of the major subpopulations of cells of the lymphoid and hematopoietic systems possesses a characteristic and distinctive set of receptors on its cell membrane (cf. reviews of Seligmann, Preud'Homme, and Brouet, 1973; Siegal and Good, 1977). Thymus-derived (T) lymphocytes, which are centrally involved in cell-mediated immune responses, bear receptors for and spontaneously form "rosettes" with sheep erythrocytes (E-rosettes) (Jondal, Holm, and Wigzell, 1972; Fröland, 1972), as well as for C-reactive protein (Mortensen, Osmand, and Gewurz, 1975), and for the mitogenic plant lectins phytohemagglutinin (PHA) and concanavalin A (Con A), to which they respond in vitro with a complex series of biochemical changes culminating in mitosis (the lymphoblastoid response). Bone marrow-derived (B) lymphocytes may exhibit several surface markers. Most often, they are recognized by their capacity to synthesize immunoglobulin (usually IgM), which is demonstrable both in the cytoplasm (CIg) and on the cell surface (SIg) by immunofluorescence staining techniques (Rabellino et al., 1971). Individual B-lymphocytes may bear more than one type of immunoglobulin heavy chain, but are restricted to a single type of light chain (Gearhart, Sigal, and Klinman, 1975). Thus, the detection of both kappa and lambda light chains in lymphocyte populations is indicative of their polyclonal nature, whereas the presence of only one class of light chain in certain lymphoid neoplasms constitutes strong evidence of their monoclonal B-lymphocytic derivation (Levy et al., 1977). B-lymphocytes may also bear receptors for the Fc fragment of IgG, enabling them to bind aggregated IgG (Dickler and Kunkel, 1972) and to form IgG-EA rosettes with sheep erythrocytes coated with IgG antibody (Jaffe et al., 1975). Finally, they may possess two distinctively different receptors for complement, detected by the formation of IgM-EAC rosettes with sheep erythrocytes coated with IgM antibody and the C_{3b} or C_{3d} component, respectively, of complement (Eden, Miller, and Nussenzweig, 1973; Okada and Nishioka, 1973; Ross et al., 1973). The C_{3b} complement receptor appears to lie in close proximity to a B-lymphocyte receptor for attachment of and infection by the EB virus (Jondal and Klein, 1973; Jondal et al., 1976). Although B-lymphocytes are not stimulated by PHA and Con A, they are capable of responding to other mitogens, notably pokeweed mitogen (PWM) and lipopolysaccharide (LPS) (Miller, Gartner, and Kaplan, 1978).

Monocytes and macrophages do not synthesize immunoglobulin, and reportedly lack the C_{3d} complement receptor (Griffin, Bianco, and Silverstein, 1975). Instead, they bear independent Fc and complement (C_{3b}) receptors, and thus form both IgG-EA and IgM-EAC rosettes (Huber et al., 1968; Griffin, Bianco, and Silverstein, 1975; Reynolds et al., 1975). Unlike lymphocytes, macrophages also ingest many of the sheep erythrocytes bound to their surfaces during rosette tests. Two other distinctive characteristics of monocytes and macrophages are their capacity to synthesize and secrete lysozyme (muramidase; Cohn and Wiener, 1963; Osserman and Lawlor, 1966), and, at least in the guinea pig, to exhibit rosette-like interactions with T-lymphocytes (Lipsky and Rosenthal, 1973). It is of interest that such "lymphocyte rosettes" have been demonstrated on Sternberg-Reed cells in Hodgkin's disease (Fig. 3.8) (Pretlow, 1978).

Several lines of evidence have given rise to the hypothesis that Sternberg-Reed and Hodgkin's cells may be derived from transformed lymphocytes. Their ultrastructural resemblance to transformed lymphocytes led Dorfman et al. (1973) to put forth this suggestion, which gained support from the observation in infectious mononucleosis of transformed lymphocytes morphologically indistinguishable from Sternberg-Reed cells (Tindle, Parker, and Lukes, 1972; Lukes and Collins, 1974). Similar conclusions had also been reached by Order and Hellman (1972) and by De Vita (1973) during the formulation of hypotheses concerning the pathogenesis of Hodgkin's disease. It was therefore of interest to ascertain whether the surface markers of Sternberg-Reed and Hodgkin's cells were indeed lymphocytic in nature.

The available information on the surface marker characteristics of Sternberg-Reed and Hodgkin's cells is still limited and inconsistent. Several investigators have observed positive staining reactions for SIg and CIg in such cells in suspensions prepared from involved lymph nodes and spleens (Leech, 1973; Payne et al., 1976), as well as in diffusion chamber cultures (Boecker et al., 1975), suggesting that these giant cells may be transformed B-lymphocytes. Kadin et al. (1974) noted positive surface fluorescence with antisera to chronic lymphatic leukemia cells, which are known to be derived from B-lymphocytes, whereas antithymocyte sera yielded no reaction. Conversely, positive immunofluorescence staining reactions for IgG were observed in normal macrophages and reticulum cells but not in Sternberg-Reed cells, in cell suspensions from three involved lymph nodes and from a cytologically positive pleural effusion studied by Biniaminov and Ramot (1974). Stuart, Williams, and Habeshaw (1977) also failed to detect SIg on these cells by immunofluorescence. Shevach et al. (1973) detected IgG-EA rosette formation (a monocyte-macrophage trait) by Sternberg-Reed cells in frozen tissue sections from three patients with Hodgkin's disease. Sternberg-Reed cells from the peripheral blood, in a patient with a preter-

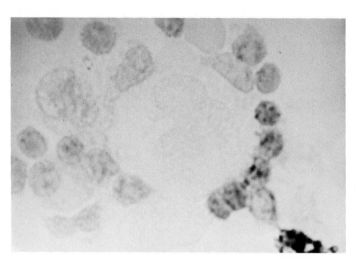 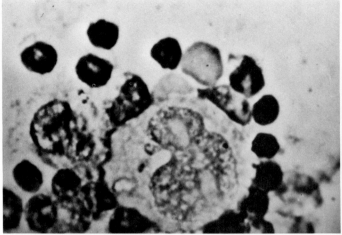

A **Figure 3.8** *A*, bright field photomicrograph of typical "lymphocyte rosette" purified from a cell suspension of in- *B*
volved tissue from a patient with Hodgkin's disease. The small lymphocytes rosetted around the large Sternberg-
Reed cell contain a brown precipitate from the immunoperoxidase procedure. There is an adjacent mononuclear
Hodgkin's cell. The cells are counterstained with methyl green. *B*, photomicrograph of the same cells viewed with
phase contrast. ×600. (Reprinted by permission of the author from the paper by Pretlow, 1978.)

minal leukemic phase studied by Hayhoe et al.
(1978), were SIg-positive, and 17 percent formed
IgG-EA rosettes; no E-, IgM-EA, IgM-EAC (complement), or M-rosette formation was observed.

Garvin et al. (1974) used an immunohistochemical technique to detect CIg in fixed sections of the
involved spleen and lymph nodes of a patient with
Hodgkin's disease. They observed intense staining
for IgG, but none for IgM, in cells interpreted in
serial hematoxylin-eosin or Schiff–methylene
blue-stained comparison sections as Hodgkin's and
Sternberg-Reed cells. They concluded that "their
content of IgG supports a lymphoid origin, presumably of the B-cell variety" for these cells.
However, Ioachim, Schmidt, and Keller (1976) detected the presence of IgM, rather than IgG, on
the surface of Sternberg-Reed cells by the immunoperoxidase technique. Taylor (1976) applied the
immunoperoxidase technique to the study of 45
cases of Hodgkin's disease, using antibodies specific for kappa and lambda light chains of immunoglobulin. In 18 of 30 cases of the nodular sclerosis subtype, 7 of 9 of the mixed cellularity type, and
1 of 5 of the lymphocyte depletion type, he observed both kappa and lambda light chains in individual Sternberg-Reed and mononuclear Hodgkin's cells. Kappa chain alone was detected in 4
cases of nodular sclerosis and 2 of mixed cellularity, whereas lambda alone was seen in 3 cases of
nodular sclerosis. No immunoglobulin light chains
were detectable in any of 4 cases of the lymphocyte
predominance type, 4 of 5 cases of lymphocyte de-

pletion type, and 5 of 30 cases of nodular sclerosis.
Similar observations with respect to the lacunar
cells of nodular sclerosing Hodgkin's disease were
made by Anagnostou et al. (1977). Schmitt et al.
(1977), using the immunoperoxidase method,
tested a F(ab)-peroxidase human anti-Ig conjugate
as well as specific antisera to differentiation antigens present on the surfaces of B-lymphocytes and
T-lymphocytes in an electron microscopic investigation of material from a Hodgkin's disease lymph
node. Sternberg-Reed cells were easily identified
on electron microscopy and revealed no SIg, CIg,
or lymphocyte differentiation antigens. Thus,
whereas Garvin et al.; Ioachim, Schmidt, and
Keller; and Taylor had all interpreted their observations as indicative of the B-lymphocyte origin of
Sternberg-Reed cells, Schmitt et al. concluded that
these cells are not derived from lymphocytes. Landaas, Godal, and Halvorsen (1977) observed positive immunoperoxidase stains for IgG in 15 of 42
formalin-fixed lymph node biopsies from patients
with Hodgkin's disease of different types. From
the finding that 13 of these 15 contained both
kappa and lambda light chains, they inferred that
the immunoglobulin in these cells was not a monoclonal biosynthetic product.

The validity of interpretations based on immunofluorescence and immunohistochemical approaches depends, of course, on several considerations. The accurate identification of Hodgkin's and Sternberg-Reed cells and their differentiation from histiocytes and "immunoblasts" (anti-

gen-transformed lymphocytes) in cell suspensions and smears may be quite difficult. The use of antibody to whole, unfractionated human immunoglobulin rather than to purified human IgM by some of these investigators may have yielded false-positive reactions for IgG due to binding of antigen-antibody complexes or aggregates at Fc receptor sites (Winchester et al., 1975). Such receptors are present not only on B-lymphocytes but also on monocytes and macrophages. The immunohistochemical method used on fixed sections by Garvin et al. (1974), though clearly valid for the intracellular detection of IgG, is a static rather than a dynamic technique, and thus does not distinguish between the intracellular synthesis of IgG, as would be expected of a lymphocyte-derived cell, and the internalization of IgG from the extracellular environment by monocytes or macrophages. The same limitation applies to the immunoperoxidase studies of kappa and lambda light chains by Taylor (1976) and by Anagnostou et al. (1977).

This question has now been decisively resolved by Kadin et al. (1978). These investigators first examined suspensions of viable Hodgkin's and Sternberg-Reed cells from 12 patients with Hodgkin's disease, using immunofluorescent reagents for surface and intracellular gamma, alpha, and mu heavy chains and kappa and lambda light chains. The Sternberg-Reed and Hodgkin's cells revealed IgG, kappa, and lambda, but no IgM or IgA on their surfaces. Although IgG was detected in all 12 cases, it was present in only 30 to 50 percent of the

giant cells. When living cells were first stained and examined for SIg, then washed, fixed in acetone, and restained for CIg, it was found that many of the Hodgkin's giant cells showed intracellular immunoglobulin in the absence of SIg. Whenever SIg was detected, however, CIg of the same type was also present within the same cell. Both kappa and lambda light chains were found within Sternberg-Reed and Hodgkin's cells in each of the twelve cases examined. When individual giant cells were examined by double-label immunofluorescence, it was found that every Hodgkin's cell that contained CIg contained *both* kappa and lambda light chains (Fig. 3.9). Kadin et al. then incubated the Hodgkin's cells at 37C in medium containing fluorescein-conjugated aggregated human IgG. Control observations were made on similarly incubated normal peripheral blood mononuclear cells. At the end of one hour, aggregates were bound and internalized by nearly all normal monocytes. Although Sternberg-Reed and Hodgkin's cells had a lesser affinity than monocytes for IgG aggregates, after two hours there was evidence of both cell surface binding and ingestion of fluorescent aggregates by them. It was concluded that the immunoglobulin found in Sternberg-Reed and Hodgkin's cells is not synthesized by these cells; instead, it is ingested by them following its attachment to the cell membrane.

The observations of Kadin et al. (1978) on cellular material freshly obtained from the involved tissues of patients with Hodgkin's disease are conso-

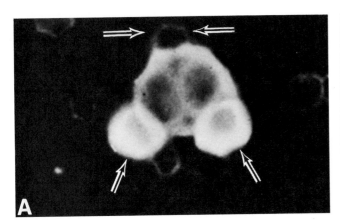
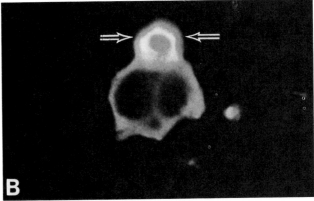

Figure 3.9 Composite ultraviolet photomicrograph showing double-label immunofluorescent cytoplasmic staining of Hodgkin's disease cells, using F(ab')₂ fragments of antibodies to lambda and kappa conjugated with fluorescein (*A*) and tetramethylrhodamine (*B*), respectively. There is polyclonal staining (for both kappa and lambda light chains) of a binucleate Sternberg-Reed cell, surrounded by three plasma cells, two of which (lower arrows, *A*) stain monoclonally for lambda whereas the third (arrows, *B*) stains monoclonally for kappa. Fainter monoclonal staining of adjacent lymphocytes can also be seen. (Reprinted by permission of the authors and the *New England Journal of Medicine,* from the paper by Kadin et al., 1978.)

nant with the results of recent studies on Hodgkin's and Sternberg-Reed cells in long-term culture in vitro. Kaplan and Gartner (1977) found that essentially all of the cultured giant cells possessed both Fc and complement (C_{3b}) receptors, as detected by the formation of IgG-EA and IgM-EAC_{3b} rosettes, and showed no fluorescent staining reaction for surface IgM with human IgM-specific antibody. About 30 percent of the acetone-fixed cells in one case stained positively for intracellular IgG, whereas intracellular IgM was not detected. Of particular relevance to the distinction between lymphocytes and macrophages was the fact that the giant cells were actively phagocytic for the sheep erythrocytes bound during rosette formation (Fig. 3.10), and that they secreted lysozyme into the supernatant culture fluids (Table 3.2). These characteristics strongly indicate that the Hodgkin's and Sternberg-Reed cells are derived from macrophages or closely related cells of the mononuclear phagocyte system (van Furth, 1975), rather than from transformed lymphocytes. The

Table 3.2 Lysozyme Activity of Hodgkin's Disease Spleen Cell Culture Supernatants

Culture and data of sampling	Lysozyme[a] (μg/ml)
Case 10, 4/8/76, flask culture	5.5
Case 14, 4/8/76, flask culture	17.0
Case 15, 4/6/76, Petri dish culture	6.5
Case 15, 6/1/76, after LB cell overgrowth	4.0
Case 19, 6/1/76, flask culture	5.8
Case 20, 6/2/76, flask culture	27.0
Case 20, 6/2/76, flask culture	14.0
Case 20, 6/3/76, Petri dish culture	54.0
Case 21, 6/3/76, Petri dish culture	30.0
Case 23, 6/14/76, explant culture	9.5
Case 23, 6/15/76, flask culture	12.5
Medium control[b]	2.8

Source: Reproduced from the paper by Kaplan and Gartner (1977).

[a] Assays performed by the lyso-plate method of Osserman and Lawlor (1966) in the laboratory of Dr. Elliott Osserman, Columbia University Presbyterian Medical Center, N.Y.

[b] It was anticipated that the complete culture medium, which contained 10% human serum, could have significant lysozyme activity.

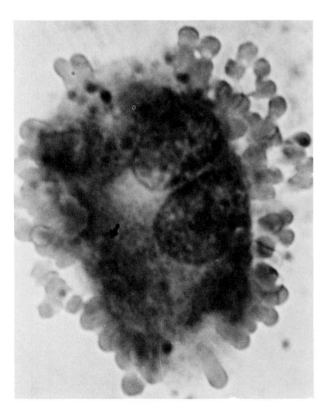

Figure 3.10 IgM-EAC rosette on a binucleate giant cell from a four-week culture of Hodgkin's disease spleen. Note that some sheep erythrocytes have been phagocytized (arrow). Wright-Giemsa, × 1900. (Reprinted by permission of the *International Journal of Cancer,* from the paper by Kaplan and Gartner, 1977.)

HuT$_{11}$ cell line established by Roberts et al. (1978) was highly phagocytic and strongly positive for nonspecific esterase, but failed to secrete lysozyme or to form IgG-EA or IgM-EAC rosettes.

Tissue Culture Studies. Attempts to characterize the pleomorphic cell population of Hodgkin's disease lymph nodes in terms of the sequence of events observed in tissue culture began with the work of Mankin (1936), Meier et al. (1937), and Lewis (1941). Regrettably, these pioneering efforts have more historical than scientific value, since they entailed poorly controlled exposure of human cells to the unknown influence of heterologous (primarily chicken) sera and tissue extracts and relied almost entirely on such nonspecific criteria as morphology for the identification and genealogic derivation of cell types. For example, Lewis (1941) attempted to relate cells morphologically identified in vitro as "Dorothy Reed cells" to normal precursors on the basis of their properties of locomotion in time-lapse motion pictures. She observed that the freely migrating small "Dorothy Reed cells" moved with a characteristic writhing motion similar to that of normal myeloblasts, and that the large "Dorothy Reed cells," which were more sluggish, resembled the "megalokaryocyte." Accordingly, she concluded that these cells were of myeloid, rather than lymphoid or monocytoid, origin.

Of the many controversies which such tissue culture studies have engendered, the most heated has revolved around the work of Grand (1944, 1949), who cultured lymph node fragments from 87 patients with Hodgkin's disease, 25 with lymphosarcoma, 21 with leukemia, 15 with nonspecific lymphadenitis, and 23 from normal controls, using the double cover slip and Carrel flask methods and a medium containing chick embryo extract and, in some instances, autogenous human serum. He noted the appearance during the first few days of incubation of sluggish, nonphagocytic giant cells which, in his opinion, resembled the Sternberg-Reed cells seen in histologic sections. These cells were described as having 6 to 20 or more nuclei of varying size and shape scattered irregularly within the cell, or occasionally arranged in a horseshoe or ring pattern around central granular inclusions. Of particular significance was his claim that these cells occurred only in cultures of Hodgkin's nodes and not in those derived from normal nodes or other pathologic states, and that the granular inclusion bodies occurred in cultures of normal node tissue only in response to the addition of supernatant fluids from the Hodgkin's node cultures and not similar fluids from cultures of other lymphomas, metastatic carcinoma, leukemia, adenitis, or normal nodes. He also ruled out the possibility that the responsible agent might have been a contaminant derived from the chicken plasma and tissue extracts in his medium, since the same medium was employed for his control cultures. He concluded that the agent was probably viral in nature.

However, these claims have not been substantiated by other investigators. Rottino (1949) cultured nodes from 23 patients with Hodgkin's disease and from 28 patients with other conditions. He states that "typical Sternberg-Reed cells were indubitably identified in cultures of only a few Hodgkin's disease nodes . . . They could be distinguished quite easily from the multinucleated giant cells. It quickly became apparent that the giant cell in question is not peculiar to any specific disease affecting the node, since it occurred in cultures of hyperplastic nodes and tuberculous nodes, as well as in cultures of Hodgkin's disease nodes and lymphoma of other types." In contrast to Grand, he observed that the giant cells were actively phagocytic and therefore classified them as foreign body giant cells. Essentially, the same conclusions were reached by Hoster and Reiman (1950) and by Siegel and Smith (1961). Moreover, the latter carefully documented the presence of cytoplasmic inclusions in normal and other types of

neoplastic nodes, as well as in those from patients with Hodgkin's disease, and concluded that there was no evidence that they are of viral origin. Sykes et al. (1962) distinguished two types of inclusions in cultures of leukemic and lymphomatous nodes: (a) a granular type occurring within vacuoles in the perinuclear area (presumably the type originally noted by Grand), which are apparently associated with the phagocytosis of cellular debris, and (b) an amorphous type, which stains blue with May-Grünwald-Giemsa and brilliant red with the fluorescent dye, Coriphosphine O, in which they had seen unidentified virus particles in preliminary electron microscopy studies.

Investigations purporting to demonstrate the successful cultivation of Hodgkin's and Sternberg-Reed cells must satisfy at least two essential requirements: (1) serial passage, with evidence of active replication rather than mere maintenance, of morphologically acceptable cells, and (2) proof, by criteria more rigorous than morphology alone, that the cells in culture are indeed derived from the neoplastic giant-cell population of Hodgkin's disease. Cultures of mixed morphology have been maintained for variable periods by modern techniques, but could not be serially passed or adequately characterized (Sykes et al., 1962; Trujillo, Drewinko, and Athearn, 1972; Pretlow et al., 1973). Other cultures in which cells began to replicate actively and could be serially passed (Pontén, 1967; Ito et al., 1968; Shiratori et al., 1969; Sinkovics et al., 1969; zur Hausen et al., 1972; Tsubota, 1972; Brieux de Salum et al., 1973) are now recognizable, in light of more recent investigations (Nilsson and Pontén, 1975) as probable instances of the overgrowth of the culture by lymphoblastoid cells derived from B-lymphocytes naturally infected with EB virus. We are left, then, with a handful of studies which merit more detailed description and analysis.

The organ culture technique devised by Jensen, Gwatkin, and Biggers (1964) was used by Young, Eisinger, and Sanders (1970) to grow tissue fragments of an involved node from a patient with clinical stage IVB Hodgkin's disease. They obtained a cell line which could be subcultured repeatedly and maintained in monolayer culture for more than six months. The adherent cells of the monolayer were pleomorphic, often markedly elongated giant cells with polyploidy and large nucleoli. In focal areas, their shape became rounded, and they then tended to form irreversible clusters. Stained preparations of cells which had lost their attachment to glass revealed cells interpreted as "protomacrophages, macrophages and cells morphologically similar to Reed-Sternberg cells." The cells were intensely phagocytic, and histochemical examination revealed high levels of acid phosphatase and nonspecific esterase. Accordingly, they were interpreted as malignant histiocytes. In a later publication by the same group (Eisinger et al., 1971), similar monolayer cultures of attached, randomly oriented cells from a total of ten patients with Hodgkin's disease are described. After achieving confluence, the cells could be serially passed at weekly intervals for at least seven or eight passages. Cells stored at $-78C$ at earlier passages again gave rise to attached monolayer cultures when thawed. However, the only indication that some of the cultured cells may have been neoplastic was the fact that inoculation of 10^6 cells of one culture line into the cheek pouches of 12 cortisonized weanling Syrian hamsters resulted in the appearance in 6 of the animals of small tumors which, however, again regressed after one to two weeks. Cytogenetic studies provided no evidence of aneuploidy or the presence of clones with distinctive marker chromosomes. Of 50 fully analyzed karyotypes, 38 were normal, and no consistent structural or numerical abnormalities were noted among the remaining 12. At least two of the cultured lines were eventually overgrown by lymphoblastoid cells.

Kadin and Asbury (1973) also placed fragments of involved splenic tissue from patients with Hodgkin's disease in modified organ culture and then subcultured the resultant cellular outgrowth. It is thus not surprising that they observed adherent cells with features closely resembling those described by the Sloan-Kettering Institute group. However, the binucleate giant cells illustrated in their report are morphologically more convincing candidates for identification as Sternberg-Reed cells than those illustrated by Eisinger et al. (1971). Moreover, Kadin and Asbury succeeded in demonstrating that bi- and multinucleate cells in their cultures, in addition to large mononuclears, were capable of DNA synthesis, as detected by radioautography of cells labeled with tritiated thymidine. Although their cultures could be serially passaged for as long as eight months, they did not succeed in establishing permanent lines of these cells. Their report makes no mention of either cytogenetic or heterotransplantation studies to demonstrate that the cultured cells were neoplastic.

Primary explant cultures from positive spleens were also prepared by Long et al. (1973, 1974a) and passaged weekly in RPMI-1640 medium supplemented with 30 percent gamma-irradiated fetal calf serum. They described the emergence of a heterogeneous population of "adherent, pleomorphic, spindle-shaped and round cells with numerous multinucleate giant cells." After 8 to 10 weekly passages, monolayers of "irregularly contoured reticular and polygonal cells" predominated; after 15 to 20 passages, stellate and round cells interspersed with occasional multinucleate cells persisted in the adherent monolayers. In two cultures, a striking morphological alteration occurred, with the emergence in suspension culture of nonadherent rapidly proliferating round cells, some of which were bi- or multinucleate. The monolayer cells formed weakly adherent spontaneous (E) rosettes with sheep, rabbit, human, and guinea pig erythrocytes, but lacked thymus-specific antigens and surface or cytoplasmic immunoglobulins, and failed to form IgG-EA or IgM-EAC rosettes (Long et al., 1977c). Although it was reported that the monolayer cells did not phagocytize latex particles or neutral red dye, subsequent studies using fresh human complement demonstrated convincingly that they did indeed have the capacity to phagocytize bacteria and other particulate material (Fig. 3.11; J. C. Long, personal communication). Cytogenetic studies revealed aneuploid karyotypes with numerous structural chromosome abnormalities in both the monolayer cells and the suspension cultures derived from them. Subcutaneous inoculation of four cell lines into athymic, *nude* mice yielded successful "takes" in 36 of 43 mice, whereas freshly biopsied tissues involved by Hodgkin's disease failed to take (Zamecnik and Long, 1977). Both monolayer and suspension culture cells

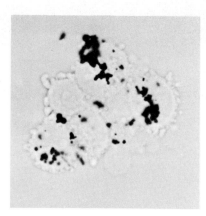

Figure 3.11   Phagocytosis of iron particles by cells from passage 24 of a culture established from a Hodgkin's disease spleen. × 160. (Previously unpublished phase contrast photomicrograph reproduced by courtesy of Dr. John C. Long, Massachusetts General Hospital, Boston.)

contained abundant lysozyme activity; both acid and alkaline phosphatase activity were also demonstrated, as was chymotrypsin-like activity (Long et al., 1977c). These investigators concluded that the cells of their monolayer and suspension cultures may be neoplastic monocytes.

Convincing evidence of clonal derivation of aneuploid giant cells bearing marker chromosomes was obtained by Boecker et al. (1975) by an in vivo culture technique. They grew cells from malignant pleural effusions of two near-terminal patients with a diagnosis of lymphocyte depletion Hodgkin's disease in diffusion chambers implanted intraperitoneally in heavily irradiated mice, and subcultured by transferring the cells to new diffusion chambers in new hosts every 11–15 days. Growth curves plotted from serial cell counts indicated an initial decrease in total cell number, followed after 4–5 days by an exponential increase with cell doubling times of 48 and 72 hours, respectively. Although the first culture was apparently lost after 11 days, the second was maintained through at least 50 days. In case 1, 14 percent of the cells on day 0 and 16 percent on day 11 were aneuploid. Giemsa banding revealed a translocation between chromosomes 3 and 13; in addition, two markers, one submetacentric, the other subacrocentric, were consistently seen in all metaphases. In case 2, 93 to 100 percent of metaphases were near triploid (55–77 chromosomes) at days 0, 11, and 50, and contained as many as 17 markers, the most consistent of which were a large submetacentric and two subacrocentrics. In both cases, the EBNA test for detection of the EB virus genome in the fresh pleural effusion cells was negative. Cells from the fresh effusions and from the diffusion chamber cultures were examined by the spontaneous E rosette test and by indirect immunofluorescence for surface immunoglobulin, using an antiserum prepared in rabbits against human immunoglobulins G, A, and M. Whereas the E-rosette test was entirely negative, 86 percent (case 1) and 70 percent (case 2) of the cultured tumor cells showed bright membrane fluorescence, even after 50 days in culture, suggesting that they were of B-lymphocyte origin. The validity of this excellent study rests, however, on the correctness of the original histopathologic diagnosis of lymphocyte depletion Hodgkin's disease. It is well known that this infrequent subtype may be extremely difficult to distinguish from diffuse histiocytic lymphoma (reticulum cell sarcoma), a neoplasm which is often of B-lymphocyte derivation and in which the occurrence of malignant pleural effusions is far more common than it is in Hodgkin's disease. Indeed, in a subsequent report by the same group (Gallmeier et al., 1977) of the establishment in diffusion chamber culture of a third cell line from a malignant pleural effusion in a patient with an initial diagnosis of lymphocyte depletion Hodgkin's disease, the diagnosis was changed to non-Hodgkin's lymphoma on later review by two additional pathologists.

Kaplan and Gartner (1977) studied the behavior in vitro of cell suspensions and tissue fragments from the involved spleens of 25 patients with Hodgkin's disease and, for comparison, from about 50 control spleens, using a variety of liquid culture techniques. Supplementation of the medium with human serum was found to be essential for propagation of the Hodgkin's giant cells, which grew in culture as round or elongated adherent cells with diameters ranging from 20 to more than 75 μm (Fig. 3.12). These cells often exhibited a strong tendency to adhere to one another, forming clusters (Fig. 3.13) similar to those mentioned by Young, Eisinger, and Sanders (1970). Although most were mononuclear, a substantial though variable fraction (usually 10 to 20 percent) were binucleate, and 1 to 2 percent contained three or more nuclei. Their nuclei were very much larger than those of typical type B macrophages (Cohen and Cline, 1971), which they resembled in certain other respects. Many of the cells had morphologic features strikingly similar to those of Sternberg-Reed cells, with two or more nuclei and large, often huge, nucleoli (Fig. 3.14). Confirming the observation of Kadin and Asbury (1973), the incorporation of tritiated thymidine into the DNA of binucleate and multinucleate cells, as well as of mononuclears, was readily detected by radioautography (Fig. 3.15). Moreover, in colchicine-treated cultures, mitotic figures were occasionally seen in both nuclei of binucleate cells (Fig. 3.3), as well as in giant mononuclears. An analysis of 70 countable mitotic figures in one case revealed that all were aneuploid; 63 were hyperdiploid, with a mode of 53 chromosomes; 6 were hypotetraploid, with chromosome numbers in the 77–91 range (Fig. 3.16); and one was hyperoctoploid, with approximately 190 chromosomes (Fig. 3.17). Another attribute of neoplasia, heterotransplantability, was demonstrable when cultured cells from six of eight different cases were inoculated intracerebrally into congenitally athymic, nude mice. After latent periods of 28 to 95 days, histologic examination revealed interstitial infiltrates composed of mono-, bi-, and occasional multinucleate cells, many of

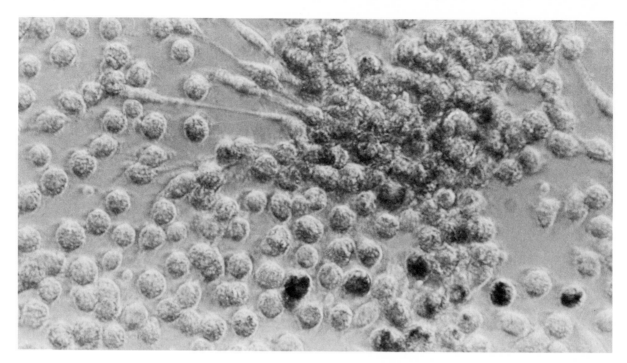

Figure 3.12 Eight-week culture of cells from a spleen involved by nodular sclerosing Hodgkin's disease, growing on a sparse fibroblastic feeder layer. The enormous size of the round or somewhat elongated, tightly adherent Hodgkin's giant cells may be appreciated by comparison with the size of the few surviving lymphoctyes. Note that some of the giant cells still contain India ink added to the culture five weeks earlier. Phase contrast, ×250. (Reprinted by permission of the *International Journal of Cancer*, from the paper by Kaplan and Gartner, 1977.)

which bore a striking resemblance to Sternberg-Reed cells (Fig. 3.18), invading the brain substance and the meninges (Fig. 3.19). Indirect immunofluorescence staining of frozen sections confirmed the human origin of the infiltrating cells. Cells recovered from the nude mouse brain were again successfully grown in vitro, revealing morphologic features identical to those observed in primary cultures. No takes were observed after more than 200 days in control nude mice inoculated with cultures of normal human spleen macrophages.

The cultured giant cells exhibited active though variable phagocytic activity for India ink and for antibody-coated sheep erythrocytes (Fig. 3.9). As indicated in the preceding section, nearly all of the large, adherent cells possessed both Fc and complement receptors, as revealed by their capacity to form IgG-EA and IgM-EAC$_{3b}$ rosettes, respectively. In contrast, they failed to form either E- or IgM-EAC$_{3d}$ rosettes and revealed no evidence of surface immunoglobulin by indirect immunofluorescence with a goat anti-human IgM-specific serum. Culture supernatants from seven different cases all revealed significantly elevated concentrations of lysozyme (Table 3.2). In the only case tested, 30 percent of the cultured giant cells were

positive for nonspecific esterase. It was concluded that the cultured giant cells were indeed derived from the Hodgkin's and Sternberg-Reed cell populations on the basis of their morphology and their manifestly neoplastic character, and that their adherent behavior in culture, their phagocytic activity, their capacity to secrete lysozyme, and their surface markers all argue strongly for their origin from the macrophage or other closely related cells of the mononuclear phagocyte system, rather than from transformed lymphocytes.

Attempts to obtain permanently established lines, using several variations in technique, including liquid overlay or semisolid agar or methylcellulose substrates, were not successful. Subsequently, however, secondary cultures of these giant cells recovered from the nude mouse brain were established as permanent cell lines (Fig. 3.20) after subcultivation in 3 percent agarose-coated flasks (H. S. Kaplan, unpublished).

Roberts et al. (1978) obtained a morphologically heterogeneous cell line (HuT$_{11}$) and four clonal sublines from a lymph node of a patient with stage IIA mixed cellularity Hodgkin's disease. The cells were aneuploid, with chromosome numbers ranging from 37 to 190, and heterotransplantable in

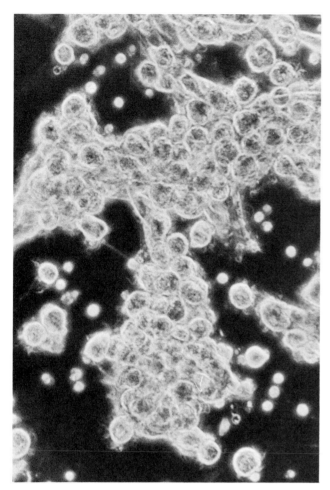

Figure 3.13 Grapelike clusters of mutually adherent Hodgkin's giant cells in a three-week-old culture. Small numbers of lymphocytes persist. Phase contrast, ×250.

the hamster cheek pouch. As indicated in the preceding section, they displayed certain features indicative of monocyte-macrophage derivation, such as phagocytic activity and strongly positive cytochemical staining reactions for nonspecific esterase, but were negative for others, such as the capacity to secrete lysozyme.

Miscellaneous. Sternberg-Reed cells have been identified in thoracic duct lymph and in the peripheral blood. Engeset et al. (1968, 1969) cannulated the thoracic duct in an initial series of four patients and a later series of ten patients with Hodgkin's disease and examined smears and filter specimens stained with May-Grünwald-Giemsa. Typical Sternberg-Reed cells were observed in seven of their ten cases (Fig. 3.21).

Their case no. 10 is of particular interest. This patient, a 51-year-old female with fever of un-

known origin, presented no palpable lymph nodes suitable for biopsy, and a right supraclavicular biopsy had been unrevealing. During the course of thoracic duct catheterization, some slightly enlarged lymph nodes were encountered behind the clavicular head of the sternomastoid muscle on the left, and histologic examination of these scalene nodes revealed Hodgkin's disease of the mixed cellularity type. In addition, Sternberg-Reed and other pathologic Hodgkin's cells were observed in both the smears and filter specimens in this case (Fig. 3.22).

The development of Sternberg-Reed cell leukemia is a rare manifestation in Hodgkin's disease. Mavor and Adams (1967) describe the clinical features, and Sinks and Clein (1966) the hematologic and cytologic features of a most remarkable, though diagnostically controversial case (also cited above in the section on cytochemistry) involving an elderly patient in whom cells interpreted as Sternberg-Reed cells became apparent in the peripheral blood two months before death. A blood sample taken 24 hours before death revealed a white blood cell count of 140,000 per cubic millimeter, of which 92 percent were interpreted as Sternberg-Reed cells! Other isolated instances have been noted by Scheerer et al. (1964) (associated with lactic acidosis), Ouyang et al. (1966), Capron and Menne (1969), Thuot et al. (1973), and Hayhoe et al. (1978). Bouroncle (1966) found Sternberg-Reed cells in the routine peripheral blood smears of two patients with advanced, generalized disease among a total Hodgkin's disease population of 890 patients. In a more intensive, systematic study of 135 cases, in which smears of leukocyte concentrates from the peripheral blood were examined at serial intervals during the course of the disease, she found "abnormal cells" in 50 (37 percent), 25 of which showed typical Sternberg-Reed cells (Figs. 3.23, 3.24). She also observed both "abnormal" cells and Sternberg-Reed cells in blood samples obtained from the splenic vein in three cases in which the spleen was surgically removed because of gross involvement or associated hemolytic blood disorders. Although "abnormal" cells were found mainly during periods of disease activity, they occurred also during clinical remission in occasional cases. Sternberg-Reed cells appeared in the peripheral blood only in patients with generalized, advanced disease and were frequently associated with intra-abdominal involvement. In 18 of the 25 cases in which Sternberg-Reed cells were detected, they were not seen until four months to one day prior to the time of death. The morphologic ap-

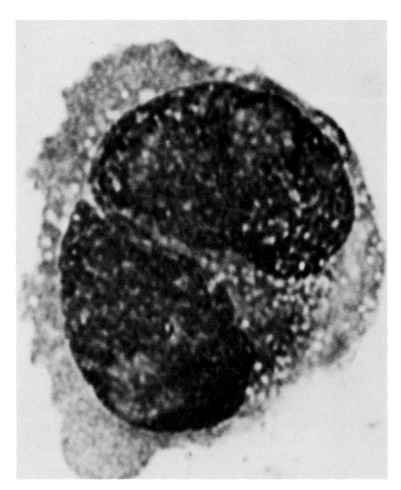

Figure 3.14   Binucleate giant cell from three-week culture of tissue fragments from an involved spleen. The huge nucleoli stain less intensely than the nuclear chromatin in this Wright-Giemsa cytocentrifuge preparation. ×2275. (Reprinted by permission of the *International Journal of Cancer,* from the paper by Kaplan and Gartner, 1977.)

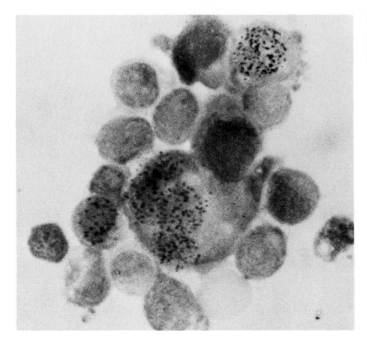

Figure 3.15   Radioautograph after incubation with ³H-thymidine, showing a giant cell with four nuclei, all of which are labeled, and two labeled mononuclear cells. ×1200.

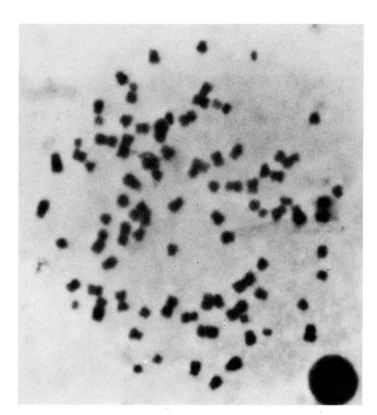

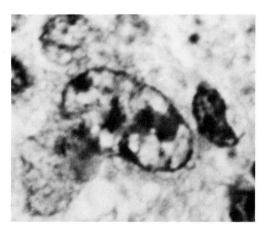

Figure 3.16 Hypotetraploid mitotic figure with 86 chromosomes in a colcemid-treated two-week culture of cells from a malignant pleural effusion which developed preterminally in a patient with stage IVB Hodgkin's disease. Other mitotic figures in the same culture contained up to 181 chromosomes. × 3,000.

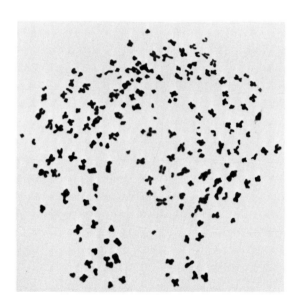

Figure 3.17 Hyperoctoploid giant cell with more than 190 chromosomes in a colchicine-treated eight-week culture of tissue fragments from an involved Hodgkin's disease spleen. × 1500. (Photomicrograph made by Philip Horne, Department of Pathology, Stanford University Medical Center.)

Figure 3.18 Classical binucleate Sternberg-Reed cells in nude mouse brain heterotransplant of a three-month culture of Hodgkin's disease spleen cells. Hematoxylin and eosin, × 1950. (Reprinted by permission of the *International Journal of Cancer*, from the paper by Kaplan and Gartner, 1977.)

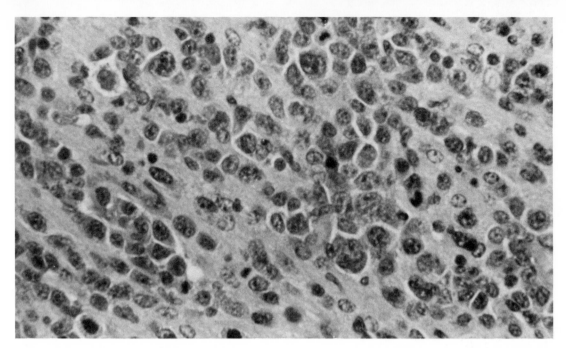

Figure 3.19 Infiltration of the nude mouse brain by cells from a three-month culture of Hodgkin's disease spleen tissue fragments. Occasional binucleate cells and mitotic figures may be seen, but the pleomorphic stromal cell population usually present in biopsies of Hodgkin's disease is of course absent. Hematoxylin and eosin, ×750.

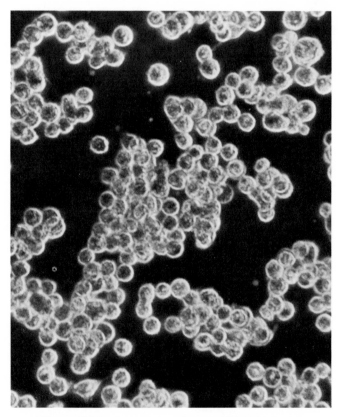

Figure 3.20 Secondary culture of Hodgkin's giant cells recovered from a nude mouse brain heterotransplant and permanently established in liquid culture in 3 percent agarose-coated flasks, in which these normally adherent cells tend to detach and form nonadherent clusters. Phase contrast, ×500.

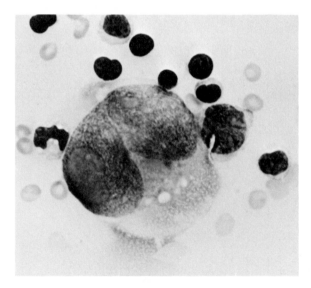

Figure 3.21 Smear preparation, stained with May-Grünwald-Giemsa, of the thoracic duct lymph of a patient with stage III nodular sclerosing Hodgkin's disease. Note the huge, binucleate Sternberg-Reed cell surrounded by normal erythrocytes and lymphoid cells, and one smaller, mononuclear Hodgkin's cell (×400). (Reprinted, by permission of the authors and the *International Journal of Cancer,* from the paper by Engeset et al., 1969.)

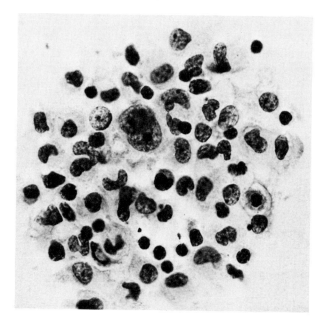

Figure 3.22 Filter specimen of thoracic duct lymph from a patient with stage III mixed cellularity Hodgkin's disease. A sheet of lymphoid and reticulum cells surrounds a binucleate Sternberg-Reed cell. Papanicolaou stain, ×380. (Reprinted, by permission of the authors and the *International Journal of Cancer,* from the paper by Engeset et al., 1969.)

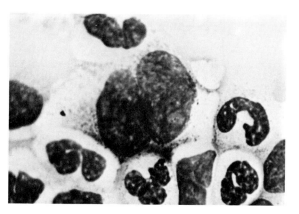

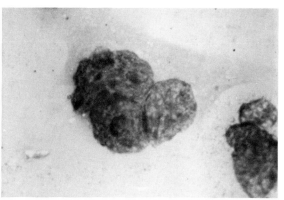

Figure 3.23 Sternberg-Reed cells in leukocyte concentrates of peripheral blood of patients with Hodgkin's disease. *Top,* mononuclear and indented, bilobate cell in same field; *bottom,* multinucleated Sternberg-Reed cell. Wright's stain, ×2400. (Reprinted, by permission of the author and Grune and Stratton, Inc., from the paper by Bouroncle, 1966.)

pearance of Sternberg-Reed cells in the peripheral blood was essentially identical with that in thoracic duct lymph (Engeset et al., 1969) or in lymph node imprints examined with phase contrast (Hoffmann and Rottino, 1950).

In a series of papers, Halie and his colleagues (1972a,b, 1974a,b) described the presence of several kinds of abnormal mononuclear cells in the peripheral blood buffy coats of patients with Hodgkin's disease. Some of these were monocytes, others were dark basophilic lymphoid cells, designated by Crowther et al. (1967a,b) as "immunoblasts," and still others were large, moderately basophilic "blast-like" cells 15–40 μ in diameter, with a nucleus of variable shape, nucleoli which were large when present, somewhat reticulated chromatin, and finely structured, moderately basophilic cytoplasm. Although the first two categories of atypical cells could be found with varying frequency in the buffy coats of normal individuals or patients with viral infections, the third category of moderately basophilic blast-like cells were not observed except in patients with Hodgkin's disease. Moreover, such cells were found in the peripheral blood of patients whose spleens were shown at staging laparotomy to be involved; patients whose spleens lacked "macroscopic or microscopical signs

of abnormal infiltration" also lacked the moderately basophilic blast-like cells. Accordingly, Halie et al. concluded that these cells were indicative of hematogenous dissemination of Hodgkin's disease, and thus constituted an indication for the use of systemic chemotherapy rather than radiotherapy in the treatment of patients presenting this manifestation.

These views have been sharply criticized by Aisenberg (1972), Kesselman, Sasyniuk, and Hryniuk (1973), and Schiffer, Levi, and Wiernik (1975). The last-named investigators studied a series of 33 previously untreated patients with Hodgkin's disease, 12 normal controls, and 8 individuals with viral infections of the upper respiratory tract. Unlike Halie et al., they coded the stained peripheral blood buffy coat smears from the patients and both groups of controls and examined them "blind." Abnormal cells detected on smears were marked and reevaluated by two of the authors together

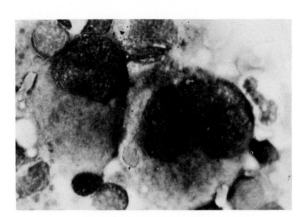

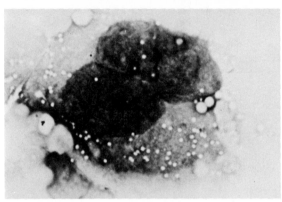

Figure 3.24 Hodgkin's cells in leukocyte concentrates of splenic vein samples from patients with Hodgkin's disease. *Top,* mononuclear and indented, bilobate cell in same field; *bottom,* multinucleated Sternberg-Reed cell. Wright's stain, ×2400. (Reprinted, by permission of the author and Grune and Stratton, Inc., from the paper by Bouroncle, 1966.)

before the code was broken. All of the types of cells described by Halie et al. were again encountered, including both cells of the "immunoblast" type and the moderately basophilic, blast-like cells. Such cells were present in 28 of 33 patients with Hodgkin's disease, but their presence was not correlated with the presence or absence of spleen involvement. Although such cells were not seen in normal individuals, "large cells with basophilic cytoplasm, often indistinguishable from those in the patients with Hodgkin's disease," were found in 5 of 8 subjects with viral infection. Cells in mitosis and giant "platelet" fragments similar to those seen in Hodgkin's disease were also present, but atypical histiocytic cells and Sternberg-Reed cells were not seen. Finally, Schiffer et al. were unable to establish any correlation between the presence or absence of the moderately basophilic cells and response to radiotherapy. They challenged the validity of the claim of Halie et al. that this group of cells is fundamentally different from the category of large, non-

specific basophilic cells, and suggested that both types of basophilic cells represent varying degrees of differentiation of the same or similar cells. Schiffer et al. concluded that these cells do not represent circulating tumor cells, but are more likely "reactive" cells responding to some stimulus associated with the malignant process.

Stromal Cells. Hodgkin's cells rarely occur, even in the most malignant forms of Hodgkin's disease, in essentially solidly packed sheets. Instead, they tend to occur singly, or in small clusters, seldom in direct contact with one another, completely surrounded by a much larger mass of stromal cells of various types. Thus, the Hodgkin's cells usually comprise only a small fraction of the volume of an enlarged lymph node. The obliteration of normal lymph node architecture typically seen in Hodgkin's disease is due predominantly to the immigration and proliferation within the node of several classes of normal or reactive stromal cells, in varying proportions. The principal cell types observed include lymphocytes of various sizes, occasional tranformed lymphocytes ("immunoblasts"), histiocytes ("reticulum cells"), eosinophils, plasma cells, and fibroblasts. Since the cytologic features of all of these cell types are well known, they will not be described here.

Rosenthal (1936) was the first to call attention to the apparent relationship between the relative abundance of lymphocytes in biopsies from patients with Hodgkin's disease and the rate of progression and prognosis of the disease. Since that time, the central role of the lymphocyte in both humoral and cell-mediated immune responses has been firmly established. In the light of modern developments in tumor immunology, Rosenthal's observation has come increasingly to be interpreted as an expression of the host immune response to presumptive tumor-specific antigens associated with the Hodgkin's cells.

This view is reinforced by the observation (Cooper et al., 1968; Peckham and Cooper, 1969; Schiffer, 1973) that a high proportion of the transformed lymphocytes, and also a variable proportion of small to medium-sized lymphocytes, in lymph nodes involved in Hodgkin's disease are actively synthesizing DNA, as measured by their capacity to incorporate tritiated thymidine. It is well established that antigens may trigger a powerful lymphoproliferative response, causing normally nonproliferating small lymphocytes to undergo a dramatic series of morphologic and biochemical changes in the process of transition to DNA-synthesizing, mitotically active immunoblasts. As Peckham and Cooper (1969) point out, the possibility that this lymphocytic proliferative activity represents an immune response gains in plausibility from the fact that overall growth rate of lymph nodes involved by Hodgkin's disease is generally rather slow, despite the fact that the labeling index of the lymphoid cells in their cases was extremely high and comparable to that seen in some lymphocytic and histiocytic lymphomas. They suggest further that the well-documented spontaneous fluctuations in size of diseased lymph nodes in some patients is entirely consistent with a benign, self-limiting cell proliferation, such as that seen in lymph nodes in which an immune response is occurring. In such instances, although the rate of division is high, this is offset by a very high cell death rate and a high rate of cell loss into the blood stream. A similar situation is encountered in infectious mononucleosis.

Crowther, Fairley, and Sewell (1967b) have reported that the peripheral blood of untreated patients with Hodgkin's disease contains an increased number of large lymphocytes ("immunoblasts") capable of DNA synthetic activity, an increased number of hyperbasophilic medium-sized lymphocytes, and occasional plasma cells. All three of these peripheral blood changes are also seen normally after antigenic challenge, suggesting the possibility that an immunologic reaction may be occurring in patients with Hodgkin's disease. Their data suggest also that the degree of abnormality of the peripheral blood lymphocyte population tends to parallel disease activity. The presence of such cells has also been noted by others (Halie et al., 1972a; Schiffer et al., 1975).

Finally, Saksela and Pontén (1968) were able to establish two lymphoblastoid clonal culture lines, from lymph nodes involved by Hodgkin's disease, which actively synthesized immunoglobulin (IgG) continuously in culture for 11 to 18 months. Whether the progressive depletion of the lymphocyte population in affected lymph nodes during the course of Hodgkin's disease and the peculiar deficiencies in cell-mediated immunoresponsiveness which are so characteristically observed in patients with the disease are consequences of a sustained immunologic war between the host lymphocyte population and the Hodgkin's cells, as has been suggested by Kaplan and Smithers (1959), Order and Hellman (1972), and De Vita (1973), is not yet clearly established. Some of the relevant investigations of these questions are presented more fully in Chapter 6.

The role of the normal histiocyte in the stromal cell reaction is much more controversial. Although lymph node biopsies containing an abundance of normal histiocytes were found by Lukes and Butler (1966) to be associated with a prognosis almost as favorable as that in lymphocyte-rich biopsies, Lohmann (1965) suggested that an abundance of reactive histiocytes was an unfavorable prognostic indicator. Coppleson et al. (1973), in an analysis of the prognostic significance of various cell types, found that the presence of either malignant or benign-appearing histiocytes in great numbers was associated with an unfavorable outcome, whereas the converse was true when lymphocytes were plentiful. All of these studies, however, include many cases diagnosed in the pre-lymphangiography era and treated by long obsolete methods. Similar investigations on more recent case material might be expected to resolve some of the residual controversies and to provide data more relevant to current management. Lennert and Mestdagh (1968) have described a progressive form of Hodgkin's disease in older patients in which an "epithelioid-cell" variant of the normal histiocyte is said to be a prominent feature.

It may well be that different types of histiocytes account for these disparities. Possibly histochemical studies, such as those carried out by Dorfman (1961, 1964) and by Peckham and Cooper (1969), would be helpful in drawing meaningful distinctions among different classes of histiocytes. Peckham and Cooper (1969) found that the esterase-positive histiocytes did not label with tritiated thymidine and had a normal diploid DNA content; they were thus clearly not a part of the Hodgkin's cell population, nor did they appear to be involved in a proliferative response comparable to that observed in the lymphocytic cells.

The role of the eosinophils, plasma cells, and fibroblasts is obscure. Fibroblasts are responsible for the laying down of bands of collagen in the nodular sclerosing form of Hodgkin's disease, which has a favorable prognosis. Conversely, however, the presence of fibroblasts or of diffuse, noncollagenous fibrosis in lymph nodes, associated with a depletion of lymphocytes, has been associated with a particularly unfavorable prognosis (Lukes and Butler, 1966). In rare instances, the fibroblastic proliferation may be so extensive as to resemble well-differentiated fibrosarcoma, in which case correct diagnosis requires a particularly painstaking and meticulous search for the sparse Sternberg-Reed cells that may be present (Rappaport, 1966, fig. 203).

In addition to these cellular infiltrates, necrosis is a not uncommon feature of Hodgkin's disease lymph node biopsies, particularly in the more aggressive histopathologic forms. Its extent varies greatly, from minute foci of fibrinoid necrosis to large areas of deeply eosinophilic, granular tissue destruction containing ghostly remnants of necrotic cells. Necrosis is often even more impressive at autopsy, suggesting that it may, in part, be a secondary consequence of treatment, as well as an integral part of the cellular interactions occurring in the disease process. Foci of necrosis are frequently surrounded by unusual concentrations of Hodgkin's cells.

Histopathologic Classification

Historical and General Considerations. The effort by pathologists to delineate morphologically and prognostically meaningful histopathologic subcategories within the broad rubric of Hodgkin's disease began about fifty years ago with the introduction by Ewing (1928) of the term "Hodgkin's sarcoma" for an infrequent, rapidly fatal form of the disease characterized microscopically by an abundance of pleomorphic, obviously neoplastic variants of the Sternberg-Reed cell. At the opposite end of the prognostic spectrum, Jackson (1937) described cases morphologically resembling Hodgkin's disease but characterized by a remarkably indolent, benign course, to which he initially gave the name "early Hodgkin's disease." This was later modified to "Hodgkin's paragranuloma" by Jackson and Parker (1944b, 1947). The existence of this entity has been challenged by other pathologists, and it has been redescribed under a variety of other names; lymphoreticular medullary reticulosis (Robb-Smith, 1947), benign Hodgkin's disease (Harrison, 1952), and reticular lymphoma (Lumb, 1954).

The delineation of these subtypes led to the histopathologic classification of Jackson and Parker (1944b). Their designation of three subcategories (paragranuloma, granuloma, and sarcoma) remained essentially unmodified for some twenty years, but its utilization was limited because, as explained below, it failed to pass the test of practical clinical utility. Meanwhile, at the Armed Forces Institute of Pathology in Washington, where large numbers of cases of Hodgkin's disease from military files were available for review, a new subcategory, nodular sclerosing Hodgkin's disease, began to be recognized through the work of Smetana and Cohen (1956) and more explicitly that of Lukes and his colleagues (Lukes, 1963; Lukes and Butler, 1966; Lukes, Butler and Hicks, 1966). Another subtype, the nodular (follicular) variant of the lymphocyte predominance form of Hodgkin's disease, emerged from the pathologic archives of the same institution through the now classic work of Rappaport, Winter, and Hicks (1956) on classification of the follicular lymphomas. Concurrently, increased emphasis was given to the importance of the relative abundance of lymphocytes, reviving a viewpoint originally stated by Rosenthal (1936), in a paper which also contains the first known (but never widely used) histopathologic classification.

These contributions crystallized into a practical new classification, which was proposed for international adoption at a conference on "Obstacles to the Control of Hodgkin's Disease," held in Rye, New York, in September 1965 (Lukes, Craver, Hall, Rappaport, and Rubin, 1966). The Rye classification has been widely adopted in major centers in the United States, Canada, South America, and western Europe, and a series of reports analyzing the intercorrelation among the Rye histopathologic types, clinical stage, propensity for extralymphatic relapse, and prognosis have strongly endorsed its utility (Franssila et al., 1967; Keller et al., 1968; Landberg and Larsson, 1969; Gough, 1970; Johnson, Thomas, and Chretien, 1970; Correa and O'Conor, 1973; Correa et al., 1973; Strum, 1973). Nonetheless, it would be premature to consider that the last word has been written on the subject of histopathologic classification of Hodgkin's disease. Indeed, as the first edition of this book was being written, Cross (1969) proposed a new classification, which appears not to have been widely accepted in the intervening years, however, and is therefore not presented here in detail. There are still problems of interpretation to be resolved in the Rye scheme, particularly at the borderlines between categories. It is reasonable to anticipate that further refinements of analysis and the introduction of more sophisticated histochemical, cytochemical, and electron microscopic techniques will continue to provide new insights into this complex and difficult subject.

The Jackson and Parker Classification.

Paragranuloma. It was stated by Jackson and Parker (1944b) that the paragranuloma form is usually clinically localized to a single peripheral lymph node or group of lymph nodes. This was true of nine of the ten cases reviewed by Wright (1956), and even his tenth case was limited to bilateral involvement of the neck. However, all of these reports antedated the utilization of lymphangiography and, more recently, of laparotomy with splenectomy and retroperitoneal node biopsy in the staging of Hodgkin's disease (cf. Chapter 4). On the basis of our experience at Stanford University Medical Center with laparotomy, splenectomy, and retroperitoneal node biopsy, it appears that a substantial fraction of our lymphocyte predominance cases (the Rye classification category which includes the paragranulomas) have occult involvement of the retroperitoneal nodes and/or the spleen (Kadin, Glatstein, and Dorfman, 1971).

Another feature of the paragranuloma cases is their indolent course and remarkable longevity. Lennert and Hippchen (1954) reported an average survival of 15 years in their cases. A number of instances of 20- to 30-year survival, with occasional clinical reactivation responding readily to minimal treatment, are well documented. Although transition to the Hodgkin's granuloma form is not infrequently observed in subsequent biopsies, Jackson and Parker stated that some cases apparently remained stable, with the morphology of paragranuloma persisting in repeated biopsies over many years.

The histologic picture is dominated by the virtually complete effacement of the normal lymph node architecture by densely packed small, mature lymphocytes (cf. Fig. 3.25). Sternberg-Reed cells are variable in number but usually rather sparse. When they are not readily detected, the erroneous diagnosis of lymphocytic lymphosarcoma (lymphoma, well-differentiated lymphocytic type) is likely to be made. In some instances, there are also foci of slightly larger lymphoblast-like cells and of histiocytes. Eosinophils are sometimes present, and plasma cells and mast cells are not uncommonly seen. Although Jackson and Parker initially reported that plasma cells may be numerous, Rappaport (1966, p. 1957) states that "the presence of more than occasional plasma cells and eosinophilic or neutrophilic granulocytes may indicate the progression of the disease into Hodgkin's granuloma; such progression is part of the natural evolution of Hodgkin's paragranuloma and may occur after varying periods of time." Invasion of the capsule and necrosis do not occur in the paragranuloma form.

Although Jackson and Parker stated that mitotic figures in the large Hodgkin's cells are not numerous in paragranuloma, Harrison (1952) found such mitoses in each of his six cases. Wright (1956) stated that in his ten cases mitoses were encountered quite frequently in these cells and that one

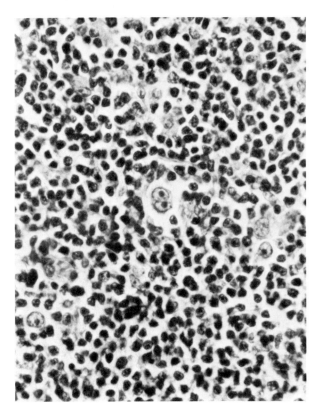

Figure 3.25   Rye lymphocytic predominance form of Hodgkin's disease; this example is also typical of the paragranuloma group of Jackson and Parker. The stroma is moderately densely packed with small to medium-sized lymphocytes. A binucleate Sternberg-Reed cell is seen in the center, and mononuclear Hodgkin's cells are present near the left and right margins of the figure. Hematoxylin and eosin stain, ×510.

tripolar mitosis was seen. Both Harrison (1952) and Wright (1956) failed to find any examples of paragranuloma in a review of cases that came to autopsy. In view of the morphologic transition of progressive cases to the granuloma form, this is hardly surprising. However, it apparently led Harrison to the erroneous conclusion that paragranuloma is a benign, nonprogressive condition, for which he preferred the name "benign Hodgkin's disease." The occurrence of aneuploidy in paragranuloma, previously mentioned (Table 3.1), suffices to establish its malignant nature.

Granuloma. This heterogeneous category is also usually first encountered in lymph nodes, although it may occasionally be localized to the gastrointestinal tract or other extralymphatic structures. It is the morphologically classical form of Hodgkin's disease, in which variable numbers of Sternberg-Reed cells and other types of Hodgkin's cells are intermingled with a remarkably variegated and pleomorphic stromal cell population (cf. Fig. 3.32).

The stromal elements usually include lymphocytes, plasma cells, mature neutrophilic and eosinophilic granulocytes, normal histiocytes, and fibroblasts, and the overall appearance is frequently dominated by these inflammatory and reactive elements. Although eosinophils are regularly present, their number varies widely; occasionally, they may be present as dense collections of so-called eosinophilic microabscesses.

The numbers of normal, nonneoplastic histiocytes also vary considerably. Occasionally, focal aggregations of these cells form nodular granulomas that may closely resemble the noncaseating tubercles of sarcoidosis. Rappaport (1966) and Strum (1973) have described a variant in which the presence of numerous histiocytes with abundant vacuolated cytoplasm ("foam cells") may simulate a xanthomatous lesion, and another extremely rare variant in which scattered Sternberg-Reed cells were found in a proliferating fibroblastic stroma histologically resembling well-differentiated fibrosarcoma.

Both necrosis and fibrosis are characteristically observed in the granuloma form (Fig. 3.33). As indicated above, necrosis may vary in extent from microscopic foci to areas large enough to be visible with the naked eye. The latter are often infarctlike, and the ghostly outlines of dead and dying cells may be partially preserved within them. Neutrophilic granulocytes, histiocytes, Hodgkin's cells, and occasionally foreign-body giant cells of the Langhans type are often present at the periphery of these necrotic areas, which are subsequently organized by the ingrowth of fibroblasts and converted to dense, sometimes hyalinized connective tissue scars.

In time, sequential biopsy specimens are likely to reveal a progressive increase in the number of neoplastic Hodgkin's cells and a gradual disappearance of inflammatory elements, particularly of lymphocytes, leading in some instances to an appearance morphologically indistinguishable from that of Hodgkin's sarcoma. Vascular invasion is observed occasionally in these transitional instances (Rappaport, 1966, figs. 201 and 202), as well as in the overtly sarcomatous form.

Sarcoma. Jackson and Parker observed that this form was more likely to occur in the deep than in the peripheral nodes; it involved the retroperitoneal nodes in nineteen of their twenty-seven cases. It is a highly malignant, invasive, and rapidly disseminating form, the neoplastic character of which, unlike that of the granuloma form, has never been seriously debated. Microscopically, there is an abundance of mononuclear Hodgkin's cells, about two to three times the size of small lymphocytes, with a round nucleus and large nucleoli (Figs. 3.35, 3.36). Classical Sternberg-Reed cells also occur but are highly variable in number. Although areas of necrosis are not infrequently observed, there is a striking paucity of the inflammatory stromal cell component. Only scattered lymphocytes and histiocytes are seen, and neutrophilic and eosinophilic granulocytes and plasma cells are rarely found.

It is of interest that Jackson and Parker were aware of the relationship of the smaller, mononuclear cells to Sternberg-Reed cells; indeed, they refer to them as "undifferentiated forms of Reed-Sternberg cell." As is indicated in the preceding section on cytology, there is now evidence indicating that these cells are the most actively proliferating neoplastic component in Hodgkin's disease and that the Sternberg-Reed cell is a more sluggishly proliferating derivative.

Comment. The Jackson and Parker classification correlates well with prognosis, at least on superficial analysis. Hodgkin's granuloma has a prognosis intermediate between that of the paragranuloma and the sarcoma types. In a series of 377 cases reviewed by Lukes (1963), median survival was 11.2 years for the paragranuloma cases, 3.2 years for granuloma, and 0.6 year for sarcoma. Smetana and Cohen (1956) noted a mortality of only 28 percent at 7 years for paragranuloma, as compared with 83 percent in Hodgkin's granuloma. Instances of five-year survival of pedigreed sarcoma cases are quite rare.

However, the Jackson-Parker classification suffers from a major drawback, which has severely limited its practical clinical utility. Cases of Hodgkin's disease are not distributed in roughly comparable numbers in the three categories; instead, the distribution is profoundly skewed, with the great bulk of cases falling in the granuloma category and essentially negligible numbers in the paragranuloma and sarcoma groups. Of the 377 cases reviewed by Lukes (1963), 344 (91 percent) were classified as granuloma, 30 (8 percent) as paragranuloma, and 3 (1 percent) as sarcoma. In other series, the frequency of the sarcoma form has been as high as 3 to 5 percent and that of paragranuloma up to 10 to 12 percent; even so, at least 80 percent of all cases remain in the granuloma category. In addition, the Jackson and Parker classification has been criticized by Haas (1953), who claimed that many transitional forms may be found in different lymph node chains and extranodal tissues at autopsy and therefore that the three categories are artificial entities. A more valid criticism is that the large granuloma category, on closer analysis, is seen to be quite heterogeneous, erroneously grouping together subcategories with widely different prognoses.

The Rye Classification. The modified histopathologic classification initially proposed by Lukes (1963) and subsequently described in detail by Lukes and Butler (1966); Lukes, Butler, and Hicks (1966); and Lukes (1971) comprised six categories: (a) lymphocytic and/or histiocytic, nodular; (b) lymphocytic and/or histiocytic, diffuse; (c) nodular sclerosis; (d) mixed; (e) diffuse fibrosis; and (f) reticular. This classification evolved out of the following general observations: (1) There is an inverse relationship between the frequency of lymphocytes and that of abnormal reticulum cells of the Sternberg-Reed cell type (Hodgkin's cells); (2) Two distinctive types of connective tissue proliferation may be observed: a disorderly, finely fibrillar type which, when extensive, was designated as "diffuse fibrosis," and another form, "nodular sclerosis," characterized by true collagen deposition in interconnecting bands of varying width around nodules of lymphoid tissue; (3) There is an association between diffuse fibrosis and depletion of the lymphocyte population of the stroma; and (4) In addition to the classical Sternberg-Reed cells and other Hodgkin's cells, a new type of atypical "lacunar" Hodgkin's cell was characteristically found in nodular sclerosis and perhaps also, in some instances, in the lymphocytic and/or histiocytic types.

The distribution of their 377 cases among the six categories was considerably more uniform than that obtained with the Jackson and Parker classification. Their six categories, listed in the order above, were found to contain 6, 11, 40, 25, 12, and 5 percent, respectively, of their cases. There was also a good correlation with prognosis; median survival in the same sequence was 12.4, 7.4, 4.2, 2.5, 0.9, and 2.3 years, respectively.

Nonetheless, it was felt that six categories would be deemed unacceptably complex by most pathologists. Accordingly, an effort was made at the Rye conference to simplify this classification. After some discussion, this was accomplished by the simple expedient of combining the nodular and diffuse forms of the lymphocytic and/or histiocytic type and the diffuse fibrosis and reticular types. The first of these combined categories, in which lymphocytes and/or histiocytes are abundant, was designated "lymphocytic predominance," and the second combined category, in which lymphocytes are sparse, was designated "lymphocytic depletion" (Lukes, Craver, Hall, Rappaport, and Rubin, 1966). The interrelationships among the Jackson and Parker; the Lukes, Butler, and Hicks; and the Rye classifications are indicated schematically in Table 3.3.

Lymphocytic Predominance. Although its name stresses the lymphocytic component of the stroma, it should be clearly understood that this category also includes those relatively infrequent instances in which normal histiocytes are the predominant stromal cell type and lymphocytes are a relatively minor component.

The principal group of cases reassigned to this category are those formerly designated as paragranuloma, in which small lymphocytes dominate the stromal reaction and normal histiocytes are sparse. In addition, the nodular form of paragranuloma first described by Rappaport, Winter, and Hicks (1956) is included within this rubric, as are the cases of histiocytic predominance and certain others formerly assigned to the granuloma group.

Sternberg-Reed cells are seldom numerous and may be so sparse as to remain undetected, thus leading to errors in diagnosis. In contrast, a peculiar Hodgkin's cell variant may occasionally be relatively numerous. These are bizarre polyploid cells with folded, overlapping nuclear lobes, delicate lacy chromatin, and small nucleoli. Eosinophilic and neutrophilic granulocytes and plasmocytes are extremely sparse or absent, and little or no fibrosis is seen (Fig. 3.25).

In the relatively infrequent nodular form, cellular proliferation tends to be aggregated in large, poorly delineated nodules, which are usually composed almost entirely of lymphocytic stroma, although in rare instances histiocytes are the predominant stromal cell type in this form as well (Fig. 3.26). The Hodgkin's cells tend to be concentrated near the centers of the nodules but are seldom in contact with one another. As in the case of the diffuse varieties, typical Sternberg-Reed cells are often rare. When diagnostic Sternberg-Reed cells are not observed, the nodular variant of lymphocytic predominance Hodgkin's disease is likely to be erroneously diagnosed as nodular (follicular) lymphoma, whereas the diffuse form is likely to be mistaken for well-differentiated lymphocytic lym-

Table 3.3 Interrelationships of the Major Histopathologic Classifications of Hodgkin's Disease

Jackson and Parker	Lukes, Butler, and Hicks	Rye	Distinctive features	Relative frequency, percent
Paragranuloma - - - -	{ Lymphocytic/histiocytic, diffuse Lymphocytic/histiocytic, nodular } - -	Lymphocytic predominance	Abundant stroma of mature lymphocytes and/or histiocytes; no necrosis; Sternberg-Reed cells may be sparse	10–15
Granuloma - - - - - - -	Nodular sclerosis - - - - - - -	Nodular sclerosis	Nodules of lymphoid tissue separated by bands of doubly refractile collagen; atypical "lacunar" Hodgkin's cells in clear spaces within the lymphoid nodules	20–50
	Mixed - - - - - - - - - - - - -	Mixed cellularity	Usually numerous Sternberg-Reed cells and mononuclear Hodgkin's cells in a pleomorphic stroma of eosinophils, plasma cells, fibroblasts, and necrotic foci	20–40
Sarcoma - - - - - - - - -	{ Diffuse fibrosis Reticular } - - - - - - - - -	Lymphocytic depletion	Sternberg-Reed cells usually, though not always, abundant; marked paucity of lymphocytes; diffuse nonrefractile fibrosis and necrosis may be present	5–15

phoma of the diffuse variety, or even for Waldenström's macroglobulinemia.

Lennert and Mestdagh (1968) made a detailed study of 50 atypical cases of Hodgkin's disease, the biopsy specimens of which were consistently remarkable for their high concentration of epithelioid cells (histiocytes). Within this group, they were able to delineate a new and distinctive subgroup characterized by massive infiltrations of focally aggregated epithelioid cells. Typical Sternberg-Reed cells were often absent, but it was always possible to discover atypical variants of such cells. Although plasma cells were often abundant, fibrosis did not occur, even after treatment. This unusual lesion, for which they proposed the name "epithelioid cell lymphogranulomatosis," differed from the histiocytic variant of the "L and H" type of Lukes and Butler in that it was observed most frequently in middle-aged and older patients and that its prognosis was neither unusually favorable, as in the "L and H" type, nor particularly unfavorable. There is disagreement among hematopathologists as to whether this is truly a variant of Hodgkin's disease or a peculiar non-Hodgkin's lymphoma; if it is indeed a form of Hodgkin's disease, it is not clear that it fits appropriately within any of the four categories of the Rye classification.

Nodular Sclerosis. Excellent descriptions of this histologic type have been presented by Lukes (1963), Lukes and Butler (1966), Hanson (1964), and Lukes (1971). It is characterized by the replacement of part of the lymph node parenchyma by interconnecting bands of collagenous connective tissue encircling nodular areas of lymphatic tissue (Figs. 3.27, 3.28). The connective tissue bands may be identified as collagen by virtue of their birefringence in polarized light (Fig. 3.29).

A wide range of variation in the extent of collagen deposition is observed, sometimes even within the same lymph node. At one end of the spectrum, an entire lymph node may be virtually obliterated by the sclerotic process, with only faint residual evidence of a nodular pattern still visible. At the other extreme is the variant which Lukes and Butler (1966), Strum and Rappaport (1971a) and Kadin, Glatstein, and Dorfman (1971) have termed the "cellular phase of nodular sclerosis," in which col-

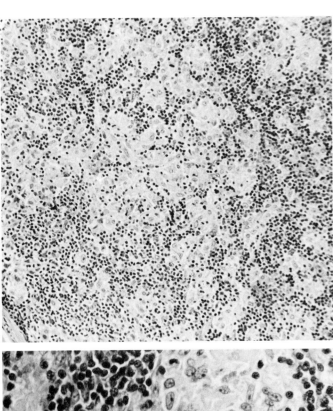

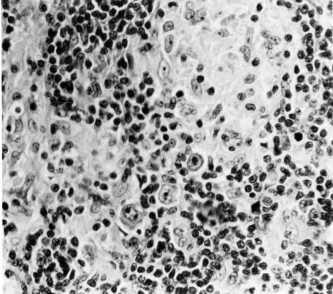

Figure 3.26 "L and H" variant of lymphocyte predominance type Hodgkin's disease. The stromal elements are comprised almost entirely of lymphocytes and "epithelioid" histiocytes. A cluster of Hodgkin's cells may be seen in the lower figure. Hematoxylin and eosin stain, ×320. (Reprinted, by permission of the author and the *Journal of Clinical Pathology*, from the paper by Cross, 1969.)

lagen deposition is either minimal or sometimes entirely lacking and a nodular pattern correspondingly difficult to discern (Fig. 3.30).

The most distinctive cellular feature in nodular sclerosis is an unusually large "lacunar" variant of the Hodgkin's cell. Its abundant, pale eosinophilic, amphophilic, or clear cytoplasm tends to retract away from adjacent cells during formalin fixation, thus giving rise to the appearance of a giant cell residing in a lacunalike clear space (Fig. 3.2). That this is, at least in part, an artifact is suggested by

the fact that it is much less apparent in Zenker-fixed tissue. The nuclei of these cells are prominently lobated, and the lobes may be numerous. The nuclear chromatin is delicate and seen within it are nucleoli which, unlike those of classical Sternberg-Reed cells, are usually small to medium in size. It is primarily the presence of this distinctive variant which, in the view of Lukes and Butler (1966), permits recognition of the relationship of the "cellular phase," despite the absence of nodules and of sclerosis, to the more overt forms of nodu-

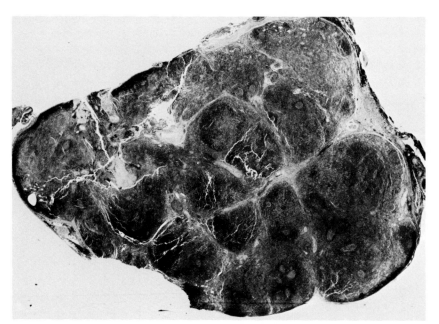

Figure 3.27   An example of nodular sclerosis with minimal collagen deposition. Thin, interconnecting bands encircle and separate nodules of lymphatic tissue of varying size. Hematoxylin and eosin stain, ×3. (Reprinted, by permission of the Editor of *Cancer,* from the paper by Keller et al., 1968.)

lar sclerosing Hodgkin's disease. Nonetheless, an unequivocal diagnosis of Hodgkin's disease of the nodular sclerosing type still requires the visualization of classical binucleated or multinucleated forms with large to huge nucleoli.

The stromal reaction in the lymphatic nodules and elsewhere within the lymph node may be predominantly lymphocytic or a mixture of lymphocytes, eosinophilic and neutrophilic granulocytes, and variable numbers of histiocytes. Occasionally

focal or even massive necrosis is seen. Individual nodules of lymphatic tissue apparently tend to undergo obliterative fibrosis. During this process the numbers of mature granulocytes increase, while lymphocytes decrease in number. Small vessels then extend into the interior of the nodule from the collagenous bands at its periphery, followed by the invasion of fibroblastic cellular connective tissue and finally the deposition of new collagen. A single lymph node may show all stages of the pro-

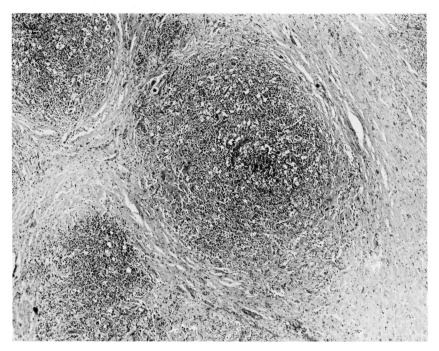

Figure 3.28   Nodular sclerosing Hodgkin's disease. The collagen bands are heavier and the lymphatic nodules smaller in this example. Some areas within the lymphatic nodules have a "salt-and-pepper" appearance due to the presence of "lacunar" Hodgkin's cell variants lying in clear spaces. Hematoxylin and eosin stain, ×105.

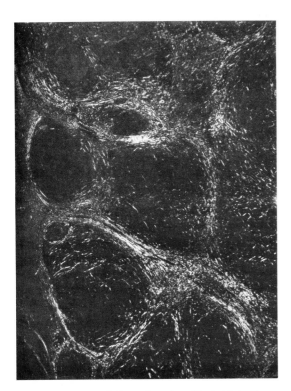

Figure 3.29 Nodular sclerosing Hodgkin's disease examined with polarized light revealing the typical birefringence which identifies the material in the connective tissue bands as collagen. (Photograph courtesy of Dr. Charles Bieber, Department of Pathology, Stanford University Medical Center.)

cess, from the "cellular phase" at one end (Fig. 3.30) to obliteration of one or more nodules at the other (Fig. 3.31).

Mixed Cellularity. This histologic type represents the residue of cases that remain when parts of the Hodgkin's granuloma category are reallocated respectively to the lymphocyte predominance, nodular sclerosis, and, in small measure, to the lymphocyte depletion categories. In this sense, mixed cellularity may be considered the lineal descendent of Hodgkin's granuloma.

The highly cellular and pleomorphic stroma is composed of a mixture of normal histiocytes, neutrophilic and eosinophilic granulocytes, plasma cells, lymphocytes, and fibroblasts in varying proportions (Fig. 3.32). Fibrosis of variable degree is often present, but collagen deposition is not seen. Focal necrosis is often observed but is seldom extensive (Fig. 3.33). Sternberg-Reed cells and other Hodgkin's cells are often numerous and readily detectable. The stromal infiltrate tends to replace and obliterate the entire lymph node, including the lymphatic sinusoids and follicles. However, in

isolated instances, focal involvement, replacing only a portion of a lymph node, may be seen.

Since the mixed cellularity type occupies an intermediate position between the lymphocyte predominance and the lymphocyte depletion categories, it is not surprising that differentiation of borderline cases may be difficult; in such instances, it is to be expected that the interpretations of different pathologists will disagree, and even that of the same pathologist reviewing the same specimen at a later date may occasionally prove inconsistent (Coppleson et al., 1970).

Lymphocytic Depletion. This rubric brings together the former diffuse fibrosis and reticular types. This was deemed a valid amalgamation because both types are characterized by a profound depletion of lymphocytes and of other reactive stromal

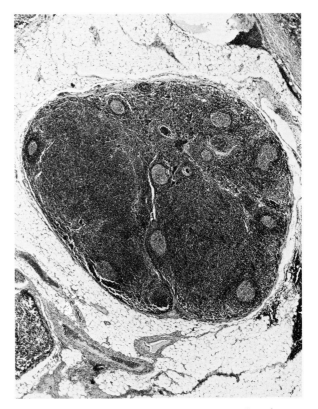

Figure 3.30 "Cellular phase" of nodular sclerosing Hodgkin's disease focally involving a splenic hilar lymph node, with partial preservation of the follicular pattern and nodal architecture. Hyperlobated cells and characteristic Sternberg-Reed cells were seen in lacunae at higher magnification, but there are no collagen bands. Hematoxylin and eosin stain, ×22. (Reprinted, by permission of the authors and the Editor of *Cancer*, from the paper by Kadin, Glatstein, and Dorfman, 1971.)

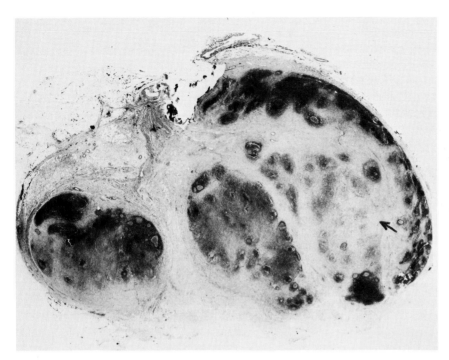

Figure 3.31 Advanced nodular sclerosis in a lymph node. The extent of collagen deposition may be compared with that seen in Figure 3.27. Obliterative fibrosis of the lymphatic nodules has progressed further in some areas than in others; in particular, a large nodule on the right (arrow) has been invaded by blood vessels and later by fibrosis and collagen deposits extending from the periphery, leaving multiple, small fragments of the original nodule. Hematoxylin and eosin stain, ×3. (Reprinted, by permission of the Editor of *Cancer,* from the paper by Keller et al., 1968.)

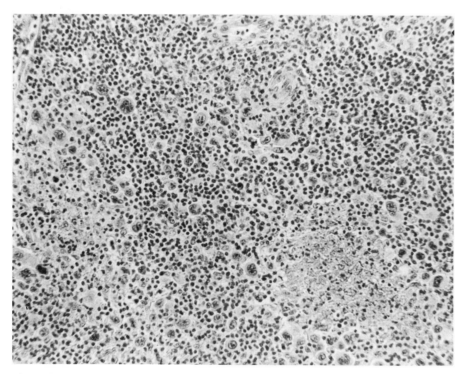

Figure 3.32 Mixed cellularity form of Hodgkin's disease, typical of the majority of cases formerly assigned to the granuloma category of Jackson and Parker. Sternberg-Reed cells are rather abundant, and the stromal elements are pleomorphic. Note the zone of necrosis at the lower right, partially surrounded by Hodgkin's cells. Hematoxylin and eosin stain, ×170.

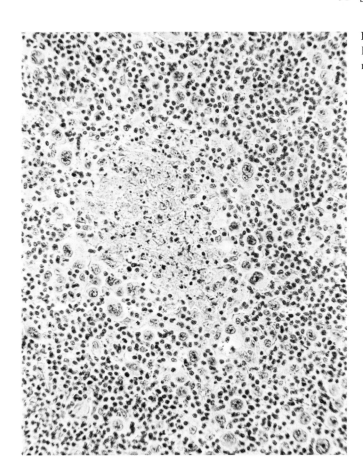

Figure 3.33 Focal necrosis in mixed cellularity Hodgkin's disease. Sternberg-Reed cells are again numerous. Hematoxylin and eosin stain, ×170.

elements. In diffuse fibrosis (Fig. 3.34), a disorderly distribution of reticulin fibers is seen, associated with the deposition of amorphous proteinaceous fibrillar material, which resembles precollagen, but lacks the birefringent character of true collagen. In some instances, cellular fibroblastic proliferation may be seen in association with the amorphous, noncellular material. There are no associated collagen bands. The process is not uniform throughout the lymph node, and small islands of cellular infiltrate may persist which are often predominantly composed of Sternberg-Reed cells. More often, however, such cells are not numerous and may even be difficult to discover, particularly in patients who have had biopsy or come to autopsy after extensive prior chemotherapy and radiotherapy.

The reticular form of lymphocytic depletion (Figs. 3.35, 3.36) is appreciably more cellular, has much less disorderly fibrosis, and is dominated by the presence of numerous Sternberg-Reed cells and the relative depletion of other cellular elements, particularly, as the name implies, of lymphocytes. It includes lesions of the Hodgkin's sarcoma type, in which the Hodgkin's cells are ex-

tremely numerous, pleomorphic, and "malignant-looking," as well as other instances in which an abundant population of more classical Sternberg-Reed cells is associated with stromal cell depletion. Areas of necrosis are commonly found, and a single lymph node may exhibit diffuse fibrosis in one portion and the reticular type of lymphocyte depletion in another, suggesting that the two types are closely related. In a detailed study of 13 cases (10 diffuse fibrosis, 3 reticular), Neiman, Rosen, and Lukes (1973) noted a distinctive clinicopathologic pattern characterized by rapidly progressive disease with fever, bone marrow involvement with pancytopenia and lymphocytopenia, and abnormalities of hepatic function often associated with hepatic, splenic, retroperitoneal node, and other subdiaphragmatic sites of involvement. Paradoxically, six of the cases had no peripheral lymphadenopathy. Survival from the time of initial presentation ranged between 0.5 and 10 months, with a median of only 5.5 months. However, in a later analysis of 39 cases (20 reticular, 19 diffuse fibrosis), 11 patients were found to have survived three years or longer, with a median survival time of 25.1 months in the reticular subtype and 22.4

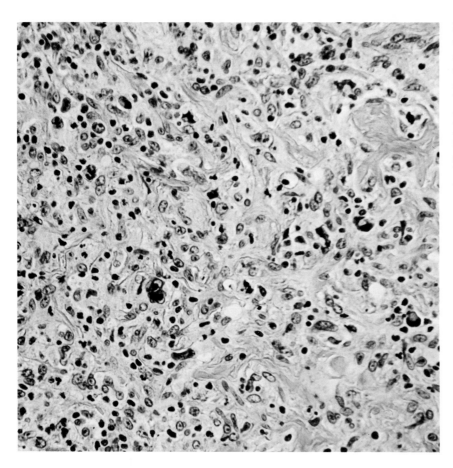

Figure 3.34 Diffuse fibrosis form of the Rye lymphocytic depletion type of Hodgkin's disease. Irregularly arranged, disorderly fibrous deposits (non-birefringent) are evident, and there is a striking paucity of lymphocytes. One binucleate Sternberg-Reed cell is seen slightly to the right of center, but such cells are sparse. Hematoxylin and eosin stain, ×315.

months in the diffuse fibrosis subtype (Bearman, Pangalis, and Rappaport, 1978).

Correlation of Histopathology with Other Parameters. An important indicator of the validity and utility of any histopathologic classification is the degree to which its various subcategories can be shown to exhibit meaningful correlations with other, nonmorphologic features of the disease. In this section, an attempt has been made to summarize much of the published data correlating histopathology with age, sex, anatomic distribution of involved sites, frequency of occurrence of vascular invasion and of noncontiguous dissemination, clinical stage, and prognosis. This subject has also been reviewed by Strum (1973) and by Patchefsky et al. (1973).

Age and Sex. As had already been mentioned in Chapter 2, the data from several countries on age-specific incidence rates for Hodgkin's disease reveal a characteristically bimodal curve, with the first peak in the 15- to 34-year range, followed by a distinct trough, and then a second peak in the group 50 years of age and over. The first peak is a striking and distinctive feature of Hodgkin's disease. Most other types of malignant neoplasms tend to predominate either in the pediatric age group or in middle-aged and elderly individuals, sparing the adolescent and young adult period.

Age-frequency distributions from most reported series of cases of Hodgkin's disease also tend to exhibit peaks in the 20- to 30-year age range, and in the 45- to 55-year group. When cases are classified according to histopathologic type, certain further distinctions in age distribution become apparent.

Jackson and Parker noted that virtually all of their patients with Hodgkin's sarcoma were over 40 years of age, and this is confirmed in the series reported by Hanson (1964), in which the median age of the eight sarcoma patients was 57 years, with only one patient under 45. In contrast, the paragranuloma cases are almost equally distributed across the first seven decades. Thus, it is the large, heterogeneous granuloma category which, though also broadly distributed, is responsible for the two characteristic peaks.

Data on age distribution of cases in which the Rye histopathologic classification was used have been presented by Franssila et al. (1967), Keller,

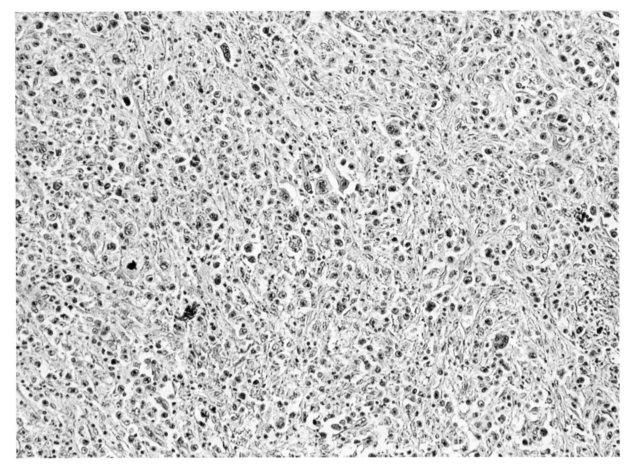

Figure 3.35   Reticular form of the Rye lymphocytic depletion type; this example is also consistent with the sarcoma type of Jackson and Parker. Lymphocytes are sparse, but Sternberg-Reed and other Hodgkin's cells are numerous, often multinucleated, and may exhibit hyperchromatic nuclei and pleomorphism. Hematoxylin and eosin stain, ×320.

Kaplan, Lukes, and Rappaport (1968), Landberg and Larsson (1969), and Dorfman (1971). The age distribution of the four histologic types observed in a series of 179 Stanford cases by Keller et al. may be seen in Figure 3.37. The numerically small lymphocyte predominance and lymphocyte depletion groups appear to be broadly distributed, differing only in the tendency for the lymphocyte predominance group to include cases in the earlier decades of life. There is a striking peak in the 15- to 25-year age range for nodular sclerosis, whereas that for mixed cellularity appears to occur distinctly later, between 25 and 45 years of age.

The data of Franssila et al. reveal essentially similar age frequency distributions for the four categories. The series reported by Landberg and Larsson (1969) is not entirely comparable with the first two series, since it contained a remarkably high proportion (47 of 149, or 31 percent) of patients 60 years of age or more. Nonetheless, the same

tendency for nodular sclerosis cases to be concentrated in the young adult age range is also apparent in this study.

Although males predominate over females in a ratio of approximately 1.5:1 in virtually all large series of cases, this ratio is reversed in the nodular sclerosis category. Representative data on this point from four published studies are summarized in Table 3.4. Three other series (Smetana and Cohen, 1956; Lukes and Butler, 1966; Cross, 1969) are drawn from military populations and are thus not suitable for estimates of sex ratio. Nonetheless, Lukes and Butler were also able to note a predilection for the occurrence of nodular sclerosing Hodgkin's disease in female patients. It is of interest that this reversal of sex ratio in nodular sclerosis is not seen before the age of puberty (Strum and Rappaport, 1970b).

Rather striking differences in the proportion of cases classified as nodular sclerosis are reported by

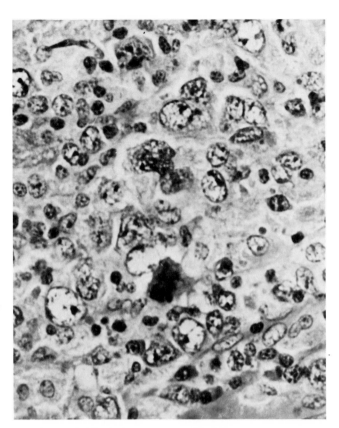

Figure 3.36 Reticular type of lymphocyte depletion Hodgkin's disease. Lymphocytes are sparse, and Hodgkin's cells of widely varying size and morphology predominate. Hematoxylin and eosin stain, ×320. (Reprinted, by permission of the author and the *Journal of Clinical Pathology,* from the paper by Cross, 1969.)

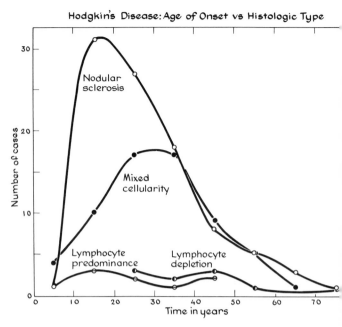

Figure 3.37 Age distribution of Hodgkin's disease by histologic type (Rye classification). (Reprinted, by permission of the Editor of *Cancer,* from the paper by Keller et al., 1968.)

various authors (Table 3.5). These discrepancies may be due in part to lack of comparability among the reported groups with respect to age and sex distribution, ethnic background, and socioeconomic status, but they are almost certainly also due to disagreement concerning histopathologic interpretation among the various pathologists concerned. This was particularly well documented in a detailed analysis of 272 cases of verified Hodgkin's disease from several cities in North America, Europe, and Australia retrospectively reviewed by an

international panel ("the Paris Panel") of expert hematopathologists. They found that the nodular sclerosis (NS) type had been significantly underdiagnosed by the original pathologists (Table 3.6); only 77 (28 percent) of the cases were originally interpreted as NS, but fully 181 (66 percent) were so interpreted by the Paris Panel (Chelloul et al.,

Table 3.4 Proportion of Males to Females in Nodular Sclerosing Hodgkin's Disease

Reference	Males	Females	Male-female ratio
Hanson, 1964	15	22	0.68
Keller et al., 1968	42	50	0.84
Landberg and Larsson, 1969	15	16	0.93
Dorfman, 1971	74	63	1.17

Table 3.5 Relative Frequency of Nodular Sclerosis in Different Series

Author	Number of cases	Cases classified as nodular sclerosis	
		No.	%
Lukes and Butler, 1966	377	149	40
Hanson, 1964	251	37	15
Franssila et al., 1967	97	45	46
Keller et al., 1968	176	92	52
Cross, 1968	242	29	12
Landberg and Larsson, 1969	149	31	21
Wiljasalo, 1969	123	68	55
Johnson et al., 1970	131	52	40
Kadin, Glatstein, & Dorfman, 1971	117	85	73
Chelloul et al., 1972	417	288	69
Kirschner et al., 1974	91	75	83

Table 3.6 Comparison between Original Histologic Diagnosis and That Given by the Paris Panel

Panel	Original diagnosis[a]				
	LP	NS	MC	LD	Total
	65	77	125	5	272
LP	10	1	5	—	16
NS	32	75	74	—	181
MC	23	1	40	2	66
LD	—	—	6	3	9

Source: Data of Chelloul et al. (1972).

[a] LP, lymphocyte predominance; NS, nodular sclerosis; MC, mixed cellularity; LD lymphocyte depletion.

1972). Large series of cases from urban populations in different parts of the world all contained a consistently high proportion of cases of the NS type (Table 3.7). In a study of Hodgkin's disease in Finland, Franssila et al. (1977) found that 53 percent of males and 83 percent of females had NS histology. In contrast, the proportion of cases of this type among the native populations of developing countries is reportedly very much lower (Correa and O'Conor, 1973). A striking example is found in a study of the histologic types of Hodgkin's disease encountered in a series of 227 cases from Nigeria, of which only 10 (4.4 percent) were interpreted as being of the nodular sclerosis type (Edington, Osunkoya, and Hendrickse, 1973).

Anatomic Distribution of Sites of Involvement. Lukes and Butler (1966) noted that their lymphocytic and histiocytic proliferation (Rye lymphocytic predominance) cases tended to involve a single peripheral node or group of nodes, most commonly in the cervical region. In contrast, they stated that "In the nodular sclerosing type, lymph node involvement appears to be limited primarily to an inverted triangular region that includes the anterior-superior mediastinum, the scalene, supraclavicular, and lower cervical regions." In their stage I cases, nodular sclerosing disease was associated with mediastinal involvement fifteen times more often than in all other types combined. Of Hanson's thirty-seven cases of nodular sclerosing Hodgkin's disease, thirty-six (97 percent) had enlargement of cervical lymph nodes, and thirty-two (87 percent) had radiographic evidence of mediastinal lymphadenopathy. Hanson also stated that "at onset, there was no extension of the disease below the thorax in any patient with nodular sclerosing Hodgkin's disease."

However, diagnostic evaluation of the extent of disease in these two series did not include either lymphangiography or staging laparotomy and biopsy. As will be discussed in detail in Chapter 4, these two diagnostic procedures have revealed Hodgkin's disease in the retroperitoneal nodes, spleen, splenic hilar nodes, and less often the liver, in a very high proportion of instances. It is now clear that, although nodular sclerosing Hodgkin's disease often does indeed tend to involve the mediastinum, involvement is by no means confined to structures above the diaphragm when a more complete and meticulous diagnostic evaluation is routinely carried out.

At Stanford University Medical Center, where the procedure of routine staging laparotomy, splenectomy, and biopsy was first introduced, data on a large number of cases with respect to the correlation between histopathologic type and sites of

Table 3.7 Relative Frequency of Nodular Sclerosing (NS) Hodgkin's Disease in Different Parts of the World

Country	City	Total no. classified	No. with NS type	Percentage of NS type
U.S.A.	Los Angeles	8	4	50
U.K.	London	59	35	59
	Manchester	26	17	65
France	Paris	84	54	62
Switzerland	Geneva	26	18	69
Norway	Oslo	49	33	70
Denmark	Aarhus	54	37	70
Holland	Leiden	25	18	72
Canada	Hamilton	28	23	82
Australia	Melbourne	58	49	85
Totals		417	288	69

Source: Slightly modified from the data of Chelloul et al. (1972).

subdiaphragmatic involvement have now been compiled by Kadin, Glatstein, and Dorfman (1971) and by Dorfman (1971). As may be seen in Tables 3.8 and 3.9, nodular sclerosis was the single most common type of lesion encountered in the spleen and retroperitoneal nodes, although the proportion of all nodular sclerosis cases in which intra-abdominal involvement was demonstrated was significantly smaller than that observed in lymphocyte predominance or mixed cellularity.

In a number of instances in which nodular sclerosis was observed in the initial peripheral node or mediastinal biopsy, the pattern observed in the spleen and splenic hilar nodes revealed neither the collagenous bands nor the distinctive "lacunar"

Hodgkin's cell on which the diagnosis of the nodular sclerosing type depends (Fig. 3.38). In other instances, however, the histologic appearance in the splenic nodules and/or splenic hilar nodes was essentially indistinguishable from that in the original biopsy.

The mixed cellularity and lymphocyte depletion types are seldom localized to a single site or region at the time of biopsy. Instead, they are likely to be widespread within the lymphatic system, with a propensity for retroperitoneal node involvement. Moreover, as noted by Keller et al. (1968), they exhibit a significantly greater likelihood of involvement of extralymphatic organs and tissues (cf. Chapter 7). The high incidence of hepatosplenic

Table 3.8 Anatomic Distribution and Type of Hodgkin's Disease Occurring below the Diaphragm in 51 Untreated Patients

	Lymphocyte predominance	Nodular sclerosis	Mixed cellularity	Lymphocyte depletion	Unclassified	Total
Spleen (117)[a]	2	27	12	0	3	44
Accessory spleen (8)	0	1	0	0	0	1
Splenic hilar lymph nodes (17)	1	6	2	1	1	11
Para-aortic lymph nodes (115)	3	21	5	0	0	29
Mesenteric lymph nodes (25)	1	0	0	0	0	1
Liver (117)	0	0	0	0	9	9
Bone marrow (117)	0	0	0	0	4	4

Source: Data of Kadin, Glatstein, and Dorfman (1971).
[a]Numbers in parentheses = total number of specimens examined.

Table 3.9 Mediastinal and Abdominal Involvement by Histologic Type of Initial Biopsy

Histologic type	Involvement				
	Mediastinal[a]	Abdominal[b]	Abdominal and mediastinal	Peripheral lymphadenopathy only	Total
Nodular sclerosis	48	12	21	4	85
Mixed cellularity	3	8	4	4	19
Lymphocyte predominance	0	6	0	7	13
Lymphocyte depletion	0	0	0	0	0
Total	51	26	25	15	117

Source: Data of Kadin, Glatstein, and Dorfman (1971).
[a]Without abdominal disease.
[b]Without mediastinal disease.

and bone marrow involvement and the paradoxical paucity of peripheral lymphadenopathy in the lymphocyte depletion type have been previously mentioned (Neiman, Rosen, and Lukes, 1973). Lukes and Butler (1966) suggested that host-resistance factors ("state of the host") may be the common denominator between histopathologic type and clinical extent of disease. It is likely that a more definitive picture of the relative frequency of involvement of various anatomic sites by the different histopathologic types will emerge as additional centers report large series of cases in which cases have been classified according to the Rye criteria and staged routinely with the aid of lymphangiography and laparotomy with splenectomy and biopsy. For the present, however, the most complete data available are those drawn from the Stanford experience (Fig. 3.39); these are also discussed and analyzed in Chapter 7.

Clinical Stage. The evolution of clinical stages from the three-stage classification originally proposed by Peters (1950) is detailed in Chapter 8. There is little doubt that a correlation exists between histopathologic type and the extent of disease at the time of initial diagnostic evaluation. Differences observed among the various reported series are in part attributable to differences in staging procedures and in part to differences in the age and sex distribution of the population sampled.

Lukes and Butler (1966) related histopathologic type to the three-stage Peters clinical classification (cf. Chapter 8). Approximately 70 percent of their lymphocytic and histiocytic proliferation (lymphocytic predominance) cases were of stage I extent; nodular sclerosis and mixed cellularity cases were

about evenly distributed among the three stages, and there was a clear predominance of stage III cases in the diffuse fibrosis and reticular groups. Essentially the same findings were reported by Landberg and Larsson (1969), with the exception that a smaller proportion of nodular sclerosis and mixed cellularity cases were limited to stage I extent, and a higher overall proportion of their cases were in stage III, perhaps reflecting the considerably greater proportion of patients in this series (31 percent) who were over 60 years of age.

Keller et al. (1968) correlated the Rye histopathologic classification with the Rye four-stage clinical classification (cf. Chapter 8), as well as with the frequency of systemic symptoms, in a series of 179 cases, most of which had been staged with the aid of lymphangiography, with the results given in Table 3.10. More recently a series of our cases routinely evaluated with the aid of lymphangiography and laparotomy with splenectomy and biopsy and staged according to the Ann Arbor clinical classification proposed by Carbone et al. (1971; cf. Chapter 8) has been analyzed in relation to the Rye histopathologic type observed in the original biopsy. These data are summarized in Table 3.11.

The general tendency for lymphocyte predominance to be limited to stage I in a considerable proportion of all cases is again evident, as is the relatively high proportion of nodular sclerosis cases limited to stage II. As might have been anticipated, however, with increasingly elaborate diagnostic evaluation there has been a reallocation of a significant proportion of cases to stages II$_E$, III, and IV, as otherwise occult disease has been discovered below the diaphragm and in extralymphatic sites. Essentially similar findings emerged from a study

Table 3.10 Distribution of Histologic Types According to Anatomic Stage and Systemic Symptoms

Histopathologic type (Rye)	Anatomic stage (Rye)				Systemic symptoms			
	I and II		III and IV		Absent (A)		Present (B)	
	No.	%	No.	%	No.	%	No.	%
Lymphocytic predominance	8	89	1	11	9	100	0	—
Nodular sclerosis	63	69	29	31	60	65	32	35
Mixed cellularity	37	57	28	43	35	54	30	46
Lymphocytic depletion	3	30	7	70	3	30	7	70

Source: Modified from Keller, Kaplan, Lukes, and Rappaport (1968).

Table 3.11 Hodgkin's Disease: Ann Arbor Clinical Stage (Carbone et al., 1971) versus Rye Histopathologic Type

Clinical stage	Histologic type					Totals
	Lymphocytic predominance	Nodular sclerosis	Mixed cellularity	Lymphocytic depletion	Unclassified or unknown	
I	6	8	1	1	0	16
I_E	0	0	0	0	0	0
All Stage I	6	8	1	1	0	16
II	10	47	8	0	3	68
II_E	0	12	0	0	0	12
All Stage II	10	59	8	0	3	80
III	3	4	1	0	0	8
III_E	0	1	0	0	0	1
III_S	1	28	12	1	2	44
III_{ES}	0	6	0	0	0	6
All Stage III	4	39	13	1	2	59
IV	0	20	4	0	1	25
All Stage IV	0	20	4	0	1	25
TOTALS:	20(7.8%)	126 (70%)	26 (14.4%)	2	6	180

Source: Stanford University Medical Center data; based in part on the study by Kadin, Glatstein, and Dorfman (1971). All of these patients were previously untreated and were staged with the aid of lymphangiography, laparotomy, and splenectomy.

by Berard et al. (1971) of a series of 191 patients seen at the National Cancer Institute between 1964 and 1968. Of 34 cases classified as lymphocyte predominance, 15 (44 percent) had stage I, and 10 (29 percent) had stage II disease. In the nodular sclerosis group, 43 of 65 cases (66 percent) were in stage II. The mixed cellularity type was more uniformly distributed by stage, with 30 of 62 cases (49 percent) in stages III and IV. Finally, fully half (13 of 26) of the lymphocyte depletion cases were in stage IV.

Noncontiguous Dissemination, Extralymphatic Relapse, and Vascular Invasion. The manner of spread of Hodgkin's disease is a complex subject, which is discussed in detail in Chapter 7. Systematic mapping of involved lymphatic and extralymphatic sites, both at the time of initial diagnostic evaluation and at the time of first relapse, has suggested that the great majority of cases of Hodgkin's disease spread contiguously from one chain of lymph nodes to others with which direct connections via lymphatic channels exist. Noncontiguous spread, including dissemination to extralymphatic sites such as the liver or bone marrow, has been seen initially in only some 10 percent of our total series of cases (Kaplan, 1962; Rosenberg and Kaplan, 1966; Kaplan, 1970).

Keller et al. (1968) analyzed the relationship between the Rye histopathologic types and the frequency of noncontiguous spread. At the time of initial staging, 26 of 176 cases showed noncontiguous spread, 17 within the lymphatic system and 9 to extralymphatic sites such as the liver or marrow. Eighteen of these 26 instances were scored as mixed cellularity or lymphocytic depletion type. Similarly, when the first site of extension of disease after completion of the initial course of treatment was considered, noncontiguous distributions were observed in 19 of 75 cases, of which 12 were of the mixed cellularity or lymphocyte depletion types. When these figures were related to the numbers of cases of each histologic type at risk, it was apparent that noncontiguous spread occurred about 2.5 times more often in mixed cellularity and lymphocytic depletion than in lymphocytic predominance and nodular sclerosis.

The frequency of noncontiguous spread, as manifested in extralymphatic sites of initial relapse, has also been analyzed by Johnson, Thomas, and Chretien (1970) in a series of 151 consecutive patients with Hodgkin's disease routinely evaluated and staged with the aid of lymphangiography and initially treated with radiotherapy. Of a total of 35 relapses, 15 occurred in extralymphatic sites (bone, 6; liver, 6; lung, 2; and pericardium, 1). There was again a strong indication that extralymphatic spread had occurred preferentially in the

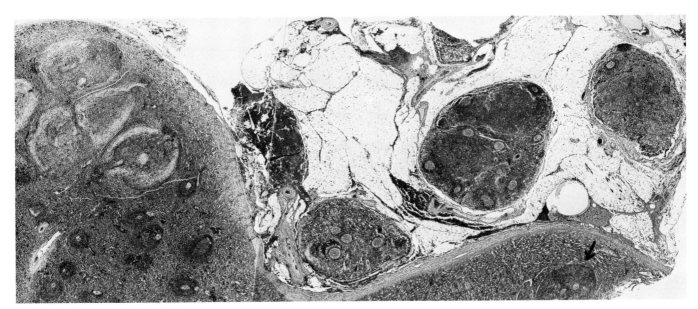

Figure 3.38 Focal involvement of the spleen and three splenic hilar lymph nodes by nodular sclerosing Hodgkin's disease. Sclerosis is prominent around the splenic nodules at upper left, but is absent in the splenic lesion at lower right (arrow) and in the lymph nodes. The latter show varying degrees of involvement and of retention of the normal follicular pattern. Hematoxylin and eosin stain, ×9. (Reprinted, by permission of the authors and the Editor of *Cancer,* from the paper by Kadin, Glatstein, and Dorfman, 1971.)

mixed cellularity and lymphocytic depletion types, particularly in those instances in which constitutional symptoms such as fever, night sweats, and/or generalized pruritus had been present initially (Table 3.12).

The occurrence of vascular invasion in Hodgkin's disease was first described many years ago by Dorothy Reed (1902) and has been noted intermit-

tently since that time (Rappaport, 1966). Its potential significance in relationship to the spread of the disease has been emphasized by Rappaport and Strum (1970); Strum, Allen, and Rappaport (1971); and Strum (1973). Employing paraffin sections stained for elastica by Weigert's method, they made a systematic search for vascular involvement in biopsy specimens from 100 randomly selected

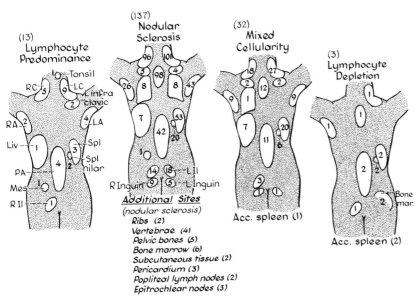

Figure 3.39 Anatomic distribution of lesions by histopathologic type, based on the composite evidence provided by physical examination, radiography, and pathologic findings in biopsy and laparotomy specimens. Numerals indicate the number of cases of each histologic type in which the indicated lymph node chain, organ, or tissue was involved. RC, LC = right and left cervical-supraclavicular nodes; RIl, LIl = right and left iliac nodes; RA = right axillary node; LA = left axillary node; PA = paraaortic node; Mes. = mesenteric node; Spl = spleen; Liv = liver. (Reprinted, by permission of the author and the Editor of *Cancer Research,* from the paper by Dorfman, 1971.)

Table 3.12 Extranodal Relapse after Primary Treatment of Hodgkin's Disease versus Histopathologic Type, Anatomic Extent, and Systemic Symptoms

Histopathologic type (Rye)	Anatomical stage (Rye)		Systemic symptoms	
	I and II	III	Absent (A)	Present (B)
Lymphocytic predominance	0/30[a]	0/4	0/29	0/5
Nodular sclerosis	4/45	0/7	2/39	2/13
Mixed cellularity	4/28	3/6	2/21	5/13
Lymphocytic depletion	2/7	2/4	1/6	3/5
Total	10/110	5/21	5/95	10/36

Source: Modified from Johnson, Thomas, and Chretien (1970).
[a]Number of extranodal relapses/number of cases at risk.

cases of Hodgkin's disease, and discovered ten instances of blood vessel invasion (Figs. 3.40, 3.41).

It is perhaps more than an interesting coincidence that they observed vascular invasion in their random sample in the same proportion of cases (10 percent) as was observed to exhibit noncontiguous initial sites of involvement in another series (Kaplan, 1970). Retrospective studies have yielded con-

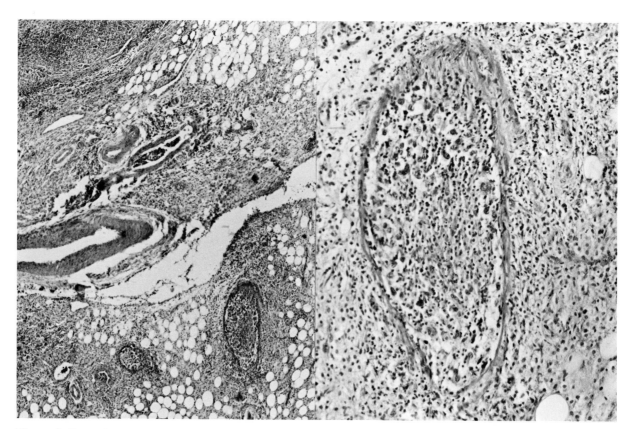

Figure 3.40 *Left,* pericapsular fat tissue surrounding a lymph node showing Hodgkin's disease. The intravascular presence of Hodgkin's tissue is readily evident in this routinely stained section. Both involved vessels are veins. Hematoxylin and eosin stain, ×35. *Right,* higher magnification of the larger of two involved vessels. Hematoxylin and eosin stain, ×125. (Reprinted, by permission of the authors and the Editor of *Cancer,* from the paper by Rappaport and Strum, 1970.)

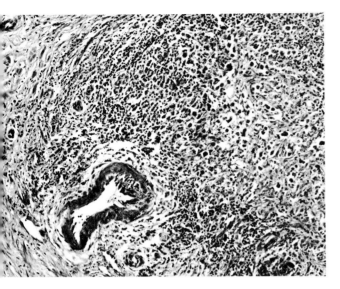

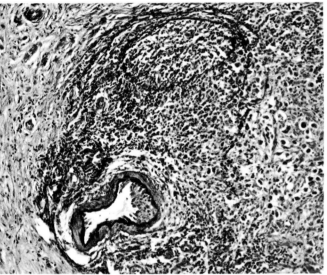

Figure 3.41 *Top,* nodular sclerosing Hodgkin's disease in a lymph node biopsy. Note the artery to the left of center; the outline of the accompanying vein, almost obliterated by invading Hodgkin's tissue, is not recognizable in this hematoxylin and eosin preparation, but is revealed by the Weigert elastica stain (*bottom*). Some of the elastic fibers have been spread apart. × 160. (Reprinted, by permission of the authors and the Editor of *Cancer,* from the paper by Strum, Hutchison, Park, and Ráppaport, 1971.)

flicting evidence on this point. Lamoureux et al. (1973) found no evidence of vascular invasion in a reexamination, with special stains, of the original node biopsies of 12 patients (of a series of 136) with initial stage I or II disease in whom extranodal dissemination had occurred. A review of 89 lymph node biopsies from 71 patients with Hodgkin's disease of all stages, and of other tissues of 19

of these patients who later came to autopsy, revealed a much higher frequency of vascular invasion in the autopsy material (79 percent) as compared with the original biopsies (19 percent), suggesting that vascular invasion is more likely to occur as the disease progresses (Naeim, Waisman, and Coulson, 1974). An indication that vascular invasion in the spleen, rather than in lymph nodes, may be important with respect to dissemination and survival emerged from a study by Kirschner et al. (1974). Whereas vascular invasion in lymph nodes, encountered in 4 (4.4 percent) of 91 lymph node biopsies, was not associated with extranodal dissemination, vascular invasion in the spleen, detected in 7 (16 percent) of 44 spleens removed at laparotomy, was often associated with spread to the liver and bone marrow, and with a grave prognosis. Strum (1973) also noted that all patients with definite or suspicious vascular invasion in the spleen had proven involvement of the liver. Additional data are needed from systematic surveys of this type in a number of other major centers, since the interrelationships among vascular invasion, noncontiguous spread, and extralymphatic relapse may well have important implications at the therapeutic level.

The relationship between histologic type and the occurrence of vascular invasion observed in the random-sample study by Rappaport and Strum (1970) is summarized in Table 3.13. Subsequent observations, including an updated analysis by Strum (1973), have been in good general agreement with the original data. Naeim, Waisman, and Coulson (1974) found vascular invasion in 4 of 7 lymph node biopsies (57 percent) with lymphocyte

Table 3.13 Vascular Invasion versus Histopathologic Type

Histopathologic type (Rye)	Number of cases in random sample	Vascular invasion	
		No.	%
Lymphocytic predominance	6	0	—
Nodular sclerosis	38	3	7.9
Mixed cellularity	39	1	2.6
Lymphocytic depletion	14	6	42.8
Unclassifiable	3	0	—
Totals	100	10	10.0

Source: Modified from data of Rappaport and Strum (1970).

depletion histology, 6 of 23 (26 percent) with mixed cellularity, 2 of 41 (4.8 percent) with nodular sclerosis, and 0 of 6 with lymphocyte predominance. The 7 instances of vascular invasion encountered by Kirschner et al. (1974) in 44 involved spleens were distributed as follows: lymphocyte depletion, 2 of 3; mixed cellularity, 2 of 10; and nodular sclerosis, 3 of 31. Thus, although the risk of vascular invasion is clearly highest in lymphocyte depletion, it is by no means limited to this histopathologic type.

Prognosis. Inasmuch as prognosis was one of the criteria utilized in the construction of each of the histopathologic classifications, it is not surprising that all of them correlate to some extent with prognosis. Representative five-year survival data for each of the various classifications are summarized in Table 3.14. The relationship between prognosis and histopathologic type is also evident in survival curves (Fig. 3.42), such as those published by Hanson (1964), Franssila et al. (1967), Keller et al. (1968), Landberg and Larsson (1969), and Kaplan (1973, 1976). Although the data of Kaplan (1976) presented in Table 3.14 clearly indicate the dramatic improvement in overall prognosis that has occurred during the past several years, relative differences in prognosis still persist. Glatstein (1974) has pointed out that the prognostic importance of histopathologic type is decreasing as overall prognosis improves. Consistent with this view, Fuller et al. (1977) found that histopathologic type had little influence on prognosis in laparotomy-negative patients with stage I and II disease. Additional, recent data bearing on this point are presented in Chapter 12.

Data on median survival time in cases classified according to the Jackson-Parker and the Lukes-Butler histopathologic classifications have been presented by Lukes and Butler (1966) and by Dalla Pria (1967). These data clearly indicate that one of the important byproducts of the recognition by Lukes et al. (1963, 1966) of the nodular sclerosis category was the extraction of this relatively favorable group of cases from the larger, much more heterogeneous, and less prognostically favorable granuloma category. This is well brought out by the data presented by Hanson (1964). In his entire granuloma group, there were 65 five-year survivors among 176 cases (37 percent), but the nodular sclerosing subgroup (23 cases) accounted for 20 of these survivors (87 percent); these differences are maintained at ten years (Table 3.15).

Since histopathologic type and clinical stage are mutually interdependent, the question has been raised whether histopathologic type is correlated with prognosis directly or whether this correlation is merely a secondary consequence of the relationship with clinical stage, which has long been known to be closely correlated with prognosis. This question is answered in part by the data analyzed by Keller et al. (1968), who found a distinct difference in prognosis by histologic type when only anatomic stage I and stage II cases were considered (Fig. 3.43). These data strongly suggest that histopathologic type influences prognosis independently of the anatomic extent of disease, despite the fact that these two parameters are mutually interdependent.

Variability and Progression of Histopathologic Type. Custer and Bernhard (1948) claimed that transitions occur not infrequently among the different types of malignant lymphoma. Specifically, they reported instances in which patients with initial biopsies interpreted as follicular (nodular) lymphoma came to autopsy with typical disseminated Hodgkin's granuloma and, conversely, instances of Hodgkin's disease that apparently underwent transition to reticulum cell sarcoma.

This challenge to the theory of the histogenetic unity of the malignant lymphomas has been criticized by Rappaport (1966). He pointed out that, in all probability, some of the patients initially given a diagnosis of follicular lymphoma or lymphocytic lymphosarcoma and dying with disseminated Hodgkin's disease in reality had Hodgkin's disease of the nodular or diffuse lymphocytic predominance type, in which Sternberg-Reed cells were so sparse as to have been undetected in the section on which the original diagnosis was made. If Rappaport's interpretation is correct, as seems likely, these instances would represent progression from one histopathologic type of Hodgkin's disease to another, rather than a major transition from one type of malignant lymphoma to another. Rappaport concludes that "no evidence is available that the occasional coexistence of these types of malignant lymphomas is more than a coincidence."

On the other hand, he considers the transition of one variant of Hodgkin's disease into another as part of the "natural and expected evolution of these lymphomas." This view is also upheld by Lukes and Butler (1966), who concluded that "a lymphocytic proliferation, associated with small numbers of histiocytes and Reed-Sternberg cells, may be the initial manifestation of Hodgkin's disease as Stage I disease. It may persist for a variable period of time, possibly depending upon the effectiveness of the lymphocytic proliferation . . . The appearance of eosinophils, noncollagenous connective tissue, and increased numbers of Reed-Sternberg cells presents the features of the lesion designated the mixed type, which appears to herald the onset of a changing host response and the beginning of disseminated disease . . . The next phase in the evolution of the histologic process appears to be the depletion of lymphocytes, which may occur at varying rates and is associated with either the appearance of diffuse fibrosis or marked increase in the number of Reed-Sternberg cells." They regard the nodular sclerosing type of Hodgkin's disease as a separate problem and consider that its evolution is still not clearly established, although "the natural tendency of the nodules to undergo sclerosis is readily apparent. The individual

Table 3.14 Survival versus Histopathologic Type in Hodgkin's Disease

Reference	No. of 5-year survivors/ total no. of patients	Percent
A. Jackson and Parker Classification		
Jackson and Parker (1947)		
Paragranuloma	15/28	53
Granuloma	18/136	13
Sarcoma	0/32	0
Smetana and Cohen (1956)		
Paragranuloma	27/35	77
Granuloma	84/308	27
Sarcoma	0/5	0
Wright (1960)		
Paragranuloma	18/19	95
Granuloma	43/157	27
Sarcoma	1/10	10
Hanson (1964)		
Paragranuloma	15/16	94
Granuloma	65/176	37
Sarcoma	0/8	0
B. Rye Classification[a]		
Franssila et al. (1967)		
LP	5/9	55
NS	21/45	47
MC	1/32	3
LD	0/11	0
Landberg and Larsson (1969)		
LP	9/18	50
NS	17/31	55
MC	17/80	21
LD	1/20	5
Gough (1970)		
LP		58
NS		45
MC		18
LD		8
Kaplan (1976)		
LP		90
NS		87
MC		71
LD		45

[a] LP = Lymphocytic predominance
NS = Nodular sclerosis
MC = Mixed cellularity
LD = Lymphocytic depletion

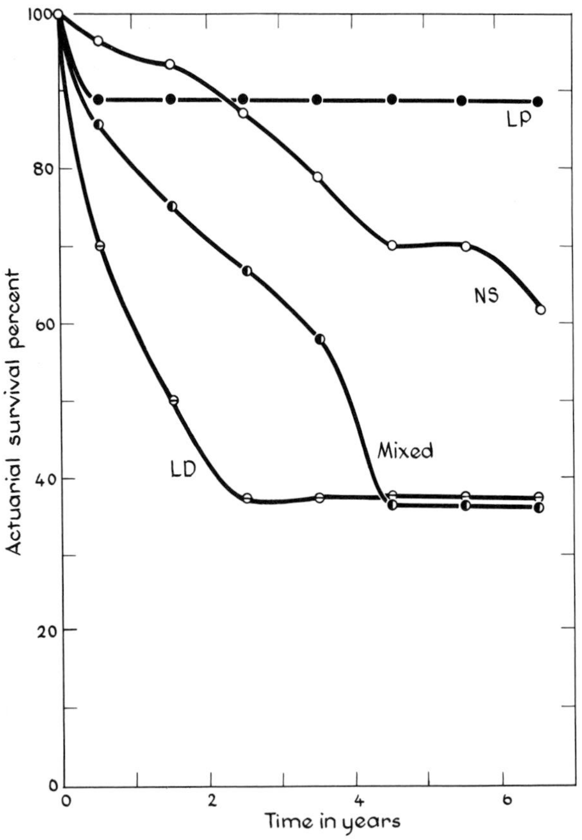

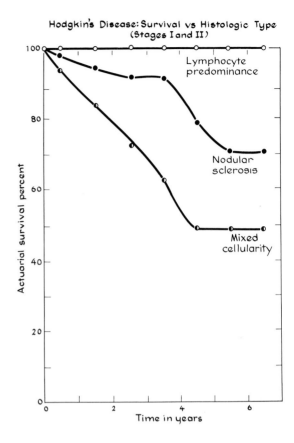

Figure 3.42   Actuarial survival in 176 cases of Hodgkin's disease according to histologic type (Rye classification; LP = lymphocytic predominance; NS = nodular sclerosis; MC = mixed cellularity; LD = lymphocytic depletion). The survival of the nodular sclerosis and mixed cellularity groups at five years is significantly different (p < .02). (Reprinted with slight modifications, by permission of the Editor of *Cancer,* from the paper by Keller et al., 1968.)

Figure 3.43   Actuarial survival in 111 cases of Hodgkin's disease first seen with Rye stage I or II disease, according to histologic type (Rye classification). The lymphocytic depletion group is omitted, since it comprised only three cases, with one death. The survival of the nodular sclerosis and mixed cellularity groups is significantly different at three years (p < .02). (Reprinted, by permission of the Editor of *Cancer,* from the paper by Keller et al., 1968.)

nodules appear to evolve from a predominantly lymphocytic proliferation with distinctive, abnormal reticulum cells scattered through the central portion of the nodules to total sclerosis that is almost completely devoid of cellularity. The initial modification of the cellular nodule begins with the occurrence of proliferating vessels from the periphery of the nodules, associated with gradual loss of lymphocytes, often in association with infiltration of numerous mature granulocytes and marked increase in abnormal reticulum cells."

It may also be asked whether Hodgkin's disease necessarily progresses at the same rate in different lesions in various parts of the body. If not, it would be expected that biopsies from lymph nodes in different areas would reveal different histologic patterns with considerable frequency. Moreover, if the histologic type in any given lymph node re-

mains reasonably constant, then the most extensive lesions would be expected to reflect the earlier histologic patterns, whereas microscopic degrees of involvement in other areas might reflect early transitions to more advanced patterns. In a detailed study of sequential biopsy material, Strum and Rappaport (1971a) found that the histologic subtypes of Hodgkin's disease tend to remain constant over long periods of observation in the great majority of cases. Concordance of early and later histologies was observed in 50 (82 percent) of 61 patients who had two lymph node biopsies and in 12 (75 percent) of 16 patients with three or more biopsies. Constancy of type was highest in nodular sclerosis (51 of 55, or 93 percent), intermediate in mixed cellularity (5 of 7, or 71 percent), and least in lymphocyte predominance (5 of 13, or 38 percent). Progression, when it occurred, was almost al-

Table 3.15 Differences in Prognosis of Nodular Sclerosis and Remainder of Granuloma Category

Histopathologic type	No. of 5-year survivors/ total no. of patients (%)	No. of 10-year survivors/ total no. of patients (%)
Nodular sclerosis	20/23 (87)	9/16 (56)
Remainder of granuloma category	45/153 (29)	10/143 (7)
Total granuloma category	65/176 (37)	19/159 (12)

Source: Data of Hanson (1964).

ways toward a prognostically more unfavorable histopathologic type. Thus this definitive study provides no support for the view that nodes showing more than one histologic type can often be found in the same patient.

As a consequence of the routine utilization of laparotomy with splenectomy and biopsy at Stanford University Medical Center, additional histologic material from a series of 185 cases has become available for comparison with the original biopsies (Kadin et al., 1971; Dorfman, 1971). In 82 (95 percent) of 86 instances in which involvement in the abdomen was documented, the same histopathologic type was observed in both the initial peripheral node biopsy and the subdiaphragmatic lesions. However, Farrer-Brown et al. (1971) reported discordant histologic types in the original biopsy and the spleen in 55 percent of their laparotomy series. Where transitions were observed, the more aggressive histopathologic types were usually encountered in the intra-abdominal sites, suggesting that these either had occurred later in time or had progressed at a more rapid rate than those in the peripheral nodes.

Special Topics

Histogenesis of Hodgkin's Disease. Many pathologists have had the experience of examining lymph node biopsies which revealed gross distortion of architecture and a diffuse proliferation of lymphocytes or histiocytes but in which no Sternberg-Reed cells could be detected, even on multiple sections. It has not been at all uncommon for the same patient to be seen later with new lymphadenopathy, biopsy of which has revealed Hodgkin's disease. No clear link has yet been established between the initial seemingly benign lymph node enlargement, to which the name "reactive hyperplasia" is usually given, and the subsequent overt lymphogranulomatous process. If "reactive hyperplasia" is indeed a preoplastic, prodromal form of Hodgkin's dis-

ease in certain instances, it would constitute a formidable challenge to the pathologist, since there is seemingly no morphologic distinction between this type of "reactive hyperplasia" and that which occurs in a variety of nonspecific inflammatory states (Dawson, Cooper, and Rambo, 1964).

Lennert (1958) studied biopsy materials submitted over a period of six years with the particular aim of establishing a distinction between nonspecific inflammatory conditions and the earliest stages of development of Hodgkin's disease in lymph nodes. He concluded that among the very earliest changes indicative of Hodgkin's disease is a "reticulocytosis", involving proliferation and change in morphology of the preexistent normal reticular cells toward the appearance observed in instances of paragranuloma. This process seemed to originate principally in the pulp and perivascularly, rather than in the sinuses or germinal centers of the lymph node. Epithelioid cell (histiocyte) proliferation was observed in 71 percent of his paragranuloma cases, in which lymphatic hyperplasia was also a prominent feature. He considered the presence of an unusual abundance of eosinophilic granulocytes strongly suspicious in early borderline cases. Plasma cell hyperplasia was also a contributory early feature in the presence of reticulum cell proliferation but was not considered by Lennert to be diagnostically significant by itself. Finally, he considered perilymphadenitis a suspicious sign when it was associated with localized occurrence of large reticular cells and eosinophilic infiltrate.

Strum and Rappaport (1970a) have recently called attention to the significance of focal involvement of lymph nodes in the diagnosis and staging of Hodgkin's disease. They observed six cases in which there was only minute focal involvement in lymph nodes, with the rest of the lymph node architecture essentially normally preserved. They stressed the importance of cutting multiple "semiserial" sections to detect the diagnostic foci.

Elsewhere in the same lymph nodes, the observation of focal obliteration of subcapsular sinuses, foci of inflammatory cells, atypical "malignant-appearing" histiocytes, and/or increased deposition of collagen should, in their view, alert the pathologist to search with particular care in the remaining tissue from a lymph node biopsy. Since most of their patients had disseminated involvement in other sites, focal involvement of this type in a lymph node is not necessarily an indication of early localized disease but may instead provide some indication of the earliest changes in lymph nodes to which the disease has only recently metastasized. Similar observations have been made by Kadin, Glatstein, and Dorfman (1971) and Henry (1971).

Thymus. Thomson (1955) suggested that Hodgkin's disease arises as an epithelial neoplasm of the thymus and disseminates secondarily to lymph nodes. This view was later refuted by Marshall and Wood (1957), who found gross thymic lesions in only 26 percent of 86 patients with terminal Hodgkin's disease, and by Patey (1963), who performed thymectomies on five patients and found histologic evidence of Hodgkin's disease in only two of the five resected thymic specimens. Nonetheless, peculiar lesions of the thymus, to which some pathologists (Lowenhaupt and Brown, 1951; Lattes, 1962) have variously referred as "granulomatous thymoma" or "mixed tumors of the thymus," have long been recognized. Castleman (1955), in his fascicle on tumors of the thymus gland, argued that these lesions represent Hodgkin's disease of the thymus. This view has received strong support from Katz

and Lattes (1969), in a review of twenty-four cases, and Fechner (1969), who studied an additional three cases. In these instances, the presenting lesion involved the thymus (Fig. 3.44) but not the mediastinal or peripheral lymph nodes, and the histologic pattern was generally similar to that of the nodular sclerosing form of Hodgkin's disease (Fig. 3.45). Sternberg-Reed cells were often extremely sparse and frequently atypical (Fig. 3.46). Hassall's corpuscles were often observed in the centers of the nodular sclerosing lymphatic nodules. Sheets of squamous-like epithelioid cells and cystic structures lined with columnar cells, presumably derived from thymus epithelium, were also sometimes seen (Fig. 3.45).

Spleen and Splenic Hilar Nodes. The frequent occurrence of Hodgkin's disease in spleens of normal weight and size (Fig. 3.47) is probably the most striking discovery emerging from the routine utilization of staging laparotomy with splenectomy and biopsy (Glatstein et al., 1969, 1970; Enright et al., 1970). Instances have now been observed in which minute, focal lesions were present in the spleen. The smallest lesions encountered were only 1 to 3 mm. in diameter. Such lesions, which were confined to the white pulp, were comprised of a mixture of lymphocytes, variable numbers of atypical histiocytes, and at least one diagnostic Sternberg-Reed cell. Larger, grossly visible nodules extended to involve the red pulp. The presence of such nodules in considerable numbers was sometimes consistent with spleens of grossly normal size (Fig. 3.48).

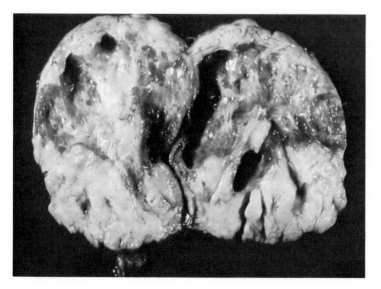

Figure 3.44 Gross specimen of thymic tumor mass containing multiple cystic spaces. The histologic pattern was typical of nodular sclerosing Hodgkin's disease; such lesions were formerly erroneously designated "granulomatous thymomas."

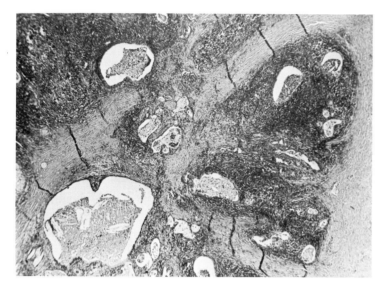

Figure 3.45 Thymus involved by nodular sclerosing Hodgkin's disease. Note how the lymphatic tissue is carved up into nodules and islands by bands of dense collagenous connective tissue. The epithelial-lined cystic structures are a distinctive feature of such lesions when they occur in the thymus. Hematoxylin and eosin stain, × 36. (Reprinted, by permission of the authors and the Editor of *Cancer,* from the paper by Katz and Lattes, 1969.)

In a series of 185 patients subjected to laparotomy with splenectomy and biopsy, involvement of the spleen was documented in 78 instances, of which 53 showed the nodular sclerosing pattern (Kadin, Glatstein, and Dorfman, 1971; Dorfman, 1971). The degree of sclerosis varied considerably in the spleen specimens studied by Kadin, Glatstein, and Dorfman (1971). Sclerosis was visible to the naked eye in 12, but was seen only on microscopic examination in 11; 4 others had no fibrosis but were classified in the nodular sclerosis group on the basis of the concept of a "cellular phase" of this lesion, characterized principally by the presence of the atypical lacunar type of Hodgkin's cell (Fig. 3.2). Splenic hilar node involvement without spleen involvement was noted in 4 of 185 cases (Dorfman, 1971); the overall frequency of splenic

hilar node disease in this study was 31 of 185 (16.7 percent).

Liver. Although gross involvement of the liver is common in the later stages of Hodgkin's disease and at autopsy, microscopic evidence of liver involvement was detected in only 9 of 117 patients subjected to needle and wedge biopsy of the liver during staging laparotomy (Kadin et al., 1971). The observed foci were usually too small to permit histopathologic classification according to the Rye categories (Fig. 3.49). However, in two subsequent instances nodules in the liver have been of sufficient size to permit recognition of the nodular sclerosis pattern. The incidence of liver involvement in other laparotomy series has ranged from 5 to 11 percent (Bagley et al., 1972; Dorfman, 1971;

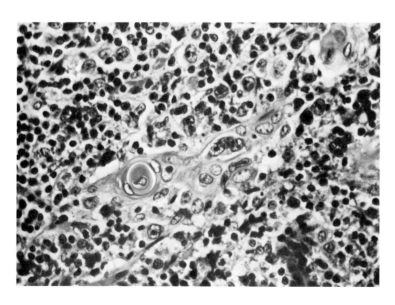

Figure 3.46 Higher magnification of such a lesion, showing atypical Sternberg-Reed-like cells within an island of thymic epithelium. Hematoxylin and eosin stain, × 480. (Reprinted, by permission of the authors and the Editor of *Cancer,* from the paper by Katz and Lattes, 1969.)

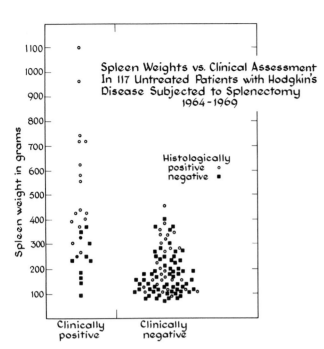

Figure 3.47 Spleen weight and histologic evidence of spleen involvement versus preoperative clinical assessment based on palpable or radiographic enlargement of the spleen; the unreliability of the clinical evaluation is obvious. (Reprinted, by permission of the authors and the Editor of *Cancer,* from the paper by Kadin, Glatstein, and Dorfman, 1971.)

Barge and Potet, 1971; Kaplan et al., 1973). In a selected series of 37 patients with multiple liver biopsies at peritoneoscopy, De Vita et al. (1971) found liver involvement in 6 (16 percent).

Inasmuch as benign epithelioid granulomas and other inflammatory reactions are not uncommonly observed in the liver and are localized to the portal triads, as is early microscopic involvement by Hodgkin's disease, a serious problem of interpretation arises in those instances in which diagnostic Sternberg-Reed cells are not discernible in the cellular infiltrate (Givler et al., 1971; Lukes, 1971). Although a *primary* diagnosis of Hodgkin's disease is certainly not warranted in such instances, most pathologists are in agreement that liver biopsies which reveal atypical, malignant-appearing histiocytes, including mononuclear Hodgkin's cells with malignant nucleoli, and a polymorphous infiltrate in patients in whom there is a previously well-established biopsy diagnosis of Hodgkin's disease can appropriately be interpreted as "consistent with Hodgkin's disease of the liver" (Dorfman, 1971; Lukes, 1971; Rappaport et al., 1971; Abt et al., 1974).

Conversely, a negative liver biopsy should not be given undue weight, particularly in patients with

known involvement of the spleen and documented abnormality of one or more liver function tests or evidence of inhomogeneity of uptake on a radioisotopic liver scan. It should be kept in mind that the liver is a huge organ and that either needle or wedge biopsies, except when taken under direct vision at laparotomy from a grossly suspicious lesion, represent at best a very tiny sample of the liver volume. In general, it has been our experience that the yield of wedge biopsy is appreciably greater than that of needle biopsy, and there have been almost no cases in which the needle biopsy has been positive and the wedge biopsy negative.

Bone Marrow. The histologic criteria for the diagnosis of Hodgkin's disease in the bone marrow are similar to those for the liver. In the absence of diagnostic Sternberg-Reed cells, mononuclear Hodgkin's cells with prominent nucleoli, seen in a pleomorphic or fibrous stroma, may suffice. Fi-

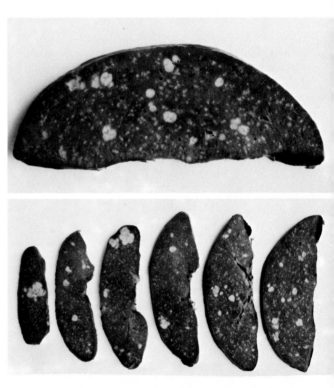

Figure 3.48 *Top,* cross-section through the midplane of a spleen of normal size and weight (110 gm.), showing multiple lesions of Hodgkin's disease of the nodular sclerosing type; *bottom,* sections through other planes of the same specimen, revealing the great multiplicity and irregularity of size and distribution of the nodular lesions. (Photomicrograph at top reprinted, by permission of the authors and the Editor of *Cancer,* from the paper by Kadin, Glatstein, and Dorfman, 1971.)

with radioactive indium chloride (^{111}InCl$_3$) have been helpful in some patients in revealing regions of abnormal uptake as a guide to site selection for biopsy (Gilbert et al., 1976a).

Of a total of 130 consecutive patients, 5 were excluded from laparotomy by the finding of bone marrow involvement in the needle biopsy (and 8 others were excluded for medical or other reasons). Despite the fact that all of the remaining 117 patients subjected to laparotomy and repeat bone marrow biopsy had had a negative needle marrow biopsy, four additional instances of marrow involvement were detected in the contralateral open surgical biopsies. Involvement in all of these was focal, but identifiable Sternberg-Reed cells associated with an appropriate stromal reaction were observed in all instances. Abundant reticulin formation was demonstrated by silver impregnation

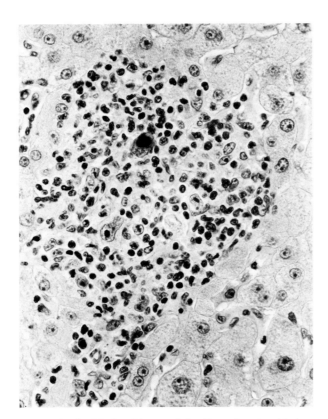

Figure 3.49 Wedge biopsy of the liver showing histiocytes with prominent nucleoli, surrounded by lymphocytes. Characteristic Sternberg-Reed cells are not seen. This was interpreted as evidence of hepatic involvement in a patient with histologically diagnostic Hodgkin's disease elsewhere. Hematoxylin and eosin stain, ×390. (Reprinted, by permission of the authors and the Editor of *Cancer,* from the paper by Kadin, Glatstein, and Dorfman, 1971.)

brosis alone is suspicious enough to warrant another marrow biopsy from a different site (Dorfman, 1971; Lukes, 1971; Rappaport et al., 1971; Strum, 1973). As in the case of the liver, microscopic involvement of the bone marrow is frequently focal in nature (Fig. 3.50). This fact renders the conventional marrow aspiration virtually useless in Hodgkin's disease (Grann et al., 1966; Rosenberg, 1968, 1971; Webb et al., 1970). Indeed, the sampling problem is formidable, even with needle biopsy. This point is well documented in our earlier experience at Stanford, where all patients with a biopsy diagnosis of Hodgkin's disease were routinely screened by Westerman-Jensen or Jamshidi (Jamshidi and Swaim, 1971) needle biopsy of marrow from the iliac crest. If this was negative, a staging laparotomy was performed, together with open surgical biopsy of the marrow from the opposite iliac crest. Bone marrow scans

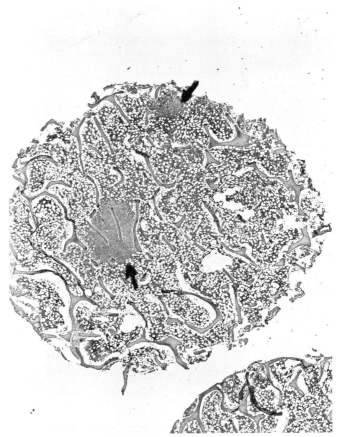

Figure 3.50 Cross-section of open surgical iliac crest bone marrow biopsy showing two discrete focal areas of involvement by Hodgkin's disease (arrows) in an otherwise normal marrow. Hematoxylin and eosin stain, ×9. (Reprinted, by permission of the authors and the Editor of *Cancer,* from the paper by Kadin, Glatstein, and Dorfman, 1971.)

technique in these foci of Hodgkin's disease. In the series of 185 patients included in the report by Dorfman (1971), there were 8 positive open bone marrow biopsies (4.3 percent). The noncaseating epithelioid granulomas (Fig. 3.51) observed at times in the bone marrow, liver, spleen, or lymph nodes (Kadin, Donaldson, and Dorfman, 1970; Brincker, 1970; Goldman, 1970; Zarembok et al., 1972) should not be erroneously interpreted as indicative of involvement of the affected organ or tissue by Hodgkin's disease. Indeed, there is evidence that such granulomas are associated with a significantly more favorable prognosis (O'Connell et al., 1975a; Sacks et al., 1978a).

Body Fluids. Invasion of the pleura, peritoneal cavity, and central nervous system are relatively rare and usually late, preterminal events in Hodgkin's disease. When effusions occur or neurological manifestations appear, it is sometimes possible to identify diagnostic Sternberg-Reed and Hodgkin's cells by cytologic examination (Billingham et al., 1975). Cells of very similar morphology are seen in body fluids with much greater frequency in certain of the non-Hodgkin's lymphomas, notably diffuse histiocytic lymphoma (formerly known as reticulum cell sarcoma), sometimes leading to the erroneous diagnosis of Hodgkin's disease of the lymphocyte depletion type. Sternberg-Reed cells have also been detected in the thoracic duct lymph of patients with para-aortic node involvement (Engeset et al., 1973).

Differential Diagnosis and Overall Diagnostic Accuracy

It is widely believed that the error of histopathologic diagnosis of Hodgkin's disease is quite high. Indeed, skeptics have dismissed many cases of long-term disease-free survival as instances of probable erroneous diagnosis. Support for this view may be found in the data of Symmers (1968), who reviewed the biopsy slides of 600 cases originally interpreted by other pathologists in Great Britain as Hodgkin's disease. Of these, only 317 (53 percent) were confirmed! Inflammatory and other nonneoplastic reactive conditions accounted for the greatest number (192, or 32 percent) of the erroneous diagnoses, and other malignant neoplasms were diagnosed in 69 (11.5 percent). The converse error, in which the diagnosis of Hodgkin's disease was missed initially, was encountered by Symmers in 85 cases. The diagnostic error was greater for the "indolent type" (paragranuloma) than in the "ordinary type," or granuloma (33 and 13 percent, respectively).

However, a detailed review of two groups of precoded biopsy slides by three different expert pathologists suggested that the diagnostic error may be substantially less in patients seen and treated at major radiotherapy centers and cancer hospitals. Group I comprised 201 cases from the files of several centers in which death from Hodgkin's disease had occurred during the first ten years after treatment, whereas Group II included 194 patients, from the same centers, who were still alive after

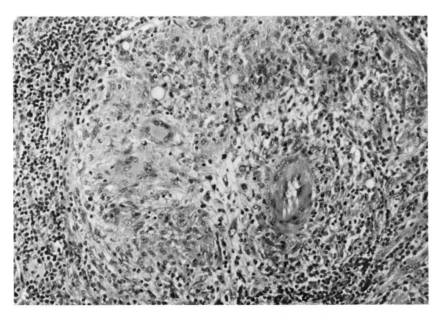

Figure 3.51 Noncaseating epithelioid cell granuloma in Malpighian corpuscle of the spleen. Hematoxylin and eosin, ×240. (Reprinted, by permission of the authors and the Editor of *Cancer,* from the paper by Sacks et al., 1978a.)

more than ten years (Lukes, Gompel, and Nezelof, 1966). The original biopsy slides in a total of 55 cases were found to be equivocal or uninterpretable. Of the remaining 340 cases, the diagnosis of Hodgkin's disease was rejected in 13 of 179 in Group I and 10 of 161 in Group II, for a diagnostic error of 7.2 and 6.2 percent, respectively. The interpretations of the three pathologists were in complete accord in 154 of the Group II biopsies examined, in partial disagreement in 25, and in open disagreement in only 9. In another study, a detailed review of 158 biopsies from 141 borderline cases, in which the histologic diagnosis was tested against the subsequent clinical course of the patient, yielded correct diagnoses in 143, or 90.5 percent (Dawson, Cooper, and Rambo, 1964). Chelloul et al. (1972), in a retrospective analysis of 515 cases, rejected the diagnosis of Hodgkin's disease in 69 (13.4 percent); of these, 15 were diagnosed as other types of malignant lymphomas, and the remaining 54 were nonneoplastic lesions.

In the study reported by Keller et al. (1968), 179 biopsies were reviewed by three pathologists and classified according to the Rye classification. There was initial complete agreement not only on the diagnosis of Hodgkin's disease but also on the specific histologic type in 120 cases (67 percent), and two of the three pathologists agreed in 45 additional cases, for a total of 92 percent. There was complete disagreement among all three on only two cases in the series.

A national cooperative clinical trial (Nickson, 1966) has made all initial biopsies available for review by a single consultant pathologist (Dr. Henry Rappaport) after a prior diagnosis of Hodgkin's disease by the staff pathologists of the many participating institutions. Major disagreements have been recorded in only 10 (3.9 percent) of the 255 cases doubly reviewed to date (Dr. H. Rappaport, personal communication). Four of these were interpreted by the consultant pathologist as other types of malignant lymphoma or unclassified neoplasm, three as consistent with but not diagnostic of Hodgkin's disease, and only three as benign lesions (reactive follicular hyperplasia, and viral and granulomatous lymphadenitis). Moreover, there was again a generally high degree of concordance in the interpretation of histopathologic type (Table 3.16). Extensive additional data on observer disagreement in histopathologic classification have recently been presented by Coppleson et al. (1970), Dorfman (1971), and Correa et al. (1973).

Finally, in a study by Kadin et al. (1971), concordance in the classification of original biopsies and intra-abdominal histologic manifestations of Hodgkin's disease between two different pathologists was recorded in over 90 percent of instances. It would therefore appear that, in the hands of experienced pathologists in major medical centers, overall diagnostic accuracy and the ability to differentiate consistently among the various histopathologic subtypes are both gratifyingly high.

Many errors in diagnosis are attributable to technically unsatisfactory biopsy slides. The many tech-

Table 3.16 Interpathologist Disagreement in the Interpretation of Histopathologic Type in Hodgkin's Disease

Interpretation of the contributing pathologist	Interpretation of the consultant pathologist[a]						
	LP	MC	NS	LD	Uncl.	Total	Subtotal
Paragranuloma		6				6	
Granuloma	2	21	19	3	3	48	
Sarcoma	2					2	
Uncl.	1	5	1			7	63
LP		6	3			9	
MC	1		9	1	1	12	
NS		6				6	
LD		2	1			3	
Total	6	46	33	4	4	93	30

Source: Unpublished data provided by Dr. Henry Rappaport, Consultant Pathologist of Record to the National Cooperative Clinical Trial on the Radiotherapy of Hodgkin's Disease (Nickson, 1966).

[a]Abbreviations: LP = Lymphocytic predominance; MC = mixed cellularity; NS = nodular sclerosis; LD = lymphocytic depletion; Uncl. = unclassified. Some of the "contributing pathologists" from the participating institutions in which the biopsies were initially interpreted preferred to use the Jackson-Parker classification. Concordance of interpretation was observed in all of the other 162 cases in the series.

nical pitfalls in histologic processing of lymphoid tissues have been stressed by Butler (1969). Differential diagnosis is seldom a problem in meticulously processed and sectioned biopsy material if classical Sternberg-Reed cells are observed. It is true that several groups (Lukes, Tindle, and Parker, 1969; Strum, Park, and Rappaport, 1970; McMahon, Gordon, and Rosen, 1970; Agliozzo and Reingold, 1971; Salvador, Harrison, and Kyle, 1971) have reported the observation of cells indistinguishable from Sternberg-Reed cells in various other malignant and benign conditions, including several instances of infectious mononucleosis, and that these reports have caused some consternation among pathologists. Moreover, in the study reported by Symmers (1968), 20 of 283 patients given erroneous diagnoses proved to have infectious mononucleosis. However, the presence of an abundance of "transformed" lymphocytes and of the serologic abnormalities characteristic of infectious mononucleosis should ordinarily lead to a correct diagnosis in such cases. Criteria for the histopathologic diagnosis of infectious mononucleosis have been detailed by Salvador, Harrison, and Kyle (1971) and Tindle, Parker, and Lukes (1972). Accordingly, the problem cases are primarily those in which diagnostic Sternberg-Reed cells are not seen, or in which the pathologist must stretch the diagnostic criteria for such cells to include borderline examples.

Entities to be kept in mind include certain other malignant lymphomas and a variety of benign reactive and inflammatory conditions. In some instances of Hodgkin's disease of the nodular lymphocytic predominance variety, typical Sternberg-Reed cells may be sufficiently sparse to be missed in the initial section. Unless the pathologist suspects Hodgkin's disease and obtains additional sections through the same lymph node in a further search for Sternberg-Reed cells, such cases are not unlikely to be erroneously diagnosed as follicular (nodular) lymphocytic lymphomas. Similarly, in the diffuse type of lymphocytic predominance, Sternberg-Reed cells may not be present in every section, and unless one or more of such cells are seen, an erroneous diagnosis of diffuse lymphocytic lymphoma is likely.

The benign conditions to be differentiated from Hodgkin's disease and other malignant lymphomas include the hydantoin pseudolymphomas; infectious mononucleosis; dermatopathic lymphadenopathy; toxoplasmosis; rheumatoid lymphadenitis; secondary syphilis; herpes zoster; postvaccinial lymphadenitis (Bichel, 1976); allergic granulomatosis; rubeola; proliferative myositis; and a variety of nonspecific inflammatory reactions (Symmers, 1968; Butler, 1969; Strum, 1973), including those seen in heroin addicts (Geller and Stimmel, 1973). Immunoblastic lymphadenopathy is a recently recognized hyperplastic disorder of the immune system which may closely resemble Hodgkin's disease (Lukes and Tindle, 1975).

Regression of lymphadenopathy after discontinuation of hydantoin medications was a constant feature of the early reported cases of hydantoin pseudo-lymphoma (Saltzstein et al., 1958; Saltzstein and Ackerman, 1959). However, cases of true Hodgkin's disease and other malignant lymphomas, in which clinical progression and even death ensued despite cessation of hydantoin therapy, have now been reported by Saltzstein (1962), Hyman and Sommers (1966), Bredesgaard (1966), and Gams et al. (1968). Thus, it is no longer justifiable to rely on a history of epilepsy treated with one or more of the hydantoin drugs in distinguishing between true and pseudo-lymphomas. The dilemma is further compounded by the fact that morphologic differentiation may in some cases be virtually impossible. Although the Hodgkin's-like lesions in some cases of pseudo-lymphoma have usually lacked classical, diagnostic Sternberg-Reed cells (Krasznai, 1966), the lymph node biopsy from the case reported by Doyle and Hellstrom (1963) revealed sparse "very large atypical reticulum cells of the Reed-Sternberg type," measuring up to 35 μ in diameter. They had lobulated nuclei, and some were mirror-image binucleate forms. The fact that nucleoli were relatively small or absent permitted exclusion of most of these cells, but fairly prominent nucleoli were present in a few, which could therefore have been deemed diagnostically acceptable Sternberg-Reed cells. In a comprehensive review of the literature, Gams, Neal, and Conrad (1968) concluded that there are as yet no consistent histologic or clinical criteria on the basis of which reliable differentiation of benign and malignant lymphoid reactions in hydantoin-treated patients can be made.

Postvaccinial lymphadenitis appears one or more weeks after smallpox vaccination (Hartsock, 1968). The enlarged nodes usually develop in the ipsilateral axillary, infraclavicular, or supraclavicular region and may be locally painful and tender. Although the history of recent vaccination should call attention to the correct diagnosis, it was overlooked in fourteen of the twenty cases reviewed by

Hartsock. An essentially identical lymphadenitis may occur in lymph nodes draining skin reactions due to herpes zoster and perhaps to other unidentified viruses (Butler, 1969). Histologically, the most conspicuous cellular elements are the atypical histiocytes ("activated reticulum cells") which proliferate throughout the lymph node pulp. They are large mononuclear cells, with nucleoli and abundant cytoplasm; occasionally, the nucleus may be indented and the nucleoli large enough to closely resemble a Sternberg-Reed cell (cf. fig. 6 in Hartsock, 1968). Mitotic figures, eosinophils, and plasma cells are often present, whereas reactive follicles are seldom prominent until two weeks or more after vaccination.

The lymphadenopathy caused by toxoplasmosis was formerly known as "lymphohistiocytic medullary reticulosis" (Robb-Smith, 1947) or "subacute nuchal and cervical lymphadenitis" (Piringer-Kuchinka, 1953; Piringer-Kuchinka, Martin, and Thalhammer, 1958). After the discovery of the etiologic agent, its association with these lymphoid reactions was elucidated by Saxén and Saxén (1959). It is characterized by hyperplasia of sinusoidal histiocytes, follicles, and pulp. Focal collections within follicles of reactive histiocytes having abundant pink-staining cytoplasm, small nuclei, and very small nucleoli are diagnostic. Although histiocytic proliferation may also be a feature of the lymphocytic predominance type of Hodgkin's disease, follicular hyperplasia is rare and the histiocytes do not infiltrate the follicles that may be present. Finally, diagnostic Sternberg-Reed cells would not be expected to occur in toxoplasmosis.

Problems of differentiation from infectious mononucleosis, as stated earlier, are unlikely to arise in typical cases. Occasionally, however, the disease may present with lymphadenopathy in the absence of fever, splenomegaly, or sore throat, and lymph node biopsy is performed, revealing diffuse proliferation of large "transformed" lymphocytes throughout the pulp. These cells, though usually mononuclear, contain large nucleoli; occasionally, they may fulfill all of the diagnostic criteria for the identification of Sternberg-Reed cells (Tindle, Parker, and Lukes, 1972). Reactive follicles are usually seen. Once the diagnosis of infectious mononucleosis is entertained, serologic confirmation is readily available.

Allergic granulomatosis is an extremely rare condition manifested in one or more nodes by proliferation of histiocytes, tiny stellate areas of necrosis, and infiltration of eosinophils. Although the histiocytes are normal-looking, and cells resembling true Sternberg-Reed cells are not seen, the presence of histiocytes, eosinophils, lymphadenopathy, and a sometimes gravely ill patient may combine to suggest the erroneous diagnosis of Hodgkin's disease.

Histologic changes often occur in lymph nodes that fill with oily contrast medium during lymphangiography (Dominok, 1964). They are nonspecific inflammatory infiltrations with foreign body giant cells and dilated oil-filled sinuses. After some months, vascularization and fibrosis may supervene. Differentiation from Hodgkin's disease should present no problems, even when, as sometimes happens, both processes occur in the same lymph node.

The commonest differential diagnostic problem is the heterogeneous collection of conditions which express themselves in lymph nodes as reactive follicular hyperplasia (Butler, 1969). Reactive follicles of varying size and shape, sharply demarcated from the surrounding lymphoid tissue, contain undifferentiated reticular cells, histiocytes, and large, normal lymphocytes, which contrast with the small, mature lymphocytes of the pulp. Active phagocytosis is often seen in the histiocytes within the reactive follicles, with nuclear debris in the abundant pale cytoplasm of these cells giving a "starry sky" appearance that is also a prominent feature in the Burkitt lymphoma. The reactive follicles typically contain an increased number of normal mitotic figures. Although the differentiation from nodular lymphoma and the nodular variety of lymphocytic predominance Hodgkin's disease is usually easily made, a troublesome small group of borderline cases may lead to diagnostic error. When a series of such problem cases were studied in depth by Dawson, Cooper, and Rambo (1964), it was found that 4 of 37 reactive nodes showed complete obliteration of the normal architecture, confirmed by reticulin stains; partial obliteration was seen in 17 others. Conversely, 2 of 106 lymphoma nodes maintained the normal architecture virtually intact. Reactive follicles were absent in 5 of 37 reactive nodes, unassociated with known hypogammaglobulinemia, whereas typical reactive follicles were normally distributed in 5 of 106 lymphoma nodes. One or more reactive follicles were seen in 23 of the lymphoma nodes. Phagocytosis was a useful criterion, since it was consistently present in the reactive nodes, but in only 4 of 42 lymphoma nodes with pseudofollicles. All nodes in which the predominant cells in either the pulp or the sinuses were large lymphocytes, lymphoblasts, or atypical reticulum cells were examples of malignant lymphoma. Conversely, diagnostic Sternberg-Reed cells were not seen in any of the reactive nodes. The authors concluded that these and other criteria can lead to the correct diagnosis in about 90 percent of all cases but that no single criterion can be relied upon absolutely.

Gross Pathology

As observed at autopsy, or occasionally in surgical lymph node dissections, gross involvement of lymph nodes by Hodgkin's disease characteristically produces confluent, irregularly lobulated nodular masses, distributed along the major lymph node chains that follow the major vessels in the neck, the supraclavicular fossa, the mediastinum, the para-aortic and iliac vessels, and/or the inguinal and femoral node groups. The contiguity of such massive involvement is entirely consistent with the contiguity of spread of the disease during life (cf. Chapter 7). Direct extension of disease from the mediastinum and hilar lymph nodes into the pulmonary parenchyma and invasion of the pericardium and pleural surfaces are not infre-

quently also observed. Gross nodulation is commonly present in both the spleen and liver, and involvement of the bone marrow has been observed in a very high proportion of cases in some series (Steiner, 1943; Hashimoto and Hanazato, 1961). Widespread dissemination to the spleen, liver, pancreas, kidney, and adrenals was also evident in a series of 36 autopsied cases from Uganda, of which 28 (78 percent) were of the lymphocyte depletion subtype (Dhru and Templeton, 1972). Westling (1965) has tabulated the anatomic sites of involvement in his own series of cases in which autopsy was performed, as well as in the two large series reported by Uddströmer (1934) and by Jackson and Parker (1947). These data are presented in Table 3.17.

In striking contrast to the relative frequency of involvement of various anatomic sites observed at autopsy is the distribution observed at the time of initial diagnostic evaluation in previously untreated patients with a biopsy diagnosis of Hodgkin's disease. In a large series of consecutive previously untreated cases, all of which were evaluated with the aid of lymphangiography and laparotomy with splenectomy, the anatomic distributions of involved sites indicated in Chapter 7 were observed.

Table 3.17   Anatomic Sites of Involvement at Autopsy

Finding	Westling (1965), 45 cases Percent	Uddströmer (1934), 192 cases Percent	Jackson-Parker (1947), 98 cases Percent
Mediastinal adenopathy	64.4	61	74.5
Pulmonary lesions of Hodgkin's disease	28.9	33	36.7
Pleural effusions	31.1	—	—
Pleural nodal lesions or infiltrations	6.7	12	10.2
Pericardial infiltrates	4.4	7	2.0
Cardial infiltrate	2.2	2	—
Splenic lesions of Hodgkin's disease	68.8	63	59.2
Hepatic lesions of Hodgkin's disease	57.7	36	52.0
Retroperitoneal lymphadenopathy	75.5	68	55.1
Renal lesions of Hodgkin's disease	15.5	7	17.3
Skeletal lesions	33.3	11	35.7
Jejunal lesions	2.2	8	8.2
Duodenal lesions	2.2	8	5.1
Gastric lesions	2.2		13.3

Source: Modified from Westling (1965), table 11.

Comparison of these data with those of the three autopsy series in Table 3.17 supports the conclusion that involvement of the liver, bone marrow, and abdominal viscera occurs late in the course of the disease. An additional discussion of these data is presented in Chapter 7, with particular emphasis on the patterns of associated involvement of different anatomic sites, their relationship to histopathologic type, and their implications for the mode of dissemination of the disease.

Presenting Manifestations

Detection by the Patient of a Lump, Swelling, or Mass. The great majority of patients with Hodgkin's disease first seek medical attention after they become aware of an unusual lump, mass, or swelling. Ultmann and Moran (1973) have estimated, on the basis of their own data and that in the literature, that Hodgkin's disease is first manifested in the lymph nodes in 90–93 percent of all cases. Of these, 60–80 percent present in the cervical nodes, 6–20 percent in the axillary nodes, and 6–12 percent in the inguinal region. In most instances, the enlarged nodes are not painful or tender, and the patient's attention is called to them by chance, perhaps while bathing or shaving. Not infrequently, masses or lymph nodes may grow to quite large size before they become noticeable (Figs. 4.1, 4.2).

Fist-sized masses in the axilla may ultimately interfere with adduction of the arm; large conglomerate chains of lymph nodes on one or both sides of the neck may interfere with buttoning the collar of a shirt or fastening the top of a dress. Vague fullness or discomfort in the abdomen may lead a patient to palpate the abdomen deeply enough to feel a mass. In other instances, diffuse puffy swelling, rather than a discrete palpable mass, may signal the presence of lymph node enlargement, especially in the supraclavicular or infraclavicular area.

Although most such lymph node enlargements are painless, the association of pain and tenderness with lymph node enlargement is by no means inconsistent with the diagnosis of Hodgkin's disease. In some instances, involved cervical-supraclavicular lymph nodes may be painless, but the patient's attention is called to them coincidentally by the

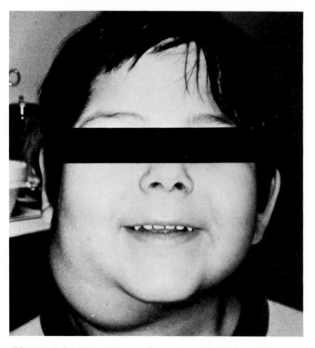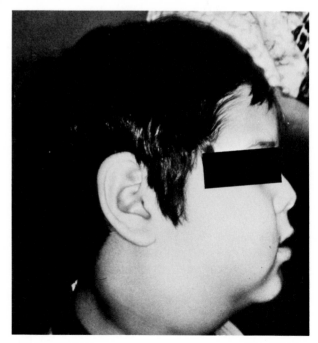

Figure 4.1　Huge mass of confluent lymph nodes in the right upper and mid-cervical region in a four-year-old boy with Hodgkin's disease.

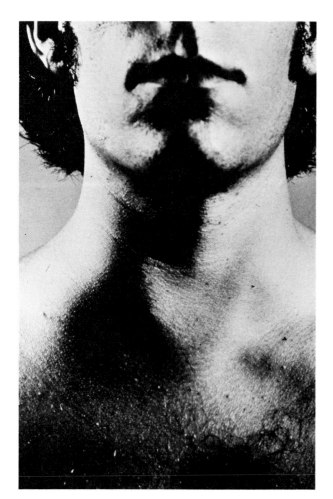

Figure 4.2 Lymphadenopathy in the right lower cervical-supraclavicular region in this 20-year-old male patient is visually evident as a bulging contour obliterating the usual concavity of the supraclavicular fossa.

pain and tenderness experienced in nearby banal inflammatory nodes associated with coexisting upper respiratory tract infections. Infrequently, pain experienced soon after the ingestion of an alcoholic beverage may first alert the patient to the presence of enlarged lymph nodes.

The apparent rate of growth of lymph node masses exhibits remarkable variation. It is not uncommon for patients who are apparently reliable historians to report that a mass has literally become apparent overnight. Such a dramatic onset is likely to bring the patient to a physician very promptly thereafter. In the great majority of cases, however, patients state that they have noted the enlarged lymph nodes for some appreciable period of time, ranging from a few weeks to several months, and occasionally, even years. In these instances, the rate of growth of lymph nodes is described as indo-

lent, sometimes almost imperceptible. There are well-documented instances of waxing and waning in the size of lymph node masses, occasionally associated with cycles of tenderness or fever. Constitutional symptoms, when present, tend to be exacerbated during periods of rapid lymph node enlargement, and exhibit spontaneous remissions concurrently with diminution in size of the enlarged nodes.

Constitutional Symptoms. Fever was present in 27 percent of our patients with Hodgkin's disease at the time of initial diagnosis. It is usually low grade, smoldering in character, and often initially ascribed to other intercurrent illnesses until its persistence leads to medical investigation. Often, the patient experiences only night sweats, without awareness of the fever with which they are usually associated. A small but important group of cases are those in which high swinging fever, often accompanied by drenching, debilitating night sweats, is the dominant and sometimes the only initial clinical manifestation of Hodgkin's disease. The diurnal fluctuations are often extreme, with temperatures ranging up to 40–41C. during the late afternoon and evening, and falling precipitously to normal or subnormal levels during the early morning hours (Fig. 4.3). The cyclic bouts of high fever described by Pel (1887) and Ebstein (1887), each lasting one to two weeks and separated by afebrile periods of similar duration, are classically characteristic of the disease but are seldom seen except in patients with far advanced disease. Significant hemolysis may occur in association with Pel-Ebstein fever. Storgaard and Karle (1975) found that the mean loss of hemoglobin during a fever period was 14 percent in a series of 19 febrile patients among a total of 104 patients with Hodgkin's disease. They suggested that increased red blood cell destruction occurring during periods of high fever was the most likely explanation for the observed hemolysis.

Hodgkin's disease should always be given careful consideration in the differential diagnosis of fever of unknown origin. When, as is often the case, peripheral lymphadenopathy amenable to biopsy is not present in such cases, it should be remembered that significant fever in Hodgkin's disease is almost always associated with the presence of intrathoracic and/or intraabdominal lymph node involvement. The presence of mediastinal lymphadenopathy is readily detectable by radiographic examination of the chest. In contrast, the detection of retroperitoneal lymphadenopathy, silent

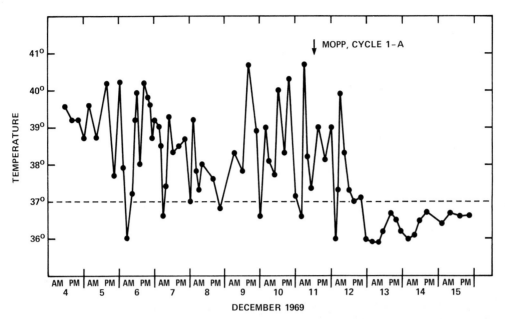

Figure 4.3 Temperature chart of a 12-year-old boy with stage IV$_L$B nodular sclerosing Hodgkin's disease, illustrating the profound diurnal fluctuations commonly seen in febrile patients. There was a dramatic lysis of his fever within 48 hours of the initiation of his first cycle of MOPP combination chemotherapy, accompanied by rapid regression of massive lymphadenopathy and splenomegaly (see Fig. 10.2).

except as a cause of fever, represented a far more difficult diagnostic problem until the advent of lower extremity lymphangiography.

The pathophysiologic mechanisms underlying recurrent fever are not well understood. Some authorities believe that fever is prevalent only in those patients whose lymph nodes exhibit appreciable degrees of necrosis, suggesting that the fever may be a secondary consequence of tissue breakdown and resorption. Sokal and Shimaoka (1967) have detected the occurrence in the urine of patients with febrile Hodgkin's disease of a pyrogen of the endogenous type usually associated with the breakdown of polymorphonuclear granulocytes.

Young and Hodas (1971a,b) noted that plasma and urine samples from such patients contain a number of low-molecular-weight proteins not found in normal body fluids nor in those of afebrile control patients with other forms of neoplastic disease. Most prominent among these low-molecular-weight proteins was a relatively cationic protein demonstrable by polyacrylamide gel electrophoresis in the presence of urea. Using similar techniques, Young et al. (1975) were successful in demonstrating in the plasma of febrile patients with Hodgkin's disease a characteristic protein electrophoretically identical to that previously seen in urine. Densitometric tracings of the gel patterns of plasmas from febrile and afebrile individuals revealed the presence of a doublet protein (DP) band

in the febrile plasmas which was absent in plasmas from normal individuals (Fig. 4.4). There was a statistically significant correlation between the severity of pyrexia and the plasma content of DP in patients with active Hodgkin's disease (Fig. 4.5). Overall, the DP content of plasmas from febrile patients exceeded by a wide margin that of afebrile patients with active Hodgkin's disease. Moreover, there was some indication that persistence of elevated levels of plasma DP following treatment might be related to disease activity; only one of ten patients in complete unmaintained remission for more than two years had detectable DP in the plasma. Although plasma DP content did not always correlate with diurnal fluctuations in temperature, defervescence and induction of clinical remissions by radiotherapy and/or chemotherapy were associated with decreases in plasma content of DP, sometimes within as short an interval as 48 hours. In contrast to the response to specific therapy, treatment with nonspecific antipyretic medications produced no apparent change in plasma levels of DP. However, the protein synthesis inhibitor cycloheximide dramatically reduced plasma DP levels and body temperature within hours of the time of drug administration (Young and Dowling, 1975; Young et al., 1975). Amlot, Slaney, and Williams (1976) detected elevated plasma levels of the C3 component of complement in 11 of 18 patients with Hodgkin's disease. They noted that it was of

cell concentrates from the peripheral blood of 24 patients with Hodgkin's disease, they found such cells to be present in only 1 of 28 tests on afebrile patients, whereas neoplastic cells were detected in 9 of 19 febrile patients. They also suggested that

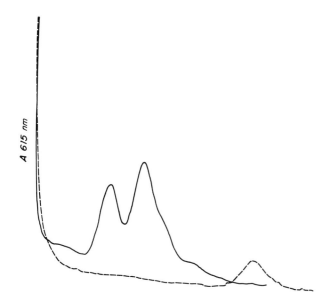

Figure 4.4   Contrasting densitometric tracings illustrating the presence of a DP band in plasma from a febrile patient with Hodgkin's disease (solid line) and the relative absence of a more distal band present in plasma from a normal individual (broken line). The sample onlay was 10 μl. (Reprinted by permission of the authors and the Editor of *Cancer Research*, from the paper by Young et al., 1975.)

higher molecular weight than normal ("macromolecular C3"), a finding which they interpreted as indirect evidence of the presence of immune complexes. Since this abnormality was present in all 9 of their febrile patients, they suggested that circulating immune complexes and fever may be pathophysiologically linked.

The release of a pyrogen from spleen and lymph node cells of patients with Hodgkin's disease during short-term incubation in vitro has been observed by Bodel (1974). Spleen cells from patients with nonmalignant diseases did not release pyrogenic material under similar culture conditions. Pyrogen production occurred whether or not the spleens from patients with Hodgkin's disease were pathologically involved by the disease, but was not well correlated with the actual occurrence of fever in individual splenectomized patients. Pyrogen production was prolonged and required protein synthesis.

Hoerni, Chauvergne, and Parsi (1970) have suggested that the fever of Hodgkin's disease may be analogous to that occurring during immune reactions following tuberculin administration in sensitized animals. They predicted that fever should correlate with vascular invasion by Sternberg-Reed and Hodgkin's cells. In a study of 47 white blood

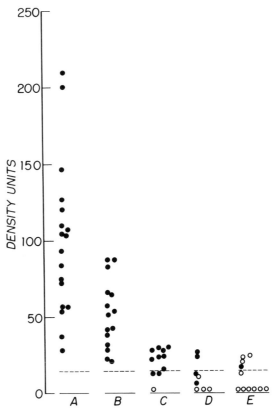

Figure 4.5   Scattergram of densitometric analyses of plasma DP content in Hodgkin's disease patients. ●, visible doublet present in the gel; ○, vague staining present without definable doublet; each entry is the mean of duplicate determinations with a S.E. < ± 0.10. Sample onlay, 10 μl. ----, lower limit of precision of the method. *A*, severe pyrexia, temperature ≥ 38.2 C PO daily while on prednisone, ≥20 mg/day; *B*, moderate pyrexia, temperature ≥ 38.2 C PO without prednisone, but/or suppressed by prednisone ≥ 30 mg/day; *C*, active Hodgkin's but afebrile, mean temperature ≤37.4 C PO for 10 days and no temperature > 37.9 C; *D*, suppressed Hodgkin's disease, afebrile in complete or partial remission on chemotherapy; *E*, inactive Hodgkin's disease, afebrile in complete remission without therapy for six months to five years. Clinical staging at the time of study or at most recent time of active disease, Groups A and B: all stage IVB. Group C: stage IIA, 5; stage IIIA, 7; stage IVA, 1. Group D: stage IIA, 1; stage IIIA, 1; stage IIIB, 1; stage IVB, 5. Group E: stage IA, 1; stage IIA, 5; stage IIIA, 4; stage IVB, 1. (Reprinted by permission of the authors and *Cancer Research*, from the paper by Young et al., 1975.)

fever may precede or accompany the occurrence of dissemination of disease. Although the evidence presented by these investigators of an association between vascular invasion and dissemination of Sternberg-Reed cells and the occurrence of fever is of considerable interest, their interpretation that these events are associated with an immunological reaction is not supported by any published evidence. Indeed, it is difficult to comprehend why the prognosis of febrile patients should be less favorable than that of afebrile patients if fever were indeed due to an immunological reaction against the tumor. Nonetheless, further investigations of this interesting hypothesis are undoubtedly warranted.

Night sweats occur as a consequence of the nocturnal defervescence of fever and may be experienced by patients who are unaware of being febrile. In their more florid form, they may indeed be dramatic. Some patients describe sweats which soak not only their nightgowns or pajamas but the bed linens as well, sometimes requiring changing of garments and bed linens one or more times during the night. Conversely, minimal expressions of this symptom are known to occur in some otherwise normal individuals, for which reason their significance may be exceedingly difficult to evaluate.

Pruritus may occur early in the course of Hodgkin's disease in 10–15 percent of all patients (Ultmann, Cunningham, and Gellhorn, 1966), and it has been reported that 85 percent of patients may experience pruritus at some time during the course of the disease (Hoster et al., 1948). It is usually generalized in character and often severe enough to induce intensive scratching leading to the production of multiple excoriations, often blood-encrusted, on the trunk and/or extremities. Occasionally, severe generalized itching may be the only symptom, and associated excoriations the only outward sign of the disease; such patients are usually referred to the care of a dermatologist, who must then be alert to this possibility in his differential diagnosis. The diagnostic problem may be further complicated by the coexistence of dermatoses which in themselves constitute an adequate explanation for the itching and thus tend to divert suspicion from the possibility of Hodgkin's disease. Bluefarb (1959, 1967) has described prurigo-like papular lesions, urticaria with erythematous lesions, erythema multiforme, erythema nodosum-like lesions, eczematoid and psoriasiform lesions, erythroderma and exfoliative dermatitis, bullous and pemphigoid lesions, edema (often secondary to lymphatic obstruction), and trophic lesions in patients with Hodgkin's disease. In rare instances, Hodgkin's disease has reportedly been associated with pemphigus (Naysmith and Hancock, 1976). Hodgkin's disease may also be complicated by a generalized ichthyosis of the skin, sometimes related to exposure to contact allergens, and often accompanied by severe generalized itching. In a small proportion of patients, itching is relatively localized, rather than generalized, usually on the upper or lower extremities, and is then less likely to be appreciated as a significant constitutional symptom until, retrospectively, the patient reports that it has disappeared during a course of radiotherapy or chemotherapy. The pathophysiologic mechanisms underlying the generalized pruritus of Hodgkin's disease are obscure. However, since itching is known to be caused by a number of tissue breakdown products such as bradykinin, kallikrein, and histamine, Newbold (1970) has suggested that pruritus in Hodgkin's disease may be due to an autoimmune reaction in which such substances are activated by the products of tumor cytolysis.

Pain in one or more chains of enlarged lymph nodes almost immediately after the imbibition of alcohol is a dramatic symptom which may occasionally be the presenting manifestation in Hodgkin's disease (Bichel, 1959; James, 1960; Brewin, 1966; Atkinson et al., 1976a). Although it appears to have some degree of specificity for this disease, the fact that it occurs in a small minority of cases severely limits its diagnostic value. Bichel (1972) has suggested that the alcohol intolerance syndrome in Hodgkin's disease may be disappearing, perhaps reflecting a change in the natural history of the disease. He notes that the incidence in a series of Danish patients studied in 1953 was 15 percent, and that recorded by James (1960) was 17.1 percent. Brewin (1966), in a study of 192 patients with Hodgkin's disease, reported alcohol intolerance in 31 percent. More recently, Bichel carefully examined the case records of 76 patients who came to autopsy during the years 1956–1968, all of whom had been carefully questioned about the occurrence of alcohol intolerance, and found that the symptom had been detected in only 7 (10 percent). In a new study initiated in 1970, he carefully questioned 30 consecutive patients admitted with Hodgkin's disease and observed alcohol intolerance in only 1 (3.3 percent). The symptoms of alcohol intolerance were detected in 27 (5.3 percent) of 506 patients with Hodgkin's disease treated at the Royal Marsden Hospital between 1963 and 1972 (Atkinson et al., 1976a). In our series of patients at

Stanford University Medical Center, the observed frequency of this symptom complex has been only 1.6 percent. Alcohol intolerance is associated with a low male-female sex ratio, with mediastinal lymphadenopathy, and with nodular sclerosis (Atkinson et al., 1976a). The decreasing incidence of this symptom complex may reflect the fact that an increasing proportion of patients with Hodgkin's disease is now detected at an earlier stage in the evolution of the disease.

The pain associated with alcohol ingestion varies greatly in character and severity; some patients describe it as sharp and stabbing, others as dull and aching, or merely as a sense of malaise and discomfort. In any case, the association with alcohol intake is usually clear enough to lead the patient to discontinue the use of alcohol in any form. Commonly, the pain begins within a few minutes after an alcoholic drink is swallowed, and lasts anywhere from a few minutes to a few hours. An interesting feature of the pain is that it is usually experienced in the immediate vicinity of one or more sites of clinically evident lymphadenopathy. This association was noted in 86 percent of the series of patients studied by Atkinson et al. (1976a). Pain in the same sites may be induced by the intravenous injection of ethyl alcohol (Hall and Olson, 1955). Pain has been observed to disappear after successful treatment and to signal an impending relapse in patients in whom other manifestations of recurrent disease have not yet become clinically apparent (Cheson, 1978). The pain is occasionally associated with nausea and even with vomiting; sometimes these symptoms occur instead of pain. The pathophysiologic mechanism of alcohol intolerance in Hodgkin's disease is unknown.

Presenting manifestations in Hodgkin's disease may also include symptoms related to various hematologic complications, including autoimmune hemolytic anemia (Bowdler and Glick, 1966; Cazenave et al., 1973) and thrombocytopenic purpura (Doan, Bouroncle, and Wiseman, 1960; Rudders, Aisenberg, and Schiller, 1972; Godeau et al., 1975). Thrombocytopenic purpura has also been observed as an initial manifestation of relapsing disease (Weitzman et al., 1977c). Patients may also complain of a variety of other constitutional symptoms of less specific significance, including anorexia, generalized weakness and malaise, and fatigue, often accompanied by weight loss. They not infrequently first seek medical attention because of such nondescript symptoms. Such cases are particularly difficult and challenging diagnostic problems because the same symptoms are commonly

encountered in a host of other illnesses, including the widely prevalent psychosomatic disorders.

Symptoms of Specific Organ System Involvement. A small group of patients first seek medical attention because of pain or other symptoms induced by involvement of specific tissues or organs. Headache, congestion and redness of the face, subcutaneous edema involving the face, the neck, and even the thorax and upper extremities, and difficulty in breathing may all indicate the existence of a superior vena caval obstruction caused by massive mediastinal lymphadenopathy. Although this is appreciably less common in Hodgkin's disease than in bronchogenic carcinoma or the lymphocytic lymphomas, well-documented cases nonetheless do occur and may be the presenting manifestation of the disease. In such instances, a careful physical examination will usually reveal engorgement of the neck veins, indicative of increased venous pressure, and radiographs of the chest will reveal the mediastinal mass. Hypertrophic osteoarthropathy has also been described as a presenting manifestation in occasional patients with mediastinal lymphadenopathy due to Hodgkin's disease (Shapiro and Zvaifler, 1973; Molyneux, 1973; Peck, 1976) and has been observed to regress following successful treatment (Atkinson et al., 1976b).

Involvement of bone is seldom seen at the time of initial diagnosis. Its presence should be suspected in patients who complain of localized, deep, often severe and unremitting pain, usually unrelated to alcohol intake and generally similar in character to that experienced by patients with metastatic cancer involving the skeletal system. Radiographs will usually reveal osteoblastic infiltration, although lytic destruction also occurs (see Chapter 5). Radioisotopic studies with ^{99m}Tc will reveal increased uptake localized in one or more bony areas, usually corresponding closely with the sites of pain.

Pain in the low back, often radiating down one or both lower extremities, may be a presenting manifestation of the spinal cord compression syndrome produced by infiltration of the extradural space. Such patients usually also complain of numbness or other paresthesias and weakness progressing to paralysis in the affected extremities. Since this unusual primary manifestation can progress to permanent paralysis unless promptly diagnosed and treated, and since it responds dramatically and completely when radiotherapy is instituted sufficiently early, the cord compression syndrome should be regarded as a medical emergency calling for an immediate careful neurologic examination, spinal tap for pressure measurements and determination of spinal fluid protein concentration, and myelography, which should be performed even in the absence of positive fluid findings when paralytic manifestations are progressive. In the rare instances in which no prior tissue diagnosis of Hodgkin's disease has been made, laminectomy and biopsy are essential to establish the diagnosis, after which prompt local radiotherapy is indicated. Intracranial Hodgkin's disease is a relatively uncommon manifestation at any time during the course of the disease and is quite rare as a presenting manifestation. Cuttner, Meyer, and Huang (1979) have described the clinical features in six patients and reviewed 28 previously published cases. Visual loss was the presenting symptom in a patient with intracranial Hodgkin's disease (Miller and Iliff, 1975).

Involvement of the abdominal viscera may give rise to a variety of symptoms. Massive retroperitoneal lymphadenopathy may obstruct the inferior vena cava, giving rise to ascites and/or edema of the lower extremities. Icterus is occasionally observed due either to infiltration of the liver or to a rare associated complication, intrahepatic cholestasis. Steatorrhea and chronic malabsorption syndrome have been reported as the major presenting symptoms in rare instances of primary Hodgkin's disease involving the small intestine (Teitelman and Brill, 1960; Ramot et al., 1965; Bernier et al., 1967), although histiocytic and lymphocytic lymphomas are more commonly encountered in such instances.

Fortuitous Detection in the Asymptomatic Patient. Many patients with Hodgkin's disease are asymptomatic adolescents or young adults who have been in apparently perfect health prior to the detection of significant peripheral lymphadenopathy on a routine physical examination performed prior to military induction or to employment. In other instances, the physical examination may be unrevealing but a routine radiographic examination of the chest, performed as a part of the preinduction or pre-employment examination, reveals an unsuspected mediastinal mass. Such instances are by no means rare and convey some impression of the insidious character which the disease may have, particularly in young patients. Occasionally, Hodgkin's disease remains undetected during life, and is diagnosed only at the autopsy table, either as an incidental finding in patients dying of other conditions or as the previously unsuspected cause of the patient's fatal illness.

Diagnostic Evaluation of the Extent of Disease

Introduction. The responsible physician's diagnostic responsibility does not end when a competent pathologist makes a biopsy diagnosis of Hodgkin's disease in his patient. The full extent of involvement is more likely than not to be greater than the lymphadenopathy first detected on physical examination or conventional radiography. It is therefore extremely unwise to proceed immediately with local treatment on the assumption that no other sites of disease exist. Instead, a meticulous and thorough diagnostic evaluation of every patient should be carried to completion prior to the delineation of a treatment plan. In those instances in which symptoms of an emergency nature are present, such as superior vena caval obstruction or the cord compression syndrome, brief courses of radiotherapy and/or chemotherapy may be instituted to afford temporary palliation and to prevent more serious sequelae, after which it is again safe to proceed with the diagnostic evaluation.

Our routine diagnostic study of all patients with a biopsy diagnosis of a malignant lymphoma includes all of the procedures listed below:

Careful history and physical examination
Radiographic examination of the chest and skeletal system
Tomography of the mediastinal and hilar lymph nodes and both lungs when chest radiography is positive or suspicious
Lower extremity lymphangiography
Trephine needle bone marrow biopsy
Laparotomy (if needle marrow biopsy is negative) with splenectomy and biopsies of the para-aortic nodes and liver and open bone marrow biopsy.
Complete blood cell count
Urinalysis
Stool guaiac test
Liver function tests

In addition to this basic routine, other procedures are selectively utilized. Careful rhinolaryngologic examination, with particular attention to the lymphoid tissues of Waldeyer's ring, is often rewarding in patients with lymphocytic and histiocytic lymphomas, but these structures are seldom involved in Hodgkin's disease. Inferior vena cavography and computed tomography may be valuable when lymphangiography fails to fill the para-aortic nodes, particularly the upper right lumbar group. Barium studies of the upper and lower gastrointestinal tract are selectively indicated in patients with Hodgkin's disease who have significant gastrointestinal symptoms and should be part of the routine investigation for most patients with other types of malignant lymphomas. Biopsy of the liver, either by the percutaneous needle technique or at laparoscopy (Scholten, 1968; De Vita et al., 1971a; Casirola, Ippoliti, and Marini, 1973; Beretta et al., 1976), or laparotomy, is indicated when hepatic enlargement and/or abnormal liver function tests cannot otherwise be explained. Radioisotopic bone scans employing ^{99m}Tc may be extremely helpful in the localization of Hodgkin's disease involving bone, even in instances in which conventional radiographic examination is apparently negative (Harbert and Ashburn, 1968; Schechter et al., 1976). In some instances, radioisotopic scans with ^{111}InCl$_3$ (Gilbert et al., 1976a) or ^{99m}Tc sulfur colloid (Ultmann and Moran, 1973) may delineate abnormal areas of uptake in the bone marrow for selective needle marrow biopsy. We have not hesitated to obtain additional excisional biopsies of suspicious lymph nodes in sites which would have altered the clinical staging classification and treatment plan; specifically, we have obtained left scalene node biopsies in selected patients whose left cervical-supraclavicular nodes were clinically negative. Bronchial brush biopsy has been useful in selected cases presenting with mediastinal and hilar lymphadenopathy (Variakojis, Fennessy, and Rappaport, 1972; Harlan, Fennessy, and Gross, 1974). Finally, laparotomy with splenectomy and biopsy of the para-aortic lymph nodes and the liver (Enright, Trueblood, and Nelsen, 1970) has been performed on most of our patients with Hodgkin's disease, initially on a selective basis (Glatstein et al., 1969), and more recently on a routine basis (Glatstein et al., 1970; Rosenberg and Kaplan, 1970). The impressive yield of positive findings is described further on in this chapter and in Chapters 7 and 8.

History. A carefully taken routine medical history, with appropriate emphasis not only on the presenting complaints but also on a detailed review of systems, will usually suffice to elucidate all of the significant symptoms of a patient with Hodgkin's disease. However, certain points deserve special emphasis.

Certain constitutional symptoms, notably fever, night sweats, and significant weight loss are associated with a significantly poorer prognosis and often indicate the presence of widespread disease. Accordingly, particular care should be taken not only to inquire whether fever, night sweats, and/or weight loss were actually experienced by the patient, but also to ascertain whether they were ascribable to the Hodgkin's disease per se, or

merely coincidental, perhaps associated with an intercurrent acute infectious process, digestive disturbance or other unrelated condition.

The classical cyclic Pel-Ebstein fever is so typical as to be virtually diagnostic (Reimann, 1977), but it is rarely encountered in patients who first present themselves with previously untreated Hodgkin's disease. Instead, they are likely to have a low grade (perhaps up to 38.0–38.5 C.) irregular, smoldering, often poorly documented febrile process. Not infrequently, the patient will have had the impression of having had a "cold," though on careful questioning the typical symptoms of catarrh, nasal congestion, rhinorrhea, and postnasal drip may be lacking. In other instances, the fever may first have been noted during the course of a brief intercurrent infectious illness, but the clue that it is relevant is its persistence after all other manifestations of the intercurrent illness have cleared. It is often helpful, in borderline situations, to ask the patient to record his or her evening temperature daily during the one to two week interval usually required for the diagnostic evaluation. Irregular, low grade temperature elevations during this interval may resolve the physician's doubts concerning the significance of earlier febrile episodes.

Severe, florid night sweats are such a dramatic experience that few patients, when questioned appropriately about them, will have any difficulty in recalling their occurrence, their severity, or their approximate duration. Not infrequently, however, the patient may give a much more equivocal response, recalling only slight dampness of the skin around the neck and precordium on awakening either during the night or in the morning. It is probably best not to give undue weight to such an equivocal and dubious symptom. Nonetheless, we have observed occasional instances in which minimal and localized nocturnal perspiration disappeared during or shortly after definitive radiotherapy, suggesting in retrospect that it may well have been both real and relevant. In taking a history from women who are in menopause, either natural or artificially induced, physicians should be alert to the possibility that the patient may confuse ordinary "hot flashes", which occur both day and night, and are seldom accompanied by appreciable real perspiration, with true night sweats, which occur only during sleep.

Tell-tale evidence that the patient with Hodgkin's disease has generalized pruritus is often immediatedly evident in the form of cutaneous excoriations and blood-encrusted scabs, which are often seen on the upper and lower extremities, frequently also on the trunk, but rarely on the face or neck. Itching may be so severe as to interfere with sleep, appetite, and general well being, although this is unusual. Caution should be observed in ascribing significance to mild or moderate itching which is confined to the upper or to the lower extremities, although we have observed occasional instances in which such localized itching disappeared during the course of radiotherapy and was therefore deemed in retrospect to have been relevant to the patient's Hodgkin's disease. Some patients may give a history of longstanding eczema or other dermatoses which may adequately explain generalized itching (Bluefarb, 1967). Careful questioning about recent use of potentially allergenic drugs and medications taken more or less concurrently with the onset of the itching may also be revealing.

The bizarre pain associated with alcohol intake has been described above. When severe, this symptom also impresses itself deeply on the patient's consciousness and is readily and vividly recalled on questioning. However, patients who have not experienced sharp pain localized in large lymph nodes, but only a dull ache, vague discomfort, or perhaps merely a sense of nausea after intake of small quantities of alcoholic beverages may not recall these symptoms when questioned about alcohol intolerance. Some patients state that they do not drink alcoholic beverages. Further questioning may then reveal that they formerly consumed alcoholic beverages but stopped because they had developed aching, discomfort, or nausea. Alcohol intolerance occurs in such a small proportion of untreated patients that its prognostic significance has never been fully elucidated. In the series of patients studied by Atkinson et al. (1976a) the median survival of patients with alcohol intolerance was slightly longer than that of the much larger series of patients without this symptom complex. Thus, alcohol intolerance remains primarily a clinical curiosity rather than a guide to management or prognosis.

Hodgkin's disease is seldom associated with early weight loss. Accordingly, when careful questioning elicits a history of involuntary weight loss exceeding 10 percent of the normal body weight, the presence of extensive disease should be strongly suspected. Significant weight loss is a prognostically unfavorable manifestation (Tubiana et al., 1971). Fatigue, weakness, and malaise, though ordinarily trivial and nonspecific, may have the same sinister connotation when they are of manifest severity.

The review of systems may disclose specific symptoms having important implications regarding sites of involvement by the disease. For example, we have seen patients whose complaint of aching left shoulder and/or scapular pain, sometimes aggravated on deep breathing or coughing, was later explained at laparotomy by direct invasion of the hemidiaphragm from an extensively involved spleen. Swelling and edema of the feet, ankles, and lower extremities may signal the presence of massive para-aortic node involvement with secondary compression or occlusion of the inferior vena cava and/or the renal veins. Unilateral chest pain aggravated on deep breathing and coughing should prompt a search for pleural or rib involvement on the affected side. Certain symptoms should alert the physician to the possible presence of a life-threatening manifestation of the disease which requires emergency evaluation and treatment. Relevant examples already mentioned include the superior vena caval obstruction syndrome and the spinal cord compression syndrome.

As indicated in Chapter 3, the various histopathologic forms of Hodgkin's disease exhibit wide disparities in their rate of progression, and both histopathology and rate of progression correlate closely with prognosis. When the patient is aware of having enlarged peripheral lymph nodes in one or more sites, it is useful to inquire concerning their duration, relative rate of growth, and time intervals between onset of enlargement at the respective sites. In relatively favorable cases, it is usual for patients to state that the enlarged lymph nodes have been evident for months, occasionally even years, growing very slowly if at all. Others give a history of the almost explosive appearance of lymphadenopathy. Lymph nodes that have been noticeably enlarged for a short time, and have continued to grow rapidly in size from the time when they were first noted, generally betoken aggressive disease. Some patients report fluctuation in size of involved lymph nodes, sometimes associated with tenderness during the periods of rapid enlargement. Cycles of lymph node enlargement are occasionally associated with simultaneous cyclic bouts of high swinging fever of the Pel-Ebstein type.

Physical Findings. The usual careful and thorough physical examination need be modified only by greater emphasis on a search for peripheral lymphadenopathy. The physician must keep in mind the anatomic distributions of all of the major lymph node chains and palpate with great care and persistence for enlarged nodes in the preauricular, occipital, submaxillary and submental, anterior and posterior cervical, supraclavicular, infraclavicular, axillary, epitrochlear, iliac, inguinal and femoral areas bilaterally. Each site in which abnormal nodes are encountered should be carefully noted on an anatomic body diagram, and the size of the node or conglomerate mass of nodes should be measured and recorded for future reference. Although most abnormal nodes are readily palpable, relatively small pathologic nodes, particularly those occurring in the axillary, infraclavicular, and supraclavicular areas, not infrequently escape detection.

In our experience, the axillary and cervico-supraclavicular areas are best examined with the patient sitting in the erect position, though in rare instances one can more readily palpate nodes in the axilla with the patient in a supine position. This is particularly true in heavily muscular young male patients. It is a common error to examine the axilla while the patient holds the upper extremity in a slightly abducted position. Under these conditions, the patient must flex and set a number of muscles traversing the axilla to maintain the arm position. It is important that the soft tissues of the axillary regions be maximally relaxed, a condition that may be achieved by asking the patient either to let the arm fall passively to the adducted position after the physician's examining hand has been placed high in the axilla or to raise the arm to the horizontal position and then relax it by resting the hand on the shoulder of the examining physician.

The presence of infraclavicular nodes can sometimes be detected by careful inspection, which may reveal a loss of the normal concavity of the infraclavicular and pectoral area. Gentle palpation in such instances will readily disclose one or more enlarged lymph nodes underlying the swollen area. Although such nodes are usually near the midclavicular line, they may occur farther laterally and then often escape detection because they are mistakenly considered part of the muscle mass anteromedial to the shoulder joint.

In the supraclavicular area, nodes are occasionally missed when they lie so far medial that they are not palpated when the examiner's hand moves downward along the lateral aspect of the neck. This error may be avoided by compressing the anterior-inferior edge of the sternocleidomastoid muscle between the thumb and index finger. Small pathological nodes lurking behind the clavicle are often made accessible to palpation by turning the patient's face far to the opposite side, with the chin maximally elevated, and manipulating the ipsilateral shoulder backward and downward, or by the Valsalva maneuver (Kuiper and Papp, 1969).

The consistency of involved lymph nodes in Hodgkin's disease, and in most other malignant lymphomas, is typically firm but not stony hard; instead, the firmness has a distinctly resilient quality, often suggestive of the feeling of a solid rubber ball. Such "rubbery" nodes are seldom tender or painful to palpation, although we have seen well documented exceptions in which tenderness was so pronounced as to make differentiation from bacterial infection or other inflammatory processes quite difficult.

Great caution must be exercised to avoid overinterpreting every palpable lymph node as being involved by Hodgkin's disease. The location of a palpable node, the age of the patient, and relevant features of the history and physical examination must be taken into account when the physician attempts to assess whether a given node is clinically significant. Lymph nodes in the submandibular area and the upper half of the neck, in both the anterior and the posterior cervical chains, are within the drainage pathway for the commonplace bacterial and viral infections of the throat and upper air passages. Although their tenderness during the acute, active phases of the infection is a helpful feature in evaluation, they may remain enlarged, but no longer tender, for an appreciable interval after the infection has resolved. Careful questioning for a history of recent upper respiratory tract infection may suggest that such nodes are probably not relevant. In contrast, lymph nodes in the lower half of the neck and in the supraclavicular fossa are seldom affected by acute upper respiratory tract infections; palpable enlargement of such nodes in a patient with Hodgkin's disease is therefore much more likely to be clinically significant. Small firm lymph nodes are often palpable in the axilla and groin; these sites drain chronic inflammatory reactions of the hands and feet, which are commonplace sequelae of accidental or occupational trauma, fungal infections, etc. Usually these are only a few millimeters to perhaps one centimeter in diameter. They are typically nontender, and often described as "shotty." In some instances, a mass of lymph nodes in the groin may be mistaken for a hernia, in which case the diagnosis may not be suspected until progressive growth of the lymph node mass clarifies its true nature. The converse is equally true; hernias may be mistaken for involved lymph nodes in patients already known to have a malignant lymphoma and are sometimes the cause of errors in staging and in treatment. The characteristically resilient, "rubbery" firmness of lymph nodes involved by Hodgkin's disease is usually sufficiently distinctive to permit the experienced observer to distinguish them from chronic inflammatory lymphadenopathy or other benign conditions. Whenever an enlarged lymph node is palpated in a site whose involvement would significantly influence either staging or treatment, it is a wise policy to subject such a node to excisional biopsy and histologic examination, even though a firm histologic diagnosis of Hodgkin's disease has already been established on biopsy material obtained from some other site.

The inadequacy of physical examination relative to radiographic examination in the detection and evaluation of intrathoracic disease is well known. Nonetheless, the physical examination can provide important clues when Hodgkin's disease involves structures within the thorax. Compression of the superior vena cava by massive mediastinal adenopathy reveals its presence by such signs as facial edema and engorgement of the veins in the neck and the upper anterior chest. Invasion of the pericardium may give rise to a friction rub, or to significant effusion, accompanied by diminished auscultatory intensity of the heart sounds, and when tamponade supervenes, by paradoxical pulse. Small pulmonary parenchymal infiltrates are usually silent on physical examination, but large infiltrations affecting entire segments or lobes of the lung yield the typical physical signs of pulmonary consolidation or of cavitation. Pleural involvement may be heralded by friction rubs or by areas of dullness over significant volumes of pleural fluid. In occasional instances, we have observed and palpated localized masses in the thoracic wall, usually anteriorly in or near the midline, replacing the sternum and invading the presternal soft tissues, or, more commonly, parasternal in location, filling one of the intercostal spaces, most often the second. Such masses are usually due to soft tissue and/or sternal invasion adjacent to involved internal mammary lymph nodes.

Moving on to the upper abdomen, the physical examination should be oriented toward the detection of hepatosplenomegaly. Palpation of the spleen should be attempted with the patient first in the supine position and then turned obliquely up onto the right side. Minimal degress of splenic enlargement detected by palpation may sometimes be confirmed by conventional radiography, or by radioisotopic spleen scans, using ^{99m}Tc or ^{111}In colloid. Enlargement of the liver is seldom massive except in patients in the preterminal stages of the disease. In our experience, hepatomegaly has not been a sensitive or reliable indicator of hepatic involvement. Patients with biopsy-proved infiltration of the liver have in many instances exhibited no evidence of hepatomegaly, whereas significant degrees of hepatic enlargement in others have proved to be due to other causes, such as hepatitis (Glatstein et al., 1969). The significance of palpable enlargement of the liver is of course greatly enhanced when the palpated liver edge is firm and nodular. Radioisotopic scans of the liver may reveal filling defects when nodules of appreciable size are present.

Very large masses of involved lymph nodes in the upper retroperitoneal area or the mesentery are occasionally palpable through the anterior abdominal wall, and grossly enlarged iliac nodes are frequently detectable on deep palpation of the abdomen along the line parallel to and 2 to 3 cm. superior to the inguinal fold. However, palpation is at best a highly insensitive method for detection of intra-abdominal lymphadenopathy; reliance must be placed instead on roentgenologic methods such as lower extremity lymphangiography, inferior vena cavography, and computed tomography. Finally, a careful neurologic examination of each patient is indicated for the detection of paresis, paralysis, abnormal reflexes, and other signs indicative of the cord compression syndrome, or the rare instances of intracranial Hodgkin's disease.

Laboratory Findings. The complete blood cell count can provide important clues to the status of the patient with Hodgkin's disease (Simmons, Spiers, and Fayers, 1973). The hematologic parameters are likely to be within normal limits in the great majority of recently diagnosed, previously untreated cases. Nonetheless, significant abnormalities of the white blood cell count, the platelet count, and the red blood cell, hemoglobin, and packed cell volume (PCV) levels are not at all uncommon. Peripheral blood cell values in 100 randomly selected previously untreated cases from our Stanford experience are presented in Table 4.1. The abnormal values are summarized in Table 4.2. It may be noted that only one patient, with stage IIIB disease, had a hemoglobin level less than 10.0 gm percent. However, 12 percent of this series of patients were anemic as defined by a packed cell volume less than 35 percent. Leukocytosis, with a white blood cell count exceeding 10,000 per mm^3, occurred in 27 percent of the series, whereas leukopenia, defined by a white blood cell count less than 5,000 per mm^3, occurred in only 5 percent. Absolute lymphocyte counts less than 1,000 per mm^3 were noted in 19 percent. The

Table 4.1 Hematologic Data on Admission in 100 Randomly Selected, Previously Untreated Patients with Hodgkin's Disease

Final stage	Case	Hemo-globin* (gm. %)	Packed cell volume (%)	White blood cells (per mm.^{3})	Lymphocytes (%)	Mono-cytes (%)	Eosinophiles (%)	Absolute lympho-cytes/mm.^{3}	Erythrocyte Sedimentation Rate (mm./hr.)
	1. J.B.	13.3	39.5	5700	48.0	7	8	2736	10
	2. R.R.	12.9	39.3	8100	27.3	8	8.3	2211	—
	3. R.J.	16.2	46.8	9550	19.5	3.5	2	1862	7
	4. T.S.	14.6	44.5	5700	10.0	6	4	570	—
	5. J.C.	16.2	47.5	9100	33.0	4	1	3003	—
	6. K.G.	13.9	44.5	5930	26.6	6.3	2.3	1577	23
	7. O.W.	13.4	39.5	5600	52.0	2	2	2912	15
I-A	8. W.G.	14.4	45.0	8700	27.0	7	8	2349	—
	9. P.G.	12.5	43.0	5300	38.0	8	—	2014	—
	10. R.B.	14.4	44.0	8400	22.0	7	1	1848	—
	11. I.A.	15.5	47.0	5700	34.0	15	6	1938	—
	12. J.B.	15.0	45.0	7500	34.0	—	4	2550	—
	13. L.B.	12.2	39.5	5800	31.0	2	—	1798	—
	14. G.L.	10.6	36.5	9000	20.0	3.5	4.5	1800	55
	15. H.B.	13.2	40.2	7200	26.0	6	6	1872	36
	16. J.A.	14.6	42.7	5600	32.0	3	5.5	1792	
	Means:	13.9	42.8	6930				2052	
I-B	17. R.C.	14.0	45.5	6350	24.5	3.5	8	1556	—
		—	—	—				—	
	18. R.G.	14.6	43.8	7950	20.5	8	1.5	1630	6
	19. P.M.	14.8	44.5	12500	15.0	4	11	1875	—
	20. J.D.	15.0	47.0	9600	30.0	3	—	2880	7
	21. I.J.	13.1	39.5	8600	15.0	9	1	1290	—
	22. J.M.	13.2	39.8	6500	15.0	6.5	7	975	43
	23. R.S.	10.7	35.0	8500	22.0	6	—	1870	37
	24. G.P.	13.9	39.0	12600	8.0	1	1	1008	37
	25. D.M.	13.9	45.0	6200	38.0	7	6	2356	8
	26. J.D.	12.3	38.0	5400	26.5	7	2.5	1431	11
	27. R.O.	12.4	37.7	11700	28.5	6	7	3349	19
	28. A.I.	13.5	42.0	7300	30.0	3	4	2190	10
	29. C.D.	13.1	40.5	8400	13.0	—	3	1092	32
	30. D.K.	12.4	38.0	8200	38.0	2	3	3116	28
	31. W.F.	15.4	45.0	8000	28.0	2	2	2240	—
	32. G.D.	10.9	38.0	14000	10.0	3	1	1400	—
	33. W.H.	13.7	42.5	9300	15.0	3	1	1395	3
II-A	34. L.K.	12.5	36.5	4900	17.0	2	6	833	31
	35. D.C.	14.4	43.1	5700	38.0	3	2	2116	7
	36. T.B.	14.5	45.5	5200	20.0	7	2	1040	16
	37. S.H.	14.2	41.6	5930	19.3	5.3	8.7	1144	—
	38. S.P.	13.6	42.0	8900	16.0	5	2	1424	28
	39. M.N.	11.2	36.0	10300	11.0	5	4.5	1133	48
	40. W.H.	15.9	47.0	6800	25.0	9	3	1700	4
	41. G.W.	14.2	43.3	7300	30.0	6	1	2190	—
	42. D.S.	12.9	40.5	7000	66.0	12	12	4620	—
	43. B.M.	13.7	39.5	8500	19.0	3	3	1615	15
	44. R.C.	15.2	44.2	8700	13.5	12.5	3.5	1175	3
	45. G.B.	14.4	41.8	10300	13.5	3	3	1391	40
	46. S.D.	12.7	39.0	9500	8.5	3	1.5	808	40
	47. H.A.	14.7	44.2	11800	18.0	4.5	1	2124	—
	48. D.B.	14.9	44.0	8500	27.0	6	3	2295	—
	49. D.B.	14.2	43.0	12000	14.0	2	2	1680	—
	50. P.S.	10.3	34.0	9000	12.0	5	4	1080	—
	Means:	13.0	41.2	8640				1772	

(*Continued*)

Table 4.1 (Continued)

II(E)-A	51. M.C.	11.0	36.0	22800	22.0	5	—	5016	—
		—	—	—				—	
	52. D.B.	11.8	37.0	8650	15.5	3	1.5	1341	48
	53. S.N.	12.0	39.0	9200	20.0	5	1	1840	—
	54. D.P.	14.7	42.3	6450	8.5	4.5	4	548	19
	55. J.F.	12.2	37.0	12000	15.0	4	4	1800	54
	56. E.K.	11.9	38.5	2800	24.0	14	6	672	43
	57. M.R.	11.7	36.0	5800	7.0	9	6	406	52
	58. T.K.	13.4	37.5	11700	9.0	4	—	1053	—
	59. A.R.	10.8	34.5	5200	6.5	13	10	338	—
	60. K.K.	11.8	34.7	5400	19.0	8	2	1026	—
II-B	62. G.B.	13.8	43.1	7100	20.0	6	1	1420	65
	63. B.H.	13.3	40.4	7700	16.0	2	40	1232	—
	64. C.L.	10.5	34.0	11800	2.0	6	3	236	—
	65. A.S.	13.7	42.5	16500	15.0	7	—	2475	—
	66. D.W.	15.0	46.3	5500	24.5	3.5	2	1348	6
	67. K.W.	11.3	35.5	12500	13.0	4	1	1625	—
	68. J.H.	11.2	34.8	12200	9.0	7	1	1098	—
	69. D.S.	11.4	37.5	20000	14.5	2	1	2900	46
	70. D.W.	12.4	38.0	8500	13.0	3	1	1105	—
	Means:	12.4	38.4	8960				1248	
II(E)-B	71. B.V.	11.3	37.5	11800	8.0	1	10	944	17
	72. G.J.	13.3	41.9	20300	9.5	9	1.5	1929	—
	Means:	12.3	39.7	16050				1436	
III-A	73. C.C.	11.3	35.1	9300	16.3	7.6	2.8	1516	53
	74. C.Z.	13.3	41.0	7800	17.0	6	—	1326	14
	75. B.H.	13.6	42.5	9600	23.0	8	2	2208	44
	76. M.E.	12.2	39.0	11900	13.0	3	21	1547	—
	77. H.C.	15.7	47.0	6200	14.0	8	—	868	9
	78. P.R.	13.9	43.2	11500	18.0	5	6	2070	40
	79. G.M.	12.7	41.0	3200	4.0	3	1	128	—
	80. J.M.	15.2	46.0	9100	17.0	4.5	3	1547	10
	81. B.O.	11.2	35.5	3500	12.0	3	8	420	53
	82. M.R.	15.6	50.5	7200	17.0	10	2	1224	—
	83. M.B.	10.3	34.0	9100	26.0	7	1	2336	—
	Means:	13.2	41.3	8040				1381	
III-B	84. G.C.	11.9	37.2	10300	17.0	8	4.5	1751	—
	85. E.A.	12.8	37.8	14800	17.5	4.5	4	2590	50
	86. L.G.	15.3	47.7	7500	13.5	9	2	1013	—
	87. P.F.	16.1	48.0	5700	18.0	16	1	1026	19
	88. R.B.	14.6	48.0	8100	5.0	6	2	405	—
	89. J.B.	13.7	42.5	13400	16.0	6	8	2144	—
	90. E.S.	10.6	31.0	13000	18.0	1	—	2340	—
	91. F.B.	8.6	27.0	12400	4.0	3	4	496	—
	92. M.K.	11.0	34.7	9900	15.5	6	3	1535	15
	93. T.B.	11.1	34.5	2400	18.5	8	3	444	—
	Means:	12.6	38.8	9750				1374	
IV-A	94. D.K.	13.0	43.7	7900	12.0	7.5	3	948	45
	95. D.D.	12.7	40.7	6000	14.0	4	8	840	25
	96. P.F.	10.8	34.8	11250	8.5	2	3	956	49
	Means:	12.2	39.7	8380				915	
IV-B	97. M.W.	14.1	46.5	18600	11.0	4	—	2046	10
	98. N.G.	11.2	36.2	11100	17.0	2	3	1887	33
	99. M.A.	12.1	38.0	18500	7.0	5	32	1295	52
	100. L.M.	10.4	34.2	7400	29.5	2	10.5	2183	55
	Means:	11.9	38.7	13900				1853	

relative frequency of abnormal findings tended to increase with clinical stage. Erythrocyte sedimentation rate (ESR) values were available in 54 patients of this series, and were elevated (> 30 mm/hr) in 26 of these (48 percent), again in association with clinical stage.

It has been claimed that leukocytosis of significant degree is an unfavorable prognostic sign, associated with relatively advanced or aggressive forms of the disease. Yet, paradoxically, there is also evidence that leukopenia carries similar connotations. Patients with initial leukopenia may also be somewhat more difficult to treat to completion with total lymphoid radiotherapy.

The platelet count is seldom remarkable at the time of diagnosis. However, occasional cases have been reported in which thrombocytopenic purpura has been a presenting manifestation of Hodgkin's disease (Rudders, Aisenberg, and Schiller, 1972; Godeau et al., 1975). It has also been stated that a sudden, marked increase in the platelet count, often accompanied by an increase in the erythrocyte sedimentation rate, may herald the invasion of a new chain of lymph nodes, and that the platelet count tends to return to normal during remission (Barry, Laroche, and Delâge, 1966). Idiopathic thrombocytopenic purpura occurs in occasional patients, and apparently has little or no prognostic significance (Antonio and Sherwood, 1976; Cohen, 1978). However, cases have been reported in which thrombocytopenic purpura was the first manifestation of relapsing disease (Hamilton and Dawson, 1973).

Anemia is perhaps the most serious, though the least common, initial hematologic abnormality and should alert the physician to a particularly searching scrutiny of the hematopoietic system for a satisfactory explanation. Anemia occurs with greater frequency during the later course of the disease in patients who fail to enter remission and in those who develop one or more relapses after initially successful treatment. In about 10 percent of the series of patients studied by Ultmann, Cunningham, and Gellhorn (1966) a hypochromic microcytic anemia was observed, due in some instances to chronic blood loss secondary to nonspecific gastrointestinal lesions. Other cases have been attributed to impaired mobilization of iron from tissue stores and to defective reutilization of red blood cell iron. Serum iron levels in such instances are low, whereas the unsaturated iron-binding capacity is normal. Low serum iron levels (< 70 μg/100 ml) are considered by some investigators to be a prognostically unfavorable "biological sign" (Teillet,

Boiron, and Bernard, 1971). Whereas red blood cell life span is usually normal (Lanaro, Bosch, and Frías, 1971), release of stored iron from the reticuloendothelial system may be impaired (Beamish et al., 1972).

Autoimmune hemolytic anemia is not uncommon during the later course of the disease (Eisner, Ley, and Mayer, 1967; Jones, 1973) and has even occurred in rare instances as an initial manifestation (Bowdler and Glick, 1966). Cyclic bouts of hemolytic anemia synchronous with Pel-Ebstein fever have also been reported (Ranløv and Videbaek, 1963; Storgaard and Karle, 1975). The ^{51}Cr red blood cell survival test, the Coombs test, and the level of urobilinogen excretion are all valuable indicators of hemolytic processes (Giannopoulos and Bergsagel, 1959; Cline and Berlin, 1963). Such abnormalities may respond dramatically to steroid therapy or to splenectomy. Occasionally, anemia may be associated with folic acid deficiency (Ultmann, 1966). Much more serious are the instances in which anemia and low hemoglobin values are attributable to inadequate production of red blood cells rather than their excessive destruction, since the single most common cause of this manifestation is marrow infiltration by Hodgkin's disease. Yet, in some patients, repeated bone marrow biopsies may be necessary to demonstrate that such infiltration actually exists.

The differential white blood cell count is also usually normal in the patient with previously untreated Hodgkin's disease, though a monocytosis of moderate degree is not infrequently noted (Table 4.1). Increased numbers of monocytes are regularly detectable in smears of leukocyte concentrates, in which Sternberg-Reed cells may also occasionally be seen (Bouroncle, 1966). An association between fever and the presence of Sternberg-Reed cells in the peripheral blood was noted by Hoerni, Chauvergne, and Parsi (1970). They observed such cells by the leucoconcentration technique in 9 of 19 examinations in which fever was concomitantly present, and in only 1 of 27 in which it was absent, in a series of 24 patients with Hodgkin's disease. An absolute lymphocytopenia below 1,000 lymphocytes per cubic millimeter is of much more serious import, usually indicating the presence of advanced and/or relatively aggressive disease (Aisenberg, 1965; Brown et al., 1967). Conversely, the presence of an abnormally high concentration of large lymphoid cells resembling immunoblasts has been reported (Crowther et al., 1967a; Halie et al., 1972a; Schick et al., 1973). The significance of this observation is discussed in Chapter 6. Significant eosinophilia is seen in occasional patients (Tauro, 1966; Table 4.1); in adults it may reflect a coexisting allergic condition, whereas, in children it may indicate the presence of a coexisting viscerolarva migrans. There is no convincing evidence that eosinophilia is correlated with prognosis (Westling, 1965).

The erythrocyte sedimentation rate (ESR) is a highly nonspecific indicator of disease activity. It is often elevated in patients with previously untreated Hodgkin's disease (Tables 4.1 and 4.2), and such elevations, in the series reported by Westling (1965), were a harbinger of a significantly decreased probability of survival. This inverse correlation with prognosis has been confirmed by the data of several other institutions (Musshoff et al., 1976; Le Bourgeois and Tubiana, 1977). When elevated initially, ESR values usually fall slowly to normal levels in patients who exhibit an apparently complete remission in response to specific therapy and may again become elevated prior to or during clinical relapse (Ultmann, Cunningham, and Gellhorn, 1966). In a series of 68 patients with clinical stages I and II Hodgkin's disease studied by Le Bourgeois and Tubiana (1977), ESR values above 30 mm/hr occurred in 80 percent of patients with relapsing disease. Conversely, relapses were detected in 90 percent of those cases in which the ESR was elevated. The average delay between observation of an elevated ESR and the detection of relapse was 4.5 months. In view of its nonspecificity, however, isolated fluctuations of the ESR should not be given undue weight, and in no instance should a new course of treatment be instituted solely on the basis of a renewed elevation of the ESR. We have seen tragic cases in which chemotherapy was begun and carried to the point of severe and occasionally fatal bone marrow toxicity for presumed but undocumented relapses of

Hodgkin's disease for which no evidence other than a renewed elevation of the ESR was ever sought. In some of these, no evidence of Hodgkin's disease was found at autopsy; such cases must be regarded as iatrogenic deaths.

When the ESR has been followed serially from the time of initial diagnosis through the course of treatment and on into the subsequent followup period, a renewed and sustained elevation of the ESR should be taken as a signal for careful evaluation of the patient (Le Bourgeois and Tubiana, 1977). Smoldering infections, pregnancy, and other possible causes of elevation of the ESR should be carefully searched for, and relapse of Hodgkin's disease should not be considered likely until a reasonable search for other causes has proved negative. Concurrently, consideration should be given to possible sites in which new manifestations of Hodgkin's disease may silently have redeveloped. Appropriate diagnostic studies aimed at the detection of the disease in such sites should then be undertaken. In particular, it is often rewarding to perform lymphangiography, liver scans and function tests, and repeat bone marrow biopsy in a search for otherwise inapparent sites of relapsing disease. Only when positive and unequivocal evidence of renewed tissue involvement by Hodgkin's disease has been obtained should specific therapy be reinstituted.

It has also been claimed (Koch et al., 1957; Pagliardi et al., 1960, 1963; Jensen et al., 1964; Auerbach, 1965) that serum copper (ceruloplasmin) and zinc values reflect the activity of Hodgkin's disease. However, lack of specificity is again evident, since a multitude of other infectious and nonspecific disease conditions can also cause elevation of the serum copper and diminution of the serum zinc concentration. Where multiple serum determinations during the course of the disease have

Table 4.2 Summary of Hematologic Abnormalities on Admission in 100 Randomly Selected, Previously Untreated Patients with Hodgkin's Disease

Hematologic abnormality	Clinical stage				% all cases
	I	II	III	IV	
Hgb < 10.0 gm.%	—	—	1/21	—	1
PCV < 35.5%	0/17	5/55	5/21	2/7	12
WBC > 10,000/mm.³	0/17	16/55	7/21	4/7	27
WBC < 5,000/mm.³	0/17	2/55	3/21	0/7	5
Absol. lymphocytes < 1,000/mm.³	1/17	9/55	6/21	3/7	19
ESR > 30 mm./hr.	2/6	14/31	5/10	5/7	48

Source: Stanford University Medical Center data (Kaplan).

been made and levels have fallen to normal after treatment, a renewed elevation of the copper level has been reported to carry the same significance in respect to possible relapse as a renewed elevation of the ESR (Hrgovcic et al., 1968, 1975; Warren et al., 1969; Mortazavi et al., 1972; Cappelaere et al., 1975; Thorling and Thorling, 1976). Similar claims have been made with respect to elevation of the leukocyte alkaline phosphatase (Martinez-Maldonado et al., 1964; Bennett et al., 1968; Jaffe and Bishop, 1970; Simmons, Spiers, and Fayers, 1973), of serum haptoglobin levels (Krauss et al., 1966a), of serum protein-bound hexose (Goulian and Fahey, 1961) and hexosamine (Spiers and Malone, 1966), and to decreased levels of bradykininogen (Eilam et al., 1968), all of which have been reported to correlate with activity or relapse of Hodgkin's disease but which are also subject to fluctuation in a variety of other disease conditions and thus are best utilized serially during the course of the disease, if at all. With the exception of the serum copper, all of these indicators have to date proved less sensitive than the much simpler and less expensive ESR, and there is no convincing evidence that any of them is more specific. Ray, Wolf, and Kaplan (1973) found that in previously untreated patients, all of whom, by definition, have "active" disease, elevated levels of serum copper and ceruloplasmin occurred in approximately one-half of the cases, and of muramidase and leukocyte alkaline phosphatase in a substantially smaller fraction (Table 4.3).

Serial determinations of the serum copper level were made in a sample population of 50 patients with Hodgkin's disease of all stages treated and subsequently followed at Stanford University Medical Center from 1971 through 1975. This group included 37 males and 13 females (3 of whom started taking contraceptive pills some months after completion of treatment). The initial serum copper value was elevated in 45 (90 percent) of these 50 patients. The data are suggestive of a trend toward an increasing proportion of elevated values among patients with advanced stage disease and among those with constitutional symptoms and extralymphatic lesions, confirming correlations noted in previous studies by Hrgovcic et al. (1975) and by Thorling and Thorling (1976). Serial determinations of the serum copper level are particularly useful in the 6- to 12-month period immediately following completion of radiotherapy and/or combination chemotherapy, since the ESR tends to rise and to remain elevated for many months as a consequence of treatment and is of

Table 4.3 Selected Laboratory Indices versus Clinical Stage, Histologic Type, and Treatment in Hodgkin's Disease

Procedure	Total group	Clinical stage					Symptoms		Histologic type[a]				Pre-therapy abnormals	Post-therapy values
		I	II	II_E	III	IV	A(−)	B(+)	NS	MC	LP	LD	Mean and (range)	Mean and (range)
Ceruloplasmin (normal 280–570)	14/27 (52)[b]	1/2	3/9	3/6	4/7	3/3	6/14	8/13	11/21	3/5	0/1	—	840 (580–1170)	410 (300–500)
Muramidase	8/31 (26)	0/3	2/13	3/6	1/8	2/3	2/19	6/12	7/25	1/4	0/1	0/1	—	—
Leukocyte Alkaline Phosphatase (normal 50–150)	6/31 (19)	0/3	1/14	3/7	1/8	1/3	3/19	3/12	5/25	1/5	0/1	—	180 (150–270)	130 (120–200)
Erythrocyte Sedimentation rate	16/22 (73)													

Source: Stanford University Medical Center data compiled by Ray, Wolf, and Kaplan (1973).
[a] NS = nodular sclerosis, MC = mixed cellularity, LP = lymphocytic predominance, LD = lymphocytic depletion.
[b] Number of abnormally elevated values/total number tested and (percent abnormal).

little help during this interval as a prognostic indicator. Conversely, the serum copper falls to normal levels and remains normal in successfully treated patients (Fig. 4.6), whereas failure of the serum copper values to return to normal following treatment, or a transient fall followed by a renewed elevation during the first 12 months after treatment (Fig. 4.7) usually denotes impending relapse. Additional data on the use of serial serum copper values as a prognostic indicator are presented in Chapter 12.

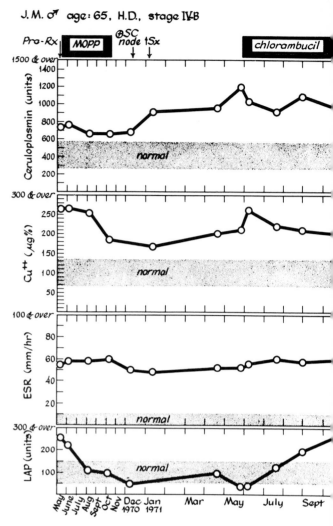

Figure 4.7 Correlation between laboratory indicators and clinical course in a 65-year-old male with stage IVB nodular sclerosing Hodgkin's disease. (Reprinted, by permission, from the paper by Ray, Wolf, and Kaplan, 1973.)

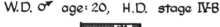
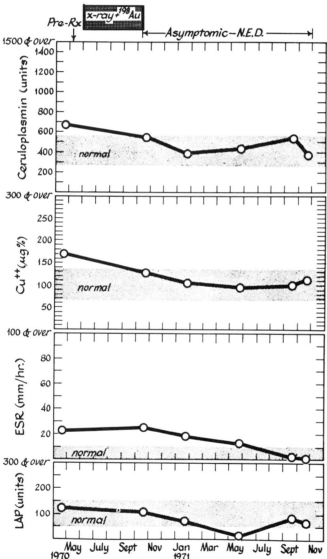

Figure 4.6 Sequential laboratory values, illustrating the relation between laboratory indicators and clinical course in a 20-year-old male with stage IVB nodular sclerosing Hodgkin's disease. (Reprinted, by permission, from the paper by Ray, Wolf, and Kaplan, 1973.)

Hypercalcemia, usually associated with hypophosphatemia and elevated levels of serum alkaline phosphatase, may occur in patients with extensive involvement of the skeletal system (Moses and Spencer, 1963; Linke, 1965; Ultmann, Cunningham, and Gellhorn, 1966). Nephrocalcinosis has been observed to develop in some of these patients. Hypercalcemia constitutes a medical emergency, and immediate measures should be taken to bring down the serum calcium levels in such instances. Elevated serum uric acid levels have also been observed in occasional cases (Primikirios, Stutzman, and Sandberg, 1961). Conversely, abnormally low serum uric acid concentrations have been reported in occasional patients with advanced Hodgkin's disease (Bennett et al., 1972; Kay and Gottlieb, 1973). Low serum iron levels, usually with normal unsaturated iron-binding capacity, may occur in the presence of anemia (Giannopoulos and Bergsagel, 1959) and have been considered by some clinicians to be a useful index of disease activity (Teillet, Boiron, and Bernard, 1971). Elevated levels of serum ferritin have been detected by serologic and radioimmunoassay methods (Bieber and Bieber, 1973; Jones et al., 1973; Sarcione, Stutzman, and Mittelman, 1975; Jacobs et al., 1976; May and Hancock, 1977). Lactic acidosis associated with the presence of large numbers of Sternberg-Reed cells in the peripheral blood was a feature of the unusual case described by Scheerer et al. (1964), and elevated blood pyruvate levels have been reported (Maneche, 1966). The syndrome of inappropriate antidiuretic hormone secretion has also been noted in association with Hodgkin's disease (Spittle, 1966; Cassileth and Trotman, 1973).

Serum protein abnormalities are not uncommon but are seldom of differential diagnostic import. Albumin synthesis may be decreased, leading to reduced serum albumin levels (Waldmann et al., 1963), whereas the α_1-, α_2-, and β_2-globulins are often increased at some time during the course of the disease (Arends et al., 1954; Neely and Neill, 1956; Goulian and Fahey, 1961; Malpas and Hamilton Fairley, 1964; Irunberry and Colonna, 1970). Hypo-γ-globulinemia was rare in the series studied by Hoffbrand (1964, 1965) but may develop later in the course of the disease (Ultmann, 1966). Cryomacroglobulins have been reported in rare instances (Krauss and Sokal, 1966), but monoclonal macroglobulinemia was not noted in any of the 205 cases studied by Moore et al. (1970). Several studies have indicated that immunoglobulin levels and antibody production are usually within normal limits, except in severely debilitated patients with far-advanced Hodgkin's disease (Barr and Hamilton Fairley, 1961; Aisenberg and Leskowitz, 1963). In a series of fifty patients studied serially during the course of their disease, Irunberry and Colonna (1970) noted increased levels of IgG, IgA, and IgM in 32, 19, and 14 percent, respectively, of samples drawn during relapse and in a smaller proportion of samples during remission. Serum complement levels are not infrequently increased, especially during relapse (Rottino and Levy, 1959; Balzola et al., 1964; Irunberry and Colonna, 1970). Isolated reports have appeared in which disease activity appeared to be correlated with elevated levels of serum proteins rich in hydroxyproline (LeRoy,

Carbone, and Sjoerdsma, 1966) and of C-reactive protein (Wood et al., 1958; Pecori et al., 1959). The latter observation is perhaps relevant to the immunologic abnormalities seen in Hodgkin's disease (cf. Chapter 6), since it has been demonstrated that C-reactive protein can bind to T-lymphocytes and thus alter their functional responses (Mortensen, Osmand, and Gewurz, 1975). Child et al. (1978) have examined the clinical significance of several of these acute phase reactive proteins.

The metabolism of amino acids may also be disturbed in some patients with Hodgkin's disease. In particular, abnormalities of tryptophan metabolism and a deficiency of plasma pyridoxal phosphate have been detected in patients with untreated Hodgkin's disease (Chabner et al., 1970; Muggeo et al., 1970; Gailani et al., 1974). It has been suggested that these abnormalities may be related to the impairment of cell-mediated immunity which is so often seen in Hodgkin's disease (De Vita et al., 1971b).

The routine urinalysis may be expected to be normal in virtually all patients with previously untreated Hodgkin's disease. Primarily, it serves as a useful baseline level against which subsequent abnormalities may be evaluated. However, cytologic identification of Sternberg-Reed cells in the urine sediment has been reported (Sano and Koprowska, 1965). Involvement of the kidneys is extremely uncommon in previously untreated patients; indeed, it is relatively infrequent even in patients dying of the disease (Martinez-Maldonado and Ramirez de Arrelano, 1966). Involvement of the lower urinary tract is even less common (Piquet-Gauthier et al., 1965). We and others have, however, seen occasional cases in which massive infiltration of the para-aortic lymph nodes has compressed the renal veins, with associated massive proteinuria, edema, and hypoproteinemia simulating the nephrotic syndrome (Brodovsky et al., 1968; Piessens and Zeicher, 1970; Ghosh and Muehrcke, 1970). Moreover, extremely interesting though rare cases have been reported in which lipoid or amyloid nephrosis has occurred in patients with Hodgkin's disease (Rohmer and Sacry, 1948; Sherman et al., 1955; Winawer and Feldman, 1959). Abel and Good (1966) cite a case in which an acid α_1-glycoprotein was excreted in large amounts in the urine. Abnormalities of pyrimidine metabolism, reflected in high urinary levels of pseudouridine, were detected in several patients with Hodgkin's disease, usually in association with constitutional symptoms, mixed cellularity or lymphocyte depletion histology, and other prognostically unfavorable manifestations (Pinkard et al., 1972). Increased urinary excretion of tryptophan metabolites, with an abnormal tryptophan loading test, has also been reported (Crepaldi and Parpajola, 1964).

For several years, we routinely obtained a diversified battery of liver function tests, including several serum enzymes, in all patients with Hodgkin's disease. However, analysis of a series of patients subjected to liver biopsy at laparotomy revealed that most of these tests had not been sensitive or reliable indices of hepatic involvement (Glatstein et al., 1969; Lipton et al., 1972; Abt et al., 1974). With the exception of those patients who present the rare complication of intrahepatic cholestasis (Bouroncle, Old, and Vazques, 1962), jaundice is a late manifestation which is seldom observed until involvement of the liver is extensive and clinically obvious by other criteria (Levitan et al., 1961). Thus, determinations of total and direct serum bilirubin levels are seldom helpful in the evaluation of the recently diagnosed, previously untreated case. The only two laboratory procedures which have been reasonably rewarding have been the bromsulphthalein retention test and the serum alkaline phosphatase. Since the latter is also elevated in patients with bone or bone marrow disease, the liver is not the only site that is incriminated when sustained and progressive increases in serum alkaline phosphatase levels are noted. The frequency of serum alkaline phosphatase elevation in untreated patients increases with clinical stage: 14 percent in stage I and II, 65 percent in stage III, and 81 percent in stage IV. The hepatic isozyme was the principal factor in such elevations, only 10 percent of which were due to the bone isozyme (Aisenberg et al., 1970). In the presence of fever, an increase in the serum alkaline phosphatase is a much less reliable indicator of organic disease.

Effusions into the pleural, peritoneal, and pericardial spaces are often due to direct invasion of these spaces by Hodgkin's disease, but in many other instances they are due to simple mechanical transudation of fluid secondary to obstructive phenomena in lymphatic vessels and lymph nodes or to nonspecific inflammatory conditions. Unfortunately, aspiration of such fluids seldom yields definitive diagnostic information. Elevated protein levels in effusions are generally regarded as indicative of neoplastic infiltration. However, we have seen several documented instances in which pleural effusions containing more than 4 gm. of protein per 100 cc. have permanently regressed without specific therapy. Although the cytology of such aspirated fluids should always be carefully

studied in smears and histologic sections of centrifuge-sedimented pellets, diagnostic Sternberg-Reed cells are seldom detectable, and their appearance in such effusions may be mimicked by mesothelial and other cells (Melamed, 1963). Accordingly, a firm diagnosis of pleural involvement usually requires tissue biopsy samples obtained either with the Cope needle or by thoracotomy. Cytologic examination of sputum or bronchial washings is occasionally successful in demonstrating Sternberg-Reed cells (Suprun and Koss, 1964). Billingham et al. (1975), using carefully defined cytologic criteria, succeeded in identifying Sternberg-Reed cells in 1 of 18 cerebrospinal fluids, 6 of 21 pleural effusions, and 1 of 2 peritoneal effusions in 41 of our patients with advanced, often pre-terminal Hodgkin's disease.

Indications for Radiographic and Radioisotopic Examination. This section presents some general comments, in the context of the general diagnostic evaluation of the patient with untreated Hodgkin's disease, concerning the clinical settings in which various types of radiographic and radioisotopic examinations may be expected to be clinically useful and helpful. Details of interpretation of specific abnormalities observed on radiographs or scans are reserved for Chapter 5. In case of doubt, the clinician should consult with the diagnostic roentgenologist or the specialist in nuclear medicine for assistance in the selection of the most appropriate procedure.

Roentgenologic examinations of the chest and of the skeletal system are essential components of the diagnostic evaluation of all patients with Hodgkin's disease. Lymphangiography is almost in this routine category but should not be performed until the chest radiographs have been examined, since the hazards of pulmonary oil embolization, which are ordinarily trivial, may be quite serious in the patient with diffuse chronic pulmonary disease, whether specifically related to Hodgkin's disease or not. In such patients, and in individuals with severe asthma or well-documented allergic reactions to iodinated organic compounds, lymphangiography may be deemed hazardous enough to be contraindicated. Each such case should be individually evaluated in consultation with the diagnostic roentgenologist. In addition, the demonstration of para-aortic and/or iliac lymph node involvement by lymphangiography, which is so vitally important in patients under consideration for definitive radiotherapy, is of appreciably less significance in those patients demonstrated to have involvement in sites such as the bone marrow or both lungs, which would dictate a shift from radiotherapy to chemotherapy.

In addition to conventional radiographic examinations of the chest, tomograms may be extremely useful in selected situations. For example, the detection of minimal degrees of mediastinal adenopathy as well as the selective demonstration of hilar, as distinguished from mediastinal, lymphadenopathy is often best accomplished with tomograms in the frontal or lateral projections. Tomograms of the lung fields may reveal small nodules that are not apparent, even on retrospective examination, in the conventional chest roentgenogram. Evidence presented in Chapter 7 indicates that pulmonary infiltration by Hodgkin's disease is seldom observed at the time of initial diagnosis except in association with hilar and/or mediastinal adenopathy. Lateral films with the patient in the decubitus position are often helpful in demonstrating the presence of free pleural effusions, particularly when large effusions accumulate in the diaphragmatic pleural space, simulating elevation of the diaphragm by enlargement of the liver on the right side, or by subphrenic processes on the left. Lateral and oblique films of the thorax may also reveal enlargement of the internal mammary lymph nodes presenting as serpentine indentations along the inner aspect of the thoracic wall adjacent to the sternum. Echocardiograms and angiocardiograms, either with carbon dioxide or with opaque media, may be useful in the detection of pericardial effusions. Radioisotopic angiocardiography with ^{99m}Tc has been recommended as a rapid and simple diagnostic procedure for the detection of pericardial effusions (Kriss, 1969).

Lymphangiography is by far the most sensitive and reliable roentgen diagnostic technique for the detection of lymphomatous involvement in the para-aortic and/or pelvic lymph nodes, with an overall diagnostic accuracy in a number of studies to date of approximately 80 to 90 percent. Nonetheless, there is a small but significant proportion of cases in which the lymphangiogram is technically unsatisfactory, either because difficulty is encountered in cannulating the peripheral lymphatics or because filling of the upper para-aortic lymph nodes is incomplete. In these instances, as well as in cases in which lymphangiography is contraindicated for one of the reasons cited above, computed tomographic (CT) scans now provide a noninvasive alternative diagnostic procedure of almost equally high resolution (Redman et al., 1977; Marshall et al., 1977; Breiman et al., 1978; Lee et

al., 1978). Moreover, CT scans may reveal adenopathy in the celiac and mesenteric lymph nodes, which are not visualized by lymphangiography. Inferior vena cavography and intravenous urography may also be helpful. Frontal, oblique, and lateral projections may reveal anterolateral displacement of the inferior vena cava and irregular pressure defects along its posterior surface due to retroperitoneal lymphadenopathy. Since the inferior vena cava courses slightly to the right of the midline, the cavogram is useful only for the detection of enlarged nodes on the right side. Thus, a normal inferior vena cavogram does not exclude the possibility of lymphadenopathy to the left of the midline in the upper or mid-lumbar region. On the subsequent intravenous urogram films, enlarged lymph nodes may indent and displace one or both ureters. Unfortunately, displacement of the inferior vena cava or of a ureter requires a relatively marked degree of enlargement of lymph nodes for its demonstration and is thus a relatively insensitive diagnostic criterion. Localization of gallium (^{67}Ga) citrate in tissues involved by Hodgkin's disease, initially reported by Edwards and Hayes (1969), has proven to be a useful adjunctive diagnostic procedure in selected cases, but is much less reliable below than above the diaphragm (Hoffer et al., 1973; Horn, Ray, and Kriss, 1975; Seabold et al., 1976; Johnston et al., 1977). Glees et al. (1977) investigated the usefulness of another new diagnostic technique, grey-scale ultrasonography, in a series of 52 patients. The ultrasonic scan was considered suggestive of spleen involvement in 7 of 9 cases in which laparotomy confirmation was later obtained; however, 3 of 11 histologically negative spleens were considered positive preoperatively, and 2 of 9 with negative scans were found to contain Hodgkin's disease. The procedure was also capable of demonstrating significantly enlarged porta hepatis, celiac, upper para-aortic, and mesenteric lymph nodes, but had insufficient resolution to detect hepatic lesions with acceptable reliability. Brascho, Durant, and Green (1977), in a study of 336 ultrasound scans in 179 patients with Hodgkin's disease or other lymphomas, reported that the procedure yielded correct interpretations regarding retroperitoneal node involvement in 87.5 percent, and that individual lymph nodes ≥ 2 cm in diameter were detectable.

Involvement of the gastrointestinal tract is quite uncommon in previously untreated patients with Hodgkin's disease, in striking contrast to the situation in the other types of malignant lymphoma. Accordingly, barium radiographic examinations of the gastrointestinal tract are indicated only on a selective basis in those patients with significant gastrointestinal symptoms. Nonetheless, as indicated in Chapter 5, lesions due to Hodgkin's disease have been described in the esophagus, the stomach, the small intestine, the colon, and even the rectum.

It is often possible to evaluate the size of the spleen, and thus to confirm or refute the clinical impression of its palpability, on the conventional roentgenogram of the abdomen, as well as on films in which the contours of the stomach or splenic flexure of the colon are visualized with air, gas, or barium. The size of the liver and the spleen may also be demonstrated with the aid of radioisotopic scans. The liver is usually studied with rose bengal-^{131}I or with ^{99m}Tc; the spleen is best delineated with ^{99m}Tc or ^{111}In colloid, or with organic mercury ([197]Hg) compounds (Parmentier et al., 1969). Scintigraphy with ^{75}Se-selenite has also reportedly been useful in selected patients (Killander, Lindblom, and Lundell, 1977). In one remarkable case studied by Chaudhuri et al. (1972), involvement of the spleen was associated with extensive splenic accumulation of [87m]Sr. Although such scans are readily able to demonstrate the overall size of these organs, their resolving power for the demonstration of intrahepatic or intrasplenic lesions is relatively poor (Lipton et al., 1972; Silverman et al., 1972; Milder et al., 1973). When discrete filling defects in the liver and spleen are not demonstrated on scans, it should not be considered that the possibility of hepatic or splenic involvement by Hodgkin's disease has been eliminated.

Any patient with localized, persistent, deep pain suggestive of osseous involvement deserves detailed, localized, roentgenographic investigation of the painful region, even when it has been included on the previous conventional films of the skeletal system. Well-collimated films of the affected area, and in some instances tomograms, may bring out detail that is not readily visualized on larger films. Where conventional radiography is negative or equivocal, radioisotopic bone scans may succeed in demonstrating localized foci of pathologically enhanced uptake (Harbert and Ashburn, 1968; Schechter et al., 1976).

Contrast myelography is indicated, often on an emergency basis as an immediate sequel to the spinal tap and pressure measurements, in patients presenting a history and neurologic findings suggestive of the spinal cord compression syndrome. The timing of the myelogram should be individualized and requires careful clinical judgment. In instances in which the symptoms are not classical and their rate of progression is indolent, and particularly where the neurologic examination and pressure measurements are negative or equivocal, it may be desirable to defer myelography and to observe the patient carefully for additional developments. In other instances, however, in which the history or neurologic findings are more convincing or the rate of progression more rapid, it may be best to proceed with myelography immediately even when the pressure measurements are not obviously abnormal.

In rare instances, patients may present symptoms suggestive of cerebral involvement either by Hodgkin's disease or by one of its poorly understood complications, multifocal leukoencephalopathy. In addition to the usual neurologic examination and electroencephalography, conventional roentgenograms of the skull and computed tomographic scans or radioisotopic brain scans may be indicated. If these are not successful in clarifying the problem, it may be necessary to proceed with invasive roentgenologic procedures such as carotid arteriography, pneumoencephalography, or ventriculography.

Surgical Diagnostic Procedures. Excisional node biopsy is of course essential for the initial diagnosis of Hodgkin's disease in virtually all instances. In patients with mediastinal lymphadenopathy in whom no enlarged peripheral nodes are palpable, blind biopsy of the scalene nodes on one or both sides may be rewarding; otherwise, mediastinal nodes may have to be obtained by mediastinoscopy (Bilgutay et al., 1969; Redding, Anagnostopoulos, and Ultmann, 1971) or by transsternal mediastinal exploration. In addition to the initial biopsy, additional excisional biopsies of suspicious lymph nodes should be performed whenever such nodes are so located that the definitive demonstration of their involvement by Hodgkin's disease would alter the staging or the treatment of the patient.

Bone marrow biopsy either by the open surgical technique, usually along the lateral aspect of the iliac crest, or with a Jamshidi needle (Jamshidi and Swaim, 1971), is essential in all patients with Hodgkin's disease. Drill biopsy is preferred by some authorities as a convenient and rapid method of obtaining an organized tissue sample of bone marrow for histologic sectioning. Although those lymphomas which tend to involve the bone marrow diffusely may be detected by simple bone marrow aspiration, experience has amply demonstrated that aspiration is seldom successful in Hodgkin's disease (Grann, Pool, and Mayer, 1966; Rosenberg, 1968, 1971a; Webb et al., 1970; Weiss, Brunning, and Kennedy, 1975; cf. also Table 4.4). This is due to the fact that involvement of the marrow by Hodgkin's disease, particularly in its early stages, is focal in character (cf. Fig. 3.45), and thus subject to an inherently large sampling error. Even generous open surgical biopsies of the bone marrow leave serious room for doubt when they are negative in patients who have advanced disease and severe constitutional symptoms. However, Sternberg-Reed cells have readily been morphologically recognizable in the occasional instances in which the sternal marrow aspirate is positive (Varadi, 1960; Yang and Palmer, 1963).

Thoracotomy may be required in an occasional patient for biopsy of mediastinal adenopathy, when no enlarged peripheral nodes are available for biopsy, or for biopsy of pleural or pulmonary nodules. Open pleural biopsy may sometimes be deferred until at least one attempt to obtain a positive pleural biopsy with the Cope needle has been made in instances of pleural effusion. Where exploration of the mediastinum is performed primarily for diagnostic purposes and conglomerate masses of enlarged lymph nodes are encountered, it is seldom possible to effect a complete resection, and postoperative radiotherapy is indicated in any event for all such cases that prove to be due to Hodgkin's disease, and for virtually all other neoplasms as well. Accordingly, major attempts at resection are seldom warranted and simple diagnostic removal of representative tissue samples for histopathologic diagnosis is usually the wisest procedure.

Biopsy of the nasopharynx revealed unequivocal evidence of Hodgkin's disease in 4, and suggestive changes in 3 more, of 45 patients studied by Björklund et al. (1975). Similar observations have been noted by Michaels and Todd (1976), who suggested the possible desirability of performing nasopharyngeal biopsies routinely in a consecutive series of patients to ascertain the true frequency of involvement in the lymphoid tissues of Waldeyer's ring. However, it is noteworthy that almost all of the biopsy-verified cases in both of these series had symptoms specifically referable to the nasopharynx. Moreover, although the Waldeyer's ring region has been irradiated prophylactically in only a small fraction of our patients with Hodgkin's disease, subsequent development of relapses in the nasopharyngeal area has been quite rare in our experience, suggesting that nasopharyngeal biopsy would have an unacceptably low yield if performed routinely. Accordingly, we continue to recommend that this procedure be used selectively in patients with localizing symptoms or with suspicious findings on mirror examination of the nasopharynx.

Laminectomy is usually indicated for decompression in patients with Hodgkin's disease presenting symptoms, neurologic abnormalities, and myelographic findings indicative of compression of the spinal cord by epidural disease, particularly in rapidly progressive cases. In the rare instances in which this is the initial presenting manifestation and no prior tissue diagnosis of Hodgkin's disease exists, biopsy of the epidural lesion is essential to establish the diagnosis. Laparoscopy with liver needle biopsy under direct observation has been recommended prior to laparotomy with splenectomy

Table 4.4   Bone Marrow Involvement in 11 of a Group of about 200 Patients with Hodgkin's Disease[a]

Case	Initials	Bone marrow aspirate	Bone marrow biopsy	Fever	Alkaline phosphatase	Liver biopsy	Anemia
1	B.R.U.	−	+	No	↑	−	Yes
2	C.A.S.	−	+	Yes	↑	−	Yes
3	B.E.R.	−	+	Yes	↑	−	Yes
4	D.I.P.	−	+	Yes	↑	Equivocal	Yes
5	F.L.E.	−	+	Yes	↑	−	Yes
6	F.A.L.	−	+	Yes	↑	−	No
7	S.C.H.	−	+	Yes	↑	None	Yes
8	G.R.A.	+ (clot)	None	Yes	↑	None	Yes
9	B.U.S.	−	+	Yes	↑	−	Yes
10	S.E.S.	−	+	No	↑	−	No
11	A.V.I.	−	+	Yes	Normal	−	No

Source: Stanford University Medical Center data, slightly modified from the paper by Rosenberg (1968).
[a]Symbols: + = positive; − = negative; ↑ = increased.

on the ground that positive liver biopsies thus obtained would obviate the need for the more extensive surgical procedure (Scholten, 1968; De Vita et al., 1971a).

Laparotomy with splenectomy and biopsy of the para-aortic nodes, the liver, and the iliac crest bone marrow was first used at Stanford University Medical Center in 1961. Initially, this procedure was performed on a selective basis in patients with untreated Hodgkin's disease who had: (1) an equivocal or unsatisfactory lymphangiogram; (2) splenomegaly accompanied by a negative or equivocal lymphangiogram; or (3) suspicious clinical hepatomegaly or abnormal liver function tests (Glatstein, et al., 1969). Histologic evidence of involvement by Hodgkin's disease was documented in a surprisingly high proportion of the resected spleens, many of which had not been clinically palpable preoperatively (Table 4.5). The procedure also proved useful in providing biopsy confirmation of involvement of upper lumbar para-aortic nodes in instances in which the lymphangiogram had been negative or equivocal (Table 4.6), and in providing larger specimens of liver tissue, obtainable in some instances from areas of visible hepatic abnormality. There were no major complications or deaths in this initial selected series of sixty-five cases.

Accordingly, we decided to undertake a study of the value of routine laparotomy with splenectomy and biopsy in a series of unselected cases of previously untreated Hodgkin's disease (Glatstein et al., 1970; Rosenberg and Kaplan, 1970; Kaplan et al., 1973). Data on a larger series of 100 consecutive patients (Table 4.7) again indicated a remarkably high yield of clinically unsuspected positive findings in the spleen, and to a lesser extent in the lymph nodes and the liver, and these findings have been confirmed and extended as the Stanford experience with staging laparotomy has grown to encompass more than 800 consecutive, previously untreated patients (cf. Chapters 7 and 8). Patients presenting with left-sided or bilateral lower cervical-supraclavicular adenopathy were initially found to have a significantly higher frequency of abdominal involvement than those in whom lower cervical-supraclavicular node enlargement was confined to the right side, and mediastinal adenopathy seemed to be inversely correlated

Table 4.5 Histologic Findings in Splenectomy Specimens of 65 Selected Patients with Hodgkin's Disease

Histologic evidence of Hodgkin's disease in spleen	Systemic symptoms	Preoperative clinical assessment of spleen		
		Positive	Negative	Totals
Positive	Absent	6	8	14 ⎫ 34
Negative	Absent	12	8	20 ⎭
Positive	Present	18	8	26 ⎫ 31
Negative	Present	2	3	5 ⎭
Totals		38	27	65

Source: Stanford University Medical Center data, slightly rearranged from the paper by Glatstein et al. (1969).

Table 4.6 Para-aortic Node Biopsy Findings versus Lymphangiographic Interpretation in 58 Selected Patients with Hodgkin's Disease

Biopsy evidence of Hodgkin's disease	Systemic symptoms	Interpretation of lymphangiogram			
		Positive	Normal	Equivocal	Totals
Positive	Absent	12	1	1	14
Negative	Absent	3	10	5	18
Positive	Present	11	2	2	15
Negative	Present	2	4	5	11
Totals:		28	17	13	58

Source: Stanford University Medical Center data, slightly rearranged from the paper by Glatstein et al. (1969). Six of the 65 patients in this series did not have biopsy, and one did not have a lymphangiogram.

Table 4.7   Results of Laparotomy in 100 Consecutive Untreated Patients with Hodgkin's Disease

Site	Preoperative assessment	Systemic symptoms absent	Systemic symptoms present	Total
Liver	Clinically positive	0/4[a]	1/11	1/15
	Clinically negative	1/53	1/32	2/85
Spleen	Clinically positive	2/6	6/10	8/16
	Clinically negative	11/51	9/33	20/84
Abdominal nodes	Positive lymphangiogram	8/11 (1)[b]	10/12	18/23 (1)
	Negative lymphangiogram	5/33 (4)	2/24 (1)	7/57 (5)
	Equivocal lymphangiogram	3/13 (1)	1/7	4/20 (1)

[a]Number with histologic evidence of Hodgkin's disease/number examined; Stanford University Medical Center data (Rosenberg and Kaplan, 1970).

[b]Figures in parentheses are numbers with positive splenic hilar nodes, but negative para-aortic node biopsy.

with subdiaphragmatic disease (Glatstein et al., 1970). However, some of these correlations have not been substantiated by our subsequent accrued experience, as detailed in Chapter 7.

The technical aspects of the staging laparotomy procedure have been fully described by Enright, Trueblood, and Nelsen (1970), Ferguson et al. (1973), and Cannon and Nelsen (1976). Surgical exposure of the upper para-aortic lymph node chains reveals the anatomical landmarks seen in Figure 4.8 (Cannon et al., 1975). In young female patients, it has been possible to move one or both ovaries either to the midline (Fig. 4.9; Trueblood

et al., 1970) or laterally over the iliac wings (Nahhas et al., 1971), where they may be shielded during subsequent radiotherapy of the pelvis. Staging laparotomy, when performed by surgical teams with adequate experience, has been associated with postoperative morbidity well within acceptable limits for a diagnostic procedure.

There were only 6 significant complications in a series of 68 consecutive cases (Enright, Trueblood, and Nelsen, 1970). With increasing experience, the frequency of complications decreased appreciably; among 291 consecutive staging laparotomies, Slavin and Nelsen (1973) encountered only 8 major

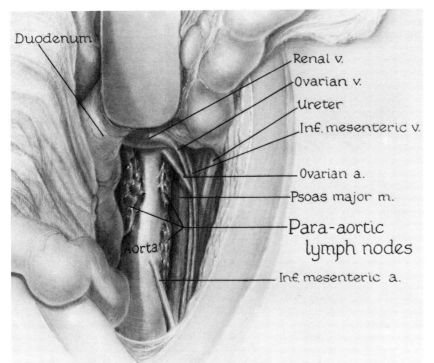

Figure 4.8 Exposure and important anatomic landmarks for para-aortic lymph node biopsy. (Reprinted, by permission, from the paper by Cannon et al., 1975.)

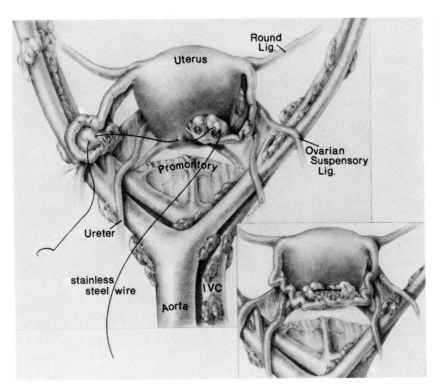

Figure 4.9 Simplified technique of posterior midline oophoropexy with single wire suture. (Reprinted, by permission, from the paper by Cannon et al., 1975.)

complications (3.7 percent). It is important to defer the staging laparotomy, in patients with bulky or massive mediastinal adenopathy, until substantial regression has been achieved with mantle field radiotherapy to avoid complications due to intubation anesthesia. Acute life-threatening complications occurred in 5 of 74 intubation anesthesias in untreated patients with mediastinal and/or hilar adenopathy, versus 0/24 in patients who had received mantle field irradiation (Piro, Weiss, and Hellman, 1976). Obstruction of the superior vena cava and bronchi during intubation anesthesia under these circumstances was also reported by Tonnesen and Davis (1976). There have been no deaths to date at Stanford in those patients in whom the procedure was performed purely for diagnostic purposes (Cannon and Nelsen, 1976). An acceptably low operative mortality has also been the general experience elsewhere. Desser, Moran, and Ultmann (1973), in a literature survey, collected data on more than 400 staging laparotomies, with an associated operative mortality less than 0.5 percent, and Gazet (1973) encountered a mortality of about 1 percent in an analysis of 1,558 splenectomies from 24 published laparotomy series. This is in striking contrast to the very appreciable mortality recorded in a number of publications when splenectomy was performed for anemia or pancytopenia believed due to hypersplenism

(Strawitz et al., 1961; Rousselot et al., 1962; Schultz et al., 1964). One such fatal instance occurred in one of our affiliated teaching hospitals. It is therefore important to recognize that the hazard of splenectomy done as part of the diagnostic evaluation is by no means comparable to that of therapeutic splenectomy undertaken for hypersplenism.

Concern has been expressed about the hazard of late deaths due to sepsis following splenectomy, especially in children. Splenectomized children appear to be at significantly increased risk of fulminant bacterial sepsis due to *Streptococcus pneumoniae* and *Hemophilus influenzae*. In a survey of 1,170 individuals who were splenectomized for Hodgkin's disease at 12 different institutions, Desser and Ultmann (1972) encountered 16 instances of serious infection, 6 of which proved fatal (a late mortality rate of 0.5 percent). A questionnaire study of children with Hodgkin's disease by Rosenstock, D'Angio, and Kiesewetter (1974) turned up 2 deaths due to sepsis in 374 laparotomies, and a retrospective national survey by the Children's Cancer Study Group (Chilcote et al., 1976) yielded 20 episodes of bacterial sepsis in 18 of 200 children splenectomized for Hodgkin's disease, with 10 deaths.

The possibility that treatment, rather than splenectomy per se, may have been responsible for at least a significant proportion of these infectious complications was not examined in these studies. Weitzman and Aisenberg (1977a) reviewed the experience at the Massachusetts General Hospital in a total of 119 patients under age 65 who had been splenectomized for Hodgkin's disease. There were 3 instances of fulminant bacterial sepsis, 2 of which were fatal, among 14 patients who had been treated with total lymphoid irradiation and MOPP combination chemotherapy. However, none of the remaining splenectomized patients, who had been treated with radiotherapy alone, MOPP alone, or less extensive irradiation plus MOPP, developed episodes of sepsis.

At Stanford University Medical Center, Donaldson, Glatstein, and Vosti (1978) analyzed bacterial infections in 181 children with Hodgkin's disease. Of these, 60 had not been splenectomized; their bacterial infection rate was 2.8 percent among those treated with radiotherapy and 23.1 percent among those treated with chemotherapy ($p < .05$). Among the 121 splenectomized children, the corresponding rates were 1.4 and 18.3 percent, respectively ($p < .05$). Although there was no difference in the overall frequency of bacterial infections that could be attributed to splenectomy, it was nonetheless true that all of the 15 episodes of bacterial meningitis due to *Streptococcus pneumoniae* and *Hemophilus influenzae* occurred in 14 children who had been splenectomized.

Some investigators have relied on the prophylactic use of penicillin in splenectomized children with Hodgkin's disease, but the experience of Ertel, Boles, and Newton (1977) suggests that this approach is not without pitfalls. They observed 9 episodes of life-threatening bacterial sepsis, 3 of which proved fatal, among 4 of 20 children 3 to 16 years of age who had been splenectomized for Hodgkin's disease. One 3-year-old child was supposed to be getting monthly penicillin but had not had any antibiotic for six weeks and died of pneumococcal sepsis on the way to the hospital. A 16-year-old boy recovered from one bout of bacterial sepsis but died during another episode that developed 28 days after his last penicillin injection. A 13-year-old boy died of *Pseudomonas* infection while under treatment for sepsis due to β-hemolytic *Streptococcus*. The fourth child, though still alive, had developed a pneumococcal meningitis two days after penicillin administration and had had several other episodes of severe infection despite prophylactic penicillin every four weeks. Doubt about the efficacy and desirability of prophylactic penicillin injections has led other investigators to become interested in the possibility of active immunization against the more widely prevalent types of *Streptococcus pneumoniae* with polyvalent pneumococcal polysaccharide vaccines that have now become available (Hilleman et al., 1978) and have been shown to increase antibody titers significantly in splenectomized children (Ammann et al., 1977). Accordingly, a prospective study has been undertaken at Stanford University Medical Center in which pediatric patients with untreated Hodgkin's disease are being given this vaccine prior to staging laparotomy with splenectomy; antibody titers in the first 17 patients are now pending.

Experience with the use of the vaccine in splenectomized patients who have already been treated has been discouraging. Siber et al. (1978) reported on antibody responses in 53 patients and 10 normal controls given such a vaccine. The mean antibody concentrations measured three weeks later were 1,566 ng of protein nitrogen per ml in controls; 963 ng/ml after subtotal lymphoid irradiation ($p < .05$); 658 ng/ml after MOPP or similar chemotherapy ($p < .05$); 377 ng/ml after subtotal irradiation plus chemotherapy ($p < .01$); and only 283 ng/ml after total lymphoid irradiation plus chemotherapy ($p < .001$). Thus it may prove essential to vaccinate such patients prior to treatment, and perhaps also prior to splenectomy, as we are currently doing with our pediatric patients at Stanford.

Other experimental approaches to the hazard of bacterial sepsis following splenectomy are discussed in Chapter 13. Although the problem is a real one, it is important to place it in proper perspective. The striking gains in survival and freedom from relapse that have been achieved (Chapter 12) in the decade since staging laparotomy was introduced by Glatstein et al. (1969) are undoubtedly due in part to the improved accuracy of staging and its impact on therapeutic strategies (Rosenberg, 1971b; Piro, Hellman, and Moloney, 1972), and these gains far outweigh in importance the small, though by no means negligible, risk of late death due to bacterial sepsis.

Many other institutions have now adopted the procedure of staging laparotomy, with results that closely parallel the Stanford experience (Lowenbraun et al., 1970; Veronesi et al., 1972; Ferguson et al., 1973; O'Connell et al., 1974; Poulsen et al., 1977; Sandusky et al., 1978). On the basis of the very high yield of diagnostic information which this procedure has provided to date and the low risk of associated complications or mortality, we believe that laparotomy with splenectomy, biopsy of the para-aortic lymph nodes, and liver biopsy has become an essential part of the routine diagnostic evaluation of patients with Hodgkin's disease, with the exception of the elderly or severely debilitated, or those with a positive bone marrow or liver needle biopsy or other evidence of stage IV disease. With increasing experience, it may become possible to further refine the indications for laparotomy and splenectomy with respect to such variables as age, sex, sites of peripheral adenopathy, presence of constitutional symptoms, and histopathologic type, and to predict those parameters for which the highest expectation of diagnostic yield would obtain.

Subsequent Clinical Course

It is undeniably true that the first course of treatment offers the patient with Hodgkin's disease his or her best chance for cure (cf. Chapter 12). Erroneous or incomplete diagnostic evaluation of the initial extent of the disease can seal the doom of a potentially curable patient just as inexorably as inappropriate selection or inept utilization of a treatment modality. For this reason, we have placed great stress on the initial diagnostic evaluation and clinical staging classification of previously untreated patients.

However, skillful long-term followup care is almost equally important. The well-informed and alert physician can anticipate the sites of relapse that are most likely to occur in a given patient. Their early detection during the followup period, at a time when such new manifestations are still amenable to definitive therapeutic management, may make it possible to salvage patients whose disease would otherwise have progressed to the point where only palliative treatment could be offered. Even in the latter situation, decisions about the timing of the initiation of palliative treatment, the selection of a treatment modality, the evaluation of response, and the subsequent series of decisions concerning the need to discontinue administration of one type of drug and to initiate the use of another can exert a tremendous influence on the quality of life achieved during the palliative period and can offer significant prolongation of useful life in many instances. Thus, optimal management of the subsequent course of the disease requires keen clinical judgment in the skillful application of this additional body of knowledge. This section presents a summary of the available information concerning the diagnostic aspects of the subsequent course, with reference not only to the manifestations of the disease itself but also to some of the major complications with which it may be associated. Therapeutic decisions relevant to the various clinical manifestations discussed here are reserved for detailed discussion in subsequent chapters.

The Followup Examination. It is now well established that initial relapses of Hodgkin's disease tend to occur predominantly during the first two years after completion of the first course of treatment (Kaplan, 1962, 1968b; Prosnitz et al., 1969; Spittle et al., 1973; Musshoff et al., 1976; Weller et al., 1976). Accordingly, it is a wise policy to adjust the frequency of followup examinations to the anticipated probability of relapse. It has been our policy to see patients with Hodgkin's disease routinely at intervals of one to two months for the first six months after completion of therapy; every two to three months during the second six months; every three to four months during the second and third year; every six months during years four and five; and yearly thereafter. Patients are of course instructed not to wait for their next regular appointment but to return immediately if unusual and sustained new symptoms and/or signs should develop during an interval between visits.

The followup examination should consist of a brief interval history, with emphasis on the occurrence of unexplained fever, night sweats, generalized pruritus, unplanned weight loss, pain, or other specific symptoms; a limited physical examination aimed particularly at the detection of peripheral lymphadenopathy and/or hepatosplenomegaly; a complete blood cell count, erythrocyte sedimentation rate, serum copper, and serum alkaline phosphatase; and surveillance X-ray films of the chest (posteroanterior and lateral views) and abdomen (anteroposterior view only). The new X-ray films should be carefully compared with the corresponding films of at least the last previous visit and, in instances of suspected change, with those of several serial prior visits. The usefulness of serial determinations of the erythrocyte sedimentation rate and serum copper in the assessment of prognosis and the detection of incipient relapse has been discussed earlier, in the section on laboratory findings (pp. 130–132), as has the serious hazard of accepting a single abnormal laboratory value, without other supporting evidence, as an adequate indication for the renewed institution of specific therapy.

It is of great importance to document relapses,

preferably by biopsy of accessible enlarged nodes or other lesions, and to avoid leaping prematurely and without substantiation to the conclusion that any new symptom necessarily signifies relapse. When a suspicious symptom or sign occurs in a patient who is not acutely ill, it is a wise policy to defer judgment and to ask the patient to return for another followup examination after a relatively short interval, usually one to four weeks. Not infrequently, it will be found that a suspiciously enlarged, firm node has again regressed or that a nondescript radiographic shadow or infiltrate is no longer present. Interval enlargement of residually opacified para-aortic or iliac nodes is usually best documented on at least two serial surveillance films and may require laparotomy and biopsy for confirmation. In the absence of other evident loci of recurrent disease, the liver and the bone marrow should be considered as possible sites of new involvement in patients who develop sustained interval fever, night sweats, or an elevated sedimentation rate. No general rules can be laid down, except that any suspicious or unequivocal new manifestation, in a patient whose Hodgkin's disease has apparently been under control, deserves hospitalization and a full-scale diagnostic evaluation, with histologic proof of the existence of new disease whenever possible, before a new course of treatment is instituted. Recently, posttreatment laparotomy has been proposed by Sutcliffe et al. (1978) as a way of documenting complete remissions or, alternatively, of detecting clinically occult disease persisting in the abdomen following radiotherapy and/or chemotherapy. Herman and Jones (1977) have stressed the importance of systematic restaging, including lymph node, bone marrow, and liver biopsies, and even laparotomy in selected patients, to document apparently complete remissions following intensive combination chemotherapy.

Relapse, Recurrence, and Extension of Hodgkin's Disease. The word recurrence is often used indiscriminately to refer to any new manifestation of disease as well as the reappearance of disease in previously treated areas. Such usage contributes to ambiguity and misinterpretation and impedes systemic analysis of the course of the disease. Accordingly, it seems appropriate to define carefully the precise meaning with which certain words will be used throughout this book. Several years of experience have demonstrated that the terminology suggested in a prior publication (Kaplan, 1966a), has been useful and unambiguous, and it has been in-corporated into the series of definitions set forth here.

A *relapse* is a new manifestation of disease appearing after completion of a course of radiotherapy and/or chemotherapy. The terms *recrudescence* and *new manifestation* are used interchangeably with relapse. A relapse may involve a *true recurrence,* a *marginal recurrence,* or an *extension* of disease, or, occasionally, the simultaneous occurrence of combinations of these. *True recurrence* is defined as the reappearance of lymphadenopathy or other evidence of activity in a treated field as the *first* new manifestation of Hodgkin's disease after an initial course of radiotherapy; it constitutes evidence that the dose applied was not tumoricidal. *Marginal recurrences* are those which appear at or immediately adjacent to the margins of radiotherapeutic fields; they indicate an inadequate appreciation of the local extent of disease. *Extensions* are defined as new manifestations of disease in discontinuous, previously untreated areas; they reflect the limitations of the diagnostic methods available for the evaluation of the initial clinical extent of disease. Extensions do not imply that spread of disease from one of the initial sites of known involvement occurred during or after irradiation; rather they imply that at least microscopic involvement of the site(s) of extension must have been present, but remained undetected and thus untreated, at the time of the initial diagnostic evaluation.

It should be noted that the term recurrence as used here applies only to previously treated disease. Since chemotherapeutic agents are systemically distributed and presumably reach all sites of involvement, any new manifestation of disease in a patient treated with chemotherapy would constitute a recurrence rather than an extension. True recurrences after radiotherapy refer only to those instances in which disease reappears in a treated field prior to any manifestation of disease appearing elsewhere. When disease recurs in a treated field after one or more extensions of disease to previously untreated areas, its interpretation is ambiguous; it may represent a true recurrence of incompletely eradicated disease in the original treatment field, but it could equally well represent an instance of *retrograde recurrence* or "reseeding" from one of the sites of extension back to a chain of lymph nodes from which the original disease had in fact been eradicated by prior radiotherapy.

Recurrence rates, defined as the number of true recurrences per treatment field at risk multiplied by 100, are of great importance in assessing the efficacy of various dose levels of radiotherapy, as dis-

¬cussed in Chapter 9. Specific clinical examples in which true recurrence and extension of disease occurred are described in the Appendix.

Contiguity of Extension of Hodgkin's Disease via Lymphatic Channels. It has long been appreciated that after radiotherapy of one or more enlarged chains of lymph nodes, new manifestations of disease are often observed in the next adjacent lymph node chain. This observation became the basis for the advocacy by Gilbert (1939), Peters (1950, 1966), and others of "prophylactic" or "segmental" irradiation of chains of lymph nodes beyond those known to be affected by the disease. Systematic investigations undertaken with the aid of lymphangiography and other advanced diagnostic methods have now made it clear that the concept of contiguity applies with equal force not only to the initial sites of involvement in previously untreated patients but also to the first sites of extension of disease after completion of an initial course of radiotherapy (Rosenberg and Kaplan, 1966; Kaplan, 1970). Detailed discussion of the evidence bearing on this concept is reserved for Chapter 7.

After local radiotherapy of lymphadenopathy initially apparently confined to one axilla, the next sites of extension are likely to be the ipsilateral infraclavicular, supraclavicular, or low cervical lymph node chains; occasionally, retrograde spread to the ipsilateral brachial or epitrochlear node is observed. The most likely sites of extension after local irradiation of lower cervical-supraclavicular adenopathy include the mediastinum, the ipsilateral axillary, infraclavicular, submandibular, or preauricular nodes, the contralateral lower cervical-supraclavicular nodes, and/or the upper lumbar para-aortic nodes and spleen (Kaplan, 1970). When disease confined to one inguinal or femoral region has been treated, the next site of extension is likely to be the ipsilateral iliac nodes and/or the para-aortic nodes.

Disease initially confined to the para-aortic lymph nodes has a considerable propensity to appear next in the spleen and splenic hilar nodes. However, we have also observed several instances in which, following radiotherapy of all of the lumbar para-aortic nodes, extension of disease was next observed in one or both iliac chains, presumably by retrograde spread via lymphatic channels in which the normal direction of flow was reversed by obstruction at the lumbar para-aortic level. The disease may also spread from the para-aortic chains upward via the thoracic duct to reach the supraclavicular nodes in a manner essentially simi-

lar to that by which intra-abdominal carcinomas spread to the "Virchow node" in the left supraclavicular chain.

Stage I Hodgkin's disease confined to the mediastinal nodes is seen infrequently; accordingly, a clear pattern of spread from the mediastinal nodes has not yet been established. Certainly, one direction of spread is centripetally into the hilar lymph nodes on one or both sides, following which the pulmonary parenchyma is at risk of becoming involved. However, we have seen three instances of so-called granulomatous thymoma (nodular sclerosing Hodgkin's disease of the thymus) which were first treated at another institution by surgical resection and later, after they had recurred, by local radiotherapy. In these cases, extension of disease beyond the thorax appeared first in the supraclavicular nodes on one or both sides, and subsequently in the upper lumbar para-aortic lymph nodes. We have also observed several instances in which the supraclavicular nodes were the first site of extension after local radiotherapy of mediastinal adenopathy.

Infectious Diseases Complicating Hodgkin's Disease

Patients with Hodgkin's disease are susceptible to infection by bacterial, fungal, viral, and other agents due both to the impairment of cell-mediated immunity which is integral to the disease itself and to the immunosuppressive effects of radiotherapy and/or chemotherapy (Chapter 6). Infection is not common at the time of initial presentation, except perhaps in severely debilitated patients with advanced, symptomatic disease. However, infectious complications which develop later are often superimposed upon and sometimes mask relapsing disease. Patients who have been treated extensively with a succession of chemotherapeutic regimens for multiple relapses are particularly prone to infections that may be difficult to control with antibiotics and not infrequently are the proximate cause of death.

At one time, tuberculosis was an almost invariable finding at autopsy (Sternberg, 1898). In recent years, a diversified spectrum of opportunistic organisms which attack the compromised host (Remington, 1972) have been identified, including *Pneumocystis carinii, Toxoplasma, Cryptococcus, Corynebacterium equi, Nocardia, Coccidioides immitis, Candida albicans,* and *Aspergillus niger* (Cheever, Valsamis, and Rabson, 1965; Casazza, Duvall, and Carbone, 1966; Cox and Hughes, 1975; Hughes,

Feldman, and Sanyal, 1975; Deresinski and Stevens, 1975; Tucker, Pemberton, and Guyer, 1975; Whiteside and Begent, 1975; Carpenter and Blom, 1976; Krick and Remington, 1976; Young and De Vita, 1976; Hancock and Henry, 1977). The lung is the organ most often affected, but involvement of the kidneys, the central nervous system, and the skin are also common. Treatment is discussed in Chapter 11.

Herpes zoster-varicella is the most prevalent viral infection in patients with Hodgkin's disease. It has been reported to occur in about 10 to 15 percent of patients who are untreated or have had only local or regional radiotherapy, and the attack rate increases to 40 percent or more in splenectomized patients who have been treated with combination chemotherapy, with or without radiotherapy (Goffinet, Glatstein, and Merigan, 1972; Wilson, Marsa, and Johnson, 1972; Monfardini et al., 1975; Schimpff et al., 1975a; Tognella et al., 1975b; Goodman et al., 1976a; Reboul, Donaldson, and Kaplan, 1978). Patients who are severely debilitated and those who have received intensive chemotherapy are at serious risk of developing the much more life-threatening disseminated form of the disease, which may be manifested not only in the skin but also in the lungs, eyes, esophagus, central nervous system, and other visceral sites. Human leukocyte interferon has recently been reported to have yielded encouraging results in preventing dissemination (Merigan et al., 1978a). Thorling and Thorling (1974) have described striking changes in serum copper levels during and after herpes zoster.

Fulminant sepsis, pneumonia, meningitis, and intravascular coagulopathy due to *Streptococcus pneumoniae* or to *Hemophilus influenzae* are known to occur with increased frequency in young children who have been splenectomized, and have been observed in significant numbers of patients with Hodgkin's disease who have undergone staging laparotomy with splenectomy (Desser and Ultmann, 1972; Weitzman and Aisenberg, 1977a; Donaldson, Glatstein, and Vosti, 1978). There is increasing evidence that susceptibility in such patients is also a function of prior intensive chemotherapy. This complex topic has been considered in greater detail in the section on surgical diagnostic procedures.

Chapter 5

Roentgenologic and Isotopic Diagnosis

Introduction

The roentgenologic examination is an invaluable diagnostic tool at many stages in the clinical evaluation and management of patients with Hodgkin's disease (Fisher, Kendall, and Van Leuven, 1962). It is an essential component of the initial diagnostic workup for the evaluation of extent of disease and clinical staging; examinations during treatment enable the radiation therapist or chemotherapist to observe the response of tumor masses; periodic roentgen examinations at serial followup visits permit the early detection of extension or recurrence of disease; and selective roentgenologic examinations in symptomatic patients may assist materially in assessing the significance of such symptoms as cough, dyspnea, chest pain, localized bone pain, and weakness or paralysis of the extremities. Radioisotope scanning procedures, in particular bone and spleen scans and studies of active bone marrow distribution, are also becoming increasingly useful in the diagnostic evaluation of patients with the lymphomas.

In the initial diagnostic workup, it has been our practice to utilize certain roentgenologic examinations routinely. Initially, our routine roentgenologic study included: (1) conventional roentgenograms of the chest (posteroanterior and lateral views), supplemented in selected cases by tomography; (2) a skeletal survey (lateral skull, lateral dorsal spine as seen on the chest film, and anteroposterior lumbosacral spine, pelvis, and upper femora); (3) lower extremity lymphangiography, (4) inferior vena cavography; (5) intravenous urography; and (6) barium examination of the stomach, small intestine, colon, and rectum. Over a period of several years, it became clear that the yield of positive barium examinations of the gastrointestinal tract at the time of initial admission of patients with Hodgkin's disease is too low to warrant their routine use. Routine examination of the skeletal system at the time of admission is also asso-

ciated with a low yield and might well be eliminated in asymptomatic patients. Inferior vena cavograms have given way to computed tomographic scans in those patients in whom the lymphangiogram is either equivocal or technically unsatisfactory. The intravenous urogram, which was formerly obtained routinely as a by-product of the inferior vena cavogram, is now performed only in patients with clinical signs or symptoms suggestive of urinary tract invasion or obstruction and in those infrequent cases in which elective vena cavography is still utilized. Thus our current minimal routine is limited to the chest examination and lymphangiography.

The roentgenologic examinations that we consider essential at each followup examination after completion of the initial course of treatment are conventional posteroanterior and lateral views of the chest and an anteroposterior view of the abdomen; the latter may be omitted after the lymphangiographic contrast medium opacifying the retroperitoneal nodes has been so depleted that it is no longer diagnostically adequate. At that time, unless there is known active disease elsewhere, repeat lymphangiography is generally indicated, after which the routine abdominal film may be resumed on subsequent followup examinations. Lymphangiography may be safely repeated two, three, or more times during the critical first five years of followup to provide reliable surveillance of the otherwise silent retroperitoneal and pelvic nodes (Perez-Tamayo et al., 1963; Steiner et al., 1970; Castellino et al., 1973b). These roentgenologic examinations play a major role in surveillance of the treated patient; in an analysis of 442 patients with Hodgkin's disease treated with curative intent at Stanford University Medical Center, Castellino et al. (1973a) found that the diagnosis of relapse in 130 patients with documented relapsing disease was initiated by the roentgenologic findings alone in 35 percent of the entire series, and that both clinical and roentgen findings contributed jointly to the diagnosis of relapse in an additional 30 percent of cases.

Thorax

Mediastinal Lymph Nodes. Mediastinal lymphadenopathy is particularly common in Hodgkin's disease and especially so in young female patients with the nodular sclerosing type of the disease; conversely, the mediastinal nodes are commonly spared, at least in the initial stages of the disease, in the lymphocytic and histiocytic lymphomas, except in preadolescent children. Involvement may occur in any of the radiographically identifiable lymph node chains within the thorax (Fig. 5.1). However, there are striking differences in the relative frequencies of involvement of different chains among patients with Hodgin's disease, and a distinctly different pattern of involvement in patients with non-Hodgkin's lymphomas (Fig. 5.2; Filly, Blank, and Castellino, 1976). The adenopathy may range in size from barely perceptible enlargement of an isolated lymph node to huge conglomerate masses compressing the trachea, bronchi, or great vessels centrally and displacing the upper lung bilaterally on one or both sides (Fig. 5.3*A*). Occasionally, the contour of the mediastinum is not greatly altered and involvement is manifested only as an increase in the transverse width of the superior mediastinum (Fig. 5.4), usually due to expansion of lymph nodes in the right paratracheal region. When the expanding lymph nodes coalesce in such a manner

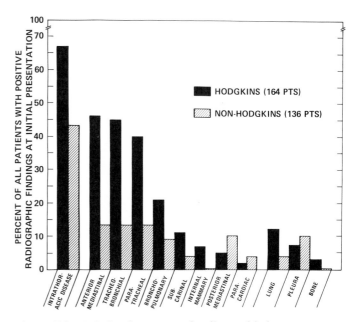

Figure 5.2   Relative frequency of radiographic involvement of various intrathoracic sites in 164 untreated patients with Hodgkin's disease and 136 untreated patients with non-Hodgkin's lymphomas. Note the striking difference in the frequency of mediastinal adenopathy observed in the two groups. (Reprinted, by permission of the authors and *Radiology,* from the paper by Filly, Blank, and Castellino, 1976a.)

as to present a relatively smooth convex contour, differential diagnosis from aneurysm may be difficult and may necessitate angiocardiography or aortography (Fig. 5.5). In most instances, however, careful study of the roentgenograms will reveal a lobulated, scalloped contour (Fig. 5.6) at the points of junction of individual large lymph nodes, whereas an aneurysm would be expected to present a single, uninterruptedly convex, smooth contour. Moderate enlargement of lymph nodes may present a contour which is initially mistaken for an aortic knob. Adequately exposed films will reveal the presence of a contour additional to that of the aortic knob; the latter can be identified clearly by following the lateral edge of the descending aorta upward (Fig. 5.7).

Serial chest roentgenograms are of great importance in the radiotherapy of large mediastinal masses. They permit the radiotherapist to follow the rate of regression and thus enable him to initiate treatment with very wide fields encompassing all of the original tumor volume, to deliver a moderate fraction of the planned total dose, and then to interrupt treatment ("split course technique") to permit regression to occur (Fig. 5.3). When serial chest films taken at approximately weekly intervals

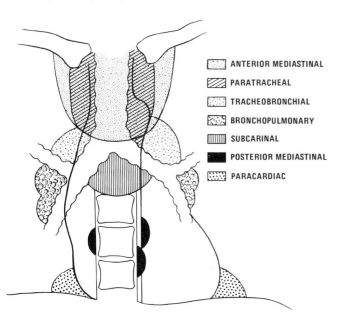

Figure 5.1   Diagrammatic representation of the anatomical relationships of several of the major mediastinal and hilar (bronchopulmonary) lymph node chains. (Reprinted, by permission of the authors and *Radiology,* from the paper by Filly, Blank, and Castellino, 1976a.)

Figure 5.3 *A*, huge mediastinal mass, composed of a conglomeration of enlarged lymph nodes, in a 19-year-old male with nodular sclerosing Hodgkin's disease. Note the slightly lobulated contours. *B*, *C*, and *D*, serial chest films after a dose of 4,400 rads had been delivered to the mantle field by the "split course technique" (cf. Chapter 9), revealing slow but ultimately complete regression of the mass, with no clinical or X-ray evidence of pulmonary fibrosis. *E* and *F*, chest X-ray examination in 1975. The cardiomediastinal silhouette is entirely normal. Note the calcified lymph node in the lateral view (arrow). The patient remains relapse-free more than 12 years post-treatment.

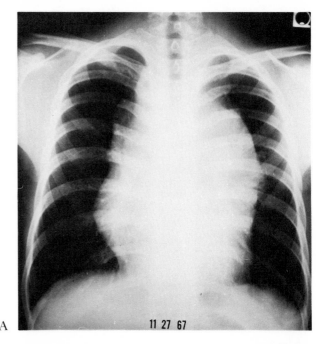

A

B

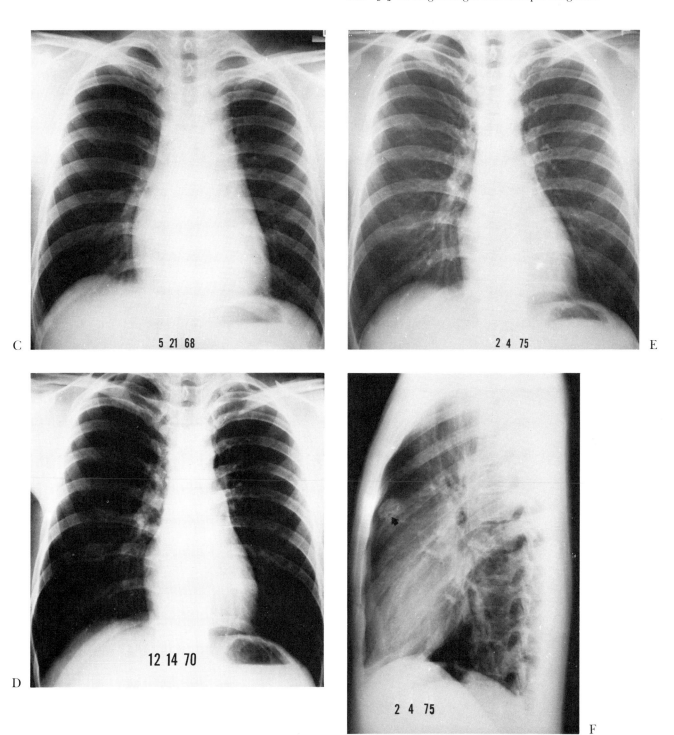

C

5 21 68

E

2 4 75

D

12 14 70

F

2 4 75

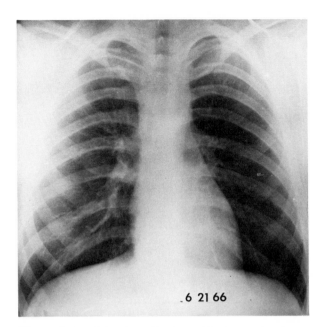

6 21 66

Figure 5.4 Minimal mediastinal widening at the thoracic inlet, with a slight increase in density over the aortic knob, are the only signs of mediastinal involvement in this 15-year-old male patient.

reveal that tumor regression has reached its nadir, radiation therapy can then be resumed and carried to completion using much narrower fields which effectively protect a much greater volume of the lung (cf. Fig. 9.48). When massive collagen deposits are present in patients with nodular sclerosis, regression after the initial moderate dose of radiation may be too sluggish to permit treatment to be completed with reduced fields within a reasonable time (Fig. 5.8). In such instances, we have sometimes had recourse to interim chemotherapy to further reduce the size of the mediastinal mass without contributing to the hazard of radiation pneumonitis (cf. Figs. 11.54 and 11.55, Chapter 11).

Thymus. In frontal projections, thymic masses usually present a rather typical configuration, particularly on the right side, where the lower edge of the thymus may project laterally beyond the cardiovascular silhouette, giving it a "sail-like" appearance (Fig. 5.9). On the left, unless thymic enlargement is massive, the thymic silhouette tends to blend with the contour of the left ventricle and the appearance is thus less specific. However, the lateral film in such instances clearly delineates a mass in the anterosuperior mediastinum, projecting into the retrosternal clear space in front of the heart (Figs. 5.9D, 5.10). An anterior location of a medias-

tinal mass should always suggest the possibility that it may be of thymic origin.

Thymic involvement by lymphomas is much more frequently encountered in children than in adults, in whom the tracheobronchial lymph nodes of the middle mediastinum are preferentially involved. Occasionally, however, so-called granulomatous thymomas are the presenting feature in adolescent or young adult patients. These tumors, long the subject of controversy, are now regarded by most authorities as a special form of nodular sclerosing Hodgkin's disease (Fechner, 1969; Katz and Lattes, 1969). We have observed examples of granulomatous thymoma in which extension of involvement to the supraclavicular, cervical, and upper para-aortic retroperitoneal lymph nodes has

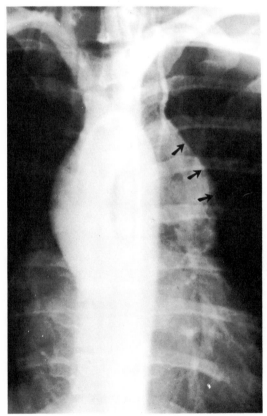

Figure 5.5 This 24-year-old asymptomatic female patient was found to have a smooth, nonlobulated anterior-superior mediastinal mass on chest roentgenogram. The aortogram seen here demonstrates that the mass does not communicate with the aorta and is thus not an aneurysm. Accordingly, a mediastinal exploration was performed, revealing a nonresectable "granulomatous thymoma," a term now considered synonymous with nodular sclerosing Hodgkin's disease of the thymus.

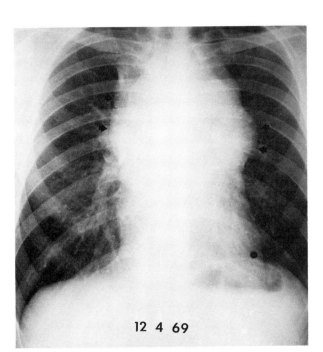

Figure 5.6 Contrast the distinctly lobulated, nodular contour, particularly on the left, of this large mediastinal mass with the smooth contour in the preceding illustration.

occurred. Whenever these extrathoracic sites have been biopsied, their microscopic appearance has been indistinguishable from that of Hodgkin's disease.

Hilar Lymph Nodes. Hilar lymph node enlargement is seldom encountered in the absence of mediastinal lymphadenopathy (Fig. 5.11). The converse is not true, however; mediastinal adenopathy was observed in 206 of 340 consecutive untreated patients with Hodgkin's disease, of whom only 39 also had unilateral or bilateral hilar lymph node enlargement (Chapter 7). The disparity is also evident, though not as great, in the data of Filly, Blank, and Castellino (1976; Fig. 5.2). In many instances, tomography may be required to detect minor degrees of hilar lymphadenopathy or to distinguish hilar nodes from larger mediastinal masses (Figs. 5.12, 5.13, 5.14). Subcarinal lymph node masses may sometimes be clearly visualized on conventional films (Fig. 5.15), but tomograms are needed in doubtful cases. We have also detected pulmonary parenchymal lesions by whole-lung tomography which were not visible, even in retrospect, on the conventional chest roentgenogram; similar instances have been documented by Davidson and Clarke (1968). In an analysis of 243 previously untreated patients with Hodgkin's dis-

ease and non-Hodgkin's lymphomas, Castellino, Filly, and Blank (1976) found that tomography provided additional information in 21.4 percent of all patients, but in only 1.2 percent did these additional findings alter the stage of the patient. In an additional 3.3 percent, the tomograms provided information that influenced the technique of radiotherapy. Thus, tomography may be an extremely useful adjunct to the conventional chest roentgenogram, but it is best used selectively to elucidate suspicious findings on the conventional roentgenogram.

Sarcoidosis often involves both the hilar lymph nodes and the mediastinum and may thus present an occasional problem in differential diagnosis. However, in sarcoidosis the hilar lymph nodes are typically rather large and multiple and the mediastinal component is relatively smaller and usually confined to the right paratracheal area (Fig. 5.16).

It may seem of little importance to be specifically concerned with the recognition of hilar, as opposed to mediastinal, lymphadenopathy since the

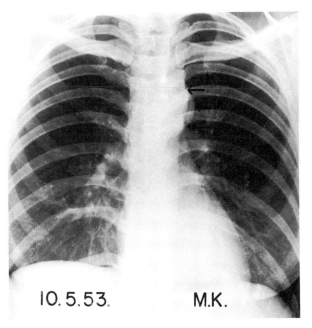

Figure 5.7 This 29-year-old female patient was found to have rubbery lymph nodes, 1 to 2 cm. in diameter, in both supraclavicular fossae. A chest film at another hospital was reported to be normal but on review appeared suspicious in the region of the aortic knob. A repeat chest film one week later revealed the double contour (arrows) in the left superior mediastinum, at the level of the aortic knob, indicative of minimal but definite mediastinal adenopathy. This patient remains relapse-free more than 25 years after radiation therapy for clinical stage II-A disease.

Figure 5.8   Slow regression after radiotherapy of massive mediastinal adenopathy due to nodular sclerosing Hodgkin's disease in a 17-year-old female patient. *A* and *B*, posteroanterior and lateral films on 1/16/67, prior to the initiation of treatment; *C*, posteroanterior film on 3/17/67, at the completion of treatment, delivering 4,400 rads to the mediastinum; *D*, posteroanterior film on 11/20/67, showing further partial regression of the mass; *E* and *F*, posteroanterior and lateral films two years later (11/14/69), showing essentially complete disappearance of the mass, with some residual distortion of the mediastinal contour. Slow regression in cases such as this is probably due to the very large mass of collagen present in the involved lymph nodes. The cellular component of the disease, contained in the nodules of lymphatic tissue, probably responds rapidly, but its response is masked by the much slower resorption of the huge collagen deposits.

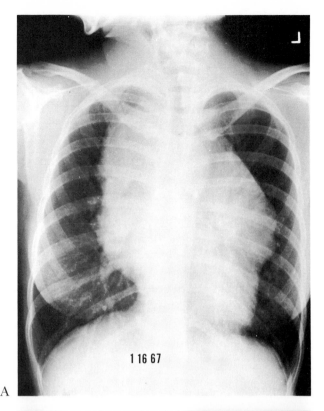

A

B

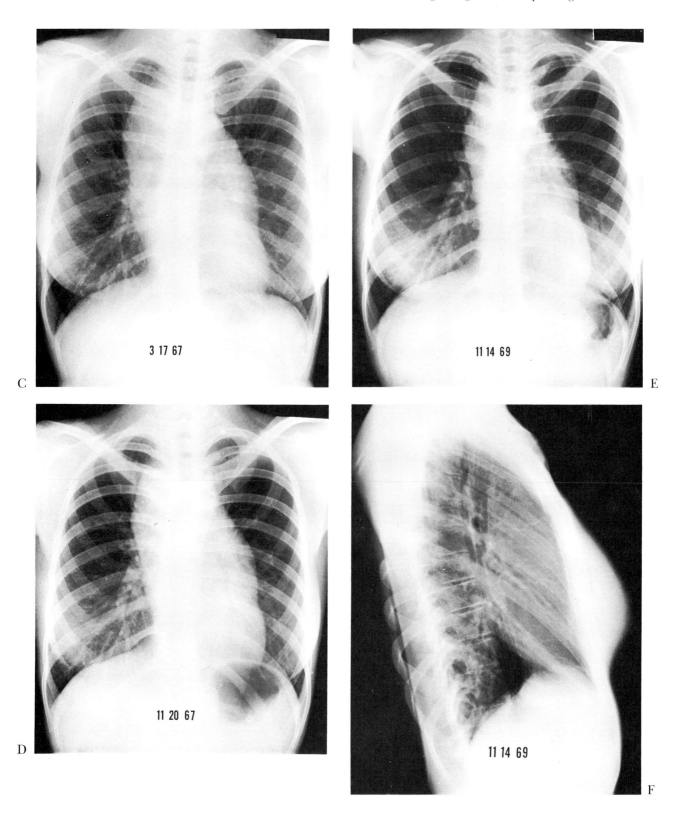

C

3 17 67

D

11 20 67

E

11 14 69

F

11 14 69

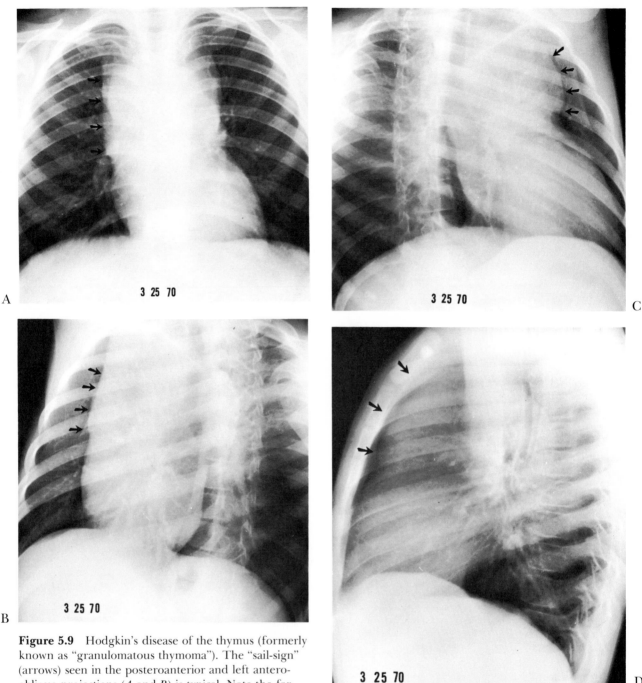

Figure 5.9 Hodgkin's disease of the thymus (formerly known as "granulomatous thymoma"). The "sail-sign" (arrows) seen in the posteroanterior and left antero-oblique projections (*A* and *B*) is typical. Note the far anterior position of the mass in the right antero-oblique and lateral views (*C* and *D*).

hilar nodes are ordinarily encompassed within the radiotherapeutic fields delineated for mediastinal involvement. However, the important point about the detection of hilar lymph nodes in Hodgkin's disease, and perhaps also in patients with the other lymphomas, is that they are commonly a precursor of pulmonary parenchymal involvement. Pulmonary parenchymal involvement by Hodgkin's dis-

ease has rarely been observed in the untreated patient in the absence of concomitant ipsilateral hilar and/or mediastinal lymphadenopathy. Such a case is illustrated in Figure 5.17 (Dhingra and Flance, 1970). Strickland (1967), in a review of 200 cases of intrathoracic Hodgkin's disease, noted that "in none of these cases did the peripheral deposit occur before glandular enlargement." Once the

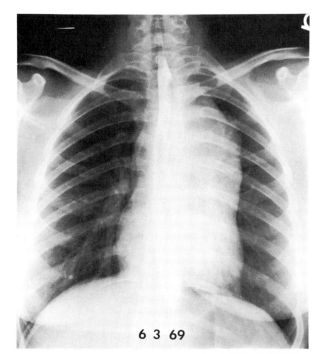

6 3 69

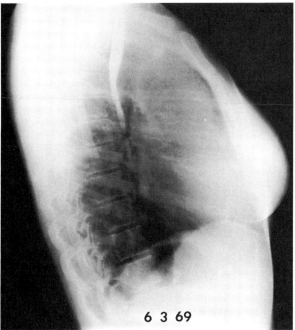

6 3 69

Figure 5.10 The anterior position of this superior mediastinal mass, as seen in the lateral view (*bottom*), is typical of the location of thymomas. This tumor, which was partially resected, proved to be another example of "granulomatous thymoma," now considered synonymous with nodular sclerosing Hodgkin's disease of the thymus. There was direct invasion of the pericardium along the inferior margin of the tumor, rendering complete surgical extirpation impossible.

hilar lymph nodes are involved, the risk of subsequent pulmonary involvement is high. Peters (1966) and Carmel and Kaplan (1976) have advocated prophylactic irradiation of one or both lung fields when hilar lymph node enlargement is manifest (cf. Chapter 9).

Lungs. Lymphomatous lesions involving the pulmonary parenchyma may present a variety of roentgenologic appearances (Fisher, Kendall, and Van Leuven, 1962; Stolberg et al., 1964). Peripheral lesions are more often multiple than solitary; when solitary lesions are detected on conventional films, whole lung tomograms often reveal additional, smaller lesions in other parts of the same and/or the opposite lung (Figs. 5.18, 5.19, 5.20). Solitary lesions are seldom massive, and, except in instances of Hodgkin's sarcoma, growth of peripheral lesions is usually relatively slow. They are generally somewhat less spherical and more irregular in outline than carcinomatous metastases and also less likely to be uniform in size. In some instances, peripheral lesions may have a very ill-defined infiltrative character (Fig. 5.20*A*; cf. also Simon, 1967), which may be exceedingly difficult to differentiate from inflammatory disease due to secondary infection, to which patients with Hodgkin's disease and other lymphomas, particularly after extensive treatment, are notoriously susceptible. When differential diagnosis is not otherwise possible, such lesions should be biopsied, either by percutaneous needle technique under fluoroscopic control, or by open thoracotomy.

Involvement of a pulmonary lobule, or less commonly of an entire lobe, may also be encountered. Such instances are often due to occlusion of the tributary bronchus by an enlarged lymph node, with a combination of atelectasis and lymphedema in the parenchyma of the lobule or lobe causing a uniform increase in its density. When the density is primarily due to atelectasis, associated with bronchial occlusion, diminution in volume of the affected lobe is usually apparent on conventional films, and overexposed films or tomograms reveal occlusion or absence of air-filled bronchi ramifying within it (Fig. 5.23). However, there may also be a component of actual tumor infiltration into the atelectatic lobe, or sufficient lymphedema to prevent its collapse. Such lobular or lobar consolidations may subsequently undergo central necrosis, and, after reestablishing communication with a bronchus, may be partially evacuated, leaving behind an irregular thick-walled cavity, usually containing an air-fluid level (Figs. 5.17, 5.19*B*, 5.21,

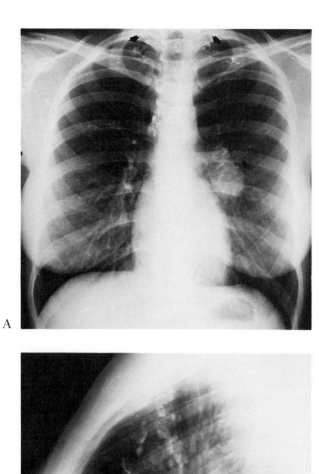

A

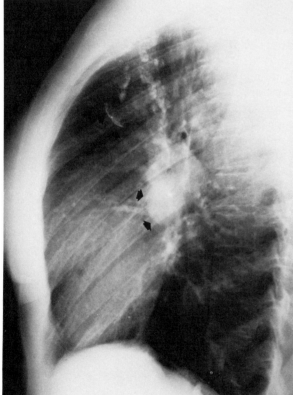

B

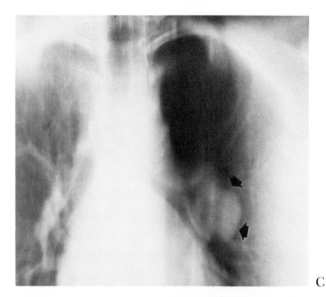

C

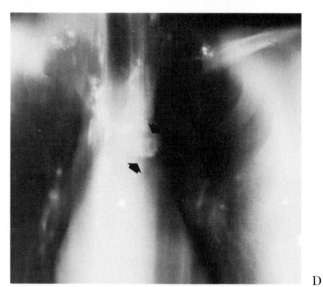

D

Figure 5.11   *A*, this posteroanterior chest film reveals discrete left hilar lymphadenopathy, but the mediastinal silhouette is apparently normal. A lymphangiogram has been performed, opacifying lymph nodes in the superior mediastinum and the right as well as the left supraclavicular fossa. *B*, the hilar mass is again well seen in the lateral view. However, the presence of concomitant mediastinal lymphadenopathy is revealed by a crescentic contour of lymphangiographic contrast material in the anterior superior mediastinum (arrows). *C* and *D*, tomograms again delineate the hilar and nearby left superior mediastinal lymph node masses.

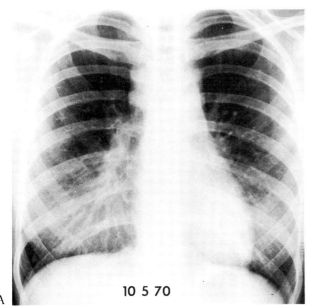

A

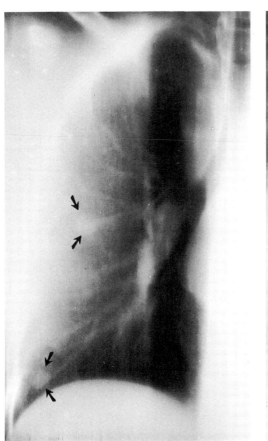

B

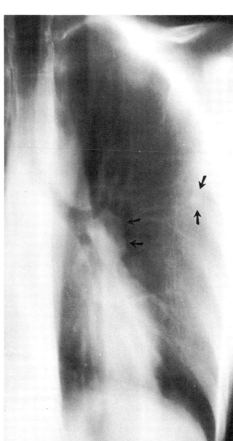

C

Figure 5.12 Casual inspection of the conventional chest film (*A*) of this 15-year-old female patient suggests that there is a moderate degree of widening of the superior mediastinum and no other significant abnormality. However, tomograms (*B* and *C*) revealed bilateral hilar adenopathy, which is distinctively nodular on the left (arrows). In addition, two parenchymal lesions were clearly apparent in the right lung, and a third in the left mid-lung; of these, only the two in the right lung could be discerned on careful reexamination of the conventional film.

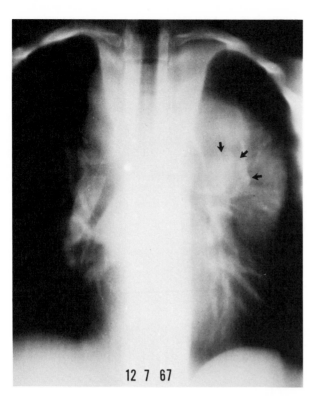

Figure 5.13   Mediastinal tomogram of the mass illustrated in Figure 5.3, revealing the presence of a smaller mass of hilar lymph nodes behind the main mediastinal mass.

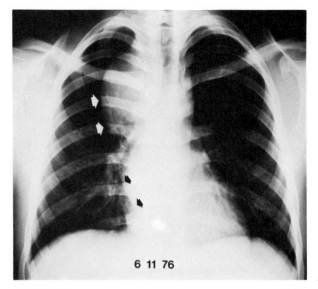

A

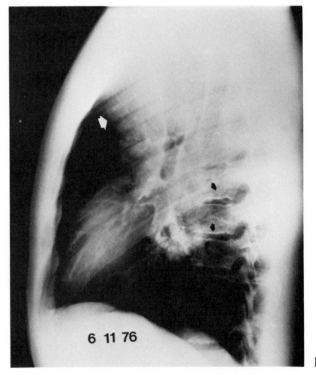

B

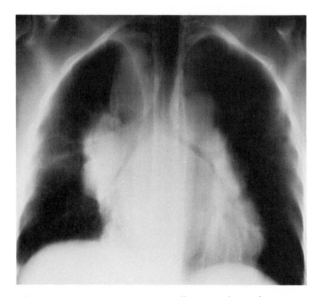

Figure 5.14   Tomogram revealing massive enlargement of the hilar (bronchopulmonary) lymph nodes bilaterally, in addition to superior mediastinal lymphadenopathy. Note the compression and splaying of the major bronchi.

Figure 5.15   *A*, in addition to the large mass which is clearly silhouetted in the right superior mediastinum (white arrows), the inferolateral margin of a subcarinal lymph node mass can be seen through the right cardiac silhouette (black arrows). *B*, in the lateral view, the superior mediastinal mass is seen to be anterior in location (white arrow), and the subcarinal mass is clearly delineated behind the upper part of the heart (black arrows).

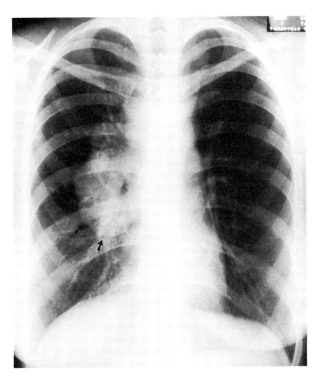

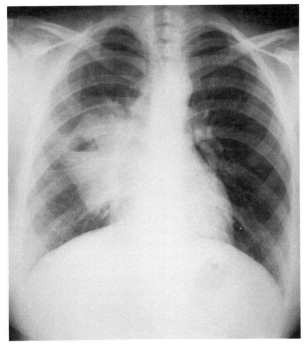

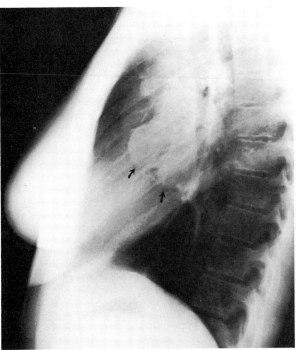

Figure 5.16 The asymmetrical distribution of lymph node enlargement in this case of nodular sclerosing Hodgkin's disease in a 17-year-old girl is limited predominantly to the right paratracheal and right hilar groups of nodes. This asymmetrical distribution is reminiscent of sarcoidosis and might well have been mistaken for it.

Figure 5.17 Primary Hodgkin's disease of the lung, with consolidation and cavitation. At exploration, the mass was found to be resectable, and a right middle and upper lobectomy was performed. There were no involved hilar nodes in the specimen, and no mediastinal adenopathy was palpable at operation. Despite the fact that extensive subsequent diagnostic studies revealed no evidence of Hodgkin's disease elsewhere, disseminated disease later appeared and progressed to a fatal termination. Rare instances of primary Hodgkin's disease of the lung probably arise within lymphoid nodules at the segmental bronchial bifurcations; in most instances, pulmonary involvement is accompanied by or preceded by hilar and mediastinal involvement. (Reproduced with the permission of I. Jerome Flance, M.D.)

5.22). Infrequently, pulmonary cavities due to Hodgkin's disease may be thin walled, like those of tuberculosis. Differential diagnosis is aided by the fact that these usually respond promptly to specific chemotherapy or to modest doses of X-irradiation.

Diffuse unilateral or bilateral lymphangitic infiltration of the lungs, similar to that commonly observed in cancer of the breast, is seen more often in chronic lymphatic leukemia than in the lymphomas. However, in some cases of Hodgkin's disease we have seen a lymphangitic infiltrative component associated with the presence of fluffy, irregular, nodular peripheral deposits (Fig. 5.24).

In patients treated with radiation therapy for mediastinal adenopathy, radiation reactions commonly appear in the paramediastinal pulmonary

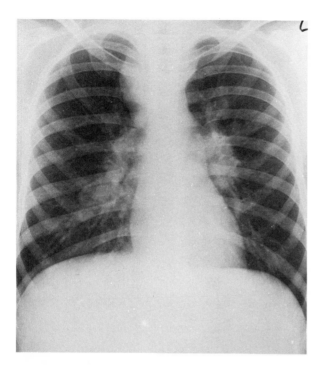

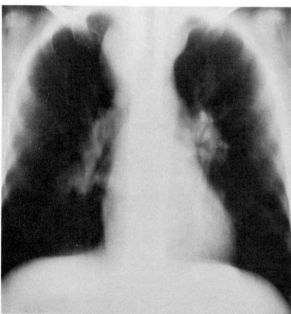

Figure 5.18   Mediastinal, bilateral hilar, and pulmonary parenchymal involvement in the left upper lobe are all visible on the posteroanterior conventional film, but additional pulmonary parenchymal nodules were demonstrated in both lungs by tomography.

parenchyma, beginning about two to three months after the completion of treatment, often associated with the development of a hacking cough and occasionally of dyspnea. At their inception, such pulmonary radiation reactions may be manifested radiographically by an accentuation and coarsening of the bronchovascular pattern in the affected zone, often with an increase in linear strands and irregular, fluffy, ill-defined infiltrates (Fig. 5.25). On serial examinations, these tend to coalesce, in part due to a progressive diminution in volume of the affected lung segments as the lesion changes progressively from an essentially inflammatory to a progressive fibrotic and contractile process. It is important that such pulmonary radiation reactions not be misinterpreted, particularly in their acute phases, as new areas of pulmonary parenchymal involvement by the lymphoma so that the patient is not subjected needlessly to additional irradiation or chemotherapy. Usually, the differential diagnosis will be readily apparent from the fact that the areas of parenchymal involvement conform closely to the contour and size of the radiotherapy fields used in the treatment of the previous mediastinal adenopathy (cf. Chapter 9). The temporal sequence of events may also be helpful in evaluation, since pulmonary radiation reactions usually appear within two to six months after completion of a course of radiotherapy. Lesions appearing during this interval should be observed for a time before the institution of antilymphoma treatment, unless they are clearly outside the margins of the radiotherapy fields.

An even more serious problem in differential diagnosis, as mentioned above, is that posed by the multiplicity of secondary infections to which patients with Hodgkin's disease and other lymphomas are so susceptible. Tuberculosis, once so commonly associated with Hodgkin's disease, is still of sufficient importance to necessitate the usual diagnostic tests for the presence of the tubercle bacillus in patients with lymphomas who develop unilateral or bilateral parenchymal infiltrates or thin-walled cavities (Fig. 5.26). However, in an increasing proportion of cases in recent years, a variety of "opportunistic" pathogens including *Coccidioides immitis, Monilia, Aspergillus, Histoplasma,* and *Pneumocystis carinii* have been isolated from such secondary pulmonary inflammatory lesions (Casazza et al., 1966; Remington, 1972; Krick and Remington, 1976; Kauffman et al., 1978; cf. Figs. 5.27, 5.28, and 5.29). Aspiration biopsy of such infiltrates was used successfully to recover the causative organism in 16 of 25 attempts in 21 high-risk

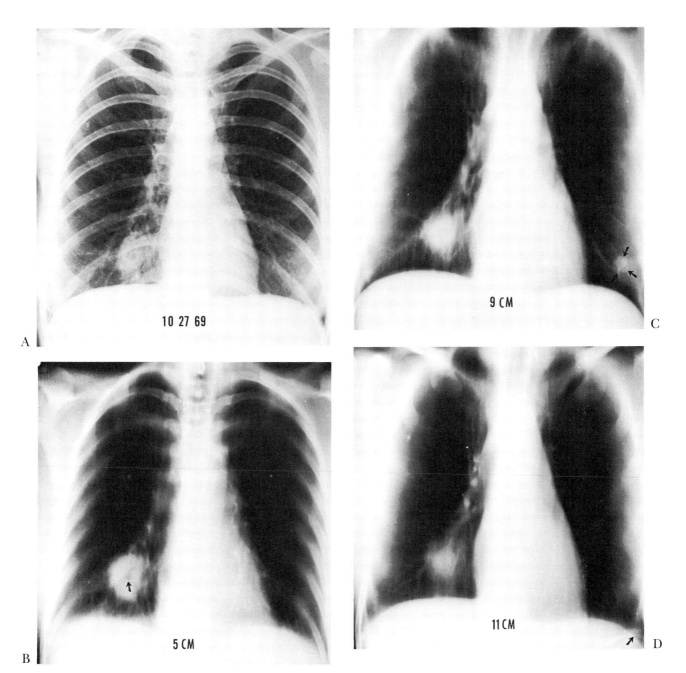

Figure 5.19 A nodular, lobulated mass containing a small pocket of air is seen at the right base of the conventional film, but tomograms clearly reveal several additional nodules in both lungs.

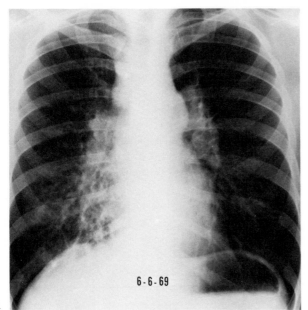

A

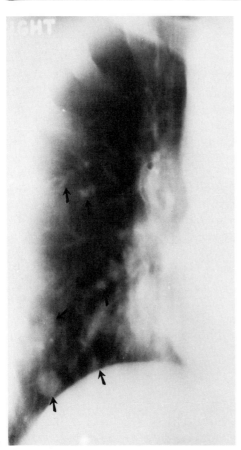

B

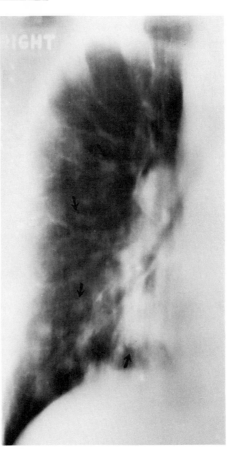

C

Figure 5.20   In addition to mediastinal and bilateral hilar adenopathy, an irregular strandlike infiltration is seen in the right lower lung field, somewhat resembling a pneumonitis. Tomograms revealed multiple additional nodular lesions in the right lung and two small nodules on the left as well.

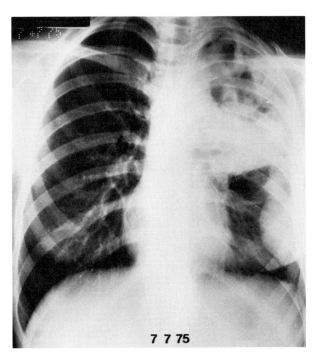

7 7 75

Figure 5.21   Hodgkin's disease involving most of the left upper lobe with extensive central necrosis and cavitation. A small nodular density is also present at the superior aspect of the right hilum (arrows).

patients, including several with Hodgkin's disease and other lymphomas (Bandt, Blank, and Castellino, 1972).

Pleura. Unilateral or bilateral pleural effusions, occasionally chylous in nature, are commonly observed as a presenting manifestation in patients with massive mediastinal lymphadenopathy due to Hodgkin's disease (Fig. 5.30), as well as later in the course of the illness. Usually they exhibit the classical roentgenologic manifestations of pleural effusion: blunting and obliteration of the costophrenic angle and displacement of the aerated lateral lung margin from the medial cortical margin of the ribs by fluid ascending in the pleural space along the lateral thoracic wall (Fig. 5.31A). In lateral roentgenograms, the posterior costophrenic sulcus, and less often the anterior sulcus as well, is obliterated, and pleural fluid is seen to ascend, particularly along the posterior thoracic wall, between the lung and the rib margin. Fluid may also enter the pleural spaces of the interlobar fissures. On the right side, the minor fissure is usually relatively horizontal and pleural effusions entering it thus project edgewise and are sharply delineated in the frontal view. In contrast, fluid in the major fissure on either side is projected obliquely as a diffuse,

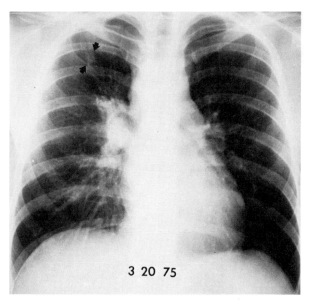

3 20 75

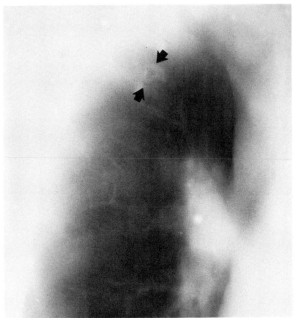

Figure 5.22   Mediastinal and right hilar lymphadenopathy associated with direct extension from the right hilar region upward into the right upper lobe. In addition, a parenchymal nodule is present in the right first interspace which, despite its small size, has already undergone central necrosis and cavitation, best seen on the tomogram (arrows).

hazy density over the lower two-thirds to three-fourths of the lung field. The true state of affairs is clearly revealed in the lateral film, where effusions into either the major or the minor fissure are projected on edge, and their anatomic relationships made evident (Fig. 5.31B).

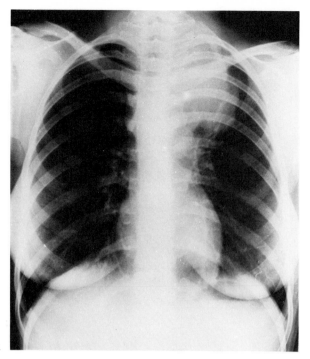

A

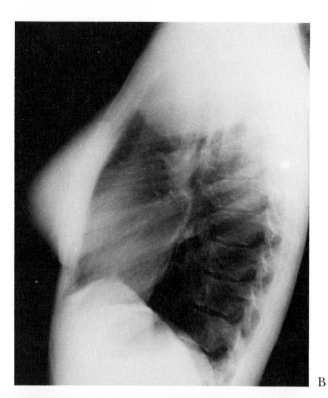

B

Figure 5.23   This large mass was initially thought to be due entirely to mediastinal adenopathy encroaching upon and displacing the left upper lobe. However, tomography clearly reveals compression and abrupt occlusion of a bronchus entering the lateral aspect of the mass, proving that this portion of the mass is in the lung parenchyma.

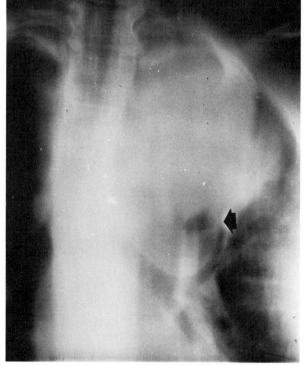

C

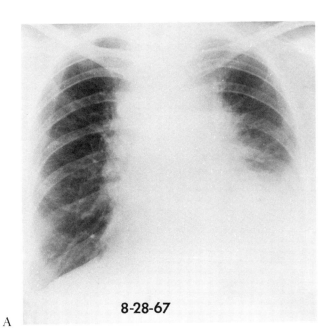

A

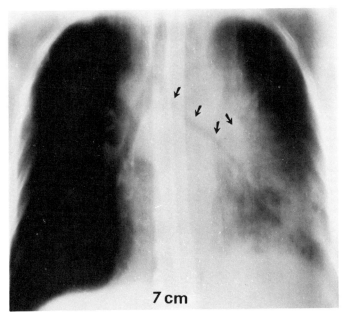

B

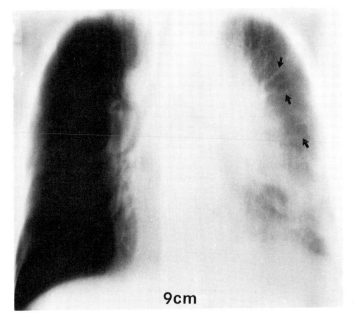

C

Figure 5.24   *A*, diffuse lymphangitic infiltration of the left lung by Hodgkin's disease extending directly outward from massive mediastinal and hilar adenopathy. There is a left-sided pleural effusion, and biopsy with the Cope needle confirmed the presence of pleural invasion. Coarse, nodular pulmonary infiltrates are also apparent at the left base in the 7 and 9 cm. tomograms (*B* and *C*). Note the compressed left main and upper lobe bronchi (arrows, *B*).

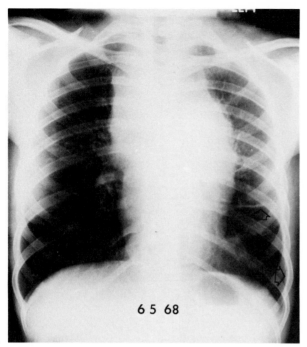

A

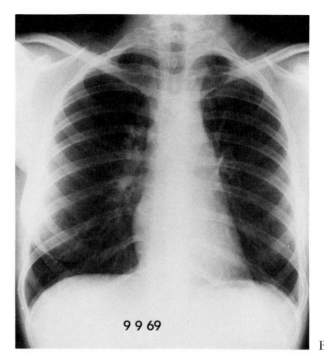

B

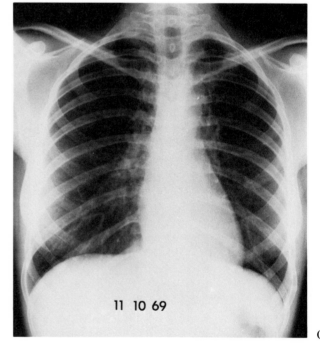

C

Figure 5.25   The pretreatment film of 6/5/68 (*A*) reveals mediastinal and hilar adenopathy, as well as minimal left pleural reaction seen just inside the rib margin and a horizontal line resembling the appearance of disk atelectasis in the left lower lung field, which on tomography led to the discovery of a solitary, subpleural pulmonary parenchymal nodule; *B*, film of 9/9/69 reveals strandlike infiltration in the left upper lung field due to postirradiation fibrosis; *C*, film of 11/10/69 reveals further contraction of the fibrotic process medially toward the mediastinum. The fact that the mediastinal mass extends so low on the left should alert the physician to the strong possibility, even in the absence of pericardial effusion, that the epicardium has been invaded.

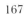

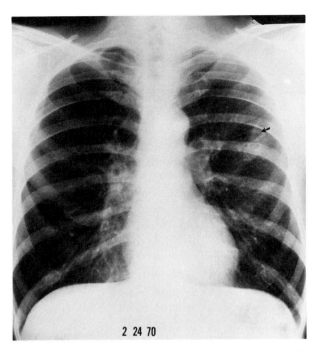

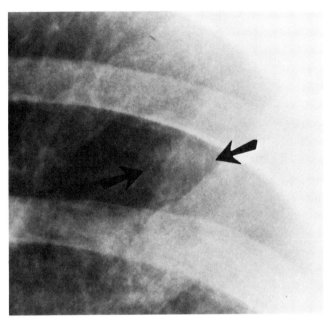

Figure 5.26 Left upper lobe infiltrate due to tuberculosis in a patient with stage III Hodgkin's disease. The absence of mediastinal or hilar adenopathy suggested that the parenchymal lesion was likely to be infectious, rather than part of the neoplastic process. Sputum smears and gastric washings revealed tubercle bacilli, and therapy with streptomycin and isonicotinic acid amide was begun.

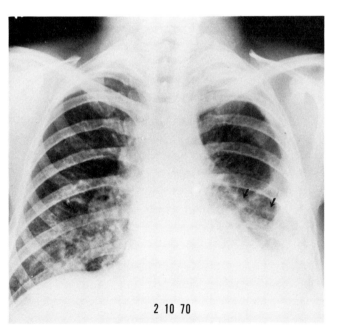

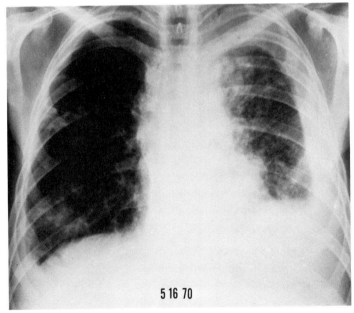

Figure 5.27 Progressive pulmonary infection in a patient with far-advanced, uncontrolled Hodgkin's disease. Fluid levels could be seen in thin-walled cavities in the right lung on the examination of 5/16/70. At autopsy, most of the left lung and multiple segments of the right lung were consolidated and the presence of cavities in the right lung was confirmed. Cultures established the presence of *Monilia* bilaterally and of *Pneumocystis carinii* in the infiltrations at the right base.

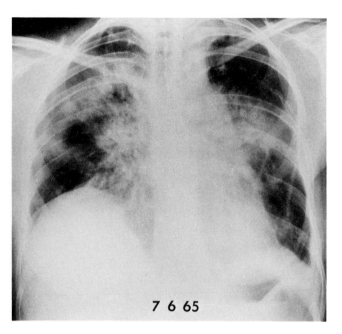

7 6 65

Figure 5.28 Complex pulmonary roentgenographic patterns in a 32-year-old patient who had been treated several years earlier for Hodgkin's disease involving the cervical, supraclavicular, and mediastinal nodes, with subsequent fibrosis and widening of the mediastinum. She later developed bilateral pulmonary extensions; these initially responded well to a succession of single chemotherapeutic agents but ultimately progressed and required local irradiation, which was followed by additional fibrosis and scarring. Preterminally she developed a bilateral infiltrative process due in part to recurrent Hodgkin's disease and in part to infection by *Pneumocystis carinii*. This case illustrates the difficulties of roentgen interpretation in a situation in which the manifestations of the primary disease, of secondary infection, and of the reaction and fibrosis resulting from treatment are all superimposed.

Minimal effusions may cause a barely perceptible thickening of the pleura (Fig. 5.25A), whereas massive effusions may compress and partially obliterate the underlying lung. In other instances, a pleural effusion may, for reasons still not well understood, form a fluid layer of uniform thickness between the diaphragmatic pleura and the overlying lung, without the telltale curvilinear obliteration of the lateral costophrenic angle, giving a very misleading appearance of elevation of the diaphragm. An important clue to the correct diagnosis of this atypical "layered" type of effusion is the fact that, when it occurs on the left side, the air bubble in the fundus of the stomach, usually separated from the lung only by the normal thickness of the diaphragm, will be seen to be displaced farther from the lung, indicating either that the di-

aphragm is of abnormal thickness or that fluid is present above or below it (Fig. 5.31A). A lateral decubitus film will cause the pleural fluid to run out into the lateral pleural space and thus establish the diagnosis conclusively; the decubitus view is also useful in chronic cases to distinguish free fluid from pleural thickening and fibrosis (Fig. 5.31C). Infrequently, pleural involvement may take the form of discrete nodules or plaques of soft tissue density between the lung and the thoracic wall (Fig. 5.32). These are usually apparent only for a limited time, after which their outlines are obliterated by the development of effusion. In doubtful cases, diagnostic thoracentesis followed by the introduction of air or carbon dioxide may clearly reveal their presence.

It is of considerable importance to ascertain, whenever possible, whether a pleural effusion associated with a mediastinal mass is merely a transudate due to compression of intrathoracic vessels by the mediastinal mass or involves an actual invasion of the pleural cavity by the neoplasm. Unfortunately, roentgenologic examination alone cannot provide the answer to this question, and laboratory analysis of the pleural fluid obtained at thoracentesis has, in our experience, not been as helpful as might have been anticipated. In a number of instances in which pleural effusions regressed and disappeared after radiotherapy directed to the mediastinum alone, and were thus identified retrospectively as having been transudates, the pleural fluid was characterized by high specific gravity and protein content.

Heart and Great Vessels. Lymphomas may directly invade the heart, particularly the pericardium and epicardium, and are usually accompanied by pericardial effusion. Although cardiac involvement is usually a late manifestation, we have observed several instances in which cardiac involvement by direct extension from a mediastinal mass has been present at the time of admission (Figs. 5.25A, 5.33). In rare instances, the mediastinal tumor, extending downward toward the diaphragm, may be so closely applied to the heart as to give a false impression of cardiac enlargement; indeed, the cardiomediastinal silhouette may resemble that seen in certain forms of congenital heart disease (Fig. 5.34).

We have also observed epicardial nodules and plaques of Hodgkin's disease, sometimes associated with pericardial effusion, appearing within several months to two years after the completion of radiotherapy for massive mediastinal Hodgkin's

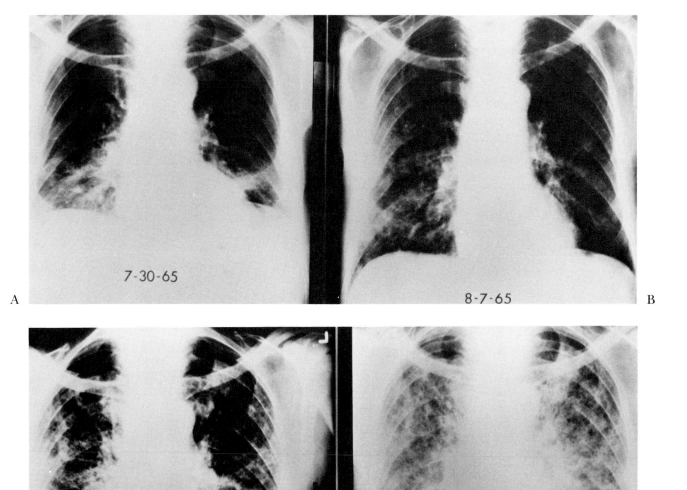

Figure 5.29 Rapid evolution of *Pneumocystis carinii* pneumonitis following chemotherapy. (Reprinted by permission of the author and *Hospital Practice*, from "The Compromised Host" by J. S. Remington, 1972.)

disease; in each such instance, the epicardial plaque or nodule appeared just outside the margins of the radiotherapy field, suggesting that microscopic invasion of the epicardium had already occurred at the time of initial treatment (Fig. 5.35). Involvement of small lymph nodes on the medial superior surface of the diaphragm (Fig. 5.36) may also give rise to epicardial masses of variable size at the right or left cardiophrenic angles (Fig. 5.37); such instances may, but need not, be accompanied by pericardial invasion (Castellino and Blank, 1972; Crowe, 1975). As a result of such observa-

tions, our radiotherapy fields have now been altered, as described in Chapter 9, to encompass the entire cardiac silhouette, up to a dose of approximately 1,500 rads, in all patients with demonstrable mediastinal adenopathy.

When pericardial effusion is suspected, ultrasonic echocardiography may be of great assistance in establishing the diagnosis conclusively (Cohn et al., 1967). The intravenous use of carbon dioxide or conventional angiocardiography may also be helpful. Another simple and safe procedure, isotopic angiocardiography using ^{99m}Tc, has also be-

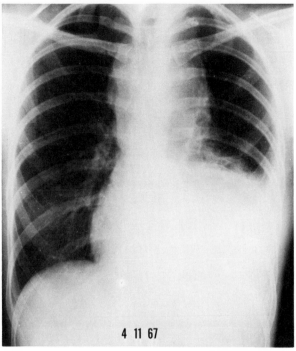

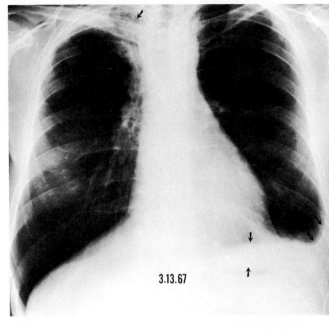

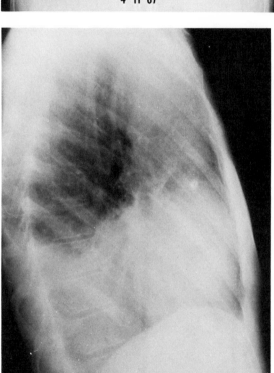

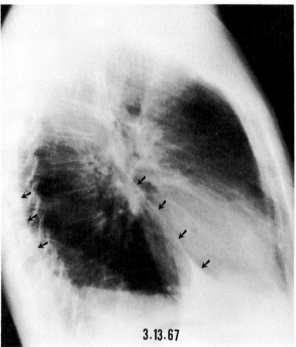

B

Figure 5.30 Extensive left pleural effusion associated with mediastinal lymphadenopathy. Cope needle biopsy revealed Hodgkin's disease invading the pleura. The patient has not had a relapse for more than twelve and one-half years after intensive radiotherapy directed at the mediastinum, the left lower lung field, and the mediastinal, diaphragmatic, and lower parietal pleura.

Figure 5.31 Pleural effusion which appeared in an otherwise disease-free 46-year-old male patient who had been treated two years previously for stage IIA Hodgkin's disease involving the neck and mediastinum; although the fluid obtained on thoracentesis contained 5 gm. per 100 cc. of protein, the pleural effusion resolved spontaneously. In the posteroanterior view (*A*), note the increased separation between the base of the left lung and the air bubble in the stomach, as well as the curvilinear obliteration of the left costophrenic sulcus; similar obliteration of the sulcus anteriorly and posteriorly is evident in the lateral view (*B*); the fact that this density is due to free fluid rather than to chronic pleural thickening is evident from its change in position, as demonstrated on the decubitus film (*C*).

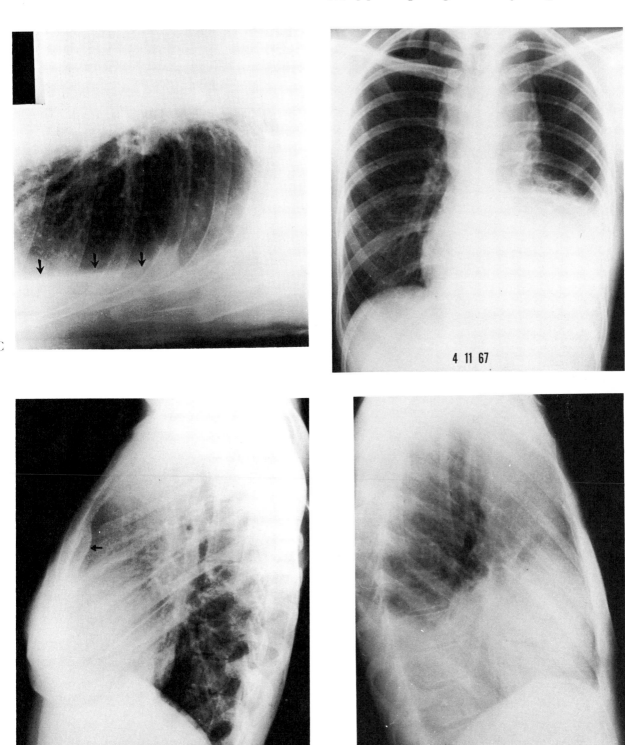

C

Figure 5.32   Lateral film showing a soft tissue mass along the anterior-superior chest wall, due either to pleural involvement or, in the absence of pleural effusion, to enlargement of internal mammary lymph nodes and invasion of the soft tissues of the anterior chest wall.

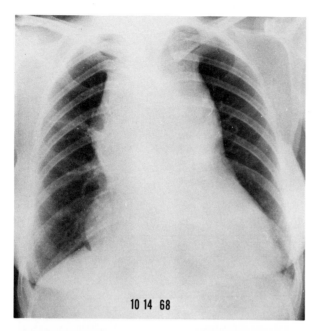

10 14 68

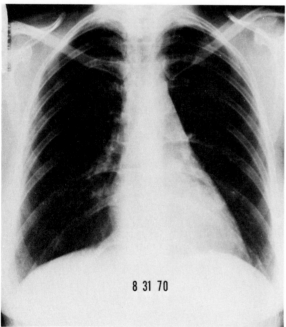

8 31 70

Figure 5.33 *Top*, cardiomegaly due to pericardial invasion and effusion, extending directly from massive mediastinal lymphadenopathy. The small, bilateral pleural effusions were low in protein content and were believed to be transudates. *Bottom*, appearance nearly two years later, after total lymphoid radiotherapy followed by six cycles of quadruple drug ("MOPP") chemotherapy (cf. Chapter 10).

come available for the diagnosis of pericardial effusion (Kriss, 1969). Retrosternal lymphomatous masses have also been detected by ultrasonic echocardiography (Tingelstad, McWilliams, and Thomas, 1976).

When pericardial effusion or nonspecific cardiomegaly become apparent roentgenologically at some interval after radiotherapy in patients with lymphomas, the possibility that one may be dealing with a radiation carditis or pericarditis must be considered. This complication was initially documented in approximately 7 percent of our cases after intensive megavoltage radiotherapy to the cardiomediastinal region (Cohn, et al., 1967; Stewart, et al., 1967), and in a higher percentage in other series (Pierce, Hafermann, and Kagan, 1969). Fortunately, it was possible to devise modifications of radiotherapeutic technique (Chapter 9) which have greatly reduced its frequency. In some instances there have been few or no associated symptoms and the cardiomegaly has spontaneously regressed without specific treatment (Fig. 5.38). In other instances, the classical signs of constrictive pericarditis and of cardiac tamponade have become apparent and have necessitated surgical intervention and pericardial decortication for relief (Fig. 5.39). It is of great importance to entertain the possibility of radiation carditis or pericarditis in such instances, since an incorrect diagnosis of cardiac or pericardial infiltration by the lymphoma, if treated with supplementary local irradiation, may well fatally aggravate the radiation carditis (Fig. 5.40).

Malignant lymphomas involving mediastinal lymph nodes, even when massive, are less likely to cause superior vena caval obstruction syndrome than is bronchogenic carcinoma. However, superior vena caval obstruction does occur in some instances, accompanied by the classical physical signs of plethora in the head, neck, and upper extremities, engorgement of the jugular veins, and evidence of elevated venous pressure. In the more chronic cases, the development of a collateral venous circulation will also be apparent, accompanied roentgenologically by fullness of the outline of the azygos vein. Although other clinical evidence will usually establish the diagnosis, upper extremity angiography may be required in selected cases. The angiogram may also assist the radiotherapist in delineating the extent of the compressed venous segment for the purpose of outlining radiotherapy treatment fields.

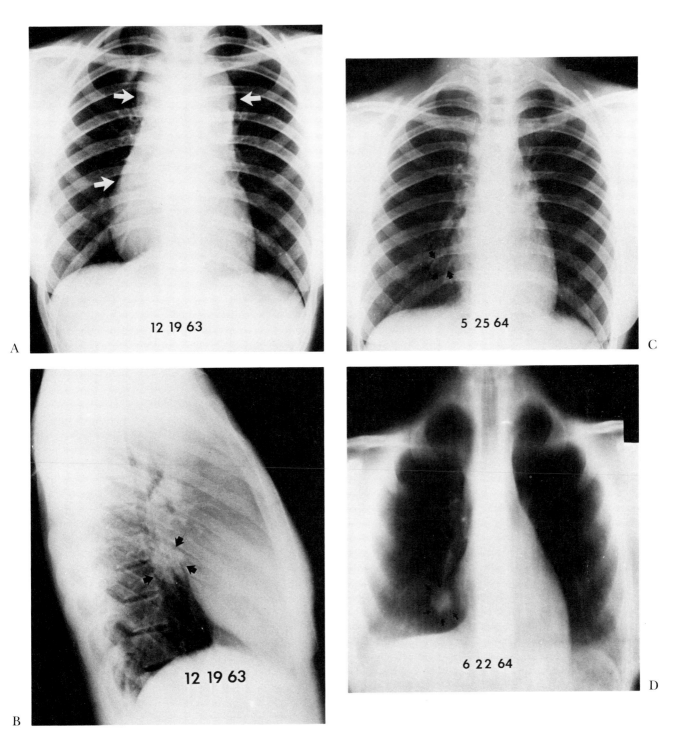

Figure 5.34 The mediastinal mass in this case has extended downward along the right atrial contour, following that contour so perfectly as to convey a misleading impression of cardiac enlargement. Cases of this type are sometimes mistakenly interpreted as congenital heart disease. The presence of associated right hilar disease is evident in the lateral view (B); on the film of 5/25/64 (C), a few months after radiotherapy, the marked change in cardiomediastinal silhouette is evident. In addition, a faint nodular density is seen in the right middle lobe near the heart, which is more distinctly visualized on the tomogram (D). This case thus illustrates the tendency for pulmonary parenchymal disease to develop ipsilaterally in patients with prior hilar adenopathy.

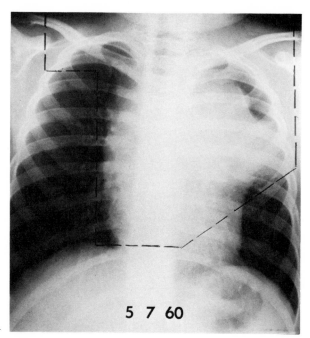

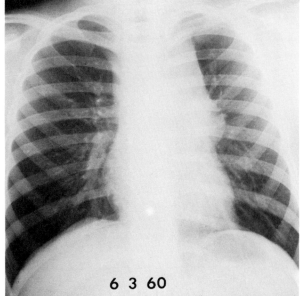

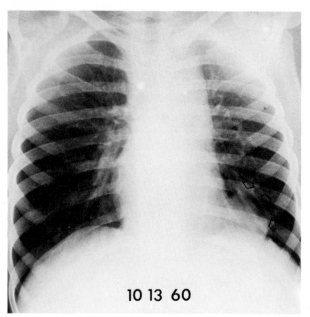

A

B

C

Figure 5.35 Extension of mediastinal Hodgkin's disease downward along the pericardium. *A*, chest film on admission (5/7/60) reveals massive mediastinal lymphadenopathy extending laterally almost to the left chest wall. The outlines of the radiotherapy field are indicated by the dashed line. *B*, repeat chest film on 6/3/60, soon after completion of radiotherapy; regression of the mass is almost complete, but minimal tenting of the left diaphragm is now present. *C*, chest film of 10/13/60 reveals a new mass (arrows) at the left cardiophrenic angle, just outside the margins of the treatment field outlined in *A*. Although this mass responded well to supplemental treatment, new foci of involvement appeared in the abdomen, and the patient ultimately died of uncontrolled Hodgkin's disease in April 1965. Such masses usually arise from enlargement of involved diaphragmatic lymph nodes (Fayos and Lampe, 1971; Castellino and Blank, 1972) and may or may not be accompanied by actual invasion of the pericardium.

Esophagus. As might be expected, the esophagus is often displaced posteriorly and sometimes also laterally by large mediastinal masses. However, direct invasion of the esophagus (Fig. 5.41) appears to be quite uncommon even at autopsy, although the diagnosis has been made during life in rare instances (Surks and Guttman, 1966; Hambly and Blundell, 1968). In a review of the literature to that date, Portmann, Dunne, and Hazard (1954) noted only two cases of apparently "primary" Hodgkin's disease of the esophagus, as contrasted with fifty-two, forty-five, and eight cases in which the stomach, small intestine, and colon, respectively, were involved. Symptoms of esophagitis may occur in patients with lymphomas, either as a transient reaction to radiation therapy or, in severely ill and debilitated patients with advanced disease, as a result of secondary monilial or other fungus infections. In either case, the only roentgenologic manifestation is coarsening and irregularity of the mucosal folds of the esophagus.

Thoracic Cage and Soft Tissues. Strickland (1967) has described a "truncated wigwam" appearance as characteristic of direct involvement of the sternum or of the retrosternal space by Hodgkin's disease. Destruction of the sternum and infiltration of the

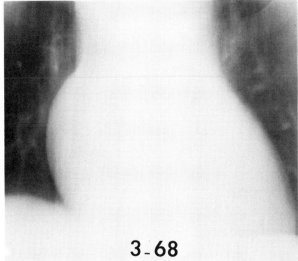

Int. mammary group
Prepericardiac group
Lat. pericardiac group (Juxtaphrenic)

Phrenic nn.

Esoph   IVC
Aorta

Figure 5.36 Diagrammatic representation of diaphragmatic lymph nodes as seen from behind (modified from Rouvière). (Reprinted by permission of the authors and the *American Journal of Roentgenology,* from the paper by Castellino and Blank, 1972.)

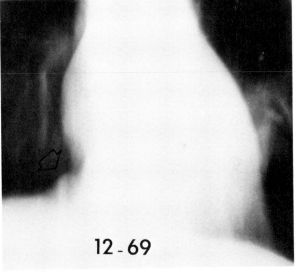

3-68

12-69

A

B

Figure 5.37 *A,* pretreatment anteroposterior tomogram is normal. *B,* post-treatment anteroposterior tomogram, showing appearance of a right cardiophrenic angle mass (arrow) as well as an infiltrate in the lingula of the left upper lobe. (Reprinted by permission of the authors and the *American Journal of Roentgenology,* from the paper by Castellino and Blank, 1972.)

presternal soft tissues is usually readily apparent on the lateral chest roentgenogram, as well as on lateral or oblique detail films or tomograms of the sternal region (Figs. 5.42, 5.43, 5.44).

At times, massive enlargement of an infraclavicular or internal mammary node is associated with extensive invasion of adjacent tissues, which, in addition to producing a clinically evident soft tissue mass, may be manifested roentgenologically as a diffuse increase in density over the upper lung field (Fig. 5.45*A*). In such instances, the lordotic view may reveal protrusion of the mass into the thorax (Fig. 5.45*B*) and tomograms may demonstrate destruction of the adjacent ribs (Fig. 5.45*C*) and even transpleural invasion of the lung parenchyma (Fig. 5.45*D*). Despite the extent of such an invasive process, response to intensive radiotherapy may be excellent (Fig. 5.45*E*).

Figure 5.38   Development and spontaneous resolution of radiation-induced pericarditis with effusion. The pretreatment chest film of 5/2/68 (*A*) reveals moderate bilateral superior mediastinal lymphadenopathy. The film of 1/3/69 (*B*), several months after completion of radiotherapy, reveals widening of the mediastinal silhouette due to paramediastinal fibrosis and slight cardiomegaly. The pleural effusion at the left base is secondary to radiation therapy directed to the spleen. By 2/17/69, massive cardiomegaly and bilateral pleural effusions are apparent (*C*), associated with anterior chest pain, fever, moderate dyspnea, and the physical findings of cardiac tamponade. Pericardiocentesis on 2/23/69 confirmed the presence of pericardial effusion, and a film (*D*) made after air injection revealed fluid levels and slight thickening of the epicardium (arrows). The patient was placed on bed rest and was given diuretics, with prompt, complete, and sustained disappearance of the effusion, as seen on the films of 3/24/69 (*E*) and 1/12/70 (*F*).

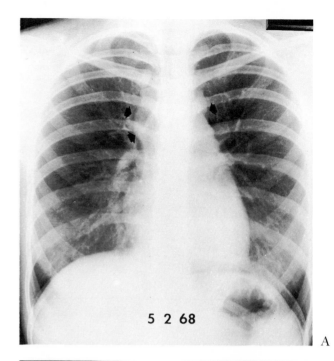

A

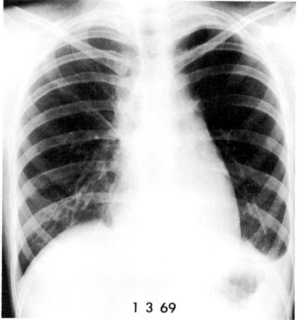

B

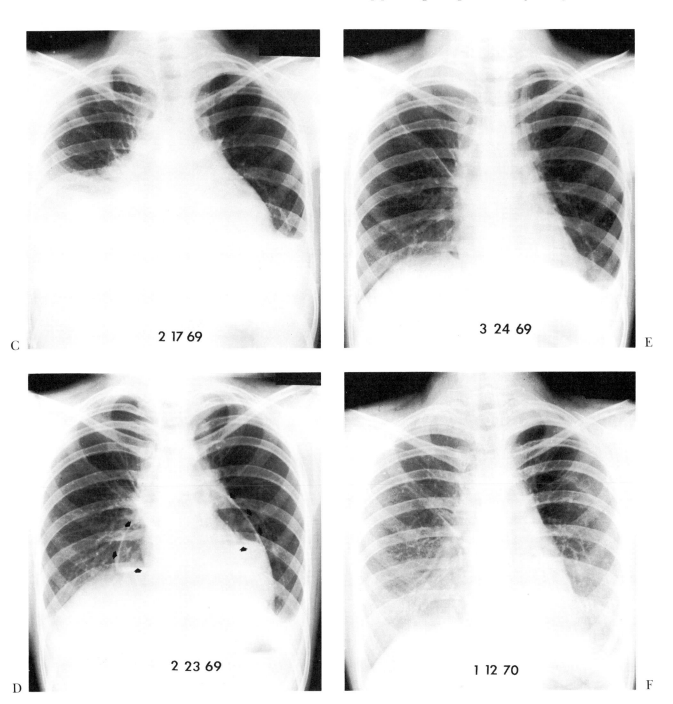

C   2 17 69

E   3 24 69

D   2 23 69

F   1 12 70

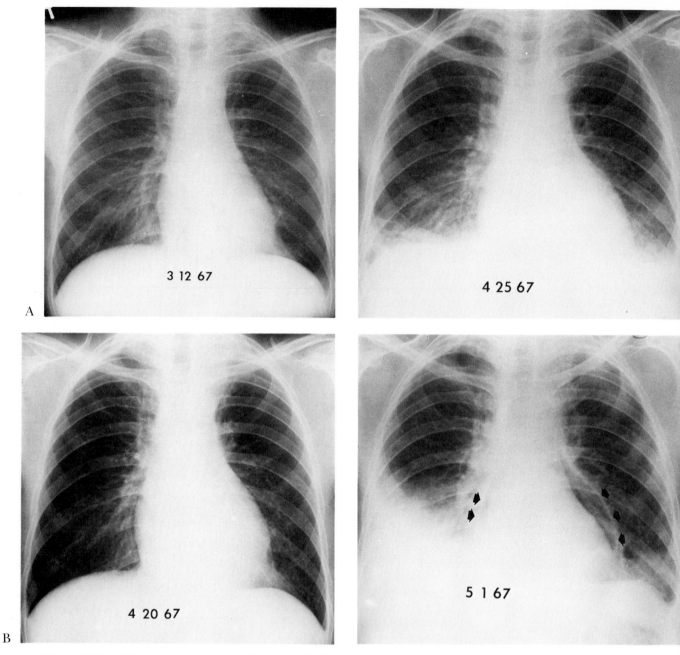

Figure 5.39   This 33-year-old male patient was initially treated in November 1965, for stage IIB Hodgkin's disease involving the mediastinal, bilateral cervical-supraclavicular, and bilateral axillary nodes. About one year later, surveillance films of the abdomen revealed progressive enlargement of the upper lumbar para-aortic lymph nodes, and a distinct bulge appeared along the left lower cardiac silhouette indicative of invasion of the pericardium, just outside of the radiotherapeutic field. Accordingly, he was given radiation to the mediastinum and para-aortic region, and the ini-

tial film (*A*) of 3/12/67, made about two months after completion of his second course of mediastinal irradiation, revealed complete regression of the mass involving the pericardium. However, by 4/20/67 (*B*), diffuse cardiomegaly had become evident, increasing rapidly during the next five days (*C*), associated with the development of pleural effusions, and the diagnosis of radiation pericarditis with effusion was made. Pericardiocentesis with injection of air was performed on 5/1/67 (*D*), revealing the moderately thickened epicardium and an air-fluid level within the pericardial sac.

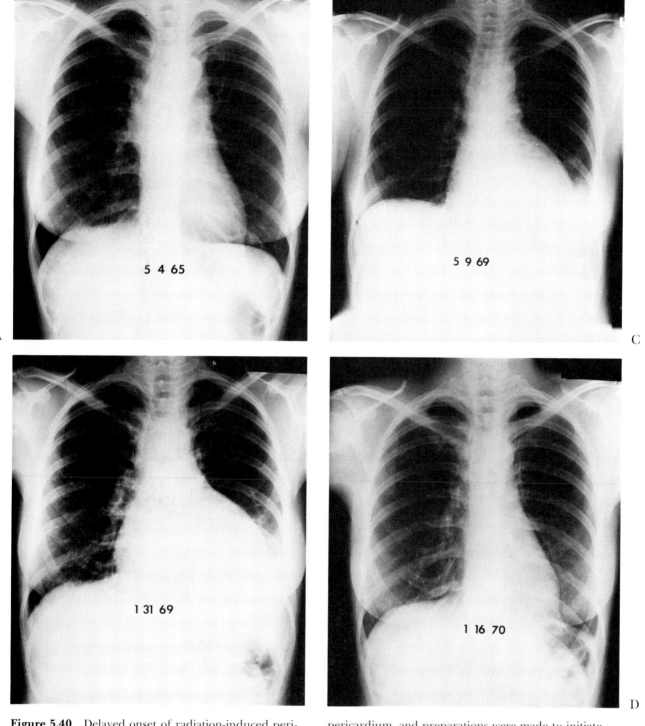

A

B

C

D

Figure 5.40 Delayed onset of radiation-induced pericarditis, apparently triggered by the cessation of steroid therapy. This 25-year-old female patient was initially treated in May 1965 for stage IIA Hodgkin's disease involving the cervical and mediastinal lymph nodes (*A*). About six months after completion of radiotherapy, she was given chronic steroid treatment by her personal physician for an unrelated medical condition and continued receiving steroid for about three years, after which the dose was rapidly tapered. Soon thereafter, pressure symptoms developed in the chest, and she became short of breath. A repeat chest film was made on 1/31/69 (*B*) and was interpreted as revealing recurrent Hodgkin's disease, possibly invading the pericardium, and preparations were made to initiate treatment with alkylating agents. However, she returned to Stanford for consultation, and investigation demonstrated no evidence of Hodgkin's disease and suggested instead that the pericardial effusion was most likely due to radiation pericarditis, which had been suppressed for nearly four years by the chronic steroid medication. Steroid treatment was reinstituted, and great care was taken to taper the dose very slowly over a period of many months, with gradual and complete response (*C* and *D*). Left pleural thickening is evident on the final film of 1/16/70, but the cardiac silhouette is normal.

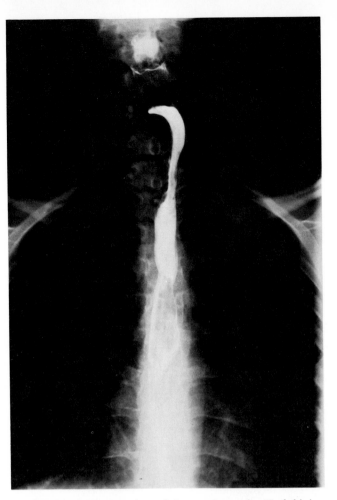
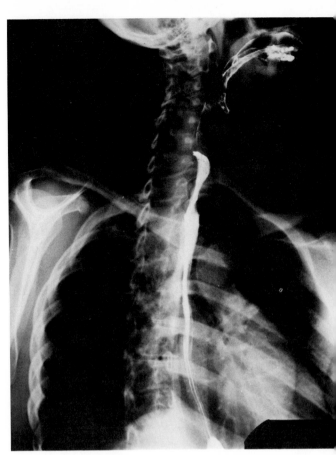

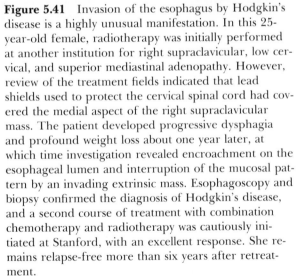

Figure 5.41 Invasion of the esophagus by Hodgkin's disease is a highly unusual manifestation. In this 25-year-old female, radiotherapy was initially performed at another institution for right supraclavicular, low cervical, and superior mediastinal adenopathy. However, review of the treatment fields indicated that lead shields used to protect the cervical spinal cord had covered the medial aspect of the right supraclavicular mass. The patient developed progressive dysphagia and profound weight loss about one year later, at which time investigation revealed encroachment on the esophageal lumen and interruption of the mucosal pattern by an invading extrinsic mass. Esophagoscopy and biopsy confirmed the diagnosis of Hodgkin's disease, and a second course of treatment with combination chemotherapy and radiotherapy was cautiously initiated at Stanford, with an excellent response. She remains relapse-free more than six years after retreatment.

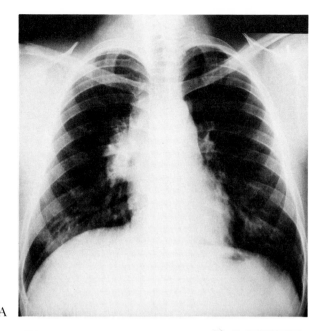

A

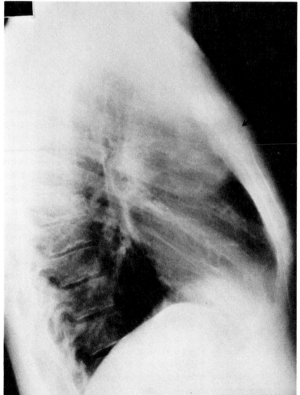

B

Figure 5.42   Invasion of the sternum and of the pre-sternal soft tissues by Hodgkin's disease in a 21-year-old male patient. The posteroanterior view (*A*) reveals the "truncated wigwam" appearance described by Strickland (1967). The presence of a soft-tissue mass anterior to the sternum and of pleural reaction immediately behind it are evident in the lateral view (*B*), as well as in the detail film (*C*), which reveals destruction of a sternal segment.

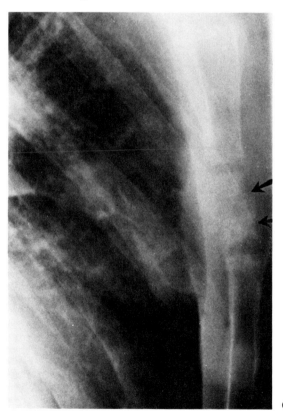

C

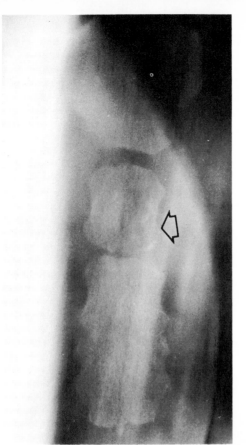 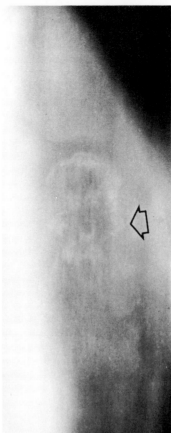

Figure 5.43 This 25-year-old female patient was first seen with a large presternal and parasternal soft-tissue mass, as well as supraclavicular and mediastinal adenopathy due to nodular sclerosing Hodgkin's disease. The tomograms clearly reveal the destructive process involving the sternum.

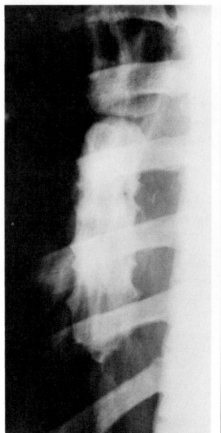 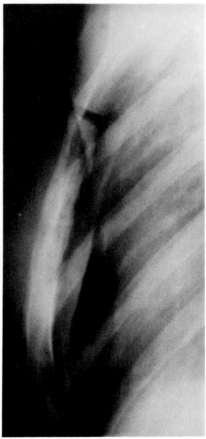

Figure 5.44 Osteoblastic infiltration of the body of the sternum, with infiltration of the presternal soft tissues seen in the lateral view.

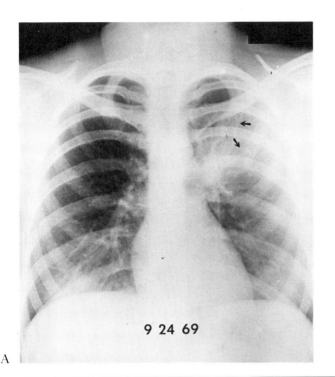

Figure 5.45 Extensive soft-tissue and bony invasion of the anterior thoracic wall by an infraclavicular lymph node mass in a 28-year-old female patient with nodular sclerosing Hodgkin's disease. In the posteroanterior view (*A*) the soft-tissue mass produces a diffuse increase in density over the left upper lung field; in the apical lordotic view, however, it is apparent that most of the mass involves the anterior chest wall, protruding inward along the subpleural space to encroach on the lung. Tomograms at several levels (*C, D, E*) reveal destruction of the first and second ribs anteriorly, as well as direct invasion of the left upper lobe of the lung extending down toward the left hilar lymph nodes. This patient was treated with radiotherapy, using a modified mantle technique (Chapter 9) which included tangential oblique beams directed toward the anterior chest wall mass. The chest wall mass and all other signs of disease gradually regressed completely within a few weeks after the completion of radiotherapy. The patient also received adjunctive combination chemotherapy and remains relapse-free more than ten years later.

A

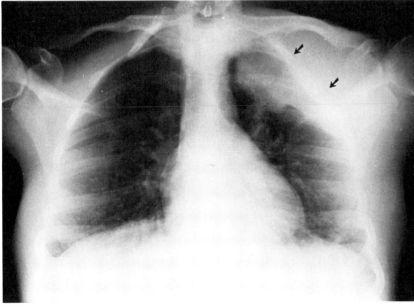

B

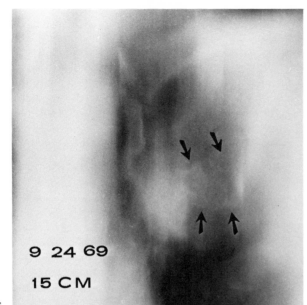

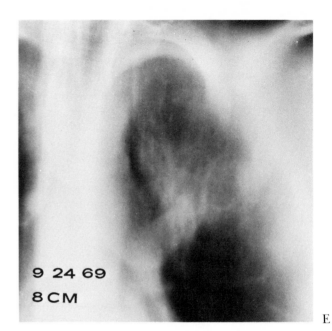

C

E

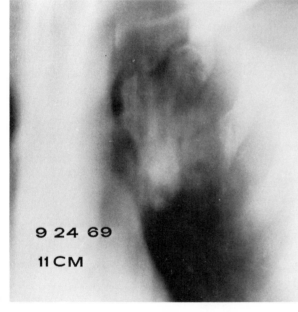

D

Abdomen

Retroperitoneal and Pelvic Lymph Nodes. It has long been known that the retroperitoneal and pelvic lymph nodes are not palpable unless they are rather massively enlarged. For many years the only roentgenologic methods available were intravenous urography and inferior vena cavography, both dependent on displacement of normal structures (ureters or vena cava, respectively) by large masses of nodes, and thus, relatively insensitive.

A new era dawned in 1952, when the British surgeon Kinmonth first described the technique of lower extremity lymphangiography. It entailed cannulation of the lymphatics on the dorsal surface of each foot, followed by the injection of radio-opaque contrast material. Kinmonth was investigating lymphedema and therefore utilized water-soluble contrast media, which did not remain in the lymph nodes of the groin, pelvis, or abdomen long enough to yield satisfactory images. The missing element was supplied when Bruun and Engeset (1956) independently developed the technique of lymphadenography, involving the direct intranodal injection of iodized oils. These media were observed to move from the injected node via efferent lymphatics to other regional lymph nodes, which were well opacified for sustained periods of time. Modern lymphangiography is the hybrid product of these two techniques, coupling dorsal pedal lymphatic cannulation with the introduction of oily contrast media of low viscosity. It was not long before it began to be used for the detection of retroperitoneal node involvement by the malignant lymphomas (Hreshchyshyn et al., 1961).

The procedure, which has been described in detail by a number of authors (Wallace et al., 1961; Fuchs, Davidson, and Fischer, 1969) entails insertion of fine-gauge needles or cannulas into the lymphatics of the dorsum of each foot through small incisions, after the lymphatics have been visualized by the subcutaneous injection of an appropriate particulate dye. The low viscosity contrast medium (Ethiodol) is then slowly injected under gravity or carefully regulated pump pressure, while filling of the lymphatics of the lower extremities and the pelvis is monitored fluoroscopically. Radiographs of the abdomen and pelvis are taken initially at the time of injection, primarily to record the size and course of the pelvic and para-aortic lymphatic vessels (Fig. 5.46) and the thoracic duct (Fig. 5.47). Additional radiographs are performed twenty-four hours after injection, at which time the lymphatic trunks have largely cleared and details of the opacified texture of the femoral, inguinal, iliac, and lumbar para-aortic lymph nodes have become apparent (Figs. 5.48, 5.49, and 5.50).

Although embolization of iodized oil to the lung occurs in all cases and is apparent on the twenty-four hour chest film as a diffuse, granular increase in pulmonary parenchymal density, it is ordinarily such a slow and gradual process as to elicit few or no respiratory symptoms. Nonetheless, the potential hazard may be serious in patients with extensive bilateral chronic inflammatory or fibrotic disease of the lungs, in whom lymphangiography is generally contraindicated. The procedure is also usually contraindicated in patients with a specific history of severe prior reaction to organic iodine-containing compounds and should be carried out with special caution, if at all, with emergency supplies of epinephrine and intravenous antihistaminics immediately at hand, in patients with asthma or other major allergic manifestations (Fischer, 1969).

The contrast medium is slowly carried away by macrophages over a period which varies from several months to as long as two or more years, thus making possible serial reexamination of the retroperitoneal and pelvic lymph nodes at intervals after the original lymphangiography. Fabian, Nudelman, and Abrams (1966) studied the persistence of diagnostically adequate opacity in serial postlymphangiogram films. They found that opacity sufficient for diagnostic purposes persisted for as long as one year in about 50 percent and for two years in about 12 percent of the cases.

Normally the opacified pelvic and retroperitoneal lymph nodes vary considerably in size (Fig. 5.48) but rarely exceed 2.6 cm. in greatest diameter. The para-aortic nodes usually lie within 2.0 cm. of the vertebral column in oblique and lateral views (Fig. 5.49). The opacified normal nodes exhibit a finely granular but essentially homogeneous texture (Fig. 5.50), although irregular filling defects of variable size are not infrequently observed in the inguinal and lower iliac nodes, and sometimes also in the lumbar para-aortic nodes, due to deposits of fat in the hila of these nodes (Figs. 5.50C, 5.51). Whereas metastases from epithelial tumors typically produce irregular filling defects, often of quite large size, infiltration of lymph nodes by the malignant lymphomas is usually more diffuse. In its earliest stages, such infiltration causes minimal separation of the focal, punctate deposits of opaque medium, resulting in a slight coarsening of the granular texture of the lymph node. As this process progresses and the opaque deposits are further separated, a highly characteristic "foamy" or reticulated pattern appears in the involved lymph nodes (Fig. 5.52), usually but not invariably associated with their enlargement (Figs. 5.53, 5.55). With further growth of the neoplastic deposits, the opaque medium may be crowded out of portions of a lymph node entirely, yielding more or less discrete filling defects, around which a thin rim of opaque material (the "rim sign") may persist at the margin of the lymph node (Figs. 5.54, 5.56, 5.57). Incomplete filling is the rule in extremely large, conglomerate lymph node masses (Fig. 5.57), often associated with displacement, tortuosity, and delayed emptying of the lymphatic trunks, filling of collateral channels, and other signs of lymphatic obstruction (Fig. 5.58). Some of the supraclavicular lymph nodes near the site of emptying of the thoracic duct into the left subclavian vein may also become

opacified. In such instances, we have occasionally observed foamy patterns indicative of involvement by lymphoma in the left supraclavicular lymph nodes which, even on reexamination, were not clinically palpable (Figs. 5.59, 5.60). Occasionally, cervical, supraclavicular, and even mediastinal nodes may opacify, presumably due to displacement, compression, and partial occlusion of the thoracic duct (Figs. 5.61, 5.62).

Some roentgenologists have claimed that it is possible to distinguish Hodgkin's disease from the other malignant lymphomas and even to differentiate nodular sclerosis from the other Rye histopathologic types on the basis of the lymphangiogram, applying such criteria as the relative uniformity of node enlargement in the pelvic versus the para-aortic nodes, the relative coarseness of the foamy pattern, and the number and size of filling defects (Davidson, 1969; Wiljasalo, 1969;

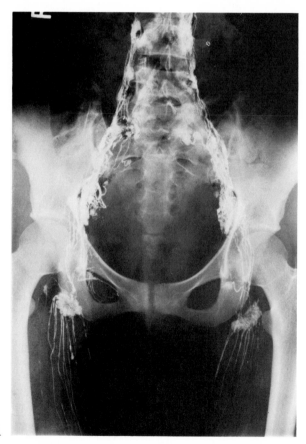

A

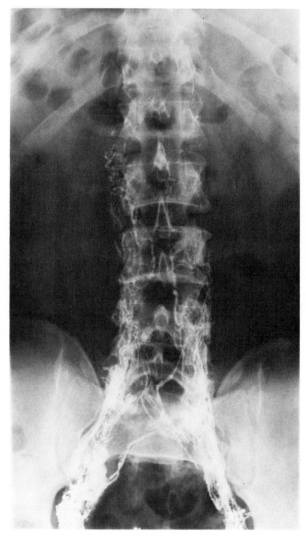

B

Figure 5.46 Normal lower-extremity lymphangiogram films during the filling phase immediately after intralymphatic injection of the oily contrast medium, revealing lymphatic vessels in the pelvic (*A*) and intra-abdominal para-aortic areas (*B*). Note the normal course of the vessels in the oblique and lateral views (*C, D, E*).

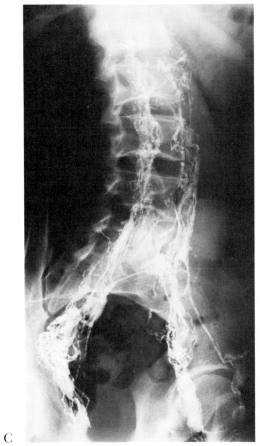

C

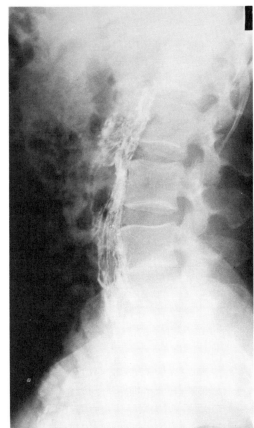

D

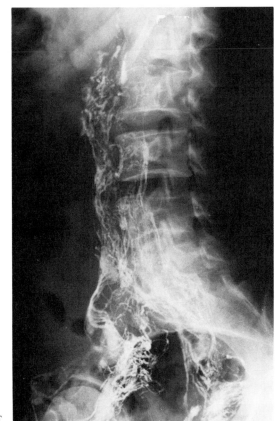

E

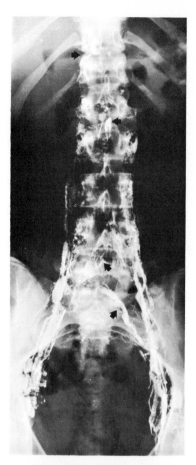

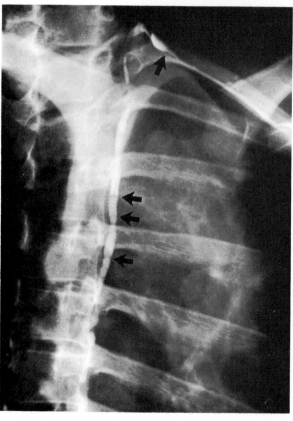

Figure 5.47 Normal lower-extremity lymphangiogram during filling. *Top*, anteroposterior abdominal film revealing the presence of normal lymphatic vessels proceeding obliquely from the right to left and from left to right in the lower lumbar para-aortic region, thus providing communication between the para-aortic lymph node chains on one side and the iliac nodes on the opposite side; *bottom*, thoracic duct visualized during the initial postinjection phase, clearly revealing the presence of several delicate valves.

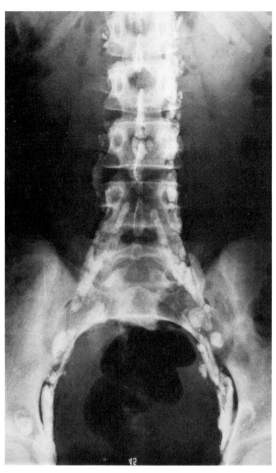

A

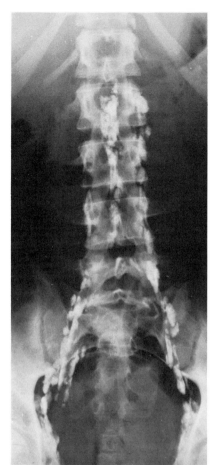

C

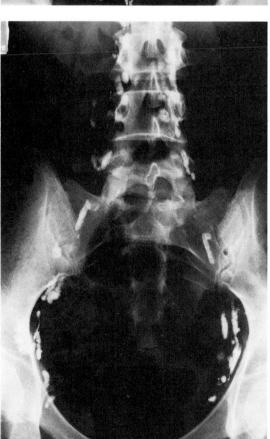

B

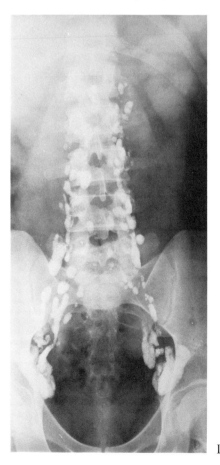

D

Figure 5.48 Normal 24-hour lymphangiogram films of four different patients to indicate the normal variation in size and distribution patterns of the pelvic and para-aortic lymph nodes. In one instance (C), some of the lymphatic vessels in the femoral region were still opacified; although retention of the contrast medium in the vessels at 24 hours is often regarded as a sign of obstruction, the small size of the lymph nodes in this case provides no support for this interpretation and suggests that this is a normal variation.

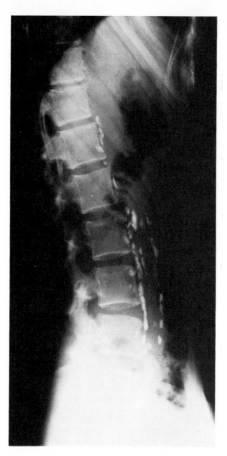

Figure 5.49   Normal 24-hour lymphangiogram in the lateral projection, revealing the linear distribution of para-aortic lymph nodes immediately adjacent to the anterior surfaces of the lumbar vertebral bodies.

Figure 5.50   Normal 24-hour lymphangiogram films in the anteroposterior (*A*), left postero-oblique (*B*), and right postero-oblique (*C*) projections. Note the stellate filling defect (arrow) in one of the lumbar para-aortic nodes, as seen in the right postero-oblique view; the very smooth outline of the filling defect is consistent with the presence of a fat deposit in the hilum of this node, a finding much more frequently encountered in the iliac, inguinal, and femoral nodes.

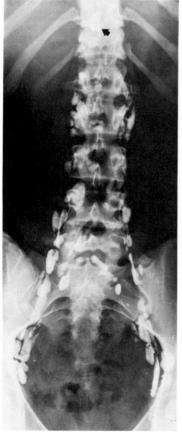

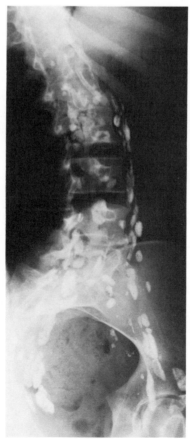

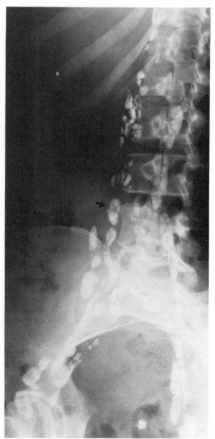

A   B   C

Schellinger et al., 1974; Gordon, Stoker, and Macdonald, 1976). Whether or not this is so, such a roentgenologic diagnosis would not in any case be acceptable in lieu of a biopsy. The essential task of the lymphangiographer is to visualize the pelvic and abdominal nodes as completely as possible, to detect abnormal nodes if they are present, and to differentiate whenever possible between lymphomatous involvement and other types of disease affecting the nodes.

Several studies have demonstrated conclusively that the diagnostic sensitivity of lymphangiography far exceeds that of inferior vena cavography, intravenous urography, or clinical palpation for the detection of lymphomatous involvement of the retroperitoneal or pelvic lymph nodes (Baum et al., 1963). In a study of our case material, Takahashi and Abrams (1967) found that lymphangiography had an overall diagnostic accuracy of 81 percent in a series of 206 proved cases of malignant lymphoma, and Wiljasalo (1969) reported an overall diagnostic accuracy of 74 percent. Most of the diagnostic error consisted of "false positive" interpretations. In approximately 10 to 15 percent of our cases to date, the roentgenographic features of the opacified lymph nodes have been diagnostically equivocal. Where the lymphangiogram was equivocal because of incomplete filling of the para-aortic lymph nodes on the right side, we formerly selectively performed inferior vena cavography, occasionally with positive results (Fig. 5.63). Today, however, computed tomographic (CT) scans have become the preferred diagnostic procedure in this circumstance.

We have not hesitated to recommend laparotomy and surgical biopsy of lymphangiographically suspicious lymph nodes. Data on our patients routinely subjected to laparotomy and para-aortic node biopsy confirm the infrequency of false negative interpretations (Glatstein et al., 1970; Rosenberg and Kaplan, 1970; Kaplan et al., 1973). Careful correlation of the histologic findings with the lymphangiographic interpretation in a series of 197 consecutive patients with Hodgkin's disease and 114 other patients with non-Hodgkin's lymphomas was performed by Castellino, Billingham, and Dorfman (1974). Their data on Hodgkin's disease are presented in Table 5.1. It may be seen that there were no false negatives. Thus, a negative in-

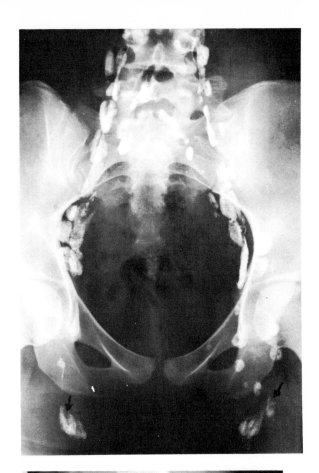

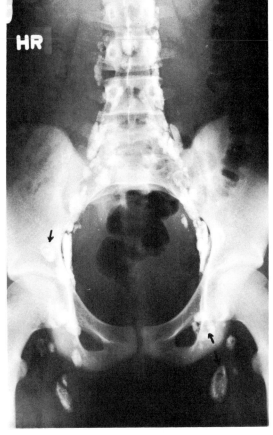

Figure 5.51 Filling defects due to fat deposits in femoral, inguinal, and iliac nodes in two otherwise normal lymphangiographic examinations.

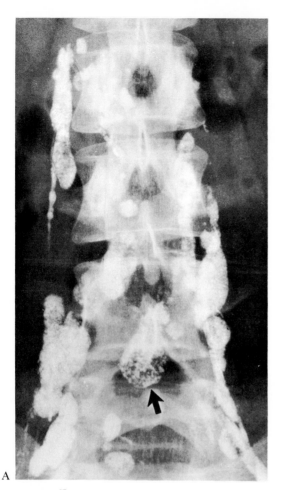

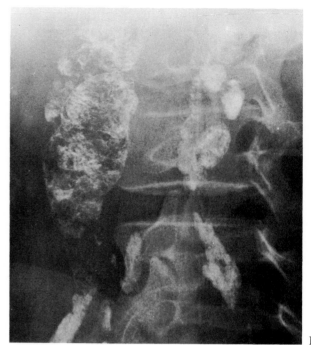

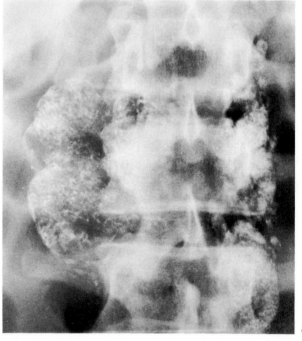

Figure 5.52 Changes due to lymphomatous infiltration of the para-aortic lymph nodes. *A*, coarse reticulated pattern in a single low lumbar para-aortic node,
with suspicious but less definite changes in other
nearby nodes, were the sole evidence of stage III involvement in this 17-year-old female with Hodgkin's
disease otherwise confined to the mediastinum and cervical-supraclavicular regions; *B*, right postero-oblique
magnification film in 12-year-old patient with stage IV
Hodgkin's disease reveals a striking contrast between
the small, essentially homogeneously opacified, normal
nodes and the huge involved nodes containing a typically "foamy" reticulated pattern, interrupted in some
places by filling defects; *C*, variation in degree of
coarseness of "foamy" pattern in different involved
nodes, some of which also contain larger filling defects.

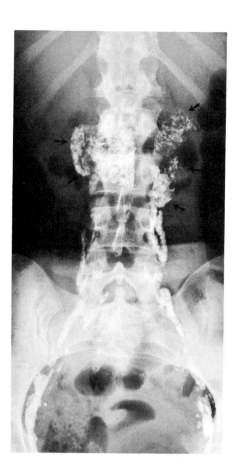

Figure 5.53 Positive lymphangiogram in a 25-year-old patient with nodular sclerosing Hodgkin's disease. Note again the striking contrast between the enlarged foamy upper lumbar para-aortic nodes and the normal lower lumbar and pelvic nodes.

Figure 5.54 Abnormality of several upper lumbar para-aortic nodes is clearly evident in the oblique projections in this case and much less apparent on the anteroposterior projection.

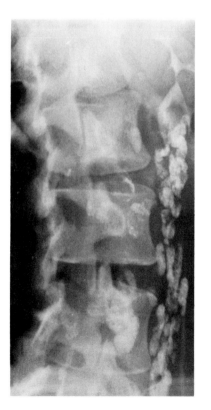
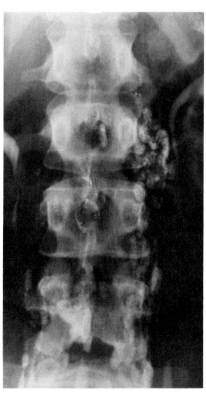
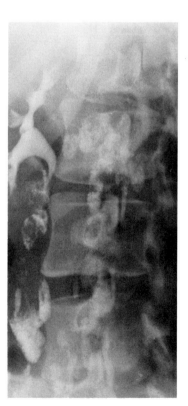

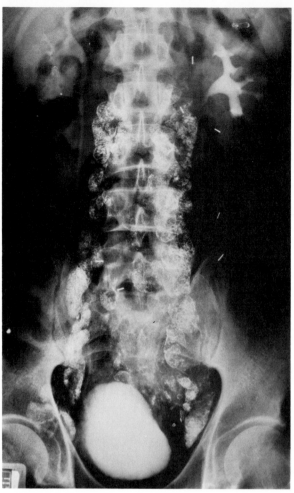

Figure 5.55 Lymphangiogram and intravenous urogram in a patient with Hodgkin's disease. Enlargement and distortion of the internal architecture are evident in virtually all of the pelvic, para-aortic, and paracaval lymph nodes in this patient. Note that the huge left iliac lymph nodes have displaced and distorted the superior aspect of the urinary bladder. Nonetheless, despite the extensive lymphadenopathy, relatively little displacement of the ureters and no obstruction of the upper urinary tract were seen.

Figure 5.56 Anteroposterior (*left*) and left postero-oblique (*right*) lymphangiographic films in a 62-year-old female patient with stage IV lymphocytic depletion Hodgkin's disease involving the bone marrow. Note the relatively small size of the lymph nodes and the presence of multiple filling defects, many of these producing "rim signs." Extraperitoneal biopsy of an iliac node confirmed the diagnosis of Hodgkin's disease originally established by bone marrow biopsy in this unusual case. This lymphangiographic appearance is not unusual in older patients with Hodgkin's disease.

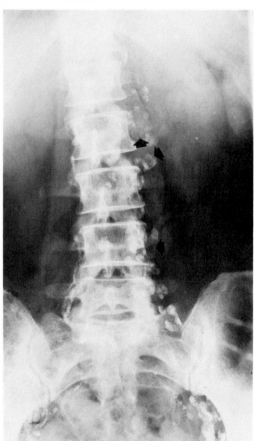

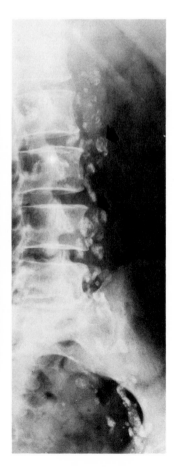

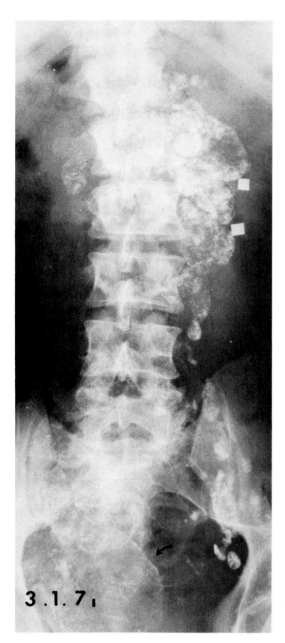

Figure 5.57 Massive lymphadenopathy is present in the right iliac and left upper para-aortic lymph node chains, and involvement of multiple other smaller nodes is also present. The incompleteness of filling and the distinctive "rim sign" along the medial border of the right iliac mass (arrow) are noteworthy.

terpretation of a lymphangiogram was associated with 100 percent accuracy. However, this was achieved at the expense of a 25 percent false positive rate, yielding an overall accuracy of 92 percent for the entire series of 197 consecutive patients. In a later analysis of 390 consecutive patients (R. A. Castellino, personal communication), overall accuracy remained 92 percent, with a false negative

rate of 2 percent and a false positive rate of 21 percent.

The remarkably high accuracy of the lymphangiographic method in Hodgkin's disease is evident from these data and from similar data on smaller series of patients studied by Glees et al. (1974), Martire (1974), and Kademian and Wirtanen (1977). Nonetheless, it is important to be aware of several sources of interpretative error. In 16 of 18 instances of false positive diagnosis documented by Castellino et al. (1974), the lymph nodes which appeared abnormal on the lymphangiogram were found to contain nonspecific "reactive changes," including fibrosis, sinus histiocytosis, reactive follicular hyperplasia, amorphous hyaline deposition, and vascular transformation which distorted the internal nodal architecture (Fig. 5.64). Parker, Blank, and Castellino (1974) have also called attention to the fact that a number of benign conditions may simulate the lymphangiographic appearance of lymphoma. Sayoc and Howland (1974) have illustrated the lymphangiographic findings in mesantoin-induced pseudolymphoma; although the initial findings were indistinguishable from those observed in true lymphomas, followup studies revealed a gradual restoration of lymph node size and architecture to normal after discontinuation of anticonvulsant medication.

Extensive experience with lymphangiography has made it clear that the abdominal or pelvic lymph nodes are in fact involved in approximately 30 percent of cases which would, by other clinical criteria, have been deemed to be in clinical stage I and in 40 to 60 percent of those that would have been categorized as clinical stage II (Baum, Bron, Wexler, and Abrams, 1963; Lee, Nelson, and Schwarz, 1964; Bourdon et al., 1966; Davidson and Clarke, 1968; Davidson, 1969; Wiljasalo, 1969; Kaplan et al., 1973). Thus, the routine use of lymphangiography has made it possible to increase the accuracy of clinical staging of the lymphomas to a very significant degree. For this reason, different series of cases clinically staged with and without the aid of lymphangiography cannot properly be intercompared.

The usefulness of the lymphangiogram does not end when the initial twenty-four hour films have been reviewed. The radiotherapist can delineate treatment fields encompassing the lymphangiographically opacified lymph nodes of the pelvis and para-aortic region with some confidence that all of the significant lymph nodes are indeed within the field. This makes it possible to reduce field sizes to a minimum and thus to spare bone marrow, as

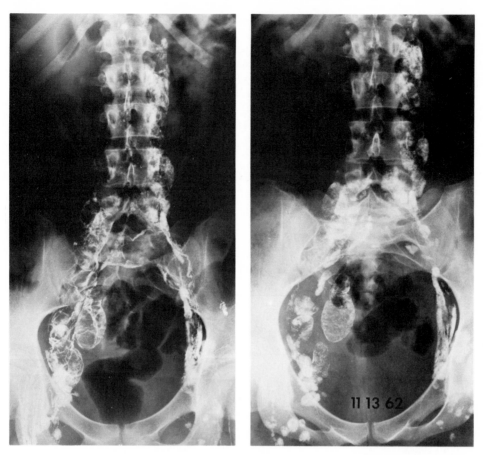

Figure 5.58 The initial lymphangiographic film during injection of the contrast material (*left*) shows displacement, tortuosity, and deviation of the lymphatic vessels in the right pelvis and right lower lumbar region; on the 24-hour film (*right*), grossly enlarged foamy lymph nodes are seen in these areas, and there is no filling of lymph nodes high on the right above the point of obstruction, at which the contrast material was shunted to the left side.

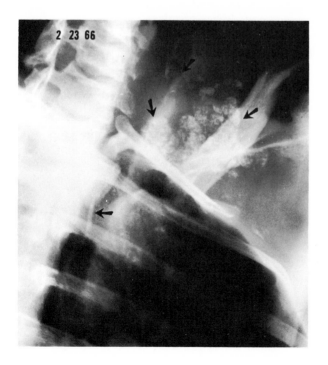

Figure 5.59 Lymphangiographic demonstration of abnormal left supraclavicular lymph nodes. This 18-year-old male patient was first seen with a large mass in the right groin. Lymphangiography revealed enormous lymph node masses in the right iliac region and abnormal nodes of smaller size in the lumbar para-aortic chains. The thoracic duct emptied into a number of clearly enlarged, foamy, reticulated lymph nodes in the left supraclavicular area, which were not palpable either before or after lymphangiographic examination.

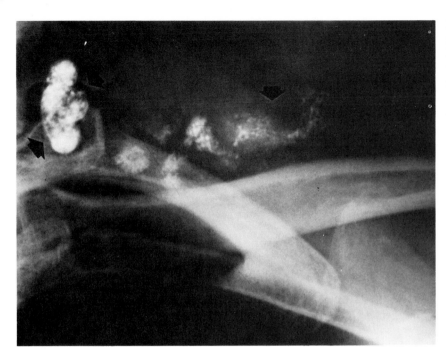

Figure 5.60 Filling defects in multiple left supraclavicular lymph nodes demonstrated on the 24-hour lymphangiogram film. These obviously involved nodes were not palpable even after the lymphangiogram had revealed their presence.

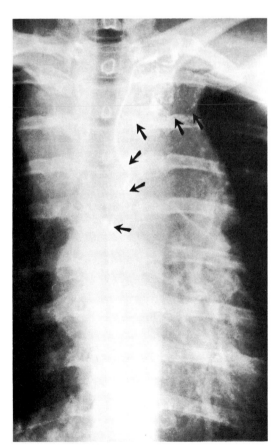

Figure 5.61 Tortuosity and displacement of the thoracic duct by mediastinal lymphadenopathy, with opacification of several large, foamy superior mediastinal nodes.

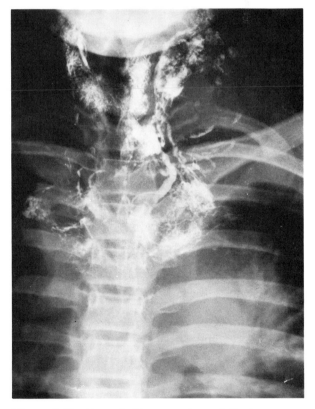

Figure 5.62 Remarkable tortuosity and displacement of the thoracic duct, with filling of collateral lymphatic vessels and retrograde filling extending into the neck on both sides, associated with the presence of massive mediastinal and left cervical-supraclavicular lymphadenopathy.

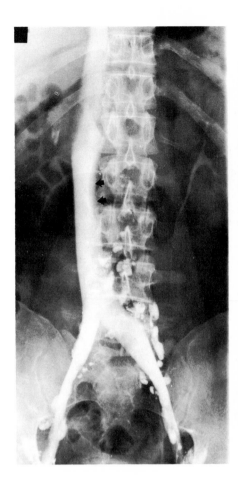 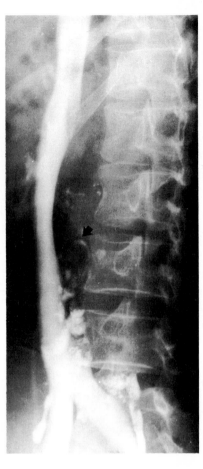

Figure 5.63 Positive inferior vena cavagram, with a long crescentic indentation of the posterolateral caval silhouette, in a region in which incomplete filling of the upper lumbar paracaval lymph nodes on the right side had resulted in incomplete visualization by lymphangiography. *Left,* anteroposterior view; *right,* right postero-oblique view.

well as to protect the kidneys and other vital structures in the abdomen. Moreover, as has been pointed out by MacDonald, Laugier, and Schlienger (1968), the response of lymph nodes to radiation therapy or to chemotherapy can be followed serially during and after treatment, thanks to the persistence of the opaque medium in the nodes (cf. Chapters 9 and 10).

Finally, in a significant proportion of cases in which no lymphangiographic evidence of abnormality is detected initially, serial followup films (aptly termed "surveillance" films by Davidson,

Table 5.1 Lymphangiographic-Histologic Correlation in Hodgkin's Disease

Histologic Diagnosis	Lymphangiographic Diagnosis			Total
	Normal	Benign Changes	Lymphoma	
Normal	97	0	2	99
Benign Changes	0	14	12	26
Lymphoma	0	0	41	41
Total	97	14	55	166

Source: Stanford University Medical Center data, reprinted by permission from the paper by Castellino, Billingham, and Dorfman (1974). The total number of cases analyzed was 197; of these, 18 had no opacified nodes removed at laparotomy, and 13 had nodes excised which were not those of diagnostic interest, leaving a net total of 166 for analysis. There were no false negatives, and 14 false positives, for an overall accuracy of 92 percent.

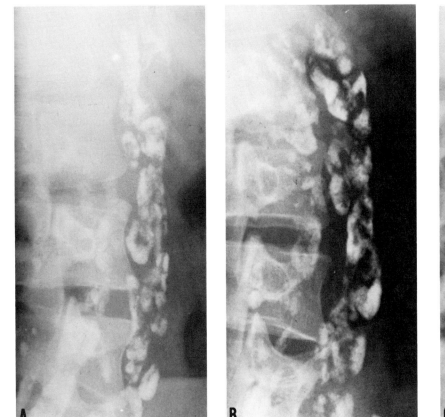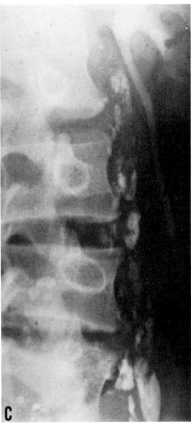

Figure 5.64 Left posterior oblique projections of the para-aortic lymph nodes in three different young adult males with nodular sclerosing Hodgkin's disease. The visualized lymph nodes in each case are quite similar in appearance, demonstrating distinct filling defects in somewhat globular but normal-sized lymph nodes. Since such lymphangiographic changes are not uncommonly seen when a lymph node is involved with Hodgkin's disease, these were interpreted as representing involvement by lymphoma. The nodes in *A* did indeed contain tumor; those in *B*, sinus hyperplasia; those in *C*, vascular transformation and fibrosis, each causing obliteration of portions of the sinusoidal system. (Reprinted by permission of the authors and *Investigative Radiology,* from the paper by Castellino, Billingham, and Dorfman, 1974.)

1969) may reveal a gradual and progressive change in size, contour, and texture of one or more lymph nodes (Figs. 5.65, 5.66, 5.67, and 5.68; Fabian, Nudelman, and Abrams, 1966; Mac-Donald, Laugier, and Schlienger, 1968). Although some of these instances are no doubt ascribable to progressive growth of an initially microscopic lymphomatous deposit, retrospective analysis occasionally reveals that small filling defects or other abnormalities were present in the affected nodes on the original films. Estimates of the "doubling time" of such enlarging nodes as measured on serial films have been utilized as a rough index of their growth rate (MacDonald et al., 1968).

Thus, a single lymphangiographic examination contributes in multiple ways over a considerable period of time to the clinical management of patients with malignant lymphomas (Cook et al.,

1966). Moreover, it is entirely feasible to perform a second lymphangiogram on a patient in whom the opaque material from the previous examination has disappeared and in whom new symptoms or signs indicative of a possible spread of the lymphomatous process to the abdominal or pelvic lymph nodes have developed; in many cases, the second (or third) lymphangiogram has revealed striking evidence of interim spread of disease (Figs. 5.69, 5.70, 5.71). The technical difficulty and hazards of such a second lymphangiogram do not appear to differ in any way from those of the first, and diagnostic accuracy is apparently similar (Perez-Tamayo, Thornbury, and Atkinson, 1963). In an analysis of 99 patients with Hodgkin's disease who had repeat lymphangiography, Castellino, Fuks, Blank, and Kaplan (1973) found that 28 (30 percent) had an abnormal second lymphangiogram al-

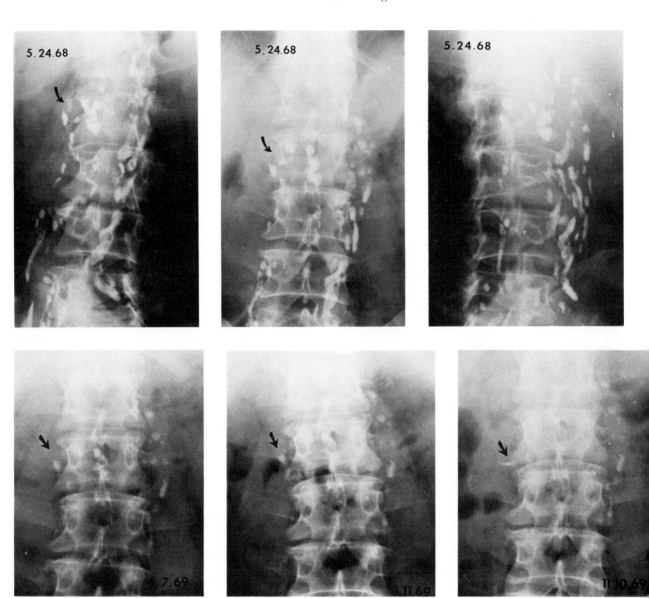

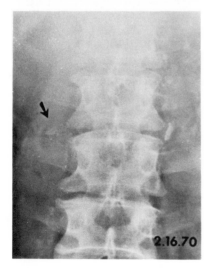

Figure 5.65 Evolution of para-aortic lymphadenopathy on serial surveillance films. Note the small, incompletely filled right upper lumbar para-aortic node (arrow) on the initial lymphangiogram film of 5/24/68. Although this examination was initially interpreted as normal, it is clear in retrospect that this lymph node contained significant filling defects, although it was not enlarged. Note that on the next film, of 4/7/69, this node has disappeared, although the small lymph node immediately beneath it is still unchanged; by 8/11/69 the adjacent node has begun to tilt laterally and is slightly displaced downward relative to its former position and is finally compressed into a flat, horizontal line on the film of 11/10/69. Unfortunately, none of these serial changes were noted at the time, and it was not until this node had virtually completely disappeared, on the examination of 2/16/70, that the sequence of serial progressive changes was recognized. Exploratory laparotomy and biopsy confirmed the presence of Hodgkin's disease in these lymph nodes.

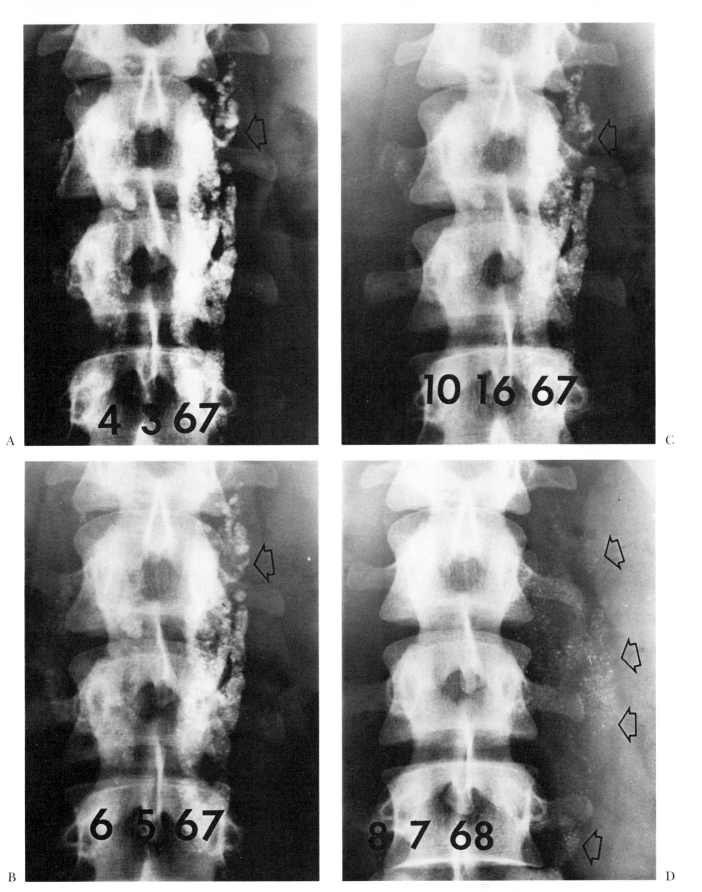

Figure 5.66 Development of para-aortic lymphadenopathy on serial surveillance films. The initial lymphangiographic examination (*A*) of 4/3/67 was interpreted as within normal limits, and the minimal changes in the upper lumbar para-aortic nodes seen in retrospect on the films of 6/5/67 (*B*) and 10/16/67 (*C*) were not regarded at that time as significant. The patient became pregnant near the end of 1967, and surveillance films of the abdomen were therefore discontinued for several months; the next surveillance film, made on 8/7/68 (*D*), a few weeks after delivery, revealed marked progression of the lymphadenopathy.

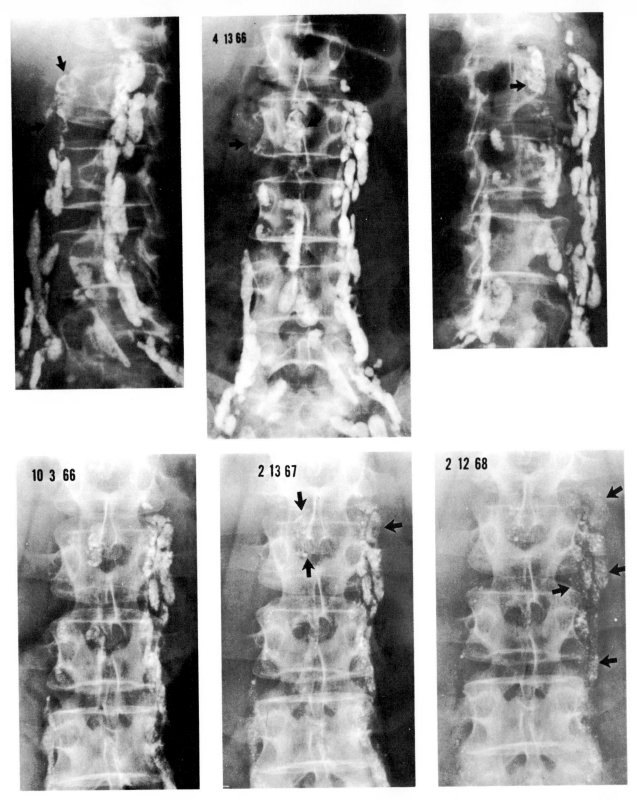

Figure 5.67 Progressive involvement of upper lumbar para-aortic lymph nodes on serial surveillance films. The initial lymphangiographic examination of 4/13/66 (*top*) was not regarded as abnormal, despite the presence of enlargement, rim signs, and filling defects in right upper lumbar para-aortic nodes (arrows), which in retrospect were clearly abnormal from the beginning. Serial surveillance films (*bottom*) reveal a disappearance of the abnormal nodes on the right on the film of 10/3/66, with slight enlargement of the node overlying the body of the second lumbar vertebra; this node is distinctly more enlarged on the film of 2/13/67 (arrows), and now a node high on the left has begun to exhibit a filling defect and minimal enlargement (arrow); finally, on the film of 2/12/68, enlargement and a stippled, foamy appearance are present in many additional nodes of the left para-aortic chain (arrows). Involvement of these nodes by Hodgkin's disease was confirmed by laparotomy and biopsy.

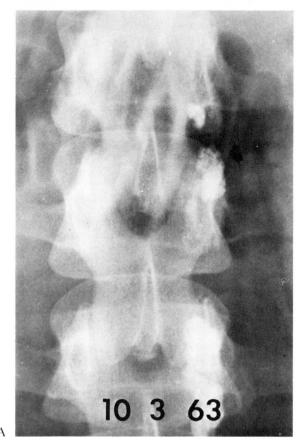

A

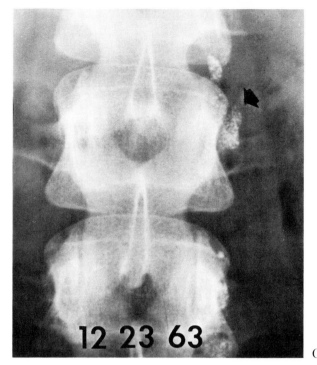

C

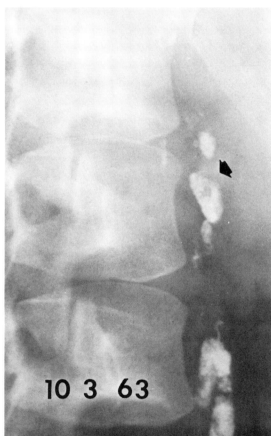

B

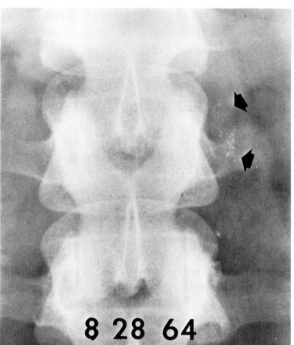

D

Figure 5.68 Progressive involvement of lumbar para-aortic nodes on serial surveillance films. The initial anteroposterior (*A*) and left postero-oblique (*B*) films of 10/3/63 were regarded as within normal limits, although in retrospect one small node is incompletely filled and distinctly suspicious. This node reveals a slight but distinct change, which was not appreciated at the time, on the surveillance film of 12/23/63 (*C*). The patient was then lost to followup for a time, and the next surveillance film of 8/28/64 (*D*) reveals distinct further progression of the localized lymphadenopathy.

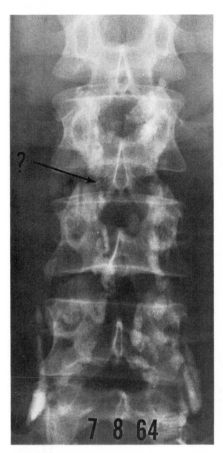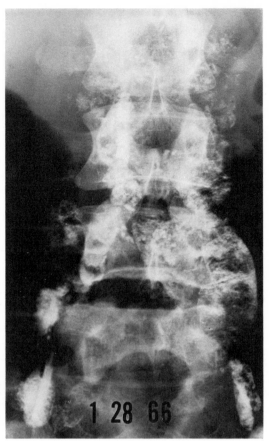

Figure 5.69 Para-aortic and iliac lymphadenopathy revealed by a second lymphangiogram. The initial lymphangiogram of 7/8/64 (*left*) was regarded as normal, although in retrospect a very slightly stippled pattern is apparent in the midlumbar node indicated by the arrow and question mark. The patient was given radiation to nodes above the diaphragm and returned with fever and anemia in January 1966, at which time a second lymphangiogram (*right*) revealed massive enlargement of the para-aortic and iliac lymph node chains, and a positive bone marrow biopsy.

though the initial study had been normal. In 22 of these, subsequent lymph node biopsy provided histologic confirmation of the interval development of involvement in the para-aortic and/or iliac chains. However, we have observed several false positive instances in which enlargement and a coarse, somewhat foamy pattern became evident in the para-aortic or iliac lymph nodes, either on a followup film or in a repeat lymphangiogram. Laparotomy and biopsy of such nodes revealed only engorgement of the sinusoids with iodized oil and a nonspecific reactive process in the node parenchyma (Fig. 5.72). The diagnostic clue which has now been recognized in such instances is that mul-

tiple lymph nodes in the para-aortic and/or iliac chains all exhibit a similar degree of enlargement and reticulation; in contrast, developing lymphomatous involvement is likely to affect the nodes in a chain selectively and unequally (Steiner et al., 1970; Castellino et al., 1974a).

A development of considerable potential interest was the discovery by Edwards and Hayes (1969) that gallium (^{67}Ga) citrate selectively localized in involved lymph nodes of a patient with Hodgkin's disease. The reliability of this new isotopic procedure in routine clinical use has now been subjected to critical evaluation. Increased activity in the para-aortic and mesenteric lymph node chains, inter-

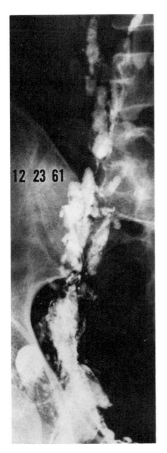
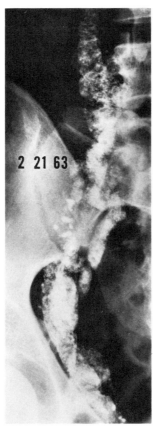

Figure 5.70 Lymphadenopathy detected on a second lymphangiogram. The initial examination of 12/23/61 (*left*) was regarded as within normal limits, and the patient was given radiation to nodes above the diaphragm. He returned in January 1963, with fever, anemia, and weight loss, and a second lymphangiogram (*right*) was performed on 2/21/63, revealing diffuse enlargement and foaminess in the para-aortic and right iliac lymph node chains, with an associated sclerotic bone lesion in the right ilium adjacent to the sacroiliac joint.

B   C

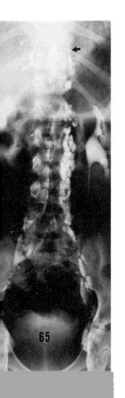
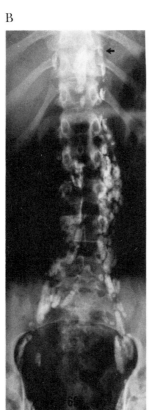
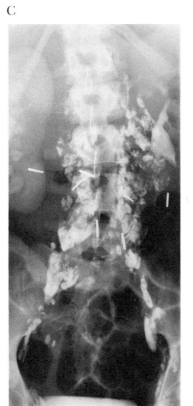

Figure 5.71 Spread of Hodgkin's disease to the lumbar para-aortic nodes detected by a third lymphangiogram. On admission in 1965, this 9-year-old boy had an apparently normal lymphangiogram (*A*). An incidental finding was the congenital abnormality of the right ureteropelvic junction with hydronephrosis of the right kidney. A repeat lymphangiogram was performed in 1969 and again was interpreted as within normal limits (*B*). However, the patient developed low-grade fever and anemia in 1973, and a third lymphangiogram revealed massive enlargement of multiple lymph nodes in the para-aortic and paracaval chains (*C*).

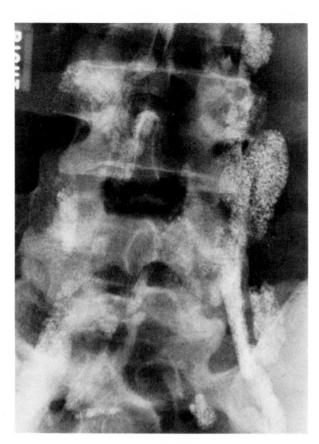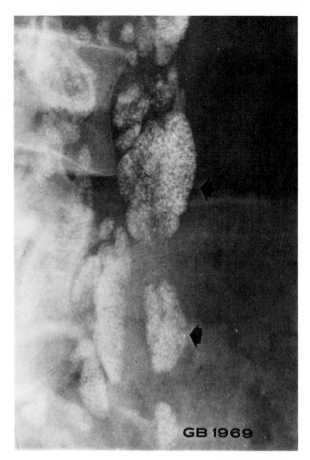

Figure 5.72 False positive second lymphangiogram associated with an intercurrent viral illness. This 20-year-old male had been treated with radiation to a mantle field for stage IA Hodgkin's disease and was apparently free of disease until nearly two years later, when he returned with fever, night sweats, and weakness of two weeks' duration. A repeat lymphangiogram revealed diffuse moderate enlargement of para-aortic and pelvic lymph nodes and a distinct increase in coarseness and reticulation of the node texture, as seen here in the anteroposterior (*left*) and left postero-oblique (*right*) views. Laparotomy was performed, and several lymph nodes were removed which revealed only reactive hyperplasia. The patient's febrile illness cleared spontaneously and is thought in retrospect to have been an intercurrent viral infection. We have seen several such instances of the development of slight enlargement and increased degree of reticulation in the para-aortic lymph nodes, either on surveillance films after an initial lymphangiogram or on a second lymphangiogram; the principal clue that these are false positive changes due to reactive hyperplasia rather than to Hodgkin's disease is provided by the uniformity and diffuseness of the change. In contrast, Hodgkin's disease would tend to involve lymph nodes in a more focal and initially limited way and would be unlikely to involve all of the lymph nodes of the para-aortic chain to an essentially equal degree (Steiner et al., 1970; Castellino et al., 1974a).

preted as indicative of involvement by Hodgkin's disease, has been confirmed at subsequent staging laparotomy in several such instances (Turner et al., 1972). Moreover, the overall accuracy of detection of sites of active disease observed by two different groups of investigators was 79 percent (Kay and McCready, 1972; Turner et al., 1972). However, the procedure was most reliable in lymph node areas above the diaphragm, in which physical examination and conventional chest radiography are readily able to provide definitive information. Horn, Ray, and Kriss (1976) found that ^{67}Ga scinti-

graphy yielded true positive information in 51 of 83 supradiaphragmatic sites of involvement (61 percent), and false negative interpretations in 32 of these instances (39 percent); conversely, true positive interpretations were rendered in only 23 (40 percent) of 58 infradiaphragmatic sites involved by Hodgkin's disease and other lymphomas; 35 other such sites (60 percent) yielded false negative interpretations. Thus, the test is least reliable where it is most needed, in lymph node sites below the diaphragm. Nonetheless, in selected instances, this procedure may provide extremely valuable data, particularly in patients who have been previously treated and who now present clinical manifestations suggestive of relapsing disease.

Essentially similar results have been reported with bleomycin labeled with [57]Co (Rasker et al., 1975) or [111]In (Lilien et al., 1975). Para-aortic lymphadenopathy has also been detected on scintigrams performed with ^{99m}Tc-pertechnetate-labeled sulfur colloid (Fairbanks et al., 1972) and with radionuclide-labeled immunoglobulin (Order et al., 1975). Uptake of ^{75}Se-selenomethionine or selenite in lymphomatous nodes has also been reported (Herrera et al., 1965; Spencer et al., 1967; Killander, Lindblom, and Lundell, 1977). Although occasionally useful in the assessment of intra-abdominal lymph node disease, these radioisotopic methods do not have the resolution or the diagnostic accuracy of conventional lymphangiography with iodized vegetable oil contrast media.

Two new noninvasive diagnostic techniques, ultrasonography and computed tomography, have begun to play a significant role in the assessment of intra-abdominal involvement by Hodgkin's disease and the other malignant lymphomas. Glees et al. (1977) were able to detect involvement of the spleen by grey-scale ultrasonography in 7 of 9 histologically verified cases; of 11 negative spleens, 3 were interpreted as positive on the ultrasonic scans, for an overall accuracy of 75 percent. In the presence of gross enlargement of both the left and right para-aortic or paracaval lymph node chains, the cross-sectional scans provided by ultrasonography reveal a dumbbell-shaped sonolucent area draped over the prevertebral vessels. When enlargement of these lymph node chains is unilateral, a mass may be seen adjacent to the aorta or inferior vena cava. Lymph node masses in the porta hepatis and mesenteric lymph nodes are also readily identifiable (Fig. 5.73), as are enlarged lymph nodes displacing the kidney (Asher and Freimanis, 1969; Damascelli et al., 1969; Filly, Marglin, and Castellino, 1976b; Brascho, Durant, and Green, 1977). However, whereas lymphangiography can detect abnormalities of architecture even in lymph nodes which are not significantly enlarged, ultrasonography depends on the detection of enlarged lymph nodes and has a lower limit of resolution, with presently available apparatus, that would not permit the detection of lymph nodes less than 1.5–2.0 cm in diameter. It is thus not surprising that Damascelli et al. (1969) found that the echographic examination failed to reveal para-aortic lymphadenopathy in 10 of 38 patients studied. Nonetheless, the method remains useful in selected pa-

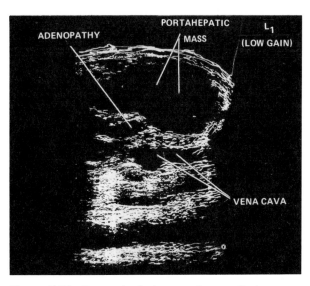

Figure 5.73   Parasagittal ultrasound scan of a large lymph node mass involving the porta hepatis chain, seen in longitudinal section of the upper abdomen. (Reprinted by permission of the authors and *Cancer*, from the paper by Filly, Marglin, and Castellino, 1976.)

tients, including those in whom lymphangiography is contraindicated.

The technique of computed tomography, originally developed for scanning of the brain and meninges, has now been extended to the remainder of the body, and rapid technological advances have greatly increased the resolution and decreased the time required for body scans. A series of 11 patients (10 with lymphomas, 1 with seminoma) suspected of having para-aortic lymph node involvement were studied with a six-second scanner by Marshall et al. (1977). Four patients had both a normal lymphangiogram and a normal CT scan, and one other patient with a normal CT scan had reactive hyperplasia at lymphangiography, confirmed at staging laparotomy. The remaining 6 patients had abnormal lymphangiograms. In 3 of these 6, the CT scan yielded significant additional information. Similar observations have been reported in other studies (Redman et al., 1977; Breiman et al., 1978; Lee et al., 1978; Pilepich et al., 1978). The resolution of the CT scans was clearly superior to that of ultrasonographs and was capable of displaying a single lymph node of normal size. Representative examples are illustrated in Figures 5.74 and 5.75. It appears likely that CT scans will become a useful addition to the diagnostic armamentarium, playing a complementary role to lymphangiography. Their greatest usefulness is in the delineation of lymphadenopathy in lymph nodes which fail to fill with lymphangiographic

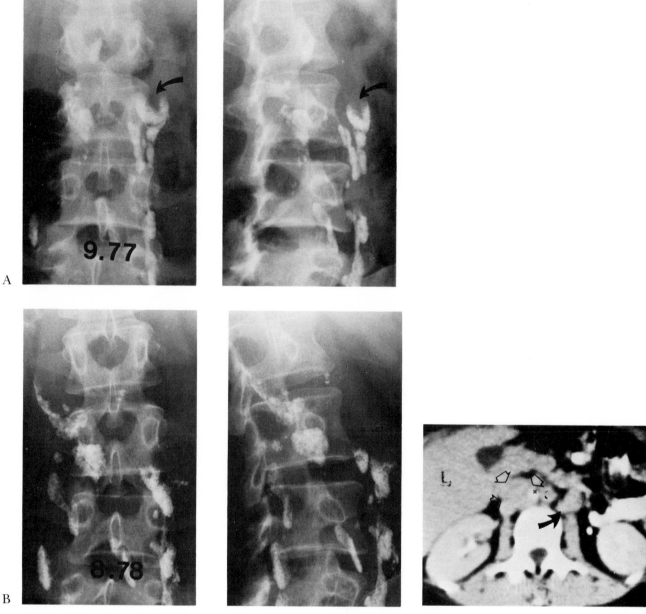

Figure 5.74   Demonstration by computed tomography of adenopathy in nonopacified retroperitoneal nodes, in addition to involvement detected by lymphangiography. This patient had an initial lymphangiogram (*A*) at another hospital in September 1977 which was interpreted as negative, but which, on review at Stanford in August 1978, revealed a filling defect (arrow) in an upper lumbar para-aortic node. A second lymphangiogram was performed (*B*), which disclosed enlargement, distortion, and displacement of several para-aortic and paracaval nodes. The CT scan (*C*) at the level of the kidneys reveals the aorta (a), liver (L), an opacified para-aortic node (x), and nonopacified masses involving the right paracaval nodes (open arrows) and the left para-aortic nodes (solid arrow). (Courtesy of Dr. Ronald A. Castellino, Division of Diagnostic Radiology, Stanford University Medical Center.)

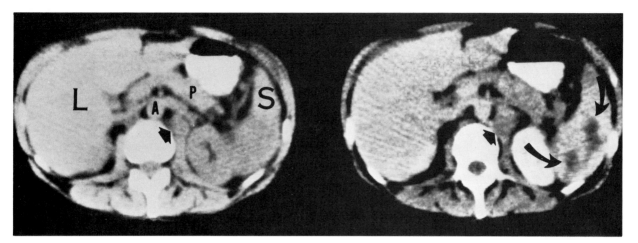

Figure 5.75 Computed tomographic scan of the upper abdomen before (left) and after (right) injection of contrast medium. The spleen (S) reveals ill-defined areas of decreased density posteriorly in the initial scan, which are revealed as zones of radiolucency (long arrows) after contrast enhancement. There is also thickening of the pancreas (P), and a left para-aortic mass (short arrow). At laparotomy, the presence of Hodgkin's disease in the pancreas and in large nodular foci in the spleen was confirmed. (Courtesy of Dr. Edward Drasin, Herrick Hospital, Berkeley, California.)

contrast material either because of lymphatic obstruction or because of their anatomic location in nonvisualized sites such as the celiac, porta hepatis, and mesenteric chains. It is also possible that CT scans will at least occasionally succeed in revealing tumor nodules in the spleen.

Spleen. Enlargement of the spleen is readily apparent on conventional radiograms of the abdomen, and in some instances, particularly those in which the spleen grows relatively more in thickness than in length, splenomegaly may be detected roentgenologically even when the spleen is not clinically palpable. However, in some instances the presence of gas in the overlying splenic flexure of the colon and in the adjacent gastric fundus may partially obscure the margins of the spleen, making its size difficult to assess. In such instances, the use of cleansing enemas and of effervescent powders or liquids to distend the stomach may reveal the splenic outline with greater clarity.

Recently it has been found that a number of radioisotope-tagged organic and colloidal preparations are deposited preferentially in the spleen and liver, thus making it possible to delineate splenic size and contours by conventional isotope "scanning" techniques. Spleen scans are relatively simple and innocuous procedures, which may be repeated serially to follow changes in size of the spleen as a function of time (Parmentier et al., 1968). In a study of liver-spleen scans in 108 patients with Hodgkin's disease, Milder et al. (1973) reported that splenomegaly detected by the radio-isotopic scan was associated with advancing stage and tumor involvement of the spleen and liver. All 13 spleens measuring over 15 cm on scan were positive for tumor. In addition to gross enlargement, lymphomas involving the spleen may produce focal filling defects in the spleen scan indicative of the presence of tumor nodules (Fig. 5.76). Chaudhuri et al. (1972) have reported an interesting example of this kind, in which several filling defects appeared in the spleen following accumulation of ^{87m}Sr sulfur colloid. Milder et al. also detected filling defects which correlated with the presence of tumor in the splenectomy specimen in seven patients. In combination with the physical examination and lymphangiogram, they found that the scan enabled accurate prediction of splenic involvement in 43 percent of their cases. A much less favorable experience with spleen scans was reported by Silverman et al. (1972), who found scintigraphic abnormalities in 8 of 11 patients with histologically normal spleens, and normal scintigrams in 7 of 20 patients with documented involvement of the spleen. Only 3 of the 6 spleens estimated by scintigraphy to be enlarged proved to contain Hodgkin's disease. Moreover, such scans do not approach the degree of resolution required to detect the small nodules which have been present in many of our splenectomy specimens. Colloidal thorium dioxide (Thorotrast) also yields consistently diagnostic opacification of the spleen on conventional radiographs, and the resolution of such splenic images is superior to that of spleen scans, but concern about the late hazards associated with

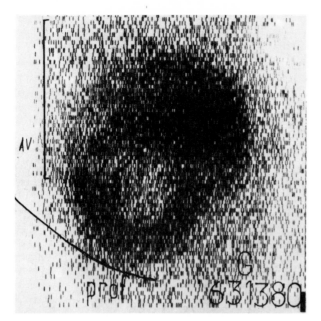

Figure 5.76 Large, irregular filling defect due to Hodgkin's disease involving the spleen, as seen in a spleen scan performed with [197]Hg-bromo-mercuri-hydroxy propane (courtesy of Dr. A. Laugier, Institut Gustave Roussy, Villejuif, France). Although such spleen scans are useful for detecting splenic enlargement and changes in spleen size with treatment and can readily detect very large filling defects such as this, they do not have the resolving power necessary to detect the small splenic lesions which have so frequently been observed in splenectomy specimens obtained during routine laparotomy (Glatstein et al., 1969, 1970).

the alpha ray emission of the thorium has limited the use of this material.

The use of selective splenic arteriography has been proposed by Markovits, Gasquet, and Parmentier (1968), who noted a bizarre "cerebriform" pattern of dilated vascular channels in the splenic pulp in a fifteen-year-old boy in whom the presence of intrasplenic Hodgkin's disease was confirmed by laparotomy and splenectomy. At Stanford, this procedure was performed in a series of 33 consecutive patients (Castellino et al., 1972). In addition to delineating the course of the splenic vessels, the procedure opacifies the splenic pulp for a brief interval, yielding a "splenogram" on one or more of the rapid serial films which are routinely obtained (Fig. 5.77). Against the homogeneous background density of the normal splenogram, it has in some instances been possible to discern discrete filling defects (Fig. 5.78). Distortion of the intrasplenic arterial arborization pattern has also been noted. However, the value of this technique appears to be limited. In none of the

patients studied by Castellino et al. (1972) was there neovascularity, encasement, truncation, or stretching of vessels in relation to sites of documented tumor, suggesting that the arterial phase is diagnostically insensitive. Conversely, the nonhomogeneity of the tissue phase occurred frequently in normal as well as in involved spleens. This finding was confirmed by Madsen and Davidsen (1973), who reported that only two of ten patients with filling defects in splenic angiograms actually had splenic involvement. Similar observations have been reported by Jonsson and Lunderquist (1974). On the basis of these exploratory studies, the use of splenic angiography in the diagnostic assessment of patients with Hodgkin's disease and other malignant lymphomas has been largely abandoned.

Computed tomographic scans readily reveal enlargement and abnormalities of contour of the spleen and may also disclose adenopathy in the adjacent splenic hilar nodes (Fig. 5.79), but the capacity of this new technique to detect intrasplenic filling defects due to nodules of tumor has been disappointing in our experience, despite occasional exceptions, such as the case illustrated in Figure 5.75.

Liver, Gallbladder, and Pancreas. The oblique curvilinear caudad surface of the liver is often distorted on roentgenographic projection, making the estimation of hepatic size from conventional abdominal roentgenograms rather unreliable. In some instances, layering of pleural fluid over the right hemidiaphragm may be mistaken for the upward displacement of the hemidiaphragm by a greatly enlarged liver; lateral decubitus films clarify such situations by revealing a shift of the fluid into the lateral pleural space. Occasionally, where metastatic deposits in the liver are relatively few in number and massive in size, they may locally alter the contour of the liver on conventional films and thus reveal their presence. Ordinarily, however, other techniques must be employed to opacify the liver and thus to reveal alterations in its internal structure indicative of metastatic tumor involvement. From the standpoint of resolution, colloidal thorium dioxide (Thorotrast) consistently yields hepatograms of the highest diagnostic quality, but its use has been seriously limited in recent years for the reasons given above. As a substitute for Thorotrast, emulsions of iodized oily media administered intravenously to experimental animals have yielded satisfactory hepatograms but are not without significant hazards. More recently, efforts

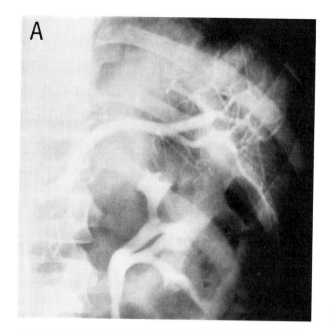

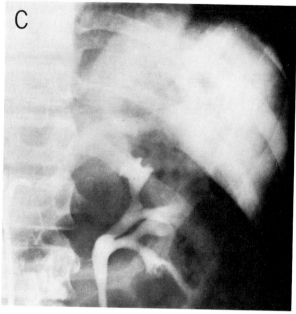

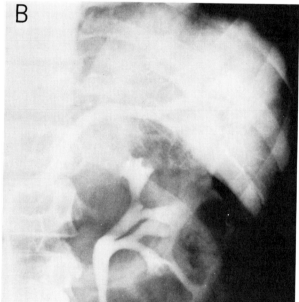

Figure 5.77 Normal splenic arteriogram and splenogram after selective percutaneous catheterization of the splenic artery (Castellino et al., 1972). *A*, splenic arteriogram; *B*, arterial phase, and *C*, venous phase of splenogram.

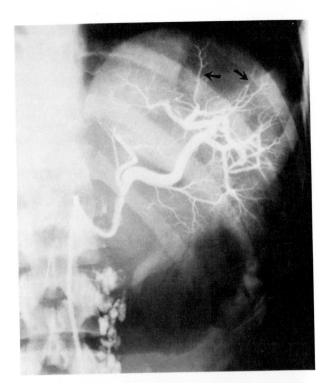

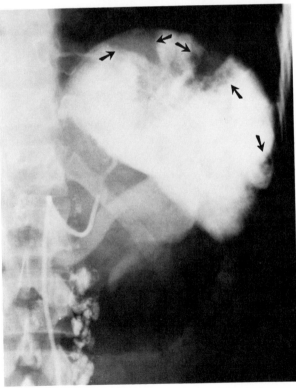

Figure 5.78 Splenic arteriogram (*top*) and splenogram (*bottom*) revealing splaying of the arborizing splenic vessels and several discrete filling defects (arrows) during the splenogram phase. Involvement of the spleen by Hodgkin's disease was confirmed at laparotomy, but it was not possible to demonstrate that the radiographically visualized filling defects conformed precisely to the nodules of tumor found in the spleen.

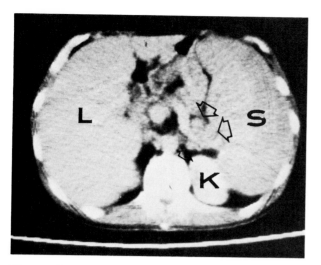

Figure 5.79 Computed tomographic scan of the upper abdomen in a patient in whom lymphangiography was medically contraindicated. The patient had been treated to a mantle field eight years earlier for CS IIA Hodgkin's disease, and returned with fever and aching lumbar pain. The spleen (S) is greatly enlarged but reveals no discrete filling defects, despite the fact that it was extensively replaced by small nodules of tumor at surgery. Note the enlarged splenic hilar and pancreatic nodes (arrows). L, liver; K, left kidney. (Courtesy of Dr. Ronald A. Castellino, Division of Diagnostic Radiology, Stanford University Medical Center.)

have been made to develop iodized organic contrast media capable of opacifying the liver after oral administration.

An alternative approach has been the development of radioisotopic scans of the liver, using materials like ^{131}I-labeled rose bengal, which enters the parenchymal cells of the liver, or particulate colloids, such as radiogold (^{198}Au), chromic radiophosphate (^{32}P), or technetium (^{99m}Tc), which are selectively deposited in the Kupffer cells of the liver sinusoids. Metastases of epithelial tumors to the liver often produce large, discrete filling defects in the pattern of such hepatic scans, thus enabling their detection. However, isotopic scans of the liver have proved of less diagnostic utility in the malignant lymphomas, where diffuse permeation of the substance of the liver by deposits of near-microscopic dimensions is the rule and large, nodular metastases are much less frequently encountered (Figs. 5.80, 5.81). Thus, in the series of patients studied by Milder et al. (1973), mottled uptake, filling defects, or both were observed in 11 of 20 biopsy-positive livers; however, these abnormalities were also present in 27 of 101 biopsy-negative livers. Hepatic size on scan correlated even less well

with the presence or absence of lymphomatous involvement. Lipton et al. (1972) found that focal filling defects on the liver scan were consistently associated with hepatic involvement, but this type of abnormality was so infrequent as to be of little clinical value. Thus, although liver scintigraphy has been recommended as a routine diagnostic procedure in the clinical assessment of patients with Hodgkin's disease (Smithers, 1970a; Hardin and Johnston, 1971), the level of reliability of the procedure as documented by subsequent clinical pathologic correlation in series of patients submitted to staging laparotomy with routine liver biopsy has been decidedly unimpressive.

The gallbladder and the external bile ducts may be readily visualized with any of a number of iodized organic compounds. Occasionally, the cholecystogram may reveal the presence of enlarged lymph nodes at the hilus of the liver by virtue of displacement of the bile ducts or of the gallbladder. Direct involvement of the gallbladder by lymphomas is quite rare.

Gross enlargement of the head of the pancreas by tumor may be revealed roentgenographically by a widening of the barium-filled duodenal loop and its displacement from the antrum of the stomach. However, the body and tail of the pancreas cannot be delineated by conventional roentgenologic techniques. Experimental attempts have been made to develop scanning procedures for the pancreas, using radioactive selenomethionine. The results obtained with computed tomography have been decidedly more impressive, however (Fig. 5.75). In patients with malignant lymphomas, apparent enlargement of the pancreas is most often, in fact, due to enlargement of the neighboring upper lumbar para-aortic and celiac lymph nodes.

Stomach. Whereas involvement of the stomach, small intestine, and colon by other types of lymphomas is by no means uncommon, involvement of the stomach is seldom a presenting manifestation of Hodgkin's disease. We have encountered no instances of gastric involvement at the time of initial diagnosis in over 1,000 consecutive, previously untreated patients with Hodgkin's disease.

In a review of all gastrointestinal studies on patients with Hodgkin's disease seen at the Mount Sinai Hospital in New York during the five-year period 1959 to 1964, Bloch (1967) found that 190 of 455 patients had had an upper gastrointestinal tract barium examination. Roentgenologic evidence of gastric involvement was observed in 14 of these (7.4 percent), of which 10 were subsequently

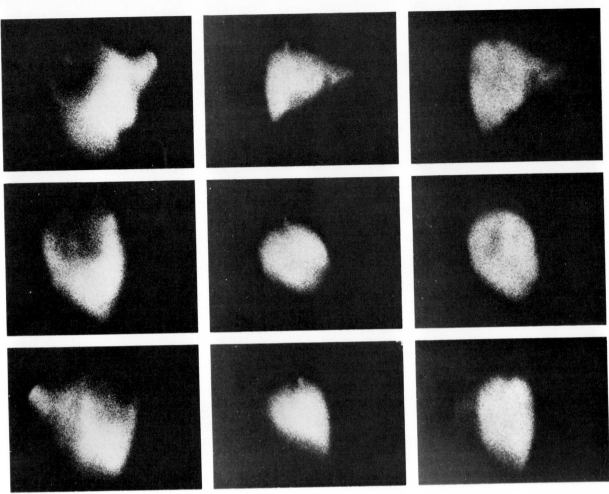

Figure 5.80 Liver scan with ⁹⁹ᵐTc sulfur colloid in July 1975 (*left*) revealed massive filling defects in the upper pole of the right lobe of the liver about four years after treatment with total lymphoid radiotherapy and colloidal radioactive gold for stage III$_S$B lymphocyte depletion Hodgkin's disease. Percutaneous needle biopsy of the liver was positive. The patient was treated with MOPP combination chemotherapy with an excellent response documented on the repeat examination of April 1977 (*middle*). However, in a third scan in January 1978 (*right*), faint irregular filling defects are again discernible in the right lobe of the liver which were considered highly suspicious of recurrent disease. *top panels,* anterior view; *center panels,* right lateral view; *lower panels,* posterior view. (Courtesy of Drs. Joseph P. Kriss and Michael Goris, Division of Nuclear Medicine, Stanford University Medical Center.)

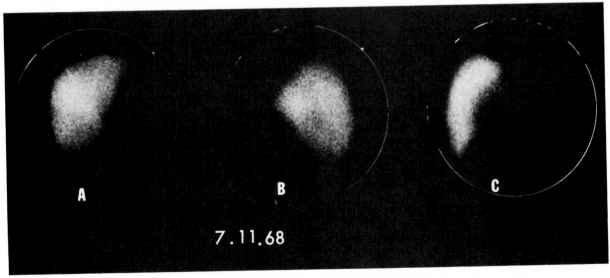

Figure 5.81 Gamma camera scintigram of the liver performed with ⁹⁹ᵐTc colloid, revealing profound distortion and irregularity of the liver due to massive nodular infiltration by Hodgkin's disease.

confirmed at laparotomy or postmortem examination. Most of these patients were in the relatively advanced stages of the disease.

All of the lymphomas produce essentially similar roentgenologic features when they do involve the stomach. Perhaps the most common manifestation is a solitary mass projecting into the lumen as a filling defect, usually associated with demonstrable ulceration (Fig. 5.82). In some instances, there is little or no mass, and the ulcer is then difficult to differentiate from a simple peptic ulcer, although some degree of infiltration of the gastric wall adjacent to the ulcer margins is usually present. In other instances, a lymphoma may infiltrate diffusely along a large proportion of the gastric wall, enlarging and sometimes stiffening the rugal folds (Fig. 5.83). Although peristaltic mobility and flexi-

bility of the stomach is usually diminished in this type of diffuse infiltration, instances have been observed in which flexibility is so well preserved that differentiation of the giant rugal fold pattern from that sometimes seen in nonspecific gastritis may be exceedingly difficult. Less frequently, multicentric lesions occur; Bloch describes one case in which four separate discrete ulcers were visualized in the distal half of the stomach (Fig. 5.84). Finally, the stomach is sometimes secondarily invaded by tumor extending from adjacent lymph node masses.

Small Intestine. Involvement early in the course of the disease is quite uncommon in Hodgkin's disease. Although jejunal and even duodenal involvement have been reported (Riederer, 1965), the region most commonly involved is the distal ileum, usually with extension of the infiltrate across the ileocecal valve to involve the cecum as well. Isolated case reports of apparently primary Hodgkin's disease of the appendix (Faerberg et al., 1965; Nagata et al., 1966) suggest that the disease may originate in or spread to the lymphatic tissue of the appendix and then secondarily invade along the walls of the adjacent distal ileum and cecum.

The roentgenologic appearance of small intestinal involvement is essentially the same for all types of malignant lymphomas. The infiltrated segments of small bowel are characteristically rather long. The mucosal pattern may be partially preserved but distorted and coarse in pattern (Fig. 5.85), or it may be entirely obliterated due to ulceration. The wall of the small intestine is usually appreciably thickened, and motility through the affected segment may be demonstrably impaired and sometimes associated with chronic diarrhea or even a sprue-like syndrome (Bickel and Rutishauser, 1942; Bernier et al., 1967). Not infrequently, multiple discontinuous zones of involvement are demonstrable; this finding, together with the great length of some of the affected segments, should suggest the diagnosis of lymphoma of the small intestine. Much less frequently, the lesions are short, with sharply outlined, overhanging margins similar to the classical "napkin-ring" pattern of the carcinomas, from which it is then difficult or impossible to distinguish them.

Colon and Rectum. Although primary Hodgkin's disease of the colon and rectum have been described in the literature (Portmann, Dunne, and Hazard, 1954; Shapiro, 1961; Levitan, 1966), such instances are rare. Even secondary involvement of

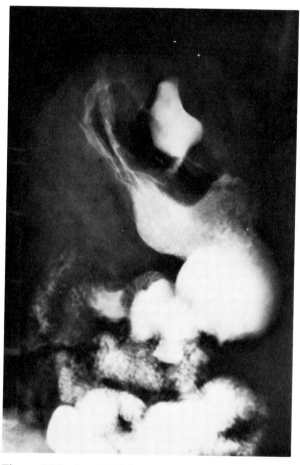

Figure 5.82 Localized form of Hodgkin's disease of the stomach. A smoothly demarcated mass occupies most of the fundus of the stomach. A large central diamond-shaped ulceration is noted within this tumor. This has the appearance of a large submucosal tumefaction. (From Bloch, 1967. Reprinted with the permission of the author and the *American Journal of Roentgenology, Radium Therapy and Nuclear Medicine.*)

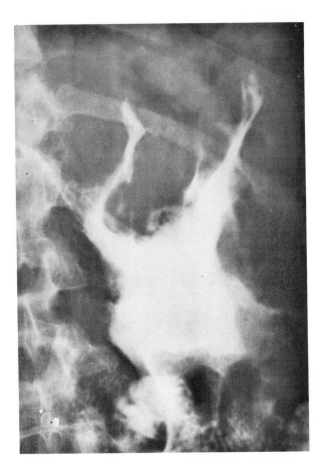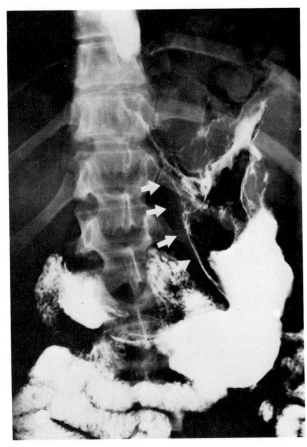

Figure 5.83 Nodular form. *Left,* barium outlines enormously thickened nodular rugal folds in the fundus of the stomach. No discrete ulcerations are noted. *Right,* in the prone projection air and barium outline the markedly altered rugal folds of the fundus of the stomach. The thickened infiltrated wall of the upper body and lower portion of the fundus of the stomach is noted along the lesser curvature (arrows). (From Bloch, 1967. Reprinted with the permission of the author and the *American Journal of Roentgenology, Radium Therapy and Nuclear Medicine.*)

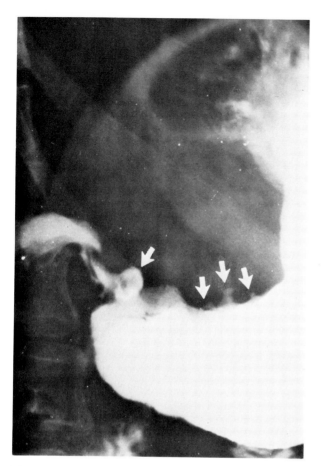

Figure 5.84 There are at least four niche-like ulcerations along the lesser curvature of the stomach (arrows). This is associated with restricted distensibility of the distal portion of the lesser curvature and narrowing of the antrum. The finding of such an infiltrated area with numerous separate ulcerations suggests the possibility of a lymphoma. (From Bloch, 1967. Reprinted with the permission of the author and the *American Journal of Roentgenology, Radium Therapy and Nuclear Medicine*.)

the colon and rectum by Hodgkin's disease during the early phases of the disease is uncommon, no such instances having been encountered in over 200 consecutive, previously untreated patients in our experience. In contrast, lymphosarcoma and reticulum cell sarcoma involving the colon and rectum were appreciably more common. In a study of 69 cases of malignant lymphoma of the colon, Wychulis et al. (1966) encountered 22 cases of reticulum cell sarcoma, 16 of small-cell lymphosarcoma, three of large-cell lymphosarcoma, four of Hodgkin's disease, one of follicular lymphoma, and 23 of mixed-cell type. They divided their cases into two groups: those in which there was apparent involvement of the colon only (50 cases), and those

which were associated with lymphomatous involvement elsewhere, either previously or simultaneously (19 cases). Regional lymph node involvement was found histologically in 25 of 48 specimens from Group I cases and in 12 of 16 Group II cases. In most of the instances in which the lesion was detected by barium enema examination, the preoperative roentgenologic diagnosis was carcinoma, although the diagnosis of lymphoma was correctly suspected in a few cases.

The roentgenologic features are usually similar to those in the small intestine. A relatively long segment or irregular infiltration of the wall of the colon or rectum, ulceration and narrowing of the lumen, and impaired flexibility and peristaltic activity of the affected segment are the most common manifestations. Not infrequently, however, the lesion produces an appearance closely simulating that ordinarily seen with carcinomas of the large bowel (Levitan, 1966). In some instances, large pelvic lymph node masses may invade the sigmoid and lower descending colon extrinsically, producing an irregular asymmetrical filling defect, which at least for some time does not completely encircle the bowel wall. Meadows (1965) has described a remarkable case of Hodgkin's disease of the colon presenting as disseminated sclerosis with associated ulcerative colitis.

Kidneys and Ureters. By far the most common roentgenologic manifestation is simple displacement of one or both ureters by enlarged lymph nodes in the lumbar para-aortic area or pelvis (Fig. 5.86). Actual narrowing and obstruction of the ureters is seen much less frequently (Fig. 5.87), usually in instances in which the lymphadenopathy is massive. However, intrinsic involvement of the ureter has been described (Braun et al., 1972). Occasionally, lymph node masses may compress and partially occlude one or both renal veins (Fig. 5.88), leading to the development of the nephrotic syndrome (Brodovsky et al., 1968; Ghosh and Muehrcke, 1970). In one of the most remarkable cases in our series, the presenting manifestation was blurring of vision and severe headache due to malignant hypertension induced by compression of the left renal artery (Fig. 5.89).

Infiltration of one or both kidneys by lymphoma is common at postmortem examination but is seldom diagnosed during life (Richmond et al., 1962). Typically, such involvement is bilateral and diffuse, the kidneys being distinctly enlarged, and is often associated with diminution in function and diffuse narrowing of the collecting system.

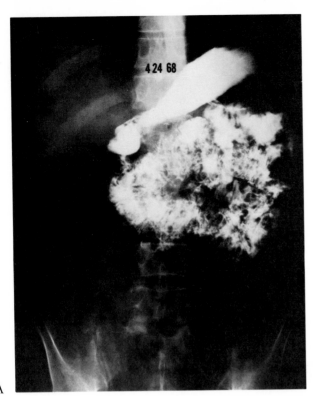

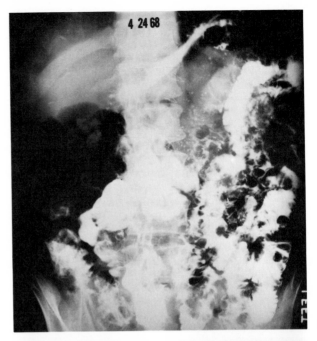

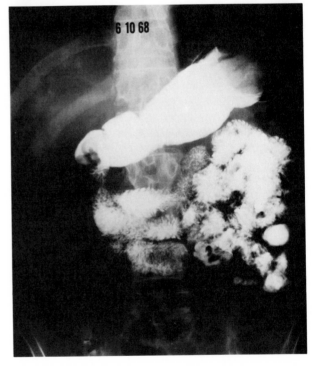

Figure 5.85 Biopsy-proved Hodgkin's disease of the small intestine. This 45-year-old male developed crampy abdominal pain, nausea, and vomiting in November 1967 and soon thereafter noted night sweats, fever, and pedal edema. A laparotomy was performed in March 1968, and biopsy of the small intestine revealed Hodgkin's disease. He was then transferred to the Peter Bent Brigham Hospital, Boston, where a barium study on 4/24/68 revealed a diffusely abnormal small bowel pattern, with loss of the valvulae conniventes, marked thickening and coarsening of the mucosal folds, irregularity of the lumen, and impaired motility (*A* and *B*). He also had left supraclavicular and axillary adenopathy, a biopsy-proved skin lesion on his back, and an osteolytic lesion of the left scapula. He was treated with chemotherapy and radiotherapy, receiving 2400 rads in 29 days to the entire abdomen, with marked symptomatic and radiographic improvement (*C*). (Photographs of the X-ray films and clinical history provided by Ann M. Lewicki, M.D., Department of Diagnostic Radiology, Peter Bent Brigham Hospital, Boston.)

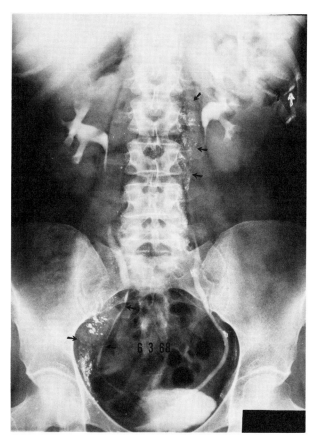

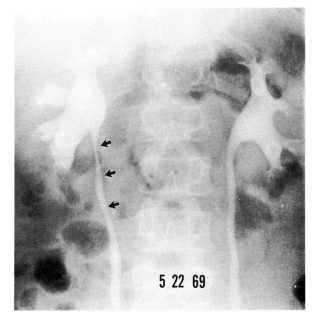

Figure 5.86 Intravenous urogram, revealing deviation of the right lower ureter by a mass of enlarged right iliac nodes and of the left upper ureter by enlarged lumbar para-aortic nodes (arrows).

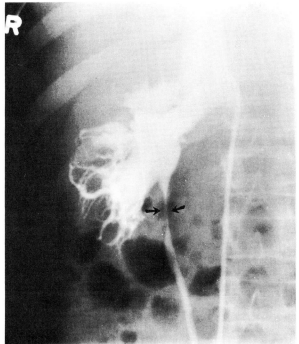

Figure 5.87 This 15-year-old boy had been treated four and one-half years earlier for stage I Hodgkin's disease involving the right neck. He remained apparently well on serial followup examinations, although in retrospect, it is clear that he should have had a repeat lymphangiogram for continued surveillance of the lumbar para-aortic nodes, since all of the opaque medium from the original examination had disappeared. He was readmitted with a two-week history of the nephrotic syndrome, characterized by lower-extremity edema, ascites, rapidly increasing weight, shortness of breath due to the development of pleural effusions, and profound proteinuria. Intravenous urography revealed caliectasis and slight lateral displacement of the right kidney and upper ureter by a soft tissue mass (*top*). An inferior vena cavagram and selective renal vein study were performed, revealing a normal right renal vein but a distinct area of constriction of the right upper ureter on the film seen here (*bottom*).

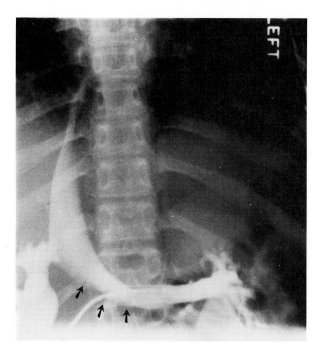

Figure 5.88 Left renal vein injection in the case described in Figure 5.87, revealing elevation and compression of the inferolateral margin of the left renal vein by an enlarged lymph node mass. The combination of compression of the left renal vein and obstruction of the right ureter was apparently sufficient to elicit the nephrotic syndrome in this case. The presence of enlarged lymph nodes in this region was confirmed at laparotomy, and radiotherapy directed to the region of the upper lumbar para-aortic lymph nodes resulted in rapid and complete disappearance of the ascites, pleural effusions, and lower-extremity edema.

Discrete nodules or mass lesions of the kidneys due to Hodgkin's disease are sometimes observed antemortem (cf. Fig. 10.3), though undoubtedly less often than would be the case if urography and/or renal arteriography were routinely employed in the investigation of advanced cases (Kyaw and Koehler, 1969; White and Palubinskas, 1970; Pick et al., 1971). Radioisotope scans of the kidneys may also indicate impaired function of one or both kidneys but would not be expected to have sufficient resolution to detect nodular disease unless of massive extent. Renal enlargement may also be due to amyloidosis, which occurs in about 5 percent of patients during the course of unsuccessfully treated Hodgkin's disease (Kiely, Wagoner, and Holley, 1969; Ultmann and Moran, 1973) and is accompanied by the nephrotic syndrome in over half of all cases (Brandt, Cathcart, and Cohen, 1968).

Bladder. Primary involvement of the urinary bladder by the malignant lymphomas is exceedingly

rare. In contrast, secondary invasion or compression of the bladder by extrinsic pelvic lymph node masses (Figs. 5.55, 5.90) is encountered not infrequently in the late stages of any of the lymphomas (Piquet-Gauthier et al., 1965). In such instances, the roentgen appearance is essentially indistinguishable from that seen when the bladder is infiltrated from the outside by carcinomatous lesions. Asymmetric displacement and compression of the bladder by an extrinsic soft tissue mass may be seen, often with some irregularity of the wall of the bladder as delineated on the cystogram, sometimes associated with gross ulceration.

Uterus, Tubes, and Ovaries. No instances in which radiologic examination has contributed to the diagnosis of Hodgkin's disease involving these structures have come to our attention.

Male Genitalia. Although involvement of the scrotum and testes has been recorded, no characteristic roentgenologic features have been described.

Peritoneal Effusions (Ascites). The malignant lymphomas not infrequently invade the peritoneal serous surfaces, more often than not rather late in the course of the disease, and then elicit a diffuse peritoneal effusion. The roentgen features do not differ from those of other types of ascites: a diffuse increase in density of the abdomen associated with a separation of the intestinal loops by intervening fluid, variable though usually moderate collection of gas in both the small and the large bowel due to secondary ileus, and variable degrees of obliteration of the properitoneal fat lines.

Skeletal System

Secondary involvement of the skeletal system by the malignant lymphomas is more often than not multiple rather than solitary. Such involvement is seldom encountered in the early stages of any of the lymphomas. We have seen only four instances of bone involvement at the time of initial diagnosis in a series of 340 consecutive untreated patients with Hodgkin's disease. However, later in the course of the disease, bone involvement becomes increasingly prevalent (Horan, 1969).

In a survey of 951 patients with proved Hodgkin's disease seen at the Christie Hospital in Manchester from 1940 to 1958, Granger and Whitaker (1967) observed 92 (9.6 percent) with radiologically demonstrable bone lesions. Perttala and Kijanen (1965) encountered 48 cases (10.6 percent)

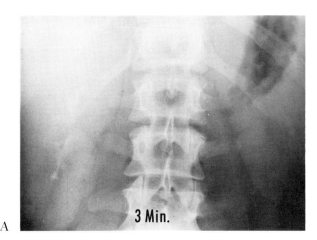

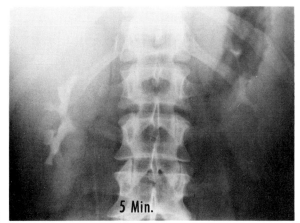

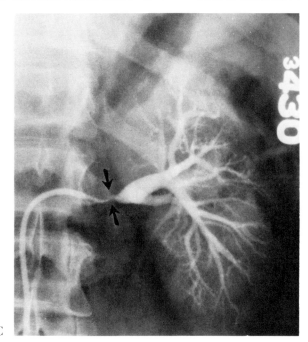

Figure 5.89 Hodgkin's disease presenting as malignant hypertension due to unilateral renal artery compression. The patient, a 26-year-old male, had noted enlarged nodes on both sides of the neck for at least two years but did not consult a physician until he suddenly developed blurred vision and pounding headaches. Ophthalmoscopy revealed splinter hemorrhages and marked arterial constriction; no pulse could be felt in either forearm, but blood pressure in the lower extremities was 240/160 and 280/180 mm. Hg. Intravenous urography revealed delayed excretion on the left side at three minutes (*A*) and reduced concentration at five minutes (*B*), without evidence of ureteral obstruction or caliectasis. Selective renal arteriography (*C*) revealed marked constriction of a short segment of the left main renal artery, which was found at laparotomy to be encased in a hard mass of lymph nodes. The spleen and splenic hilar nodes were also grossly involved and were resected; microscopic examination revealed nodular sclerosing Hodgkin's disease, as did a cervical node biopsy. The patient's pulseless state was attributed to compression of the subclavian arteries by lymph node masses, but arterial biopsy to exclude Takayasu's syndrome was deemed too hazardous, so there is no proof of this point. The patient was treated with total lymphoid radiotherapy and antihypertensive medications. He died of complications of hypertension nearly eight years later without an intervening relapse of Hodgkin's disease.

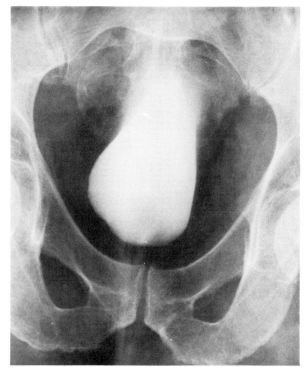

Figure 5.90 Compression and elongation of the urinary bladder by massive bilateral iliac node involvement by nodular sclerosing Hodgkin's disease in a 57-year-old male.

in a series of 453 cases in Finland; among the 470 cases reviewed by Musshoff, Busch, and Kaminski (1964), bone involvement was noted in 66 (14 percent). Although routine skeletal surveys yield an occasional asymptomatic case of radiologically evident bone involvement, most instances are discovered when roentgenologic examinations are performed because of local bone pain. The data of Granger and Whitaker (1967) suggest that bone involvement is a very unfavorable prognostic sign; the interval from the first roentgen evidence of bone lesion to death was less than two years in about 60 percent of cases, less than three years in nearly 80 percent, and the five-year survival was only 4.2 percent. Similarly, the data of Perttala and Kijanen (1965) indicate a five-year survival after detection of the osseous lesion of only 9.7 percent. However, these reports antedate the era of high-dose, total lymphoid radiotherapy and cyclic combination chemotherapy. In our experience and that of others (Musshoff and Boutis, 1968; Peters, Hasselback, and Brown, 1968), solitary lesions in bone, if treated intensively, have had no adverse influence on prognosis, and even widespread bone disease, treated with both radiotherapy and combination chemotherapy, may be compatible with long-term relapse-free survival. This subject is addressed again in relation to staging (Chapter 8) and prognosis (Chapter 12).

The osseous lesions of Hodgkin's disease may be lytic, sclerotic (osteoblastic), or mixed. In the Granger-Whitaker study, 261 lesions (75 percent) were lytic, of which 27 were associated with periosteal reaction; 47 (13.6 percent) were sclerotic, of which 6 were associated with periosteal reaction; and 18 (5.2 percent) were mixed, of which one was associated with periosteal reaction. Periosteal reaction was observed alone in 20 instances (5.8 percent). It is believed that Hodgkin's disease and other lymphomas affect bone in two ways: by hematogenous spread to the bone marrow, with subsequent growth from within the bone; and by extrinsic pressure from involved lymph nodes, leading to sclerosis of the "ivory vertebra" type (Fig. 5.91, 5.92) with or without anterior marginal erosion of vertebrae, para-vertebral soft tissue masses, and other evidence of direct invasion of bone (Fig. 5.93). Predominantly lytic lesions are often found in the long bones (Fig. 5.94), whereas those in the skull may be of either the lytic or the sclerotic type (Figs. 5.95, 5.96). Lesions in the sternum may also be either lytic (Figs. 5.42, 5.43) or sclerotic (Fig. 5.44). Occasionally, localized expansion and lysis simulating the appearance of cysts or other benign lesions of bone may be seen, especially in the ribs (Fig. 5.97). Combined lytic and sclerotic lesions in the long bones may simulate chronic osteomyelitis (Figs. 5.98, 5.99).

Recently, favorable experiences have been reported with bone scanning after the administration of ^{85}Sr, ^{99m}Tc, or other bone-seeking radioactive isotopes for the detection of skeletal involvement by Hodgkin's disease (Harbert and Ashburn, 1968; Schechter et al., 1976). Sites of abnormality are revealed as focal areas of increased uptake and deposition of the isotope (Figs. 5.100, 5.101). In several instances in our experience, such foci have been detected by this technique at a time when conventional roentgenographic films of the same region were either negative or equivocal. Serial scans may be useful not only in detecting bone lesions initially but in following their response to treatment (Fig. 5.101). In contrast to these bone-seeking radionuclides, it has been reported that radioactive indium chloride (^{111}InCl$_3$) is taken up selectively in bone marrow, in a distribution very similar to that of radioactive iron (Lilien et al., 1973). Gilbert et al. (1976a,b) have assessed the value of ^{111}InCl$_3$ bone marrow scans in 26 untreated and 102 previously treated patients with Hodgkin's disease and other lymphomas. The indium scans were reliable in evaluating the presence or absence of normal marrow elements in various regions of the skeleton (Fig. 5.102) and were helpful in selected patients in detecting focal areas of impaired uptake, needle biopsy of which revealed extensive replacement by Hodgkin's disease (Fig. 5.103). However, only 58 percent of patients who had documented lymphoma in marrow biopsies had decreased indium uptake at the biopsy site. Thus, marrow scintigraphy must be regarded as a relatively insensitive test for marrow invasion or replacement by lymphoma, though it may be useful in selected patients as a guide to the selection of needle biopsy sites, as well as in the detection of marrow aplasia or regeneration (Fig. 5.104).

Central Nervous System

The most common manifestation of central nervous system involvement by the malignant lymphomas is the syndrome of spinal cord compression by extradural tumor infiltration (Eggleston and Hartmann, 1968). Such lesions, when detected early, respond dramatically to decompression by laminectomy and postoperative radiotherapy. However, localization of the level of the lesion on neurologic evidence alone is sometimes unreliable.

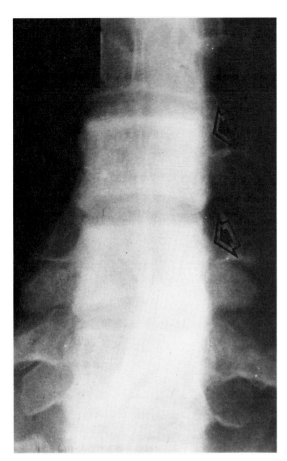

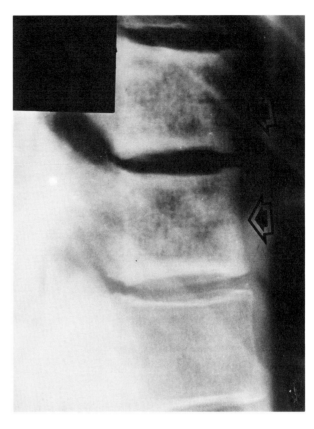

Figure 5.91   Typical "ivory vertebrae" due to Hodgkin's disease. These lesions in the dorsal spine of a 24-year-old female must have been present initially, but were not apparent, even in retrospect, on the initial roentgenogram; instead, progressive sclerosis developed some months after completion of radiotherapy to her massive mediastinal disease, with treatment fields encompassing this segment of the dorsal spine.

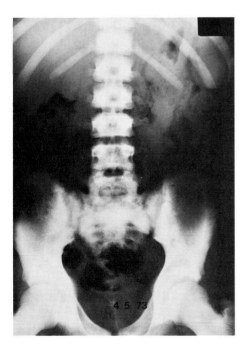

Figure 5.92   Remarkable osteoblastic involvement of the bodies of all of the dorsal lumbar vertebrae, the sacrum, the pelvis, both femora, and multiple ribs in a 14-year-old boy with nodular sclerosing Hodgkin's disease. The spleen is apparently enlarged. The patient was treated with MOPP combination chemotherapy, entered complete remission, and remains relapse-free more than six years later.

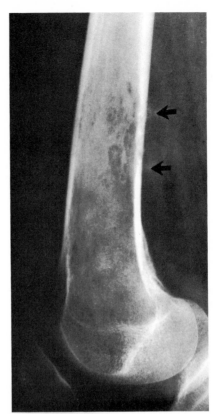

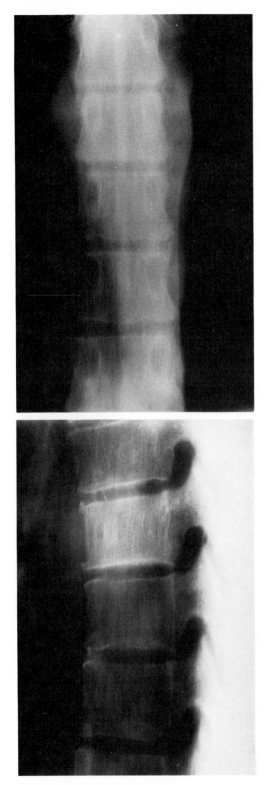

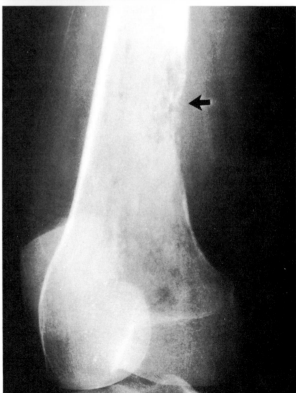

Figure 5.93 Early sclerotic changes in a dorsal vertebra, associated with paravertebral soft tissue mass and erosion of the anterior border of the vertebra, as seen in the lateral projection.

Figure 5.94 Irregular lytic femoral lesions in an 18-year-old female with rapidly progressing Hodgkin's disease.

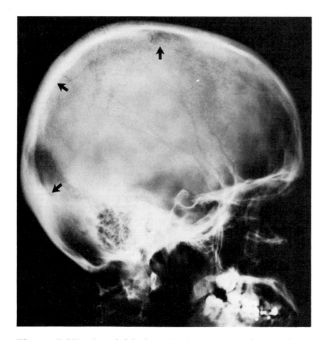

Figure 5.95 Cranial lesions in the same patient as in 5.94. Note that the lesion in the anterior parietal region is predominantly lytic in character, whereas the posterior parietal and posterior occipital regions exhibit sclerotic changes, with obliteration of the diploic layer.

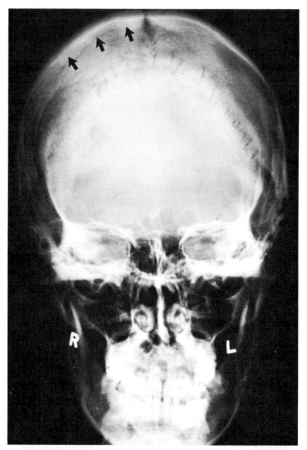

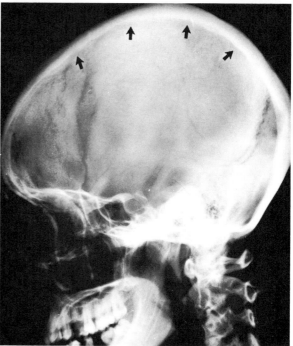

Figure 5.96 Sclerotic infiltration of the skull, with obliteration of the diploic layer and diffuse thickening of both the inner and the outer tables.

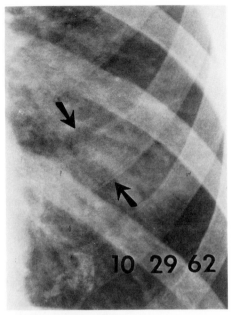

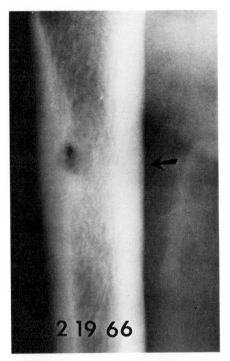

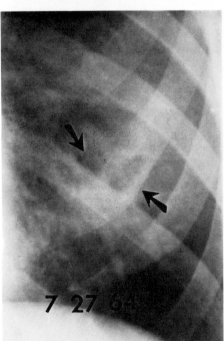

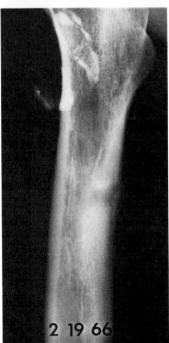

Figure 5.97 Unusual lesion due to biopsy-proved Hodgkin's disease in the left anterior fifth rib. On the initial film of 10/29/62 (*top*), there is a slight break in the cortex along the superior margin of the rib, associated with a diffuse increase in coarseness of its trabecular pattern, which was not regarded at the time as abnormal. However, by 7/27/64 (*bottom*), the lesion had progressed to diffuse irregular lytic change, somewhat resembling a cystic lesion of the rib. Because there was no other evidence of disease at the time, biopsy was performed, revealing the presence of Hodgkin's disease.

Figure 5.98 An unusual femoral lesion, somewhat resembling localized chronic osteomyelitis, which developed later in the patient in Figure 5.97.

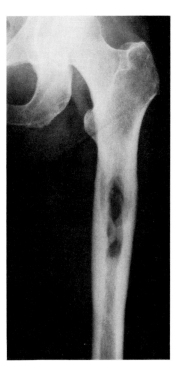
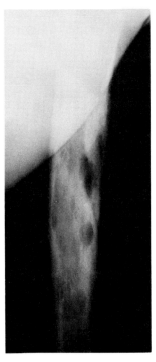

Figure 5.99 A more extensive femoral lesion presenting a mixture of rather discretely outlined lytic areas and sclerosis and thickening of the cortex, somewhat resembling osteomyelitis, in a patient with stage IV Hodgkin's disease.

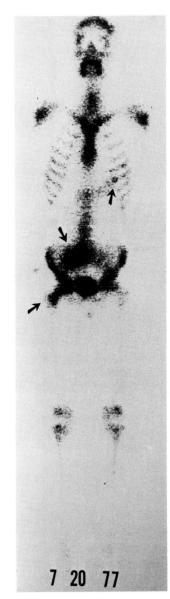

Figure 5.100 Relapse in the skeletal system detected by a positive ^{99m}TcMDP bone scan. This 19-year-old male had been treated with multiple cycles of MOPP combination chemotherapy and adjuvant radiation therapy for stage IVB Hodgkin's disease with documented liver and bone marrow involvement. After a brief complete remission, he returned complaining of pain in the low back and right hip, and the bone scan revealed areas of abnormal uptake in the right upper femur, the right sacroiliac region, and probably also in a left anterior rib (arrows). (Courtesy of Drs. Joseph P. Kriss and Michael Goris, Division of Nuclear Medicine, Stanford University Medical Center.)

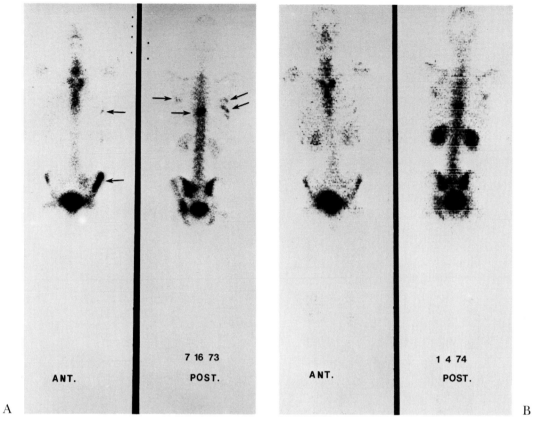

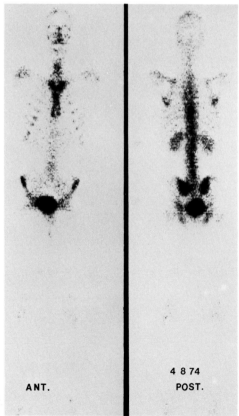

Figure 5.101 Multiple osseous lesions in the ribs, dorsal spine, and left ilium (arrows) were detected by a ^{99m}TcEHDP bone scan in July 1973 in this 35-year-old male with stage IV_0B Hodgkin's disease. He was treated with combined modality therapy (total lymphoid irradiation and MOPP combination chemotherapy, alternating technique) with gradual, apparently complete clearing of the bone lesions on repeat scans in January and April 1974, and has remained relapse-free for more than five years. (Courtesy of Drs. Joseph P. Kriss and Michael Goris, Division of Nuclear Medicine, Stanford University Medical Center.)

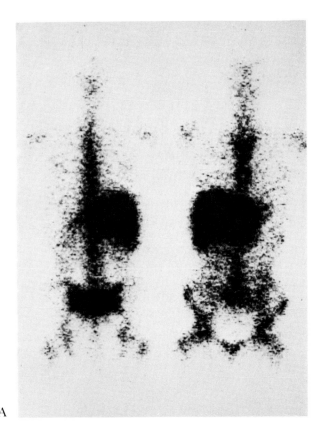

A

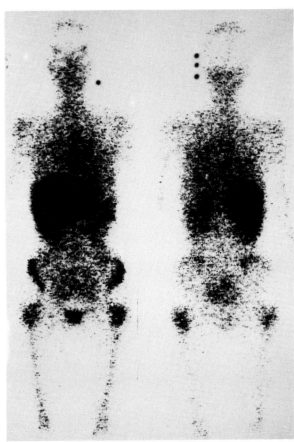

B

Figure 5.102 *A*, normal ^{111}InCl$_3$ bone marrow scan in a female patient with stage III$_S$A Hodgkin's disease. *B*, repeat scan three months later, immediately after completion of total lymphoid and hepatic irradiation. Note the decreased uptake over the irradiated regions, especially in the distribution of the "inverted-Y" subdiaphragmatic field, and the markedly increased uptake in areas of compensatory marrow activation in unirradiated regions, especially the cranium, lateral pelvis, femora, and humeri. (Courtesy of Drs. Joseph P. Kriss and Michael Goris, Division of Nuclear Medicine, Stanford University Medical Center.)

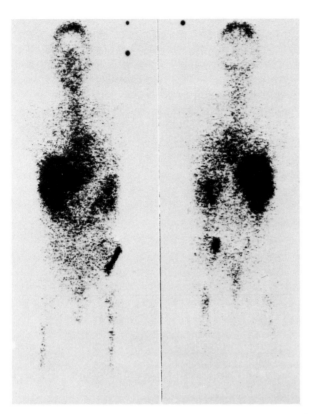

Figure 5.103 Abnormal ^{111}InCl$_3$ bone marrow scan in a 52-year-old male patient with stage III$_S$B Hodgkin's disease who had been treated with total lymphoid irradiation and ^{198}Au gold colloid. About one year later, he developed fever and anemia. A Jamshidi needle biopsy was performed in the left anterior superior iliac crest, revealing an intensely hyperplastic bone marrow and no evidence of tumor. The bone marrow scan revealed an isolated area of increased uptake in the left iliac crest, in the region of the biopsy, and markedly decreased uptake in the right pelvis and in focal, "moth-eaten" areas in both femora. Accordingly, a repeat needle biopsy was performed in the right iliac crest, revealing extensive replacement of the marrow by Hodgkin's disease. (Courtesy of Drs. Joseph P. Kriss and Michael Goris, Division of Nuclear Medicine, Stanford University Medical Center.)

In such instances, myelography may be extremely useful in delineating the exact anatomic location of the extradural lesion, and occasionally in revealing the presence of multiple lesions, and thus preventing errors in selection of the level at which laminectomy is to be performed. Myelography should be considered as a virtual emergency procedure in such instances to avoid unnecessary delay in diagnosis and treatment and to prevent the progression of paralysis to an irreversible state. Typically, the myelographic appearance of an extradural lesion produced by a malignant lymphoma is a rather smoothly tapering constriction of the iodized oil-filled subarachnoid space, which, in some instances, is asymmetrical in contour (Fig. 5.105, 5.106).

Actual invasion of the brain by Hodgkin's disease is rare; Marshall, Roessman, and Van den Noort (1968) were able to collect only twelve such cases from the world literature, to which they added two cases of their own. The number of reported cases has now grown to thirty-four (Cuttner, Meyer, and Huang, 1979). In the more slowly evolving cases, the typical roentgen signs of increased intracranial pressure may be seen: separation of the sutures in younger patients, accentuation of the convolutional markings of the skull in a slightly older age group, associated with demineralization of the dorsum sellae. Focal lesions are rarely demonstrable on conventional skull radiographs but may now be readily demonstrated by

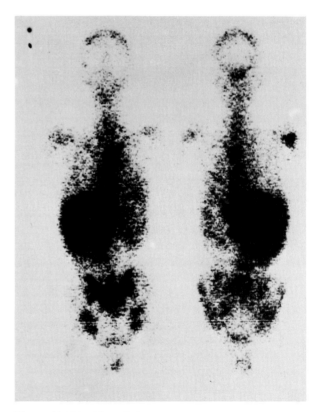

Figure 5.104 ^{111}InCl$_3$ bone marrow scan revealing remarkable regeneration of the bone marrow in a young male patient who had been treated with total lymphoid irradiation about eight years earlier and with multiple cycles of MOPP combination chemotherapy for a documented relapse in the liver six years earlier. (Courtesy of Drs. Joseph P. Kriss and Michael Goris, Division of Nuclear Medicine, Stanford University Medical Center.)

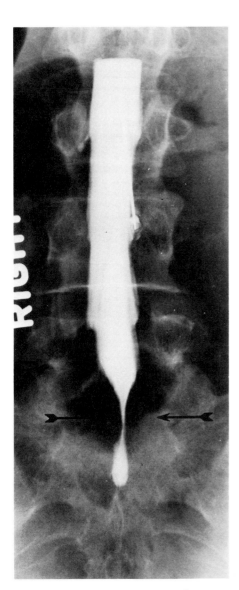

Figure 5.105 Myelogram revealing an extradural mass compressing the lower spinal canal at the L_5-S_1 intervertebral space. Concurrently, this patient had a massive relapse of his nodular sclerosing Hodgkin's disease in the right iliac nodes, with compression of the urinary bladder.

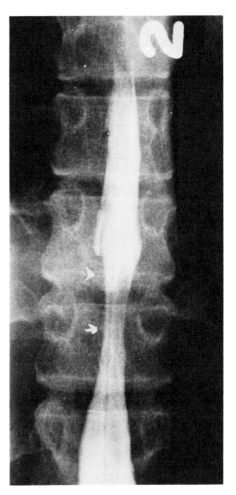

Figure 5.106 Myelogram demonstrating two sites of epidural spread in a young adult male patient treated initially with local radiotherapy for CS IIA lymphocyte predominance Hodgkin's disease. He later relapsed in the left iliac nodes and in the bone marrow and was treated with additional radiotherapy and MOPP chemotherapy with an apparently complete remission. However, he relapsed again one year later and developed progressive central nervous system involvement despite ABVD combination chemotherapy. The myelogram reveals compression of the spinal canal by a mass at the T_9-T_{10} level and a complete obstruction at T_7.

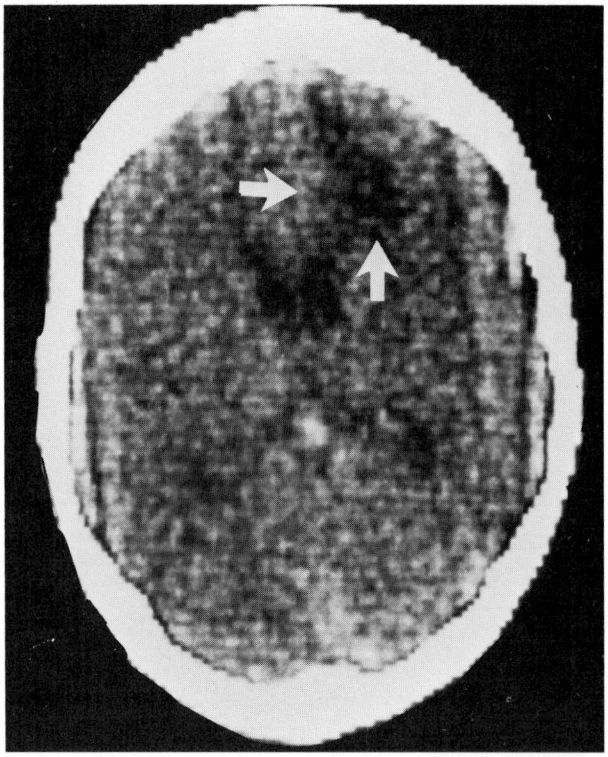

Figure 5.107   Computed tomographic scan revealing a focal radiolucent area (arrows), which proved to be due to a rare intracerebral metastasis of Hodgkin's disease. (Courtesy of Dr. William H. Marshall, Jr., Division of Diagnostic Radiology, Stanford University Medical Center.)

computed tomography (Brant-Zawadzki and Enzmann, 1978; Fig. 5.107). In selected patients, such special procedures as air encephalography, ventriculography, or radioisotopic scans of the brain (Thompson and DeNardo, 1969; Fig. 5.108) and carotid or vertebral anteriography (Fig. 5.109) may be indicated. Meningeal and epidural tumor masses are most conveniently detected by computed tomography (Fig. 5.110). Multifocal leukoencephalopathy, a rare and bizarre complication of Hodgkin's disease and leukemia, usually exhibits no specific roentgenologic features.

Miscellaneous

Lymphomatous involvement of the structures of Waldeyer's ring is usually apparent on direct inspection and palpation, but occasionally basal and lateral views of the skull will reveal the extent of such lesions more adequately by virtue of their encroachment on and distortion of the normal nasopharyngeal and oropharyngeal air spaces. Involvement of the paranasal sinuses is also readily demonstrable roentgenologically as a diffuse opacification of the air space of the involved sinus, often with destruction of the marginal bony cortex and invasion of the adjacent bony structures. Lateral soft tissue views of the neck will reveal involvement of the vallecula, epiglottis, or larynx, though again such lesions are more often readily apparent on indirect mirror examination of the larynx. Lymphomas arising or secondarily involving the orbit may produce proptosis and conjunctival edema. In some instances, this will be accompanied roentgenologically by expansion of the optic foramen unilaterally or by infiltration and destruction of the bony walls of the orbit.

Occasionally, lymph node masses in the anteromedial region of the neck may be difficult to distinguish from masses involving the thyroid. In such instances, radioiodine thyroid scans will assist in demonstrating that the mass is extrathyroidal in nature. Direct invasion of the thyroid gland by Hodgkin's disease, though quite rare, has been described (Roberts and Howard, 1963; Veronesi, Cascinelli, and Preda, 1966).

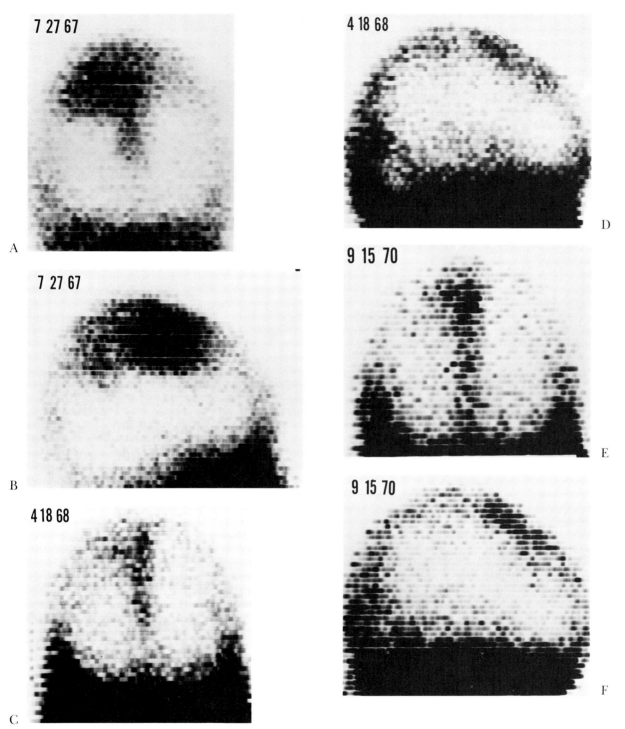

Figure 5.108 Abnormal brain scans due to Hodgkin's disease involving the meninges and right cerebral hemisphere in a 30-year-old female patient with a six-year history of active disease. *A* and *B*, initial examination of 7/17/67, revealing a diffuse increase in uptake in the right cerebral hemisphere in the anteroposterior view and in the postero-frontal, parietal, and anterior occipital regions in the lateral view. The patient was treated with whole-brain irradiation, with an excellent response which was manifest in the serial repeat brain scans of 4/18/68 (*C* and *D*) and 9/15/70 (*E* and *F*). (Reprinted with modifications, by permission of the authors and the Editor of *Cancer,* from Thompson and DeNardo, 1969.)

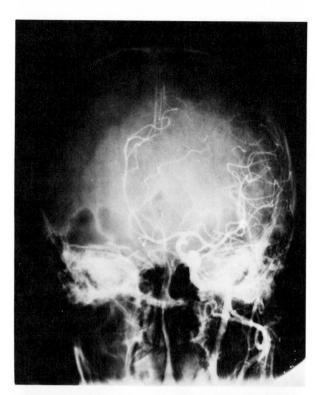

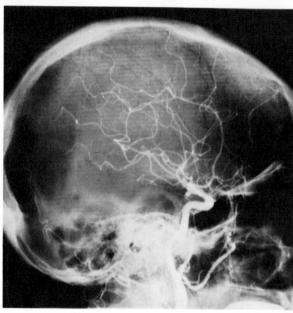

Figure 5.109   Left cerebral mass lesions due to Hodgkin's disease in a 57-year-old female patient revealed by carotid arteriography and confirmed by biopsy.

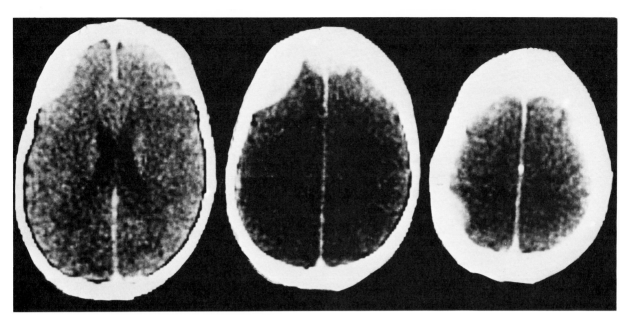

Figure 5.110   Multiple meningeal masses due to Hodgkin's disease protrude inward from the cranial contours at different levels in these computed tomographic scans. This patient also had epidural compression and obstruction of the spinal canal (Fig. 5.106). (Courtesy of Drs. William H. Marshall, Jr., and Ronald A. Castellino, Division of Diagnostic Radiology, Stanford University Medical Center.)

Chapter 6

The Nature of the Immunologic Defect

Historical Aspects

The history of Hodgkin's disease was for a time closely interwoven with that of tuberculosis. In the last two decades of the nineteenth century, these two diseases were found to coexist so often at autopsy that many pathologists found it quite plausible to accept the view of Hodgkin's disease as a granulomatous lesion, and Sternberg (1898) went so far as to propose that it was simply an atypical form of tuberculosis. This view was refuted by the work of Clarke (1901), Dorothy Reed (1902), Longcope (1903, 1907), and others (cf. reviews by Wallhauser, 1933; Hoster et al., 1948), who presented persuasive evidence that the two diseases were quite distinct and independent entities. Nevertheless, their frequent association persisted. Jackson and Parker (1947) observed tuberculosis in about 20 percent of autopsies on patients with Hodgkin's disease, and Ewing (1928), observing a similarly high incidence, commented: "In New York State where the disease is very common, tuberculosis follows Hodgkin's disease like a shadow." Although this oft-quoted remark is no longer true, thanks to public health measures aimed at the eradication of tuberculosis, Razis et al. (1959b) were still able to report a 5.1 percent incidence of tuberculosis in patients with Hodgkin's disease.

That heightened susceptibility to tuberculosis might be attributable to an immunologic defect in patients with Hodgkin's disease was independently discovered by Parker et al. (1932) and Steiner (1934). Although, as early as 1902, Dorothy Reed had noted, without further comment, that "tuberculin was given in five of the (eight) cases but without reaction," these investigators were the first to test relatively large numbers of patients systematically for their cutaneous reactivity to tuberculin. Steiner found that, contrary to the high tuberculin reactivity of the general population at that time, 27 of 33 patients with Hodgkin's disease exhibited no cutaneous reaction to 0.001 mg. of either human

or avian tuberculin, and 20 of 28 remained unresponsive despite a tenfold increase in dose. Of particular importance was the well-documented observation by both groups of investigators that the tuberculin reaction was not infrequently negative in the presence of active tuberculosis in these patients (as was also true of Dorothy Reed's case 1).

These observations were confirmed by Dubin (1947), who encountered only one positive tuberculin reaction among 38 cases of Hodgkin's disease in a region in which the frequency of positive tuberculin reactions in the general population at the time was 52 percent. However, astutely noting that the frequency of positive serologic reactions for syphilis in both white and Negro patients with Hodgkin's disease was also less than expected and that some patients with coexisting brucellosis seemed unable to make antibody against the *Brucella* organism, he postulated that the immunologic deficiency of Hodgkin's disease was not specifically restricted to tuberculosis but was generalized.

Stimulated in part by Dubin's paper, Schier and his associates (1956) conducted systematic tests of the capacity of patients with Hodgkin's disease to exhibit delayed hypersensitivity reactions to a diversified battery of natural antigens. These studies, which are described in excellent reviews by Aisenberg (1964a, 1966) and by Chase (1966), may be said to have ushered in the modern era of investigation of this subject. However, it was not until several years later, with the advent of lymphangiography and more accurate clinical staging, that it became possible to relate immunologic responses to the extent of involvement and other clinical parameters in previously untreated patients with Hodgkin's disease. New investigative pathways were opened with the recognition that lymphocytes are not all identical but fall into two broad categories: bone marrow-derived, "bursa-equivalent" (B) lymphocytes, which are responsible for antibody synthesis (humoral immunity), and thymus-derived (T) lymphocytes, which, in addition to being active in cell-mediated cytotoxic responses, modulate the immune system through their "helper" and "suppressor" functions. It was soon evident that certain responses of T-lymphocytes in vitro could be regarded as analogs or correlates of delayed hypersensitivity reactions and other cell-mediated immune responses in vivo. From such studies in vitro have come a better definition of the nature of the impairment and some indication of the underlying mechanisms involved. A general survey of the evidence available to date and of some of the interpretations stimulated by it is given in this chapter.

Delayed Hypersensitivity

Unresponsiveness to Natural Antigens. The cutaneous reaction to tuberculin is the classical example of a reaction of the delayed hypersensitivity type. Such reactions are also elicited by a variety of other bacterial and fungal antigens, as well as by contact chemical allergens. As the name suggests, they are distinguished from the immediate type of cutaneous hypersensitivity by the lapse of an interval of twenty-four to forty-eight hours or more between the time of exposure to the antigen and the local development of erythema and induration. This difference in rate of expression results in turn from the fact that the immediate type of reaction is mediated by humoral antibody which is readily and quickly delivered to the site of reaction, whereas the delayed type of hypersensitivity reaction is mediated by cells, which require time to migrate into the tissue site and there to undergo a complex series of responses, which have been described in detail by Lawrence (1956), Oort and Turk (1965), and Turk (1967).

Schier et al. (1956) studied a series of 43 patients with Hodgkin's disease and 79 "normal" controls (including patients with duodenal ulcers, diabetes mellitus, cirrhosis of the liver, and rheumatic heart disease). Whereas histamine elicited an immediate wheal reaction in all subjects of both groups, the delayed hypersensitivity response to four different antigens (purified tuberculoprotein, *Trichophyton gypseum, Candida albicans,* and mumps skin test antigen) was severely and significantly depressed in the Hodgkin's disease group relative to the controls. They concluded that patients with Hodgkin's disease exhibit a generalized unresponsiveness or anergy to antigens of the delayed-reacting type, possibly resulting from a defect in the production or transport of the cellular antibodies concerned in this type of tissue immunity; and they suggested that this type of immunologic defect might explain

the susceptibility of patients with Hodgkin's disease to tuberculosis and other indolent infections.

Schier et al. observed no correlation between these skin test responses and the severity or duration of the disease or prior treatment with radiation, nitrogen mustard, or steroids. Lamb et al. (1962), again using a battery of antigens, attempted to assess cutaneous responses in relation to the general condition of their patients. In patients in "good condition," the incidence of anergy was as follows: controls, 3/208 (1.4 percent); Hodgkin's disease, 26/49 (53 percent); leukemia, 3/25 (12 percent); non-Hodgkin's lymphomas, 1/20 (5 percent); and carcinoma, 0/27 (0 percent). Anergy was appreciably more common among patients in "poor condition," occurring in 7 of 8 such patients with Hodgkin's disease (88 percent), 5 of 10 with leukemia (50 percent), 13 of 21 with non-Hodgkin's lymphomas (62 percent), and 12 of 31 with carcinoma (38 percent). They suggested that the high incidence of anergy in the Hodgkin's disease patients in good condition, as compared with the other groups, might indicate that anergy is a primary attribute of the disease process itself, rather than a secondary consequence of nutritional deficiencies, cachexia, or inanition. Similar data were obtained by Sokal and Primikirios (1961).

At the National Cancer Institute, Brown et al. (1967) studied a series of 50 previously untreated patients with Hodgkin's disease, in all of whom the disease was staged with the aid of lymphangiography and other modern diagnostic measures. They compared the responses of these patients to several antigens of the delayed type with those of a group of controls which included 17 healthy individuals and 26 patients with mycosis fungoides (Table 6.1). Responsiveness to each of the five antigens employed was reduced among the Hodgkin's disease patients, and only 28 of 50 (56 percent) gave a positive response to one or more of the antigens, as compared with 25 of 25 controls (100 percent).

However, the reactions of the patients with stage I Hodgkin's disease were comparable to those of normal controls; thus, 5 of the 8 stage I patients (63 percent) had a positive reaction to two or more intradermal antigens versus 17 of 25 (68 percent) among the controls. Responsiveness decreased appreciably with increasing anatomic extent of disease (Table 6.2). One or more intradermal tests were positive in 7 of 8 stage I patients, but in only 13 of 24 stage II, 3 of 7 stage III, and 5 of 11 stage IV patients.

The Bethesda studies were later extended to en-

Table 6.1 Skin Test Reactivity in Hodgkin's Disease

	Patients		Controls	
Antigen tested[a]	No. positive/No. tested	% positive	No. positive/No. tested	% positive
DNCB	57/90	67	41/43[b]	95
Mumps	50/73	69	22/25	88
Candida albicans	23/99	23	13/25	52
Histoplasmin	11/100	11	4/10	40
PPD	10/101	10	6/25	24
Coccidioidin	0/59	0	—	—
Any one or more intradermal	66/100	66	25/25	100
Any two or more intradermal	23/102	23	17/25	68

Source: Data of Brown et al. (1967) and Young et al. (1972, 1973b).

[a] PPD, purified protein derivative of tuberculin; DNCB, dinitrochlorobenzene; sensitizing dose, 2%; challenge doses, 0.05 and 0.1%; interval to challenge, 14 days; all sensitized prior to the initiation of treatment.

[b] Includes 26 patients with mycosis fungoides.

compass a total of 103 patients with untreated disease, with generally similar results (Young et al., 1972, 1973b). Positive reactions to mumps antigen were observed in 50 (69 percent) of 73 patients tested, as compared with 22 (88 percent) of 25 normal controls, and did not vary significantly with stage of disease. Responses to the other intradermal antigens tested occurred less frequently in both patients and controls (Table 6.1) and tended to decline with advancing stage. Skin test reactivity was inversely correlated with constitutional symptoms when patients with stage I and II or stage III and IV disease were considered together. All of the 7 patients who were completely anergic (unresponsive to all tests) had systemic symptoms. Somewhat lower response rates (59 and 66 percent, respectively) were observed in the series of 27 patients studied by Winkelstein et al. (1974) and the series of 52 patients reported by Case et al. (1976).

Much lower rates of response to intradermal antigens (purified protein derivative of tuberculin, coccidioidin, histoplasmin, blastomycin, *Candida albicans* extract, and mumps skin test antigen) were observed in two successive Stanford studies. In the first of these, a total of 185 patients was studied from 1964 through 1968 (Kaplan, 1970). This series included 28 patients with untreated stage I disease, of whom only 12 (43 percent) responded to mumps antigen, and very few responded to any of the other antigens (Table 6.3). The second series was initiated in 1969, and by January 1972 had accrued 154 previously untreated patients, all staged with the aid of lymphangiography and laparotomy with splenectomy (Eltringham and Kaplan, 1973). Only 51 of 151 evaluable patients (34 percent) responded to one or more of these intradermal antigens, and a positive reaction to mumps antigen was obtained in only 40 (26 percent) of 151 patients (Table 6.4). In agreement with the observations of

Table 6.2 Relationship of Clinical Stage to Skin Test Reactivity

		Number and (percent) reactive with		
Clinical stage	Number of cases	DNCB	Intradermal antigen(s)	Both
I	8	8 (100)	7 (87)	7 (87)
II	24	17 (71)	13 (54)	9 (38)
III	7	4 (57)	3 (43)	2 (29)
IV	11	6 (54)	5 (45)	3 (27)

Source: Data of Brown et al. (1967); DNCB = dinitrochlorobenzene.

Table 6.3 Response to Intradermal Antigens in 28 Stage I Cases

Antigen	Number positive	Percent positive
Mumps	12	43
Candida albicans	5	18
Tuberculin (PPD)	0	—
Coccidioidin	1	4
Blastomycin	0	—
Histoplasmin	2	7

Source: Data of first Stanford University Medical Center series (Kaplan, 1970).

Table 6.4 Delayed Hypersensitivity Responses in Hodgkin's Disease: Responses to Individual Intradermal Antigens

Stage	No. positive/No. tested						One or more intradermal antigens[a]
	PPD	Blastomycin	Mumps	Candida	Histoplasmin	Coccidioidin	
IA, IIA, II$_E$A	1/67	0/41	21/67	2/67	3/67	2/66	24/67 (36)
IB, IIB, II$_S$B, II$_E$B	1/24	1/13	5/24	1/24	4/24	2/23	9/24 (38)
IIIA, III$_S$A, III$_E$A, III$_{ES}$A	0/28	0/16	3/28	2/28	1/28	2/25	4/28 (14)
IIIB, III$_S$B, III$_{ES}$B	0/17	0/11	6/17	0/17	1/17	1/16	7/17 (41)
IVA, IVB	1/15	0/12	5/15	0/15	3/15	2/15	7/15 (47)
Totals	3/151	1/93	40/151	5/151	12/151	9/145	51/151 (34)

Source: Data of second Stanford University Medical Center series (Eltringham and Kaplan, 1973).

[a] Number positive/Number tested and (% positive).

Young et al. (1972) on mumps antigen, there was no significant influence of clinical stage on response rate. Moreover, unresponsiveness did not appear to occur more frequently among patients with constitutional symptoms. Reactivity to blastomycin was so low that it was dropped from the test battery during the study, and a new antigen, streptokinase-streptodornase (SK-SD) was tested at a concentration of 5 units/0.1 ml. Some of the nonresponders were retested at a tenfold higher concentration. The results, which are presented in Table 6.5, reveal that only 6 (10.3 percent) of 58 untreated patients with Hodgkin's disease reacted to 5 units of SK-SD, whereas 93 percent of age- and sex-matched controls had previously been shown to respond (Gaines, Gilmer, and Remington, 1973). Only 1 of the 6 SK-SD responders was among the group of 19 patients who had reacted to one or more of the other intradermal antigens. Of particular relevance was the observation that 8 additional patients, out of a group of 29 who failed to react to 5 units of SK-SD, were capable of a response when retested with 50 units.

Table 6.5 Delayed Hypersensitivity Responses in Hodgkin's Disease: Results of Intradermal Testing with SK-SD

Response to other intradermal antigens	No. positive to SK-SD/ No. tested	
	5 units	50 units
Positive	1/19	2/10
Negative	5/39	6/19
Totals	6/58	8/29

Source: Data of second Stanford University Medical Center series (Eltringham and Kaplan, 1973).

Other investigators have now reported similar observations. Faguet (1975) noted anergic responses to a battery of skin test antigens in 21 (60 percent) of 35 untreated patients. Ziegler, Hansen, and Penny (1975) tested 27 patients with untreated Hodgkin's disease with *Candida,* mumps, tuberculin, and SK-SD and observed anergy in 4 (35 percent) of 14 stage I–IIIA and in 9 (69 percent) of 13 stage IIIB–IV patients. In a series of 42 patients with stage II–IV disease, Bobrove et al. (1975) noted positive responses to intradermal antigens in 22 (58 percent) of 38 patients tested. Holm et al. (1976) were able to obtain positive responses to tuberculin in only 12 (39 percent) of 31 patients, whereas 16 of 17 (94 percent) of their controls responded.

Active Sensitization with Chemical Allergens. Skin testing with the natural antigens such as tuberculin unfortunately does not distinguish between true anergy in a previously sensitized individual and the lack of response in individuals never previously exposed to the antigen. It has long been known that a number of chemical agents, on contact with the skin, have the property of inducing delayed hypersensitivity reactions essentially indistinguishable from those induced by tuberculin. The agent most extensively studied is 2,4-dinitrochlorobenzene (DNCB); dinitrofluorobenzene (DNFB) and paranitrosodimethylaniline have also been used to a limited extent. The advantage of this approach is that both the fact of exposure to the agent and the timing of that exposure are under the control of the investigator.

Rostenberg et al. (1956) and Epstein (1958) initiated studies with these compounds in patients with malignant lymphomas and leukemias. Soon thereafter, Fazio, Calciati, and DePaoli (1962) demonstrated an excellent correlation between the DNCB response and tuberculin reactivity in a series of 12 patients with Hodgkin's disease. Only two of these were tuberculin-positive, and the same two were the only DNCB-reactive patients in the group. Levin et al. (1964) noted a similar, though somewhat less perfect, correlation between tuberculin reactivity and DNFB responses in a series of healthy subjects, patients with non-neoplastic disease, and patients with various types of cancer and malignant lymphoma. They observed positive responses to DNFB in only 2 of 19 patients with malignant lymphomas (11 percent), as contrasted with 12 of 16 (75 percent) in healthy controls.

Aisenberg (1962) was the first to attempt a systematic correlation between disease activity and immunologic responsiveness to DNCB in Hodgkin's disease. He studied a series of 37 patients, in 25 of whom the disease was active. Anergy to DNCB was demonstrated in all of 40 tests in the 25 patients with active cases, despite the fact that 14 were rated as being in good to excellent general health at the time of testing, and the disease was apparently localized (stage I or stage II) in 8. In contrast, 14 of the 20 tests performed on patients with inactive disease were positive, one was equivocal, and only 5 were negative (anergic). Of particular interest was the observation of the transition from anergy to normal reactivity in two patients after they had been in remission following local radiotherapy for a period of more than two years, and the reverse transition back to the anergic state concomitantly with the development of relapse in one of these. Aisenberg concluded that the immunologic defect manifested by anergy to DNCB and other delayed hypersensitivity antigens is an early manifestation of Hodgkin's disease and is closely correlated with disease activity.

Unfortunately, these early studies were carried out prior to the availability of lymphangiography and thus could not be correlated reliably with clinical stage. Several series of patients have now been studied with the DNCB technique after careful clinical staging with the aid of lymphangiography and other modern diagnostic procedures. In striking contrast to all of the earlier reports, Brown et al. (1967) observed positive responses to sensitization with DNCB at a concentration of 2.0 percent (2,000 μg/0.1 ml) in 35 (70 percent) of 50 patients with previously untreated Hodgkin's disease. These response rates remained substantially unchanged after the study had been extended to encompass a total of 103 patients (Young et al., 1972,

1973b). Most of the patients who responded to DNCB also reacted to one or more of a series of intradermal natural antigens (Table 6.1). Nonetheless, the incidence of anergy to DNCB was significantly greater among patients than among controls. However, inasmuch as all of their eight patients with documented stage I disease reacted positively to DNCB and seven of the eight reacted to at least one intradermal antigen, the Bethesda group suggested that the development of anergy is probably a secondarily acquired manifestation associated with advancing anatomic extent of involvement, rather than a concomitant of the initial phase of Hodgkin's disease.

A series of 185 patients in whom the disease was similarly evaluated and staged were tested with 2.0 percent DNCB at Stanford University Medical Center from 1964 through 1968 (Kaplan, 1970). An extremely high incidence of anergy to DNCB was observed, even in patients with stage I disease (Table 6.6). At the same sensitizing concentration (2.0 percent), negative reactions to challenge with DNCB were observed by De Gast, Halie, and Nieweg (1975) in 20 of 30 patients (67 percent), including 2 of 5 with stage I disease, and by Case et al. (1976a) in 24 of 50 patients (48 percent), including 3 of 8 with stage I disease.

Careful comparison of the technical details of the test procedure, as performed at Bethesda, at Stanford, and by Aisenberg, revealed a number of differences in the sensitizing dose, the locus of sensitization, the challenge dose, and the time interval to challenge, some of which may well have accounted for the differences in results observed in these three series. However, there was one other important difference: none of the Bethesda patients had received either radiotherapy or chemo-

Table 6.6   DNCB Responses versus Clinical Stage in Hodgkin's Disease

Stage	Total no. tested	Positive reactions	
		No.	%
I	33	12	36
II	87	15	17
III	40	4	10
IV	25	2	8
Totals:	185	33	18

Source: Data of first Stanford University Medical Center series (Kaplan, 1970). Patients were sensitized with 2% DNCB, and challenged on the opposite arm three or more weeks later with 0.1% DNCB.

therapy prior to the time of sensitization, and 43 of them were also challenged prior to treatment. Although sensitization was also routinely performed prior to treatment in most of the Stanford patients, many of them had received a substantial fraction of their planned course of radiotherapy at the time of first challenge. Evidence discussed in a later section of this chapter strongly suggests that the high incidence of anergy to DNCB observed in this series of patients might well have been due, at least in part, to the effects of local radiotherapy.

Accordingly, a new series of biopsy-proved, previously untreated patients with Hodgkin's disease, in whom staging was accomplished with the aid of lymphangiography and laparotomy with splenectomy and para-aortic node and liver biopsy, have been studied with a modified technique aimed at enhancing the sensitivity of the DNCB response. A battery of intradermal, natural antigens was used simultaneously as before. Patients were assigned at random to one of three different sensitizing concentrations of DNCB: 100, 500, and 2,000 $\mu g/0.1$ ml (0.1, 0.5, and 2.0 percent). All sensitizations and intradermal antigen tests were performed prior to treatment; the initial challenge with two different doses of DNCB (0.1 and 0.01 percent) was applied after an interval of about two weeks and, as in the Bethesda studies, prior to the initiation of radiotherapy. The results observed in a series of 84 consecutive patients (Table 6.7) indicate that the 0.5 percent sensitizing dose is able to

reveal minor degrees of immune deficiency that are likely to be masked at the 2.0 percent concentration (Eltringham and Kaplan, 1973). This is most clearly evident in patients with localized (stage IA and IIA) disease: whereas 10 (67 percent) of 15 such patients responded at the 2.0 percent level (a response rate not significantly different from that observed by the Bethesda group), only 4 (25 percent) of 16 patients responded after sensitization with 0.5 percent DNCB. Overall, only 10 (26 percent) of 39 patients with Hodgkin's disease of all stages responded to the lower DNCB sensitizing dose, a response rate very significantly lower ($p < 0.001$) than that in healthy young adult controls (24 of 29, or 83 percent).

Data on a new Stanford series of 531 consecutive previously untreated patients of all stages are presented in Table 6.8. In general, these results confirm the earlier findings of Eltringham and Kaplan (1973). However, the much larger study population permits the detection of modest but highly significant differences in response as a function of the extent of disease and the presence or absence of constitutional symptoms. Thus, there were 113 positive responses (36.3 percent) among the 311 patients with stages I and II as contrasted with 56 positive responses (25.5 percent) among the 220 patients with stages III and IV ($\chi_1^2 = 7.02$, $p < 0.01$). Among the asymptomatic patients, 128 of 355 (36.1 percent) responded, as compared with 41 (23.3 percent) of 176 patients with constitu-

Table 6.7   Response of Normal Control Subjects and Patients with Untreated Hodgkin's Disease to Intradermal Antigens and to Different Concentrations of Dinitrochlorobenzene (DNCB)

Group and stage (Stanford, 1970)	No. positive/No. tested		
	0.1% concentration[a]	0.5% concentration	2.0% concentration
Controls	3/16 (19)[b]	24/29 (83)	26/27 (97)
Stages IA, IIA, II$_E$A	0/5 —	4/16 (25)	10/15 (67)
IIB, II$_E$B	— —	1/5 (20)	1/8 (12)
IIIA, III$_S$A, III$_E$A	0/6 —	2/6 (33)	2/4 (50)
IIIB, III$_S$B, III$_{ES}$B	0/3 —	2/8 (25)	— —
IVA, IVB	0/2 —	1/4 (25)	0/2 —
Subtotals, all A's	0/12 (0)	6/22 (27)	12/19 (63)
Subtotals, all B's	0/4 (0)	4/17 (24)	1/10 (10)
Totals	0/16 (0)	10/39 (26)	13/29 (45)

Source: Stanford University Medical Center data (Eltringham and Kaplan, 1973).

[a] A randomizing procedure was used to allocate patients to one of three different sensitizing concentrations of DNCB. Challenge concentrations were 0.1% and 0.01%; the lower concentration gave very few positive reactions and has been omitted from the data presented here. Both sensitization and challenge were performed before initiation of treatment in all cases.

[b] Number of positive reactions/number treated and (percent positive). The differences in response rates of patients and controls at the 0.5% and 2.0% sensitizing concentrations of DNCB are highly significant ($p = < .01$).

Table 6.8   Response to First DNCB Challenge in Untreated Patients with Hodgkin's Disease

Stage	No. negative	No. positive	Total no. tested	Percent positive
IA	33	21		
I_EA	—	—		
IB	1	2		
I_EB	1	—		
All I's	35	23	58	39.7
IIA	85	65		
II_EA	23	9		
$II_{ES}A$	1	—		
II_SA	—	2		
All IIA's	109	76	185	41.1
IIB	40	9		
II_EB	13	3		
$II_{ES}B$	—	—		
II_SB	1	2		
All IIB's	54	14	68	20.6
All II's (A + B)	163	90	253	35.6
IIIA	8	6		
III_EA	1	1		
$III_{ES}A$	7	2		
III_SA	54	20		
All IIIA's	70	29	99	29.3
IIIB	7	2		
III_EB	5	1		
$III_{ES}B$	9	1		
III_SB	30	10		
All IIIB's	51	14	65	21.5
All IIIB's (A + B)	121	43	164	26.2
IVA	15	2	17	11.8
IVB	28	11	39	28.2
All IV's	43	13	56	23.2
All Cases	362	169	531	31.8
All A's	227	128	355	36.1
All B's	135	41	176	23.3

$\left.\begin{array}{l}\text{All A's } 36.1 \\ \text{All B's } 23.3\end{array}\right\} \chi^2_{(1)} = 8.53,\ p < .01$

Source: Stanford University Medical Center data (Kaplan); DNCB sensitizing concentration 500 μg/0.1 ml (0.5%); challenge concentration 100 μg/0.1 ml (0.1%) applied approximately 14 days later.

tional symptoms ($\chi_1^2 = 8.53$, $p < 0.01$). The fact that intradermal skin tests with SK-SD (Table 6.5) also revealed a dose-dependent difference in reactivity lends weight to the view that the impairment of cell-mediated immune reactions, such as delayed hypersensitivity, in patients with Hodgkin's disease is not an all-or-none phenomenon, but a more subtle, continuous gradient of immunologic deficit which is present, in some degree, even in patients with earliest manifestations of the disease.

Passive Transfer of Hypersensitivity. It has been known for some years that sensitivity to tuberculin can be transferred from one individual to another by the injection of living white blood cells from the sensitized donor (Lawrence, 1949). This technique was successfully utilized by Urbach et al. (1952) to induce tuberculin reactivity in six tuberculin-negative patients with sarcoidosis. The Minnesota group (Kelly et al., 1960; Good et al., 1962) were the first to attempt cellular transfer to patients with

Hodgkin's disease from donors sensitive to various microbial antigens or to DNCB. Using donors whose blood type matched that of the recipients, they injected the white blood cells from 500 ml. of blood subcutaneously into normal subjects and patients with Hodgkin's disease. The recipients were then challenged with the corresponding antigen 48 hours later. Whereas such transfers were successful in 22 of 23 normal individuals, they failed in all of the 13 patients with Hodgkin's disease.

Fazio and Calciati (1962) injected approximately 0.5 ml. of packed buffy coat white blood cells from known tuberculin-sensitive donors, diluted 1:10 with saline and injected partly intradermally and partly subcutaneously into 7 patients with Hodgkin's disease and 10 normal subjects, all of whom had previously been shown to be tuberculin negative. Both groups were challenged 18 to 24 hours later with 0.05 mg. of old tuberculin intradermally, and the reaction was scored after 24 hours. Tuberculin sensitivity was successfully transferred to all of the 10 normal subjects but to only 1 of the 7 patients with Hodgkin's disease, the one exception being a feeble reaction. Similar tests were performed by Rodriguez Paradisi et al. (1969), who reported successful transfer of tuberculin sensitivity in only one of four patients with far-advanced Hodgkin's disease. Müftüoğlu and Balkuv (1967) injected an average total of 30×10^6 lymphocytes subcutaneously into each of 44 recipients. They succeeded in converting 9 of 10 normal subjects and 9 of 12 others with cancer, leukemia, or lymphosarcoma. In striking contrast, only 1 of 22 patients with Hodgkin's disease developed a positive tuberculin reaction after cellular transfer. Somewhat greater success has been claimed by Khan et al. (1975) in the passive transfer of responsiveness to patients with Hodgkin's disease in remission by injection of transfer factor from normal donors. Paradoxically, R. A. Smith et al. (1973) reported that transfer factor prepared from the peripheral blood leukocytes of a tuberculin-positive patient with inactive Hodgkin's disease succeeded, whereas transfer factor from a normal tuberculin-positive donor failed in converting the peripheral blood lymphocytes from three tuberculin skin test–negative patients with Hodgkin's disease to tuberculin-positive responses in vitro, using the macrophage migration inhibition assay.

An interesting, though as yet unconfirmed, extension of the passive transfer approach has been reported by Han (1973, 1974). He extracted ribonucleic acid (RNA) by the hot phenol method from the peripheral blood lymphocytes or spleen cells of three donors: one normal individual (B.D.), with strongly positive SK-SD, monilia, and mumps skin test responses; a patient with stage II Hodgkin's disease in remission (G.D.), who had become tuberculin skin test–positive after BCG vaccination; and a patient (P.M.) with active stage II Hodgkin's disease and positive skin tests for SK-SD and mumps. All three donors were trichophyton skin test–negative. The extracted "immune" RNA, after dilution and sterilization, was injected intradermally into 24 patients with Hodgkin's disease (19 in remission and 5 with active disease, 2 of whom were receiving concurrent chemotherapy), as well as 20 patients with other types of malignant neoplasms. Skin test responses were converted to positivity to tuberculin in all of the 13 tuberculin-negative patients with Hodgkin's disease who received "immune" RNA from donor G.D. RNA from donor B.D. or P.M. succeeded in converting the SK-SD, monilia, and mumps responses in 7 of 9, 3 of 7, and 3 of 5 patients, respectively. Serial tests on 4 successfully converted patients revealed that the converted state disappeared quickly in 1, but persisted for one to five months or longer in the other 3. Some indication of specificity of the responses was inferred from the fact that none of the patients were concurrently converted to trichophyton positivity. Ribonuclease treatment of "immune" RNA reportedly abolished its capacity to transfer tuberculin reactivity in three patients, whereas RNA incubated with deoxyribonuclease (to which RNA is insensitive) remained active when tested in two patients.

Delayed Homograft Rejection

The capacity of organisms to reject grafts of foreign tissues is an immunologic response which shares with delayed hypersensitivity the property of being mediated by cells rather than by humoral antibody. It is thus not surprising that the immunologic defect in Hodgkin's disease is also expressed as a decreased capacity for homograft rejection. Kelly et al. (1958) applied full-thickness skin homografts in 15 patients and observed normal rejection in only 3 instances. Delayed rejection was observed in two of their cases, partial survival of the graft for an indefinite period of time in eight, and complete acceptance of the graft in two. Green and Corso (1958) observed delayed skin homograft rejection in four patients with Hodgkin's disease, as well as in two with lymphosarcoma and two with leukemia.

In a subsequent study, Green et al. (1960) investigated the hypothesis that Hodgkin's disease might stem from a maternal-to-fetal lymphocyte chimera, with the resultant induction of a chronic autoimmune disease state in the immunologically tolerant fetus. They applied skin grafts from the mothers of five patients with Hodgkin's disease, as well as from three unrelated donors of the same blood type as the patients with Hodgkin's disease. Although a prolonged graft survival was observed in four of their five cases, interpretation is clouded by the fact that some of their patients had received extensive radiotherapy or chemotherapy.

Miller, Lizardo, and Snyderman (1961) observed that the survival time of skin homografts was normal in six and prolonged in five other patients with Hodgkin's disease. Colombani et al. (1964) attempted to relate skin-graft survival in 12 normal subjects and in 6 patients with Hodgkin's disease to the leukocyte antigens of the donors and recipients. They observed a significantly prolonged survival time of both the most incompatible and the most compatible homografts in the patients relative to that in their normal controls.

A lymphocyte transfer technique has been developed to screen donor-recipient histocompatibility prior to organ transplantation (Gray and Russell, 1963). This is an appreciably more complex immunologic reaction than the cellular transfer of tuberculin hypersensitivity and is believed to involve reciprocal graft-versus-host and host-versus-graft reactions by immunocompetent lymphocytes (Brent and Medawar, 1964). Aisenberg (1965a),

using a slight modification of the technique of Gray and Russell, studied a total of 85 transfers of peripheral blood lymphocytes from normal individuals and patients with Hodgkin's disease into recipients with and without Hodgkin's disease. Most of the Hodgkin's disease patients were the same patients reported on in his earlier DNCB study (Aisenberg, 1962). A summary of Aisenberg's observations at 2, 7, and 11 to 14 days after cellular transfer is presented in Table 6.9. He concluded that the intracutaneous reaction of lymphocytes from donors with Hodgkin's disease is only slightly impaired relative to that of lymphocytes of normal donors at 48 hours but markedly depressed at 7 days and again at 11 to 14 days. Moreover, recipients with Hodgkin's disease had a distinct prolongation of the cutaneous transfer reaction induced by lymphocytes from normal donors, analogous to a delayed homograft rejection reaction. These studies suggest that the immunologic defect may be a complex phenomenon which resides not only in the immunologic effector cell (the lymphocyte) but also in host factors which remain to be identified.

Unfortunately, most of the patients studied in these reports were not rigorously characterized with respect to clinical stage and some had received prior or concurrent radiotherapy and/or chemotherapy. Accordingly, although the limited homograft data available to date are generally consistent with the results of delayed hypersensitivity testing, they add little to the information provided by the studies described in the preceding sections.

Table 6.9 Lymphocyte Transfer Reactions

Donor	Recipient	Time	Number of transfers	Number of patients with diameter of induration of:			
				0–2 mm.	3–5 mm.	>5 mm.	Average mm.
Normal	Non-Hodgkin's disease	48 hours	14	2	7	5	5.5
		7 days	14	1	3	10	5.1
		11–14 days	9	7	0	2	1.4
Normal	Hodgkin's disease	48 hours	33	6	10	17	5.0
		7 days	31	1	11	19	6.6
		11–14 days	22	6	2	14	4.6
Hodgkin's disease	Non-Hodgkin's disease	48 hours	10	1	4	5	5.5
		7 days	10	7	1	2	1.7
		11–14 days	7	7	0	0	0
Hodgkin's disease	Hodgkin's disease	48 hours	22	9	7	6	3.7
		7 days	21	16	2	3	1.6
		11–14 days	14	14	0	0	0

Source: Data of Aisenberg (1965a).

Tests In Vitro of Cell-mediated Immunity

Although procedures in vivo such as delayed hypersensitivity skin tests and homograft rejection studies have the merit of direct relevance to the assessment of cell-mediated immunity, they also suffer from certain serious disadvantages. They may elicit unsightly and even uncomfortable skin reactions which limit the frequency with which they can be serially repeated. They do not lend themselves to the quantitative discrimination of fine differences in degree of response. Finally, the underlying mechanisms of the immunologic deficit cannot be studied in vivo. Accordingly, investigators have sought to exploit certain lymphocyte responses in vitro as analogs or correlates of cell-mediated immune function. Among the most important of these responses are lymphoblastoid transformation induced by plant lectins and other mitogens, the mixed lymphocyte reaction, surface membrane receptor-specific binding of sheep erythrocytes (rosette formation), and the capacity of lymphocytes to bind and to become agglutinated by certain lectins and to mediate their polar migration ("capping") and shedding from the cell membrane. The application of these tests in vitro to the study of patients with Hodgkin's disease has provided a wealth of new data, some of it conflicting and difficult to interpret, but generally contributing toward a better understanding of the situation and opening the way to systematic investigation of underlying mechanisms.

Lymphoblastoid Transformation. Small lymphocytes from the peripheral blood may be induced to undergo morphologic transformation to blast-like, DNA-synthesizing, mitotically active cells after incubation in vitro with plant lectins such as phytohemagglutinin (PHA), concanavalin A (Con A), and pokeweed mitogen (PWM); with antigens such as tuberculin or vaccinia; and with antigenically foreign cells (Nowell, 1960; Elves et al., 1963; Pearmain et al., 1963; Lycette and Pearmain, 1963; Hirschhorn et al., 1963). This response provides an additional parameter with which to assess the functional state of small circulating lymphocytes from patients with Hodgkin's disease and, as such, has been studied by a number of investigators, most of whom have used either morphologic transformation or the incorporation of tritiated thymidine (^{3}H-TdR) into lymphocyte DNA as the measured endpoint. Stimulation by PHA and Con A is apparently selective for T-lymphocytes, whereas PWM primarily affects B-lymphocytes (Janossy and Greaves, 1972).

Hersh and Oppenheim (1965b) studied a total of 23 patients with biopsy-proved Hodgkin's disease, in all but 1 of whom the disease was clinically active at the time of study. Eleven patients with negative lymphangiograms were designated as having stage II disease, and the remaining 12 had stage III disease. Twelve of the patients had one or more constitutional symptoms. Although 12 patients had received prior chemotherapy, all had been without therapy for periods of two weeks to 72 months. A series of 35 control subjects, including 16 normal individuals and 19 patients with acute leukemia in complete remission, were similarly studied.

There was a striking impairment in the capacity of peripheral blood lymphocytes from patients with Hodgkin's disease to undergo lymphoblastoid transformation after incubation in vitro with PHA or vaccinia. Among the controls, transformation was observed in the PHA-stimulated cultures in a median of 70 percent of the lymphocytes, with a range of values from about 58 to 84 percent. In contrast, the median value in the patients with Hodgkin's disease was only 11 percent, and only 4 of the 29 sets of cultures from these 23 patients showed values overlapping the normal range. Moreover, whereas a median of 1.5 percent of the PHA-stimulated lymphocytes from control subjects were in mitosis, the median mitotic response in lymphocytes from patients with Hodgkin's disease was 0 percent. All differences between the patient and the control cultures were statistically significant at the 1 percent level.

Hersh and Oppenheim also observed that unstimulated lymphocyte cultures from patients with Hodgkin's disease died more rapidly than those from normal controls. After incubation for five days, only 29 percent of the cells in the unstimulated cultures from the patients were morphologically intact, as compared with a median of 56 percent among the controls.

Since a number of the patients with Hodgkin's disease had significant lymphocytopenia, seven sets of cultures were carried out with concentrated preparations of their peripheral blood lymphocytes, separated from the other white blood cells by the glass bead column technique. Culture of these lymphocyte preparations with PHA yielded essentially the same abnormal results as before, the percentage of transformed cells ranging from 0 to 65 percent, with a median of 29 percent. When the patient's cells were washed and cultured in calf serum, rather than in autologous plasma, the transformation response was not restored to normal. Conversely, resuspension of washed cells from a normal subject in the plasma of patients with Hodgkin's disease who showed impaired transformation did not interfere with the blastoid transformation response of the normal cells in two of three cases, but killed all of the normal cells in the third instance. Han (1972) observed no inhibitory effect on PHA-stimulated transformation of normal lymphocytes after incubation in sera from patients with Hodgkin's disease (with the exception of the sera from a few patients who were currently receiving cytotoxic chemotherapy for active disease).

These last observations are in disagreement with those reported by Trubowitz et al. (1966), who found that the capacity for lymphoblastoid transformation of lymphocytes from 13 patients with Hodgkin's disease was defective relative to that of normal lymphocytes but was somewhat improved when they were cultured in normal plasma (median, 40 percent) instead of autologous plasma (median, 23 percent). Moreover, control cells cultured in plasma from patients with Hodgkin's disease showed a somewhat diminished capacity for lymphoblastoid transformation relative to that of the same cells cultured in normal plasma, the difference being of borderline significance.

Several other groups (Sartoris et al., 1965; Holm et al., 1967; Lawler et al., 1967; Thomas et al., 1967; Libánský, et al., 1973; Gallmeier et al., 1973; Rühl et al., 1974; Winkelstein et al., 1974) have also observed impaired blastoid responses of lymphocytes from patients with Hodgkin's disease. Sartoris et al. (1965) found a close correlation between the capacity of lymphocytes from patients with Hodgkin's disease to respond to tuberculin stimulation in vitro and the tuberculin skin test reaction of those patients. Cavallero et al. (1966) found a similar correlation between the tuberculin skin reaction of patients with Hodgkin's disease and the response of their lymphocytes to stimulation with PHA. Gotoff et al. (1973) observed positive lymphoblastoid responses to *Candida* in 2 patients with Hodgkin's disease who were *Candida* skin test–positive, whereas 12 other patients, who were *Candida* and PPD skin test–negative, showed no response in the antigen stimulation assay in vitro. However, many of their patients were receiving radiation therapy or chemotherapy at the time of the study.

Aisenberg (1965c) utilized the incorporation of ^{14}C-labeled thymidine into the DNA of lymphocytes cultured in the presence of PHA, PPD, or foreign cells as the index of immunogenic, blastoid stimulation in vitro. Normal lymphocyte cultures showed a 50- to 300-fold increase in the rate of in-

corporation of thymidine in response to PHA. Among the 10 patients with Hodgkin's disease whose lymphocytes were similarly studied, responses to the three different stimuli were somewhat variable. Only 4 of the 10 showed normal reactivity to PHA, and only 1 reacted well to stimulation with PPD. Overall, the reactions of lymphocytes from 5 of the 10 anergic patients with Hodgkin's disease were clearly depressed, and responses were borderline in 1 other instance.

An intriguing, though as yet unconfirmed, study was reported by Fazio and Bachi (1967), who incubated lymphocyte cultures from seven anergic and two normo-responsive patients with Hodgkin's disease with PHA alone, PHA plus ribonucleic acid (RNA) extracted from biopsies of normal human lymphoid tissue, both added simultaneously, and PHA followed by the addition of RNA 24 hours later. As in earlier reports, the percentage of cells stimulated to blastoid transformation was normal in the two tuberculin-positive patients and was significantly depressed in all of the seven tuberculin-negative patients, whether or not RNA was added concurrently with PHA. However, when PHA was added first and RNA from normal human lymphoid tissue was added 24 hours later, the response of all seven lymphocyte cultures from tuberculin-negative patients with Hodgkin's disease was restored to the normal range. Unfortunately, they did not utilize controls incubated with RNA from lymph nodes involved by Hodgkin's disease or RNA from normal nonlymphatic tissues.

The first study in which the capacity for lymphoblastoid transformation in vitro was correlated with clinical stage, routinely evaluated with the aid of lymphangiography, was that of Brown et al. (1967). The mean lymphocyte response to PHA was 49 percent in 43 patients with untreated Hodgkin's disease, a highly significant decrease from the 72 percent mean value among their controls. However, the blastoid responses of lymphocytes from patients with stage I disease were all within the normal range. Diminished responses were observed in a significant proportion of cases with disease of more advanced anatomic extent, with the poorest response among the stage IV patients. There was no obvious correlation with the histopathologic type of Hodgkin's disease observed in the initial biopsies, nor was the capacity of lymphocytes to undergo transformation in vitro correlated with peripheral lymphocyte count.

De Gast, Halie, and Nieweg (1975) also noted a stage-related impairment of response to PHA in a series of 30 patients with Hodgkin's disease. Whereas normal stimulation was observed with lymphocytes from all 5 of their patients with stage I and 6 of 9 with stage II disease, distinctly subnormal responses occurred in 5 of 9 patients with stage III, and 6 of 7 with stage IV disease. Moreover, lymphocyte stimulation by an antigen, α-hemocyanin, was impaired in 11 of 15 patients. It was of interest that the DNCB skin test reaction in vivo was negative in 10 (91 percent) of the 11 patients with an impaired response to α-hemocyanin, whereas the correlation between the DNCB and the PHA tests was poor. Lymphoblastoid responses to another antigen, tetanus toxoid, failed to occur in six of nine patients studied by Fuks et al. (1976b).

Certain modifications of technique, which have permitted more detailed analysis of the PHA stimulation response, have revealed unambiguous abnormalities even in a high proportion of patients with stage I disease. Matchett, Huang, and Kremer (1973) followed the kinetics of the PHA-stimulated uptake of ^{3}H-TdR as a function of time in the peripheral blood lymphocytes of a series of 26 untreated patients, all staged with the aid of lymphangiography and bone marrow biopsy, and compared these with similar data from 20 concurrent controls. Cells from patients with Hodgkin's disease often showed good early responses at 2–3 days, especially in stages I and II, but failed to sustain them through days 4 and 5. When the daily uptake of ^{3}H-TdR by limiting concentrations of cells was used as the index of transformation, all of the patients, including those with localized disease and no symptoms, showed a striking deficiency of the blood lymphocyte response. It was concluded that "impaired lymphocyte function is inherent to Hodgkin's disease and is not a complication of far-advanced and extensive disease only." However, the great complexity of the situation is evident from the fact that response to another plant lectin, PWM, was normal in several of the patients with an impaired PHA response, and that spleen lymphocytes, unlike those from peripheral blood, showed a greater than normal ^{3}H-TdR uptake after PHA stimulation, even when incubated in autologous plasma, suggesting that the spleen may store or sequester a subpopulation of PHA-responsive T-lymphocytes. In contrast, Cohnen et al. (1973c) noted parallel (and generally impaired) responses to both PHA and PWM in 7 of 8 patients with Hodgkin's disease.

Levy and Kaplan (1974) investigated the stimulation by PHA of protein (instead of DNA) synthesis in peripheral blood lymphocytes. This assay system, which measures the uptake of tritiated leucine (^{3}H-Leu) into protein after incubation of cells with a range of concentrations of PHA, has one important advantage over the standard ^{3}H-TdR uptake assay: it is much faster, requiring only 20 hours for completion, so cell viability can be preserved in the absence of serum, a significant perturbing factor in the ^{3}H-TdR assay, with the result that precision and reproducibility are enhanced. Levy and Kaplan studied 37 normal subjects and 44 consecutive untreated patients with Hodgkin's disease staged with lymphangiography, bone marrow biopsy, and (in those with negative marrow biopsies) laparotomy with splenectomy. Stimulation of normal donor lymphocytes was strongly PHA concentration-dependent, with a peak at 1 μg/ml. The response of lymphocytes from the patients was very significantly lower than normal ($p < 0.01$) at all but the highest PHA concentrations tested (Fig. 6.1). When the results were considered separately for patients with limited (stages I and II) versus advanced (stages III and IV) disease, a significantly greater degree of impairment ($p < 0.01$) was evident in the advanced group at all PHA concentrations from 1 to 10 μg/ml (Fig. 6.2). There was appreciable overlap of individual responses, and five patients (four with limited disease) had stimulation ratios at or above the mean for the normal donors. Nonetheless, 85 percent of patients with limited disease had stimulation ratios below the normal mean, and the mean for the entire limited-disease group was very significantly below normal ($p < 0.01$). Thus, as Eltringham and Kaplan (1973) had observed after the use of an optimized sensitizing dose of DNCB, the increased sensitivity and precision of this modified PHA stimulation assay was able to detect a defect in lymphocyte function even in patients with stage IA disease. These results remained unchanged after the study had been extended to include 132 patients with untreated Hodgkin's disease (Fuks et al., 1976b). Moreover, adaptation of the same assay method to stimulation by Con A revealed a similar impairment of response to that lectin in 18 patients. Levy and Kaplan (1974) observed that the correlation of the test results in vitro with those of concurrent DNCB and natural antigen skin tests was poor, suggesting that these tests may measure different aspects of the T-lymphocyte response, or may involve different subpopulations of lymphocytes. Several possible mechanisms were postulated for impaired lectin stimulation of lymphocytes from patients with Hodgkin's disease.

Independent confirmation of the existence of a concentration-dependent defect in lymphocyte response to PHA has been provided by other investigators. Ziegler, Hansen, and Penny (1975) studied

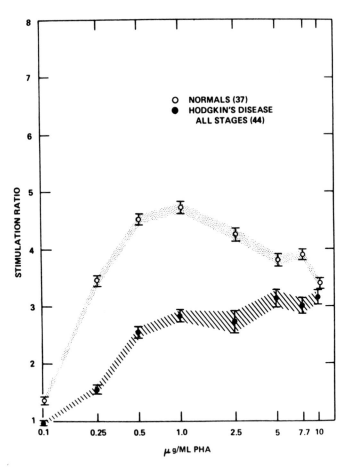

Figure 6.1 Phytohemagglutin (PHA) stimulation of protein synthesis in peripheral blood lymphocytes, expressed as the stimulation ratio—the ratio of ^{3}H-leucine counts per minute in the PHA-stimulated culture to counts per minute in the unstimulated control culture for each subject at each PHA concentration. The data from 37 normal controls and from 44 patients with Hodgkin's disease are pooled and presented as the mean ±S.E. at each PHA concentration. Stimulation ratios differ significantly ($p < 0.01$) at each PHA concentration up to 10 μg/ml. (Reprinted by permission of the *New England Journal of Medicine,* from the paper by Levy and Kaplan, 1974.)

27 similarly staged patients with untreated Hodgkin's disease, using a broad range of PHA concentrations in the conventional ^{3}H-TdR uptake assay. Two distinctive patterns of abnormality were observed: a reduced response at all doses of PHA, seen in 9 patients (33 percent), 6 of whom had advanced disease, and a reduced response evident only at low doses of PHA, seen in 7 additional patients (26 percent), 6 of whom had advanced disease. Impairment of the PHA response correlated well with both anergy and lymphocytopenia in their study. Faguet (1975) also reported significant

impairment of the blastoid response over the concentration range 1.6–6.4 μg PHA-protein per 10^6 lymphocytes in a series of 35 patients with untreated Hodgkin's disease; deficient responses were noted in 74 percent of these, including many of those with localized (stage I and II) disease. There was some correlation with skin test response in vivo: 91 percent of anergic patients failed to respond normally to PHA, whereas only 50 percent of those with positive reactions to one or more of the skin test antigens failed to do so. Case et al. (1976a) also observed impaired lymphocyte re-

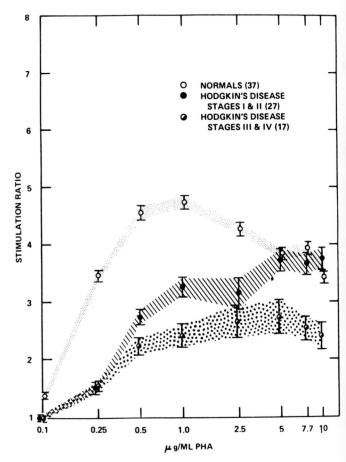

Figure 6.2 Phytohemagglutinin (PHA) stimulation ratios (means ±S.E.) of lymphocytes from normal subjects, patients with Hodgkin's disease stages I and II, and patients with Hodgkin's disease stages III and IV. Significance of difference between normal and stages I and II is $p < 0.01$ at PHA concentrations of 0.1 to 2.5 μg/ml; between normal and stages III and IV, $p < 0.01$ at concentrations of 0.1 to 10 μg/ml; and between stages I and II and III and IV, $p < 0.01$ at concentrations of 1.0, 5.0, 7.7, and 10.0 μg/ml. (Reprinted by permission of the *New England Journal of Medicine* from the paper by Levy and Kaplan, 1974.)

sponses to a range of concentrations of PHA, Con A, and PWM in 58 percent of a series of 52 untreated patients, including 15 (52 percent) of 29 with stage I and II disease.

In addition to their response to plant lectins, normal lymphocytes from sensitized donors also exhibit blastoid transformation responses to specific skin test antigens. Although such tests have been performed in relatively few patients with untreated Hodgkin's disease, the limited available data are again indicative of impairment of this type of cell-mediated immune response. Gaines, Gilmer, and Remington (1973) found that the lymphocytes of 3 patients with positive *Toxoplasma* dye test titers, as well as those of 20 with negative

titers, failed to respond to *Toxoplasma* antigen in vitro (Fig. 6.3). The same investigators noted negative lymphoblastoid transformation responses to SK-SD in vitro in the lymphocytes from 22 of 23 untreated patients, including all 6 of those with positive skin test reactions to 5 or 50 units of the antigen (Fig. 6.4). In contrast, Holm et al. (1976) noted a close correlation between the lymphoblastoid response to 2.5 μg tuberculin (PPD) and the skin test reaction to tuberculin in vivo in a series of 31 patients with Hodgkin's disease. Only 1 of the

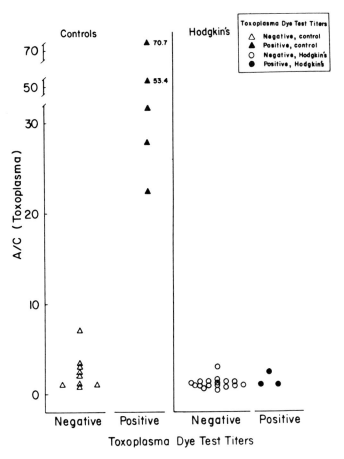

Figure 6.3 Impaired lymphocyte transformation responses to *Toxoplasma* antigen in Hodgkin's disease. Note that the antigen/control (A/C) stimulation ratios for all three patients with positive *Toxoplasma* dye test titers were in the same range as those of patients and normal individuals with negative titers, whereas the responses of five normal controls with positive dye test titers were all markedly elevated. (Reprinted by permission from the paper by Gaines, Gilmer, and Remington, 1973.)

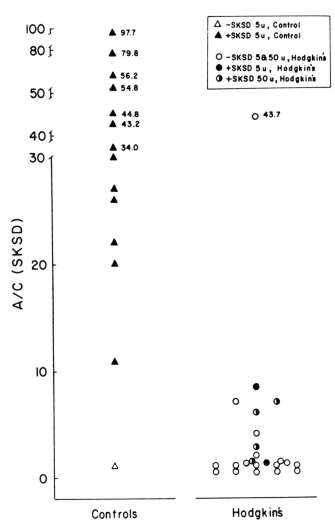

Figure 6.4 Impaired lymphocyte transformation responses to SK-SD in Hodgkin's disease. Note that the antigen/control (A/C) stimulation ratios of all but one of the 23 patients were in the range 0–10, whereas the A/C ratios of all but 2 of the 14 normal controls exceeded 20. Several of the patients failed to respond even to a tenfold increase in antigen concentration. (Reprinted by permission from the paper by Gaines, Gilmer, and Remington, 1973.)

12 PPD skin test–positive patients had an impaired lymphocyte response to the antigen in vitro; conversely, only 1 of 19 patients who were skin test–negative had a normal lymphoblastoid response to PPD. There was a further correlation between the mean diameter of the skin reaction and the level of incorporation of ^{14}C-TdR in lymphocytes stimulated by 2.5 μg PPD. Of interest was the fact that impairment of response was relatively independent of stage. Thus, deficient responses in vitro to PPD were observed in 7 (47 percent) of 15 patients with stage I and II disease, and in 11 (55 percent) of 20 patients with stage III and IV disease. Normal lymphocyte responses in vitro to PPD and to streptolysin 0 had previously been reported by Heine and Stobbe (1967), but the fact that 17 of the 20 patients they studied had previously been treated with radiation, drugs, or both, clouds the interpretation of their data.

Mixed Lymphocyte Reaction. The lymphoblastoid and cytotoxic reactions observed when lymphocytes from genetically different donors are mixed (Hirschhorn et al., 1963) are generally regarded as analogs in vitro of the lymphocyte transfer reaction. The mixed lymphocyte reaction (MLR) is therefore widely used to screen potential organ transplant donors. Lang et al. (1972, 1974) reported that peripheral blood lymphocytes from 2 (22 percent) of 11, and later, 7 (22 percent) of 32 untreated patients yielded negative MLR tests. Rühl et al. (1975) found that the capacity of lymphocytes from 30 patients with Hodgkin's disease to respond in the MLR test was significantly impaired, whereas their capacity to stimulate responses by normal lymphocytes was intact or only slightly reduced. In contrast, Björkholm et al. (1975c) found that the stimulatory capacity of lymphocytes from 39 untreated patients with Hodgkin's disease was severely impaired, whereas their mean capacity to respond was not significantly different from that of normal controls, although impaired responses were noted with lymphocytes from 10 of the 39 patients. The same group (Holm et al., 1975) also studied another parameter of lymphocyte response to foreign cells in vitro. They found that the capacity of lymphocytes from 23 untreated patients to lyse foreign cells in the presence of PHA or of specific antibodies to the foreign cells was impaired in some patients but was higher than normal in others. There was some degree of correlation with the percentage of lymphocytes bearing receptors for complement. Twomey et al. (1976) studied 12 patients

with Hodgkin's disease, of whom 5 had been previously treated and 1 other was cachectic (group A), and the remaining 6 (group B) were untreated and in good to fair general condition. Lymphocytes from all 6 patients in group A and 1 patient in group B failed to stimulate normal lymphocytes in the one-way MLR test. Fuks et al. (1976b) tested lymphocytes from nine untreated patients (three stage IA, two IIA, two IIB, one IIIA, and one IIIB) as stimulator cells in one-way MLR assays with responder cells from unrelated normal individuals and observed positive responses in eight instances (89 percent). However, five of these responses were only weakly positive. Conversely, the peripheral blood lymphocytes of these patients were found to respond adequately when stimulated either by normal donor cells or by cells from other patients with Hodgkin's disease; positive reactions were observed in 20 (95 percent) of 21 such random combinations (Fig. 6.5). Thus, although the number of patients in whom the mixed lymphocyte reaction has been studied is still rather small, the capacity of lymphocytes from untreated patients (except perhaps for those with far-advanced disease or cachexia) to stimulate and/or to respond to lymphocytes from other, unrelated individuals in the one-way MLR test appears to be within normal limits or only slightly impaired.

E-Rosette Formation. The binding of uncoated, antibody-coated, or antibody plus complement-coated sheep erythrocytes to specific surface membrane receptors of different subpopulations of lymphocytes to form E-, EA-, and EAC-rosettes, respectively, has been discussed in the section on surface markers in Chapter 3. The capacity to form spontaneous (nonimmune) E-rosettes appears to be a specific property of human T-lymphocytes, which possess a surface membrane receptor with binding affinity for uncoated sheep erythrocytes (Fröland, 1972; Jondal, Holm, and Wigzell, 1972; Wybran, Carr, and Fudenberg, 1972). Human T-lymphocytes also possess specific surface membrane differentiation antigens which react in cytotoxic assays with appropriately absorbed anti-human thymocyte sera (R. W. Smith et al., 1973; Bobrove et al., 1974). When the E-rosette test and the cytotoxic assay were both applied to Ficoll-Hypaque gradient purified suspensions of peripheral blood mononuclear cells from the same normal donors (Table 6.10), the percentages of T-lymphocytes determined by the two methods were consistently in very close agreement (Bobrove et al., 1975).

Figure 6.5 Mixed lymphocyte reaction (MLR) of peripheral blood lymphocytes from various combinations of normal individuals and patients with untreated and treated Hodgkin's disease. The data express the activity of ³H-thymidine incorporated into the cells per culture. The striped area indicates the control nonresponder ranges. (Reprinted, by permission of the *Journal of Clinical Investigation,* from the paper by Fuks et al., 1976b.)

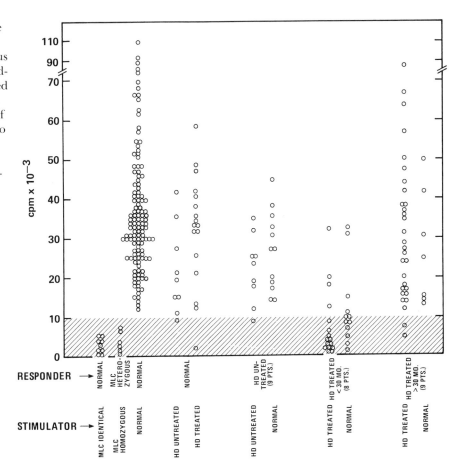

Table 6.10 Comparison of the Cytotoxic Antibody Assay and the E-Rosette Assay for Estimating Peripheral Blood T-Lymphocytes in Normal Individuals

Donors	% cytotoxicity	% E rosettes
1	66	75
2	70	65
3	66	59
4	60	50
5	54	34
6	65	49
7	55	62
8	45	46
9	70	65
10	49	50
11	68	64
12	53	55
13	65	60
14	70	64
15	53	64
16	70	71
	61 ± 2.1[a,b]	58 ± 2.6[b]

Source: Bobrove et al. (1975).

[a] Mean ± S.E.

[b] Not significantly different.

Bobrove et al. (1975) then used the E-rosette and cytotoxic assays to assess T-lymphocyte levels in 15 untreated patients with Hodgkin's disease, all but 2 of whom exhibited a lower percentage of E-rosette-forming cells (E-RFC) than the percentage detected by the cytotoxic assay (Table 6.11). The mean percentage of E-RFC in these 15 patients (42 ± 3.9 percent) was very significantly lower ($p < .01$) than the mean percentage of T-lymphocytes (63 ± 2.9 percent) estimated by the cytotoxic assay. Essentially the same results were obtained after this Stanford study had been extended to include a total of 98 normal donors and 127 consecutive patients with untreated Hodgkin's disease (Fuks et al., 1976d). The mean normal E-RFC level was 64.8 percent, with 95 percent confidence limits of 52 and 78 percent. In the patients, the mean E-RFC value (51.5 percent) was very significantly lower than normal ($p < 0.01$). Moreover, individual E-RFC values for 63 (49 percent) of the 127 patients were more than two standard deviations below the mean for normal donors. The distribution of such low E-RFC levels by stage was: stage I, 6/11 (54 percent); stage II, 28/59 (47 percent);

Table 6.11 Discrepancy between the Cytotoxic Antibody Assay and the E-Rosette Test with Respect to Peripheral Blood T-Lymphocyte Levels in Untreated Patients with Hodgkin's Disease

Donors	% cytotoxicity	% E rosettes
1. IIA	63	30
2. IIA	62	65
3. IIA	70	24
4. IIA	69	51
5. IIA	72	74
6. IIB	51	29
7. IIB	48	38
8. IIB	47	38
9. IIB	62	35
10. IIIA	71	42
11. IIIA	69	18
12. IIIA	79	57
13. IIIB	47	36
14. IVA	57	49
15. IVA	80	46
	$63 \pm 2.9^{a,b}$	42 ± 3.9^{b}

Source: Bobrove et al. (1975).

[a] Mean ± S.E.

[b] Significantly different $(p < 0.01)$.

stage III, 20/38 (53 percent); and stage IV, 9/19 (47 percent), thus revealing no correlation with the clinical extent of disease. E-RFC levels were also unrelated to the presence or absence of constitutional symptoms.

Other investigators have reported data on E-RFC levels in Hodgkin's disease. Cohnen et al. (1973a), in a study of ten patients, noted decreased E-RFC levels in seven and borderline values in three. Fröland (1972) observed normal percentages of E-RFC in six patients with Hodgkin's disease, using a different method for the preparation of rosettes. However, essentially the same method was used in a study of 19 untreated patients by Andersen (1974), who found a significant decrease in the mean percentage of E-RFC as compared with the levels observed in 21 control subjects. There was again no evident correlation with either clinical stage or constitutional symptoms. Thus, these data suggest that T-lymphocyte number or function, or both, are decreased in patients with untreated Hodgkin's disease. This question is further elucidated in a series of clinical investigations described in the section on mechanisms of impairment of cell-mediated immunity later in this chapter.

A modification of the E-rosette test developed by Wybran, Carr, and Fudenberg (1972) apparently detects a subpopulation of T-lymphocytes with high affinity receptors for sheep erythrocytes, permitting the rapid formation of rosettes after centrifugation. Such cells are referred to as active rosette-forming cells (A-RFC). In a study of 27 patients with untreated Hodgkin's disease, Lang et al. (1977) found that A-RFC levels were within normal limits. This conclusion is supported by our own data from a study of 13 patients (Fig. 6.6).

Felsburg and Edelman (1977) have reported some interesting observations on increases in A-RFC levels after challenge with specific antigen, which correlated well with skin test responses to the corresponding antigen (PPD or tularemia) in a series of normal subjects. The mean increase in A-RFC levels in 14 skin test–positive individuals was 56.1 ± 13.8 percent, whereas in 5 skin test–negative individuals, the mean percentage change in A-RFC levels was -3.1 ± 4.3 percent. Seven individuals were tested with both antigens. All three of those who were skin test–negative to PPD and positive to tularemia antigen showed a marked increase in A-RFC values after challenge in vitro with tularemia antigen, and either no response or a slight decrease in A-RFC values after challenge with PPD. The other four subjects were skin test–positive to both antigens, and three responded in vitro with a striking increase in A-RFC after challenge with both antigens. However, the fourth of these subjects anomalously failed to respond to tularemia antigen and showed a decrease, rather than an increase, after challenge with PPD. Nonetheless, these data suggest that the increased A-RFC response after challenge with specific antigen may prove to be a particularly valuable test in vitro of cell-mediated immunity, since it appears to correlate with delayed hypersensitivity responses in vivo far more consistently than has been the experience with a number of other tests in vitro.

We have applied this test in patients with untreated Hodgkin's disease (D. P. King and H. S. Kaplan, unpublished). Prior to challenge with specific antigen, A-RFC levels have been consistently normal, even in patients whose total E-RFC values were significantly reduced. Data on response to specific antigen are still fragmentary, since such tests can be applied only to those patients with Hodgkin's disease who are skin test–positive to one or more intradermal antigens. With two exceptions (Fig. 6.6), all of the patients studied to date have revealed responses entirely consistent with those reported by Felsburg and Edelman; their A-RFC values have increased significantly in response to the antigen to which they had been previously shown to be skin test–positive and were unchanged after challenge with other antigens to

NORMAL DONORS

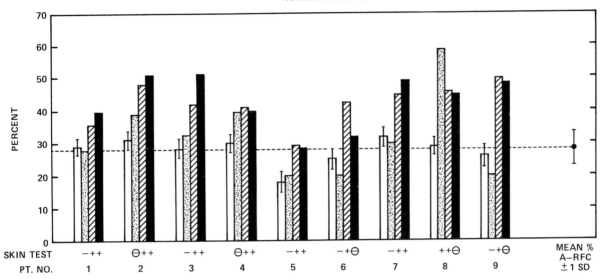

UNTREATED HODGKIN'S DISEASE DONORS

MEDIUM ONLY (±5%)
1 TU PPD ADDED   MEAN OF
0.5 CFU MUMPS ADDED   DUPLICATE CULTURES
1 U SKSD ADDED

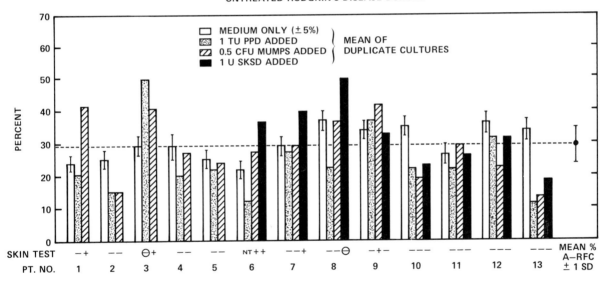

Figure 6.6 Active rosette-forming cells (A-RFC) in the peripheral blood of normal individuals and of patients with untreated Hodgkin's disease, tested after incubation with: (a) medium alone (control levels); (b) skin test antigens to which they had been shown positive (+) cutaneous responses; and (c) skin test antigens to which they had shown negative (−) cutaneous responses. Anomalous responses are circled. (Donna P. King and Henry S. Kaplan, unpublished data.)

which they were skin test–negative. The mechanism of the response is unknown, although Felsburg and Edelman have suggested the possibility that the antigen-specific lymphocytes release a soluble factor after contact with specific antigen which, in turn, is capable of altering the membrane receptors of other T-lymphocytes so that they also display an increased affinity for E-rosette formation with sheep erythrocytes. Studies in additional patients with Hodgkin's disease will be required to assess the practical usefulness of this test.

Other Responses In Vitro. Aggregation of guinea pig macrophages (peritoneal exudate cells) was observed after incubation with supernatant fluids from cultures of human peripheral blood lymphocytes from sensitized donors in the presence of specific antigen. This phenomenon provided the basis for the macrophage aggregation assay developed by Gotoff et al. (1973). Lymphocytes from normal individuals secreted macrophage aggregation factor (MAF) into the culture supernatant fluid after incubation with specific antigen. Such responses correlated with DNA synthesis by the stimulated lymphocytes in 82 percent of tests and with skin test reactions to the corresponding antigens in 84 percent of tested individuals. Unfortunately, 9 of 14 patients with Hodgkin's disease selected for study were receiving radiation therapy or chemotherapy at the time of testing. It is thus perhaps not surprising that only 21 percent reacted to one or more of the skin test antigens and that only 28 percent exhibited MAF activity. The possibility that this test in vitro may prove to correlate well with skin test reactions in vivo will not be evaluable until much larger numbers of previously untreated, meticulously staged patients with Hodgkin's disease have been studied.

Another test in vitro which has been reported to correlate well with delayed hypersensitivity responses in vivo is the leukocyte migration inhibition test (Søborg and Bendixen, 1967). Whitehead et al. (1974) adapted this test to the use of dinitrochlorobenzene (DNCB) dissolved in medium or conjugated to lymphocytes in the presence of dimethyl sulfoxide. They sensitized a series of patients with miscellaneous diseases to 2,000 μg of DNCB, and then applied skin test challenge doses of 50 and 100 μg 14 days later. Concurrently, they examined the responses of lymphocytes from the same individuals to lymphoblastoid stimulation and to migration inhibition by DNCB in vitro. DNCB failed to stimulate DNA synthesis in the lymphocytes of presensitized individuals, but, at a concentration of 1.1 μg/ml in medium, the chemical allergen yielded positive leukocyte migration inhibition tests in 23 of 26 skin test–positive patients, a false negative rate of only 12 percent, and positive responses in 2 of 18 unsensitized patients who were DNCB skin test–negative, a false positive rate of 11 percent. No published data have yet appeared on the application of this interesting test to patients with Hodgkin's disease.

Hancock, Bruce, and Richmond (1976a) applied the nitroblue tetrazolium (NBT) test and a microorganism-killing method in vitro to assess phagocytic activity and capacity of peripheral blood neutrophils to kill microorganisms in a series of 41 patients with Hodgkin's disease and 21 others with non-Hodgkin's lymphomas. The NBT score was normal or modestly elevated in all patients, and, with the exception of 6 patients with Hodgkin's

disease who exhibited a decreased capacity to kill *Candida,* all patients also showed normal or enhanced capacity to kill microorgansims in vitro. Steigbigel, Lambert, and Remington (1976) studied neutrophil, monocyte, and macrophage bactericidal functions in vitro in 29 untreated patients with Hodgkin's disease. They observed no significant impairment of these functions with respect to four different microorganisms in either neutrophils or monocytes. Macrophages from patients with Hodgkin's disease contained significantly more viable *Listeria* after 1.5 hours of incubation than normal control macrophages, most probably because of their greater phagocytic avidity. Leb and Merritt (1978) reported that monocyte chemotactic function was normal in six, and far below normal in three, of nine patients with untreated Hodgkin's disease. The low values tended to occur in patients with advanced (stage III and IV) disease. Monocyte bactericidal function tests yielded essentially similar results: essentially normal in stage II, somewhat reduced in stages III and IV. Some correlation was noted between impairment of these monocyte functions and the occurrence of anergy to all of four skin test antigens. A quite different macrophage function, the capacity to restore antigen-induced blastoid responses of glass bead column–purified populations of lymphocytes, was found to be normal in anergic patients with stage IV Hodgkin's disease (Blaese et al., 1972). It may be noted here that this result is apparently in disagreement with observations reported some years later by Williams and co-workers (Goodwin et al., 1977; Sibbitt, Bankhurst, and Williams, 1978) which are discussed in a subsequent section on suppressor cells.

Humoral Immunity

In striking contrast to the selective impairment of delayed hypersensitivity and other cell-mediated immune responses described above, patients with Hodgkin's disease, except in the far-advanced, near-terminal stages of the illness, show normal humoral antibody responses to antigens to which they have been previously exposed. Thus, Schier et al. (1956) reported normal responses to mumps vaccine in 12 patients with Hodgkin's disease. They also noted that their patients had mean levels of serum complement which were slightly higher than normal. Kelly et al. (1958) observed normal levels of mumps complement fixation antibody, of typhoid-paratyphoid agglutinin and of isoagglutinin titers in all of the patients with Hodgkin's disease whom they tested. They also observed normal to high levels of serum gamma globulins in all of eight patients examined. Hoffmann and Rottino (1950b) also observed normal antibody response to typhoid immunization in their patients with Hodgkin's disease. Antibody production in response to secondary immunization with tetanus toxoid (Barr and Fairley, 1961) and to blood group substances (Fairley and Akers, 1962) has also been reported to be within the normal range.

However, not all reports are unanimous on this score. For example, depressed antibody levels have been reported in response to *Brucella* (Dubin, 1947) and pneumococcal polysaccharide (Geller, 1953). Aisenberg and Leskowitz (1963) studied antibody formation to pneumococcal polysaccharide types 1 and 2 in a series of patients with active Hodgkin's disease in whom the existence of cutaneous anergy to DNCB had been established. They observed normal antibody formation in response to both antigens in 13 of 19 patients. Of the six who showed an impaired capacity to form both antibodies, four were in poor clinical condition and died within six months of the time of testing. However, eight of the patients who formed antibody initially showed an abnormally rapid decline in titer within six months thereafter.

The capacity of patients with Hodgkin's disease to synthesize antibodies in response to antigens to which they have never previously been exposed is somewhat more controversial. Barr and Fairley (1961) noted an impaired capacity of their patients with Hodgkin's disease to respond to primary immunization with tetanus; Greenwood, Smellie, Barr, and Cunliffe (1958) employed tetanus toxoid in ten patients with Hodgkin's disease who had never before been immunized to that antigen. Of these, six failed to respond, three responded in the subnormal range, and only one responded normally. Saslaw et al. (1961) found that 22 of 37 patients with Hodgkin's disease failed to respond to primary immunization with tularemia vaccine; in contrast, only 3 of 48 controls similarly tested failed to develop normal antibody titers. Moreover, among the 15 patients with Hodgkin's disease who did respond, the initial agglutinin titers ranged from 1:10 to 1:640, indicating that their response was of the anamnestic type.

Brown et al. (1967) tested 34 of their 50 patients intradermally with tularemia antigen and found that none had a positive skin test. Only 6 of their 50 patients had significant (1:16 to 1:32) antitularemia titers initially. Immunization with tularemia antigen elicited a median titer of 1:256 and an average increase of 6.5 tube dilutions in both their patients with Hodgkin's disease and their 12 normal controls. Only three of their patients had final titers of 1:32 or less. They observed no correlation between the tularemia antibody response and clinical stage, histopathology, cutaneous reactivity to DNCB or intradermal antigens, or lymphocyte count. Weitzman et al. (1977b) observed normal or somewhat elevated antibody titers to *H. influenzae*, type b, in 17 untreated patients. Normal titers of antibody to α-hemocyanin were found by De Gast et al. (1975) in 13 of 15 untreated patients with Hodgkin's disease; the 2 patients with low titers both had stage IV disease. However, Sybesma et al. (1973) found that 6 of 29 patients with Hodgkin's disease had an impaired capacity to produce antibodies to influenza A (Hong Kong), and Hersh (1973) noted that antibody production to keyhole limpet hemocyanin was delayed in onset, subnormal in titer, and transient in duration. Jones et al. (1976) have described a remarkable case in which a male patient with stage IA nodular sclerosing Hodgkin's disease of the right axilla had, nearly four years earlier, served as a normal volunteer in studies of antibody production to bacteriophage ØX174. His primary response was the lowest of his group of volunteers, but it was his secondary antibody response to reinoculation six weeks later that attracted attention, because his peak titer was only 1,350, more than tenfold lower than the normal peak titer range of 26,000–50,000. Thus, profound impairment of the secondary antibody response to a neoantigen antedated the earliest clinical manifestations of Hodgkin's disease in this patient by some 3.5 years. Jones et al. suggested that "immunoparesis in Hodgkin's disease may be a very early feature, and can occur in the absence of widespread distortion of lymph node architecture, splenic involvement, or immunosuppressive treatment."

Not surprisingly, investigators have differed in their interpretation of these data. Whereas Aisenberg (1964, 1966) concluded that antibody responses in patients with Hodgkin's disease are essentially normal until the terminal stages of the disease, Chase (1966) emphasized the distinction between the antibody responses of such patients to previously experienced antigens, which appear generally to be normal, and to antigens to which they have never previously been exposed, which he concluded are likely to be significantly impaired. He likened the distinction to the impairment of antibody synthesis observed in rabbits after X-irradiation (Dixon et al., 1952), in which the response was significantly impaired only when the animals were irradiated prior to the first injection of antigen, leaving animals which had been previously immunized capable of a normal anamnestic response. However, it would appear that the validity of this distinction has at least been severely shaken, if not completely refuted, by the subsequently reported data of Brown et al. (1967) cited above.

Many of the patients in the earlier reported series in whom deficient antibody responses were observed had been inadequately staged and/or treated. Accordingly, data from studies on previously untreated, meticulously staged patients, such as those of Brown et al. (1967), De Gast et al. (1975) and Weitzman et al. (1977b), must be accorded greater validity. These studies tend to support the conclusion that primary antibody production tends to be normal in patients with Hodgkin's disease till the far-advanced, near-terminal stages of disease.

Serum gamma globulins were found to lie within the normal range in eight patients with Hodgkin's disease (Kelly et al., 1958). Goldman and Hobbs (1967) studied a series of 50 cases of Hodgkin's disease and concluded that the levels of IgG tended to be slightly elevated, those of IgA were slightly reduced, and those of IgM were at or below the lower limit of normal. They found no discernible correlation with clinical stage or with prior treatment. Data on immunoglobulin levels have also been reported by Barr and Fairley (1961), Miller (1962), and De Gast et al. (1975), who noted no consistent abnormalities. However, the mean serum levels of IgG and IgA (and also of IgM in females but not in males) were significantly elevated in the series of 51 untreated patients studied by Wagener et al. (1976). It has also been reported that serum IgE levels are increased in Hodgkin's disease (Thomas et al., 1976; Amlot and Green, 1978). Goldman and Hobbs (1967) detected an α_3-globulin in 62 percent of their cases; the significance of this observation is not yet clear. Two serum IgG-M components of different light-chain types were noted in a patient with Hodgkin's disease studied by Chisesi, Capnist, and Barbui (1976). Long et al. (1977b) and Brown et al. (1978), using the sensitive Raji cell radioimmunoassay, detected elevated levels of soluble immune complexes in 34 of 90 sera from 75 patients with Hodgkin's disease. The guinea pig macrophage assay for soluble immune complexes was reportedly positive with sera from 23 of 26 patients studied by Kávai et al. (1976). Amlot, Slaney, and Williams (1976) observed increased levels of a "macromolecular" C3

component of complement, interpreted as indirect evidence of the presence of immune complexes, in nine of nine patients with, and two of nine without, constitutional symptoms. However, normal levels of C3 and C7 were observed by Lichtenfeld et al. (1976); in contrast, the levels of whole complement and C5, C8, and C9 were significantly increased in their series of ten patients with Hodgkin's disease.

A quite different type of humoral response, the capacity of cultured leukocytes to produce interferon in response to viral infection, was studied by Rassiga-Pidot and McIntyre (1974), who observed normal responses in cells from 13 patients with stage I–III disease and impaired interferon production by cells from 8 patients with stage IV disease.

Mechanisms of Impairment of Cell-mediated Immunity

The studies cited above, in vivo and in vitro, clearly indicate that most patients with Hodgkin's disease suffer from a selective impairment of cell-mediated immunity which, especially in those with limited disease, is often a subtle, relative, and stimulus-dependent defect rather than the absolute unresponsiveness implied by the older term, anergy. It is now well established that cellular, as distinguished from humoral, immune responses are mediated primarily by the thymus-dependent (T-lymphocyte) system, with the cooperation (in at least some functions) of the monocyte-macrophage system. The complexity of these responses has become increasingly appreciated as the development of tests in vitro has made possible more detailed manipulation and analysis of their components. Thus, a daunting array of possibilities confronts the investigator seeking to elucidate the mechanism(s) underlying the immunologic deficit in these patients. The available evidence from several different lines of investigation is summarized in this section.

Lymphocytopenia. As early 1914, Bunting called attention to the occurrence of lymphocytopenia in patients with Hodgkin's disease, and Wiseman (1936) presented extensive additional data confirming this observation. In the same year, Rosenthal (1936) reported that the lymphoid tissues of patients with Hodgkin's disease were often characterized by a significant depletion of lymphocytes and suggested that the relative abundance of tissue lymphocytes might be correlated with the prognosis of the disease.

Aisenberg (1965b) analyzed the lymphocyte counts in 50 consecutive fatal cases of Hodgkin's disease, both at the time of onset of the disease and again during the last six months of the patient's life. In addition, he studied lymphocyte counts in an additional 25 outpatients within a relatively short interval after the onset of their disease. The average lymphocyte count was in the normal range (1,500 to 3,000 per cubic millimeter) in only 2 of the 50 patients in the near-terminal stages of the disease, and more than three-fourths of the patients had fewer than 500 lymphocytes per cubic millimeter. This striking lymphocyte depletion late in the course of the disease contrasted with the finding of low-normal or only minimally depressed lymphocyte counts at the onset of the disease.

Brown et al. (1967) have provided data on lymphocyte counts in a series of 50 previously untreated patients with Hodgkin's disease, in all of whom the disease was clinically staged with the aid of lymphangiography and other diagnostic procedures. Nineteen of their 50 patients (38 percent) had lymphocyte counts below 1,500 per cubic millimeter. Although there was a wide disparity of values in all stages, the median counts were significantly lower in patients in stages III and IV than in stages I and II. There was no consistent relationship between lymphocyte count and histopathologic type, nor was there a clear-cut difference in lymphocyte counts in relation to the presence or absence of constitutional symptoms. All but one of their stage I patients had an absolute lymphocyte count in the normal range. This study was extended by Young et al. (1972, 1973b) to include 103 patients with untreated disease, with similar results. They observed a correlation between the peripheral lymphocyte count and skin test reactivity to DNCB and to various intradermal antigens in their patients, although here again a considerable degree of overlap and variability was apparent.

Hematologic data on 100 randomly selected, untreated patients with Hodgkin's disease (Table 4.1, Chapter 4) reveal that absolute lymphocyte counts $< 1,000/mm^3$ occurred in 19 (1 of 17 in stage I; 7 of 43 in stage IIA and II$_E$A; 2 of 11 in stage IIB; 3 of 11 in stage IIIA; 3 of 10 in stage IIIB; and 3 of 7 in stage IV). The frequency of lymphocytopenia remained stable in two later Stanford studies involving nonoverlapping patient populations; counts $< 1,000/mm^3$ were noted by Eltringham and Kaplan (1973) in 24 (17 percent) of 141 patients, and by Bobrove et al. (1975) in 9 (21 percent) of 42 patients. Similar data have been reported by Heier and Normann (1974); in their series, however, the

frequency of lymphocytopenia was directly related to advanced stage and to lymphocyte depletion histologic type. Eltringham and Kaplan (1973) and Levy and Kaplan (1974) were unable to discern any correlation between absolute lymphocyte count and DNCB skin test or PHA stimulation response, respectively. Winkelstein et al. (1974) also found that lymphocytopenia did not appear to alter the PHA stimulation response. Collectively, these data support the views of Aisenberg, who concluded that the anergy of early Hodgkin's disease is clearly not accounted for by lymphocytopenia and suggested instead that the functional capacity of lymphocytes in early Hodgkin's disease may be depressed.

T- and B-Lymphocyte Number. As has already been discussed in the section on rosette formation (Chapter 3), two distinctive attributes of T-lymphocytes have been exploited for their identification and enumeration: (1) their specific surface membrane antigens, which react with absorption-purified anti-human thymocyte sera in either a complement-dependent cytotoxic assay (R. W. Smith et al., 1973; Bobrove et al., 1974) or indirect immunofluorescence assay (Chin et al., 1973), and (2) their possession of a surface membrane receptor capable of binding sheep erythrocytes, detected by the formation of spontaneous nonimmune E-rosettes (Fröland, 1972; Jondal et al., 1972; Wybran et al., 1972). In the peripheral blood of normal donors, the percentage of T-lymphocytes detected by the cytotoxic assay and the percentage of E-rosette-forming cells (E-RFC) are in very close agreement (Bobrove et al., 1975). The marker most commonly used to identify B-lymphocytes has been their capacity to synthesize and to exteriorize immunoglobulins (usually IgM) on the surface membrane (Rabellino et al., 1971). Direct or (usually) indirect immunofluorescence tests, using antisera against whole or fractionated human immunoglobulins, are performed on living cells or on acetone-fixed cells for the detection of surface (SIg) or cytoplasmic (CIg) immunoglobulin, respectively. A small residue (normally less than 5 percent) of peripheral blood lymphocytes do not give positive reactions for either T- or B-cell markers, and are known as "null" cells.

There have been few studies to date of the percentage of T-lymphocytes in the peripheral blood of untreated patients with Hodgkin's disease. Aiuti and Wigzell (1973), using the cytotoxic assay, reported distinctly low percentages of T-lymphocytes in two and marginally low values in five other patients with Hodgkin's disease who were uncharacterized with respect to stage, histologic type, age, sex, or treatment history. However, they neglected to determine, and to correct appropriately for, the percentage of monocytes and myeloid cells in their suspensions. Since many patients with Hodgkin's disease have a peripheral blood monocytosis, contamination of the gradient-purified cell suspensions by monocytes may be very high, especially in patients with advanced disease (Bobrove et al., 1975). Failure to take such increased values into account would be expected to yield spuriously low percentages of T-lymphocytes.

Bobrove et al. (1975) quantitated the percentages of T- and B-lymphocytes and of monocytes in the peripheral blood of 22 normal donors and of 42 consecutive patients with untreated Hodgkin's disease, all staged with lymphangiography, bone marrow biopsy, and, with the exception of those with overt stage IV disease, laparotomy with sple-

nectomy. After appropriate correction for contamination by monocytes, the percentages of T-lymphocytes detected by the cytotoxic assay ranged from 61 to 90 percent (mean, 77 ± 1.9 percent) among 20 patients with stage IIA or IIB disease (Table 6.12), and from 48 to 98 percent (mean, 81 ± 2.7 percent) among 22 others with stage III and IV disease (Table 6.13). Only two of these values fell below the range observed among normal donors (65 to 91 percent, with a mean of 77 ± 1.5 percent) (Table 6.14). Except for 9 patients with an absolute lymphocytopenia ($<1,000$ lymphocytes/mm^3), absolute T-lymphocyte levels were also within normal limits. These observations were later extended to a series of 127 patients by Fuks et al. (1976d) and confirmed. As previously mentioned, Cohnen et al. (1973a), Ramot et al. (1973), Andersen (1974), and Holm et al. (1976) also noted low percentages of E-RFC in patients with untreated Hodgkin's disease, but did not per-

Table 6.12 Patients with Limited Hodgkin's Disease

Type	Stage	% cyto-toxicity	% mono-cytes and myeloid cells	% T-lympho-cytes	% B-lympho-cytes	Absolute lympho-cyte counts/ mm^3	Absolute T-lympho-cyte counts/ mm^3	Absolute B-lympho-cyte counts/ mm^3
NSHD	IIA	74	9	81	17	1,600	1,296	272
NSHD	IIA	53	33	79	12	1,809	1,429	217
NSHD	IIA	66	5	69	28	2,880	1,987	806
NSHD	IIA	62	18	76	17	1,751	1,330	298
NSHD	IIA	63	10	70	25	703	492	175
NSHD	IIA	86	3	88	26	1,680	1,478	437
NSHD	IIA	57	16	69	27	3,720	2,567	1,004
NSHD	IIA	63	13	72	25	2,232	1,607	558
NSHD	II$_E$A	48	28	77	9	1,032	795	93
NSHD	IIA	63	30	90	19	830	747	158
NSHD	IIA	70	10	77	26	2,280	1,756	593
NSHD	IIA	71	15	83	9	856	710	77
MCHD	IIA	68	5	76	24	1,530	1,147	367
NSHD	IIB	48	21	61	35	1,274	777	446
NSHD	IIB	71	18	86	8	1,877	2,474	230
NSHD	IIB	70	15	84	15	1,612	1,354	242
NSHD	IIB	62	26	83	12	1,445	1,199	173
NSHD	IIB	51	20	64	25	2,720	1,741	680
NSHD	IIB	47	ND[c]	—	17	1,452	—	247
Unclass. HD	IIB	43	38	69	28	728	502	204
		62 ± 2.4[a]	17 ± 3.9	77 ± 1.9	19 ± 1.9	$1,667 \pm 197$	$1,336 \pm 138$	364 ± 56
		$(43-86)$[b]	$(5-33)$	$(61-90)$	$(8-35)$	$(703-2880)$	$(492-2567)$	$(77-1004)$

Source: Bobrove et al. (1975).

[a] Mean $\pm$ S.E.

[b] Range.

[c] Not done.

Table 6.13 Patients with Advanced Hodgkin's Disease

Type	Stage	% cyto-toxicity	% mono-cytes and myeloid cells	% T-lympho-cytes	% B-lympho-cytes	Absolute lympho-cyte counts/mm³	Absolute T-lympho-cyte counts/mm³	Absolute B-lympho-cyte counts/mm³
NSHD	IIIA	45	35	70	27	816	571	220
NSHD	IIIA	43	36	70	23	1,274	892	293
NSHD	IIIA	67	10	74	16	1,513	1,120	242
NSHD	IIIA	77	4	80	15	3,240	2,592	486
NSHD	IIIA	71	14	83	16	5,256	4,362	841
NSHD	IIIA	66	21	83	21	1,206	1,001	253
NSHD	IIIA	10	79	48	12	1,452	697	174
NSHD	IIIA	69	24	90	17	2,376	2,138	404
NSHD	IIIA	79	14	92	10	2,058	1,893	206
NSHD	IIIA	75	19	93	12	2,295	2,134	275
MCHD	IIIA	56	20	70	33	1,786	1,250	589
NSHD	IIIB	53	40	88	12	765	673	92
NSHD	IIIB	47	27	67	18	1,008	675	181
NSHD	IIIB	28	71	96	8	548	526	44
NSHD	III$_E$B	50	31	72	25	380	274	95
NSHD	IIIB	64	42	94	10	1,539	1,447	154
NSHD	IVA	50	39	80	14	2,072	1,658	290
NSHD	IVA	80	19	98	8	1,474	1,444	118
MCHD	IVA	34	60	85	27	2,028	1,724	548
MCHD	IVA	65	29	92	12	1,330	1,224	160
NSHD	IVA	57	14	67	17	2,660	1,782	452
NSHD	IVB	78	21	90	7	290	261	20
		57 ± 39[a]	30 ± 4.1	81 ± 2.7	16 ± 1.5	1,698 ± 233	1,379 ± 197	279 ± 43
		(10–80)[b]	(4–79)	(48–96)	(7–33)	(290–5256)	(261–4362)	(20–841)

Source: Bobrove et al. (1975).

[a] Mean ± S.E.

[b] Range.

form the cytotoxic assay concurrently. Accordingly, their conclusion that patients with Hodgkin's disease often exhibit a T-lymphocytopenia remains open to challenge in light of the more extensive studies of Bobrove et al. (1974) and of Fuks et al. (1976d). The weight of present evidence supports the conclusion that T-lymphocytopenia is infrequent in patients with Hodgkin's disease and thus cannot account for the defects of cell-mediated immune function seen in this disorder.

The percentages of B-lymphocytes in the peripheral blood of 22 normal donors (Table 6.15), as detected by fluorescent staining of SIg, ranged from 13 to 30 percent with a mean of 20 ± 1.1 percent (Bobrove et al., 1975). Similar determinations in 42 patients with untreated Hodgkin's disease revealed greater variability (range 7 to 35 percent), but the mean value (19 ± 1.9 percent) for 20 patients with stage II disease (Table 6.13) was normal, and that for 22 patients with stage III or IV disease (16 ± 1.5 percent, Table 6.14) was only slightly decreased. The fact that low B-cell counts were observed in about one-half of the patients could not be correlated with their skin test reactivity, PHA responses, or E-RFC levels. These findings were confirmed by Fuks et al. (1976b) in a later study of 61 untreated patients; although the mean percentage of B-cells was normal in stages I and II, and only marginally decreased in stages III and IV, 23 patients (38 percent) had absolute B-lymphocyte values more than two standard deviations below the mean for normal donors. Normal percentages of B-lymphocytes have been reported in several smaller series of untreated patients (Gajl-Peczalska et al., 1973; Falletta et al., 1973; Cohnen et al., 1973b; Gallmeier et al., 1973; Holm et al., 1976).

There is some evidence that the proportions of T- and B-lymphocytes in certain of the involved tissues of patients with Hodgkin's disease may dif-

Table 6.14   T- and B-Lymphocytes in Normal Doners

% cyto-toxicity	% monocytes and myeloid cells	% T-lympho-cytes	% B-lympho-cytes	Absolute lympho-cyte counts/mm³	Absolute T-lympho-cyte counts/mm³	Absolute B-lympho-cyte counts/mm³
71	19	87	14	1,764	1,535	276
49	25	65	27	ND[c]	—	—
67	12	77	16	2,376	1,820	480
67	21	75	19	2,285	1,715	432
68	24	79	13	2,072	1,637	269
54	15	73	23	ND	—	—
70	13	80	14	1,914	1,530	268
65	10	72	26	1,872	1,350	471
55	16	65	25	ND	—	—
59	14	73	19	2,052	1,495	390
65	17	78	26	1,400	1,092	364
80	10	89	13	2,700	2,400	350
60	20	75	23	1,940	1,450	430
58	20	72	22	1,800	1,296	396
64	30	91	16	2,244	2,040	360
68	11	76	26	2,160	1,640	560
57	15	67	30	2,134	1,430	640
75	10	83	20	1,890	1,570	378
71	16	80	22	2,000	1,600	440
66	17	83	19	ND	—	—
70	10	79	14	ND	—	—
53	26	72	14	ND	—	—
64 ± 1.6[a] (49–80)[b]	17 ± 1.2 (10–30)	77 ± 1.5 (65–91)	20 ± 1.1 (13–30)	2038 ± 73 (1400–2700)	1600 ± 76 (1092–2400)	407 ± 25 (268–640)

Source: Bobrove et al. (1975).

[a] Mean ± S.E.

[b] Range.

[c] Not done.

fer from those expressed in the peripheral blood. Kaur et al. (1974) studied cells from the spleens of ten patients, only one of whom had received prior treatment. They found that the percentage of T-cells in these ten spleens, as measured by blastoid transformation in response to PHA, was significantly higher (mean 67 percent, range 50 to 80 percent) than that in six nonmalignant spleens studied previously (28 percent). The lowest value (50 percent) was observed in one of three uninvolved spleens, whereas the two highest values (78 and 80 percent) occurred in the two most heavily involved spleens. However, estimation of T-cell number by another marker, the capacity to form E-rosettes, yielded an appreciably lower value (51 percent), which was not significantly different from levels in the peripheral blood of the patients (56 percent) or normal controls (55 percent). The fact that the percentage of B-lymphocytes (SIg-bearing cells) in these ten spleens was significantly reduced (35 percent), compared to that in six non-malignant spleens (57 percent), supports the interpretation that there was a real shift in relative abundance of T- versus B-cells in the Hodgkin's disease spleens. It was also noted that the mean percentage of lymphocytes exhibiting spontaneous transformation in unstimulated cultures was significantly higher among cells from these spleens (6.8 percent) than in those from the peripheral blood (2.1 percent). In other studies of involved spleens from patients with Hodgkin's disease, Hunter et al. (1977) and Santoro, Caillou, and Belpomme (1977) also found significantly increased percentages of T-cells by the E-rosette test. The latter group reported that there was a smaller than normal percentage of B-cells in the spleens that were involved, and suggested that the increase in splenic T-lymphocytes may indicate a local immune reaction against Sternberg-Reed cells in involved spleens. However, the possibility that the

Table 6.15 Percent T-Lymphocytes by the E-Rosette Method in Ficoll-Purified Peripheral Blood Lymphocytes from Normal Donors and Patients with Untreated Hodgkin's Disease, before and following 24-hr Incubation in RPMI-1640 Medium Containing 20% Serum of Various Origins

Type of serum	Donors	No. of individuals tested	% E-Rosettes before Incubation[a]	% E-Rosettes following incubation in medium containing 20%[a]	
				Tested serum	Fetal calf serum
Fetal human serum	Normal	5	60.4 ± 0.87	59.4 ± 0.75	60.2 ± 0.20
	Hodgkin's disease	5	40.0 ± 8.45	62.4 ± 2.79	58.8 ± 2.13
Human AB serum	Normal	25	61.9 ± 0.59	61.6 ± 0.73	61.4 ± 0.58
	Hodgkin's disease	24	51.5 ± 3.02	49.7 ± 3.23	61.3 ± 1.33
Adult bovine serum	Normal	5	60.6 ± 0.65	60.8 ± 0.80	60.8 ± 0.37
	Hodgkin's disease	6	37.8 ± 6.67	38.5 ± 6.65	57.0 ± 1.98

Source: Fuks et al. (1976d).

[a] Mean ± S.E.

functions of T-cells in involved spleens may be impaired is suggested by the finding that their responses to PHA and Con A were significantly diminished (Willson, Zaremba, and Pretlow, 1977).

Cossman, Deegan, and Schnitzer (1977) examined involved tissues from nine patients with nodular sclerosing Hodgkin's disease by rosetting techniques and found an increased abundance of complement-receptor-bearing B-lymphocytes in the nodular infiltrates in all nine cases. In 5 of 32 patients studied by Habeshaw et al. (1976), highly abnormal levels of IgM-receptor-bearing cells, presumed to be immature T-lymphocytes, were encountered in peripheral blood, lymph node, and spleen mononuclear cell populations. An increased abundance of IgM-EA rosette-forming cells in involved spleens, and especially in nodular foci of splenic disease, was observed by Hunter et al. (1977).

Macrophage-Lymphocyte Interactions. There is now ample evidence that cooperative interactions between macrophages and lymphocytes are essential steps in both humoral antibody and cell-mediated immune responses. It is thus relevant to consider the possibility that factors which interfere with or alter such interactions might contribute to the defect of cell-mediated immunity seen in Hodgkin's disease. However, the literature to date on this subject is remarkably sparse, and that which exists provides little support for the hypothesis that impaired macrophage function, including interactions with lymphocytes, may be involved.

Sheagren, Block, and Wolff (1967) measured the rates of clearance of intravenously injected ^{125}I-labeled aggregated human serum albumin as an index of the phagocytic function of the reticuloendothelial system in patients with Hodgkin's disease. They observed a greater than normal rate of clearance, which was most marked in patients with disease of advanced extent and in those with relapsing, active disease. Increased rates of monocyte phagocytosis of IgG-coated red blood cells were noted by Urbanitz, Fechner, and Gross (1975) in three patients with stage IIB Hodgkin's disease, whereas the phagocytic activity of monocytes from seven patients with advanced (stage III and IV) disease was significantly impaired. The phagocytic activity of peripheral blood leukocytes (neutrophils and monocytes) was normal or moderately elevated in two series of patients with Hodgkin's disease studied by Hancock, Bruce, and Richmond (1976a) and Steigbigel, Lambert, and Remington (1976). Navone, Palestro, and Resegotti (1975) reported a correlation between the number of macrophages in unstimulated blood cell cultures and the degree of blastoid transformation of PHA-stimulated lymphocytes in the patients they studied. However, the finding by Blaese et al. (1972) that macrophages from anergic patients with stage IV Hodgkin's disease were active in restoring lymphocyte transformation responses in vitro to normal levels makes it quite unlikely that the fundamental immunologic deficit in such patients resides in the mononuclear phagocyte system. Other aspects of this subject are discussed in the next section on suppressor cells.

Suppressor Cells. During the past decade, there has been mounting evidence that the response of the immune system is modulated by interactions between cells with the capacity for certain positive immune response functions, such as antibody production, cytotoxic activity, or helper activity, and other cells capable of specific inhibition or suppression of immune responses. Such "suppressor cells" have been identified in some instances as a subpopulation of T-lymphocytes (Rowley et al., 1973; Dutton, 1975; Webb and Jamieson, 1976). The mechanisms whereby suppressor cells exert their specific inhibitory effects on immune function are not yet known. Perhaps because of its novelty, the concept of the suppressor cell has attracted the interest of many investigators, who have invoked the presence of such cells in a number of immunologic and other disorders. In many instances, however, such inferences have been based solely on the observation that particular immune responses were significantly augmented when a subpopulation of lymphoid cells was removed from the assay system. Convincing evidence of the existence of suppressor cells requires that immune responses be inhibited when particular subpopulations of cells are added back to the assay system, as well as the demonstration that such inhibitory effects are specific.

Twomey et al. (1975) studied the capacity of irradiated leukocytes and mononuclear cells from patients with Hodgkin's disease to stimulate mixed lymphocyte reactions (MLR) in cultures with normal responder lymphocytes. They observed that stimulation was significantly below normal with the cells from 16 of 30 patients; of the 16, all but one had stage III or IV disease and 2 had been previously treated. Further studies were carried out with the peripheral blood mononuclear cells from 5 patients with a subnormal capacity for stimulation of the mixed lymphocyte reaction. Stimulation was markedly increased when adherent cells were removed by passage through glass wool, as well as by preincubation of the cells in a protein synthesis inhibitor, cycloheximide. The authors interpreted these responses as indicative of the presence of

suppressor cells in the peripheral blood mononuclear cell population of patients with advanced Hodgkin's disease and suggested that the suppressor cells were probably lymphocytes, since removal of phagocytic cells did not alter the stimulation response. However, no experiments were performed to demonstrate resuppression when the adherent cells removed by passage through glass wool were restored to the assay system, nor was specificity demonstrated for these cells, as contrasted with similar cells from the peripheral blood of normal individuals.

Goodwin et al. (1977) have further investigated the role of suppressor cells in human peripheral blood. Glass wool–adherent cells from normal donors were shown to suppress the mitogenic responses of peripheral blood T-lymphocytes to PHA and Con A. It was postulated that the mechanism of suppression might involve the secretion of prostaglandin E_2, since suppressor cell activity could be counteracted by the addition of prostaglandin synthetase inhibitors such as indomethacin. These investigators then studied the effect of indomethacin on the PHA stimulation response of 6 patients with untreated Hodgkin's disease and of 29 normal individuals. At the concentration of PHA employed in the assay, the mean response of the peripheral blood mononuclear cells of the patients was 6,672 cpm, with a range of 4,673 to 11,050, and their stimulation indices, relative to unstimulated cells, ranged from 19 to 53, with a mean of 30; in contrast, the mean response among the 29 controls was 13,667 cpm, with a mean stimulation index of 60 ($p < 0.001$). The addition of indomethacin at a concentration of 1 $\mu g/ml$ caused a marked increase in response of the mononuclear cells from both the patients and the normal controls. The average increase was 182 ± 60 percent for the patients, versus 44 ± 18 percent for the controls. The phytohemagglutinin response of mononuclear cells from the patients could also be greatly augmented by prior removal of glass wool–adherent cells; after such restoration of the response, indomethacin had little or no further effect on the response. Mitogen-activated cultures of mononuclear cells from three patients with Hodgkin's disease produced about four times more prostaglandin E_2 than normal mononuclear cells. The authors concluded that a prostaglandin E_2-producing suppressor cell is responsible for the hyporesponsiveness to PHA in patients with Hodgkin's disease. The same group (Sibbitt, Bankhurst, and Williams 1978) later reported that the PHA response of lymphocytes from patients with Hodgkin's disease could be restored to normal by removal of glass wool–adherent suppressor cells and again inhibited by restoration of such cells to the cultures. In contrast, PHA responses of normal individuals were decreased by removal of glass wool–adherent cells. However, Blaese et al. (1972), as mentioned above, had found that the capacity of macrophages from anergic patients with stage IV Hodgkin's disease to restore lymphocyte transformation responses in vitro was apparently normal. Experiments to test the specificity of the suppressor cell effect, by reciprocal mixing of Hodgkin's lymphocytes with glass wool–adherent cells from normals, and vice versa, were apparently not performed by Sibbitt, Bankhurst, and Williams. Similar effects were noted by Schechter and Soehnlen (1978) in seven of nine patients with treated stage III or IV disease, but not in two untreated patients with stage II disease.

Additional evidence of suppressor cell activity in the mixed lymphocyte reactions of patients with Hodgkin's disease has now been reported. Engleman et al. (1978) devised a screening procedure for HLA-D specific suppressor T-cells, based on the observation that such cells are resistant to a dose of irradiation (1,000 rads) that inactivates responder cells in donor cell populations. Suppression was detected by the addition of irradiated responder cells to mixtures of unirradiated responder cells and heavily irradiated (6,000 rads) stimulator cells from four different normal donors. Of 70 patients with Hodgkin's disease thus tested, 41 (59 percent) had positive suppressor tests, whereas only one of 50 healthy donors yielded a positive test. Similar suppressor effects were reported by Hillinger and Herzig (1978) after the addition to MLR cultures of responder cells treated with mitomycin C. They observed that suppression was significantly increased among patients with active Hodgkin's disease (78 ± 4.6 percent) and among treated patients in remission (58 ± 9.3 percent). However, although mononuclear cells from normal individuals suppressed less frequently (21 ± 6.9 percent), in this test the cells of some normal individuals demonstrated suppressor activity which was fully comparable to that observed in patients with Hodgkin's disease, an observation which again raises questions about the specificity, and thus the significance, of such suppressor effects.

Alteration of Lymphocyte Surface Membranes. Alterations of the surface membrane of lymphocytes might well be expected to have a significant influence on their immune function. Lectins such as Con A have served as useful probes of alterations in the lymphocyte surface membrane, measuring such properties as binding affinity, agglutinability, and capacity for cap formation. Ben-Bassat and Goldblum (1975) studied these parameters in a series of 118 patients with Hodgkin's disease, of whom 54 were untreated, newly diagnosed patients. Cap formation was studied with fluorescein-isothiocyanate-conjugated Con A (F-Con A) in lymphocytes from both peripheral blood and fresh biopsy material, and compared with the corresponding responses of lymphocytes from normal individuals. Approximately 20–35 percent of normal lymphocytes formed caps with F-Con A. In contrast, cap formation by peripheral blood and tissue lymphocytes from patients with Hodgkin's disease was markedly reduced, in most instances falling in the range of 1–10 percent (Fig. 6.7). Almost identical results were obtained by Mintz and Sachs (1975), who noted a mean proportion of cap-forming cells of only 2.1 percent among 15 patients with active Hodgkin's disease, as contrasted with 10.6 percent in 6 patients with Hodgkin's disease in remission and 29.4 percent in a series of normal individuals. Both groups of investigators also noted an increased agglutinability of peripheral blood lymphocytes from patients with Hodgkin's disease with Con A. In a later study, Aisenberg, Weitzman, and Wilkes (1978) reported that cap-forming cell levels were below normal in 9 of 13 untreated patients with stage I and IIA disease, 6 of 8 in stage IIIA, and 8 of 8 in stages IIIB and IV. There was also some indication that these responses may be related to disease activity; capping levels were low in all of 6 patients in relapse and in only 9 of 16 in remission following treatment. These observations clearly indicate that the surface membrane of a significant subpopulation of lymphocytes in patients with Hodgkin's disease is altered with respect to lectin agglutinability and cap formation. However, no direct link has yet been established between these abnormalities and the impairment of cell-mediated immunity in these patients.

Humoral Factors. It is now well established that alteration of the T-lymphocyte surface membrane by humoral factors in serum, perhaps by masking of specific receptors, can alter or even abrogate cell-mediated immune functions. Thus, antilymphocyte antibodies and other immunoglobulins capable of attachment to the surface of T-lymphocytes are known to depress such responses as PHA

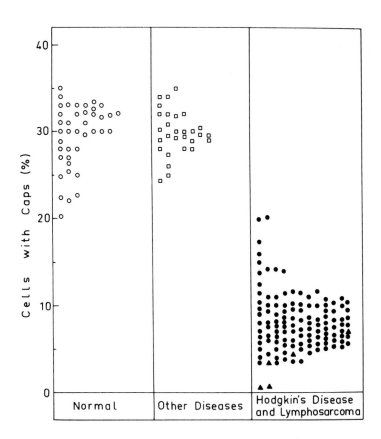

Figure 6.7   Cap formation by fluoresceinated concanavalin A bound to the surface membranes of lymphocytes from the peripheral blood of patients with Hodgkin's disease (●) and lymphosarcoma (▲), normal controls (○), and patients with other diseases (□), including 12 with fevers of undetermined etiology, 2 with polycythemia vera, 2 with pancytopenia, 1 with infectious mononucleosis, 2 with rheumatoid arthritis, 2 with multiple sclerosis, and 8 with carcinomas. (Reprinted by permission of the authors, from the paper by Ben-Bassat and Goldblum, 1975.)

stimulation, E-rosette formation, and the mixed lymphocyte reaction (Fröland, 1972; Wernet and Kunkel, 1973). Humoral immunosuppressive factors have been reported in patients with hepatic disease (Newberry et al., 1973), renal failure (Newberry and Sanford, 1971), systemic lupus erythematosus and other collagen disorders (Wernet and Kunkel, 1973; Winchester et al., 1974), and primary intracranial tumors (Brooks et al., 1972). In some of these disease states, the humoral factor has been identified as an immunoglobulin, and sometimes more specifically as an antilymphocyte antibody (Winchester et al., 1974). Grifoni and his colleagues (1968a, 1969, 1970, 1973) have described the presence of cytotoxic antilymphocyte antibodies in patients with Hodgkin's disease and more recently have reported that these antibodies can inhibit the PHA stimulation response of normal lymphocytes (Tognella et al., 1975a). Not all of the humoral immunosuppressive factors encountered in disease states have proved to be immunoglobulins, however. For example, an E-rosette inhibitory factor detected in the serum of patients with hepatitis B virus infection has been identified as a low density lipoprotein (Chisari and Edgington, 1975). C-reactive protein has also been reported to bind reversibly to T-lymphocytes and to inhibit their functional responses in vitro (Mortensen, Osmand, and Gewurz 1975).

In Hodgkin's disease, several groups of investigators have entertained the possibility that serum factors might be responsible for the inhibition of cell-mediated immune function and have searched for experimental evidence in support of this thesis. Trubowitz, Masek, and Del Rosario (1966) noted a slight increase in the lymphoblastoid response of lymphocytes cultured in normal plasma instead of autologous patient plasma, and Gaines, Gilmer, and Remington (1973) observed that plasma from untreated patients with Hodgkin's disease inhibited transformation of lymphocytes from normal donors. However, other studies have revealed either no consistent inhibitory effect of Hodgkin's disease serum or plasma on the response of normal lymphocytes (Hersh and Oppenheim, 1965b; Thomas et al., 1967) or a persistent impairment of the response of Hodgkin's disease lymphocytes regardless of whether they were tested in the presence of normal serum (Holm, Perlmann, and Johansson, 1967; Han and Sokal, 1970; Han, 1972), in the presence or absence of autologous plasma (Matchett, Huang, and Kremer, 1973), or after prolonged washing of the cells in serum-free medium (Levy and Kaplan, 1974). Han (1972) simultaneously assayed the stimulation of normal lymphocytes by PHA in the presence of normal serum versus sera from 63 patients with Hodgkin's disease and was unable to demonstrate any inhibitory effect except in the case of sera from those patients who were receiving cytotoxic chemotherapy. In brief notes giving few experimental details, Scheurlen, Schneider, and Pappas (1971) and Zorini et al. (1974) have stated that Hodgkin's disease sera inhibited the lymphoblastoid response to specific antigens and to PHA, respectively. Pappas, Pees, and Girmann (1977) studied 19 patients with Hodgkin's disease (only 5 of whom were untreated) and reported that the lymphoblastoid response of normal lymphocytes to PHA was inhibited by the sera of 9 of 11 nonsplenectomized patients, wheras the sera of 7 of 8 splenectomized patients supported normal responses by such cells. Three patients were tested before and after splenectomy; inhibitory activity was present preoperatively in the sera of two of these and disappeared following splenectomy in both cases. These studies require confirmation in larger numbers of untreated patients.

A new analytic approach was provided by the discovery that a substantial proportion of cells identifiable by the cytotoxic assay as T-lymphocytes fail to form E-rosettes (Bobrove et al., 1975; Fuks et al., 1976d). At least three possible explanations were considered: (1) a defect or decreased density of receptors on the surface of a subpopulation of T-cells, (2) the presence of "suppressor" cells, and (3) masking of receptor sites by a cytophilic antibody or other humoral inhibitor. Further investigation (Fuks et al., 1976d) provided evidence supporting the third possibility: E-rosette formation

by lymphocytes from patients with Hodgkin's disease was readily and consistently restored to normal by short-term incubation in fetal calf or fetal human sera but not in adult bovine or adult human sera (Table 6.15). There was no concomitant change in the percentage of T-lymphocytes detected by the cytotoxic assay; instead, the two assays were brought into close agreement after incubation in fetal sera. The E-rosette response was most markedly and consistently increased by such incubation in those instances in which it had been most profoundly impaired. Thus significant increases were noted in all of 32 patients with preincubation rosette levels of 50 percent or less, in 15 of 17 with initial levels in the 51–60 percent range, and in only 3 of 23 with initially normal or near-normal levels (≥61 percent). Similar observations were noted by Bentwich, Cohen, and Brautbar (1976).

Incubation of peripheral blood lymphocytes in the presence of fetal sera also restored the PHA stimulation response to normal (Fuks et al., 1976d). When the lymphocytes from 17 patients with Hodgkin's disease were tested over a range of PHA concentrations, they exhibited significantly reduced stimulation ratios, relative to those of normal donors, similar to the impaired responses previously observed by Levy and Kaplan (1974). After incubation for six to eight hours in RPMI-1640 medium containing 20 percent fetal calf serum, the PHA stimulation ratios of lymphocytes from these patients rose to the normal range, whereas those of the normal donors were unaffected (Fig. 6.8). The simplest interpretation of these observations is that fetal sera, unlike those of adults, are capable of eluting a rosette-inhibitory material

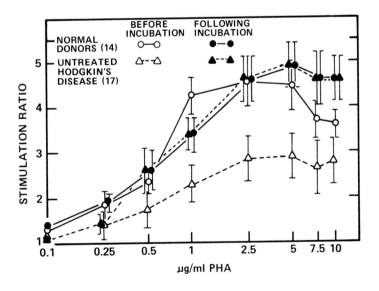

Figure 6.8 PHA stimulation of protein synthesis of peripheral blood lymphocytes from normal donors and patients with untreated Hodgkin's disease, before and after 6- to 8-hr incubation in RPMI-1640 containing 20 percent fetal calf serum. The data are expressed as the stimulation ratio—the ratio of ^{3}H-leucine counts per minute in PHA-stimulated cultures to counts per minute in unstimulated control cultures for each PHA concentration. The data for each group are pooled and presented as the mean ± S.E. of the stimulation ratios at each PHA concentration. (Reprinted by permission of the authors and the Editor of the *Journal of Immunology,* from the paper by Fuks, Strober, King, and Kaplan, 1976.)

from the surfaces of T-lymphocytes from patients with Hodgkin's disease, thus unmasking receptor sites which are then capable of functioning normally in both the E-rosette and the PHA stimulation tests.

The logical next step was to ascertain whether such a rosette-inhibitory factor could be detected in the sera of patients with Hodgkin's disease by virtue of its capacity to bind to Hodgkin's disease lymphocytes which had first been restored to normal function by incubation in fetal calf serum. Subsequent reincubation in medium containing 20 percent Hodgkin's disease serum again significantly reduced E-rosette levels in peripheral blood lymphocytes from 22 (85 percent) of 25 patients with Hodgkin's disease (Fuks, Strober, and Kaplan, 1976). E-rosette formation by these cells could be restored to normal by a second round of incubation with fetal calf serum. Hodgkin's disease serum significantly depressed the response of only 1 of 12 patients with non-Hodgkin's lymphomas and failed to depress the E-rosette levels of lymphocytes from any of 34 normal subjects or of 12 patients with various types of carcinomas. The fact that the lymphocytes of 85 percent of Hodgkin's disease patients were affected, as compared to those of only 1 (1.7 percent) of 58 other individuals, suggested that the mechanism of action of the serum rosette inhibitory factor may be specifically associated with Hodgkin's disease. However, specificity was concentration-dependent rather than absolute (Fig. 6.9); at a 20 percent concentration of Hodgkin's disease serum, rosette levels of lymphocytes from patients with Hodgkin's disease were markedly depressed and those of normal subjects were unaffected, but at concentrations exceeding 60 percent, significant depression was also observed with normal donor lymphocytes in three successive experiments.

The spleen seemed a likely tissue of origin of the serum E-rosette inhibitor in patients with Hodgkin's disease and offered the added practical advantage of being readily available for study as a result of staging laparotomy. Extracts prepared from the involved spleens (and from one uninvolved spleen) of eight patients have been tested for their capacity to inhibit E-rosette formation by lymphocytes from normal subjects and have consistently shown marked E-rosette inhibiting activity (Fig. 6.10), whereas similarly prepared extracts from the spleens of most patients with non-Hodgkin's lymphomas and from normal spleens of acute trauma victims have been devoid of such activity (Bieber, Fuks, and Kaplan, 1977). Rosette levels

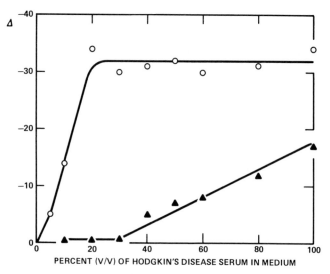

Figure 6.9 Effect of concentration of Hodgkin's disease serum (percentage, vol./vol., in culture medium RPMI-1640) on the capacity of peripheral blood lymphocytes from a normal donor (▲—▲) pretreated with fetal calf serum and of a patient with stage III mixed-cellularity Hodgkin's disease (○—○), similarly pretreated, to form E-rosettes. Lymphocytes were first incubated for 24 hours in 20 percent fetal calf serum and then incubated for an additional 2 hours in different concentrations of normal human AB or Hodgkin's disease serum. The difference in response (△) at each concentration was calculated by subtracting the percentage of E-rosette-forming cells after incubation in human AB serum from the corresponding percentage after incubation in Hodgkin's disease serum. (Reprinted, by permission of the authors and the *New England Journal of Medicine*, from the paper by Fuks, Strober, and Kaplan, 1976).

depressed by Hodgkin's disease spleen extracts could again be restored to normal levels by incubation in fetal calf serum. Lymphocytes from patients with Hodgkin's disease were not susceptible to the spleen extracts until they had first been restored by incubation in fetal calf serum; thereafter, however, incubation with Hodgkin's disease spleen extracts again profoundly depressed their E-rosette levels (Fig. 6.11).

Analysis of the active fraction indicated the presence of β-lipoprotein, C-reactive protein (CRP), and the C1q component of complement, as well as ferritin and albumin. Accordingly, additional preparations were made from seven Hodgkin's disease spleens, eight spleens from patients with non-Hodgkin's lymphomas, and two normal spleens to investigate the possibility that the E-rosette inhibitory substance might be an abnormal β-lipoprotein or lipoprotein complex. E-rosette in-

Figure 6.10 Depression of the E-RFC response of peripheral blood lymphocytes of normal donors by extracts from the spleens of eight consecutive patients with Hodgkin's disease. Similarly prepared extracts from normal donor spleens had no such effect. Data of M. M. Bieber and H. S. Kaplan. (Reprinted by permission of the Editor of *Cancer Research,* from the paper by Kaplan, 1976.)

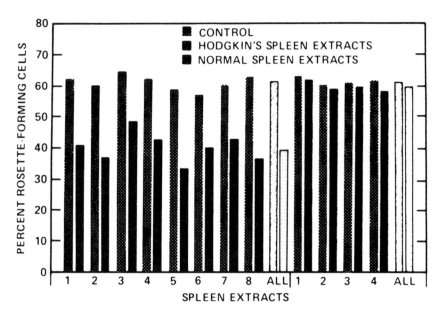

hibitory activity was found only in the low-density lipoprotein fractions after analytical flotation in the presence of potassium bromide. After further characterization, the active fractions proved to be complexes with densities between 1.050 and 1.075

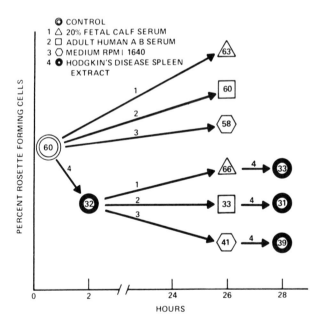

Figure 6.11 Depression of the E-RFC response of the peripheral blood lymphocytes of an individual normal donor by Hodgkin's disease spleen extract, restoration to normal levels by fetal calf serum, but not by adult human serum or RPMI-1640 medium alone, and redepression by Hodgkin's disease spleen extract. Data of M. M. Bieber and H. S. Kaplan. (Reprinted by permission of the Editor of *Cancer Research,* from the paper by Kaplan, 1976.)

g/cm^3 containing β-lipoprotein, C1q, CRP, and possibly other unidentified substances. With the exception of albumin, no other serum proteins could be identified (Bieber, Fuks, and Kaplan 1977). Similar activity was detected in serum.

In subsequent studies (Bieber et al., 1979), sera from patients with Hodgkin's disease were fractionated on sucrose gradients, yielding E-rosette inhibitory activity of higher density (>1.2 g/cm^3). It was thus possible to dissociate this activity from lipoprotein. After a second-stage potassium bromide isopycnic gradient separation, the activity was again found in the low-density fraction (1.02–1.06 g/cm^3). Thin-layer chromatography revealed that the active material is a glycolipid. Similarly fractionated normal sera were devoid of this activity. Further studies aimed at the chemical identification of the E-rosette inhibitory factor are in progress.

The possibility that ferritin might play a role in the immunodeficient responses of patients with Hodgkin's disease was first suggested by the observation of elevated serum and spleen ferritin levels in such patients by Bieber and Bieber (1973) and Jones et al. (1973). Later, the faster-migrating (F) of the two lymphocyte-associated antigens detected in the involved tissues of patients with Hodgkin's disease by Order, Colgan, and Hellman (1974) was identified as ferritin (Eshhar, Order, and Katz, 1974). More recently, Moroz et al. (1977a,b) used radioiodination of the surface proteins of peripheral blood mononuclear cells from four patients with Hodgkin's disease to demonstrate the presence of a blocking protein, which could be released from the cell surface by incubation with the antihelminthic drug, levamisole. The blocking protein reacted with antibody to human spleen ferritin but had no detectable iron and could be dissociated into subunits of 18,000 daltons molecular weight, suggesting that it is an apoferritin rather than ferritin. After treatment with levamisole and release of the blocking protein, the E-rosette response of peripheral blood lymphocytes from patients with Hodgkin's disease rose to normal levels. The possibility is not excluded, however, that some other low-molecular-weight E-rosette inhibitory substance bound to the lymphocyte surface membrane was also released by levamisole treatment concurrently with apoferritin.

The production of chemotactic factors and of inactivators of such factors has also been investigated in patients with Hodgkin's disease. Ward and Berenberg (1974) detected elevated levels of chemotactic factor inactivator (CFI), a naturally occurring regulator of inflammatory mediators, in the sera of nine patients with Hodgkin's disease. After activation of the sera with zymosan, the chemotactic activity of the Hodgkin's sera was significantly lower than that of four similarly treated normal sera. However, Rühl et al. (1974) found no evidence of significant depression of the production of a monocyte chemotactic factor in patients with Hodgkin's disease. Golding et al. (1977) studied the correlation between cutaneous delayed hypersensitivity reactions and the production of PHA-induced lymphokines such as leukocyte inhibitory factor (LIF) in 30 patients with untreated Hodgkin's disease. Both parameters were markedly depressed and displayed a 78 percent correlation coefficient. Spontaneous production of LIF-like activity was detected in supernatants of mononuclear cell cultures from 40 percent of the patients, and there appeared to be an inverse correlation between the spontaneous and the PHA-induced production of this activity. The supernatants of some unstimulated Hodgkin's disease mononuclear cell cultures were found to suppress the lymphoblastoid responses of normal cells to PHA.

Restoration of the Immune Response

Fluctuation with Disease Activity. Spontaneous fluctuations of immune status with changes in disease activity have been well documented. Sokal and Primikirios (1961) described the recovery of reactivity to tuberculin in two patients during long remissions, and Sokal (1973) recorded a remarkable instance of a patient with five distinct cycles of tuberculin negativity and positivity which coincided

with periods of reactivation and remission, respectively. Similarly, Aisenberg (1962) observed the restoration of the DNCB skin test from anergy to reactivity in two patients who had been in remission for over two years following local radiotherapy and the return to the anergic state in one of these patients during a subsequent relapse.

Several different approaches have been taken by investigators seeking to enhance the capacity of patients with Hodgkin's disease to mount cell-mediated immune responses. As has already been described in the section on passive transfer of hypersensitivity, efforts to restore skin test reactivity by inoculating anergic patients with transfer factor prepared from peripheral blood leukocytes of skin test–positive donors have yielded either negative or transient results. The greater rate of success reported by Han (1973, 1974) with "immune" RNA, also previously described, seems an approach worthy of further careful investigation, although the duration of the induced responses was limited to a few months in the most favorable case.

Vaccination. The long-known relationship between Hodgkin's disease, tuberculosis, and anergy to tuberculin has suggested the possibility that enhancement of resistance to tuberculosis by vaccination with the bacillus of Calmette-Guerin (BCG) might concomitantly stimulate immune responses in general, including those known to be deficient in patients with Hodgkin's disease.

De Marval (1940) attempted to immunize patients with Hodgkin's disease actively with preparations of BCG. Although two control groups simultaneously vaccinated with BCG became tuberculin positive, his patients with Hodgkin's disease remained tuberculin negative. Indeed, he reported that some of his patients with Hodgkin's disease (who may well, however, have had far-advanced disease) were able to withstand daily subcutaneous doses of up to 2 ml. of crude tuberculin without any apparent reaction!

Sokal and Primikirios (1961) also attempted to convert the tuberculin reaction of patients with Hodgkin's disease by BCG vaccination. Twelve of their patients with Hodgkin's disease had no constitutional manifestations, and ten of these were successfully converted to reactivity to second-strength tuberculin, whereas none of three patients with constitutional manifestations were converted. These investigations were continued by Sokal and Aungst (1969), who reported that 24 of 32 patients with advanced Hodgkin's disease (predominantly stage IV) were successfully converted to tuberculin reactivity after BCG vaccination. A quite different approach, theoretically aimed at interference with a hypothetical causative virus rather than vaccination per se, is the basis of the studies reported by Latarjet and Ennuyer (1969), involving the inoculation of patients with heavily irradiated extracts of their own diseased lymphoid tissues.

Thymus Extracts. Since the defects in cell-mediated immunity in Hodgkin's disease selectively involve the T-lymphocyte system, some investigators have suggested that the underlying mechanism might involve hypofunctionality of the thymus, which could perhaps be restored by thymus grafts or injections of thymic extracts. Rzepecki et al. (1973), in a brief letter giving few details, reported the transplantation of thymus glands from donors with myasthenia gravis to two patients with Hodgkin's disease and seven others with various forms of leukemia. They claimed "favorable effects," but presented no objective evidence to support this claim. Soon thereafter, a letter strongly criticizing this approach, and warning specifically that the use of myasthenia gravis donors might do more harm than good, was published by Papatestas, Genkins, and Kark (1973). Aiuti et al. (1975) observed an increased percentage of E-rosette-forming cells in two of three instances when lymphocytes from patients with Hodgkin's disease were incubated in vitro with pig thymus extract. The response to thymosin, a partially purified hormone-like human thymus extract, was studied by Sakai et al. (1975) in patients with malignant neoplasms, including one with stage IVB Hodgkin's disease. The E-rosette level of this patient rose from its initial level of 9.5 percent to 38 percent after incubation in vitro with thymosin. The patient was then given seven daily intramuscular injections of 100 mg thymosin. By day four, the E-rosette level had risen to 43 and 57 percent in the absence and presence, respectively, of added thymosin in vitro, and by the seventh day, the corresponding values had further increased to 54 and 65 percent.

Chemical Agents. The possibility that drugs might be used to restore immune function seems not to have been seriously entertained until it was discovered that levamisole, a widely used antihelminthic agent, was capable of stimulating lymphocytic and phagocytic function in vitro. Tripodi, Parks, and Brugmans (1973) administered levamisole orally to anergic patients with various types of neoplasms and observed the restoration of cutaneous delayed hypersensitivity reactions. The drug was first used in Hodgkin's disease by Levo, Rotter, and Ramot (1975), who reported that it converted the skin test responses of ten patients with stage IA and IIA disease in remission from negative to positive and increased their percentage of E-rosette-forming cells to normal. Followup studies on the same patients were performed six months later by Ramot et al. (1976), who found that their skin test reactivity had persisted, whereas their E-RFC had again fallen to pretreatment levels. They readministered levamisole at a daily dose of 150 mg for three days and noted a renewed increase in E-RFC to normal levels within one to four weeks in all ten patients. The response was well sustained for at least two months in four of these, partially sustained in others, and lost again within two months in two patients. Similar observations have been reported by others (Verhaegen et al., 1975; Sampson and Lui, 1976).

Ramot et al. (1976) extended their study to a total of 28 patients with Hodgkin's disease, of whom 8 had been previously untreated, and 21 normal controls, to whom the drug was given orally at the same dose level. Whereas the mean E-RFC level of the normal controls was essentially unchanged before and after treatment, that in the patients increased significantly, thus confirming the earlier observations of Levo, Rotter, and Ramot (1975). Both treated and untreated patients, irrespective of stage, are stated to have responded. As noted above, this group of investigators was later able to demonstrate that incubation with levamisole releases radioiodine-labeled proteins, one of which was later identified as apoferritin, from the surface membranes of lymphocytes from patients with Hodgkin's disease (Moroz et al., 1977a,b).

Transfer Factor; Interferon. Khan et al. (1975, 1976) administered transfer factor, at doses up to 10 units/m² intramuscularly every four weeks, to eight patients with Hodgkin's disease, four of whom were initially anergic to DNCB and a battery of skin test antigens. Five of these patients exhibited successful passive transfer of reactivity to one or more antigens and/or to DNCB. By the E-rosette test, the mean percentage of T-lymphocytes in the peripheral blood of the transfer factor–treated group was 46.3 percent, which was not significantly different from the 37.8 percent value in a control group of seven patients.

Blomgren et al. (1976) treated a patient who had lymphocyte predominance Hodgkin's disease with interferon, given intramuscularly for several months. In addition to inducing a partial remission, which is described later in this chapter, they observed a distinct improvement in the response of his peripheral blood lymphocytes to PHA, PWM, and Con A, which was evident within 1.5–2 months after the start of interferon treatment and persisted for several months.

Correlation with Prognosis

The high incidence of anergy in patients with far-advanced disease and the fluctuation of skin test reactivity concurrently with remission and relapse have suggested that the immune status of patients with Hodgkin's disease might be a prognostically useful parameter and, further, that treatment-induced restoration of the immune response might be reflected in improvement of prognosis. The weight of present evidence suggests that initial pretreatment immune responses have limited validity in this context. In contrast, the restoration of immune parameters to or toward normal following treatment, or their failure to be restored, may well have significant prognostic import.

Corder et al. (1972) and Young et al. (1973b) found that pretreatment responses to DNCB, mumps, and other skin test antigens did not correlate well with subsequent prognosis in a series of 60 previously untreated patients. Specifically, life-table analysis of the survival of 6 anergic and 20 nonanergic patients with stage III and IV disease revealed a slight increase in early deaths, but no long-term impairment of prognosis in the anergic group. In a similar analysis of patients with stage I and II disease, they concluded that no single skin test or combination of tests could be related to prognosis and survival. Although unresponsiveness to DNCB occurred in some 70 percent of our patients (Eltringham and Kaplan, 1973), five-year relapse-free survival, tantamount to permanent cure, was achieved in over 60 percent of all cases (Kaplan, 1976), clearly indicating that initial unresponsiveness is not incompatible with cure. In a followup study of 43 previously untreated patients in the Bethesda series on whom PHA-stimulated lymphoblastoid response data were available, Corder et al. (1972) also found no correlation between this test and subsequent clinical course or survival.

A more recent analysis of Stanford data on 531 patients with untreated Hodgkin's disease (R. T. Hoppe and H. S. Kaplan, unpublished) leaves open the possibility, however, that initial delayed hypersensitivity responses may have at least limited prognostic import. For example, actuarial five-year survival in pathological stages IA and IIA was 100 percent among the 97 patients who reacted positively, and only 89 percent ($p = 0.002$ by the Gehan test) among 142 patients who failed to react, to a challenge with 0.1 percent DNCB after prior sensitization with 0.5 percent DNCB. The corresponding five-year survival rates in stage IIIA were 96 and 88 percent; those in stage IIIB, 77 and 59 percent. When the cutaneous reactions to both mumps skin test antigen and DNCB were positive in stage IV (A + B), actuarial five-year survival was 75 percent; when both tests were negative, it was 51 percent. However, except for the stage IA and IIA groups cited above, these differences, though rather consistently unidirectional, were not significant at the 5 percent level.

Sokal and Primikirios (1961) observed that two patients who had a long remission from Hodgkin's disease recovered their reactivity to tuberculin. Sokal (1973) described a patient with prior tuberculosis and stage IVB Hodgkin's disease who displayed five cycles of tuberculin negativity and positivity correlated with periods of disease activity and remission, respectively, over a period of seven years. Sokal and Aungst (1969) observed a striking correlation between the response to BCG vaccination and prognosis. Seven of the 8 patients whose tuberculin responses remained negative died of Hodgkin's disease within one year, whereas only 1 of the 24 patients who developed positive tuberculin skin tests after BCG vaccination died within this time interval. The median survival of the former group was 7.5 months, whereas that of the latter group was over 30 months (Fig. 6.12). It was also of interest that the nonresponders were predominantly male, had a shorter prior duration of disease, and included the three oldest patients in the entire study. The authors suggested that the response to BCG vaccination predicted the subsequent course of these patients with advanced disease so well because the test is in itself a measure of the activity of the mechanism responsible for resistance to the disease.

The possibility that posttreatment changes in the tuberculin reaction might be useful as a prognostic index was suggested by Ciampelli and Pelù (1963). In their series of 47 patients, 8 of 23 whose tuberlin reaction was negative at the start of treatment became tuberculin-positive by the end of treatment, and 6 of these 8 were scored as having a sub-

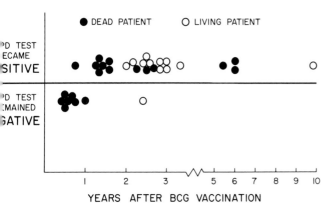

Figure 6.12 Survival of patients with advanced Hodgkin's disease after BCG vaccination, according to postvaccination tuberculin response. (Reprinted by permission from the paper by Sokal and Aungst, 1969.)

sequently "favorable" course. In contrast, 8 of 24 patients with initially positive tuberculin reactions became tuberculin negative later, and only one of these had a "favorable" course. Twelve of the 16 patients whose tuberculin reactions were positive initially and remained so after treatment had a "favorable" course. Since their cases were neither staged nor treated by contemporary methods, it is difficult to assess the validity of these data. Chang, Stutzman, and Sokal (1975) studied serial delayed hypersensitivity skin test responses before and after treatment in a series of 64 evaluable patients with active stage III or IV Hodgkin's disease, 21 of whom had received little or no previous treatment. Before the institution of multiple drug chemotherapy, 53 percent of these patients had one or more positive skin tests, and this response rate remained essentially unchanged (55 percent) during intensive chemotherapy. However, the percentage of responders rose to 79 percent during maintenance therapy and became 100 percent after discontinuation of all treatment. The pretreatment skin test responses were of no value in predicting clinical response to chemotherapy. Too few patients remained anergic after intensive chemotherapy to permit the assessment of prognosis in relation to posttreatment immune response.

The DNCB skin test data of Aisenberg (1962) have been reviewed in a previous section. The observation that positive skin tests developed after remissions of two years or more in two patients treated with local radiotherapy, and that one of these patients reverted to anergy during a subsequent relapse, suggested to Aisenberg that the DNCB response is closely correlated with disease activity and prognosis. Additional examples of

such "reversals" of the DNCB reaction during periods of remission were noted by Kaplan (1970). More recently, Fuks et al. (1976b) documented the restoration of responsiveness to DNCB during the first year after radiotherapy in 9 of 15 initially DNCB-positive patients who had become transiently anergic to the allergen at the completion of treatment. In addition, 12 (23 percent) of 52 patients who were anergic to DNCB prior to treatment later demonstrated positive reactions (Table 6.16).

Jackson, Garrett, and Craig (1970) reported on changes in the lymphoblastoid response during the course of the disease in 41 patients in whom serial determinations were performed, using uptake into DNA of ^{125}I-iododeoxyuridine (a thymidine analog) as the index of response. Unfortunately, the clinical stage of these cases had not been unambiguously established, since lymphangiography was used selectively rather than routinely. They noted a progressive, though not statistically significant, decrease in uptake of the analog with increasing clinical stage at presentation. After treatment, responses declined for several months and then returned to normal among patients in remission as well as in those with lymphadenopathy alone but failed to recover in patients with generalized disease. The authors concluded that "the altered response is a consequence of the disease rather than its cause and is capable of reversal by treatment."

DeSousa et al. (1977) studied the PHA responses of lymphocytes from 32 children with Hodgkin's disease before and at intervals from 2 to 72 months after treatment. All of the 8 children in whom relapses later occurred had a persistently low PHA response after treatment. These investigators concluded that sustained low PHA responses after

Table 6.16 Influence of Radiation Therapy on Delayed Hypersensitivity Responses to DNCB of Patients with Hodgkin's Disease[a]

Before treatment	%		After treatment	%	
Pos[b]	17/69	25	Pos	12/17	71
			Neg	5/17	29
Neg[c]	52/69	75	Pos	12/52	23
			Neg	40/52	77

Source: Fuks et al. (1976b). Reprinted by permission of the *Journal of Clinical Investigation.*

[a] Patients were sensitized with 500–2,000 µg DNCB before treatment and challenged with 100 µg 10–14 days later and at serial intervals of 3–6 months after completion of treatment.

[b] Positive delayed hypersensitivity response to DNCB.

[c] No delayed hypersensitivity response to DNCB.

chemotherapy or radiotherapy may correlate with unfavorable prognosis. However, Fuks et al. (1976b) found that PHA responses were consistently impaired for as long as ten years after total lymphoid or extended field radiotherapy in patients with Hodgkin's disease who had remained relapse-free continuously during the posttreatment interval.

Very limited information is available on other tests in vitro of immune function in relation to treatment and prognosis. Björkholm et al. (1975b) studied 33 consecutive previously untreated patients with Hodgkin's disease, of whom 13 were in clinical stage I or II and 20 were in clinical stage III or IV. They examined four parameters of lymphocyte response: the level of E-rosette-forming cells, the DNA synthesis response to Con A, the DNA synthesis response to PPD, and spontaneous lymphocyte DNA synthesis. Although the authors interpreted their data as indicating some correlation with these lymphocyte parameters, their patients reflect a skewed distribution with respect to clinical stage, histopathology, and mean age, making difficult any independent assessment of the prognostic significance of the lymphocyte responses. Thus, the 18 patients in complete remission included 10 of 13 in clinical stage I and II, as compared with only 8 of 20 in clinical stage III and IV; 12 of 15 with NS or LP histopathologic type, as contrasted with only 6 of 18 with MC or LD type; and a mean age of 32.9 years, as contrasted with 56.3 years among those with incomplete remission, relapse, or death. Subsequent extensions of these studies yielded similar conclusions (Björkholm et al., 1978). Holm et al. (1975) found that the activity of effector cells of antibody-induced lymphocyte-mediated cytotoxicity (K cells) was virtually abolished in four patients with Hodgkin's disease who died 6 to 13 months after testing and was lower among patients in incomplete remission or with relapse after treatment than among those remaining in complete remission. They noted a similar but less pronounced correlation with prognosis for PHA-induced cytotoxicity.

In a randomized clinical trial, Hoerni et al. (1974) attempted to ascertain whether nonspecific stimulation of the immune system by vaccination with BCG could improve prognosis in a series of 30 patients, 19 of whom had constitutional symptoms. Patients who had entered remission after radiotherapy and chemotherapy were assigned at random to receive either no further treatment or BCG. After a followup interval of 40 months, relapse-free survival was 79 percent in the BCG-treated group and 53 percent in the controls. Although this difference is suggestive, it falls short of statistical significance ($p > 0.10$). Moreover, although patients were randomly allocated to the two arms of the study, no stratification procedure was used, with the result that the BCG-treated group contained a substantially higher proportion of patients who had previously been treated with cyclic combination chemotherapy, whereas a greater fraction of the controls received single-drug (vinblastine) chemotherapy, a discrepancy which might well account for the observed differences in relapse-free survival in the absence of BCG. Thus, the value of nonspecific immunotherapy with BCG or other adjuvants, given as a supplement to conventional radiotherapy and/or chemotherapy, remains moot.

Blomgren et al. (1976) treated a patient with lymphocyte predominance Hodgkin's disease, classified as stage IVB (probably Ann Arbor stage II_EB from their description) with interferon (5×10^6 U daily), given by intramuscular injection, to a total dose of 1,377 million U over a period of seven months. Initially, there was partial regression of peripheral adenopathy, disappearance of pruritus and night sweats, and diminution of cough. However, progressive enlargement of the peripheral and hilar lymph nodes was again noted within a few months, and a biopsy revealed a shift to mixed cellularity histopathology. Accordingly, interferon treatment was discontinued and the patient was started on combination (CVPP) chemotherapy, on which he again entered partial remission.

Effects of Treatment on the Immune Response

The earlier literature on the immune status of patients with Hodgkin's disease is of limited value today, not only because patients had not been diagnostically evaluated and staged by modern standards, but also because many patients had received one or more courses of radiotherapy, chemotherapy, or both, with the result that the role of the disease and the role of its treatment were inextricably confounded. It has long been known that ionizing radiation and some of the radiomimetic and steroid compounds are lymphocytotoxic, but until recently there were few reports on their long-term effects on cell-mediated immune responses. The available information is briefly summarized in this section.

Many studies of patients receiving radiotherapy for various types of neoplastic disease have demonstrated that acute lymphocytopenia and the suppression of immune function become evident soon after the initiation of treatment, with partial recovery within 18–24 months in some instances. Fuks et al. (1976b) studied the immunologic responses of a series of 79 patients with Hodgkin's disease, all of whom had been staged with the aid of lymphangiography, had been treated with a singe course of local, extended-field or total lymphoid irradiation, and had been in continuous complete remission for periods of one to ten years thereafter. Ten of the patients had received several (usually six) cycles of prophylactic combination chemotherapy (MOPP) following completion of radiotherapy. Their immune responses were compared with those of 148 untreated patients and 86 normal subjects. At the completion of radiotherapy, all patients manifested severe lymphocytopenia, with a mean absolute lymphocyte count of only 503/mm³, as compared with a pretreatment mean of 1,634 ± 132 in those with stage I and II and 1,643 ± 200 in those with stage III and IV disease. However, among those in remission for 12 to 111 months posttreatment, the mean lymphocyte count was again normal (1,985 ± 182), and absolute lymphocytopenia was noted in only 7 of 26 (27 percent). Only 3 of these had had lymphocytopenia prior to treatment; conversely, 8 other patients with pretreatment lymphocytopenia later had normal lymphocyte levels. Interestingly, the percentage of monocytes in the treated patients was not significantly different from that of the normal controls. Postirradiation lymphocytopenia in patients with Hodgkin's disease has also been documented by Sutherland, McCredie, and Inch (1975), Hancock et al. (1977a,b), and Björkholm et al. (1977a).

B-lymphocytes, identified as SIg-positive cells, comprised 20 ± 1.2 percent of the total blood lymphocyte population in the normal subjects studied by Fuks et al. (1976b), with a mean absolute count of 407 ± 25/mm³. In five patients tested immediately following completion of radiotherapy, the mean absolute B-lymphocyte count was profoundly decreased (47.2 ± 31.3/mm³), but by 12 to 111 months after the completion of radiotherapy, both the mean percentage (37 ± 2.2 percent) and the mean absolute B-lymphocyte count (725 ± 66) were significantly higher (p <0.01) than those of the normal subjects, confirming an observation previously made by Engeset et al. (1973) in a small series of patients. An absolute B-lymphocytosis, defined as a value more than two standard deviations above the normal mean, was present in 16 (61 percent) of 26 patients, and one patient had a count of 1,526 B-lymphocytes/mm³.

T-lymphocytes, scored by the cytotoxicity assay on gradient-purified buffy coat suspensions corrected for monocyte number, constituted 77 ± 1.5 percent of the total lymphocyte population in normal subjects, with a mean absolute count of 1,600 ± 76/mm³. Immediately following radiotherapy, the five patients tested had a profound depletion of T-lymphocytes, with a mean of only 150 ± 134/mm³. However, in striking contrast to the relatively early B-lymphocyte recovery and overshoot, T-lymphocyte levels remained significantly depressed among 26 patients tested while in remission 12 to 111 months following completion of radiotherapy. In this group, the mean percentage of T-lymphocytes was only 41 ± 2.8 percent, and the mean absolute count of 793 ± 66 T-lymphocytes/mm³ was very significantly (p <0.01) lower than normal. Absolute T-lymphocytopenia occurred in 19 of 26 (73 percent) of these patients, some of whom had been irradiated more than eight years previously. Björkholm et al. (1977a) also observed a T-lymphocytopenia among patients in remission following radiation therapy.

Small lymphocytes which display neither T- nor B-lymphocyte surface markers are known as "null" cells. These cells, which are estimated by subtracting the combined T- and B-cell percentages, normally constitute only a small fraction (approximately 3 percent) of total peripheral blood lymphocytes. In untreated patients with Hodgkin's disease, their levels were also low but more variable (Fuks et al., 1976b). Since 90 percent of untreated patients had values of 14 percent or lower, this was taken as the upper limit of normal. Patients in remission after radiotherapy had distinctly elevated percentages (15 to 49 percent) of null lymphocytes, even as late as nine years postirradiation. The nature of this increased population of null cells is unknown, except that they did not react in the alpha-naphthyl acetate staining procedure for nonspecific esterase and therefore do not appear to be monocytes. It is possible that they represent immature forms of B-lymphocytes, T-lymphocytes, or both.

These marked changes in the relative and absolute numbers of B-, T-, null, and total circulating lymphocytes are also accompanied by functional sequelae. Levy and Kaplan (1974) reported that the lymphoblastoid stimulation responses to a range of PHA concentrations, as measured by the ³H-leucine uptake assay, were profoundly depressed (Fig. 6.13) in a series of 16 patients in con-

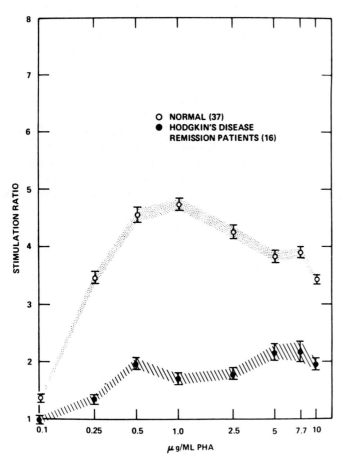

Figure 6.13 Profoundly impaired phytohemagglutinin (PHA) stimulation responses (means ±S.E.) of peripheral blood lymphocytes from patients with Hodgkin's disease in long-term remission after radiotherapy. Significance of difference from normal is $p < 0.01$ at all PHA concentrations tested. (Reprinted by permission of the *New England Journal of Medicine,* from the paper by Levy and Kaplan, 1974.)

tinuous remission for periods of two to eight years after a single course of radiotherapy. These findings were later confirmed and extended to a series of 66 patients by Fuks et al. (1976b). There was no evident correlation between followup interval and PHA response; patients observed for as long as ten years had a mean stimulation ratio (2.39 ± 0.30) which was not significantly greater than that (2.03 ± 0.28) for patients tested only one year postirradiation. Moreover, the extent of the radiotherapeutic fields and their topographic localization also bore no relation to the PHA test results. Patients whose radiation fields were entirely infradiaphragmatic had a mean stimulation ratio of only 1.78 ± 0.20, entirely comparable to that of patients who had received total lymphoid radiotherapy. Adjunctive MOPP combination chemo-

therapy did not further depress the PHA response significantly. Stimulation responses to a range of concentrations of Con A and to tetanus toxoid were also markedly impaired in patients tested during long-term, continuous remission following irradiation. After extended field radiotherapy, Sutherland, McCredie, and Inch (1975) observed a 30 percent decrease in the DNA synthesis response to PHA which lasted for about 300 days, rebounding by 1,000 days to 38 percent above the pretreatment level. Faguet (1975) also noted an increased impairment of the PHA response following radiotherapy or combination chemotherapy.

Depression of E-RFC levels after radiotherapy has been noted by Cohnen et al. (1973a) and Andersen (1974). Confirming this observation, the percentage of E-RFC in 26 patients in continuous long-term remission after a single course of radiotherapy was found to be markedly lower than normal (Fuks et al., 1976b). However, unlike the situation described earlier for E-RFC in untreated patients with Hodgkin's disease, the mean E-RFC level in the treated patients $(38.1 \pm 1.6$ percent) was comparable to (indeed, slightly higher than) their mean percentage of T-cells determined by the cytotoxic assay $(32 \pm 2.3$ percent). Moreover, incubation of the peripheral blood lymphocytes of the treated patients in the presence of fetal calf serum had no effect on the percentage of E-RFC. Taken together, these two observations indicate that the low E-RFC levels in the treated patients reflect a true depletion of T-lymphocytes in the peripheral blood, rather than the masking of a subpopulation of T-cells by a rosette-inhibiting serum factor, as is apparently the case in untreated patients. Lang et al. (1978) found that active rosette-forming cell (A-RFC) levels were also significantly decreased in a series of 21 patients previously treated with radiotherapy, chemotherapy, or both.

The capacity of peripheral blood lymphocytes from these treated patients to stimulate or respond to foreign lymphocytes in vitro in the one-way MLR test was also investigated by Fuks et al. (1976b). Lymphocytes from 12 patients in long-term remission were capable of stimulating normal MLR reactions in 92 percent of tested combinations when mixed with responder cells from unrelated normal individuals, though in 3 of 17 individual tests the responses, though positive, were weak. However, an entirely different result was seen when the one-way MLR test was run in the opposite direction (Fig. 6.14). Recent radiotherapy markedly reduced the capacity of lymphocytes from the treated patients to respond. Eight pa-

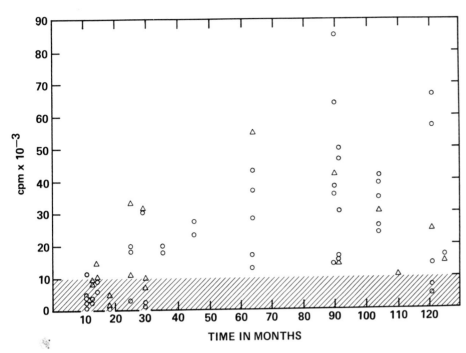

Figure 6.14 MLR of peripheral blood lymphocytes from Hodgkin's disease patients treated with radiotherapy and in complete remission 1–11 years after therapy; correlation of response with time elapsing from therapy. Stimulator cells were obtained from normal donors (△) or other treated patients (○). (Reprinted, by permission of the *Journal of Clinical Investigaion,* from the paper by Fuks et al., 1976b.)

tients tested 12 to 30 months after total lymphoid irradiation yielded positive responses in only 4 (33 percent) of 12 combinations when randomly paired with normal donor lymphocytes, and in only 4 (25 percent) of 16 combinations when paired with lymphocytes from other treated patients. As the interval of followup increased beyond two years, there appeared to be a gradual recovery of the capacity of lymphocytes from irradiated patients to respond in the MLR test. Among those treated 31–120 months earlier, there were positive responses in 35 (95 percent) of 37 tests in which responder cells from patients were mixed with stimulator cells from normal donors or other treated patients. Normal responses were observed in all but two patients who had been in continuous remission for five years or more.

Apparently full recovery of both delayed hypersensitivity responsiveness and normal immunoglobulin levels was reported by Kun and Johnson (1975) in a followup study of 69 patients with Hodgkin's disease who had been in remission for five years after intensive radiotherapy. However, Check et al. (1973) found that cutaneous responses to mumps skin test antigen were profoundly impaired for as long as ten years after irradiation. At Stanford University Medical Center, a series of 69 patients who had been sensitized with 0.5–2.0 percent DNCB were repeatedly challenged before treatment and at 3- to 6-month intervals after treatment until a positive reaction became apparent. An analysis of their responses by Fuks et al. (1976b) is presented in Table 6.16. Of 17 patients with positive pretreatment reactions, 15 (88 percent) were found to be anergic to DNCB immediately following completion of radiotherapy. Nine of these patients regained their reactivity by 4–12 months postirradiation, and a tenth individual did so at 40 months after radiotherapy. However, 5 patients remained anergic to DNCB for as long as eight years. Conversely, of the 52 patients who were initially unresponsive, 12 (23 percent) later responded positively to challenge with DNCB after they had been in complete remission for periods of one to five years or more.

The effect of chemotherapy on the immune response of patients with Hodgkin's disease has received much less detailed study. Chin et al. (1973) applied the indirect immunofluorescence technique, using a heterologous antithymocyte serum, to the detection and enumeration of T-lymphocytes in a series of 38 patients with malignant lymphomas, including 20 with Hodgkin's disease, all of whom were receiving chemotherapy at the time of study; they observed T-lymphocyte percentages in the normal range. In six patients studied by Swain and Trounce (1974), quadruple-drug chemotherapy induced a slight but significant increase in the proportion of E-rosette-forming cells. Impairment of the lymphoblastoid response to PHA during treatment with corticosteroids, antimetabolites, alkylating agents, and various combinations of these agents has been repeatedly observed in patients with Hodgkin's disease and other lymphomas (Hersh and Oppenheim, 1965a; Holm, Perlmann, and Johansson, 1967; Han and Sokal, 1970; Han, 1972). Marked depression of cutaneous delayed hypersensitivity responses was noted by Hancock et al. (1977a) following combination chemotherapy. However, the duration of impairment following either single-drug or cyclic combination chemotherapy, though generally assumed to be relatively transient, has not been established with any precision.

The influence of treatment on humoral immunity was investigated by Weitzman et al. (1977b) in a series of 44 patients with Hodgkin's disease. Untreated patients had normal antibody titers against *H. influenzae* type b (mean 396 ng/ml). Titers were unaffected by radiotherapy alone and only marginally reduced by chemotherapy alone. However, in patients receiving combined radiotherapy and chemotherapy, the mean antibody titer fell to 147 ng/ml ($p < 0.01$). IgM levels, which were normal prior to treatment, were also significantly reduced by chemotherapy, particularly in previously splenectomized patients. In contrast, the levels of IgG, IgA, and several components of complement were all normal or elevated. Hancock et al. (1977a), in a study of 85 patients before and after treatment, reported that Ig levels were unaffected in a nonsplenectomized group, but that both IgM and IgA decreased significantly in the splenectomized group, especially after combination chemotherapy.

The widespread adoption of staging laparotomy with splenectomy as part of the diagnostic evaluation of patients with Hodgkin's disease has also raised questions concerning the impact of splenectomy on susceptibility to infection and on immune function. Wagener et al. (1976) studied a series of 15 patients before and after splenectomy. They found that skin test reactivity and the MLR test were unchanged; however, in those patients with spleens weighing 240 gm or more, they noted a significant decrease in the percentage of E-rosette-forming cells, an increase in EAC rosette-forming (B) cells, and an increase in the PHA stimulation response, especially in the presence of stage III and IV disease. They concluded that splenectomy has no demonstrable untoward effect on cellular immunity. Similar conclusions were reached by Hancock et al. (1977a,b), who found that neutrophil phagocytic function was not significantly influenced by splenectomy, radiotherapy, or chemotherapy. Splenectomy also had no effect on antibody titers to the capsular polysaccharide of *H. influenzae* type b (Weitzman et al., 1977b).

Possible Tumor-Associated Antigens; Antigen-Antibody Reactions

A number of unrelated lines of investigation have yielded intriguing bits and pieces of evidence that can be interpreted as indicative of the existence of tumor-associated antigens or of various types of reactions to them in patients with Hodgkin's disease. Although some of these studies also relate to the subject matter of Chapter 2 and have been discussed there, it seemed desirable and convenient to bring together in this section the available information in this elusive and complex field.

Crowther, Fairley, and Sewell (1967a, 1967b) studied the morphology and tritiated thymidine uptake of unstimulated lymphoid cells from the peripheral blood of patients with Hodgkin's disease. Phagocytic monocytes and granulocytes were first removed from defibrinated blood by use of finely divided iron powder and methyl cellulose. A significant increase in the number of large lymphoid cells, about 20μ in diameter, was noted in the preparations from 14 of 18 untreated patients. These cells were morphologically similar to those found in efferent lymph nodes draining sites of antigenic stimulation in experimental animals. Consistent with this was the finding that tritiated thymidine uptake was increased in the lymphoid cell preparations from 15 of 17 patients, and that the label, in autoradiographs, was almost entirely confined to these large cells, an observation also made by Kuper and Bignall (1964). Crowther et al. stated that these large cells may be seen in all stages of Hodgkin's disease and that their number was not correlated with the ability of the patients to give delayed hypersensitivity reactions to tuberculin or streptokinase. Lymphoid cells "spontaneously" active in DNA synthesis have also been observed in the peripheral blood of patients with Hodgkin's disease by Huber et al. (1970, 1975), Schick, Trepel, and Begemann (1975), and Holm et al. (1976). Mitchell et al. (1973) found that those patients who showed no lymphoblastoid transformation response to PHA had the highest spontaneous uptake of tritiated thymidine. Crowther et al. suggested that these cells may reflect the occurrence of an immunologic reaction of the host against the disease. In a more recent review, Crowther (1973) has cautioned that the identity and specificity of the putative antigen against which such reactions are seemingly directed still remain to be established and that alternative interpretations of these findings are not excluded.

Various antigens have been detected in the peripheral blood and in involved tissues of patients with Hodgkin's disease. Bieber and Bieber (1973) observed an apparently abnormal ferritin in the circulation, and Jones et al. (1973) confirmed the occurrence of ferritinemia in such patients. Order and his colleagues (1971, 1972) prepared heterologous antisera against involved splenic tissues removed at laparotomy and demonstrated positive indirect immunofluorescence reactions, after appropriate absorption of these sera, with the involved spleens of 18 of 19 patients with Hodgkin's disease. However, antisera against 5 of 18 control spleens also yielded positive reactions in this system, indicating that the relevant antigens were tumor-associated rather than tumor-specific. An apparently similar or identical antigen has been described by Favre, Carcassonne, and Meyer (1977). Katz et al. (1973) and Order, Colgan, and Hellman (1974) were later able to partially purify and to separate these antigens into slow (S) and fast (F) components with respect to their electrophoretic mobility. After further purification and analysis, it was demonstrated by Eshhar, Order, and Katz (1974) that the F antigen is apparently identical with ferritin, thus providing a possible link to the earlier observations of Bieber and Bieber (1973). More recently, Moroz et al. (1977a,b) have reported that the lymphocytes of patients with Hodgkin's disease bear ferritin on their surface membranes and that it may be removed by treatment with levamisole. Sarcione et al. (1975, 1977) observed increased rates of ferritin synthesis by splenic tumor tissue and by peripheral blood lymphocytes, and an increased rate of ferritin release by peripheral blood cells.

A distinctly different tissue immunofluorescence approach was used by Denton and Field (1973). They prepared cell suspensions of fresh involved lymph node or splenic tissue and incubated these suspensions on microscope slides with sera from the same patients obtained during the active phase of their Hodgkin's disease. After careful washing, a second incubation was performed with fluoresceinated antiserum to whole human immunoglobulin, and the preparations were examined by fluorescence microscopy. Control preparations were simultaneously made, omitting the first incubation with autologous serum or using cell suspensions from uninvolved tissues. In tests on 57 involved samples and 17 control samples from 48 patients, they failed to detect membrane immunofluorescence in any instance, thus providing no evidence for the existence of autoantibodies in the sera of patients with active disease. However, Grifoni et al. (1968b) noted increased blastoid transformation when small lymphocytes from patients with Hodgkin's disease were cultured in vitro with homogenates prepared from autologous involved lymph nodes.

In a continuing series of investigations in which they used cytotoxicity tests, direct immunofluorescence, and passive hemagglutination techniques, Grifoni and his colleagues (1968a, 1969, 1970, 1973) have reported the presence of antilymph node and antilymphocyte autoantibodies and alloantibodies in the sera of many patients with Hodgkin's disease, most of whom were in stage III or IV. Marked fluctuations of antibody levels serially determined over time were noted in some patients. The antibody was found to persist even in remission. Grifoni (1973) concluded that this evidence indicates that two populations of immunocompetent cells are operative and in mutual conflict, thus providing support for the Kaplan-Smithers (1959) hypothesis that an autoimmune lymphoid reaction may play a role in the pathogenesis of Hodgkin's disease.

Longmire et al. (1973) used a radioimmunoassay before and after incubation for 10 days to quantify IgG content of leukocyte-rich cell suspensions prepared from 10 control spleens and from 22 spleens of patients with Hodgkin's disease (19 untreated), of which 11 were uninvolved, 6 lightly involved by scattered small nodules, and 5 heavily involved (>60 percent tumor tissue). The mean 10-day unstimulated IgG synthesis of the 10 normal spleens was 625 ng IgG N/20 × 10⁶ cells, whereas those of the uninvolved and the lightly involved Hodgkin's disease spleens were 3,563 and 2,750, respectively. Cells cultured from the heavily involved spleens synthesized somewhat less IgG per unit volume than the normal spleens. When these figures were multiplied by total spleen mass after determination of cell number per gram, total organ synthesis of IgG could be calculated. It was found that mean total IgG synthesis in the uninvolved Hodgkin's disease spleens was about 5.5-fold that of the normal spleens, and that for the lightly involved spleens was 11-fold higher than normal. Stimulation of secondary IgG production by the cultures in response to smallpox vaccine also revealed a greater mean response by the uninvolved and lightly involved Hodgkin's disease spleens than by normal spleens, but the 5 heavily involved spleens failed to respond. When the culture-produced IgG, cleared of aggregates by heating at 56 C for 30 minutes and ultracentrifugation, was incubated with purified homologous lymphocyte suspensions from normal subjects, followed by careful washing, the IgG produced by cultures from 4 normal spleens failed to display significant binding, whereas that from 3 Hodgkin's disease spleens showed a highly significant degree of specific binding. Longmire et al. considered these findings suggestive of a response to antigenic challenge; moreover, they concluded that a portion of the IgG produced during cultures of Hodgkin's disease spleen tissue is specific for binding sites on or associated with lymphocytes.

The only tissue culture–derived Hodgkin's disease–associated antigen described to date is that discovered and partially characterized by Long et al. (1973, 1974a, 1977a). They prepared monolayer cultures from tumor nodules of 18 Hodgkin's disease spleens, 10 normal adult spleens, and 3 normal fetal spleens and thymuses. The clarified culture supernatants were pelleted, resuspended in sucrose gradients, and the peak sedimenting in the specific gravity range 1.15–1.21 g/ml was inoculated into rabbits. The heterologous antibody thus raised was absorbed with normal human spleen, fetal calf serum, and type A-positive human erythrocytes before use. Some of the antisera were tested by agar-gel diffusion and immunoelectrophoresis against antigens from the purified 1.15–1.21 g/ml peaks, yielding positive reactions with nine of ten cultured Hodgkin's disease spleen lines, as compared with two of eight cell lines from uninvolved spleens from patients with Hodgkin's disease and three of six lines from control spleens. The antigen, which resisted solubilization with Tween-ether and migrated as a single band by immunoelectrophoresis, could not be detected in disrupted, noncultured spleen tumor tissue from patients with Hodgkin's disease. In later studies using indirect immunofluorescence, surface membrane fluorescent staining was observed in about 45 percent of viable cells from Hodgkin's spleen cultures and less than 5 percent of those

from normal cultures. Similar tests on acetone-fixed cells revealed fluorescent cytoplasmic staining of 51 percent of cells from Hodgkin's cultures versus 4–8 percent of those from normal cultures. Absorption of the antiserum with density 1.15–1.21 antigen removed its reactivity for Hodgkin's disease target cells. Corroboratory evidence was also obtained in studies with ^{125}I-radiolabeled antibody, which revealed that the quantity of antigen present on cells from Hodgkin's disease cultures was 15- to 30-fold greater than that on cells from control cultures. Although the emergence of the antigen is clearly related to propagation in vitro of the Hodgkin's disease splenic tumor tissue, the identity of the antigen remains to be established. It was clearly distinguishable from the F and S antigens described by Order et al. (1971, 1974), from the Epstein-Barr virus, and from two C-type RNA viruses, RD-114 and the Rauscher murine leukemia virus. The authors concluded that it may prove to be a viral component, a tumor or fetal antigen, or a normal tissue constituent. Subsequently, Long et al. (1977b) reported that 23 sera with elevated levels of soluble immune complexes (among a total of 90 tested sera from patients with Hodgkin's disease) all reacted with antigen-bearing cultured cells from spleens involved by Hodgkin's disease. Absorption with cultured cells removed the immune complexes and abrogated the reactivity of the sera. Paradoxically, although the antibody component from the circulating immune complexes apparently reacts with the tissue culture antigen, it has not been possible to detect the antigen in fresh Hodgkin's spleen tissue.

Hancock, Bruce, and Richmond (1976b) used a leukocyte migration inhibition technique in vitro to examine the response of leukocytes to an extract prepared from spleen tissue obtained at necropsy from a patient with Hodgkin's disease with gross splenic involvement, and the response to a similarly prepared extract from a normal spleen removed during gastrectomy. Migration was inhibited in 31 (56 percent) of 55 patients with Hodgkin's disease and 19 (49 percent) of 39 with other types of lymphomas, as compared with only 1 (4 percent) of 23 normal volunteers and 1 (4 percent) of 25 patients with nonmalignant disease. None of the patients whose leukocyte migration was inhibited by the Hodgkin's disease spleen extract showed inhibition of migration when tested with the normal spleen extract. Assessment of the significance of these findings must await additional studies with similarly prepared extracts from involved spleens of other patients with Hodgkin's disease, preferably obtained at staging laparotomy rather than at necropsy.

Summary

Immunologic investigations of increasing sensitivity and sophistication now leave little room for doubt that virtually all patients with Hodgkin's disease, including most of those with highly localized involvement, suffer from a selective, though often subtle and partial, impairment of cell-mediated immunity. This deficit is expressed in vivo by an increased susceptibility to certain types of bacterial, fungal, and viral infections and by a decreased capacity for delayed hypersensitivity reactions to intradermal recall antigens or chemical allergens. Several test responses in vitro are also impaired, including lymphoblastoid transformation by plant lectins and natural antigens, the capacity to form spontaneous, nonimmune (E) rosettes, and the capacity for cap formation after binding of certain lectins. These abnormalities have been shown to be due to functional alterations of T-lymphocytes, rather than to quantitative depletion of total, T-, or B-lymphocytes. The functional impairment of the E-rosette response is a reversible phenomenon brought about by the binding to a subpopulation of T-lymphocytes of a serum E-rosette-inhibiting factor which is also present in extracts from the spleens of patients with Hodgkin's disease. Ferritin is also reportedly synthesized at significantly increased rates by peripheral blood lymphocytes and bound reversibly to their surface membranes in such patients. Other studies in vitro suggest that suppressor cells may play a role in the impairment of certain immune responses, possibly through the secretion of humoral mediators such as prostaglandin E_2; however, specificity of suppressor cell effects in Hodgkin's disease has not been demonstrated. The possibility of restoration of the immune response in vivo has been raised by recent studies with the antihelminthic drug, levamisole, as well as by studies in vitro with indomethacin, an inhibitor of prostaglandin synthetase. Although the occurrence of immunologic impairment in early Hodgkin's disease suggests that it may well have a role in the pathogenesis of the disease, little correlation has been demonstrated between the pretreatment immune status of patients with Hodgkin's disease and their prognosis. However, posttreatment restoration of immune responsiveness appears to be associated with sustained remission, and conversely, failure of immune recovery appears to be associated with an increased risk of relapse. Investigations bearing on the possible existence of tumor-associated antigens and of antigen-antibody reactions in Hodgkin's disease are reviewed, and their possible significance in relation to the pathogenesis of the disease and of its associated immunologic deficit is assessed.

Chapter 7

Patterns of Anatomic Distribution

In this chapter are described the clinical settings in which involvement of specific organs or tissues by Hodgkin's disease is most likely to occur, the symptoms and signs associated with such involvement, and the specific diagnostic measures that may be most appropriate for documentation. The frequencies with which two (or more) specific sites are involved at time of initial diagnosis and the frequencies with which extension to specified sites occurs after local treatment of any given primary site or sites provide the basis for the hypothesis that, in the great majority of instances, Hodgkin's disease spreads nonrandomly and predictably via lymphatic channels to contiguous lymph node chains and other lymphatic structures. The hypothesis of contiguous, nonrandom, lymphatic spread is critically analyzed in relation to other hypotheses at the end of this chapter.

Specific Organ and Tissue Involvement

Lymph Nodes. For reasons that are not clear, certain chains of lymph nodes are seldom or rarely involved by Hodgkin's disease, although they are often affected in patients with other types of malignant lymphoma. Thus, the mesenteric lymph nodes were involved in only 3 of 285 consecutive cases, in striking contrast to the frequency with which the nearly lumbar para-aortic nodes participated in the disease process (Fig. 7.1). That this is not simply due to failure of detection is indicated by the consistency with which routine biopsies of the mesenteric nodes have been negative, even in patients with documented para-aortic node disease, in our experience with diagnostic laparotomy; in a consecutive series of 814 cases, mesenteric node involvement was documented in only 19 (2.3 percent). Conversely, several reports suggest that the celiac nodes are involved more often than any other single lymph node group in the abdomen; indeed, they may be involved even in the absence of splenic involvement (Mitchell et al., 1972; Irving, 1975). In a series of 81 staging laparoto-

mies in which careful lymph node mapping was undertaken by Ferguson et al. (1973), celiac node involvement was documented in 43 percent (Table 7.1). The data of Irving are in excellent agreement; celiac node involvement was observed in 35 (42 percent) of 84 patients with Hodgkin's disease submitted to staging laparotomy.

In the pelvis, the hypogastric and midline presacral nodes are rarely involved, except in instances in which there is massive enlargement of the iliac nodes. The epitrochlear nodes are involved with moderate frequency, and the popliteal nodes occasionally, in the lymphocytic and histiocytic lymphomas; yet, despite the relative frequency of axillary node involvement in Hodgkin's disease, epitrochlear node presentations are seldom observed (Weiss and Jenkins, 1977), and popliteal node involvement is exceedingly rare. Internal mammary node involvement, almost invariably associated with anterior mediastinal adenopathy, usually presents as a parasternal chest wall mass (Fig. 7.2) and may secondarily lead to invasion and destruction of the sternum (Goldman, 1971).

The lymph nodes at the hila of the lungs are affected in only about one-third of the cases in which mediastinal lymphadenopathy is present (Fig. 7.1). However, their special significance with respect to the probability of pulmonary parenchymal involvement, which is discussed in further detail below, calls for particularly careful and selective evaluation of the hilar nodes by tomography, as well as by conventional chest radiography, in all instances in which the mediastinal nodes are enlarged. Tomography is also valuable in detecting involvement of intrapulmonary lymph nodes, occasionally documented in patients with Hodgkin's disease (Fellows, Abell, and Martel, 1969). Adenopathy may also occur in the diaphragmatic nodes at the cardiophrenic angle (Figs. 5.36, 5.37; Fayos and Lampe, 1971; Castellino and Blank, 1972).

Specific symptoms may have diagnostic value as clues to the detection of involved lymph nodes in

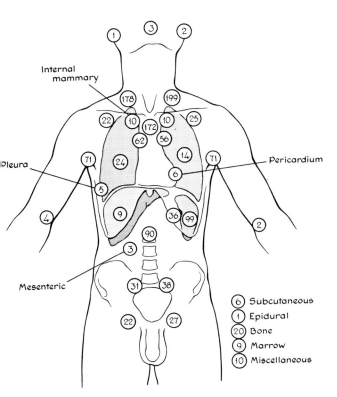

Figure 7.1 Anatomical distribution of sites of involvement in 285 consecutive, unselected, previously untreated patients with Hodgkin's disease, 272 of whom were submitted to staging laparotomy with splenectomy. (Reprinted by permission, from the paper by Kaplan, Dorfman, Nelsen, and Rosenberg, 1973.)

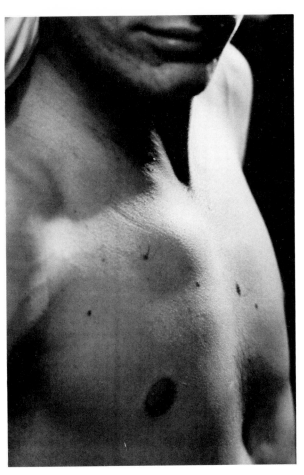

Figure 7.2 Parasternal chest wall mass due to internal mammary lymphadenopathy. (Reprinted by permission of the author and *Chest,* from the paper by Goldman, 1971.)

Hodgkin's disease. The presence of constitutional symptoms, and particularly of fever and/or night sweats, in a patient with seemingly isolated lymphadenopathy in the groin, neck, or axilla should alert the physician to a renewed, painstaking search for intrathoracic or intra-abdominal lymphadenopathy, or for involvement of such silent extralymphatic sites as the liver or bone marrow, since constitutional symptoms are rare in patients with true stage I disease confined to peripheral lymph nodes.

The local symptoms produced by lymphadenopathy are those usually attributable to pressure or obstruction. In peripheral sites, they may in-

Table 7.1 Frequency of Abdominal Lymph Node Involvement in 81 Patients with Hodgkin's Disease

Lymph node group	No. positive/No. biopsied	% positive
Portal	20/68	29
Celiac	7/16	43
Splenic	15/70	21
Mesenteric	8/68	12
Right aortic	19/77	25
Left aortic	14/79	18
Right iliac	11/76	14
Left iliac	9/76	12

Source: Data of Ferguson et al. (1973).

clude pain, edema, specific neuropathy, and even obliteration of the pulse in an extremity. In the thorax, enlarging lymph node masses may produce cough, dyspnea, transudative or chylous pleural effusions, and the signs and symptoms of the superior vena caval obstruction syndrome. Intra-abdominal lymph node masses may give rise to obstruction of the inferior vena cava, with ascites, edema of the lower extremities, and other manifestations of the nephrotic syndrome; enlargement of the lymph nodes at the hilum of the liver, which has been relatively uncommon in our experience but not that of others (Table 7.1), may cause obstructive jaundice; and the relatively rare mesenteric form of Hodgkin's disease may be reflected clinically in the presence of steatorrhea and the chronic malabsorption syndrome.

Spleen. The detection of minimal to moderate degrees of splenic enlargement by palpation is a crude and unreliable procedure, and the assessment of spleen involvement by conventional radiography, splenic arteriography, or radioisotopic scanning is little better. When splenomegaly is detected, it may not be due to Hodgkin's disease, since the spleen may also become enlarged in response to a variety of other stimuli. Conversely, small focal areas of infiltration of the spleen by Hodgkin's disease produce no detectable enlargement. Accordingly, it is not surprising that a very considerable diagnostic error is associated with the assessment of Hodgkin's disease of the spleen. The only definitive evidence is that provided by the "breadloafing" technique of gross examination of the splenic specimen removed at laparotomy (cf. Fig. 3.48) and the painstaking examination of multiple histologic sections taken from each suspicious area. In this way, lesions as small as 1 to 3 mm, in diameter have been detected (Kadin, Glatstein, and Dorfman, 1971). The data from our two series of patients subjected to laparotomy and splenectomy, which are presented in Tables 4.6 and 4.7, indicate that Hodgkin's disease is histologically demonstrable in palpably or radiographically enlarged spleens in only about 60 to 65 percent of instances; in other words, splenomegaly per se constitutes a "false positive" indication of splenic Hodgkin's disease in some 35 to 40 percent of cases (Glatstein et al., 1969, 1970; Rosenberg and Kaplan, 1970; Kaplan et al., 1973). Even more serious is the "false negative" error; gross or microscopic evidence of Hodgkin's disease was detected in one-fourth to one-third of the splenic specimens removed from patients in whom the spleen had not been clinically or radiographically enlarged (Fig. 3.47). These observations have now been confirmed by many other groups (Piro, Hellman, and Moloney, 1972; Prosnitz, Nuland, and Kligerman, 1972; Veronesi et al., 1972; Zarembok et al., 1972; Nordentoft et al., 1973; Paglia et al., 1973; Aisenberg and Qazi, 1974; Gamble et al., 1975; Irving, 1975; Sutcliffe et al., 1976).

The frequency of splenic involvement in untreated patients with Hodgkin's disease, as collated from the major published laparotomy series, is presented in Table 7.2. This composite figure of 37 percent is almost identical with that recorded in our consecutive series of 814 staging laparotomies in previously untreated patients (Kaplan, unpublished data), in which spleen involvement was documented in 314 cases (39 percent). Involvement of the spleen was strongly dependent on histopathologic type (Table 7.3), as was the likelihood of a change of stage following laparotomy. Thus, the spleen was found to be involved in 85 (60 percent) of 142 patients with mixed cellularity or lymphocyte depletion histology, and in only 226 (34 percent) of 670 patients with lymphocyte predominance, nodular sclerosis, or unclassified disease.

Confirming our previous observations (Glatstein et al., 1969, 1970; Kaplan et al., 1973), the spleen was positive in every instance in which Hodgkin's disease was demonstrated in either the liver or the bone marrow (Table 7.4). The para-aortic and splenic hilar nodes were each involved in 150 (47.8 percent) of the 314 patients with positive spleens; conversely, only 24 (4.9 percent) and 8 (1.6 percent) of the 488 patients with negative spleens had documented involvement of the para-aortic and splenic hilar lymph nodes, respectively (Table 7.4). Biopsy of selected lymph nodes at staging laparotomy has also permitted objective assessment of the accuracy of lymphangiography in the detection of retroperitoneal lymphadenopathy (Table 5.1, Chapter 5). These data almost certainly underestimate the true frequency of splenic involvement in untreated Hodgkin's disease, since almost all patients with clinical stage IV and many patients with clinical stage III disease were not submitted to staging laparotomy in most of these institutions.

Thymus. Isolated involvement of the thymus by Hodgkin's disease has long been a subject of intense taxonomic controversy among pathologists, some of whom have until recently preferred to designate such instances as a separate clinical entity, to which the name "granulomatous thymoma" has been applied (Fig. 3.44). Careful followup ob-

Table 7.2 Frequency of Spleen Involvement at Laparotomy in Untreated Patients with Hodgkin's Disease

Reference	Spleen clinically positive or suspicious		Spleen clinically negative		Total	
	No. positive/ no. removed	(%)	No. positive/ no. removed	(%)	No. positive/ no. removed	(%)
Jelliffe et al. (1970)	7/12	(58)	5/10	(50)	12/22	(55)
Lowenbraun et al. (1970)	4/6	(67)	4/6	(67)	8/12	(67)
Rosenberg & Kaplan (1970)[a]	8/16	(50)	20/84	(24)	28/100	(28)
Hanks et al. (1971)	5/6	(83)	3/8	(38)	8/14	(57)
Hass et al. (1971)	11/12	(92)	4/28	(14)	15/40	(38)
Perlin et al. (1972)	7/11	(64)	7/18	(39)	14/29	(48)
Piro et al. (1972)	12/15	(80)	11/39	(28)	33/54	(61)
Prosnitz et al. (1972)	—	—	—	—	15/40	(38)
Veronesi et al. (1972)	—	—	—	—	22/71	(31)
Zarembok et al. (1972)	6/7	(86)	9/23	(39)	15/30	(50)
Ferguson et al. (1973)	—	—	—	—	25/76	(33)
Nordentoft et al. (1973)	4/10	(40)	12/24	(50)	16/32	(47)
Paglia et al. (1973)	—	—	9/37	(24)	—	—
Aisenberg and Qazi (1974)	5/10	(50)	34/90	(38)	39/100	(39)
Gamble et al. (1975)	—	—	44/139	(32)	—	—
Irving (1975)	—	—	—	—	43/84	(51)
Sutcliffe et al. (1976)	—	—	25/68	(37)	—	—
Totals	69/105	(66)	187/574	(33)	281/755	(37)

[a] Data on unselected, previously untreated patients, including those of the earlier report by Glatstein et al. (1970).

servations on such cases have, however, demonstrated that in many instances lymphadenopathy subsequently appears in extrathoracic sites, usually in the neck and supraclavicular areas, less often in the para-aortic nodes (Fazekas, Greenberg, and Rambo, 1974). Biopsy of such secondary manifestations invariably reveals lesions which are indistinguishable from typical Hodgkin's disease, usually of the nodular sclerosing variety (Katz and Lattes, 1969; Fechner, 1969; Nickels, Franssila, and Hjelt, 1973; Keller and Castleman, 1974; Bergh et al., 1978). However, Benjamin et al. (1972) have argued that thymic neoplasms containing large mononuclear Sternberg-Reed-like cells with demonstrable periodic acid-Schiff-positive granules should be considered true thymomas.

When significant enlargement of the mediastinal lymph nodes is also present, it is seldom possible to diagnose thymic involvement without surgical exploration of the mediastinum and the removal of at least a portion of the mass for histologic examination. However, the possibility of thymic involvement, particularly in children and in adolescent patients, should be kept in mind whenever the lateral roentgenogram of the chest reveals that the mediastinal mass protrudes far anteriorly to fill

Table 7.3 Spleen Involvement and Change of Stage at Laparotomy in Relation to Histopathologic Type of Disease

Histopathologic type	No. submitted to laparotomy	Spleen positive		Stage increased		Stage decreased	
		No.	%	No.	%	No.	%
Lymphocyte predominance	45	7	15.6	6	13.3	4	8.9
Nodular sclerosis	599	211	35.2	115	19.2	61	10.2
Mixed cellularity	136	80	58.8	50	36.8	10	7.4
Lymphocyte depletion	6	5	(83.3)	1	(16.7)	1	(16.7)
Unclassified	26	8	30.8	4	15.4	2	7.7
Totals	812	311	38.3	176	21.7	78	9.6

Source: Stanford University Medical Center data on 814 consecutive, previously untreated patients with Hodgkin's disease (Kaplan). Data on histopathologic type in 2 cases was unavailable at the time of compilation.

Table 7.4 Correlation between Involvement of Spleen and of Selected Other Sites at Staging Laparotomy

Site involved[a]	Spleen			Total involved	
	Pos.	Neg.	?	No.	%
Liver	43	0	0	43	5
Bone marrow	23	0	0	23	3
Para-aortic nodes	150	24	3	177	22
Splenic hilar nodes	150	8	0	158	19
Spleen	314	488	12[b]	314	39

Source: Data from 814 staging laparotomies, July 1, 1968–Dec. 31, 1977; all *untreated* patients, unselected except for exclusion of most clinical stage IV cases (Kaplan).

[a] Biopsies were not taken routinely from the celiac, porta hepatis, mesenteric, or iliac lymph node chains; the available data reveal that 15 (60 percent) of 25 celiac and/or porta hepatis node biopsies and only 19 (5 percent) of 353 mesenteric node biopsies were positive. Positive biopsies were obtained from iliac node chains in 13 instances.

[b] One spleen had been previously removed for trauma, one was lost due to fixation error, and ten were not removed because the patients were young children.

much or all of the retrosternal space, immediately adjacent to the heart (Fig. 5.10). The frequency with which the mediastinal lymph nodes are also affected and the not-infrequent additional problem of diffuse invasion of the mediastinal areolar connective tissue make curative resection of such thymic masses rarely possible to achieve. This fact, coupled with the ease and reliability with which radiotherapeutic eradication of the thymic and mediastinal disease can be accomplished, suggests that simple biopsy rather than attempted radical resection is indicated whenever a thymic mass is encountered surgically in a patient with known or suspected Hodgkin's disease.

Tonsil and Waldeyer's Ring. The remarkably low frequency of involvement of the tonsil and the lymphatic structures of Waldeyer's ring by Hodgkin's disease (Fig. 7.1) stands in striking contrast to the frequency with which the other types of malignant lymphoma affect these structures. Here again, we see significant evidence of the biologic differences among the various forms of lymphoid neoplasia. When Hodgkin's disease of the tonsil, nasopharynx, or Waldeyer's ring does occur, it is commonly associated with involvement in the upper cervical and sometimes also in the preauricular lymph nodes on one or both sides. Accordingly, when node involvement in the latter sites is noted clinically, the physician should be alerted to the need for particularly careful examination of

the oropharynx, tonsillar fossa, and nasopharynx. A review of the literature and of their personal observations of involvement of these sites has been presented by Ennuyer, Bataini, and Hélary (1961). More recently, Todd and Michaels (1974) have reviewed 16 patients with biopsy-proved involvement of Waldeyer's ring by Hodgkin's disease in the files of the Royal Marsden Hospital and the Royal National Throat, Nose, and Ear Hospital, London, 1946–1973. Of these, 8 had disease of the nasopharynx, 7 of the tonsil, and 1 of the posterior pharyngeal wall. There was a remarkable preponderance of mixed cellularity histopathology, which was present in 7 of the 8 cases of nasopharyngeal involvement and in 6 of 7 with tonsillar disease. The lymphocyte depletion pattern was seen in 1 patient with tonsillar involvement and 1 other with posterior pharyngeal wall involvement. Of interest is the fact that there no cases with nodular sclerosing disease. Involvement was primary in and confined to lymphoid tissues of a portion of Waldeyer's ring in 4 of these patients, whereas in the remaining 12, other sites of involvement were also present. The authors stated that the course of the disease did not seem to differ from the usual course of Hodgkin's disease.

Björklund et al. (1975) performed careful examinations of the upper air passages in 76 patients, followed by biopsy of the nasopharynx in 45, of whom 7 (16 percent) had "abnormal microscopic findings." Four of these were definitively diagnosed as Hodgkin's disease; the other 3 were considered suggestive but not conclusive. The authors suggested that biopsy of the nasopharynx be added to the list of staging procedures. However, the low yield of positive biopsies makes this recommendation seem inappropriate.

Lungs. Although rare instances of primary Hodgkin's disease apparently arising within the lung have been reported (Kern, Crepeau, and Jones, 1961; Dhingra and Flance, 1970), very few such cases satisfy the requirement that there be no associated hilar or mediastinal lymphadenopathy, in the presence of which the pulmonary parenchymal lesion might well be a secondary rather than a primary manifestation. One such case is illustrated in Figure 5.17. More often, pulmonary involvement is associated with concomitant mediastinal and ipsilateral or bilateral hilar adenopathy (Fig. 7.3), or it develops at a later date in patients who have previously been treated for mediastinal and/or hilar involvement (Carmel and Kaplan, 1976). Confirming this view, Whitcomb et al. (1972) noted the

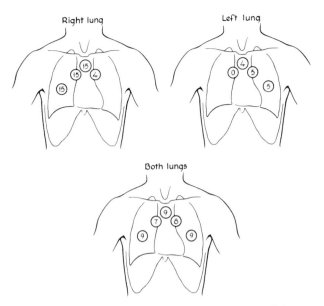

Figure 7.3 Correlation between involvement of the right or left lung (upper drawings) and involvement of the ipsilateral and contralateral hilar nodes and mediastinum. The corresponding data for bilateral pulmonary parenchymal involvement are shown in the lower drawing. The circled numerals give the frequency of involvement for each site.

presence of hilar adenopathy in all of the series of 18 previously untreated patients with Hodgkin's disease of the lung in their study.

The conventional roentgenogram of the chest should not be relied upon for detection of the pulmonary lesions of Hodgkin's disease. We have seen a number of instances in which solitary or multiple small pulmonary nodules which were clearly demonstrated on tomograms could not be seen even on careful retrospective reexamination of the conventional film (Figs. 5.12 and 5.19). The roentgenologic characteristics of Hodgkin's disease of the pulmonary parenchyma, described in Chapter 5, have been painstakingly correlated with the gross and microscopic pathology by Versé (1931), Moolten (1934), Pierce et al. (1936), Stolberg et al. (1964), and others. Although one or more discrete nodular lesions represent the most prevalent pattern, the occurrence of massive consolidation of entire pulmonary segments or lobes, often associated with cavitation, is also well documented (Perttala and Svinhufvud, 1965; Dhingra and Flance, 1970). In the later stages of the disease, diffuse lymphangitic infiltrative processes may also be observed. Differentiation from lung abscess may be difficult in isolated cases (Billingsley and Fukunaga, 1963).

The differential diagnosis of pulmonary paren-

chymal Hodgkin's disease from a variety of pulmonary infectious processes is an extremely difficult problem, which is further complicated by the fact that both Hodgkin's disease and infection may coexist in the same lung (Vieta and Craver, 1941). We have seen a number of tragic instances in which pulmonary infiltrates interpreted as due to Hodgkin's disease have been treated with a succession of chemotherapeutic agents. As one drug after another was found to be ineffective, bone marrow toxicity inexorably supervened, leading ultimately to the use of steroids, with a rapid and usually fatal exacerbation of the pulmonary process, which was usually demonstrated at autopsy to be due to bacterial, granulomatous, fungal, or parasitic infection rather than to Hodgkin's disease.

Repeated sputum culture on specific media, as well as careful examination of stained smears of the sputum, obtained if necessary by tracheal puncture, and gastric washings for the detection of tubercle bacilli, fungi, or other specific microorganisms are indicated in all cases. Unfortunately, the tuberculin, coccidioidin, and other specific skin tests are seldom helpful, since patients with Hodgkin's disease are likely to be anergic and thus to show negative reactions to cutaneous hypersensitivity tests, even when they harbor the specific infection being tested. Cytologic preparations of sputum or bronchial washings may occasionally reveal diagnostic Sternberg-Reed cells (Suprun and Koss, 1964). Bronchial brush biopsy, which provides small tissue fragments for conventional microscopic sections, has reportedly been successful in providing a diagnosis in some instances in which cytologic smears were inconclusive (Variakojis, Fennessy, and Rappaport, 1972; Harlan, Fennessy, and Gross, 1974). Where these procedures are unavailing, needle or open lung biopsy may be necessary for definitive diagnosis. This is particularly important in cases in which suspected pulmonary Hodgkin's disease constitutes the only indication for the initiation of chemotherapy and in patients already under chemotherapeutic management who show progression of a pulmonary infiltrative process at a time when their clinical response to a specific drug regimen is otherwise quite satisfactory. When pulmonary involvement is present at the time of initial diagnosis, it is likely to be of the nodular sclerosing histopathologic type, as might be expected from its association with mediastinal and hilar adenopathy. Other histopathologic types are more frequently represented among cases in which pulmonary involvement supervenes late in the course of the disease, although nodular sclerosis remains the dominant form. Nodular sclerosis was present in 26 of the 29 patients with Hodgkin's disease involving the lung studied by Whitcomb et al. (1972).

In patients who have recently undergone radiotherapy for mediastinal lymphadenopathy, a shaggy, irregular roentgenologic infiltration commonly appears in the paramediastinal pulmonary tissues, usually confined sharply to the radiotherapeutic field. Typically, this appears two to three months after the completion of radiotherapy. As it undergoes gradual resolution, the margins of the mediastinum once again become more sharply defined, though sometimes wider than previously, as the radiation reaction progresses to fibrosis over a period of several months (cf. Figs. 9.46 and 9.50). Although the experienced observer will rarely mistake radiation pneumonitis for Hodgkin's disease, physicians unfamiliar with the shapes of mediastinal radiotherapeutic fields may erroneously interpret such changes as the extension of Hodgkin's disease outward into the lungs. We have seen instances in which chemotherapy or a second course of radiotherapy was actually instituted under this erroneous impression, usually with tragic consequences.

Pleura. Invasion of the pleura by Hodgkin's disease may occur with or without pulmonary parenchymal involvement but is almost invariably associated with prior or concomitant mediastinal lymphadenopathy (Vieta and Craver, 1941). It is typically manifested in the form of a pleural effusion (Weick et al., 1973), which is usually free-flowing, although in later stages, particularly after multiple thoracenteses, it may tend to become pocketed. When the associated mediastinal adenopathy is relatively massive, as is often the case, it is exceedingly difficult to evaluate whether the pleural effusion is simply a transudate secondary to compression and obstruction of venous and lymphatic vessels in the mediastinum or is due to actual invasion of the pleural surface by the neoplastic process. In the latter case, fluid obtained at thoracentesis will usually have an abnormally high protein content. However, this criterion is unreliable; we have seen documented instances in which pleural effusions containing more than 5 gm. per 100 cc. of protein disappeared following radiotherapy to the mediastinal lymph nodes and did not reappear (cf. Fig. 5.31). Pleural effusions with low specific gravity and low protein content are probably simple transudates. Neither these nor the overtly chylous pleural effusions should be regarded, without further proof, as indicative of actual pleural invasion by Hodgkin's disease. Cytologic examination of cells pelleted from thoracentesis fluids is seldom rewarding, although diagnostic Sternberg-Reed cells can occasionally be detected by this method (Fig. 7.4). In doubtful cases, it is imperative to obtain histologic confirmation, either with the Cope needle or by open thoracotomy and biopsy. Extrapleural masses and sub-

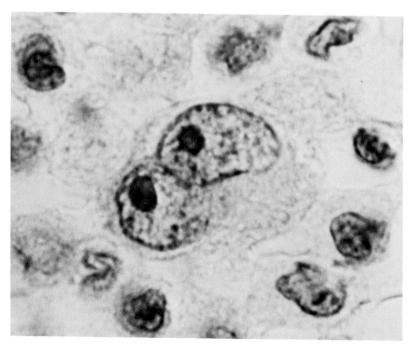

Figure 7.4 Typical binucleate Sternberg-Reed cell in the fixed, sectioned pellet of a pleural effusion which developed preterminally in a 45-year-old male with initial stage $IV_{M+}B$ Hodgkin's disease who relapsed following treatment with MOPP combination chemotherapy and other subsequent chemotherapeutic regimens. The permanent line of Hodgkin's giant cells seen in Fig. 3.20 was established from this pleural effusion material. Hematoxylin and eosin, ×2500.

pleural invasion without effusion may also occur, producing localized distortions of the mediastinal or pleural radiographic silhouette (Blank and Castellino, 1972; Castellino and Blank, 1972).

Liver. In a total of more than 800 diagnostic laparotomies performed to date, there have been no instances of liver involvement without concomitant spleen involvement (Table 7.4). We have seen one such case in consultation, however; the patient underwent laparotomy at another hospital for fever of unknown origin and a left upper quadrant mass and was found to have Hodgkin's disease of the lymphocytic depletion type involving the jejunum, the mesenteric nodes, the omentum, and the liver. The spleen, which was palpably enlarged, was removed and revealed only congestion and hyperplasia. This case suggests that the rare instances of Hodgkin's disease primary in the gastrointestinal tract may spread to the liver via the mesenteric nodes, bypassing the spleen, a spread much like that of the gastrointestinal carcinomas. Isolated reports of cases with involvement of the liver in the apparent absence of splenic involvement (Parker, 1972; Michel et al., 1973) almost invariably refer to previously treated patients in whom prior splenic involvement cannot be excluded.

We have also seen one patient (unfortunately not subjected to laparotomy) in whom clinical evidence of hepatic involvement and an equivocal liver needle biopsy were associated only with involvement of the right axilla by a large lymph node mass; although this patient later succumbed with documented liver involvement, the status of the spleen was never ascertained. Dr. Vera Peters (personal communication) has suggested that such an instance may be explained by the existence in some individuals of collateral lymphatic channels running along the right lateral thoracic wall between the liver and the right axilla. In the presence of extensive axillary lymphadenopathy, it might occasionally be possible for the disease to spread in the retrograde direction along such lymphatic channels into the liver, bypassing the usual route through the supraclavicular nodes, the thoracic duct, the para-aortic nodes, and the spleen. Sternberg-Reed cells have occasionally been detected in the hepatic sinusoids (Barge and Potet, 1971), suggesting that spread from the spleen to the liver is usually hematogenous rather than lymphatic. Studies with [198]Au gold colloid suggest that streamline flow occurs in the human portal vein (Gates and Dore, 1978); blood from the superior mesenteric vein is directed predominantly to the right lobe of the liver, whereas blood from the splenic and inferior mesenteric veins apparently tends to go predominantly to the left lobe. This may explain the observation, in eight of our laparotomy cases in which liver involvement was documented and both lobes of the liver were adequately sampled, that the left lobe was positive and the right lobe negative in six, the converse distribution occurred in none, and both lobes were positive in two. However, additional data on the relative frequency of left and right lobe involvement will be needed to validate this inference.

There is a disheartening lack of correlation between apparent hepatic size, assessed either by palpation or by radioisotopic scans, or the routine liver function tests, and biopsy evidence of liver involvement at laparotomy (Givler et al., 1971; Bagley et al., 1972; Abt et al., 1974; Belliveau, Wiernik, and Abt, 1974). Of the various liver function tests, only the bromsulphalein retention test and the serum alkaline phosphatase level were of any value whatever as clinical indicators of probable hepatic involvement (Aisenberg et al., 1970). Jaundice is seldom a presenting manifestation in patients with previously untreated Hodgkin's disease except in the rare instances in which intrahepatic cholestasis is associated with extrahepatic Hodgkin's disease (Groth et al., 1972; Perera, Greene, and Fenster, 1974). Even percutaneous needle biopsy of the liver was not without significant error, as demonstrated by subsequent wedge biopsies, and sometimes additional needle biopsies, obtained at laparoscopy (Bagley et al., 1973; Beretta et al., 1976) or at laparotomy (Glatstein et al., 1969). When laparotomy and splenectomy are negative, the chance of occult liver involvement is indeed small. Conversely, the finding of Hodgkin's disease in the splenectomy specimen constitutes presumptive evidence that microscopic involvement of the liver may also be present, even in those instances in which needle and wedge biopsies of the liver are negative. Extension to the liver has been observed even in patients with only microscopic involvement of the spleen who received total lymphoid radiotherapy without prophylactic irradiation of the liver (Hellman et al., 1978).

Bone Marrow. Involvement of the bone marrow is detectable in from 5 to 15 percent of previously untreated patients (Grann, Pool, and Mayer, 1966; Rosenberg, 1968, 1971a; Duhamel, Najman, and André, 1971; Myers et al., 1974; O'Carroll, McKenna, and Brunning (1976). It is generally associated with extensive clinical stage III or IV disease, usually attended by night sweats and/or fever. Spleen involvement is an almost invariable concomitant; in 814 consecutive staging laparotomies in previously untreated patients, bone marrow involvement was detected by open or trephine biopsy in 23 patients, all of whom also had documented spleen involvement (Table 7.4). Most of these patients had peripheral blood counts within the normal range. However, when untreated patients present with a white blood cell count below 5,000, a platelet count below 150,000, or a hematocrit below 29 percent, bone marrow involvement is usually present.

Bone marrow involvement in previously treated patients is often heralded also by the development of constitutional symptoms. When no other obvious site of disease is evident on careful diagnostic reevaluation of such patients, suspicion should focus on the bone marrow, and a repeat bone marrow biopsy should be obtained. In some instances, the sudden appearance of anemia, leukopenia, or thrombocytopenia, or various combinations thereof, may forecast the existence of marrow involvement; unless otherwise explained, these hematologic abnormalities, if confirmed by repeated blood cell counts, should also be investigated by bone marrow biopsy. The only other laboratory test that is suggestive is an elevation of the serum alkaline phosphatase level, noted in 30 of 34 cases reviewed by Rosenberg (1971a). Moreover, the heat stability of the enzyme may permit the physician to discriminate between involvement of the liver and of bone or bone marrow (Aisenberg et al., 1970).

A number of investigators (Grann, Pool, and Mayer, 1966; Rosenberg, 1968; Webb et al., 1970; Han, Stutzman, and Roque, 1971; Liao, 1971) have demonstrated conclusively that actual biopsy specimens from the bone marrow, whether obtained by open surgical procedures or with a trephine needle (Jamshidi and Swaim, 1971), are essential for the diagnosis of bone marrow involvement by Hodgkin's disease and that simple aspiration is virtually worthless for this purpose (Table 4.4). The histopathologic appearance of Hodgkin's disease involving the bone marrow has been carefully described by O'Carroll, McKenna, and Brunning (1976). Involvement of the marrow may be focal and minute (Fig. 3.50). Focal deposits were noted in 3 of the 15 cases studied by O'Carroll et al. Accordingly, the problem of sampling is very serious indeed. Thus, a single negative biopsy should not be considered to exclude marrow involvement, particularly in patients in whom sus-

tained, otherwise unexplained constitutional symptoms or hematologic abnormalities persist. In such instances, it is wise to repeat the bone marrow biopsy at a different site. Chen et al. (1977) have reported a higher yield of positive bone marrow biopsies when two trephine biopsy specimens are taken from each posterior iliac crest. Radioisotopic scans using ^{111}In Cl$_3$ (Gilbert et al., 1976a) or ^{99m}Tc polyphosphate (Ferrant et al., 1975) may be helpful in locating suspicious sites for biopsy (Fig. 5.102). However, bone marrow biopsies are occasionally positive in patients in whom radiographic examinations and radioisotopic scans have revealed no indication of marrow involvement (Ferrant et al., 1975).

Bone. As with bone marrow involvement, the clinical setting in which bone involvement may be anticipated is usually that of relatively advanced disease, often associated with constitutional symptoms. However, local invasion of bone adjacent to localized but often relatively massive adenopathy may also be seen in cases of limited anatomic extent. These two different patterns of involvement stem from the fact that Hodgkin's disease may attack skeletal structures either by direct extension, with invasion of the bone through the periosteum from contiguous diseased lymph nodes and pressure effects leading to periosteal reaction, or by hematogenous spread, in which blood-borne emboli reach the medullary cavity of bone, in much the same manner as with metastases from other types of neoplasms (Lecanet et al., 1971; Beachley, Lau, and King, 1972).

Bone involvement is generally heralded by the development of deep, aching, often quite severe pain, which is usually rather well-localized to the site at which involvement of bone is ultimately demonstrated. The serum alkaline phosphatase may be elevated when bone involvement is diffuse (Aisenberg et al., 1970) but is likely to be within normal limits in localized instances. Even where previous conventional X-ray films of the skeletal system have been negative, additional detailed examinations are indicated over the painful region in patients with otherwise unexplained pain in the vicinity of an osseous structure. Osteolytic changes are the commonest manifestation, but diffuse osteoblastic increase in bone density, though less frequent (Perttala and Kijanen, 1965), is more characteristic. Mixtures of blastic and lytic change are also seen (Lecanet et al., 1971). In some instances, periosteal reaction is prominent (Granger and Whitaker, 1967); it is important not to mistake such instances, in which involvement by Hodgkin's disease is present in bone, with the relatively rare instances in which mediastinal Hodgkin's disease is associated with hypertrophic osteoarthropathy (Molyneux, 1973; Shapiro and Zvaifler, 1973; Atkinson et al., 1976a; Peck, 1976). Various patterns of radiographic involvement are illustrated in Chapter 5. Radioisotopic bone scans may reveal focal areas of increased uptake indicative of bone involvement (Fig. 5.99), even in instances in which conventional radiographs are normal or equivocal (Harbert and Ashburn, 1968; Schechter et al., 1976). Subsequent examinations will usually reveal progressive changes in the conventional radiographs.

Except where bone involvement is widespread and involves multiple sites, involvement of bone should not be equated with involvement of bone marrow or regarded as necessarily having an unfavorable impact on prognosis (Musshoff, Busch, and Kaminski, 1964). There are many well-documented instances of long, disease-free survival in patients whose isolated bone lesions were treated appropriately with radiotherapy, suggesting that the appearance of Hodgkin's disease in a single bone is by no means an indicator of widespread dissemination to other sites. The favorable prognosis of such cases of solitary bone involvement is consistent with the fact that most of them are due to the nodular sclerosing variety of Hodgkin's disease (Fig. 3.39). Perhaps clustering of such cases accounts for the paradoxical finding (Stuhlbarg and Ellis, 1965; Beachley, Lau, and King, 1972) of longer survival among their cases with bone involvement than in the remainder of their patients, a finding which is distinctly at variance with most other reported data (Horan, 1969).

Breasts. The appearance of nodules in the subcutaneous tissues and even in the glandular substance of the breast is a relatively infrequent and usually a late manifestation (McGregor, 1960; Lawler and Riddell, 1966). It is seen most often in patients who have, or who have previously had, relatively massive axillary and/or infraclavicular node involvement on the ipsilateral side, suggesting that obstruction to lymphatic pathways may underlie the appearance of disease in the breast. The lesions may appear as small subcutaneous nodules, often in the axillary tail of the breast, occasionally under or near the areola, sometimes mimicking Paget's disease of the breast (Fig. 7.5). Sometimes the entire substance of the gland may become massively infiltrated and firm, and were it

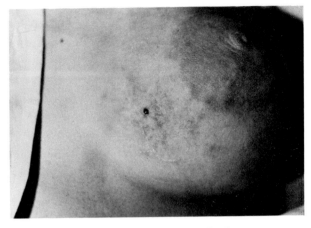

Figure 7.5 Infiltration of the skin and subcutaneous tissues of the breast in a 21-year-old female patient with stage IV Hodgkin's disease involving both pleural cavities. Induration of the subcutaneous tissues of the medial aspect of the breast developed soon after admission, probably by direct invasion through the chest wall. The small, dark, round lesion is the site of a punch biopsy which revealed the typical histologic features of Hodgkin's disease. Breast involvement has been rare in our experience and associated with a very unfavorable prognosis.

not for a preexisting diagnosis of Hodgkin's disease, differential diagnosis from carcinoma of the breast might well require biopsy. Instances have been described (Kushner, 1969) in which the process infiltrates the subcutaneous lymphatics of the breast, simulating inflammatory carcinoma both clinically and on mammography. Isard and Sklaroff (1967) have used the technique of thermography for the detection of breast lesions due to Hodgkin's disease. Although such breast lesions respond well to radiotherapy or chemotherapy, they appear, in the small number of cases that we have seen to date, to be associated with a grave prognosis.

Skin and Subcutaneous Tissues. Subcutaneous nodules are seldom seen except in patients with extensive or highly aggressive disease. Most commonly they appear in the thoracic wall, within the lymphatic drainage pathway of concurrent or prior massive axillary or infraclavicular lymph node involvement, or in the groin or flank, near areas of massive inguinal, femoral, or iliac node involvement (Benninghoff et al., 1970). They have occurred postsurgically in some instances (Jackson, Ney, and Fisher, 1959), apparently because of surgical implantation; we have seen two such cases after ill-advised attempts at radical groin dissection. The nodules are usually discrete, exhibit the typical "rubbery" consistency of Hodgkin's disease in lymph nodes, and are seldom tender or painful, unless they enlarge to the point of ulceration and secondary infection (Fig. 7.6).

Szur and his colleagues (1970) have reported three rare cases of primary cutaneous Hodgkin's disease. Multiple reddish, purplish, or fleshy nodular lesions of the skin, sometimes disappearing and reappearing spontaneously, were present in all three. Biopsies of the skin lesions revealed Sternberg-Reed cells and other typical histologic features of the disease. Survival for sixteen, six and one-half, and six years, respectively, was noted in these cases. Similar cases have been reported by Témine et al. (1965), Van der Meiren (1948), and Hövelborn (1932). However, it is likely that all of these reported cases of supposed primary cutaneous Hodgkin's disease were in reality a benign cutaneous disorder known as lymphomatoid papulosis (Macaulay, 1968). This rare disorder is readily confused with Hodgkin's disease, since biopsies of the skin reveal a dermal infiltrate of large mononuclear and occasionally multinucleate cells with hyperchromatic, lobulated or kidney-shaped nuclei, prominent nucleoli, and basophilic cytoplasm, which may at times closely resemble Sternberg-Reed cells. We have seen one such case in consulta-

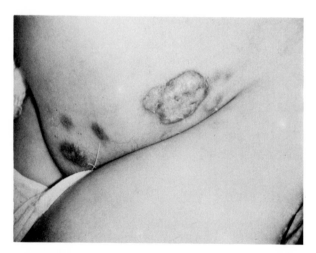

Figure 7.6 Nodules of Hodgkin's disease involving the skin and subcutaneous tissues of the left groin and supra-pubic region in an 18-year-old female with massive bilateral inguinal lymphadenopathy. The anatomic distribution of such cutaneous lesions in the areas of drainage of involved lymph nodes suggests that the neoplastic cells reach the skin from these nodes by passive retrograde flow via obstructed lymphatic vessels. (Reprinted, by permission, from the paper by Benninghoff et al., 1970.)

tion, in which the correct diagnosis was made by Dr. Ronald F. Dorfman. In one recently reported case, there was an elevated serum IgA level, and the peripheral blood lymphocytes bearing immunoglobulins were almost entirely limited to IgA-bearing cells (Prandi et al., 1977). A clinical, histopathologic, and cytologic study of the differential features of lymphomatoid papulosis, primary cutaneous Hodgkin's disease, mycosis fungoides, and Sézary's syndrome has recently been presented by Brehmer-Andersson (1976).

Other cutaneous manifestations of the malignant lymphomas have been described fully by Bluefarb (1959) and by Amblard et al. (1973). Though infrequent, the association of generalized anhidrosis, acquired ichthyosis, and exfoliative dermatitis with Hodgkin's disease has been sufficiently dramatic to warrant description by a number of authors (Markowitz and Tringali, 1962; English et al., 1963; Colomb, Plauchu, and Piante, 1969). Other nonspecific skin lesions may occur in association with Hodgkin's disease, and usually resolve when the disease is treated. These include erythema multiforme, erythema nodosum-like lesions, and eczematoid or psoriasiform lesions. Though exceedingly rare, the association of pemphigus and Hodgkin's disease has been reported (Naysmith and Hancock, 1976).

Finally, certain cutaneous disorders, or systemic disorders with cutaneous manifestations, seem to predispose to the secondary development of lymphomas, including Hodgkin's disease. One such entity is alopecia mucinosa, also known as follicular mucinosis, a curious lesion in which mucinous degeneration of the hair follicles and sebaceous glands associated with nonspecific inflammatory reaction in the dermis leads eventually to alopecia. It has been reported that lymphomas developed in over 25 percent of adult patients with this condition (Pinkus, 1964). In a more recent study, 17 percent of a series of 47 patients progressed to the development of lymphomas, most of which were mycosis fungoides, but a few developed Hodgkin's disease (Emmerson, 1969). In lymphomatoid granulomatosis, a vasculitic, angiodestructive, granulomatous and lymphoreticular proliferative process involving the skin, lungs, kidneys, and nervous system, the majority of cases proceed to the development of frank lymphomas, and approximately 70 percent of cases are fatal within five years (Liebow, Carrington, and Friedman, 1972). In one of the case reports of this uncommon entity, the secondarily acquired lymphoma was Hodgkin's disease (MacDonald and Sarkany, 1976). Dermatomyositis, which is a related disorder, has also been reported in association with Hodgkin's disease, as well as with a variety of other occult neoplasms (Arundell, Wilkinson, and Haserick, 1960).

Pericardium. Pericardial involvement almost always occurs by direct invasion from mediastinal lymphadenopathy (Fig. 7.7), usually of relatively massive extent (cf. Fig. 5.33). In rare instances, it is clinically silent and detected surgically at the time of mediastinal exploration or at autopsy (Rottino and Hoffmann, 1952). More often, it is associated with a pericardial friction rub or with cardiomegaly due to pericardial effusion (Hagans, 1950). The secondary signs of pericardial tamponade, such as paradoxical pulse and engorgement of neck veins, may be present. When the possibility of pericardial involvement is entertained, confirmation by ultrasound echocardiography is indicated. In occasional cases, pericardiocentesis with air or carbon dioxide injection or radioisotopic angiocardiography using ^{99m}Tc (Kriss, 1969) may also be desirable.

Paracardiac masses may also be present initially or develop later in the course of the disease. It is now recognized that such masses result from involvement of diaphragmatic lymph nodes at the right cardiophrenic angle and at the cardiac apex on the left (Fayos and Lampe, 1971; Castellino and

Blank, 1972; Crowe, 1975; Huber et al., 1978). One such case is illustrated in Figure 5.35, Chapter 5.

Central and Peripheral Nervous System. Hodgkin's disease may invade the epidural space by extension through the intervertebral foramina from paravertebral lymph node masses, usually in the dorsal or lumbar regions or, less often, by direct invasion from involved vertebrae. In either case, the process is clinically silent until significant compression of either nerve roots or the spinal cord itself becomes evident (Sparling, Adams, and Parker, 1947; Murphy and Bilge, 1964). Although almost any segment of the spinal cord may be affected, involvement is more common in the dorsal and lumbar regions than in the cervical spinal cord (Bickel, 1971). Pain is usually a prominent feature, limited to selective dermatomes when an isolated nerve root is affected, or experienced in the low back and radiating down the lower extremities when spinal cord compression is present (Nováková, 1978). Numbness and other paresthesias may occur instead of or in addition to pain. The condition progresses at a variable rate to weakness and paralysis of one or both lower extremities, sometimes accompanied by difficulties with sphincter control (Eggleston and Hartmann, 1968). Frequent, careful monitoring of the neuro-

Figure 7.7 Frequencies of involvement of the mediastinal and hilar lymph nodes in patients with pericardial, pleural, sternal, and internal mammary node involvement. Note that mediastinal adenopathy was present in every instance.

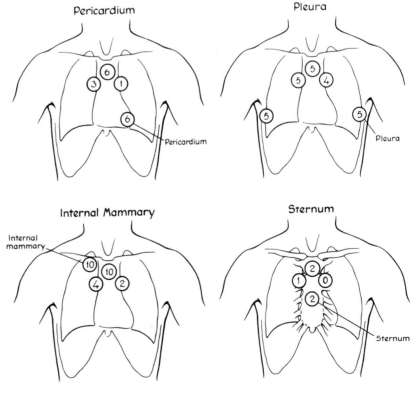

logic status is essential to avoid progression to irreversible paralysis. Complete reversibility is the rule when appropriate treatment is administered early enough. Conversely, the probability of obtaining a complete remission diminishes as the extent of neurologic deficit increases (Friedman, Kim, and Panahon, 1976). Accordingly, the condition should be dealt with as a medical emergency involving neurologic examination, diagnostic spinal puncture with particular emphasis on protein and pressure determinations, and myelography in cases with pressure findings indicative of obstruction. Myelography usually reveals complete or partial obstruction of the spinal canal (Figs. 5.104, 5.105), not infrequently associated with osteoblastic involvement of the adjacent vertebral body (Manners, 1977). Laminectomy with decompression is indicated only in rapidly progressive cases and is generally thought to be contraindicated when complete paralysis has been present for more than 48 to 72 hours or when the sites of involvement are multiple and noncontiguous (Murphy and Bilge, 1964). As soon as feasible, radiotherapy should be instituted to encompass the affected segment of the spinal cord and associated epidural mass with a generous margin. Radiation doses in excess of 2,500 rads are required to achieve optimal complete remission rates (Friedman, Kim, and Panahon, 1976). Although technically classified in Rye stage IV, epidural masses due to Hodgkin's disease usually respond well to treatment and are not necessarily associated with significant deterioration in prognosis. For this reason, epidural involvement by Hodgkin's disease is classified as an "E" lesion in the newer Ann Arbor staging classification (cf. Chapter 8). Intramedullary involvement of the spinal cord, and parenchymal infiltration of peripheral nerves, are seen only rarely, almost invariably in patients with widely disseminated disease (Parker, 1972). Impairment of peripheral nerve conduction has been documented in occasional patients (Walsh, 1971), and peripheral neuritis progressing to paralysis has been described in the brachial distribution (Pezzimenti, Bruckner, and DeConti, 1973).

Hodgkin's disease may also invade the leptomeninges or, still more rarely, the brain. Leptomeningeal involvement, characterized clinically by cranial nerve palsies, headache, papilledema, cord compression syndrome, paresthesias, and/or pain, has been documented in two of our cases, as well as in sixteen with other types of lymphoma. It was a late feature of the disease and thus associated with a distinctly unfavorable prognosis (Griffin et al.,

1971). Eosinophilic meningitis has been described in association with leptomeningeal Hodgkin's disease (Strayer and Bender, 1977). Intracranial Hodgkin's disease may elicit similar symptoms and signs; in addition, disorientation, somnolence, personality change, convulsive seizures, and hemiparesis have been reported (Santos Silva, 1965; Marshall et al., 1968; Reagan and Bennett, 1971; Brazinsky, 1973; Cambier et al., 1973; Cuttner et al., 1979). Localization may be accomplished with the aid of computerized tomographic (CT) scans (Fig. 5.106), brain scans (Fig. 5.107), or cerebral arteriography (Fig. 5.108). Response to total brain irradiation in our experience to date has been excellent (Thompson and DeNardo, 1969).

Certain paraneoplastic syndromes involving the central nervous system may occur as rare complications of Hodgkin's disease. Progressive multifocal leukoencephalopathy (PML), first described by Åström, Mancall, and Richardson (1958), is a demyelinating disease characterized by progressive disorientation and dementia, dysarthria, unsteady gait, visual disturbances, and unilateral hemiparesis progressing to become bilateral and to eventual irreversible coma, with death supervening usually in three to six months. The diagnosis has been made during life only infrequently. At autopsy, histologic examination of the brain reveals patchy areas of demyelinization with glial proliferative reactions in the white matter characterized by altered oligodendrocytes and giant astrocytes. Electron micrographic examination of the lesions reveals occasional glial cells, the nuclei of which are packed with electron-opaque viral particles, having a morphology closely similar to that of the so-called papovavirus group, of which the mouse polyoma virus and the simian vacuolating virus 40 (SV40) are the principal prototypes (ZuRhein and Chou, 1965; Silverman and Rubinstein, 1965; ZuRhein, 1969).

Subacute cerebellar degeneration has been reported in a very small number of patients with Hodgkin's disease and other lymphomas, occasionally in association with myelopathy and neuropathy (Rewcastle, 1963; Castaigne et al., 1964; Horwich, Buxton, and Ryan, 1966; Froissart et al., 1976; Trotter, Hendin, and Osterland, 1976). The onset is usually with headache, vertigo, diplopia, dysarthria, and progressive ataxia with loss of balance. The course is more variable, and remissions of variable duration have been reported, but the disease usually progresses to a fatal outcome in less than one year. Autopsy reveals atrophy of both hemispheres and the vermis of the cerebellum with absence of Purkinje cells in large areas of the cortex and diffuse ballooning of the proximal axons of some of the remaining Purkinje cells.

Granulomatous angiitis of the central nervous system is a usually fatal segmental vasculitis in which epithelioid histiocytes, multinucleated giant cells, and lymphocytes are deposited focally in the walls of arteries and veins of the cerebrum, spinal cord, or both (Rewcastle and Tom, 1962). In one recently reported case, there was a remarkable remission of the neurological disorder concomitantly with response of the Hodgkin's disease to radiotherapy (Greco et al., 1976). The Guillain-Barré syndrome (acute idiopathic polyneuritis) has also been reported in a number of instances in association with Hodgkin's disease (Lisak et al., 1977). It is characterized by the relatively rapid onset of weakness in one or both lower extremities, and occasionally also in the upper extremities, loss of reflexes, minimal sensory loss, and cytoalbuminologic dissociation on analysis of the cerebrospinal fluid. Gradual recovery is the rule, although restoration of neurologic function may be incomplete in some instances. Other rare neurologic disorders occasionally seen in association with Hodgkin's disease and other lymphomas include anterior horn cell degeneration (Somasundaram, Cho, and Posner, 1975), diffuse nongranulomatous reticular cerebral infiltration (Buge et al., 1977), and a variety of unusual infections (Ghatak, 1975).

Gastrointestinal Tract. Unlike the other malignant lymphomas, Hodgkin's disease rarely arises in the gastrointestinal tract. There were no cases with involvement of the gastrointestinal tract at the time of initial diagnosis in our consecutive series of 340 previously untreated patients (Kaplan, 1970). Even at autopsy, gastrointestinal tract involvement is encountered in only about 8 percent of all cases (Uddströmer, 1934). Nonetheless, well-documented instances of Hodgkin's disease involving the esophagus (Hambly and Blundell, 1968; Kelley, 1968), the stomach (Morano and Orecchia, 1965; Schuller et al., 1966), the small intestine (Cohen and Canter, 1959; Sternlieb et al., 1961; Bernier et al., 1967; Edwards, 1969; Kahn, Selzer, and Kaschula, 1972), the colon (Portmann et al., 1954), and even the rectum (Shapiro, 1961; Harned and Sorrell, 1976) and the appendix (Faerberg et al., 1965; Nagata et al., 1966) have been reported in the literature.

In the esophagus and stomach, the symptoms are usually those associated with ulceration or ob-

struction (Mody et al., 1965), and the roentgenologic appearance of the lesion is seldom distinguishable from that of other infiltrating or ulcerating neoplasms (Bloch, 1967). In some cases, Hodgkin's disease of the stomach may mimic the appearance of the other malignant lymphomas involving the stomach, producing "giant rugae," stiffening, and diminution of peristaltic activity due to diffuse infiltration of the gastric wall (cf. Chapter 5).

In the small intestine, involvement is most commonly encountered in the distal ileum, where it may progress to, but seldom beyond, the ileocecal valve. However, lesions have also been reported in the proximal ileum (Teitelman and Brill, 1960) and jejunum, as well as in multiple sites (Sternlieb et al., 1961). The clinical picture often closely mimics that of idiopathic sprue, with diarrhea, steatorrhea, chronic malabsorption, and severe weight loss (Eidelman et al., 1966; Bernier et al., 1967; Shreeve et al., 1968). The roentgenologic appearance in such cases is similar to that encountered in the chronic malabsorption syndrome (Fig. 5.84) and remains undetected until the time of surgical intervention or occasionally until autopsy.

Urinary Tract. Involvement of the urinary tract is seldom clinically evident during the course of the disease and may be uncommon even at autopsy, occurring in only 14 (7 percent) of the 192 cases studied by Uddströmer (1934); however, in a more recent series, involvement of the urinary tract was detected in 56 percent of autopsied cases (Richmond et al., 1962). Para-aortic or iliac adenopathy may compress or even directly invade and obstruct the adjacent ureter (Braun et al., 1972), causing a hydronephrosis, which may clear after radiotherapy to the affected nodes, as in the case cited by Fisher, Kendall, and Van Leuven (1962). Compression and distortion of the contour of the bladder, visualized by intravenous urography or cystography, may occur in the presence of massive iliac adenopathy (Figs. 5.55, 5.89). Rarely, nodular or diffuse renal enlargement may be observed in instances of metastatic infiltration of the renal parenchyma (cf. Fig. 10.3); death due to chronic renal failure may occur (Champion, Coup, and Hancock, 1976). Renal arteriography has been diagnostically helpful in some cases (cf. Fig. 5.88; Williams et al., 1969; Kyaw and Koehler, 1969; Pick, Castellino, and Seltzer, 1971).

Silent spread of the disease to the para-aortic nodes may be ushered in, in some instances, by the nephrotic syndrome, due to compression or oc-

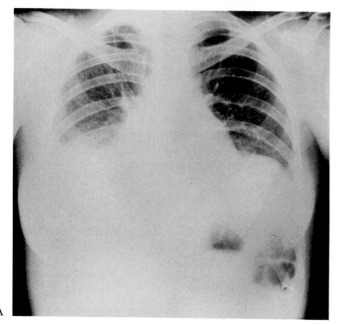

A

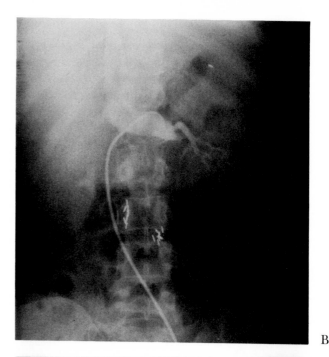

B

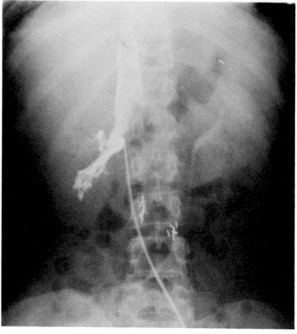

C

Figure 7.8   Lipoid nephrosis, developing seven months after completion of total lymphoid radiotherapy in a 21-year-old female with stage III Hodgkin's disease, characterized by rapid weight gain, ascites, and pleural effusion (*A*), edema of the lower extremities, severe proteinuria with waxy and hyaline casts, and a serum cholesterol level of 431 mg. per 100 cc. Selective renal venography revealed the renal veins to be patent (*B*, *C*). She responded promptly to steroids, and there was no recrudescence after use of the steroids was gradually tapered off. However, about 18 months later she developed a mass in the left upper quadrant of the abdomen, shown by biopsy to be due to Hodgkin's disease. This relapse proved refractory to treatment with combination chemotherapy, and she died about three years after the episode of lipoid nephrosis.

clusion of the renal vein on one or both sides by enlarged nodes (Brodovsky et al., 1968; Ghosh and Muehrcke, 1970). However, the nephrotic syndrome may also occur in the absence of regional involvement by Hodgkin's disease, and it is then sometimes associated with immune complex deposits in the glomeruli (Lokich, Galvanek, and Moloney, 1973; Sutherland et al., 1974; Yum, Edwards, and Kleit, 1975; Routledge, Haun, and Morris Jones, 1976). Finally, there are some instances in which no renal lesion can be detected as an explanation for the nephrotic syndrome (Plager and Stutzman, 1971; Hansen et al., 1972). Lower-extremity edema and proteinuria, with or without ascites, are the main clinical features. The intravenous urogram indicates impaired excretion and concentration of the contrast agent, and renal venography may pinpoint the site of compression (Figs. 5.86 and 5.87). In one such case in our series, there was prompt and complete clearing of lower-extremity edema, ascites, and proteinuria soon after the initiation of radiotherapy to the affected nodes. Plager and Stutzman (1971) have described cases in which repeated bouts of nephrotic syndrome occurred in the same patient, each time heralding reactivation of Hodgkin's disease. The edema and proteinuria diminished when distant lymphadenopathy was treated with local radiotherapy, as well as in response to systemic chemotherapy.

A rare complication of Hodgkin's disease is lipoid nephrosis, which may occur at a time when no other clinical manifestations of persistence or recurrence of the lymphoma can be detected (Yum, Edwards, and Kleit, 1971; Moorthy, Zimmerman, and Burkholder, 1976). The only such case in our experience to date occurred in a twenty-one-year-old female who developed rapid weight gain, decreasing urine volume, lower-extremity edema, proteinuria with hyaline and waxy casts, and a serum cholesterol level of 431 mg. per 100 cc. about seven months after completion of total lymphoid radiotherapy for stage IIIA disease. She responded very promptly to steroid therapy, which was then tapered to cessation without a recrudescence of the nephrotic process (Fig. 7.8). However, the lipoid nephrosis in this patient may also have been an early indication of impending relapse, since she developed a left upper quadrant mass of enlarged lymph nodes about 18 months later and ultimately died with disseminated Hodgkin's disease after treatment with combination chemotherapy. Finally, in some patients with Hodgkin's disease, the nephrotic syndrome may develop in association with amyloid deposits in the kidneys (Brandt, Cathcart, and Cohen, 1968; Kiely, Wagoner, and Holley, 1969; Yum, Edwards, and Kleit, 1975).

Endocrine Glands. Although the adrenal glands are sometimes encased and invaded by Hodgkin's disease at autopsy, adrenal involvement is seldom, if ever, recognizable during life. In contrast, the thyroid gland is not infrequently the seat of lymphomatous deposits or of secondary invasion from cervical node masses at autopsy, and several instances of apparently primary Hodgkin's disease of the thyroid have been reported (Rupp et al., 1962; Roberts and Howard, 1963; Veronesi et al., 1966; Reiffers et al., 1976). Diagnosis in such instances usually proceeds from the discovery of a nodular or diffuse goiter to radioisotopic scans revealing a "cold" defect and thence to surgical exploration and biopsy. Apparently primary Hodgkin's disease of the ovary has also been reported (Long and Patchefsky, 1971).

Mode of Spread of Hodgkin's Disease

Earlier misconceptions about the unpredictable, capricious distribution of lymph node involvement in patients with Hodgkin's disease were swept away with the advent of lymphangiography, which revealed that involvement of the para-aortic and iliac lymph node chains is the silent link between the upper trunk and the groin. For example, patients with palpable enlargement of lymph nodes in the neck and in one or both inguinal regions almost invariably have a positive lymphangiogram. Indeed, exceptions to this pattern have been so infrequent as to raise serious doubts about the histopathologic diagnosis of Hodgkin's disease. Similarly, extension of disease to remote lymph node chains, formerly thought to occur with a frequency sufficient to vitiate rational preventive measures (Scheer, 1963), has also been explained by lymphangiography; almost invariably, clinically unsuspected involvement of the intervening para-aortic lymph node chains was either present initially in such instances or had developed silently during the interval prior to overt distant relapse. Thus, what might be termed the "lymphangiography era" has for the first time permitted the accumulation and systematic analysis of data on large numbers of consecutive cases, all studied with the aid of lymphangiography. When laparotomy with splenectomy and biopsy of nodes, liver, and marrow was added to the diagnostic program, the principal change in frequency of involvement was that noted in the spleen (cf. Tables 4.7 and 7.2). Data on all documented sites of involvement in 160 such cases are presented in Table 7.5, and a new tabulation of sites of involvement in 86 laparotomy-staged patients with clinical and/or pathological stage I disease is presented in Table 7.6.

It has long been known by radiotherapists (Gilbert, 1939; Peters, 1950, 1966; Kaplan, 1962) that, after local radiotherapy of an involved chain of lymph nodes, the next manifestation of disease is often in one of the adjacent lymph node chains. The first systematic attempt to map sites of disease was that of Rosenberg and Kaplan (1966), who demonstrated that involvement of various chains of lymph nodes in a series of 100 consecutive, previously untreated patients with Hodgkin's disease was distinctly nonrandom; when a given chain of nodes was affected, other chains which are known to be directly connected with it via lymphatic channels were likely also to be involved, either concurrently or as the next subsequent manifestation of the disease. Rosenberg and Kaplan also noted that even extralymphatic sites such as the lung, liver, and bone marrow are more likely to be involved in

association with certain predictable patterns of lymph node involvement. These findings have now been confirmed and extended in a number of subsequent studies (Han and Stutzman, 1967; Banfi et al., 1968; Prosnitz et al., 1969; Kaplan, 1970).

Two quite different theories, the "contiguity" theory of Rosenberg and Kaplan (1966) and the "susceptibility" theory of Smithers (1969a, 1970a, 1973), have been proposed for the mode of spread of Hodgkin's disease. The contiguity theory considers Hodgkin's disease to be a monoclonal neoplasm of unifocal origin which spreads secondarily by metastasis of preexisting tumor cells, much like other neoplasms, except that spread is predominantly via lymphatic rather than hematogenous pathways. The term *contiguity* refers to the existence of direct connections between pairs of lymph node chains by way of one or more lymphatic channels which do not have to pass through and be filtered by intervening lymph node barriers. Contiguous pairs of lymph node chains, in this view, may be adjacent or quite far apart, as long as the lymphatic channel between them would permit tumor cells to pass directly from one chain to another.

Table 7.5   Anatomic Sites of Involvement in 160 Previously Untreated Patients with Hodgkin's Disease Routinely Staged with Lymphangiography, Laparotomy, Splenectomy, and Liver Biopsy[a]

Site or organ		Frequency of involvement		Site or organ		Frequency of involvement	
		No.	%			No.	%
Lymph nodes				Inguinal and femoral	R	14	9
Axillary	R	46	29		L	15	9
	L	48	30	Spleen		58	36
Infraclavicular	R	10	6	Liver		4	2
	L	15	9	Lung	R	7	4
Cervical and	R	100	63		L	2	1
supraclavicular	L	114	71		Bilat.	5	3
Mediastinal		94	59	Pericardium		4	2
Hilar	R	37	23	Pleura		3	2
	L	34	21	Bone marrow		7	4
Epitrochlear and	R	4	2	Skeletal system		13	8
brachial	L	3	2	Subcutaneous		4	2
Preauricular	R	0	—	Waldeyer ring		1	1
	L	1	1	Thymus		5	3
Para-aortic		59	37	Gastrointestinal tract		0	—
Splenic hilar		23	15	Genitourinary tract		0	—
Mesenteric		2	1	Central nervous system		0	—
Iliac	R	23	15				
	L	26	16				

[a]Staging laparotomy was not performed in five of these cases in which bone marrow and/or bilateral lung involvement was discovered preoperatively.

Table 7.6 Sites of Involvement, Histopathologic Type, and Staging Laparotomy Findings in Untreated Patients with Clinical and/or Pathological Stage I Hodgkin's Disease

	Lymph node chain clinically involved at presentation[a]							
	RA	RCS	M	LCS	LA	RIF	LIF	All sites
Total number of patients	5	26	9	41	4	5	5	95
Histopathologic type[b]								
LP	1	6	0	7	0	1	1	16
NS	2	8	9	19	3	3	3	47
MC	2	8	0	10	1	0	1	22
IF	0	1	0	3	0	0	0	4
U	0	3	0	2	0	1	0	6
Positive sites at staging laparotomy[c]								
Spleen	1	8	0	7	1	0	0	17
Splenic hilar nodes	1	1	0	2	1	0	0	5
Para-aortic nodes	0	1	0	1	0	0	0	2
Other	0	0	0	0	0	0	0	0

Source: Stanford University Medical Center data (Kaplan).

[a] RA, LA: right, left axillary; RCS, LCS: right, left cervical-supraclavicular; M: mediastinal; RIF, LIF: right, left inguinal-femoral nodes.

[b] LP: lymphocyte predominance; NS: nodular sclerosis; MC: mixed cellularity; IF: interfollicular; U: unclassified.

[c] After staging laparotomy, 18 of 86 clinical stage I cases (21%) were reclassified in pathological stage III or III$_s$; conversely, 10 clinical stage II or III cases were found to belong in pathological stage I, yielding a net total of 78 pathologic stage I cases.

Smithers suggested that Hodgkin's cells may move in and out of lymph nodes from the bloodstream, much as normal lymphocytes do (Gowans and Knight, 1964). He further postulated that there might be intrinsic differences in the susceptibility of different lymph node chains to the development of Hodgkin's disease and used a tabulation of sites of disease in stage I patients (Smithers, 1973) to estimate the relative susceptibilities of the five most common sites of involvement above the diaphragm. In the susceptibility hypothesis, emphasis is placed on the concept of Hodgkin's disease as a disorder of the entire lymphatic system, and the possibility is entertained of multifocal origin, perhaps by the spread of a causative agent rather than of preexisting tumor cells. Following involvement in a first site, the remaining lymph node sites would have an independent probability of being the next to become involved, and these probabilities are assumed to be proportional to the probabilities of initial involvement.

Specific examples of contiguity of lymph node involvement, as postulated by the contiguity theory, are illustrated in Figure 7.9 and summarized in Table 7.7. It may be noted that the axillary nodes are contiguous via lymphatic channels with the ipsilateral epitrochlear, brachial, infraclavicular, supraclavicular, and low cervical lymph node chains, but not with the contralateral cervical, supraclavicular, infraclavicular, or axillary nodes. Similarly, the inguinal lymph nodes are contiguous with the ipsilateral femoral and iliac chains and possibly with the lower lumbar lymph nodes as well but not with the contralateral iliac, inguinal, or femoral nodes; the submandibular and upper cervical nodes are contiguous with the ipsilateral preauricular, postauricular, occipital, lower cervical, and supraclavicular lymph nodes, as well as with the structures of Waldeyer's ring, but not with the ipsilateral axilla or the contralateral neck or supraclavicular area.

Because of their pivotal situation (Figs. 7.9H) the left supraclavicular lymph nodes have the greatest number of lymphatic connections with other chains, and the patterns of associated lymph node involvement when these nodes are involved by Hodgkin's disease show a correspondingly greater degree of diversity and complexity. In particular,

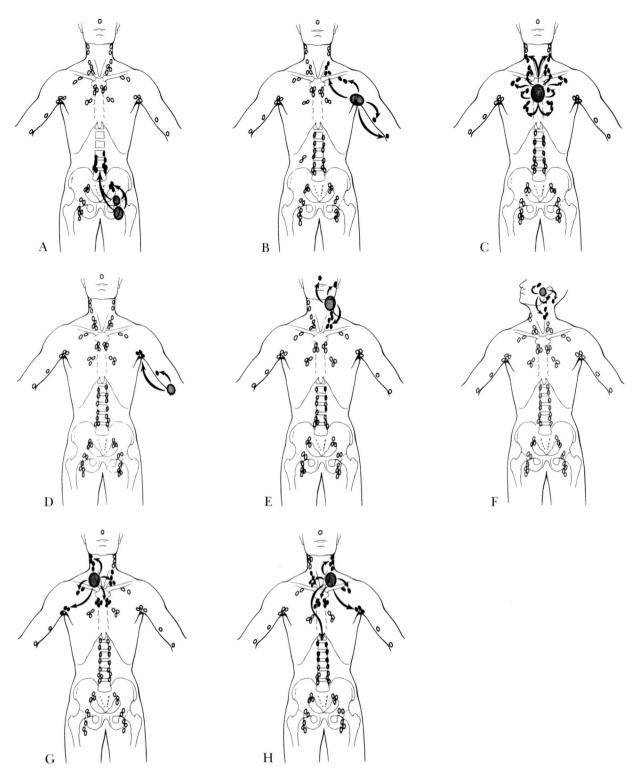

Figure 7.9   Diagrammatic representation of the pathways of contiguous extension of Hodgkin's disease from various hypothetical primary sites, as postulated by the contiguity theory. The initially involved lymph node chains are heavily encircled and stippled; the major directions of spread are indicated by the arrows, and the node chains most likely to become the sites of primary extension are solidly blackened. *A*, primary site = left inguinal-femoral nodes. *B*, primary site = left axillary nodes. *C*, primary site = mediastinal nodes. *D*, primary site = left epitrochlear nodes. *E*, primary site = left upper cervical nodes. *F*, primary site = left preauricular nodes. *G*, primary site = right lower cervical-supraclavicular nodes. *H*, primary = left lower cervical-supraclavicular nodes.

Table 7.7 Contiguity of Lymph Node Chains via Lymphatic Channels

Involved site	Contiguous nodes	Noncontiguous nodes
Left axillary[a]	Left epitrochlear, brachial, infraclavicular, and low cervical	Right cervical, supraclavicular, infraclavicular, axillary, or epitrochlear; mediastinal; para-aortic, iliac, inguinal, femoral
Left epitrochlear	Left brachial and axillary	All other chains
Left supraclavicular	Left axillary, infraclavicular, and cervical; right supraclavicular and cervical; mediastinal; upper lumbar para-aortic(?)	Right axillary; left epitrochlear; iliac, inguinal, and femoral; and Waldeyer ring structures
Left upper cervical	Left supraclavicular, lower cervical and preauricular; Waldeyer ring structures	Left axillary, brachial, and epitrochlear; right supraclavicular, lower cervical, axillary, brachial, and epitrochlear; mediastinal; and all subdiaphragmatic chains
Left preauricular	Left upper cervical, postauricular, and occipital; Waldeyer ring structures	All other sites
Anterior and middle mediastinal	Left and right supraclavicular, lower right cervical and infraclavicular; internal mammary; left and right hilar and intrapulmonary	Subdiaphragmatic, upper cervical, axillary, and epitrochlear
Lumbar para-aortic	Left and right iliac, inguinal, and supraclavicular, infraclavicular, and lower cervical; mesenteric; posterior mediastinal; splenic hilar; and spleen	Anterior and middle mediastinal, upper cervical, axillary, brachial, epitrochlear, and femoral; and Waldeyer ring structures
Left iliac	Left inguinal and femoral; lumbar para-aortic	Right iliac, inguinal, and femoral; all supradiaphragmatic sites
Left inguinal or femoral	Left iliac; lumbar para-aortic	Right iliac, inguinal, and femoral; all supradiaphragmatic sites

[a] The contiguous connections of the corresponding lymph node chains on the right side are the mirror images of those listed for the left side; however, the upper lumbar para-aortic nodes are not considered contiguous with the right supraclavicular nodes, except in the small proportion of cases (7 percent) in which the thoracic duct empties on the right side or on both sides.

stress has been placed on one special form of contiguity by Rosenberg and Kaplan (1966), Teillet and Schweisguth (1969), and Kaplan (1970). This is the association of lower cervical-supraclavicular lymph node involvement with involvement in the upper lumbar para-aortic lymph nodes and/or the spleen and splenic hilar nodes. In the contiguity theory, involvement of these sites was presumed to occur via the thoracic duct, since it was apparently associated with left-sided or bilateral supraclavicular adenopathy far more often than with right-sided supraclavicular involvement (Table 7.8), whereas the inverse relationships appeared to hold for involvement of the mediastinal and hilar nodes (Glatstein et al., 1969, and Table 7.9). However, preferential association of abdominal involvement with left-sided supraclavicular adenopathy was not observed in later laparotomy studies at other centers (Prosnitz, Nuland, and Kligerman, 1972; Zarembok et al., 1972; Nordentoft et al., 1973; Aisenberg and Qazi, 1974; British National Lym-

Table 7.8 Frequency of Subdiaphragmatic Involvement in 100 Consecutive Laparotomies in Patients with Left-Sided versus Right-Sided Cervical-Supraclavicular Node Involvement[a]

Histological findings[b]	Left side only	Bilateral	Right side only
Positive	12 (40%)	23 (46%)	1 (8%)
Negative	18	25	12
Totals	30	48	13

[a] These data, which were compiled by Dr. Eli Glatstein, are essentially similar to those in the series of 50 unselected laparotomies reported by Glatstein et al. (1970). In addition to the 91 cases accounted for above, there were 9 cases in which the cervical-supraclavicular nodes were uninvolved on either side.

[b] Histologic evidence of Hodgkin's disease in the splenectomy specimen and/or the para-aortic and splenic hilar node biopsies.

Table 7.9 Frequency of Mediastinal Involvement in 100 Consecutive Patients with Hodgkin's Disease Relative to Involvement of the Left versus the Right Lower Cervical-Supraclavicular Nodes[a]

	Cervical-supraclavicular involvement			
	Left side only	Bilateral	Right side only	Neither
Mediastinum				
Involved	16 (53%)	33 (69%)	11 (84%)	5
Uninvolved	14	15	2	4
Totals	30	48	13	9

[a] See footnote a to Table 7.8.

phoma Investigation, 1975), nor was such an association apparent in a more recent tabulation of our own data in a series of over 800 consecutive staging laparotomies (Kaplan, unpublished; Table 7.10). Thus, the transdiaphragmatic association of left-sided or bilateral supraclavicular with upper para-aortic and/or celiac node involvement can no longer be considered to provide evidence for the contiguity theory. However, subdiaphragmatic involvement continues to show an inverse correlation with mediastinal involvement; it was present in 30 of 78 patients without mediastinal involvement (38 percent) and in only 46 (28 percent) of 167 patients with mediastinal involvement ($\chi^2 = 2.96$).

The anatomic distribution of involved sites in 426 consecutive cases of previously untreated Hodgkin's disease is indicated on body diagrams grouped by final clinical stage (Figs. 7.10 to 7.25). Involvement was documented by biopsy, physical examination, radiography including routine lymphangiography, and, in some instances, laparotomy with splenectomy and biopsy of the liver, retroperitoneal nodes, and bone marrow. In the stage

II patterns illustrated in Figures 7.11 through 7.14, noncontiguous patterns were observed in only 4 of 185 cases; thus, lymph node involvement was contiguous in 98 percent of these cases.

Another analytical approach is that devised by Dr. George Hutchison (1972), who compared the observed distributions in 158 of our Rye stage II cases with expectation based on the random association of two or more sites with the probabilities given by their relative frequencies in 53 observed stage I cases. The results of his analysis of our data, presented in Tables 7.11 and 7.12, indicate that the observed patterns for two or three involved sites depart significantly from random expectation. In particular, there is an apparent deficiency of bilateral neck node involvement in the absence of associated mediastinal adenopathy, an excess of associated neck and mediastinal node involvement, and a deficiency of all noncontiguous contralateral distributions. When four involved sites were analyzed, the distributions could not be shown to differ significantly from random expectation, suggesting that by the time the disease has extended to

Table 7.10 Association of Left, Right, and Bilateral Cervical-Supraclavicular Adenopathy with Mediastinal Adenopathy and Subdiaphragmatic Involvement at Staging Laparotomy in Clinical Stage I and II Hodgkin's Disease

Cervical-supraclavicular adenopathy	Mediastinal adenopathy	Subdiaphragmatic involvement at staging laparotomy	
		No. pos./Total no.	% pos.
Left	−	8/29	28
	+	15/49	31
Right	−	9/20	45
	+	8/33	24
Bilateral	−	13/29	45
	+	23/85	27

Source: Data from a series of 814 previously untreated patients submitted to staging laparotomy, July 1, 1968–Dec. 31, 1977 (Kaplan).

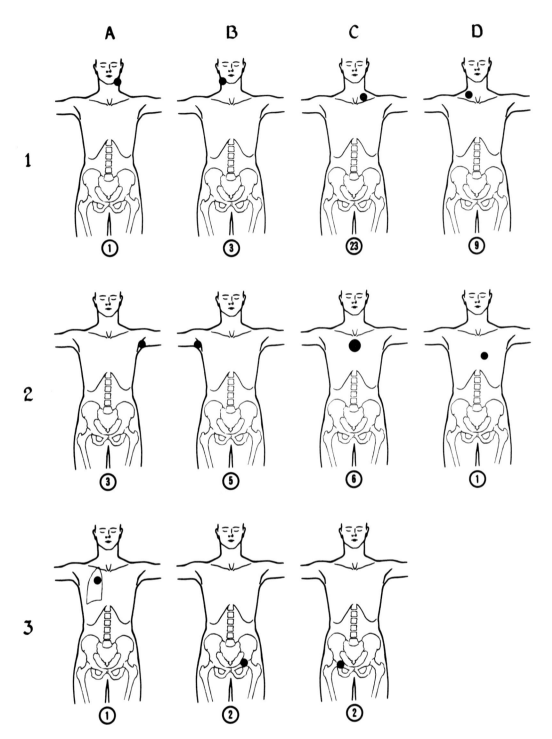

Figure 7.10 Rye stage I_1 (Ann Arbor stage I) patterns in 56 previously untreated patients. The case illustrated in position D-2 is a unique example in our experience to date of primary left hilar node disease which, on later review, was reinterpreted as diffuse histiocytic lymphoma. The encircled numeral below each diagram indicates the number of patients in whom that particular anatomic distribution was observed.

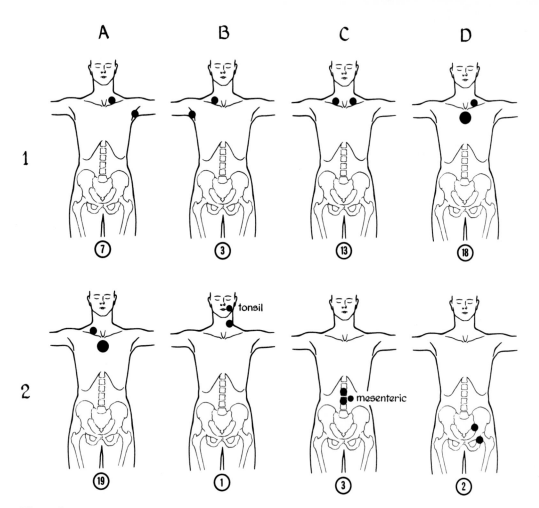

Figure 7.11   Rye stage I_2 (Ann Arbor stage II) patterns in 66 previously untreated patients. Note the frequency of patterns C-1, D-1, and A-2.

Table 7.11 Nonrandomness of Involved Lymph Node Distributions in Stage II Hodgkin's Disease

Region	All patients		Nodular sclerosing		Mixed cellularity	
	Obs.	Exp.[a]	Obs.	Exp.	Obs.	Exp.
Bilateral neck	14	24.3	3	9.8	4	4.4
Ipsilateral neck, axilla	13	9.3	3	3.8	2	1.7
Contralateral neck, axilla	0	11.7	0	4.7	0	2.1
Neck, mediastinum	44	21.6	23	8.7	7	3.9
Bilateral axillae	1	0.9	0	0.3	0	0.2
Axilla, mediastinum	0	3.8	0	1.6	0	0.6
Total, two regions	72	71.6	29	28.9	13	12.9
Bilateral neck, axilla	8	20.9	3	10.6	2	4.0
Bilateral neck, mediastinum	44	22.9	25	11.6	6	4.4
Neck, bilateral axillae	2	3.2	0	1.7	1	0.6
Ipsilateral neck, axilla, mediastinum	8	6.5	4	3.3	2	1.2
Contralateral neck, axilla, mediastinum	1	8.9	0	4.4	1	1.6
Bilateral axillae, mediastinum	0	0.4	0	0.2	0	0.07
Total, three regions	63	62.8	32	31.8	12	11.87
Bilateral neck, axillae	6	3.2	2	1.6	2	0.5
Bilateral neck, axilla, mediastinum	17	18.1	10	9.5	2	3.1
Neck, bilateral axillae, mediastinum	0	1.8	0	0.9	0	0.35
Total, four regions	23	23.1	12	12.0	4	3.95
Total, all regions	158	157.5	73	72.7	29	28.72

[a] From an analysis by Dr. George Hutchison (Harvard School of Public Health, Boston, MA.) of the random expectation of involvement of any two to four Rye stage II sites, based on their relative frequencies as sole sites of involvement in stage I cases, compared with observed frequencies in 158 of our Rye stage II cases.

Obs. = observed numbers; Exp. = expected numbers on a random basis. A similar analysis of data from a national cooperative clinical trial, the results of which are consistent with those above, has been presented elsewhere (Hutchison, 1972).

Table 7.12 Nonrandomness of Involved Lymph Node Distributions in Stage II Hodgkin's Disease[a]

Relation to other site	All patients		Nodular sclerosing		Mixed cellularity	
	Obs.	Exp.	Obs.	Exp.	Obs.	Exp.
Adjacent contiguous	57	30.9	26	12.5	9	5.6
Adjacent noncontiguous	14	24.3	3	9.8	4	4.4
Nonadjacent	1	16.4	0	6.6	0	2.9
Total, two regions	72	71.6	29	28.9	13	12.9
Adjacent contiguous	52	29.4	29	14.9	8	5.6
Adjacent noncontiguous	8	20.9	3	10.6	2	4.0
Nonadjacent	3	12.5	0	6.3	2	2.27
Total, three regions	63	62.8	32	31.8	12	11.87
Adjacent contiguous	17	18.1	10	9.5	2	3.1
Adjacent noncontiguous	6	3.2	2	1.6	2	0.5
Nonadjacent	0	1.8	0	0.9	0	0.35
Total, four regions	23	23.1	12	12.0	4	3.95
Adjacent contiguous	126	78.4	65	36.9	19	14.3
Adjacent noncontiguous	28	48.4	8	22.0	8	8.9
Nonadjacent	4	30.7	0	13.8	2	5.52
Total, all regions	158	157.5	73	72.7	29	28.72

[a] See footnote to Table 7.11.

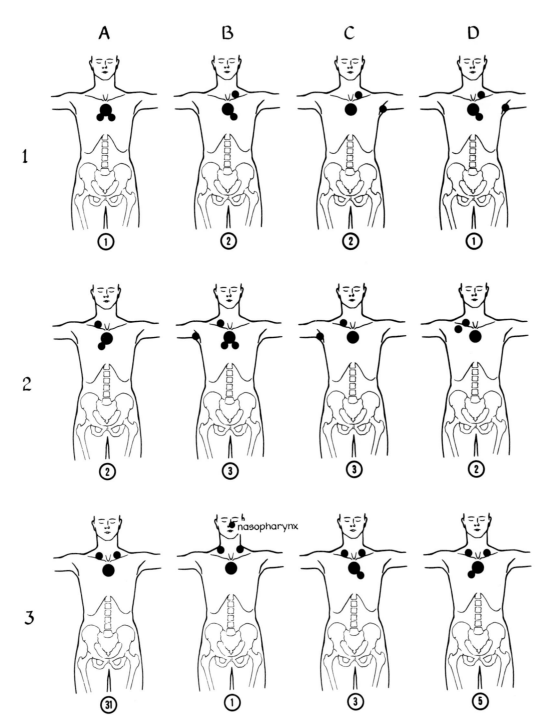

Figure 7.12 Rye and Ann Arbor stage II supradiaphragmatic patterns in 90 previously untreated patients in whom the mediastinal nodes were involved. The only noncontiguous pattern observed is that illustrated in position F-2.

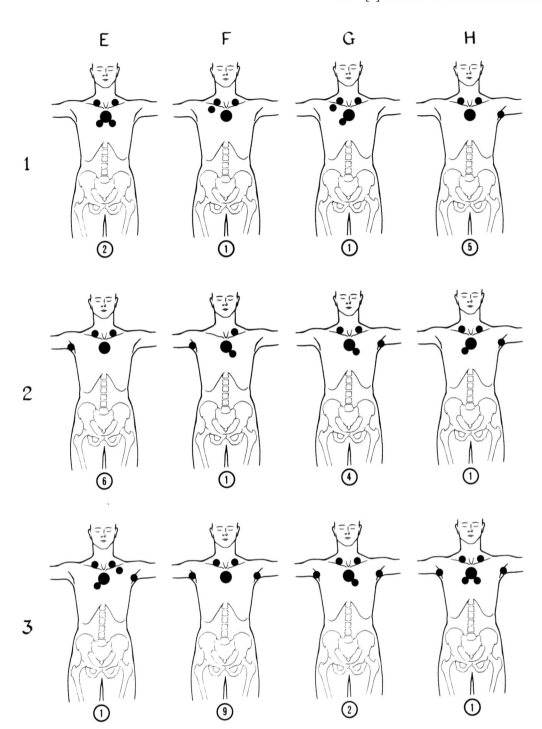

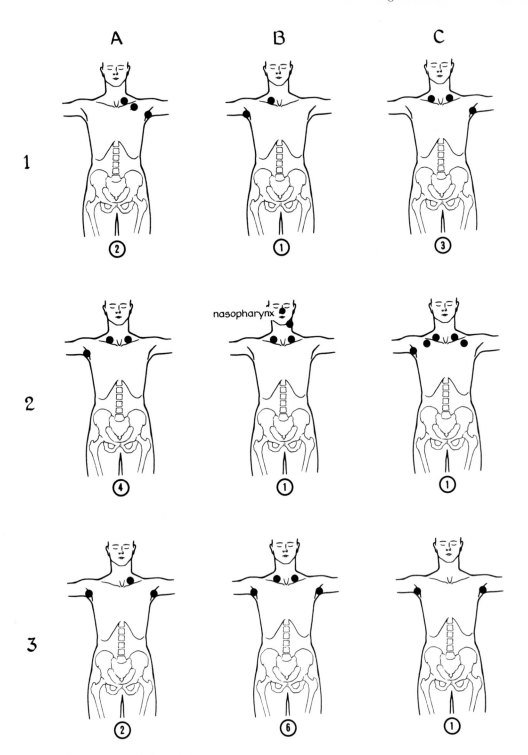

Figure 7.13   Rye and Ann Arbor stage II supradiaphragmatic patterns in 21 previously untreated patients in whom the mediastinal nodes were not involved. Three noncontiguous distributions were observed, two illustrated at position A-3 and one at C-3.

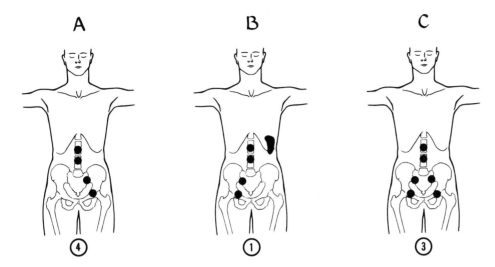

Figure 7.14   Rye and Ann Arbor stage II infradiaphragmatic patterns of involvement in 8 previously
untreated patients.

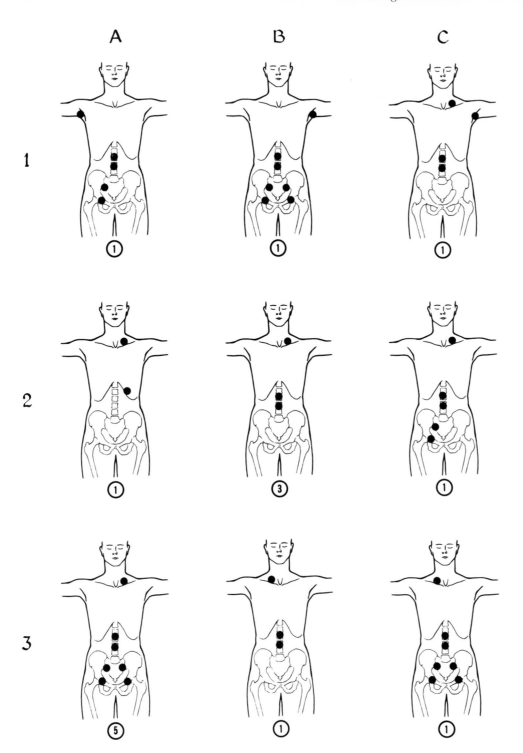

Figure 7.15 Rye and Ann Arbor stage III patterns in 24 previously untreated patients in whom neither the mediastinal nodes nor the spleen were involved.

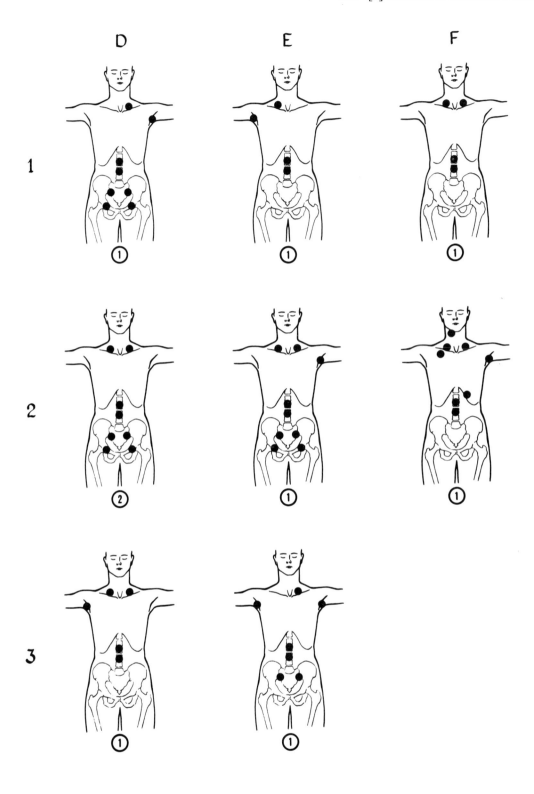

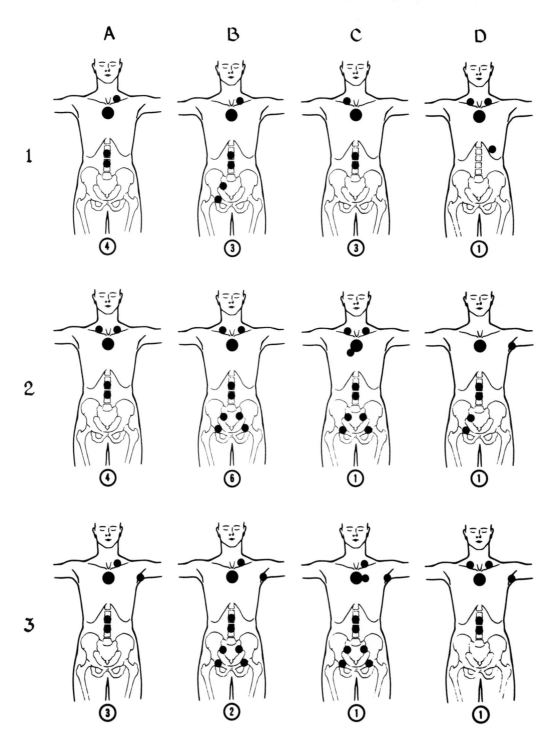

Figure 7.16 Rye and Ann Arbor stage III patterns in 43 previously untreated patients in whom the mediastinal nodes were enlarged but the spleen was apparently not involved. However, only a small proportion of these cases were staged with the aid of laparotomy and splenectomy, so the frequency of spleen involvement is almost certainly underestimated.

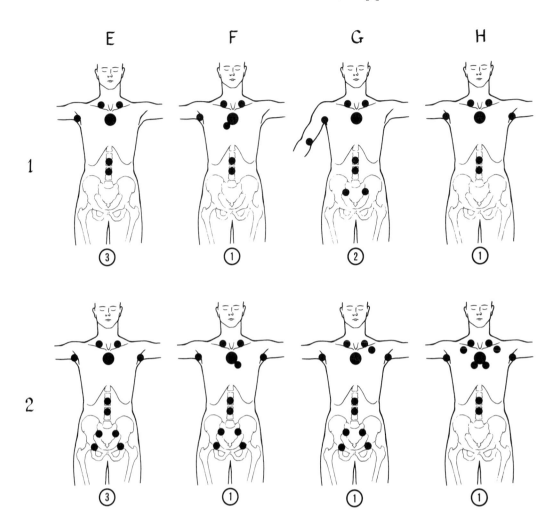

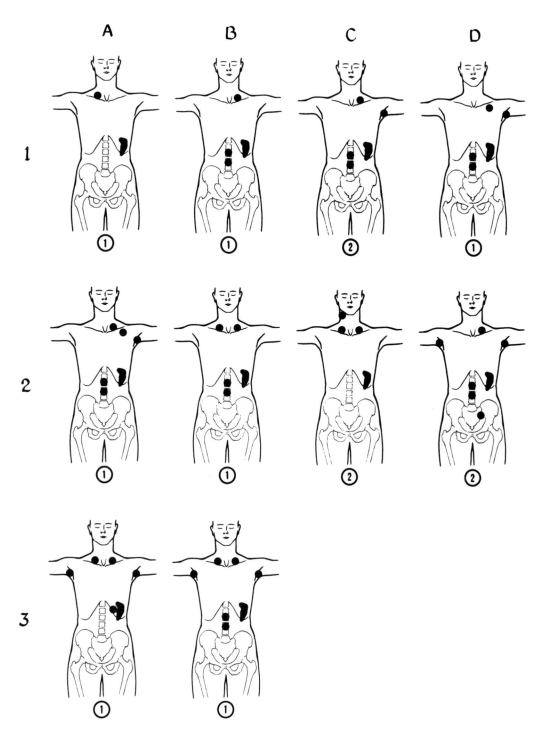

Figure 7.17   Rye and Ann Arbor stage III patterns in 13 previously untreated patients in whom the spleen was involved but the mediastinal nodes were not. Some instances of spleen involvement in the absence of retro-peritoneal node involvement may have been due to sampling error in the selection of nodes for biopsy.

four or more regions, other pathways of dissemination may begin to be utilized.

A rather similar type of analysis was applied by Lillicrap (1973) in a comparison of the predictions of the susceptibility hypothesis of Smithers with the observed patterns of spread in three different series of patients with Hodgkin's disease. For two regions of involvement, the predictions of the susceptibility theory were found to differ significantly from observed distributions in several important respects. Bilateral neck disease was observed significantly less often than predicted, whereas involvement in the neck and mediastinum was more frequent than predicted. Moreover, there were 46 instances of homolateral neck-axilla involvement, and only 2 contralateral cases, whereas susceptibility theory would have predicted an equal number of each pattern. In contrast, the observed patterns were consistent with contiguity theory in all but 8 of 212 cases. Once again, as the analysis was extended to three and four different regions of involvement, there was a slight increase in the percentage of apparently noncontiguous patterns, and a somewhat better agreement was observed with the predictions of susceptibility theory.

Modifications of the susceptibility theory were proposed by Smithers, Lillicrap, and Barnes (1974) in an attempt to make the theory more consistent with observation. Both modifications accept the concept that spread occurs via lymphatic channels, as predicted by contiguity theory. In the first model it is assumed that in a certain proportion of cases, estimated at 50 percent, spread is governed only by the intrinsic susceptibilities of the various lymph node sites, whereas in the remainder of cases, spread is dependent not only on site susceptibility but on transmission in the normal direction of lymph flow along lymphatic channels. Thus half of all instances of spread would occur by way of the lymphatic system exclusively in the direction of flow, and the other half would occur via the bloodstream, with "homing" of either tumor cells or an unidentified etiologic agent from an initial site of lymph node involvement to the bloodstream and thence selectively to other lymph node sites of high susceptibility. In a second model, they proposed that the intrinsic susceptibility of each lymph node region is coupled with spread along lymphatic channels which is twice as likely to occur in the normal direction of flow as in the retrograde direction. Although several discrepancies remain, both models exhibit an appreciably better agreement with observed patterns of two and three sites of involvement.

Different histopathologic forms of Hodgkin's disease appear to exhibit significantly different patterns of lymph node and extralymphatic distribution. Thus, the lymphocyte predominance (LP) form is often encountered in stage I cases involving upper cervical, supraclavicular, axillary, inguinal, or other peripheral, superficial lymph nodes, and seldom involves the mediastinal or hilar nodes (Kadin, Glatstein, and Dorfman, 1971). The mixed cellularity (MC) and lymphocyte depletion (LD) forms, which are more often observed in relatively advanced cases, also tend to spare the mediastinal and hilar nodes, and have a significantly greater propensity for extralymphatic and noncontiguous patterns of spread (Keller et al., 1968). Conversely, although exceptions are by no means uncommon, the nodular sclerosing (NS) form classically tends to involve the lower cervical-supraclavicular and the anterior and/or middle mediastinal nodes, with or without associated hilar node involvement (Lukes and Butler, 1966; Keller et al., 1968). Hutchison (1972) found that patterns of involvement in nodular sclerosis rarely deviated from expectation based on contiguity theory, whereas mixed cellularity was more consistent with a pattern of spread independent of the initial site of origin. There appeared to be a significant excess of instances of bilateral axillary involvement in patients with mixed cellularity disease. The greater frequency of spleen involvement in mixed cellularity and lymphocyte depletion than in lymphocyte predominance and nodular sclerosis has already been noted (Table 7.3).

The contiguity theory has also been applied to analyses of the sites of first extension of disease after local radiotherapy of initially carefully staged cases of Hodgkin's disease. In the original study by Rosenberg and Kaplan (1966), 22 of 26 extensions of disease were to contiguous lymph node chains. Our subsequent experience confirms this observation, as do the studies of Han and Stutzman (1967), Peters et al. (1968), Landberg and Larsson (1968), Prosnitz et al. (1969), and Banfi et al. (1969). The last-named authors found that the next site of involvement after initial treatment was in the adjacent lymph node chain in 72 percent of their cases. In a study of 72 cases in children, Teillet and Schweisguth (1969) found that the supraclavicular nodes were the site of initial relapse in 20 of 34 patients with onset in the upper cervical nodes; the mediastinal nodes in 14 and the para-aortic in 12 of 21 patients with onset in the supraclavicular area; the left supraclavicular nodes in one of two patients with onset in the para-aortic chain; and

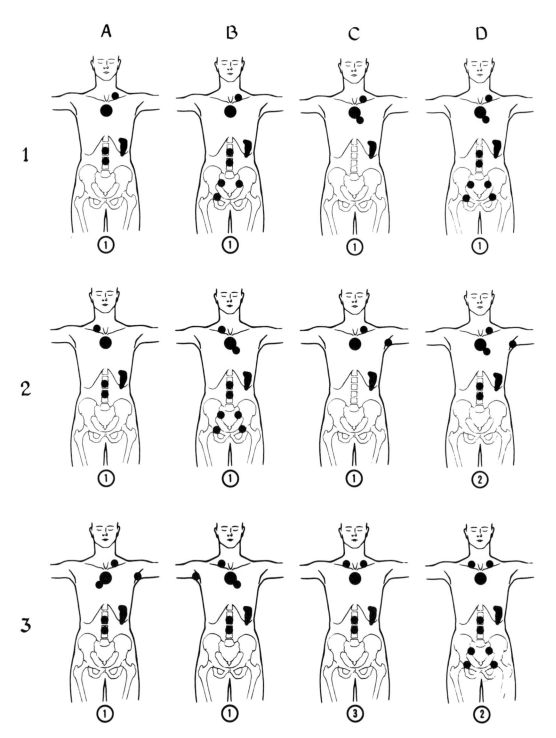

Figure 7.18   Rye and Ann Arbor stage III patterns in
32 previously untreated patients in whom both the
spleen and the mediastinal nodes were involved.

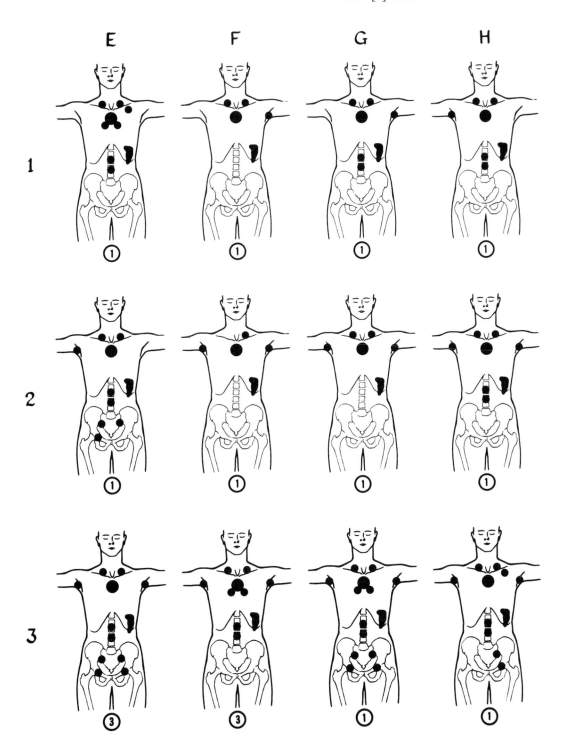

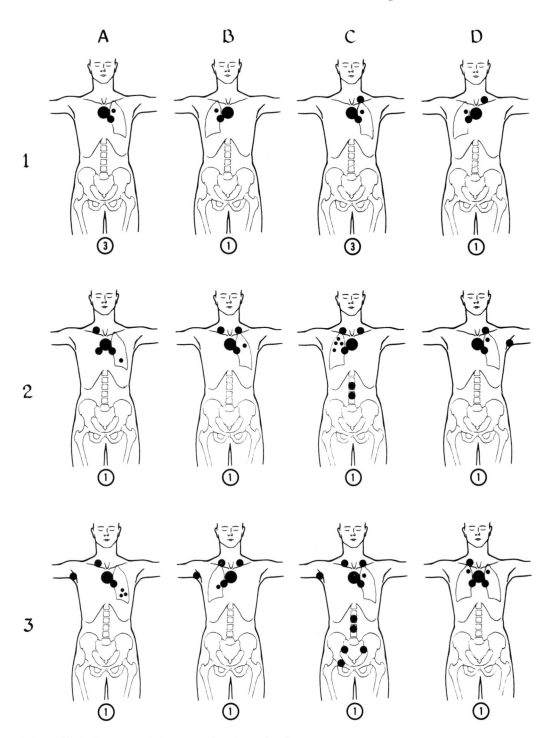

Figure 7.19   Rye stage IV patterns in 25 previously untreated patients in whom the pulmonary parenchyma was involved on one or both sides. In the Stanford (1970) and Ann Arbor staging classifications, patterns A-1, B-1, C-1, D-1, A-2, B-2, D-2, and B-3 would be designated stage II$_E$ and pattern C-3 would be designated stage III$_E$ (cf. Chapter 8). Note the correlation with mediastinal and ipsilateral hilar node involvement.

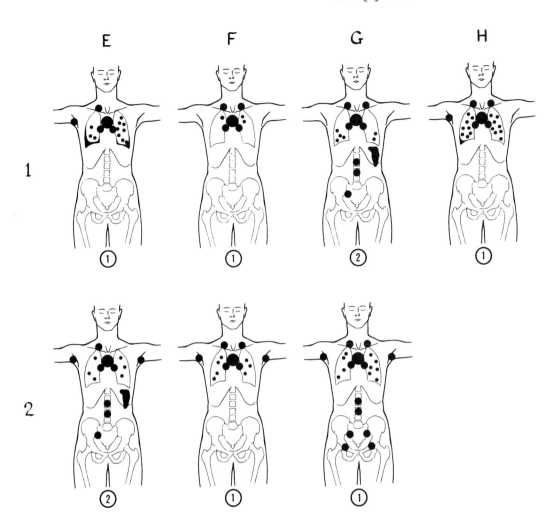

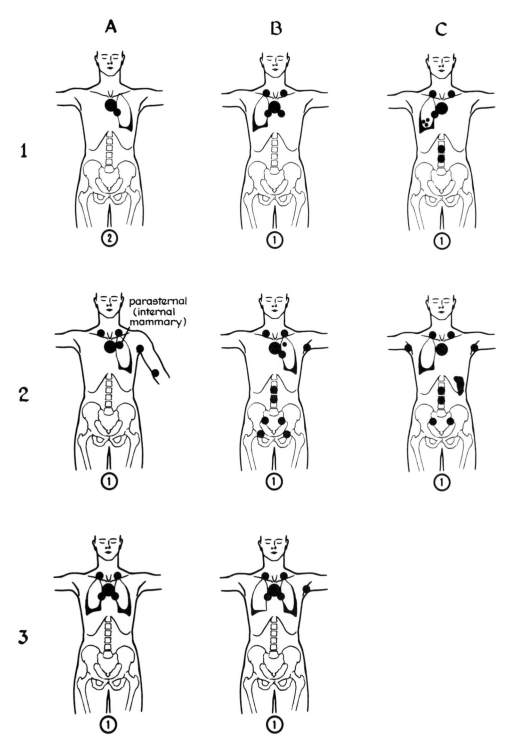

Figure 7.20 Rye stage IV patterns in 9 previously untreated patients in whom the pleura was involved. Those with only unilateral involvement would be redesignated stage II_E (patterns A-1, B-1, and A-2) or stage III_E (patterns B-2 and C-2) in the Stanford (1970) and Ann Arbor clinical staging classifications (cf. Chapter 8). Note the correlation with mediastinal node involvement.

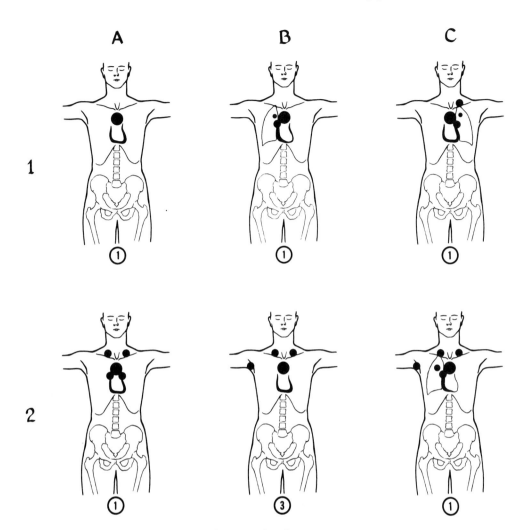

Figure 7.21 Rye stage IV patterns in 8 previously untreated patients in whom the pericardium had been invaded. All would be redesignated stage II_E in the later classifications. Note that mediastinal adenopathy was present in all cases.

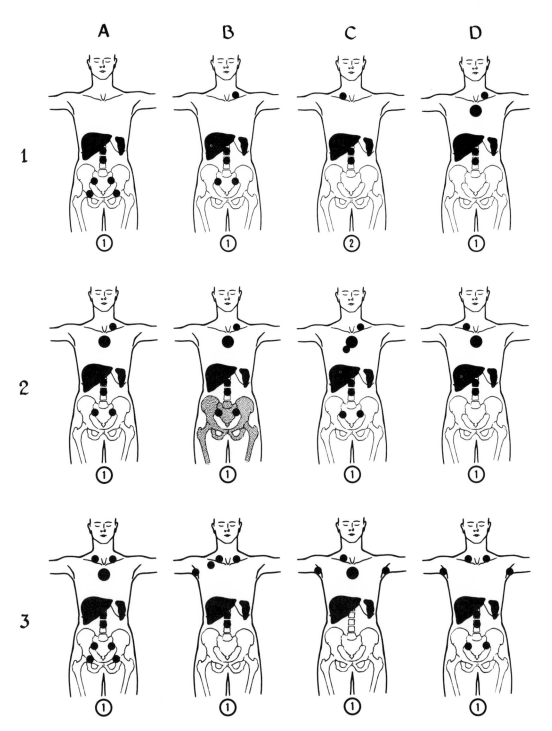

Figure 7.22 Rye and Ann Arbor stage IV patterns in 13 previously untreated patients in whom the liver was involved. Note that concomitant involvement of the spleen was documented in every case, and that para-aortic node involvement was also present in all but one instance (C-3). Bone marrow disease was also demonstrated in the patient illustrated in pattern B-2.

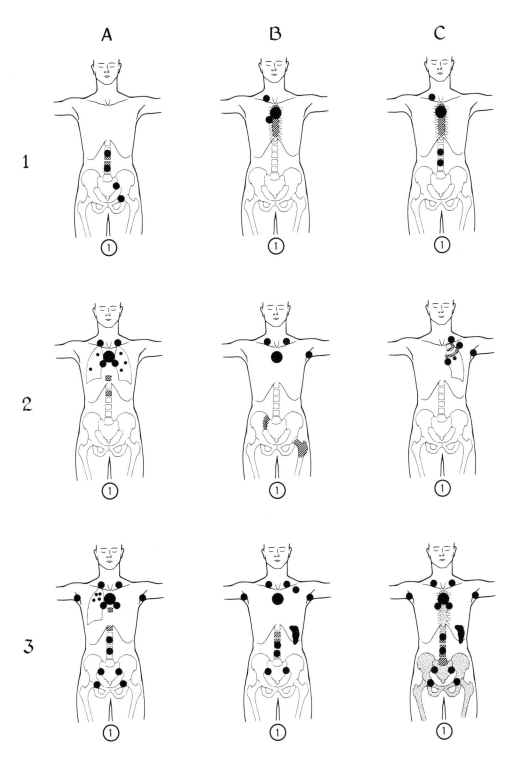

Figure 7.23 Rye stage IV patterns in 9 previously untreated patients in whom one or more bones were involved, with or without involvement of the bone marrow. Patterns A-1, B-1, and C-2 would be redesignated stage II$_E$, and pattern C-1 redesignated stage III$_E$ in the Stanford (1970) and Ann Arbor (1971) classifications.

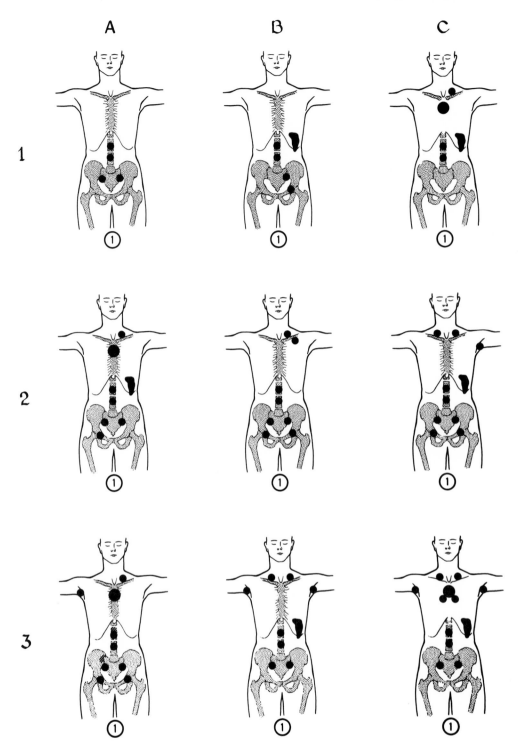

Figure 7.24   Rye and Ann Arbor stage IV patterns in 9 previously untreated patients in whom the bone marrow was involved (in addition to those cases illustrated in Figures 7.22 and 7.23).

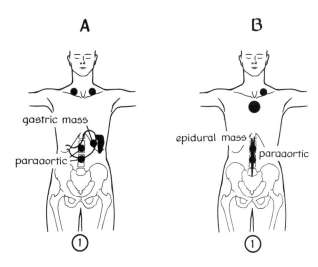

Figure 7.25 Rye stage IV patterns in which miscellaneous other extralymphatic sites were involved. On subsequent review of additional histopathologic material, the case illustrated in pattern A-1 was reclassified as a diffuse histiocytic lymphoma. The case illustrated in pattern B-1 would be considered stage III_E in the Ann Arbor classifications.

the upper cervical or axillary nodes in 9 of 14 patients whose disease first presented in both the supraclavicular and mediastinal nodes.

The frequency of later extension to the lumbar para-aortic nodes in patients with initial low cervical-supraclavicular involvement, presumably via the thoracic duct, has been conclusively documented. Among 80 such cases at risk, para-aortic node extensions occurred in 29 (36 percent) and constituted the single most prevalent site of extension in patients treated initially with local or limited-field, supradiaphragmatic radiotherapy (Kaplan, 1970). The radiographic evidence of para-aortic extension in some of these cases is illustrated in Figures 5.65 to 5.71. Smithers (1970) noted subdiaphragmatic spread in 23 percent of his cases within two years after initial treatment of supraclavicular node disease. Transdiaphragmatic extension was the first manifestation of relapse in 33 (40 percent) of 83 patients with clinical stage I and II disease analyzed by Rubin et al. (1974). In a similar study, Baldetorp, Landberg, and Svahn-Tapper (1976) noted such extensions in 31 percent of patients treated for clinical stage I and II supradiaphragmatic disease. The initial sites of involvement in 65 of our cases with documented extensions of disease after local or limited-field radiotherapy are grouped by site of extension in Figures 7.26 to 7.33.

The major common denominator in our cases

with positive histologic evidence of Hodgkin's disease in the spleen has been the involvement of one or more para-aortic lymph nodes, usually first demonstrated by lymphangiography and subsequently confirmed in most instances by biopsy at the time of laparotomy (Table 7.4). The problem of sampling error at the time of surgery is believed to account for a small proportion of cases in which the excised lymph nodes contain no evidence of Hodgkin's disease, despite a positive lymphangiogram; in some instances, metallic clips placed at the site of lymph node removal permitted the demonstration on subsequent abdominal roentgenograms that the lymph nodes which were most suspected on the lymphangiogram still remained within the abdomen after surgery. In other instances, spleen involvement has been associated with splenic hilar or celiac node involvement, with or without associated para-aortic node involvement.

Splenic involvement is extremely rare as an isolated manifestation in Hodgkin's disease (Alslev, 1956; Bacci, Bianchi, and Ferramosca, 1969; Amadini and Novi, 1975). The probability that the spleen will be involved rises sharply when the celiac, para-aortic, and/or splenic hilar lymph nodes have been affected. The lymph nodes at the hilum of the spleen and along the splenic pedicle have been involved in about half of all instances in which the spleen itself was macroscopically involved (Table 7.4). Moreover, we have observed a small number of cases in which one or more lymph nodes at the hilum of the spleen were grossly or microscopically diseased, despite the fact that the excised spleen itself was uninvolved.

Involvement of the spleen in turn poses the threat of hepatic parenchymal involvement. In Figure 7.1 it may be seen that the initial diagnostic evaluation of 285 previously untreated patients disclosed involvement of the spleen in 99 instances and of the liver in only 9. The spleen was involved in every instance in which the liver was involved; this is also apparent in the more extensive data of Figures 7.17, 7.18, and 7.22 and Table 7.4. From these data alone, it is apparent that involvement of the spleen and liver by Hodgkin's disease must entail a nonrandom, patterned association. It would thus appear that hepatic involvement is almost invariably secondary to splenic involvement. Consistent with this conclusion is the fact that the probability of liver involvement is in direct proportion to the size and weight of the involved spleen (Glatstein et al., 1969). Massive involvement of the spleen is accompanied by biopsy evidence of liver involvement in over 50 percent of cases, whereas

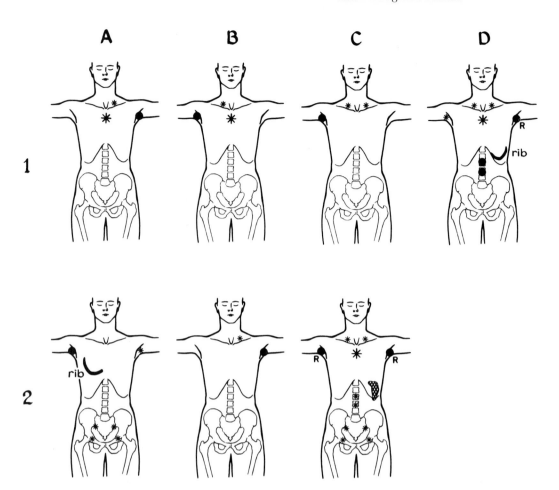

Figure 7.26 Primary axillary node extensions of disease (solid black areas) after local or limited-field radiotherapy in seven cases. Initial sites of involvement are shown by asterisks, except for the spleen, which is cross-hatched. Ipsilateral supraclavicular node involvement was present in all but case A-2.

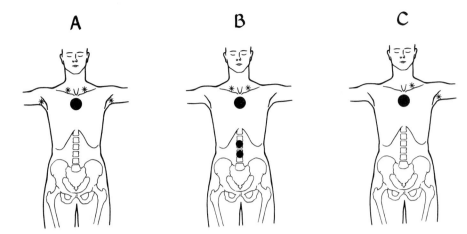

Figure 7.27 Primary mediastinal node extensions (black circles) in three cases, all with initial involvement of the supraclavicular nodes on one or both sides (asterisks). Mediastinal node extension would almost certainly have been recorded more often if the mediastinal region had not usually been included in the field of radiotherapy in such cases. Simultaneous extension to the para-aortic nodes occurred in one case.

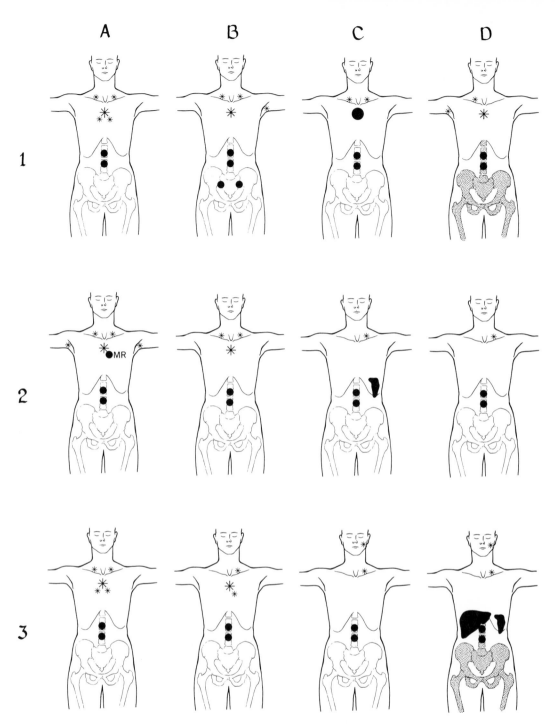

Figure 7.28 Primary para-aortic node extensions (black circles). The bone marrow (stippled) was also involved in two of these cases, the spleen in three, and the bones, the lung, and the liver in one each. One other patient (A-2) developed a marginal recurrence (MR) in the pericardium, immediately beyond the inferolateral margin of the radiotherapeutic contour used for his initial mantle field. Asterisks show initial sites of involvement. Note that prior supraclavicular node involvement on one or both sides was the common denominator for para-aortic node extension.

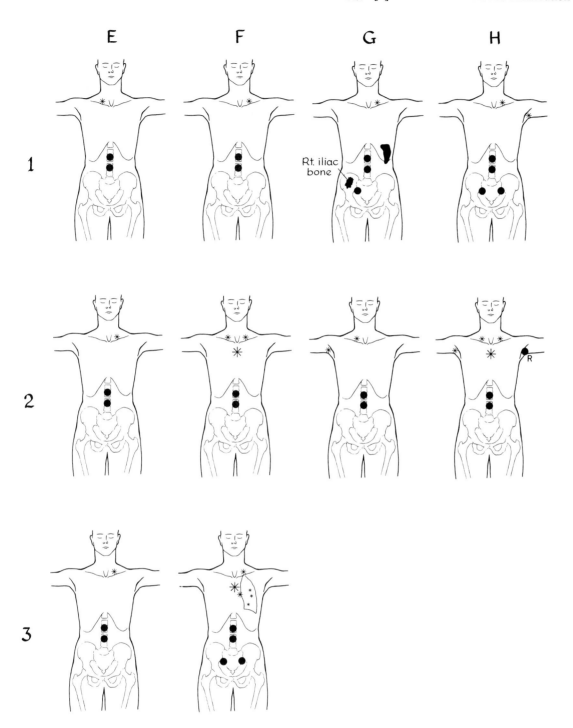

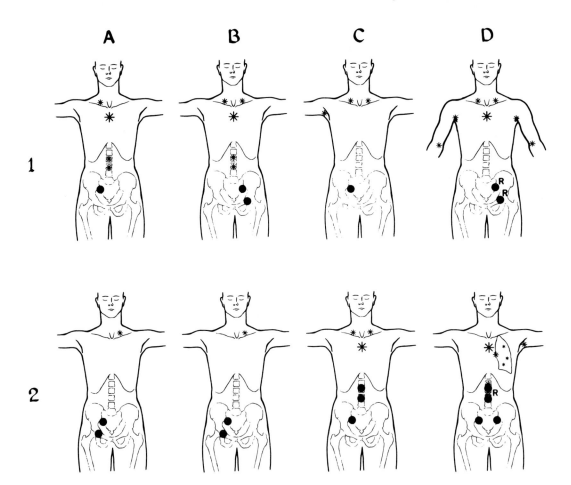

Figure 7.29   Primary inguinal and/or iliac node extensions (black circles). In one case (D-1), the term recurrence (R) might be more appropriate, since these node chains had been prophylactically irradiated four years earlier. Asterisks show initial sites of involvement. Note that para-aortic node involvement either accompanied or preceded the extensions in four of these eight cases; recurrence (R) in the para-aortic nodes was associated with iliac extension in one (D-2).

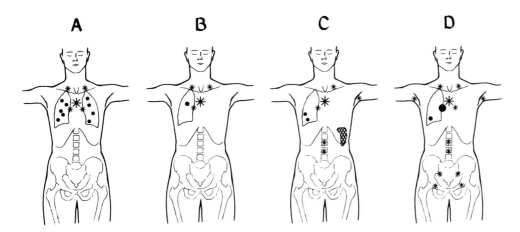

Figure 7.30 Primary extensions to the pulmonary parenchyma (black circles) in four cases, all of which were preceded (A-1, B-1, and C-1) or accompanied (D-1) by ipsilateral hilar adenopathy. Asterisks show sites of initial involvement except for the spleen, which is cross-hatched.

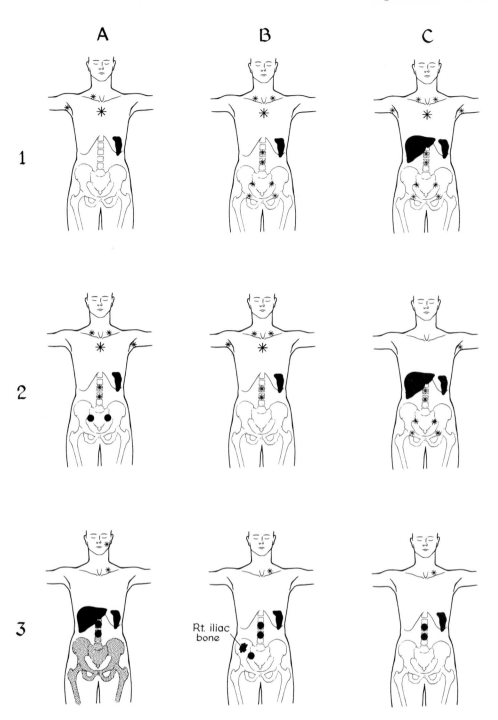

Figure 7.31   Primary extensions (black) involving the spleen, alone or with other organs, in nine cases. Stippling indicates bone marrow involvement. Such extensions were preceded or accompanied by both supraclavicular and para-aortic adenopathy (asterisks) in all but one case (A-1), in which para-aortic node involvement was not documented by biopsy but may well have been present, and one other (C-2) in which the initial presence of left axillary adenopathy strongly suggests that left supraclavicular disease, though clinically undetected, was probably also present.

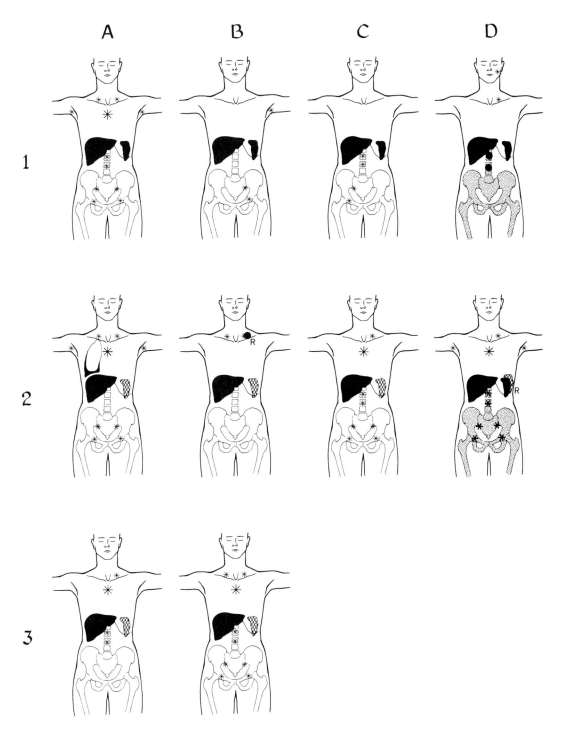

Figure 7.32   Primary extensions to the liver in ten cases. Note that all were preceded or accompanied by spleen involvement. Prior involvement of the spleen is indicated by cross-hatching, concomitant involvement by solid black; in one case (D-2), disease recurred (R) in the spleen.

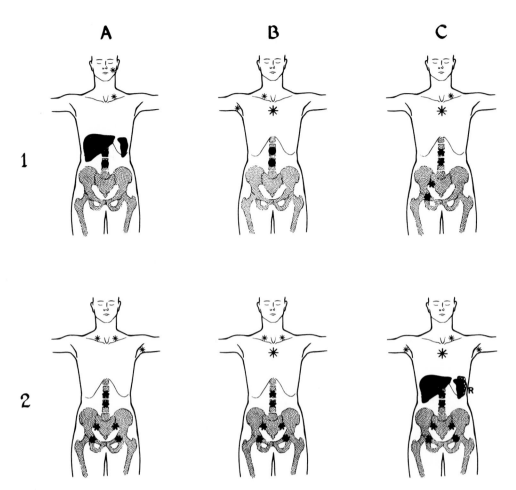

Figure 7.33   Primary extensions to the bone marrow (stippled) in six cases, in all of which there was prior (asterisks) or concomitant (black circles) para-aortic adenopathy. Prior spleen involvement is indicated by cross-hatching, associated extensions to the liver or spleen by solid black areas; case C-2 is the same as case D-2 in Figure 7.32.

positive liver biopsies are seldom obtained when spleens shown to contain Hodgkin's disease are still within or near the normal limits of size. In the selected series of laparotomy-staged cases (Glatstein et al., 1969), the combination of a palpable spleen and a positive lymphangiogram was noted in eight patients, all of whom had biopsy-documented hepatic involvement. Finally, in our earlier experience, before the implications of splenic involvement were recognized, spread of disease to the liver occurred subsequently in 15 of 34 cases (45 percent) in which prior splenic involvement had been documented (Kaplan, 1970).

As indicated in Figure 7.1, positive marrow biopsies were obtained in only 9 of 285 previously untreated patients at the time of initial diagnostic evaluation. None of these nine instances occurred in an asymptomatic patient with regionally localized disease (stages IA or IIA). Thus, the clinical setting in which bone marrow involvement may be anticipated is that of advanced disease, particularly in the presence of such constitutional symptoms as night sweats or fever. That Hodgkin's disease cannot reach the bone marrow without becoming blood-borne can hardly be doubted. Moreover, there have been rare but well-documented instances in which Sternberg-Reed cells have been detected in the peripheral blood (Bouroncle, 1966; Capron and Menne, 1969; Thuot et al., 1973; Schiffer, Levi, and Wiernik, 1975; Figs. 3.23, 3.24). Nonetheless, a pattern for the spread of the disease from the spleen to the bone marrow is suggested by the fact that the spleen was involved in all 23 of our laparotomy-staged cases with bone marrow involvement (Table 7.4). The demonstration by Bouroncle (1966) of Sternberg-Reed cells in venous blood expressed from the involved spleen during splenectomy (Fig. 3.24) is consistent with the view that spread beyond the spleen, principally to the liver and bone marrow, may well be hematogenous rather than lymphatic. Moreover, Rappaport and Strum (1970) have demonstrated direct invasion of Hodgkin's disease into the lumen of splenic blood vessels. However, the pathway by which the disease reaches the spleen itself remains controversial. Our earlier observations of the linkage between upper para-aortic and/or splenic hilar lymph node involvement and spleen involvement suggested the possibility of retrograde lymphatic spread from these nodes into the substance of the spleen. However, this view was open to the objection that the spleen does not seem to be supplied with afferent lymphatics (Rouvière, 1932). Moreover, retroperitoneal lymph node involvement cannot be demonstrated in a significant proportion of patients in whom splenic disease is encountered at laparotomy (Table 7.4).

The alternative view that spleen involvement entails hematogenous dissemination has been put forward by Halie and his colleagues (1972a,b, 1974a,b). These investigators based their conclusion on studies of peripheral blood leukocyte concentrates in patients with Hodgkin's disease. They observed "large blast-like cells up to 40 μm in diameter with a finely structured moderately basophilic cytoplasm, a nucleus varying in appearance from oval to lobulated with a somewhat reticulated chromatin network, and one or more large irregularly-shaped nucleoli" in 13 of 14 patients with Hodgkin's disease involving the spleen, in only 1 of 11 patients in whom the spleen was uninvolved, and in none of the leukocyte concentrates from normal individuals or patients with viral infections. These observations have been strongly challenged by Schiffer, Levi, and Wiernik (1975), who found large cells with basophilic cytoplasm, often indistinguishable from those in patients with Hodgkin's disease, in 5 of 8 subjects with viral infections of the upper respiratory tract. When such cells were detected in leukocyte concentrates from patients with Hodgkin's disease, there was no correlation with the presence of splenic involvement, even when many cells were detected. They concluded that the basophilic cells do not represent circulating tumor cells but are probably "reactive" to the malignant process and that there is no evidence to support the view that spleen involvement is the consequence of blood-borne dissemination. If the tumor cells of Hodgkin's disease reach the spleen only by way of the bloodstream, they must surely also lodge in the lungs, liver, and bone marrow. It would therefore be expected that patients with stage II or III disease involving the spleen who have been treated with radiotherapy alone and in whom the lungs, liver, and bone marrow remain at risk would invariably develop subsequent involvement in one or more of those sites. This expectation is flatly contradicted by the very high relapse-free survival rates of patients with stage III$_S$A disease treated with radiotherapy alone (cf. Chapter 12).

Although the pulmonary parenchyma is very often involved late in the course of Hodgkin's disease, as well as at autopsy (Uddströmer, 1934; Westling, 1965), involvement is much less frequent at the time of initial diagnosis. It was detected in only 24 (8.4 percent) of 285 consecutive, previously untreated patients (Fig. 7.1). It is of interest that both mediastinal and hilar lymphadenopathy were present in all of those 24 instances; however, one case of primary pulmonary Hodgkin's disease (Fig. 5.17) has come to our attention. When hilar adenopathy was unilateral, the associated pulmonary parenchymal lesions were invariably confined to the ipsilateral lung (Fig. 7.3).

Smithers (1969a, 1970a) has argued that carcinomas, which are known to spread via lymphatics, frequently occur as microscopic metastatic foci in lymph nodes, whereas node involvement by Hodgkin's disease is generally diffuse and tends to replace the entire node. However, well-documented instances of exactly such microscopic focal involvement of part of a node by Hodgkin's disease have now been reported by Strum and Rappaport (1970a), by Henry (1971), and by Kadin, Glatstein, and Dorfman (1971).

The probable pathway and direction of spread in cases in which both the supraclavicular and the lumbar para-aortic nodes are involved remains a particularly vexing point. That the thoracic duct serves as the conduit for cell transfer from the para-aortic lymph nodes upward to the left supraclavicular fossa is not disputed. The direction of flow in the thoracic duct is normally from the abdomen to the neck, and the duct is well provided with valves (Fig. 5.47B). Moreover, Sternberg-Reed cells and Hodgkin's cells were detected by Engeset et al. (1968, 1973) in the thoracic duct lymph of all patients with involvement of the para-aortic nodes above the fourth lumbar vertebral level (Figs. 3.21, 3.22). However, the concept that these tumor cells may sometimes travel in the retrograde direction down the thoracic duct from the supraclavicular region to the upper lumbar para-aortic lymph nodes has been much more controversial. Support for this possibility, which was formerly suggested by the greater frequency of left-sided or bilateral supraclavicular rather than right-sided supraclavicular involvement in association with para-aortic node involvement, is no longer evident in recent analyses of more extensive laparotomy data (Table 7.10). Moreover, the frequency of association of right supraclavicular involvement with subdiaphragmatic involvement is in excess of expectation in relation to the reported frequency of insertion of the thoracic duct on the right side in 5 percent, and bilaterally in 2 percent, of normal lymphangiograms (Fuchs, 1969; Figures 7.34, 7.35, and 7.36). The pressure in the duct is only a few millimeters of water, and reversal of flow was readily observed by Neyazaki et al. (1965) and by Takashima and Benninghoff (1966) after

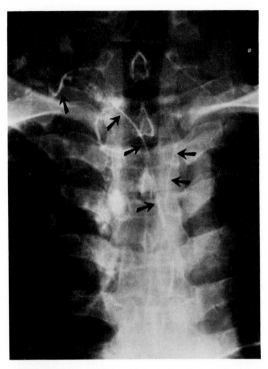

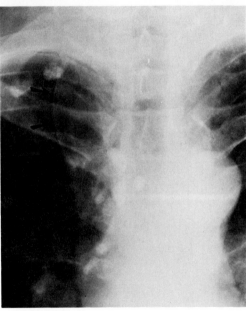

Figure 7.34 *Top*, bilateral emptying of the thoracic duct visualized during lymphangiography. The duct is single up to the level of the aortic arch and then bifurcates into two channels (arrows), the larger of which empties on the right side of the neck. *Bottom*, the presence of an azygos lobe (arrows) in this case raises the question whether these two developmental anomalies are associated. Note the opacified lymph nodes in the right supraclavicular and paratracheal regions.

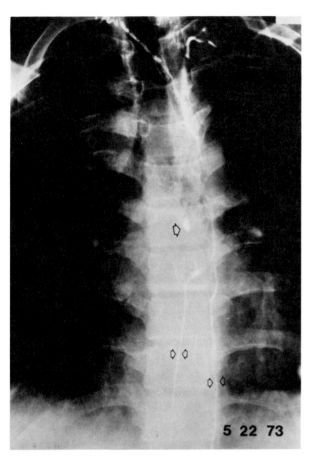

Figure 7.35 Duplication of the lower half of the thoracic duct, and bifurcation of the upper end with bilateral insertion.

Figure 7.36 Another anatomical variation of the upper end of the thoracic duct, with bifurcation and bilateral insertion.

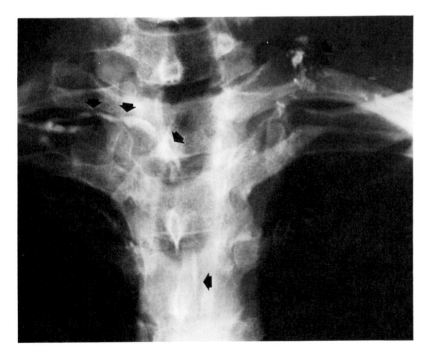

chronic ligation of the thoracic duct in dogs. Studies of side pressures in the canine thoracic duct by Browse, Lord, and Taylor (1971) reveal that the pressure gradient along the thoracic duct was often opposite to that required for forward flow. On the other hand, Dumont and Martelli (1973), after ligating and cannulating the canine thoracic duct and injecting opaque contrast materials in the retrograde direction, were able to demonstrate radiopaque material in the para-aortic lymph nodes in only 1 of 16 animals. It is of course quite possible that retrograde flow might occur more often in the thoracic duct of man, which is normally vertical, than in that of dogs, which is horizontal.

Rouvière (1932), in his classic study of the anatomy of the lymphatics in man, noted that the thoracic duct usually has two competent valves at its upper end, but that the presence of a single, incompetent valve is a not-infrequent normal variation, usually compensated by the oblique insertion of the duct through the venous wall. He comments that "the closure of the thoracic duct is not always perfect, for it is not rare to find in cadavers some blood in the terminal part of the duct." It is thus not difficult to imagine that prolonged compression and partial occlusion of the duct by enlarged lymph nodes near its insertion in the subclavian area may cause a similar reversal of flow to occur in man. This sequence of events would

account most satisfactorily for instances in which supraclavicular adenopathy is initially associated with a normal lymphangiogram and where para-aortic adenopathy does not become manifest, even on repeat lymphangiography, until long afterward: four to ten years in some of our cases (Figs. 7.37, 7.38, and 7.39; cf. also Figs. 5.65 through 5.71, Chapter 5), more than ten years in a case cited by Smithers (1970), and fifteen years in a patient with paragranuloma seen by us in consultation. Retrograde flow in obstructed lymphatics is a generally accepted explanation for cases in which involvement of central lymph node chains is later followed by lymphadenopathy in the next *distal* chain (examples: supraclavicular followed by ipsilateral high cervical or axillary, high cervical followed by ipsilateral preauricular, axillary followed by ipsilateral brachial or epitrochlear, para-aortic followed by unilateral or bilateral iliac node involvement; Fig. 7.40). It has also been invoked to account for the localization of skin and subcutaneous lesions in the areas of drainage of involved lymph node chains (Benninghoff et al., 1970). These documented examples provide precedent and plausibility for the view that at least some instances of spread via the thoracic duct, particularly those with an appropriate time sequence, occur in the retrograde direction.

In summary, although the susceptibility theory

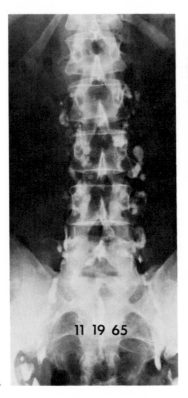 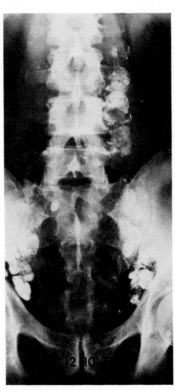

Figure 7.37 *A*, normal lymphangiogram in November 1965 in a 46-year-old male physician with stage IIA Hodgkin's disease. After completion of mantle field radiotherapy, he refused subdiaphragmatic irradiation. He remained relapse-free for about four years, but was then lost to followup until he returned in December 1971, complaining of fatigue and low-grade fever. A second lymphangiogram (*B*) revealed massive lymphadenopathy and delayed emptying of left pelvic lymphatics, indicative of partial obstruction.

A

B

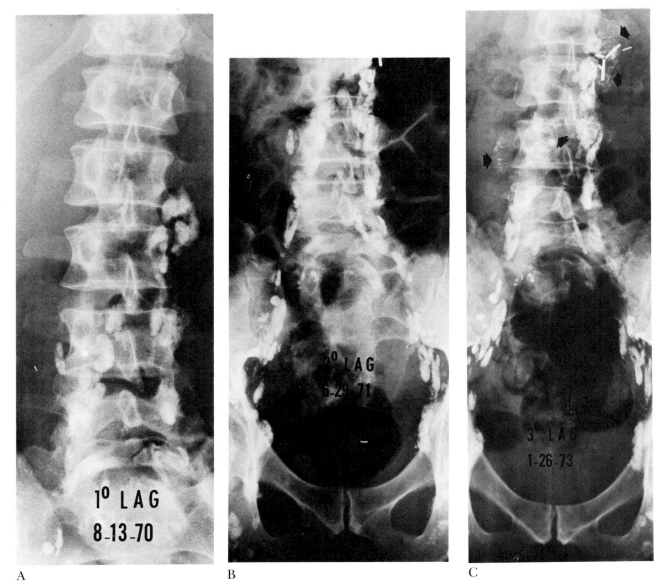

A   B   C

Figure 7.38 This 40-year-old male patient had a normal lymphangiogram (*A*) and a negative staging laparotomy in August 1970 and was treated with involved field radiotherapy for stage IIA supradiaphragmatic Hodgkin's disease. When the contrast agent had almost disappeared, a second lymphangiogram (*B*) was performed in June 1971 and was again interpreted as normal. Late in 1972, he began to have low-grade fever, and a third lymphangiogram (*C*) in January 1973 revealed enlargement and foaminess in high left para-aortic nodes and a lower right paracaval node (arrows). Biopsy confirmation of relapsing Hodgkin's disease was obtained.

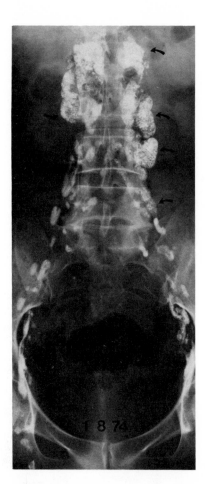

Figure 7.39   Obviously abnormal lymphangiogram in a 45-year-old woman who had been treated with involved field radiotherapy for stage IIA Hodgkin's disease nine years earlier at another institution, where the original lymphangiogram was said to have been normal.

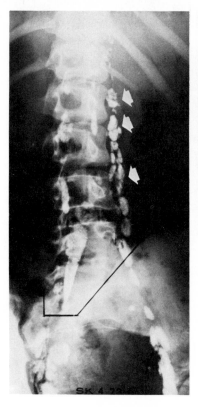
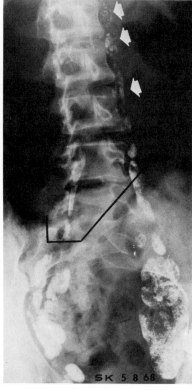

Figure 7.40   Retrograde extension into the iliac lymph nodes. This 13-year-old girl had an initial lymphangiogram in April 1965 which was interpreted as probably normal, though some small filling defects were noted in several of the left lumbar para-aortic nodes. Laparotomy was suggested for biopsy confirmation but was refused by her mother. The patient was treated to a mantle field and then, prophylactically, to a modified para-aortic field (outlined) which stopped above the pelvis to spare the ovaries. Three years later, she noted discomfort in the left pelvis, and physical examination revealed a left iliac mass which was confirmed by the repeat lymphangiogram of May 1968 and by biopsy. (Reprinted by permission of the authors and *Radiology,* from the paper by Castellino et al., 1973.)

of Smithers (1969, 1970), as subsequently modified by Smithers, Lillicrap, and Barnes (1974), remains a viable alternative, most of the evidence presented in this chapter seems consistent with the contiguity hypothesis initially proposed by Rosenberg and Kaplan (1966) and extended by Kaplan (1970). This hypothesis postulates that the vast majority of cases of Hodgkin's disease probably arise unifocally in and remain confined for a long time to the lymphatic system, and that the disease tends to spread from a given lymph node chain to others with which direct communication via lymphatic channels exists (Table 7.7). Moreover, even when dissemination occurs beyond the lymphatic system, patterns of association are frequently evident. Thus, a kind of "road map" for successive sites of involvement may be constructed (Kaplan, 1970). It may be predicted, for example, that para-aortic node involvement is associated with a high probability of spleen involvement, which in turn is commonly followed by liver and/or bone marrow involvement. Conversely, the intrathoracic sequence seems to proceed from the mediastinal to the hilar nodes on one or both sides and thence to ipsilateral (or bilateral) pulmonary parenchymal metastasis. There is evidence that these patterns are more characteristic for some histopathologic types of Hodgkin's disease than for others (Keller et al., 1968; Hutchison, 1972); in particular, the lymphocytic depletion form, in which vascular invasion is apparently most prevalent (Rappaport and Strum, 1970; Naeim, Waisman, and Coulson, 1974), appears to give rise to noncontiguous patterns, probably involving blood-borne dissemination, in a higher proportion of instances.

However, the prognostic significance of vascular invasion remains unclear. Lamoureux et al. (1973) carefully reviewed the original biopsy material in 11 of 12 patients with regionally localized Hodgkin's disease who developed extranodal dissemination following primary radiotherapy, and failed to find evidence of vascular invasion in any of these cases. Kirschner et al. (1974) found that vascular invasion involving the spleen, which was present in 7 (16 percent) of 44 spleens involved by Hodgkin's disease, was associated with hepatic and bone marrow metastasis, early relapse, and decreased survival, whereas vascular invasion observed in 4 (4.5 percent) of 91 lymph node biopsies was not attended by an increased frequency of extranodal dissemination or diminished survival. They concluded that the presence of vascular invasion in the spleen is an ominous sign. Naeim, Waisman, and Coulson (1974) observed that the average survival time in a group of patients in whom vascular invasion was not demonstrable in the original lymph node biopsies was 65.8 months, as contrasted with 21.8 months in those whose lymph node biopsies showed vascular invasion, a statistically significant difference. None of the 16 patients who lived more than five years in their series showed vascular invasion in the original biopsy material, whereas 9 of 18 patients who died less than two years after diagnosis had demonstrable vascular invasion. Additional systematic studies of the correlation between the presence of vascular invasion in biopsy material and in splenectomy specimens and the subsequent development of extralymphatic dissemination would clearly be helpful in formulating treatment policies for such patients.

Chapter 8

Clinical Staging Classification

In an excellent historical review and analysis of the problem of clinical classification, Karnofsky (1966a) pointed out that the concept that Hodgkin's disease passes through a successive series of clinical stages, with a progressively worsening prognosis, dates back at least as far as 1902, when Dorothy Reed, in her classical paper, referred to two clinical stages of the disease. "During the first stage of the disease, which may be prolonged over months, the general physical condition is apparently normal, even while the glands are increasing rapidly . . . The disease affects progressively the neighboring glands apparently following a normal lymphatic distribution," almost always beginning in the cervical area. "The second stage of the disease, marked by progressive asthenia, cachexia, and anemia, invariably develops, usually after one or more years, but occasionally after a very brief period of glandular growth . . . Irregular or continuous fever is the rule, attributable to the inflammatory nature of the disease."

Ziegler (1911) presented a more detailed analysis of the clinical course of the disease, which was reformulated by Longcope and McAlpin (1920) into seven clinical forms: localized, mediastinal, generalized, acute, larval, splenomegalic, and osteoperiostitic. From their descriptions, one might surmise that the localized, mediastinal, and generalized forms would now fit within current stages I and II. The localized form is described as follows: "The cervical nodes are most often affected. The solitary masses grow slowly for two or three years, and the disease assumes a chronic course. . . The mediastinal form represents one variety of localized form in which the mediastinal nodes are especially involved. The patient presents a remarkable picture with all the symptoms and signs of mediastinal tumor—cough, dyspnea, orthopnea, pain and other evidences of pressure." In the generalized form, "there is an extension of the localized process to neighboring groups of nodes and the disease becomes more or less generalized." Their descriptions of the acute and the larval or latent forms suggest that these might fit into current

stages IIB and IIIB. In the acute form: "death may occur within a few weeks, or at most months. In this form, the enlargement of the lymph nodes is often markedly widespread, but not very great." In the larval form: "the disease is confined more or less exclusively to the thoracic or abdominal lymph nodes. The superficial nodes may escape completely. The symptoms are varied and often indefinite. Abdominal pains, jaundice, diarrhea, or effusions into the pleural or abdominal cavities may occur. The spleen and liver are often enlarged. Fever is frequently present. Some of the most pronounced examples of remittent fever occur in this type." Their splenomegalic form, in which the disease is thought to be confined to the spleen, would today be considered of doubtful validity; the final form, involving bone and bone marrow, would fall within the group of cases which, by virtue of extralymphatic spread, are now classified as stage IV.

In the last thirty-five years, several clinical staging classifications have been proposed, based in each instance on the extent of the detectable disease and on the presence or absence of constitutional symptoms and signs. In some, symptoms have been intermingled with anatomic extent, whereas in others, anatomic extent and constitutional symptoms have been separately evaluated, the former usually being indicated by a Roman numeral and the latter by an appended alphabetical letter.

The staging classification proposed by Craver (1951) divided the disease into three categories: class 1, localized disease; class 2, regional or intermediate disease; and class 3, generalized disease. Although this was one of the first important classifications in modern times, it suffered from the fact that the terms "localized" and "regional" were subject to widely different interpretations. The greater specificity and clarity of the staging classification proposed by Peters (1950), as modified by Peters and Middlemiss (1958) to take account of constitutional symptoms, led to its prompt acceptance in almost every part of the world (Table 8.1). The more complex classification suggested by

Table 8.1   The Evolution of Clinical Staging Classifications in Hodgkin's Disease

	Peters, 1950[a]	Rye, 1965[b]	Peters et al., 1968[c]	Musshoff and Boutis, 1969[d]	Stanford classification (Rosenberg and Kaplan, 1970)
Stage I:	Involvement of a single site or lymphatic region	I_1 Disease limited to one anatomic region I_2 Disease limited to two contiguous anatomic regions on the same side of the diaphragm	*Lymph node presentation* Disease limited to one anatomic region or to two contiguous anatomic regions on the same side of the diaphragm *Extranodal presentation* Disease in extranodal site alone *or* with involvement of one contiguous group or chain of lymph nodes	Lymph node involvement on one side of the diaphragm, *with* or *without* localized, *contiguous* extralymphatic organ or tissue involvement (A: no systemic symptoms; B: systemic symptoms present)	Involvement of a single lymph node region (I) or of a single extralymphatic organ or site (I_E)
Stage II:	Involvement of two or three proximal lymphatic regions A: with no symptoms of generalized disease B: with symptoms of generalized disease	Disease in more than two anatomic regions or in two noncontiguous regions on the same side of the diaphragm	Disease in more than two anatomic regions or in two noncontiguous regions on the same side of the diaphragm Disease in a single extranodal site with involvement of two adjacent lymph node chains	Lymph node involvement on both sides of the diaphragm, including the spleen, *with* or *without* localized *contiguous* extralymphatic organ or tissue involvement (A: no systemic symptoms; B: systemic symptoms present)	Involvement of two or more lymph node regions on the same side of the diaphragm (II) or solitary involvement of an extralymphatic organ or site and of one or more lymph node regions on the same side of the diaphragm (II_E)

(*continued*)

Table 8.1 (Continued)

	Peters, 1950[a]	Rye, 1965[b]	Peters et al., 1968[c]	Musshoff and Boutis, 1969[d]	Stanford classification (Rosenberg and Kaplan, 1970)
Stage III:	Involvement of two or more distant lymphatic regions	Disease on both sides of the diaphragm but limited to involvement of lymphoid tissues (lymph nodes, thymus, spleen, and/or Waldeyer's ring)	(a) disease in single extranodal site and involvement of lymph nodes beyond limits of stage II *without* extension to other side of diaphragm (b) disease in two extranodal sites of different tissue origin (c) disease in multiple extranodal sites in same tissue of origin. *Note:* (b) and (c) are *without* lymph node involvement	Disseminated organ involvement	Involvement of lymph node regions on both sides of the diaphragm (III), which may also be accompanied by involvement of the spleen (III_S) or by solitary involvement of an extralymphatic organ or site (III_E) or both (III_{SE})
Stage IV:		Involvement of the bone marrow, lung parenchyma, pleura, liver, bone, skin, kidneys, gastrointestinal tract, or any tissue or organ in addition to the lymphoid tissue	Any lymph node region with involvement of liver, lung, or bone marrow (excluding chronic lymphatic leukemia). In Hodgkin's disease, subdivide each stage into: (a) without systemic effects of disease; and (b) with systemic effects of disease	Extension of disease beyond the limits of stage III	Multiple or disseminated foci of involvement of one or more extralymphatic organs or tissues, with or without associated lymph node involvement. In Hodgkin's disease, the clinical form is also denoted by the absence (A) or presence (B) of otherwise unexplained fever and/or night sweats

(continued)

Comment				
The first well-defined clinical staging classification. It explicitly recognized the importance of both anatomic extent and of constitutional symptoms. Its principal disadvantage was the heterogeneity of the stage III category	Main advantage of this proposal was subdivision of the Peters stage III cases into new stages III and IV, segregating the widespread lymphatic cases from those with spread beyond the lymphatic system. In practice, the criterion of "contiguity" required for the distinction between stage I₂ and certain stage II cases has proved troublesome. Moreover, many cases of localized extralymphatic disease had a relatively good prognosis, despite their being grouped here in Stage IV with other, more widely disseminated and rapidly fatal cases	This prognostic classification recognizes the distinction between *localized* and widely *disseminated extralymphatic* disease and is applicable to other lymphomas, as well as to Hodgkin's disease, but is overly complex	These authors (as well as Peters et al., 1968) present data to document the fact that survival in cases with limited lung or other localized extralymphatic involvement is not significantly different from that associated with the corresponding extent of lymphocytic disease alone, and far better than that in disseminated disease. Thus, the *redistribution of Rye stage IV* is clearly necessary. However, this classification combines the Rye stages I + II, which seems undesirable, and gives no clear guidelines on what constitutes "localized" or "contiguous" extralymphatic disease	This proposed classification attempts to combine the best features of the Rye classification and those of Peters et al, 1968, and Musshoff and Boutis, 1969. It is intended for use both in Hodgkin's disease and in the non-Hodgkin's group of lymphomas

[a] As modified by Peters and Middlemiss (1958); a similar classification was also described by Jelliffe and Thomson (1955).
[b] Rosenberg (1966); modified from Kaplan, Bagshaw, and Rosenberg (1964). All stages in the Rye classification are subclassified *A* (no systemic symptoms) or *B* (fever, night sweats, and/or generalized pruritus).
[c] Peters, Hasselback, and Brown (1968).
[d] Musshoff and Boutis (1969).

Hohl, Sarasin, and Bessler (1951) has been widely accepted only in central Europe; a modified version was proposed by Banfi et al. (1965). The simple subdivision of the disease into "localized" and "generalized" stages, used over a period of many years by Paterson, Easson, and their colleagues at Manchester, England (Paterson and Tod, 1953), has not found favor elsewhere because it confounds anatomic extent and constitutional symptoms, with the result that the patients with anatomically localized disease are classified as having generalized disease if they happen to have symptoms.

With the advent of lymphangiography and other modern diagnostic aids, it became possible to distinguish with greater precision among patients with localized versus widespread involvement. Accordingly, in the course of initiating a series of clinical trials at Stanford University Medical Center, Kaplan et al. (1964) proposed that the Peters stage III category be subdivided into two components: a new stage III, in which the disease involves lymph nodes and other lymphatic structures both above and below the diaphragm, but has not extended beyond the lymphatic system, and a new stage IV, in which the disease has extended secondarily to involve any of the extralymphatic organs or tissues. They further proposed that the Peters and Middlemiss concept of dividing certain stages into two clinical forms, A and B, depending on the absence or presence, respectively, of constitutional symptoms, be extended to all four anatomic stages. In their original proposal, a fifth stage, designated as stage 0, was suggested for those cases in which Hodgkin's disease apparently confined to a single lymph node had been completely removed at the time of excisional biopsy and no additional evidence of disease could be detected on diagnostic study. However, this situation pertains to such a small and insignificant proportion of cases that stage 0 has subsequently been dropped, and such patients are now pooled with others in stage I. The other features of this classification were incorporated, with slight modifications, into the staging classification adopted in 1965 at the International Symposium on Hodgkin's Disease, held at Rye, New York (Rosenberg, 1966). At the same meeting, agreement was reached on the lymph node chains that would be designated as "regions" for the purpose of staging (Fig. 8.1).

As clinical experience with the Rye classification has increased, certain imperfections and difficulties have become apparent. It was recognized that the correlation between anatomic extent of disease

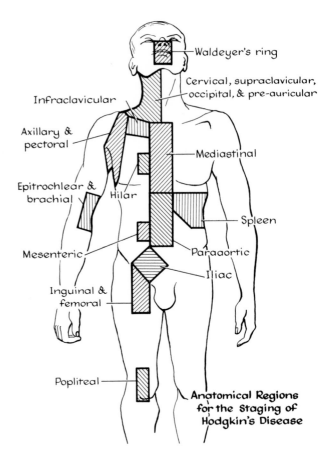

Figure 8.1 Diagram of the anatomic definition of separate lymph node regions adopted for staging purposes at the Rye (1965) symposium on Hodgkin's disease. (Reprinted, by permission, from the paper by Kaplan and Rosenberg, 1966c.)

and prognosis could be further improved if the Rye classification were modified in certain respects. The first of these is the ambiguity involved in the Rye definition of stage I disease as disease limited to a single lymph node region (I_1) or disease in two contiguous lymph node regions (I_2). The definition tends to blur the distinction between stages I and II and suffers from some ambiguity with respect to the definition of contiguity.

Musshoff and his colleagues (1968, 1970) called attention to another defect in the Rye staging classification, relating to stage IV cases. They drew a distinction between essentially localized extralymphatic organ involvement, which is more or less contiguous with involved regional lymph nodes (designated as the "p.c." type), and disseminated extralymphatic involvement (their "p.d." type). Although both of these would be subsumed under stage IV in the Rye classification, Musshoff et al. found, in a retrospective analysis of their own cases, that they had a strikingly different prognosis (Fig. 8.2*A*). Indeed, the p.c. type of organ involvement did not appear to have a significantly worse prognosis than that of lymph node disease of comparable extent (Fig. 8.2*B*). Similar data have been presented by Peters, Hasselback, and Brown (1968).

On the basis of their findings, Musshoff et al. (1968) proposed a new staging classification in which organ involvement of the "p.c." type was classified in accordance with the extent of associated lymphatic involvement. Although we believed that their three-stage classification was somewhat oversimplified, there was nonetheless a great deal of merit in their proposal. Since the Rye classification was already in relatively widespread use, it seemed desirable to retain as much of its format as possible. Accordingly, the revised Stanford (1970) clinical classification set forth in Table 8.1 (Rosenberg and Kaplan, 1970) differed from the Rye classification in only three respects, all of which were intended to improve the correlation with prognosis: (1) stage I was redefined to include only the former Rye stage I$_1$ (Fig. 8.3) and was adapted to include the rare case of primary Hodgkin's disease arising in an extralymphatic structure; the former stage I$_2$ was relegated to stage II (Fig. 8.4); (2) localized extralymphatic involvement of the p.c. type described by Musshoff et al. was classified in accordance with the extent of its associated lymphatic involvement and separately denoted by adding the suffix "E" (for extralymphatic) to the Roman numeral indicating anatomic stage. Such a case would thus be assigned to stage II if the associated lymphatic involvement were limited to one side of the diaphragm (Fig. 8.5) and to stage III if the lymphatic involvement were on both sides of the diaphragm (Fig. 8.6); (3) the new stage IV category was reserved for diffuse, disseminated forms of extralymphatic involvement (Fig. 8.7). The various earlier staging classifications are summarized in Table 8.1, and an attempt is made to suggest the approximate areas of overlap among them.

At the Workshop on the Staging of Hodgkin's Disease held at Ann Arbor, Michigan, in April 1971, an international panel of medical oncologists, radiotherapists, and pathologists agreed on a new approach to the problem of staging, as well as on a new staging classification (now known as the Ann Arbor classification), which embodies the key features of the Stanford (1970) classification. In this scheme (Carbone et al., 1971), a sharp distinction is drawn between the *clinical stage* (CS), which

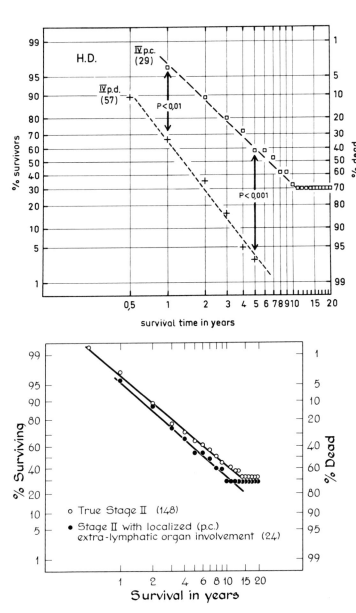

Figure 8.2 *Top,* survival data for 86 patients with Rye stage IV Hodgkin's disease, treated initially at Freiburg i. Br. between 1948 and 1967, subdivided into two groups: ("p.c."), those with localized extralymphatic sites of involvement, and ("p.d."), those with disseminated extralymphatic sites of involvement. (Reprinted, by permission, from the paper by Musshoff, 1970.) *Bottom,* survival data for a series of 172 cases of Hodgkin's disease involving two or more lymph node chains above the diaphragm, subdivided into two groups: those without extralymphatic involvement ("true" stage II, 148 cases) and those with localized ("p.c.") extralymphatic organ involvement (Rye stage IV, Ann Arbor stage II$_E$, 24 cases), treated at Freiburg i. Br., 1948–1967. (Translated, redrawn, and reproduced, by permission, from the paper by Musshoff et al., 1968.)

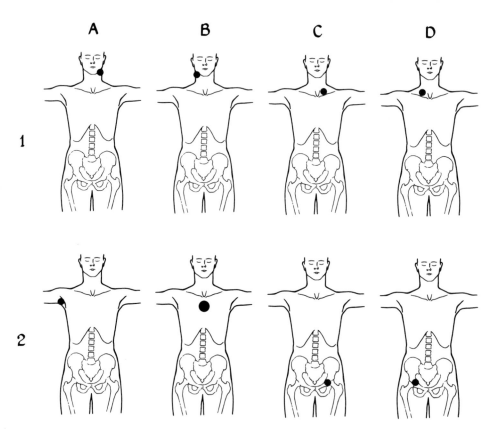

Figure 8.3 Examples of anatomic distributions in which a single anatomic region is involved. These would be classified as stage I_1 in the Rye scheme and as stage I in the Stanford (1970) and Ann Arbor (1971) classifications.

is based solely on the evidence derived from the initial biopsy, the history, physical examination, laboratory tests, radiographic examinations, and radioisotopic scans, and the *pathologic stage* (PS), which, in addition, is based upon gross and microscopic evidence derived from laparotomy or laparoscopy, splenectomy, liver biopsy, open marrow biopsy, and/or additional lymph node or other tissue biopsies. Each patient receives *both* a CS and a PS designation; for those in whom no tissue specimens other than the initial biopsy are obtained, the CS and PS are of course the same.

The Ann Arbor staging classification is presented in Table 8.2. Careful comparison with the Stanford classification (Table 8.1) will reveal the following changes: (1) in stages II and III, the less restrictive word "localized" has replaced the word "solitary" to describe limited extralymphatic disease that may appropriately be designated by the suffix "E"; (2) in stage II, it is recommended (but optional) that the number of involved sites be indicated by a subscript numeral (II_2, II_3, etc.); (3) in

stage IV, the word "diffuse" replaces "multiple," since "E" lesions need no longer be strictly solitary (it was agreed that involvement of the liver will always be considered diffuse and involvement of the bone marrow always disseminated, even when only a single focus of disease can be demonstrated in these organs); and (4) unexplained loss of 10 percent or more of body weight in the six months prior to admission has been added to the list of prognostically significant systemic symptoms which may appropriately be designated by the suffix "B."

The decision to classify extralymphatic disease in stage IV instead of in stage II_E or III_E will sometimes require the exercise of careful judgment and discretion by the physician. In general, the "E" designation is intended for extralymphatic disease so limited in extent and/or location that it can still be subjected to definitive treatment by radiotherapy. For example, direct invasion of the lung or pericardium (associated with mediastinal and/or ipsilateral hilar adenopathy), a subcutaneous chest wall mass (Fig. 7.2) secondary to invasion from an inter-

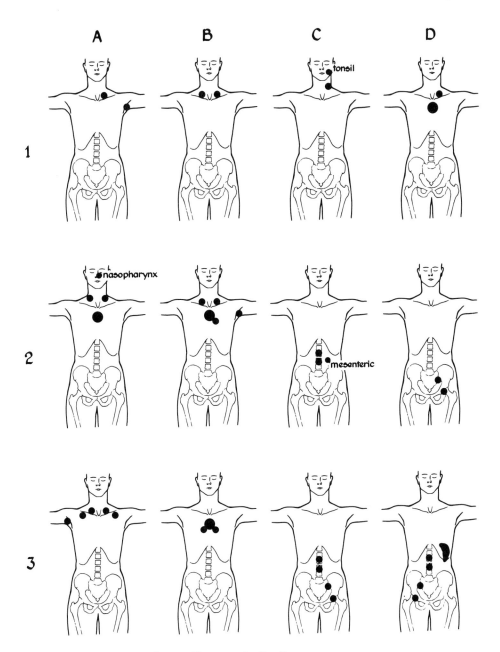

Figure 8.4   Examples of stage II anatomic distributions in the Stanford (1970) and Ann Arbor (1971) classifications. Note that A-1, B-1, C-1, D-1, C-2, and D-2 would all be designated as stage I_2 in the Rye classification.

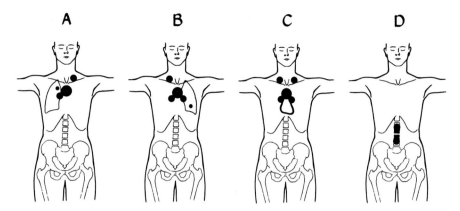

Figure 8.5   Examples of distributions involving a single extralymphatic site (lung in A-1 and B-1, pericardium in C-1, and bone in D-1), as well as one or more lymph node chains on one side of the diaphragm. Although these would all be classed as Rye stage IV cases, their favorable prognosis (Musshoff et al., 1968) supports their reallocation to stage II$_E$ in the Stanford (1970) and Ann Arbor (1971) classifications.

nal mammary or infraclavicular lymph node, sternal invasion from an anterior mediastinal mass (Fig 8.6), or other localized bone or epidural involvement in immediate proximity to involved lymph node chains are ordinarily classed as localized extralymphatic (E) disease.

The Ann Arbor classification has the additional virtue that it is readily applicable also to the non-Hodgkin's group of lymphomas, in which it is not uncommon for the neoplastic process to arise in and be confined to an extralymphatic organ or site, such as the stomach, the small intestine, the lung, the thyroid, or the skin. There are well-documented instances in which the extralymphatic lesion appears to be the primary site and in which there is no associated lymph node involvement; in others, only the regional nodes which drain the parenchymal tissue or structure are also involved. In the Rye classification, such cases would have had to be assigned to stage IV, despite their favorable prognosis. In the new classifications, they are designated as stage I cases if the extralymphatic primary site is truly solitary or as stage II if accompanied by regional lymphadenopathy.

The concept that localized extralymphatic (E) lesions do not adversely affect prognosis and should not imply dissemination of the disease has recently been challenged by Levi and Wiernik (1977a), who reported the occurrence of relapses in 9 of 11 stage II$_E$A and III$_E$A patients treated with extended field radiotherapy alone, as compared with only 14 relapses among 84 similarly treated patients with

stage IIA and IIIA disease. They reported relapses in only 1 of 7 stage II$_E$A and III$_E$A patients treated with limited field radiotherapy plus adjuvant MOPP chemotherapy, and only 2 relapses among 36 patients with stage IIA and IIIA disease similarly treated with combined modality therapy, and concluded that adjuvant chemotherapy should be employed whenever E lesions are present. However, in a recent analysis of our own data, Torti et al. (1978) found that freedom from relapse at five years in patients with E lesions treated with radiotherapy alone was slightly but not significantly less than that of similarly treated patients without E lesions, and that actuarial survival at five years was 89 percent in the former group and 91 percent in the latter. In comparable groups treated with localized radiotherapy and adjuvant chemotherapy, survival at five years was 81 percent for the group with E lesions and 89 percent for the group without E lesions, thus revealing no advantage in the prophylactic use of MOPP chemotherapy for patients with localized extralymphatic disease. We concluded that localized E lesions, when appropriately treated with radiotherapy, do not adversely affect prognosis and that there are real and significant differences in prognosis of localized versus disseminated extralymphatic involvement which validate the concepts underlying the Ann Arbor staging classification.

The string of letters and numerals used in the Ann Arbor classification will at first glance seem complicated and formidable to the reader, but a

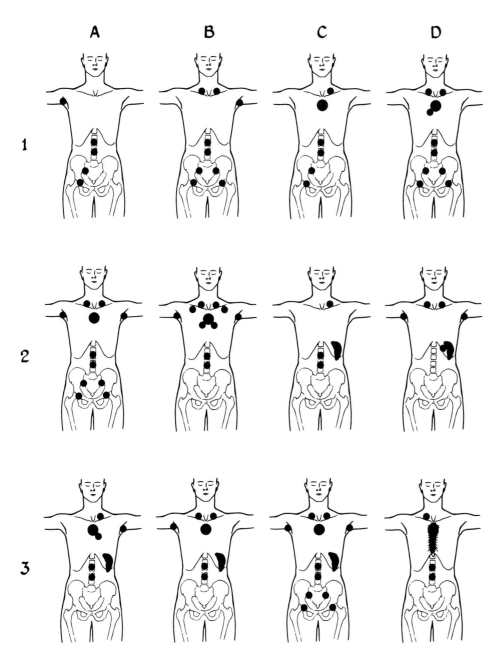

Figure 8.6 All but one of these distributions would be classed in stage III in both the Rye and the Stanford (1970) or Ann Arbor (1971) classifications. The exception is D-3, in which the presence of sternal involvement would call for reallocation to stage IV in the Rye scheme, but would remain in stage III and simply be denoted as stage III_E in the Stanford and Ann Arbor schemes.

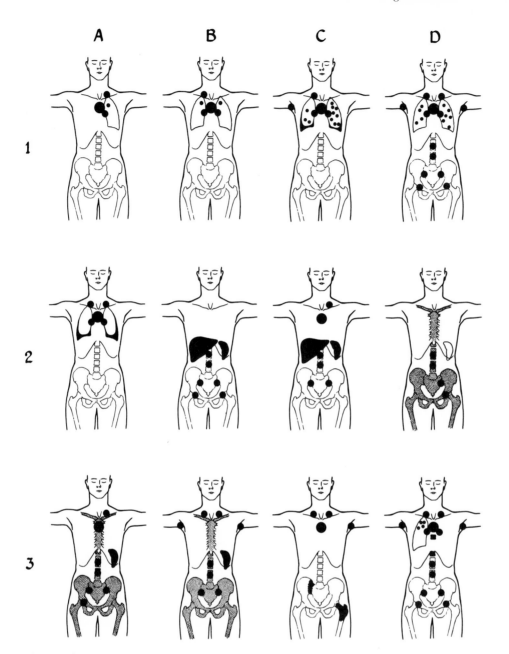

Figure 8.7   All but one of these distributions would be classed in stage IV in the Rye, the Stanford (1970) and the Ann Arbor (1971) classifications. The solitary lung nodule of A-1, associated with limited node involvement, would be designated as stage II_E in the Stanford and Ann Arbor classifications. Stippled areas indicate bone marrow involvement.

Table 8.2   Ann Arbor Staging Classification[a]

Stage	Definition
I	Involvement of a single lymph node region (I) or of a single extralymphatic organ or site (I_E)
II	Involvement of two or more lymph node regions on the same side of the diaphragm (II) or localized involvement of an extra-lymphatic organ or site and of one or more lymph node regions on the same side of the diaphragm (II_E)
III	Involvement of lymph node regions on both sides of the diaphragm (III), which may also be accompanied by involvement of the spleen (III_S) or by localized involvement of an extralymphatic organ or site (III_E) or both (III_{SE})
IV	Diffuse or disseminated involvement of one or more extralymphatic organs or tissues, with or without associated lymph node involvement

The absence or presence of fever, night sweats, and/or unexplained loss of 10 percent or more of body weight in the six months preceding admission are to be denoted in all cases by the suffix letters A or B, respectively.

[a] Adopted at the Workshop on the Staging of Hodgkin's Disease held at Ann Arbor, Michigan, in April 1971 (Carbone et al., 1971).

moment's reflection will reveal their much greater information content, precision, and lack of ambiguity. Certain letter symbols are used to indicate that tissue specimens were obtained from the following organs or tissues, with the added symbol "+" or "−" to indicate the presence or absence, respectively, of histopathologic evidence of involvement: S for spleen, H for liver (hepar), M for marrow, N for lymph nodes (para-aortic or other), L for lung, P for pleura, O for bones (osseous system). The omission of any or all of these letters from the PS designation means that no tissue specimens were obtained from the corresponding tissue or organ.

Let us consider a hypothetical asymptomatic patient with biopsy-proved Hodgkin's disease involving the left supraclavicular lymph nodes, in whom physical examination reveals no other peripheral adenopathy or organomegaly, and X-ray examination reveals only mediastinal involvement. Since only two sites of involvement (left supraclavicular and mediastinal) were clinically evident, such a patient would then be classified clinically as $CSII_2$-A, and could be compared, with respect to prognosis or other features, with other patients classified as $CSII_2$-A, regardless of differences in extent of subsequent diagnostic evaluation. However, a full description of each case also requires a PS designation. If our hypothetical patient was not subjected to laparotomy, splenectomy, open marrow or liver biopsy, or other lymph node biopsies, the PS classification would be identical to the CS, and his full staging description would be $CSII_2$-A, $PSII_2$-A; the omission of all letter symbols in the PS designation would indicate that no other tissue specimens were obtained. If a splenectomy had been performed,

together with para-aortic node, liver, and marrow biopsies, all of which were histologically negative, this additional information would be very simply conveyed thus: $CSII_2$-A, $PSII_2$-A$_{S-,\ H-,\ N-,\ M-}$. If the para-aortic node biopsy had been positive, the PS stage would change to III, and he would now be classified in $CSII_2$-A, $PSIII$-A$_{S-,\ H-,\ N+,\ M-}$. Similarly, documented spleen involvement would yield $CSII_2$-A, $PSIII$-A$_{S+,\ H-,\ N+,\ M-}$. Finally, biopsy-proved involvement of the liver or bone marrow, in addition to the spleen and para-aortic nodes, would be indicated by $CSII_2$-A, $PSIV$-A$_{S+,\ H+,\ N+,\ M-}$ or CSH_2-A, $PSIV$-A$_{S+,\ H-,\ N+,\ M+}$, respectively. The converse situation, in which additional tissue specimens fail to substantiate the involvement of certain organs or tissues initially suspected on clinical grounds, is also readily denoted. For example, the symptomatic patient with several supradiaphragmatic lymph node regions involved, and a palpable spleen which reveals no disease when removed, would be described thus: $CSIII_S$-B, $PSII$-B$_S$; the symptomatic patient with stage II adenopathy plus hepatomegaly and elevated alkaline phosphatase, but negative liver biopsies (and other tissues) at laparotomy: $CSIV_H$-B, $PSII$-B$_{H-,\ S-,\ N-,\ M-}$. A simple and convenient form for recording all of the relevant information, as well as the clinical stage and pathologic stage, has been designed (Fig. 8.8); several examples of its use for hypothetical cases are presented in Figures 8.9 to 8.12.

The major value of a staging classification is to allow meaningful comparisons of results obtained in different medical centers so that therapeutic programs can be intelligently compared and evaluated. It is essential that all reports which deal with the clinical course and therapy of malignant lymphomas carefully outline the diagnostic techniques used to arrive at a clinical staging opinion and clearly state which staging classification was used. It must be stressed that staging of patients with and without the aid of lymphangiography cannot be accurately compared, irrespective of the staging classification used. Accordingly, great care should be taken, in analyzing published data, not to confuse stage IIIA or stage IIIB cases of the present era with similarly designated cases of the prelymphangiography era. To some extent, the same point applies to certain manifestations of stage IV, since increased modern utilization of tomography, needle biopsy, and other diagnostic techniques has undoubtedly increased the accuracy with which we now detect involvement in stage IV sites such as the lung, the liver, and the bone marrow. Only thus can investigators in this field make meaningful comparisons and draw sound conclusions concerning advances in diagnosis and/or treatment with a view to making recommendations for their adoption by practicing physicians everywhere. The Ann Arbor workshop attempted to deal with this problem by specifying four categories of procedures in the diagnostic evaluation: (1) those that could properly be considered *mandatory* in all cases of Hodgkin's disease; (2) others for which the requirement is *contingent* in nature; (3) others which are *optional* as useful ancillary tests; and (4) others regarded as *promising* for clinical investigation. These are presented in Table 8.3. It will be noted that staging laparotomy with splenectomy is listed as a contingent procedure. Institutional policies obviously differ with respect to the indications for staging laparotomy in Hodgkin's disease, as discussed in Chapter 4. When the pathologic stage designation and its letter suffixes are properly used, the Ann Arbor staging classification has the major advantage that it immediately reveals whether or not a given patient has been staged with the aid of laparotomy and splenectomy. This is of importance in comparing data from different institutions because of the well-recognized change in stage distribution which results from the histopathologic examination of tissues obtained at laparotomy.

At Stanford University Medical Center, where this diagnostic procedure originated, we have followed a policy since July 1968 of submitting all previously untreated patients with Hodgkin's disease, except those with overt stage IV disease, to staging laparotomy with splenectomy. A recent tabulation of the data on 814 consecutive patients who underwent staging laparotomy from July 1968 through December 1977 (Kaplan, unpublished) clearly reveals the magnitude of the staging error when staging is based on clinical criteria alone (Table 8.4). For example, of 342 patients judged on clinical grounds to be in stage IIA, only 244 remained in stage IIA after pathologic staging; 86 were found to have stage III disease, 10 stage IV disease, and 2 were down-staged to stage I. Seventeen of 80 clinical stage IA patients proved to have occult stage III disease. An even greater percentage of patients with CSIII disease changed stage after laparotomy. Overall, the clinical assessment of stage proved to be in error in almost one-third of the entire series (257 of 814 patients; 32 percent).

In the remainder of this book, the Ann Arbor (1971) classification has been utilized whenever possible. An effort has been made to indicate the differences in prognosis and in therapeutic strategy associated with each stage and with selected types of clinical situations (cf. Chapter 12).

It is appropriate to discuss next the definitions of individual lymph node regions. Current usage is reflected in the diagrammatic representation presented in Figure 8.1, which was adopted at the Rye symposium (Rosenberg, 1966; Kaplan and Rosenberg, 1966c). However, it must be admitted that any such designation of lymph node regions is by its very nature arbitrary. It is not at all difficult to cite illogical examples. The difficulty of subdividing the cervical and supraclavicular area into two or more regions has resulted in this entire area being considered one lymph node region, despite the fact that it contains perhaps more lymph nodes than exist in a comparable volume anywhere else in the body. Thus, we have the paradox that a patient with multiple involved nodes on one side of the neck, extending from the submandibular level down to the supraclavicular fossa, is classified in Rye stage I_1 and Ann Arbor stage I. Yet, a patient with enlarged lymph nodes in the supraclavicular and the ipsilateral axillary or infraclavicular areas, which are no farther apart than the upper and lower neck, is classified in Rye stage I_2 and in Ann Arbor stage II.

Another major area containing multiple lymph nodes is the mediastinum, which, for lack of any convenient or reproducible subdivisions, is also regarded as a single region. Thus, even quite massive involvement of lymph nodes throughout the mediastinum is designated as Rye stage I_1 (Ann Arbor stage I). Since the hilar lymph nodes, for appropriate reasons, are considered as independent lymph node regions, even minimal involvement of the

Table 8.3   Recommendations for the Diagnostic Evaluation of Patients with Hodgkin's Disease[a]

A. Mandatory Procedures

1. Biopsy, with interpretation by a qualified pathologist

2. History, with special attention to the presence and duration of fever, night sweats, and unexplained loss of 10 percent or more of body weight in the six months preceding admission

3. Physical examination

4. Laboratory tests
   a. Complete blood cell count and platelet count
   b. Erythrocyte sedimentation rate
   c. Serum alkaline phosphatase

5. Radiographic examinations
   a. Chest (posteroanterior and lateral)
   b. Lymphangiogram
   c. Intravenous urogram
   d. Skeletal survey (spine and pelvis)

B. Contingent Procedures

1. Chest tomography (frontal or lateral), *if* pulmonary, hilar, and/or mediastinal involvement is present or suspected

2. Bone marrow biopsy (needle or open), *if* CS III, alkaline phosphatase elevated, anemia, or at time of laparotomy

3. Laparotomy and splenectomy, *if* decisions regarding management are likely to be influenced

4. Inferior vena cavography, *if* lymphangiogram or urogram equivocal or unsatisfactory

5. Liver biopsy (needle), *if* there is a strong clinical indication of hepatic involvement

C. Optional Ancillary Procedures

1. Radioisotopic bone scans, in selected patients with bone pain and negative or equivocal roentgenograms

2. Radioisotopic liver or spleen scans, in selected patients; limited value

3. Tests of immunologic function

4. Additional blood chemistry determinations: uric acid, calcium, copper, etc.

D. Promising Procedures for Clinical Investigation

1. Radiogallium (^{67}Ga) and radioselenium (^{75}Se) scans

2. Biological indicators of disease activity: reduced serum Fe^{++}, elevated serum Cu^{++}

[a] Adopted at the Workshop on the Staging of Hodgkin's Disease, held at Ann Arbor, Michigan (Rosenberg et al., 1971).

mediastinum and the adjoining hilar lymph nodes would be classified as Rye stage I_2 (Ann Arbor stage II); if bilateral hilar lymphadenopathy were present, the same case would be designated as stage II in both classifications.

The spleen, thymus, and Waldeyer's ring are all considered lymphatic structures. The thymus is ordinarily considered to be a part of the mediastinum and is lumped with the mediastinal lymph nodes as a single region, primarily because it is seldom possible, even at mediastinal exploration, to distinguish between thymic involvement alone and thymic plus mediastinal lymph node involvement. The Waldeyer structures and the spleen are each considered equivalent to a single lymph node region for purposes of classification. Thus, a case of Hodgkin's disease involving one tonsil or the lymphoid tissues of the nasopharynx without other evidence of disease would be classified as Rye stage I_1 (Ann Arbor stage I); the same case, together

Table 8.4   Staging Laparotomy Experience in Unselected, Previously Untreated Cases of Hodgkin's Disease[a]

Clinical stage[b]	Pathologic stage[b]				Change of stage[c]	
	I	II	III	IV	No. changed/total no.	%
IA	**63**	—	17	—	17/80	21
IB	**5**	—	1	—	1/6	16
IIA	2	**203**	77	8	87/290	30
II$_E$A	—	**41**	9	2	11/52	21
All IIA	2	**244**	86	10	98/342	29
IIB	—	**62**	16	4	20/82	24
II$_E$B	—	**16**	7	2	9/25	36
All IIB	—	**78**	23	6	29/107	27
All II (A + B)	2	**322**	109	16	127/449	28
IIIA (±E, S)	6	40	**71**	14	60/131	46
IIIB (±E, S)	1	20	**70**	22	43/113	38
All III (A + B)	7	60	**141**	36	105/244	43
IVA	—	1	2	**9**	3/12	25
IVB	—	2	4	**17**	6/23	26
All IV (A + B)	—	3	6	**26**	9/35	26
All A's	—	—	—	—	178/565	32
All B's	—	—	—	—	79/249	32
Totals	**77**	**385**	**274**	**78**	257/**814**	32

[a] Including all but selected CSIV cases seen at Stanford University Medical Center, July 1, 1968–December 31, 1977.

[b] Ann Arbor staging classification.

[c] In addition, involvement of the spleen was detected in 6 of 323 patients with PSII (A + B) disease (2%), in 42 of 70 with PSIII-A (60%), and in 40 of 71 with PSIII-B (56%). Thus, anatomical evidence affecting stage and/or treatment was obtained in a total of 344 (42%) of these 814 staging laparotomies.

with unilateral involvement of the cervical lymph nodes, as Rye stage I$_2$ (Ann Arbor stage II).

As has been mentioned, stage IV of the Rye classification encompasses an undesirable degree of heterogeneity. Although technically within Rye stage IV, localized disease involving certain extralymphatic sites may be quite compatible with a prognosis just as favorable as that of stage I or stage II (Musshoff et al., 1968; Peters et al., 1968). Examples of such "favorable" types of stage IV involvement include: disease locally invading the pericardium from the mediastinum; a single nodule in one lung or direct invasion of one lung from ipsilateral hilar lymphadenopathy; local unilateral involvement of the pleura; invasion of the epidural space from an adjacent lymph node mass with spinal cord compression; and direct invasion of the sternum from an underlying mediastinal or adjacent internal mammary node mass. In large measure, the favorable prognostic character of such Rye stage IV lesions stems from the fact that they can still be treated radiotherapeutically with doses sufficiently high to afford a reasonably good chance of their eradication, along with that of the associated lymph node disease. High doses of ra-

diation obviously cannot be employed safely to eradicate more widespread types of stage IV disease, such as involvement of both lungs, both pleural surfaces, the liver, multiple bones, multiple subcutaneous nodules, and/or the bone marrow. It is for these reasons that the new classifications concur in proposing that essentially localized extralymphatic involvement of the favorable type be staged in accordance with the extent of the associated lymph node disease and that stage IV be reserved for the more widely disseminated forms of extralymphatic disease (Tables 8.1 and 8.2).

All cases of Hodgkin's disease continue in the new classifications, as in the Rye scheme, to be subclassified as A or B to indicate the absence or presence, respectively, of constitutional symptoms. Since generalized pruritus appears to have little or no influence on prognosis (Tubiana et al., 1971), it has been dropped from the list of specific constitutional symptoms. Relative to other constitutional symptoms, pruritus tends to occur more often in female patients (Table 8.5), probably reflecting a correlated triad of nodular sclerosis, pruritus, and female sex. Certain other symptoms, such as malaise, fatigue, and generalized weakness, are so

Name _____ Age____ Sex____ Record #_____
Date of Adm. _____

Hodgkin's Disease
(Ann Arbor Classification)

Constitutional Symptoms

	+	–	?
Fever			
Night sweats			
Wt. loss >10%			

Rye Histopathological
type of Initial Biopsy

LP	NS	MC	LD	?

Clinical Staging

Physical exam.	+ R L	– R L	? R L
Axilla			
Upper cerv.			
Lower cerv. s'clav.			
Iliacs			
Ing.- fem.			
Spleen			
Liver			
Other (spec.)			

X-ray	+ R L	– R L	? R L	Not done
Lung				
Pleura				
Hilar				
Mediast.				
Pericard.				
Lymphgr.				
IVP				
Bones				
Other (spec.)				

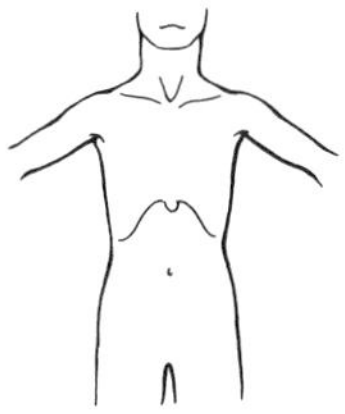

Scans	+	–	?	Not done	sq. cms
Bone					
Spleen					
Liver					
Gallium					
Other (spec.)					

Clinical Stage

Pathological Staging

	Not done	+	–	?	wt. gms
S - (spleen)					
H - (liver, hepar)					
N - (paraaortic, other nodes)					
M - (marrow)					
L - (lung)					
P - (pleura)					
O - (osseous)					

E - localized extralymphatic involvement ☐

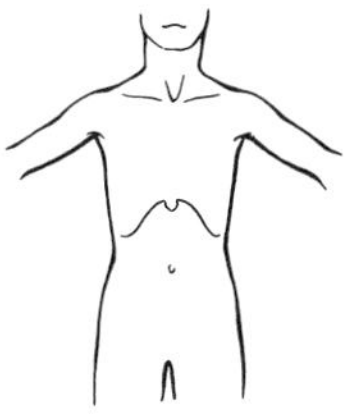

Pathological Stage

Figure 8.8 This staging form has been designed to provide a convenient and concise summary of the clinical information on the basis of which the clinical stage (CS) and pathologic stage (PS) determinations are made. The manikins are to be used to indicate graphically all anatomic sites of involvement documented during the diagnostic workup.

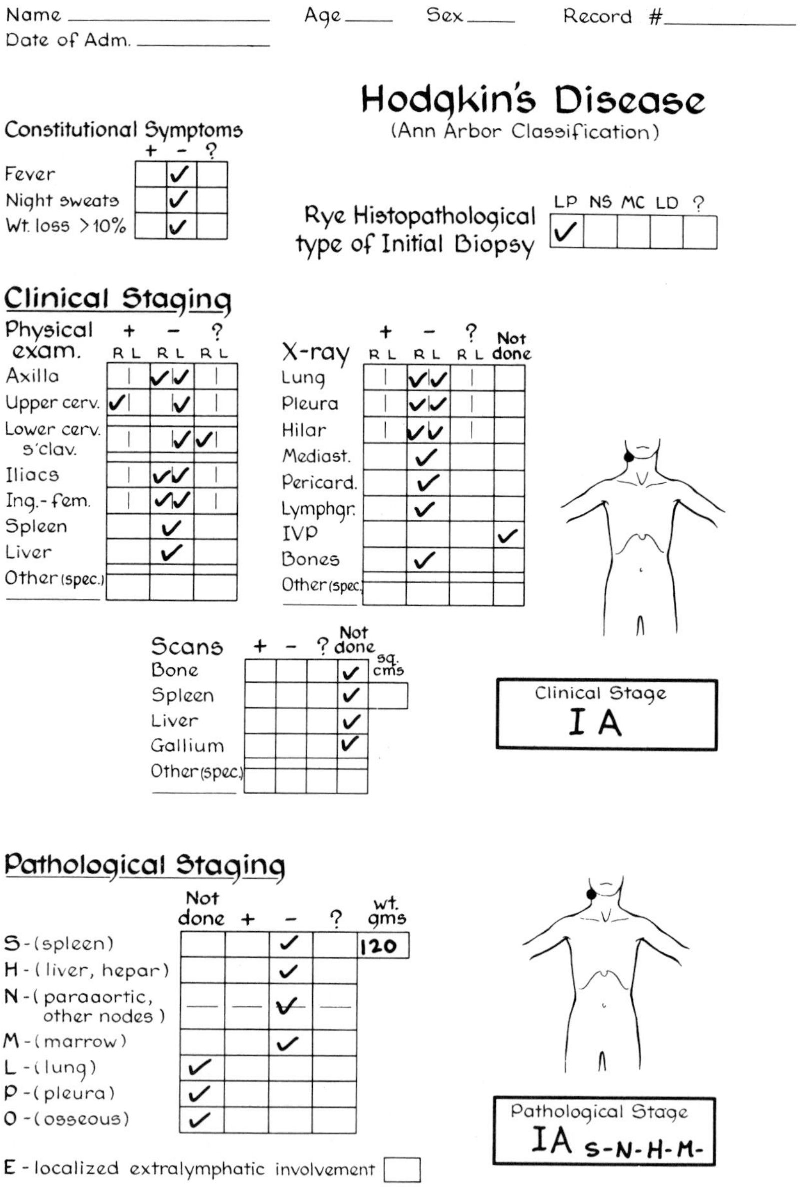

Name _____ Age_____ Sex_____ Record #_____
Date of Adm. _____

Hodgkin's Disease
(Ann Arbor Classification)

Constitutional Symptoms

	+	–	?
Fever		✓	
Night sweats		✓	
Wt. loss >10%		✓	

Rye Histopathological type of Initial Biopsy

LP	NS	MC	LD	?
✓				

Clinical Staging

Physical exam.	+ R L	– R L	? R L
Axilla		✓ ✓	
Upper cerv.	✓	✓	
Lower cerv. s'clav.		✓ ✓	
Iliacs		✓ ✓	
Ing.- fem.		✓ ✓	
Spleen		✓	
Liver		✓	
Other (spec.)			

X-ray	+ R L	– R L	? R L	Not done
Lung		✓ ✓		
Pleura		✓ ✓		
Hilar		✓ ✓		
Mediast.		✓		
Pericard.		✓		
Lymphgr.		✓		
IVP				✓
Bones		✓		
Other (spec.)				

Scans	+	–	?	Not done	sq. cms
Bone				✓	
Spleen				✓	
Liver				✓	
Gallium				✓	
Other (spec.)					

Clinical Stage
I A

Pathological Staging

	Not done	+	–	?	wt. gms
S - (spleen)			✓		120
H - (liver, hepar)			✓		
N - (paraaortic, other nodes)	—	—	✓	—	
M - (marrow)			✓		
L - (lung)	✓				
P - (pleura)	✓				
O - (osseous)	✓				

E - localized extralymphatic involvement ☐

Pathological Stage
I A S-N-H-M-

Figure 8.9 An example of the use of the staging form to record the hypothetical case of an asymptomatic patient with Hodgkin's disease of the lymphocytic predominance (LP) type which, on clinical examination, was confined to the right upper cervical region and was accordingly staged as CS I-A. Since all of the tissue specimens obtained at laparotomy and open marrow biopsy were negative, the pathologic stage remains the same, but the fact that these additional tissue specimens were obtained and that they were negative is indicated by the added suffixes: PS I-A$_{S^-,N^-,H^-,M^-}$.

Name _____ Age ____ Sex ____ Record # _____
Date of Adm. _____

Hodgkin's Disease
(Ann Arbor Classification)

Constitutional Symptoms

	+	–	?
Fever	✓		
Night sweats	✓		
Wt. loss >10%		✓	

Rye Histopathological type of Initial Biopsy

LP	NS	MC	LD	?
		✓		

Clinical Staging

Physical exam.

	+ R L	– R L	? R L
Axilla	✓ ✓		
Upper cerv.	✓ ✓		
Lower cerv. s'clav.	✓ ✓		
Iliacs		✓ ✓	
Ing.-fem.		✓ ✓	
Spleen	✓		
Liver	✓		
Other (spec.)			

X-ray

	+ R L	– R L	? R L	Not done
Lung		✓ ✓		
Pleura		✓ ✓		
Hilar		✓ ✓		
Mediast.	✓			
Pericard.		✓		
Lymphgr.			✓	
IVP		✓		
Bones		✓		
Other (spec.)				✓

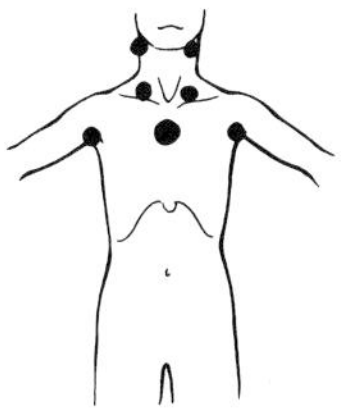

Scans

	+	–	?	Not done	sq. cms
Bone	✓				
Spleen	✓				120
Liver	✓				
Gallium				✓	
Other (spec.)				✓	

Clinical Stage
II (5) B

Pathological Staging

	Not done	+	–	?	wt. gms
S - (spleen)		✓			170
H - (liver, hepar)			✓		
N - (paraaortic, other nodes)		✓			
M - (marrow)			✓		
L - (lung)	✓				
P - (pleura)	✓				
O - (osseous)	✓				

E - localized extralymphatic involvement ☐

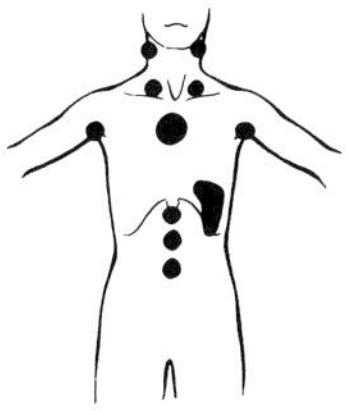

Pathological Stage
III_S B S+N+H–M–

Figure 8.10 The staging form describes the hypothetical case of a patient with "B" symptoms (night sweats and fever) accompanying his mixed cellularity (MC) type of Hodgkin's disease. Clinically, his lymphadenopathy was limited to the axilla, supraclavicular fossa, and neck bilaterally, and, by X-ray, to the mediastinum. However, the lymphangiogram was equivocal. The clinical stage was therefore CS II-B. Laparotomy, splenectomy, and biopsies revealed a positive spleen and para-aortic nodes, with a negative liver and bone marrow, making the final stage PS $III_S\text{-}B_{S+,N+,H-,M-}$.

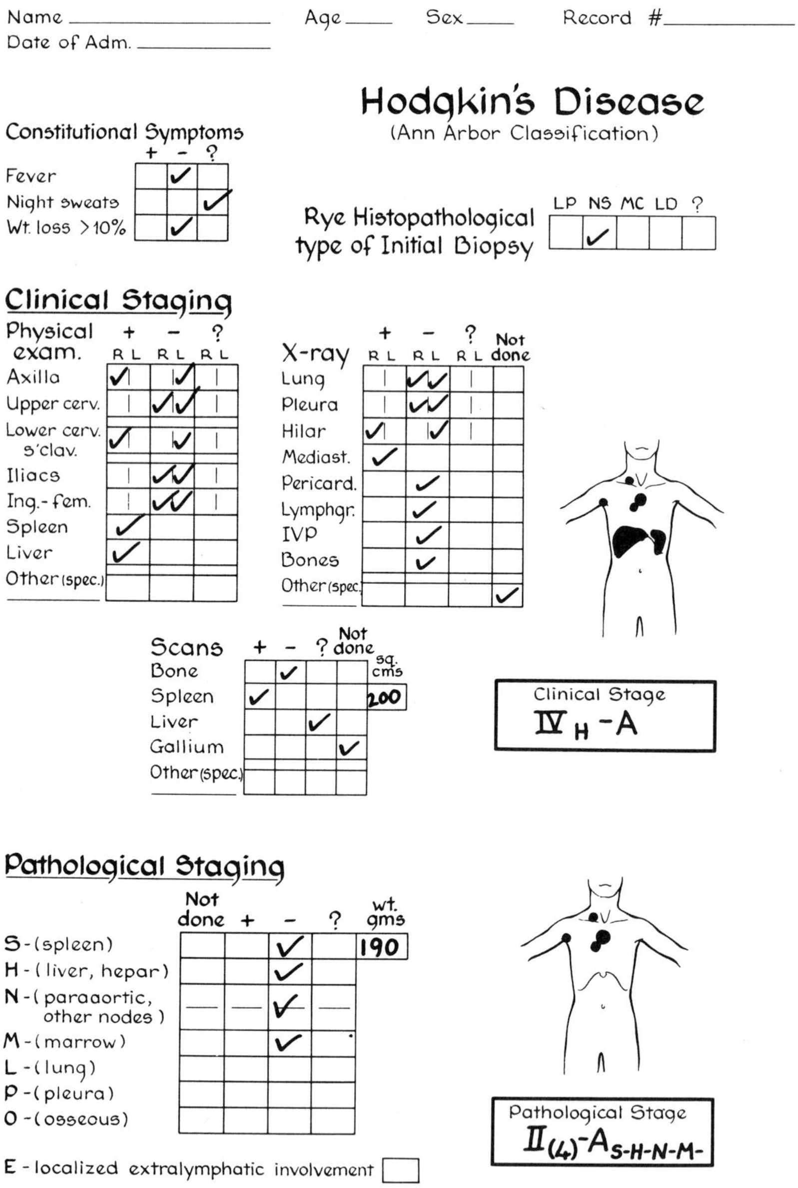

Name _____   Age ____ Sex ____   Record # _____
Date of Adm. _____

Hodgkin's Disease
(Ann Arbor Classification)

Constitutional Symptoms

	+	–	?
Fever		✓	
Night sweats			✓
Wt. loss >10%		✓	

Rye Histopathological type of Initial Biopsy

LP	NS	MC	LD	?
	✓			

Clinical Staging

Physical exam.	+ R	+ L	– R	– L	? R	? L
Axilla	✓		✓	✓		
Upper cerv.			✓	✓		
Lower cerv. s'clav.	✓			✓		
Iliacs			✓	✓		
Ing.-fem.			✓	✓		
Spleen	✓					
Liver	✓					
Other (spec.)						

X-ray	+ R	+ L	– R	– L	? R	? L	Not done
Lung			✓	✓			
Pleura			✓	✓			
Hilar	✓		✓				
Mediast.	✓						
Pericard.			✓				
Lymphgr.			✓				
IVP			✓				
Bones			✓				
Other (spec.)							✓

Scans	+	–	?	Not done	sq. cms
Bone	✓				
Spleen	✓				200
Liver			✓		
Gallium				✓	
Other (spec.)					

Clinical Stage

$$IV_H\text{-}A$$

Pathological Staging

	Not done	+	–	?	wt. gms
S - (spleen)			✓		190
H - (liver, hepar)			✓		
N - (paraaortic, other nodes)				✓	
M - (marrow)			✓		
L - (lung)					
P - (pleura)					
O - (osseous)					

E - localized extralymphatic involvement □

Pathological Stage

$$II_{(4)}\text{-}A_{S\text{-}H\text{-}N\text{-}M\text{-}}$$

Figure 8.11 An interesting example of "downstaging" as a result of the laparotomy findings is portrayed on this staging form. The patient was a young female with nodular sclerosing (NS) Hodgkin's disease, whose equivocal night sweats were not deemed sufficiently convincing to warrant classification in the "B" category. In addition to palpable lymphadenopathy in the right lower neck and axilla and radiographic evidence of enlarged right hilar and mediastinal nodes, her spleen and liver were palpable. The spleen also appeared enlarged, and the liver was thought to contain equivocal filling defects by radioisotopic scan. Accordingly, she was classed as CS IV_H-A. At laparotomy, the liver appeared grossly normal, and biopsies revealed no evidence of Hodgkin's disease. The spleen, though slightly large, was not histologically remarkable. Thus, her final stage was PS $II_{(4)}$-$A_{S\text{-},N,H,M}$.

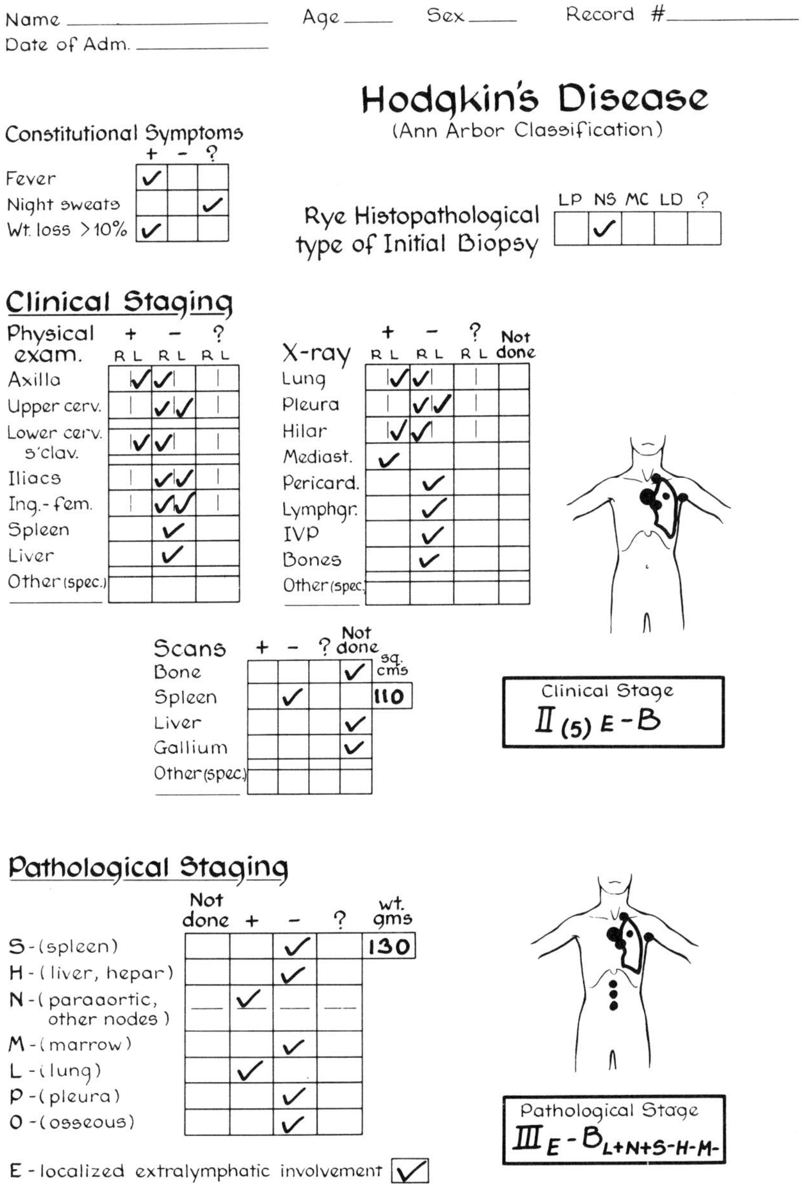

Name _____   Age _____   Sex _____   Record # _____
Date of Adm. _____

Hodgkin's Disease
(Ann Arbor Classification)

Constitutional Symptoms

	+	−	?
Fever	✓		
Night sweats		✓	
Wt. loss >10%	✓		

Rye Histopathological type of Initial Biopsy

LP	NS	MC	LD	?
	✓			

Clinical Staging

Physical exam.

	+ R L	− R L	? R L
Axilla	✓ ✓		
Upper cerv.		✓ ✓	
Lower cerv. s'clav.	✓ ✓		
Iliacs		✓ ✓	
Ing.- fem.		✓ ✓	
Spleen		✓	
Liver		✓	
Other (spec.)			

X-ray

	+ R L	− R L	? R L	Not done
Lung	✓ ✓			
Pleura		✓ ✓		
Hilar	✓ ✓			
Mediast.	✓			
Pericard.		✓		
Lymphgr.		✓		
IVP		✓		
Bones		✓		
Other (spec.)				

Scans

	+	−	?	Not done	sq. cms
Bone				✓	
Spleen	✓				110
Liver			✓		
Gallium			✓		
Other (spec.)					

Clinical Stage

$$II_{(5)E}-B$$

Pathological Staging

	Not done	+	−	?	wt. gms
S - (spleen)			✓		130
H - (liver, hepar)			✓		
N - (paraaortic, other nodes)		✓			
M - (marrow)			✓		
L - (lung)		✓			
P - (pleura)			✓		
O - (osseous)			✓		

E - localized extralymphatic involvement ✓

Pathological Stage

$$III_{E}-B_{L+,N+,S-,H-,M-}$$

Figure 8.12 This example describes a febrile patient with NS type Hodgkin's disease involving the left axillary and supraclavicular nodes clinically, and the mediastinal and hilar nodes, as well as a nodule in the adjacent left upper lobe pulmonary parenchyma, radiographically. These findings are summarized in the clinical stage designation CS $II_{(5)E}$-B. However, the finding of involvement of the para-aortic nodes at laparotomy and biopsy confirmation of the lung disease resulted in a final stage PS III_{E}-$B_{L+,N+,S-,H-,M-}$.

Table 8.5   Relative Frequency of Pruritus by Sex and Clinical Stage

Clinical stage	Pruritus						Any constitutional symptom					
	Present			Absent			Present			Absent		
	Male	Female	Ratio	Male	Female	Ratio	Male	Female	Ratio	Male	Female	Ratio
I and II	18	10	1.8	30	10	3.0	48	20	2.4	104	78	1.4
III and IV	9	17	0.5	51	23	2.2	60	40	1.5	37	38	1.0
Totals	27	27	1.0	81	33	2.5	108	60	1.9	141	116	1.2

highly nonspecific and so difficult to document that they were not considered acceptable for staging purposes in the Rye classification or in its successors. Other manifestations, such as anemia, leukocytosis, lymphopenia, anergy, or an elevated sedimentation rate are also nonspecific, though more readily documented. When due to Hodgkin's disease, significant anemia is almost invariably accompanied by fever and/or night sweats, with the consequence that it would be placed in the B category in any case. However, evidence that significant loss of body weight is an independent variable associated with unfavorable prognosis was presented at the Ann Arbor workshop (Tubiana et al., 1971). For this reason, unexplained loss of 10 percent of body weight or more was added to the list of systemic symptoms in the Ann Arbor classification (Table 8.2).

Thus, the only constitutional symptoms recognized by the Ann Arbor classification for staging purposes are otherwise unexplained fever, night sweats, and significant weight loss. When any one or more of these three symptoms is present in convincing form, the B designation is appropriately included in the staging, irrespective of the anatomic extent of the disease. Thus, for example, a patient with disease involving the inguinal, iliac,

and para-aortic lymph nodes, with fever and/or night sweats, would be classified as Ann Arbor stage IIB. The same classification would hold if the spleen were also involved, but the classification would change to Ann Arbor stage IVB if the liver were involved, in addition.

At the opposite end of the scale, the patient with lymphadenopathy limited to one supraclavicular fossa who has low-grade fever or night sweats of recent onset would be classified in Ann Arbor stage IB. However, patients with true stage I disease have constitutional symptoms so infrequently (Table 8.6) that each such instance should be regarded with skepticism and a renewed search for other sites of disease instituted, with particular emphasis on previously undetected, occult involvement of the mediastinal or para-aortic lymph nodes, the liver, and the bone marrow. Nonetheless, we have seen a small number of cases of stage I disease with constitutional symptoms, usually of relatively mild character, which disappeared after local radiotherapy directed to the sites of anatomic involvement. It would therefore appear that Hodgkin's disease localized to superficial lymph node chains does occasionally give rise to constitutional symptoms. The disappearance of mild, localized, or otherwise equivocal symptoms after treat-

Table 8.6   Constitutional Symptoms versus Clinical Stage in Previously Untreated, Biopsy-Proved Cases of Hodgkin's Disease

Clinical stage	Total		Fever		Night sweats		Pruritus		Alcohol pain		Total with one or more symptoms	
	No.	%	No.	%	No.	%	No.	%	No.	%	No.	%
I	61	13.7	1	1.4	1	1.4	4	6.6	0	—	5	8.2
II	189	42.5	41	21.7	41	21.7	27	14.3	6	3.2	55	29.1
III	116	26.1	34	29.3	27	23.3	17	14.7	0	—	48	41.3
IV	79	17.7	43	54.4	40	50.6	19	24.1	1	1.2	56	70.9
All	445	100	119	26.7	109	24.5	67	15.0	7	1.6	164	36.8

ment may retrospectively confirm the significance for staging purposes of symptoms that may initially have been difficult to evaluate.

It has been proposed by a number of groups, particularly in the European centers (Westling, 1965; Tubiana et al., 1971), that a variety of laboratory tests, including the erythrocyte sedimentation rate, leukocyte alkaline phosphatase, serum copper or zinc, absolute lymphocyte count, white blood cell count, haptoglobin, and alpha-2-globulin, be taken into consideration in assessing the clinical form of the disease. There is undoubtedly merit in this general concept, since reliance solely on a history of constitutional symptoms not infrequently confronts the clinician with the difficulty of making an arbitrary decision when symptoms are of minimal or equivocal severity or when the patient is a poor historian. It would thus be extremely helpful if these or other objective laboratory indicators could play a part in the decision. Unfortunately, as has already been discussed in Chapter 4, all of those enumerated above are nonspecific and may be abnormal in the presence of a variety of bacterial, fungal, or other infections, even when these are subclinical in severity. None-

theless, recent analyses strongly suggest that the erythrocyte sedimentation rate (Le Bourgeois and Tubiana, 1977) and the serum copper level (Thorling and Thorling, 1976) or the serum copper-zinc ratio (Bucher and Jones, 1977) do indeed have prognostic value in Hodgkin's disease. Perhaps continuing correlative studies of the relationship between such laboratory indices and prognosis will provide sufficient data to permit meaningful proposals on this point to be offered at some future international conference on the problem of clinical staging classification.

In a series of 1,225 consecutive previously untreated patients classified after the type of diagnostic evaluation described in Chapter 4, the Ann Arbor stage distribution presented in Table 8.7 was encountered. It will be noted that 150 cases (12.2 percent) were anatomically limited to a single lymph node region (stage I), and that only 10 (6.7 percent) of these (9 males, 1 female) had constitutional symptoms. There were 131 stage IV cases, comprising 10.7 percent of the total. The majority of the cases fell in stages II and III, which together constituted about 77 percent of the total. Spleen involvement was documented in a significantly

Table 8.7 Ann Arbor Stage Distribution of 1,225 Consecutive, Previously Untreated Patients with Biopsy-Proved Hodgkin's Disease

Ann Arbor stage	Males No.	Males %	Females No.	Females %
IA	101	13.6	39	8.1
IB	9[a]	1.2	1	0.2
All I (A + B)	110	14.8	40	8.3
IIA	193 (3)[b]	26.0	163 (1)	33.8
IIB	64 (4)	8.6	53 (0)	11.0
II_EA	26 (1)	3.5	36 (0)	7.5
II_EB	19 (0)	2.6	16 (0)	3.3
All II (A + B ± E)	302 (8)	40.6	268 (1)	55.6
IIIA	120 (98)	16.2	76 (45)	15.8
IIIB	90 (56)	12.1	42 (25)	8.7
III_EA	10 (8)	1.3	8 (6)	1.7
III_EB	19 (12)	2.6	9 (4)	1.9
All III (A + B ± E)	239 (174)	32.2	135 (80)	28.0
IVA	26	3.5	14	2.9
IVB	66	8.9	25	5.2
All IV (A + B)	92	12.4	39	8.1
Totals	743	100.0	482	100.0

Source: Stanford University Medical Center data, 1961–1977 inclusive (Kaplan).

[a] One of the nine was classified as stage I_EB.

[b] Numerals in parentheses indicate numbers of patients with documented spleen involvement.

Table 8.8 Pathologic Stage, Histopathologic Type, Age, and Sex Distribution of 1,225 Consecutive Untreated Patients with Hodgkin's Disease, 1961–1977

Stage	Sex	Age	Histopathologic Type[a]					Subtotals	A + B	%
			LP	NS	MC	LD	U + C			
IA	♂	0–16	9	6	1	0	2	18		
		17–49	20	21	13	0	7	61		
		50+	4	8	9	1	0	22		
			33	35	23	1	9	101		
	♀	0–16	1	0	1	0	0	2		
		17–49	2	21	1	0	5	29		
		50+	0	5	0	1	2	8		
			3	26	2	1	7	39		
			36	61	25	2	16	140		
									150	12.2
IB	♂	0–16	0	0	0	0	1	1		
		17–49	0	3	0	0	2	5		
		50+	0	0	2	0	1	3		
			0	3	2	0	4	9		
	♀	0–16	0	0	0	0	0	0		
		17–49	0	1	0	0	0	1		
		50+	0	0	0	0	0	0		
			0	1	0	0	0	1		
			0	4	2	0	4	10		
IIA	♂	0–16	6	26	6	0	1	39		
		17–49	9	117	29	1	9	165		
		50+	4	7	4	0	0	15		
			19	150	39	1	10	219		
	♀	0–16	2	28	2	0	1	33		
		17–49	4	128	13	0	9	154		
		50+	1	6	1	0	4	12		
			7	162	16	0	14	199		
			26	312	55	1	24	418		
									570	46.5
IIB	♂	0–16	0	6	0	0	0	6		
		17–49	3	49	15	1	2	70		
		50+	0	5	2	0	0	7		
			3	60	17	1	2	83		
	♀	0–16	0	11	2	0	0	13		
		17–49	0	46	1	1	5	53		
		50+	0	0	0	0	3	3		
			0	57	3	1	8	69		
			3	117	20	2	10	152		

Table 8.8 (*continued*)

Stage	Sex	Age	LP	NS	MC	LD	U + C	Subtotals	A + B	%
					Histopathologic Type[a]					
	♂	0–16	2	10	3	0	2	17		
		17–49	5	58	33	0	8	104		
		50+	1	4	4	0	0	9		
			8	72	40	0	10	130		
IIIA										
	♀	0–16	0	8	3	0	0	11		
		17–49	1	52	7	1	3	64		
		50+	2	3	2	0	2	9		
			3	63	12	1	5	84		
			11	135	52	1	15	214		
									374	30.5
	♂	0–16	0	3	4	0	1	8		
		17–49	0	55	23	7	5	87		
		50+	0	8	2	0	1	11		
			0	66	29	7	7	106		
IIIB										
	♀	0–16	0	6	3	1	0	10		
		17–49	0	28	5	0	5	38		
		50+	0	1	2	0	0	3		
			0	35	10	1	5	51		
			0	101	39	8	12	160		
	♂	0–16	0	1	1	0	0	2		
		17–49	1	13	3	0	0	17		
		50+	0	3	2	2	0	7		
			1	17	6	2	0	26		
IV-A										
	♀	0–16	0	2	1	0	0	3		
		17–49	0	9	0	0	0	9		
		50+	0	1	1	0	0	2		
			0	12	2	0	0	14		
			1	29	8	2	0	40		
									131	10.7
	♂	0–16	0	7	1	1	0	9		
		17–49	0	29	9	1	1	40		
		50+	0	6	7	1	3	17		
			0	42	17	3	4	66		
IV-B										
	♀	0–16	0	2	0	0	0	2		
		17–49	0	10	3	2	0	15		
		50+	0	5	2	1	0	8		
			0	17	5	3	0	25		
			0	59	22	6	4	91		
Totals			77 (6%)	818 (67%)	223 (18%)	22 (2%)	85 (7%)		1,225	100.0

Source: Stanford University Medical Center data, 1961–1977 inclusive (Kaplan).

[a] LP, lymphocyte predominance; NS, nodular sclerosis; MC, mixed cellularity; LD, lymphocyte depletion; U, unclassified; C, composite (Hodgkin's + non-Hodgkin's).

greater proportion of males (132 of 541, or 33.6 percent) than of females (81 of 403, or 20.1 percent) with stage II and III disease. The proportion of cases in stage I was of course somewhat reduced and that in stage II correspondingly increased, when the Rye stage I_2 cases were reallocated to the stage II category. A further breakdown of these data by age, sex, and histopathologic type is presented in Table 8.8.

It should be stressed that the data in Table 8.7 are merely indicative of the staging distribution seen in a particular university medical center and undoubtedly are subject to appreciable selection as a consequence of such factors as the general level of medical care in the area, patterns of patient referral, accessibility of the medical center via different modes of transportation, economic level of the population, and age distribution of the population (Table 8.8 and 8.9). Staging data on all cases of biopsy-proved Hodgkin's disease developing within a given time interval in the total population of a large, defined geographic area would have the distinct advantage of being essentially unselected and thus more representative. However, the only such series of cases to date is that from the province of Saskatchewan, Canada, reported by Meighan and Ramsay (1963). Unfortunately, these cases were staged prior to the general availability of lymphangiography and are thus not comparable to data obtained with the aid of lymphangiography.

Although detailed discussion of prognosis is a complex subject reserved for a later chapter, it is appropriate to comment here that all of these staging classifications satisfy one additional requirement of any good staging classification: they correlate well with prognosis. The data of Peters (1950,1961) and others established convincingly that survival in stage I and stage II cases is very

much better than that in the Peters (1950) stage III category. Whether there is a real difference in prognosis between stage I and stage II has been somewhat controversial. Such differences have been evident in the data reported from some institutions and absent in others. Since most of the earlier studies were made in the pre-lymphangiography era, the data are subject to unknown correction factors for the proportion of stage I and stage II cases that should, in reality, have been classified in stage III but in which the presence of para-aortic lymph node involvement remained undetected. It was gratifying to note that the subdivision of the former Peters stage III category into the Stanford (1964) and later Rye stages III and IV was reflected in clear and convincing differences in prognosis between stage III and stage IV (Kaplan, 1966b). Data are now presented in Chapter 12 on a consecutive series of 923 laparotomy-staged patients admitted to Stanford University Medical Center since July 1968. Although five-year survival in Ann Arbor stages I and II was similar (93.6 and 90.6 percent, respectively), ten-year survival in stage I remained high (91.5 percent), whereas that in stage II declined to 80.7 percent. The redefinition of the heterogeneous Rye stage IV cases has similarly been reflected in increased prognostic utility of the new Ann Arbor classification.

The presence or absence of constitutional symptoms, particularly of night sweats and fever, is also reflected impressively in the survival of patients staged with the aid of lymphangiography. This was evident in Ann Arbor stage I and stage II patients treated with intensive, localized-field megavoltage radiotherapy confined to areas of lymph node involvement. Those with constitutional symptoms showed a much greater propensity for the later appearance of disease in other, previously untreated

Table 8.9   Influence of Age on Clinical Stage Distribution

| Ann Arbor clinical stage | Age group, years | | | | | | Total |
| | 20 or under | | 21–40 | | 41 and over | | |
	No.	%	No.	%	No.	%	No.
IA and IIA	170	30.5	287	51.5	100	18.0	557
IB and IIB	37	22.8	101	62.3	24	14.8	162
All I and II	207	28.8	388	54.0	124	17.2	719
IIIA and IVA	66	25.7	139	54.1	52	20.2	257
IIIB and IVB	64	25.7	126	50.6	59	23.7	249
All III and IV	130	25.7	265	52.4	111	21.9	506
Totals	337	27.5	653	53.3	235	19.2	1225

sites, whereas the majority of the asymptomatic patients thus treated had no subsequent manifestations of disease elsewhere (Kaplan, 1968a; Rosenberg and Kaplan, 1970). Clear-cut differences in survival persist in the laparotomy-staged series analyzed in Chapter 12. For example, five-year survival in patients with stage IIA was 90.7 percent, that in stage IIB, 79.3 percent. The corresponding gap in stage III is even wider, 84.7 versus 66.0 percent. Thus, the presence of constitutional symptoms appears to be associated with a significantly poorer prognosis, probably because the anatomic sites of disease are more likely to be underestimated in such patients, despite careful and thorough diagnostic evaluation.

Chapter 9

Radiotherapy

Historical Perspective

It was only a few years after the discovery of X-rays that Pusey (1902) reported what was probably the first attempt to treat Hodgkin's disease and other lymphomas with the new rays. In the nearly eight decades since that time, the field of radiotherapy has undergone dramatic changes, stemming from the invention of reliable equipment which provided progressively higher beam energies, from the development of greatly improved physical techniques for beam alignment and for the accurate measurement of dose distribution in tissues and tumors, and from the painstaking collection of clinical data concerning the mode of origin and directions of spread of different types of neoplasms, making possible the rational delineation of specific treatment plans tailored to the natural history of individual types of tumors.

The early X-ray therapy equipment available during the first two decades of the century, not unlike the automobiles of that era, was highly unpredictable in performance, and the X-ray beams were not only of low energy but of low and variable intensity. In the 1920's the advent of the Coolidge tube led to the development of then-unprecedented 180 kilovolt X-ray therapy apparatus, far more reliable and long-lived in operation, and not long thereafter of additional increments of energy to 200 to 250 kv, which for many years remained the standard throughout the world. Treatment of patients with Hodgkin's disease with apparatus of this energy range will be referred to in subsequent discussions as *kilovoltage* radiotherapy. Finally, in the 1950's, the virtually simultaneous development of several new types of apparatus providing beams with energies of millions of electron volts ushered in the supervoltage, or more properly, the *megavoltage,* era of radiotherapy. These devices include Van de Graaff electrostatic generators operating at a peak energy of 2 million electron volts (MV); radioactive cobalt (^{60}Co) teletherapy units which emit gamma rays with an energy equivalent to 3 MV;

betatrons which provide beams of electrons or X-rays at energies in the 20- to 40-MV range; and linear electron accelerators which also provide both electron and X-ray beams but have been primarily used to date as X-ray sources in the 4- to 8-MV energy range (Fig. 9.1).

In the first decades of radiotherapy, no reliable physical technique for measuring beam intensity or tissue dose was available. The early pioneers in radiotherapy had to rely instead on a biologic indicator, the human erythema dose (HED), and their therapeutic doses were usually specified in fractions of an HED. In the late 1920's, radiologic physicists were able to agree internationally on a physical unit, the roentgen (r), which was defined in terms of the ionization produced in air. It soon became acceptable practice in kilovoltage radiotherapy to specify dose in terms of the exposure dose or air dose in roentgens from which, knowing the field size and dimensions of the patients, one could derive the skin dose, percentage depth dose, and tumor dose. However, air dose and skin dose have little meaning with megavoltage radiotherapy beams, as the peak dose is delivered several millimeters to several centimeters below the surface of the skin. Accordingly, a new unit, the rad, which refers to the dose of ionizing radiation actually absorbed in tissue, was adopted. Radiologic physicists have also introduced a series of refinements in treatment technique, such as multiportal, arc, and rotation therapy, differential absorbers called wedge filters for use over curved surfaces of the body, and isocentric beam alignment procedures.

The history of the development of potentially curative radiotherapy for the treatment of Hodgkin's disease mirrors these technologic and physical advances closely. The results of nineteenth-century treatment with arsenicals, iodides, various sera and other biologic preparations, and surgery, must have been dismal indeed, for, as was mentioned earlier, Senn (1903) was so impressed by the dramatic short-term responses observed in his two cases as to write of the "curative effect of the roent-

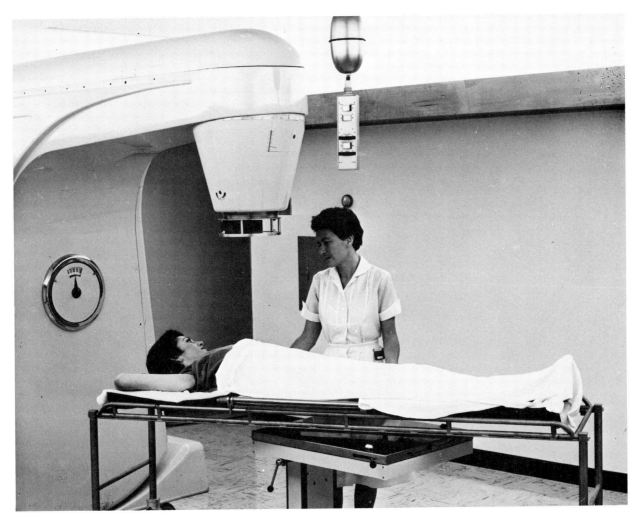

Figure 9.1   This 6 MV linear electron accelerator has been in use at Stanford University Medical Center since 1962 for all mantle and inverted-Y field treatments of patients with Hodgkin's disease and other malignant lymphomas. Its high output and variable source-skin operating distance make this type of unit particularly convenient for wide-field megavoltage radiotherapy. (Photograph courtesy of Varian Associates, Palo Alto, California.)

gen ray in the treatment of pseudoleukemia." In the next two decades, the principal techniques of treatment involved the administration of small doses to the entire trunk at weekly intervals for many weeks, or of massive single doses confined to the area of clinical involvement. Although dramatic regression of lymphadenopathy was not infrequently observed, recurrence in the treated field or extension to some previously untreated site was invariably the rule, and after several successive courses of radiotherapy to various lymph node regions, the disease appeared to become progressively more refractory to treatment, with an inevitably fatal outcome. Moreover, major complications due to severe tissue injury and even fatalities after massive doses to larger fields were relatively common. Paradoxically, the pattern of

multiple recurrences leading to a refractory state and death was not charged to the inadequacy of the radiotherapeutic techniques then available, but viewed rather as an expression of some fundamental biologic attribute of the disease itself. Thus was born the tragic myth that Hodgkin's disease is a hopeless condition, with an inexorably fatal outcome, for which many physicians continued to advocate merely palliative therapy until the last decade, when the impressive results of intensive treatment approaches finally brought about a widespread change in attitudes concerning the disease.

Gilbert (1939) and Peters (1966) have described the earliest aggressive treatment techniques introduced in the 1920's. All of these involved the use of "segmental" fields, encompassing limited segments of the body, in contrast to the total trunk and whole body exposure techniques advocated by Teschendorf (1927) and others. The method propounded by Voorhoeve (1925) and Kruchen (1929) entailed treatment to localized fields carefully confined to areas of involvement only. Voorhoeve gave what were then regarded as relatively high doses: up to 90 percent "HED" (an early, crude unit of dose) per field, fractionated over two to three days for larger fields. A typical course required two to three weeks to deliver an average dose of 70 percent HED to all fields; in some cases, such courses were repeated in three months. Schreiner and Mattick (1924) also advocated a "treatment of attack" giving depth doses of 60 to 70 percent HED in two or three consecutive days. Chaoul and Lange (1923) divided the trunk into two anterior and two posterior fields; treating one field per day, they delivered 10 percent of an HED daily to a total of 60 to 80 percent HED. A somewhat similar method was used by Sluys (1931).

However, modern radiotherapy for Hodgkin's disease really began with the work of Gilbert (1925, 1939), who was the first to point out certain clinical patterns of the behavior of the disease and to attempt to adapt his radiotherapeutic techniques to them. He rejected the sharply localized techniques of Voorhoeve and Kruchen because: "Many times I have seen, in patients recently treated for peripheral adenopathy, recurrence developing in the immediate vicinity of a field too narrowly irradiated" (Gilbert, 1939). Accordingly, he began to advocate irradiation of suspected microscopic disease in apparently uninvolved adjacent lymph node chains as well as the clinically evident sites of lymphadenopathy. In considering the problem of dose rate, he rejected the method of Chaoul and Lange (1923) because of the severe systemic toxicity it produced.

In a detailed description of their treatment technique, Gilbert and Babaiantz (1931) stressed the formulation of a systematic plan of irradiation in each case after careful clinical and roentgenologic search for all detectable sites of involvement. They emphasized that the fundamental principle of treatment is the destruction of all "granulomatous lesions" in the first course of irradiation. To this end, they advocated concentrating all initial efforts on the regions known to be invaded by the disease, after which they extended the fields of treatment, within the limits of the hematologic tolerance of the patient, to encompass those apparently healthy regions "which experience shows are more frequently invaded by the process." They illustrated

diagramatically a typical series of treatment fields for a hypothetical case of Hodgkin's disease with supradiaphragmatic involvement; from their figure, we may infer that they would have used direct lateral cervicosupraclavicular and axillary fields on each side; paired anterior and posterior oblique mediastinal fields, all presumably encompassing known sites of involvement; anterior and posterior splenic fields, upper and lower anterior transabdominal fields, and somewhat narrower upper and lower posterior abdominal fields. They gave 180 r (air dose) daily for about fifteen days to each region in succession, to a recommended depth dose of 400 to 500 r to each involved region. This required giving skin doses of 700 to 1100 r to the cervical, axillary, and other superficial lymph node regions, and the delivery of 1,000 r to each of four oblique mediastinal fields.

By the time of Gilbert's report (1939) to the International Congress of Radiology, others had begun to adopt some of his ideas. Ratkóczy (1936) recommended a tumor "sterilization" dose of at least 2,000 r in the treatment of localized, apparently unicentric Hodgkin's disease. In Toronto, as Peters (1966) has reported, a radiotherapy treatment field plan very similar to Gilbert's was used from 1928 to 1953, and Desjardins (1945) described a similar plan. However, the Toronto group used single relatively large doses of 600 to 800 r to each field in succession. With 200 kv. X-rays, this resulted in an estimated midline tumor dose of 800 to 1500 r, delivered to virtually all main lymphatic regions. In addition, the lymphatic chains actually involved by Hodgkin's disease were supplemented to tumor doses ranging from 1,500 to 4,500 r or more. From 1937 to 1953, 400 kv. apparatus was used at Toronto to deliver the higher doses to the involved areas, the treatment to other lymphatic regions continuing with 200 kv. as before.

In 1931, Gilbert and Babaiantz were able to report that of fifteen patients treated by their method, the first of whom had been treated in 1922, seven were still alive, with an average survival of 6.5 years for the living patients and 4.3 years for the entire group, a survival rate which at that time was unprecedented. Nonetheless, Gilbert (1939) seems to have had ambivalent feelings about the possibility of cure, since he states, "The aim should always be to obtain prolonged remission *equivalent to clinical cures,* remissions which can be renewed without risk on the appearance of the *inevitable recurrences* [italics inserted]."

Voorhoeve (1925) pointed out that many authors of that early era reported their survival data in rather haphazard fashion, often omitting significant numbers of patients who had not been treated with what they regarded as optimal techniques, and failed to distinguish between survival time after the onset of symptoms and survival time after the start of therapy. Even Gilbert's data (1939) were not above suspicion in this regard, and perhaps this is one of the reasons why his concepts of treatment, which have received strong affirmation in modern times, were so long neglected by all but a handful of other radiotherapists. Referring to Gilbert's then unrivaled three-year survival rate of 45.7 percent and five-year survival rate of 34.2 percent, Craft (1940) states: "Gilbert apparently does not include, in this particular series, cases which were not treated systematically, therefore his survival rates are somewhat higher than most authors report."

In fact, the first reasonably convincing evidence that the survival of patients with Hodgkin's disease is significantly prolonged by X-ray therapy, relative to that of patients receiving general supportive care but no specific treatment, was presented by Craft himself in 1940. He reviewed a series of 179 cases, 92 percent of which were biopsy proved, in which the patients had been treated with roentgen therapy at the University of Minnesota between 1926 and 1939, and compared their survival with that of 52 untreated cases discovered in the autopsy files of the department of pathology, University of Minnesota, between June 1, 1910, and December 31, 1939. His survival curves for the two series are reproduced in Figure 9.2. It will be noted that 65 of 149 treated patients (43.6 percent) survived three years or more, versus only 8 (15.4 percent) of 52 untreated patients; at five years, survival in the respective groups was 30 of 128 (23.4 percent) versus 3 of 52 (5.8 percent). By ten years all of the untreated patients were dead, whereas 5 of 45 treated patients (11.1 percent) still survived; and of the 18 treated patients at risk for thirteen years, 3 (16.7 percent) survived. Although the two groups were not entirely comparable, and were not randomly assigned, Craft concluded: "The difference between the three and five year survival rates, for the treated and the untreated groups, is very significant and attests to the therapeutic value of roentgen ray therapy. These significant differences should convince even the most dubious of the effectiveness of roentgen ray therapy in Hodgkin's disease. The patients not only live longer, but their general well-being is tremendously improved in the large majority of cases."

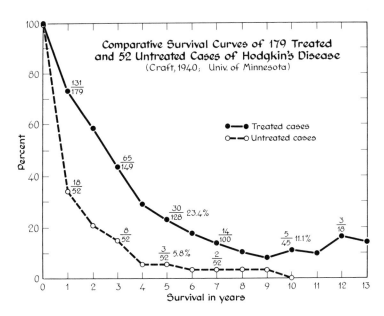

Figure 9.2 Comparative survival curves of a series of 52 patients with Hodgkin's disease who received no specific treatment and of 179 patients treated with kilovoltage X-ray therapy between 1926 and 1939 at the University of Minnesota (Craft, 1940). Note that five-year survival in the untreated group was only 5.8 percent and that all patients were dead by the tenth year.

Craft's paper remained obscure, however, and his enthusiasm was not widely shared. Most radiotherapists credit the classic paper of Peters (1950) as the first to seriously arouse widespread interest in the curative potentialities of radiation therapy for Hodgkin's disease. Reviewing a series of 113 patients treated at Toronto from 1924 to 1942, she was able to report a five-year survival of 51 percent and a ten-year survival of 25 percent for all stages; particularly impressive were the five-year survival figures of 88 percent in her stage I cases and 72 percent in her stage II cases. The doses employed ranged from 1800 to 5,000 r, depending on the site and extent of the disease, with somewhat higher dose levels in the relatively localized cases. In addition, many of the patients had received "prophylactic" irradiation to doses of 400 to 800 r to lymph node-bearing areas apparently uninvolved by disease. Several years later, Peters and Middlemiss (1958) were able to extend the period of observation on the same cases out to the twentieth year and beyond. They observed no significant decrement of survival after the tenth year and concluded: "Thus, if a patient survives ten years without recurrence, there is very little risk of a recurrence during the following twenty years." Excellent five- and ten-year survival rates after intensive kilovoltage X-ray therapy were also reported by Nice and Stenstrom (1954), Hynes and Frelick (1953), Hynes (1955), Jelliffe and Thomson (1955), Healy, Amory, and Friedman (1955), and Fuller (1967). Kaplan (1962, 1966b) presented evidence indicating that survival in stages I and II was far better after intensive than after palliative doses. Finally, Easson and Russell (1963) published a paper boldly and dramatically entitled "The Cure of Hodgkin's Disease," basing their claim for cure on the same type of evidence as had been observed by Peters and Middlemiss (1958), namely, that their observed survival rates at fifteen and twenty years were not significantly less than those at ten years. Thus, sixty years after Senn's prematurely optimistic claim that the roentgen ray had a curative effect in Hodgkin's disease, firm evidence to support this view was finally at hand.

Meanwhile, the megavoltage era of radiotherapy had been ushered in during the 1950s. Released from the limitations of kilovoltage X-ray therapy, radiotherapists were finally able to extend the therapeutic principles enunciated by Gilbert (1939) and by Peters (1950) to their logical conclusions. The Stanford 5 MV linear accelerator was one of the first such machines used for megavoltage radiotherapy of Hodgkin's disease (Brown and Kaplan, 1957; Kaplan, 1962, 1965). The highly encouraging preliminary results obtained in stage I and stage II cases (Kaplan, 1962) led the Stanford group, in that same year, to undertake the first systematic effort to extend megavoltage radiotherapy with curative intent to patients with widespread lymphadenopathy both above and below the diaphragm (stage III). This entailed the further development and refinement of linear accelerator radiotherapy techniques to permit the delivery of tumoricidal doses to virtually all lymphoid structures in the body within acceptable limits of normal tissue tolerance. A detailed description of these techniques, which have been successfully adapted to 4 MV linear accelerators by Gray and Prosnitz (1975), and to ^{60}Co teletherapy apparatus by Peters (1966), Anderson et al. (1969), Svahn-Tapper and Landberg (1971), and others, follows in the main section of this chapter.

Technical Considerations in Radiotherapy with Curative Intent

The major parameters of radiotherapeutic technique are the tumor dose and dose rate, the beam energy, the treatment distance, and the distribution, shape, and alignment of treatment fields.

Certain descriptive terms which have crept into use in the radiotherapeutic literature perhaps deserve clarifying comments. *Megavoltage* refers only to beam energy, and not to dose; *radical,* or *intensive* radiotherapy, refers to the use of relatively high tumor doses; *involved field* (IF) radiotherapy, usually employed only for localized disease, refers to treatment limited to involved lymph node chains; *"prophylactic," complementary,* or *extended-field* (EF) radiotherapy refers to the treatment of apparently uninvolved lymphatic regions; when all major lymph node regions are treated, the term *total nodal* irradiation (Johnson et al., 1970) has been used; however, since the spleen, the thymus, and sometimes also Waldeyer's ring are often treated in addition, the term *total lymphoid* irradiation (Kaplan, 1970) is perhaps more appropriate. Both terms, TNI and TLI, obviously are slight exaggerations, since some lymphoid tissues, such as the popliteal nodes, for example, are not treated. It should be emphasized that, although the techniques of intensive, extended-field megavoltage radiotherapy have been developed to relatively sophisticated levels, they are still undergoing continued refinement aimed at the elimination of sources of treatment failure and at minimization of complication rates. Accordingly, although the description given here represents, in my opinion, the most advanced state of the art today, it will inevitably undergo further modification and refinement in the years ahead.

Radiation Dose. The selection of dose levels in radiotherapy is an empirical process, in which a balance is struck between two conflicting goals: the use of a dose high enough to be maximally effective against a tumor and a dose low enough to cause little or no lasting damage in normal tissues. In practice, an optimal tumoricidal dose level is one which yields apparently permanent eradication of tumor in a high proportion of instances, with an acceptably low complication rate due to normal tissue radiation injury.

Jelliffe and Thomson (1955) and Kaplan (1962, 1966a) have suggested that the recurrence rate in each treated field is an appropriate criterion for the evaluation of the tumoricidal effect of any given radiation dose in patients with Hodgkin's disease. For purposes of analysis it is important that only *true recurrences,* as distinguished from *marginal* and *retrograde recurrences,* be scored. True recurrence has been defined (Kaplan, 1966a) as "the reappearance of lymphadenopathy or other evidence of activity in a treated field as the first new manifestation of Hodgkin's disease after an initial course of radiotherapy." Marginal recurrences, as the name suggests, are those developing at or near the margins of a radiotherapeutic field; they indicate that the local extent of disease was not fully appreciated when the dimensions of the field were established. *Retrograde recurrence,* or "reseeding," refers to the reappearance of disease in a treated field secondary to the appearance of *extensions* of disease in previously untreated areas. Recurrence rates are given as the number of true recurrences per treatment field at risk, multiplied by 100.

I have compiled (1966a) data from the world literature, as well as from Stanford University Medical Center, on true recurrence rates in Hodgkin's disease as a function of radiation dose. Such retrospective analyses are beset with numerous pitfalls, to which explicit attention was drawn. In particular, the dose rate and total treatment time were often not stated in the published reports; where the fractionation pattern was not explicitly stated, it was assumed that the widely used schedule of five treatments per week and about 200 rads tumor dose per treatment had been utilized. The composite data (Figure 9.3) indicate that recurrence rate is inversely related to dose, falling from a level of 60 to 80 percent with doses of 1,000 rads or less, to a rate of only 4.4 percent for the dose range 3,500 to 4,000 r. At the dose level of approximately 4,400 rads, delivered in 4 to 4.5 weeks, which we have employed at Stanford during the past fifteen years, there have been only four true recurrences in a total of 317 involved treatment fields at risk, a true recurrence rate of only 1.3 percent (Kaplan, 1970).

The complications observed at these dose levels are discussed in detail in a later section of this chapter. Here, it suffices to state that such doses of megavoltage X-rays, delivered to large fields encompassing multiple lymph node chains, are well tolerated by normal skin, connective tissue, and mucous membranes, and may even be delivered safely to small volumes of such vital organs as the lungs, liver, and kidneys. Accordingly, we have adopted a dose of approximately 4,000 to 4,400 rads, given at the rate of 1,000 to 1,100 rads per week, as a reasonable estimate of the optimal tumoricidal dose. Papillon et al. (1966a) recommend a minimal tumor dose of 3,500 rads but are prepared to add an additional 1,000 to 1,500 rads in relatively resistant cases; they employ a dose rate of 1,000 rads per week. Peters (1966) advocates a dose of 3,500 rads in three weeks to involved lymph nodes, and 2,500 rads in three weeks to ad-

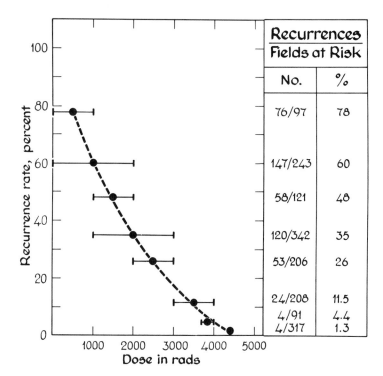

Recurrences Fields at Risk	
No.	%
76/97	78
147/243	60
58/121	48
120/342	35
53/206	26
24/208	11.5
4/91	4.4
4/317	1.3

Figure 9.3 Influence of total radiation dose (delivered at approximately 1,000 rads per week) on true recurrence rate in Hodgkin's disease. The data are those compiled by Kaplan (1966a), supplemented by the additional point at the 4,400 rad dose level (Kaplan, 1970).

jacent, apparently uninvolved lymph node chains, using ^{60}Co teletherapy.

A strong theoretical argument can be made for using the highest tumoricidal dose consistent with normal tissue tolerance. Kaplan (1966a) has pointed out that it is a reasonable assumption that the probability (P_1) of eradication of disease in any one area of involvement ($P_1 = 1 -$ Recurrence Rate) is essentially independent of the probabilities ($P_2 P_3, \ldots P_n$) of eradication in other areas of involvement. Failure to eradicate disease in any one site, even if all the rest are controlled, might well lead ultimately to the death of the patient. Accordingly, the probability of permanent cure is given by the product ($P_1 \cdot P_2 \cdot P_3 \cdot P_n$) of the individual probabilities of tumor eradication in each treated field (assuming negligible diagnostic error in the detection of involved sites).

Calculations of such probabilities for a hypothetical series of patients presenting one to five areas of involvement are given in Table 9.1. It will be seen that even at low doses there is a small but appreciable probability of cure of stage I lesions, in which only a single area of involvement is at risk.

Table 9.1   Probability of Eradication of Hodgkin's Disease in All Involved Lymph Node Chains versus Radiation Dose

No. of lymph node chains involved	Clinical stage	Theoretical "cure rate" (%)[a] if each involved lymph node chain receives a dose of:			
		1000 rads	2000 rads	3000 rads	4400 rads
1	I	40	65	83	98.7
2	II	16	42	69	97.4
3	II or III	6	27	57	96.1
4	II or III	3	18	48	94.9
5	II or III	1	11	39	93.7

Source: Slightly modified from Kaplan (1966).

[a] The theoretical "cure rate" is calculated from the recurrence rate data of Figure 9.3 on the assumptions that: (*a*) there is no diagnostic error in the detection of lymph node chain involvement, and (*b*) the probabilities of eradication of disease in different lymph node chains are mutually independent.

However, the probability of cure diminishes rapidly when two or more fields are treated with such low doses. "Thus, advocacy of palliative dose levels on the grounds that Hodgkin's disease is incurable constitutes a circular argument, since the utilization of such dose levels offers essentially no chance for cure, except in the relatively rare patients with true stage I disease" (Kaplan, 1966a). In striking contrast, as radiation doses increase to levels which afford a very high probability of tumor eradication in any one field, the rate of attrition is much less when additional fields also require treatment. Table 9.1 reveals that even the small difference in efficacy between a dose of 3,000 rads and one of 4,400 rads becomes progressively more impressive as additional fields enter into consideration. Minimization of the probability of recurrence is particularly crucial in patients with relatively advanced disease, simply because the chances of recurrence multiply as the numbers of lymph node chains involved increase. Table 9.1 indicates that there is no theoretical reason why even stage III disease presenting multiple areas of involvement of the lymphatic system might not be radiocurable in a very substantial proportion of cases, and this prediction has now been amply confirmed (cf. Chapter 12).

Is the same dose adequate to eradicate *massive* lymphadenopathy? Carmel and Kaplan (1976) analyzed data on intrathoracic recurrence and relapse rates as a function of mediastinal tumor size. The overall local recurrence rate in 106 patients with bulky to massive mediastinal adenopathy was 24 percent, whereas the rate in 271 patients with minimal mediastinal involvement was only 7 percent. For this reason, we have adopted a policy of "boosting" the dose to the mediastinum, in patients with bulky or massive mediastinal adenopathy, to a total dose of approximately 5,000 rads, usually delivered by a split course technique, to be described below. The same augmented total dose level is used for other sites of bulky or massive lymphadenopathy, as for example in the cervical-supraclavicular or axillary regions.

Conversely, is the same radiation dose necessary in the "prophylactic" treatment of apparently uninvolved lymph node chains? This is a controversial problem for which, unfortunately, no definitive data appear to exist. Nearly two decades ago, I suggested (Kaplan, 1962) that the same dose should be used for the treatment of extended fields, and this general policy has been in force for many years at Stanford. However, in recent years it has been suggested that a lower dose, on the order of 3,000 to 3,500 rads, should suffice for the eradication of microscopic disease in apparently uninvolved lymph node chains, with decreased morbidity and risk of late complications. There appears to be merit in this argument, and in recent years we have elected to reduce the dose to prophylactically treated Waldeyer fields to 3,600 rads in four weeks. A reduced dose level (3,000–3,500 rads) has also been used for apparently uninvolved pelvic lymph node chains. Excellent results have also been obtained when radiation dose was reduced to levels as low as 1,500 to 2,500 rads and then supplemented with adjuvant combination chemotherapy in pediatric patients with Hodgkin's disease and in patients with stage III and stage IV disease. These newer approaches are discussed in greater detail in Chapter 11.

Dose Fractionation Pattern. The influence of dose fractionation pattern has been studied by Scott and Brizel (1964), Friedman et al. (1967), and Seydel et al. (1967). All three groups have employed an essentially similar method, involving the plotting of a scatter diagram (Fig. 9.4 *bottom*), each point on which represents an observed instance of local control or recurrence of Hodgkin's disease in a field treated with a specified total dose over a specified time interval. Whereas Scott and Brizel (1964) and Seydel et al. (1967) used a logarithmic scale for both the total tumor dose, plotted as the ordinate, and the total treatment time plotted as the abscissa,

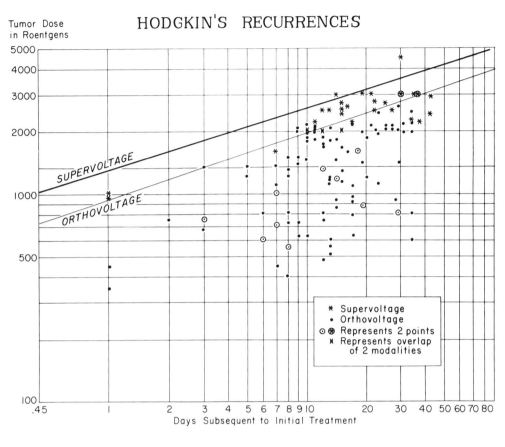

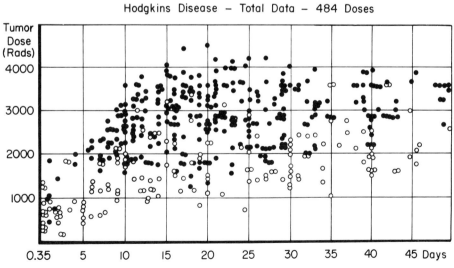

Figure 9.4   Data on dose fractionation patterns versus recurrence or local eradication of specific lymph node chains involved by Hodgkin's disease. *Top*, log-log plot of total radiation dose versus total treatment time. Note the difference of about 500 rads between the kilovoltage and the "supervoltage" regression lines. (Reprinted, by permission, from the paper by Scott and Brizel, 1964.) *Bottom*, linear scatter-gram of similarly derived data. (Reprinted, by permission, from the paper by Friedman, Pearlman, and Turgeon, 1967.)

Friedman et al. (1967) have used linear scales for both parameters. All cases included in the analysis were observed during an interval of two or more years after the completion of treatment. From the scatter diagrams, regression curves may be fitted, either by eye or by the least squares technique, to obtain an estimate of the lowest total dose, delivered over any given time interval, at which few or no recurrences would be expected. Such regression lines are curvilinear on the linear coordinate plots presented by Friedman et al., and linear on the logarithmic plots of Scott and Brizel and of Seydel et al. The results obtained by all three groups are generally similar. The required total doses for megavoltage energies are approximately 500 rads greater for any given time interval than those for kilovoltage X-rays (Fig. 9.4 *top*).

Seydel et al. (1967) made a further attempt to derive separate regression lines for "100% local control" for tumors of three different size ranges (>100 cm.^{3}, 15 to 100 cm.^{3}, and <15 cm.^{3} volume) and for "prophylactic" treatment of apparently uninvolved fields. However, the numbers of data points available for such separate assessments are too few to be considered highly reliable. In general, all three groups have the greatest number of data points at total treatment times between ten and forty days; accordingly, the regression curves are least reliable when radiation doses are given in total time intervals of less than ten days.

The lines derived by Scott and Brizel (1964) and by Seydel et al. (1967) indicate an equal (and essentially 100 percent) probability of local control of Hodgkin's disease with doses of 2,500 rads given in 10 days, 2,900 to 3,000 rads in 30 days, or 4,000 rads in 40 days. The curve for 96 percent probability of local control derived by Friedman et al. (1967) yields somewhat higher estimates: about 3,200 rads in 10 days, 3,600 in 20 days, 3,900 in 30 days, and 4,300 in 40 days. At the higher doses and longer time intervals, the 96 percent local control probability curve of Friedman et al. is in better agreement with our own observations to date, which indicate a recurrence rate of 4.4 percent at a dose of 4,000 rads given in 28 to 30 days, and of 1.3 percent at a dose of 4,400 rads given in the same time interval.

Radiotherapists desiring to deliver treatment in shorter overall time intervals may utilize these regression curves to select total doses for any given time interval that may be expected to be of comparable efficacy. However, it must be stressed again that the curves are based on substantially fewer data points at time intervals of less than ten days,

and the total doses indicated by the regression curves at such short treatment times should not be regarded with confidence.

Normal tissue tolerance is also influenced by fractionation. Le Bourgeois and Bouhnik (1976), in a study of 69 patients with stage I or II disease, found that complication rates were much higher when a dose of 4,000 rads was given in 12 exposures of 330 rads each, three times per week for 26 days, than when the same total dose was given in fractions of 200 rads each, five times per week. Normal tissue tolerance equivalent to that following 4,000 rads (200 rads five times per week) was obtained with 15 exposures to 250 rads four times per week for a total of 3,750 rads, or with 10 exposures of 330 rads three times per week to a total of 3,300 rads.

Beam Energy. As indicated in the preceding section, megavoltage X-ray dose levels must be carried slightly higher, for a corresponding level of probability of local disease control, than kilovoltage X-ray doses, as would be expected from the measured relative biologic effectiveness (R.B.E.) of about 0.9 for megavoltage X-rays. However, for biologically equivalent doses delivered to the level of the lymph node chains, particularly those in the mediastinum and para-aortic regions, kilovoltage X-rays necessarily deliver a far greater dose to the skin and subcutaneous tissues. Accordingly, tumoricidal doses may be delivered to lymph nodes in any part of the body with megavoltage X-rays with little or no evidence of cutaneous reaction, whereas the skin reactions that occur when biologically equivalent doses of kilovoltage X-rays are delivered to the same lymph node chains are almost invariably quite severe, involving a moist, exudative erythema and frequently the development of late subcutaneous fibrosis, cutaneous atrophy and telangiectasia (Fig. 9.5). In the case of the deeper lymph node chains, the cutaneous reaction associated with kilovoltage X-ray therapy is likely to be such a serious limiting factor as to prevent the delivery of desired dose levels in depth.

Another important advantage of megavoltage energies is that the edges of well-collimated beams are quite sharp and that lateral scatter is minimal, thus permitting lymph nodes in close proximity to vital structures such as the kidneys and lungs to be treated safely to high dose levels. In contrast, kilovoltage X-ray beams have a much larger penumbra, which may add very significantly to the hazard of treating lymph nodes in such sites. Finally, the depth dose provided by megavoltage beam ener-

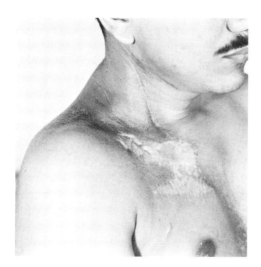

Figure 9.5 Severe subcutaneous fibrosis, lymph-edema, cutaneous atrophy, and depigmentation in the right cervical, supraclavicular, and infraclavicular regions resulting from the inappropriate use at another institution of 200 kv X-rays, following an equally inappropriate right radical neck dissection, in the treatment of CS IA Hodgkin's disease in this young adult male. Four years later, he was referred to Stanford for consultation when he developed recurrent adenopathy near the upper margin of the treatment field. Additional radiation therapy was considered contraindicated by the severity of his initial radiation injury. If he had been properly treated with megavoltage X-rays, an appreciably higher dose could have been delivered safely to a larger field extending up to the mastoid tip, with little or no visible cosmetic effect.

gies is far greater than that with kilovoltage X-rays. It is therefore a relatively simple matter, even in quite massive or obese patients, to deliver the requisite doses to the depth of the midplane of the body, as required for the treatment of mediastinal, para-aortic, or upper iliac lymph nodes.

For all of these reasons, megavoltage therapy has replaced kilovoltage therapy in the treatment of Hodgkin's disease. Within the megavoltage energy range, some types of apparatus are better adapted than others to the treatment of the lymphomas. Linear electron accelerators providing X-ray beams in the 4 to 8 MV energy range have been used very successfully for over twenty years in the treatment of Hodgkin's disease (Kaplan, 1962). The treatment techniques devised for them have now been adapted (Peters, 1966; Meurk et al., 1968; Glenn et al., 1968; Anderson et al., 1969; Svahn-Tapper and Landberg, 1971) to ^{60}Co teletherapy apparatus operating at source-skin distances of at least 100 cm. It is important to stress that ^{60}Co units operating at source-skin distances

of only 50 to 80 cm. do not provide comparable depth doses and usually have significantly greater penumbrae and inconveniently low dose rates. Although betatrons are suitable, in principle, for this type of treatment, their relatively low X-ray beam intensity renders them inconvenient in practice. For practical purposes, therefore, megavoltage radiotherapy as described in the remainder of the chapter refers to 4 to 8 MV X-rays from linear accelerators, operating at nominal source-skin distances of 100 cm., and to the gamma rays of multikilocurie ^{60}Co teletherapy units operating at nominal source-skin distances of at least 100 cm. In practice, the wide fields often employed in the treatment of Hodgkin's disease frequently require the use of actual source-skin distances of as much as 120 to 160 cm., as indicated in the next section. Accordingly, the most convenient ^{60}Co units for this purpose are those with swivel heads which can be rotated to provide longer treatment distances.

Field Size and Shape. It is highly desirable to treat multiple lymph node chains in continuity with as few fields as possible (Kaplan, 1962, 1965). This is due to the fact that the dosimetry in the vicinity of junctions between adjacent fields is more complex and difficult, and errors in dosimetry are therefore more likely to occur when multiple small fields necessarily involving multiple junctions are employed. When the error results in the delivery of inadequate dose in the deeper tissues in the plane of the junction, diseased lymph nodes lying in or near this plane would be undertreated, with a correspondingly increased likelihood of recurrence. Conversely, where errors occur resulting in overlap of dose from adjacent fields, "hot spots" may produce serious damage in underlying normal tissues in the plane of the junction. The megavoltage beams described above can readily be utilized at treatment distances of 100 to 160 cm., making it possible to encompass all of the major lymph node chains above the diaphragm in a single anterior and posterior treatment field, the "mantle" field, and all of the major lymph node chains below the diaphragm in a single "inverted-Y" field (Fig. 9.6a). Thus only a single junction is required, which occurs at a level in the body (approximately the eleventh or twelfth dorsovertebral level) at which there are relatively few lymph nodes. In some instances, poor hematologic tolerance may necessitate splitting the inverted-Y field into separate para-aortic-spleen and pelvic fields, with an additional gap at about the level of the fifth lumbar vertebra (Fig. 9.6b).

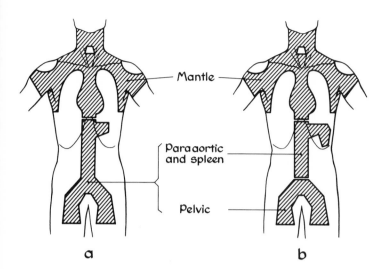

Mantle

Paraaortic
and spleen

Pelvic

a   b

Figure 9.6 Diagram of the mantle and inverted-Y fields used in total lymphoid radiotherapy of Hodgkin's disease: (*a*) two-field technique, with small extension to include the splenic pedicle, used in patients who have undergone splenectomy; and (*b*) three-field technique (with full spleen extension when the spleen is still present) used when hematologic tolerance is poor. Note the gap(s) between adjacent fields. (Reprinted by permission from the paper by Rosenberg and Kaplan, 1970.)

These large fields must be shaped to the contours of the lymph node chains which they are designed to encompass. For this purpose, contoured lead or lead-bismuth, low-melting-point alloy (Cerrobend) blocks or equivalent volumes of lead shot are used to protect normal tissues such as the lungs, kidneys, the right lobe of the liver, and most of the heart, leaving an aperture through which the megavoltage beam irradiates the desired lymph node chains. This is relatively easy to accomplish with the inverted-Y field, but is appreciably more complex and demanding for the mantle field. It is probably an acceptable compromise for small radiotherapy clinics treating a relatively small number of such cases to approximate the ideal contours by using various combinations of wide, medium-sized, and narrow lead blocks, shaped to the general contours of the lungs. However, major radiotherapy centers treating a large number of patients with Hodgkin's disease have generally found it preferable to prepare templates shaped to the contours of the mediastinal and hilar lymphadenopathy of individual patients. Weisenburger and Juillard (1977) have used upper extremity lymphangiography as an aid in localization of the axillary lymph nodes.

Our techniques at Stanford University Medical

Center for the delineation of the mantle field have undergone a very considerable evolution from the very crude treatment fields utilized initially (Brown and Kaplan, 1957; Kaplan, 1962) to the much more sophisticated optical technique devised by Earle and Bagshaw (1967), which has now been further modified and refined by our staff physicists, whose method is the one which we now employ (Page et al., 1970a and b). Their description refers to treatment with a 6 MV linear accelerator X-ray beam using opposing anterior and posterior fields which extend from the level of the diaphragm to the base of the skull.

To obtain an adequate field size of 30 to 40 cm., treatment must be given at an increased source-skin distance (SSD), usually 130 cm. Since it is not possible to elevate the treatment couch sufficiently to provide this treatment distance with the beam directed upward, all treatments are given with a downward-directed beam, and the patient is turned into the prone position for treatment of the posterior field.

The initial localization procedure is carried out on a simulator (Fig. 9.7) in which the target of a diagnostic X-ray tube occupies a position similar to that of the target of the 6 MV linear accelerator, whose geometry and mechanical motions the simulator is designed to reproduce. The initial beam-alignment procedure, subsequent treatments, and dosimetric calculations are all oriented to the same centering point for all patients, the suprasternal notch (SSN). With the patient lying on the treatment couch of the simulator, localization films are taken at the requisite SSD for both the prone and the supine treatment positions. The patient is first positioned supine on the simulator couch at the appropriate SSD required for treatment of the anterior field. The beam is centered at the SSN, and a mark is tattooed on the skin of the patient at this centering point. Two additional skin marks are then tattooed 10 cm. on either side of the midline along the shadow of the alignment crosswire, as projected by the light localizer in the simulator housing (Fig. 9.8). These lateral skin marks aid in reproducing the positions of the arms. A template table with a lucite top incorporating a steel wire coordinate grid is placed on the simulator couch, centered over the patient, and an anteroposterior radiographic localization film is then taken (Fig. 9.9).

The patient is then turned to the prone position, with the SSN in the center of the transparent Mylar section of the couch. The centering point for the posterior field is established directly oppo-

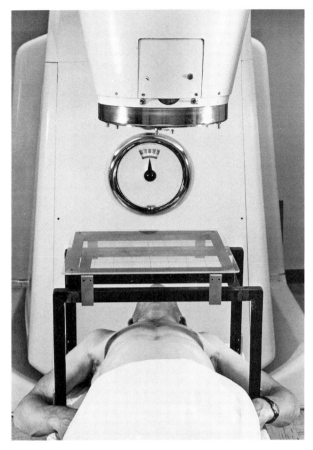

Figure 9.7 Patient supine on the simulator couch with the simulator template table in position for the antero-posterior localization films. (Reprinted by permission from the paper by Page, Gardner, and Karzmark, 1970a.)

site the SSN by rotating the simulator under the couch so that the beam is directed upward, centering the beam at the SSN, and then rotating the simulator mount 180° so that the simulator beam now points vertically downward. A mark is tattooed on the skin of the posterior thorax coincident with the center of the crosswire shadow, and two additional marks are placed 10 cm. laterally as before. The posteroanterior localization film is taken with the template table positioned above the prone patient. The patient is then permitted to rest while the films are developed.

Next, the radiotherapist outlines on each of the two radiographs the areas of lung to be shielded, as well as the contours of any desired supplementary lead blocks for the pericardial area (Fig. 9.9). Templates indicating both the shapes and the positions of the lead shields are then prepared for each field. First, the localization film is replaced in its original position on the simulator couch on the

template table. Alignment and distance are checked by lining up the radiographic images of the coordinate grid wires on the template table with their shadows projected by the light localizer. A sheet of clear X-ray film is used as the template. It is taped to the top of the template table, and the required shielding pattern and position of the crosswires are drawn onto the template with the aid of the simulator light localizer in such a way as to coincide with the outline drawn by the radiotherapist on the radiograph (Fig. 9.10).

Preliminary confirmation of the shape and location of the lead shields may be obtained by making a new set of radiographs (simulator verification films) with 1/4 mm.-thick lead sheet cut to correspond with the outline on the template and positioned accordingly. Since the template table is 5 cm. higher than the shielding table actually used during treatment, the radiographic images of the 1/4 mm.-thick lead sheet templates will correspond

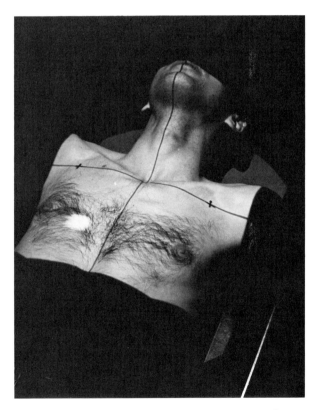

Figure 9.8 Light beam of the simulator X-ray tube housing illuminating the anterior chest wall. The projected shadow of the alignment cross-wire is centered at the suprasternal notch (SSN). Marks are painted on the skin at SSN and 10 cm. laterally in each direction, and a permanent small tattoo is placed at the SSN. (Reprinted by permission from the paper by Page, Gardner, and Karzmark, 1970a.)

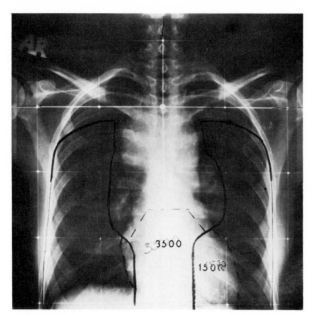

Figure 9.9 Anteroposterior simulator verification film, with the coordinate grid of the template table centered at SSN. The radiotherapist has delineated the contours of the lung-shielding blocks on the film with a wax pencil. Note the broken lines indicating that a small portion of the left lung block (the "pericardial block") is to be cut separately and omitted, when mediastinal adenopathy is present, until a dose of 1,500 rads has been delivered to the heart, after which it is reinserted for the remainder of the mantle treatment.

closely to the shadows of the 5-cm.-thick lead shielding blocks used for treatment. The radiotherapist then checks the simulator verification films to confirm that the areas actually shielded by the lead sheet patterns match those outlined on the original localization films (Fig. 9.11). Rectangular lead ingots are then cut with a heavy-duty band or sabre saw to the contours of the cleared X-ray film templates to provide the lead shielding blocks used in treatment. Typical templates and sets of lead blocks for an anterior mantle field are seen in Figure 9.12. The transparent templates are filed with the patient's chart and used routinely during radiotherapy to check the position of the lead blocks and as a part of the treatment record thereafter. We have routinely used lead blocks 5 cm. in thickness; when it has been important to reduce the transmitted dose to minimal levels, we have added an additional block to bring the total thickness to 10 cm. Kuisk (1973) has recommended the use of 7-cm.-thick lead-bismuth alloy blocks to reduce transmission of the primary beam to 1.4 percent.

When treatment starts, a final set of radiographs is made (accelerator port films), using the linear ac-

celerator X-ray beam, with the patient in the supine and prone treatment positions and the lead shielding blocks aligned for actual treatment (Fig. 9.13). Any necessary final adjustments in positioning of the treatment blocks can be made by the radiotherapist by inspection of these port films after the first treatment. Typical simulator localization and verification films and the corresponding accelerator port films for a posterior mantle field are shown in Figure 9.14, and anterior mantle port films are seen in Figure 9.15. Others have described similar localization techniques (Silverman, 1969; Schroeder, Scher, and Meurk, 1970; Carson, Hendee, and Ahluwalia, 1973; Rao and El-Mahdi, 1973). The importance of repeated verification

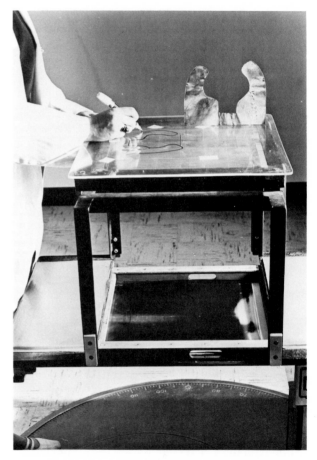

Figure 9.10 Technician drawing the prescribed lung shielding pattern on a sheet of clear X-ray film, using the coordinate grid of the template table as a guide to follow the contours drawn by the radiotherapist on the localization film, which has been replaced in the undercouch film tray. A thin lead sheet is also shown, which has been cut to the contours of the clear film template; note the pinhole perforations to indicate the outline of the pericardial block. (Reprinted by permission from the paper by Page, Gardner, and Karzmark, 1970a.)

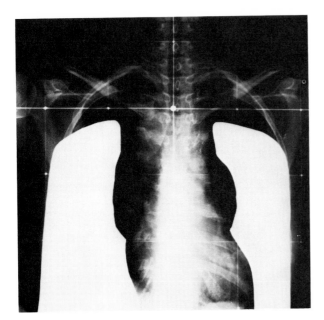

Figure 9.11 Simulator verification film made with thin lead sheet templates. The radiotherapist, after examination of this film, indicates the required adjustments in alignment and/or shape of the templates, which are then ready to be used for cutting the lead lung-shielding blocks. In this instance, the right lung block needs to be shifted medially about one centimeter to avoid unnecessary exposure of the paramediastinal lung as well as to avoid the possibility of shielding right axillary nodes.

films to assure accuracy of mantle field localization has been stressed by Marks et al. (1974a), who detected 330 localization errors among 902 treatment verification films in 99 patients undergoing mantle field treatment. The major source of error was in the shielding of the axillary region. Upper extremity lymphangiography was utilized by Weisenburger and Juillard (1977) to demonstrate that when patients are treated in the prone position, the shoulders tend to fall forward and the axillary nodes may be displaced far enough anteromedially so that they are shielded by the lung blocks. They stated that this problem may be obviated by elevation of the shoulders with sandbags during posterior mantle field treatments. Our limited experience with this refinement of technique has not been uniformly satisfactory, however.

A study by McCord et al. (1973) was more reassuring with respect to the problem of field reproducibility. In an analysis of 526 daily port verification films during mantle treatment of 24 patients, they found that the treatment shielding blocks had been placed within 5 mm. of the original plan in 60 to 70 percent of all daily treatments. Shielding of

known areas of involvement was detected in only 18 port verification films. The frequent use of port verification films is useful not only in detecting errors in shielding block placement but also in minimizing the frequency of such errors, since the

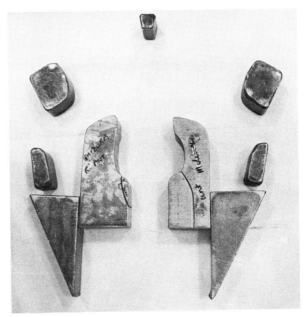

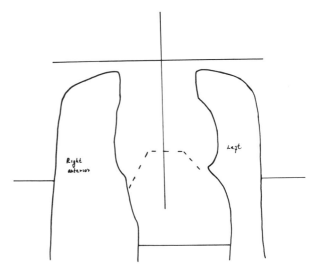

Figure 9.12 Typical clear film template and set of lead blocks for anterior mantle field treatment. Note the small segments along the lower medial aspect of both lung blocks; these are the pericardial blocks, which are omitted, when there is mediastinal adenopathy, until a dose of 1,500 rads has been delivered to the entire heart. The other blocks, from the top down, are: the laryngeal shielding block, shields for the humeral heads, cutaneous "flash" blocks positioned visually just inside the contour of the axilla to protect the axillary skin from the tangential edge of the beam, and blocks to delimit the lower limit of the axillary volume.

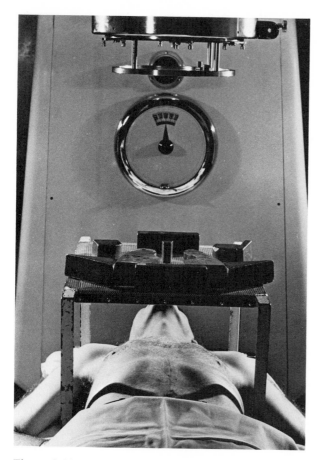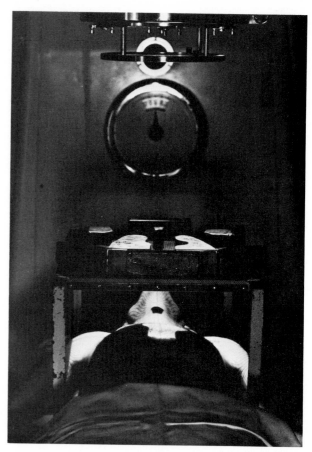

Figure 9.13   Lead shielding blocks aligned on the clear film template taped to the top of the accelerator shielding table for anterior mantle field treatment. *Left,* room illuminated; *right,* room darkened and light localizer switched on to show shadowed projection of field contours on skin surface. (Reprinted by permission from Page, Gardner, and Karzmark, 1970a.)

procedure focuses attention on the great importance of precise localization.

Other techniques of obtaining the shaped lead shields have been devised. In Leyden, Holland (Van Dorssen, Mellink, and Thomas, 1970), and in other radiotherapy clinics (Edland and Hansen, 1969), a technique has been devised in which holes cut to the desired shape in a thick polystyrene foam slab are filled immediately prior to treatment with lead shot, which can then be removed again by a suction device after treatment. Techniques of casting lead shot, or molten lead, or lead-bismuth alloy to the desired template shapes have been described by other groups (Fordham et al., 1969; Maruyama et al., 1969; Kuisk, 1973; Powers et al., 1973; Benassi et al., 1974; Luk et al., 1977). However, we find the procedure described above convenient and economical. It has the added advantage that the complete lung block may be comprised of segments, such as the pericardial block, which may be omitted or inserted at will. When the

treatment of a given patient is completed, the lead shielding blocks may be melted down in a mold once again to obtain rectangular lead ingots from which new lead shielding blocks may be cut.

A recent innovation is the "thin lung block" technique (Figs. 9.16, 9.17), which is used to deliver conventionally fractionated doses of radiation to the entire lung volume on one or both sides during mantle field treatment of patients with unilateral or bilateral hilar adenopathy. Formerly, we had treated such patients to doses of about 1,500 rads in two weeks by the simple expedient of omitting the lung block on the desired side during alternate treatments, both anteriorly and posteriorly. However, this method delivered a high dose rate (about 275 rads per day) to the lung on the days when it was treated and resulted in an unacceptably high incidence of radiation pneumonitis (cf. Table 9.10). Accordingly, since 1969, the dose rate to the lung has been reduced, initially by decreasing the daily mantle field dose until the lung irra-

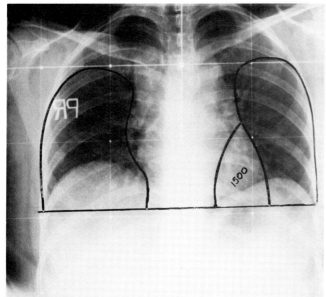

A

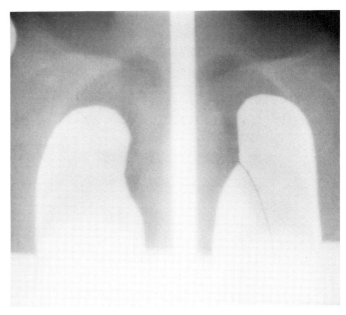

C

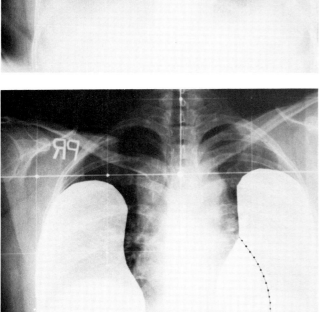

B

Figure 9.14 *A*, initial posteroanterior simulator localization film showing lung contours to be shielded for a
posterior mantle field. *B*, simulator verification film of
the same patient, with thin lead sheet patterns positioned on the clear film template on the template table
during the exposure to indicate the lung areas
shielded. *C*, port film made on the treatment couch
with the accelerator 6 MV X-ray beam; the lung and
cervicodorsal spine lead shielding blocks have been positioned on the clear film template on the accelerator
shielding table. (Reprinted by permission from the
paper by Page, Gardner, and Karzmark, 1970a.)

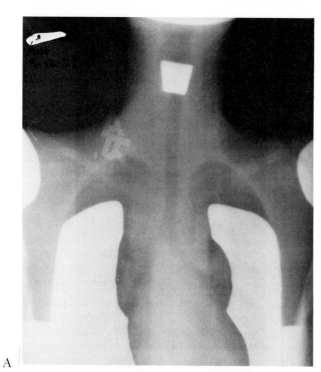

A

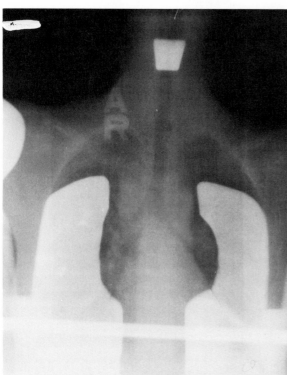

B

Figure 9.15 Typical anterior mantle field port films. Note the humeral head, axillary skin, and laryngeal shields. The laryngeal shield is omitted when massive cervical adenopathy encroaches too closely on the midline. The axillary skin shield is omitted for the first 2,000 rads when large axillary masses protrude close to the surface. The contour of the pericardial block is also apparent; these blocks are cut separately when mediastinal adenopathy is present and are omitted (*A*) until after 1,500 rads have been given to the heart. The pericardial blocks are then added (*B*) for the remainder of the mantle treatment, and an additional "subcarinal block" is inserted after 3,000–3,500 rads to conform to the dashed line in the template shown in Figure 9.12.

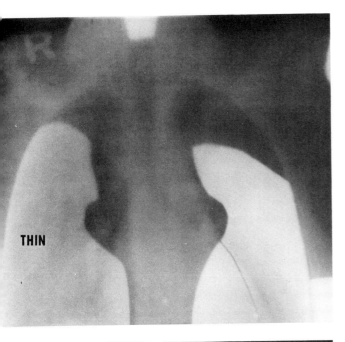

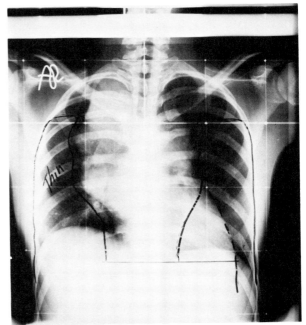

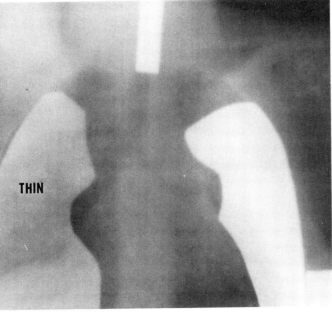

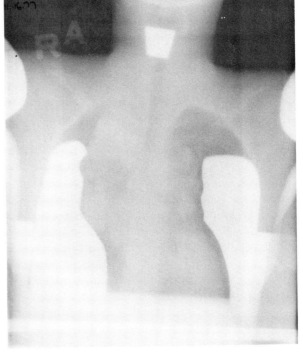

Figure 9.16 Two examples of the thin lead lung block technique, used to deliver 37 percent of the daily dose to the ipsilateral lung during the entire four-week period of mantle field treatment in patients with hilar adenopathy. The thin block is 2.1 cm., the regular block 5 cm. in thickness; the difference in penetrability is apparent on these port films. *Top,* anterior mantle; note that the left infraclavicular region has been deliberately left unshielded. *Bottom,* posterior mantle; note that the pericardial block has not yet been inserted, nor has the spinal cord shield been extended to cover the dorsal as well as the cervical region. These adjustments are made after doses of 1,500 and 2,000 rads, respectively.

Figure 9.17 Localization film (*top*) and accelerator port film (*bottom*) of another example of the use of the thin lung block technique in a patient with massive mediastinal and right hilar adenopathy. The right lung block is of reduced (2.1 cm.) thickness.

diation had been completed, and more recently by the use of reduced-thickness lead blocks which permit the transmission to the lung of approximately 37 percent of the dose that reaches the mediastinal nodes during the same exposure. Direct measurements with a phantom containing a cork lung have confirmed the calculated dose transmission and indicate that the prescribed dose is accurate to ±8 percent without correction for lung thicknesses ranging from 16 to 26 cm. (Palos et al., 1971). Thus, the prescribed total dose of 1,650 rads is given to one or both lungs in 20 fractions throughout the four-week period of mantle field treatment. There appears to have been an extremely gratifying reduction of the hazard of radiation pneumonitis (Table 9.10; cf. also Carmel and Kaplan, 1976). The development of pulmonary parenchymal Hodgkin's disease also appears to have been effectively reduced at these low dose rates (Carmel and Kaplan, 1976).

Certain other refinements in the mantle technique have been introduced in recent years. A lead block 1 to 2 cm. wide is positioned over the cervical spinal cord in the posterior treatment field throughout treatment, and this spinal cord shield is extended down to cover the dorsal spinal cord in addition, after a dose of 2,000 rads has been delivered to the midplane of the mediastinum (Fig. 9.14C). The larynx is shielded by a small trapezoidal lead block during anterior mantle treatments (Figs. 9.12, 9.15, 9.17). The skin of the axillae and the humeral heads are shielded (Fig. 9.15) during both anterior and posterior treatments. The use of axillary skin shields has eliminated the severe skin reactions which were sometimes seen previously due to high doses in the cutaneous contours tangential to the beam. These shields are omitted for the first 2,000 rads, however, when large axillary node masses are present. Special care and precision are required in mantle field irradiation of young children (Fig. 9.18).

To minimize the possibility of missing microscopic foci of pericardial invasion when mediastinal lymphadenopathy is present, the left lung shields are cut into two main sections (Figs. 9.14 and 9.15), both anteriorly and posteriorly. The lower medial section, known as the pericardial block, is drawn to the contours of the left lateral cardiac silhouette. A dose of 1,500 rads is given with the pericardial block omitted (Fig. 9.15A), after which it is reinserted for the remaining treatments (Fig. 9.15B). An additional "subcarinal" block (Fig. 9.19) is inserted after 3,000 to 3,500 rads have been delivered, to shield the area

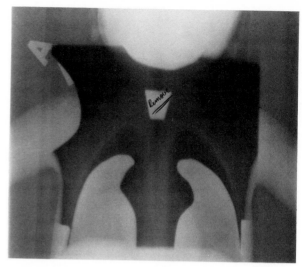

Figure 9.18   Anterior mantle port film of a 4.5-year-old child with Hodgkin's disease. The mantle technique is well tolerated by young children but demands the exercise of particular care and precision in the delineation of fields and the daily placement of shielding blocks. Note that the radiotherapist, on review of this film, has asked that the laryngeal block be removed, at least for the first 2,000 rads of treatment, due to the proximity of cervical adenopathy.

between the two lung blocks from the level of the diaphragm up to the inferior margin of the subcarinal lymph nodes (the lower edge of which is about 5 cm. below the carina), thus providing additional protection for the heart. Finally, the occasional observation of marginal recurrences in relatively low-lying infraclavicular lymph nodes has led us to revise the superior contours of the anterior lung blocks. Whereas the posterior lung blocks follow the inferior margins of the clavicles closely (Fig. 9.14), the upper margins of the anterior lung blocks are drawn well below the clavicles (Fig. 9.15), thus increasing the dose to the infraclavicular region anteriorly. When infraclavicular adenopathy is present initially, we then supplement the dose to the involved infraclavicular area with local 200 kv X-ray therapy. Conversely, there are situations, such as subdiaphragmatic stage II or high cervical stage I lymphocyte predominance disease, in which it is unnecessary to irradiate the mediastinal or hilar nodes. In these circumstances, the mantle field is reduced to a "minimantle", as shown in Figure 9.20.

The inverted-Y field used to treat the infradiaphragmatic lymphoid regions varies somewhat, depending on whether the patient has undergone splenectomy. When the spleen is present, we usually include it in the anterior and posterior

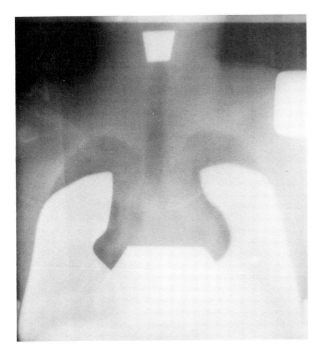

Figure 9.19 Anterior mantle field port film showing a "subcarinal" block in position, shielding the lower mediastinum and part of the heart. The cranial boundary of the block is placed about 5 cm. below the tracheal bifurcation to avoid shielding diseased subcarinal lymph nodes. The block is omitted until a dose of about 3,000 rads has been delivered to the mediastinum, after which it is used for all remaining anterior mantle treatments. This refinement in technique has virtually eliminated the hazard of radiation pericarditis, with a negligible risk of later relapse in the shielded area (Carmel and Kaplan, 1976).

para-aortic treatment field by extending the field laterally to cover part of the left upper quadrant, as indicated in Figure 9.6. It should be noted that the shape of the field is intended to provide shielding for as much as possible of the left kidney, although the course of the splenic pedicle and the nodes that lie along its path necessarily require irradiation of part of the upper pole of the left kidney. Note also that the upper lateral corner of the field is shielded to protect the left costophrenic angle. When the spleen must be treated in addition to the para-aortic nodes, it is seldom possible for the patient to tolerate treatment to both para-aortic and pelvic regions simultaneously. Accordingly, an additional junction level must be established, usually at about the lower margin of the fifth lumbar vertebra, but in any case avoiding obviously diseased lymph nodes as delineated on the lymphangiogram. The edge of this new match line is again indicated with a tattoo mark, as is routinely

done at the lower margin of the mantle field, to assist in the precise localization of the gap that must be left untreated at the skin surface if the two fields are to abut perfectly at the depth of the midplane of the body. In these instances, the pelvic field, representing the lower end of the inverted-Y, is then treated separately, usually after a short rest period, in patients who have already completed treatment to the mantle and para-aortic-splenic regions.

In patients who have had prior splenectomy as a part of their diagnostic program, a metal clip left by the surgeon at the stump of the splenic pedicle is used as the lateral margin of the small extension of the para-aortic field which is still required to encompass the residual lymph nodes along the remaining length of the splenic artery and vein (Fig. 9.21). The localization, beam alignment, and block positioning procedures are similar to those for the mantle field (Fig. 9.22). Perhaps as a consequence of the sharply increased white blood cell and platelet counts following splenectomy (Salzman and Kaplan, 1971), we have observed that patients who have undergone splenectomy can usually tolerate treatment of the entire inverted-Y field (Figs. 9.23, 9.24) down to the femoral lymph node level in a

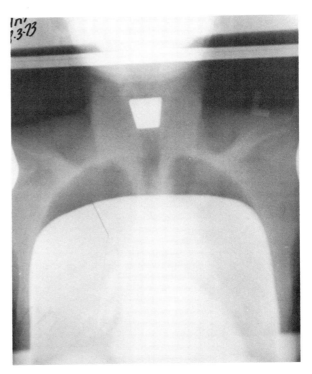

Figure 9.20 Anterior "minimantle" port film. This modification of technique is used in those clinical situations in which irradiation of the mediastinal and hilar nodes is unnecessary or otherwise contraindicated.

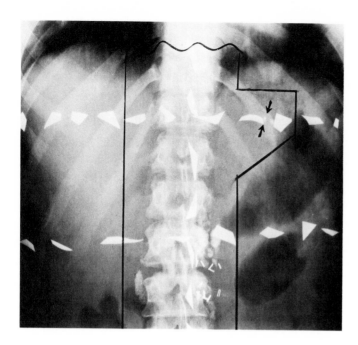

Figure 9.21   Simulator localization film on which the radiotherapist has outlined the desired margins of the upper end of an inverted-Y field. A small left lateral extension is used to irradiate the splenic pedicle, the stump of which has been marked with a metal clip (arrows) at the time of splenectomy. The wavy line at the upper end is a reminder that a "gap" between this field and the previously treated mantle field must be carefully calculated to permit the two fields to abut perfectly in the midplane.

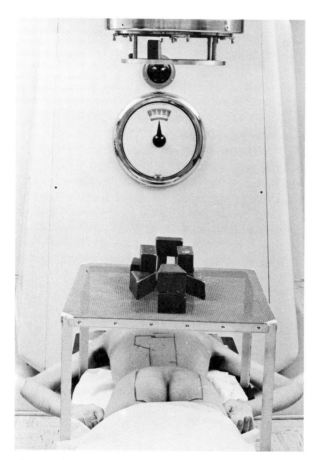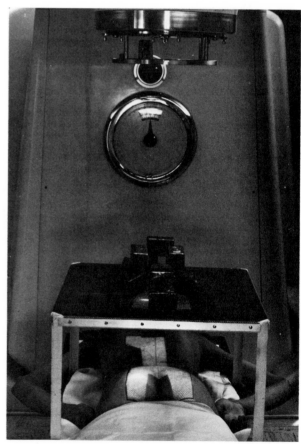

Figure 9.22   Patient in prone position for posterior inverted-Y field treatment encompassing both the para-aortic-splenic pedicle and the pelvic regions. *Left,* room illuminated, showing lead blocks in place on the shielding tray. *Right,* light localizer on and room darkened to permit checking alignment of shadow pattern with skin marks on the patient. (Reprinted by permission from the paper by Page et al., 1970b.)

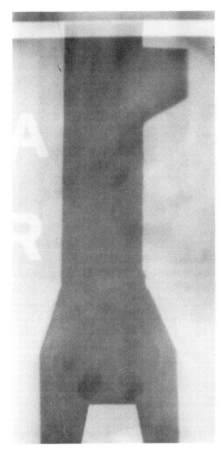

Figure 9.23 Inverted-Y port film of a seven-year-old boy with documented subdiaphragmatic disease.

single course of treatment, thus obviating the need for a junction line between the para-aortic and pelvic fields, which are now treated simultaneously in most of our cases. Patients with supradiaphragmatic stage IA or IIA disease and negative findings at laparotomy have been treated with a modified "spade" field (Fig. 9.25) which flares at its lower end to encompass the common iliac nodes, but shields the tissues of the true pelvis. Goodman, Piro, and Hellman (1976b) observed no pelvic lymph node relapses among 81 such patients treated only to a mantle and para-aortic fields. Our own experience in the treatment of a considerably large number of such patients with a mantle plus a spade field alone indicates about a 4 percent pelvic lymph node relapse rate.

Hopfan et al. (1977) and others have expressed concern about the potentially serious clinical complications which may arise from technical errors in matching adjacent fields. Several approaches to circumventing this problem have been proposed. Armstrong and Tait (1973) suggested the use of a specially shaped filter called a "penumbra genera-

tor" to reduce the magnitude of dose nonuniformity and to simplify field matching. At Stanford, we have continued to use the "gap" method described in the section on dosimetry, but, after a midplane dose of 2,000 rads has been delivered, we have taken the precaution of adding a midline posterior spinal cord block from the top of the inverted-Y or spade field down to the lower margin of the first lumbar vertebra (Fig. 9.29), thus encompassing the entire length of the spinal cord below the diaphragm and obviating any hazard of radiation myelitis. Marks et al. (1971, 1974b) devised an "extended mantle" field, in which they added the upper portion of the inverted-Y field, down to about the level of the third lumbar vertebra, to the lower margin of a classical mantle field. However, this technique seems to have been associated with an appreciably greater morbidity than we have observed with the usual mantle field. Marks et al. (1974b) reported nausea in 53 percent, vomiting in 36 percent, esophagitis in 32 percent, and dehydration of sufficient severity to require hospitalization in several of their patients. Nisce and D'Angio (1973) and Snyder (1977) have described the "3

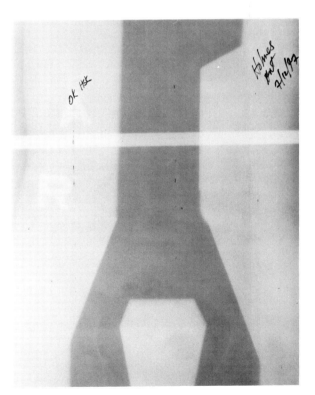

Figure 9.24 Inverted-Y port film of a 23-year-old woman with para-aortic lymph node involvement. The lower end of the field extends beyond the margin of the film. Note that the upper edge of the ovarian shielding block has been placed at the pelvic brim.

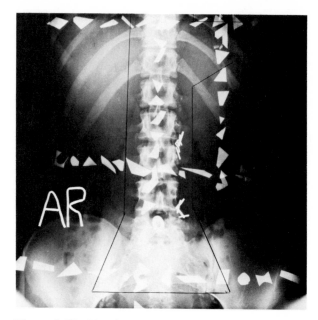

Figure 9.25 "Spade" field, which shields the true pelvis but encompasses the common iliac, para-aortic, and splenic hilar nodes, used in laparotomy-negative patients with supradiaphragmatic stage IA or IIA disease.

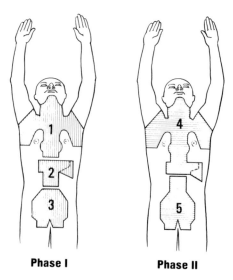

Phase I   **Phase II**

Figure 9.26 Schematic diagram of the "3 and 2" technique of total lymphoid irradiation. In phase I, three fields are treated sequentially, each receiving eight doses of 250 rads in an overall period of four and one half weeks, with no rest period between fields. Then, after a rest interval of three to four weeks, phase II is carried out through two fields with a different junction level, as shown; each field receives nine doses of 200 rads daily, again with no rest interval between fields unless required by low white blood cell or platelet counts. (Reproduced by courtesy of Dr. Lourdes Z. Nisce, Memorial Sloan-Kettering Cancer Center, New York; slightly modified from the paper by Nisce and D'Angio, 1973.)

and 2" technique developed at Memorial Hospital, New York. The course of radiotherapy is divided into two phases (Fig. 9.26). Phase I involves treatment of three different fields, with two intervening junctions. The uppermost field is a conventional mantle, followed by a para-aortic–porta hepatis–spleen field, and then a separate pelvic field. The lower margin of the pelvic field is truncated posteriorly, since only the anterior pelvic field contributes significantly to dose at the inguinal and femoral regions. Each segment receives approximately 2,200 rads in eight fractions over a two-week period in sequence. The first phase is followed by a rest period of three to four weeks, after which the second phase is initiated, delivering a total of 1,500 rads in six fractions over one to one and a half weeks to two fields, the uppermost being a conventional mantle to which a short para-aortic–porta hepatis–spleen segment has been attached, and the lower segment being a pelvic field which extends upward to encompass the lower para-aortic lymph node chains. Thus, three different junctions are used at different levels, with the result that inhomogeneities of dose at each junction tend to be decreased by the contributions from the fields treated in the other phase of the treatment program (Fig. 9.27). Morbidity with the "3 and 2" technique is reportedly low (Poussin-Rosillo, Nisce, and Lee, 1978).

Special problems are posed for the radiotherapist by documented involvement of the liver and the lymph nodes of the mesentery and transverse mesocolon in patients with Hodgkin's disease. We have developed modifications of technique to deal with each of these problems. For patients with laparotomy-documented involvement of the spleen, who are considered to have presumptive evidence of microscopic liver disease even when liver needle and wedge biopsies are negative, as well as for patients with biopsy-proven involvement of the liver, external beam treatment can be accomplished safely and effectively by a simple modification of the inverted-Y field. When such patients are submitted to the usual localization procedure, the outline of the right lobe of the liver is drawn on the anterior and posterior localization films (Fig. 9.28). It is not necessary to delineate the left lobe of the liver, since this is inevitably encompassed in the para-aortic–splenic pedicle field. The shape of the right lobe of the liver can usually be adequately delineated from conventional radiographs of the abdomen. The superior margin is

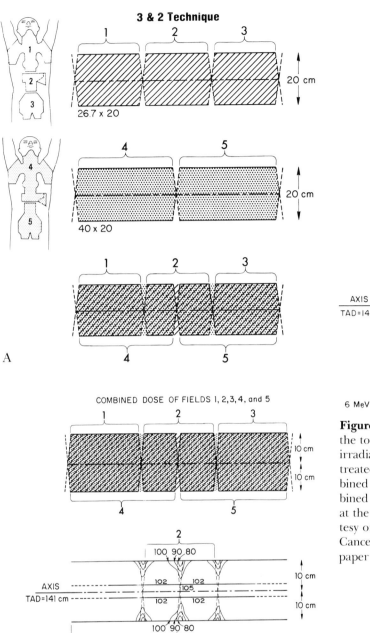

DOSE AT JUNCTION POINT OF FIELDS 4 & 5

Figure 9.27   Dosimetry of the "3 and 2" technique. *A*, the top diagram illustrates schematically the volumes irradiated in phase I; the middle diagram, the volumes treated in phase II; and the bottom diagram, the combined treatment volumes and junction zones. *B*, combined isodose distribution of all five fields. *C*, dosimetry at the junction of fields 4 and 5. (Reproduced by courtesy of Dr. Lourdes Z. Nisce, Memorial Sloan-Kettering Cancer Center, New York; slightly modified from the paper by Nisce and D'Angio, 1973.)

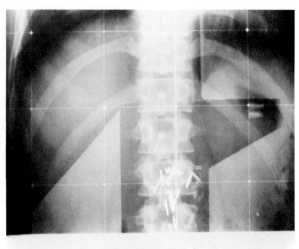

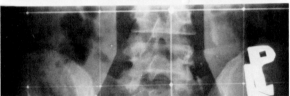

Figure 9.28   Posterior localization film for an inverted-Y field modified to encompass the right lobe of the liver, in a patient with biopsy-proven involvement of the liver. In this specific example, the radiotherapist must modify the field by moving the upper margin of the liver field downward to spare the right lung and the lower margin downward to the level at which the bowel gas pattern delineates the lower border of the liver.

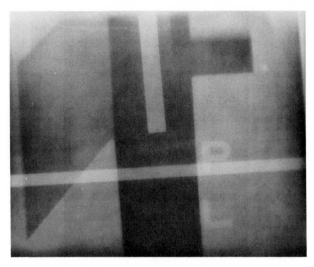

Figure 9.29   Posterior port film illustrating a hepatic–para-aortic–splenic pedicle field. The entire right lobe of the liver is irradiated through a 50 percent transmission lead block, thus receiving half the daily dose of the para-aortic nodes and splenic pedicle. Note that, as an added safeguard against miscalculation or malpositioning with respect to the junction plane between the mantle and para-aortic fields, a lead block has been inserted over the lower dorsolumbar spinal cord posteriorly after a dose of 2,000 rads has been delivered to the para-aortic midplane.

defined by the right hemidiaphragm, and the inferior margin is usually delineated by the gas-filled right colon. The liver field is then drawn on the skin of the patient, along with the para-aortic–spleen or splenic pedicle field. During treatment, a lead block of reduced thickness is placed over the right lobe of the liver (Figs. 9.29, 9.30). With our 6 MV linear accelerator X-ray beam, a lead block 13.6 mm. in thickness is sufficient to yield 50 percent transmission of the primary beam. Thus, with each treatment to the inverted-Y field, 50 percent of the midplane para-aortic dose is delivered to the right lobe of the liver, and a total dose of 4,400 rads over five weeks to the inverted-Y yields a liver dose of 2,200 rads in the same interval. Hematologic tolerance with this technique has been quite good, and there has been little if any added morbidity (Schultz, Glatstein, and Kaplan, 1975).

The other technical modification, known informally as the "three-way upper abdomen technique" (Goffinet et al., 1976) was devised primarily for patients with non-Hodgkin's lymphomas, in

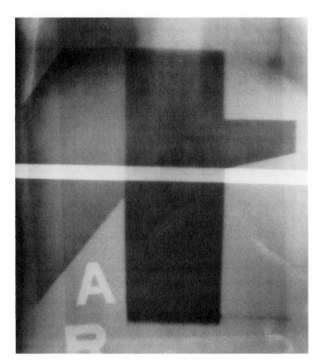

Figure 9.30   Anterior hepatic–para-aortic–splenic pedicle field port film with a 50 percent transmission lead block in place over the right lobe of the liver.

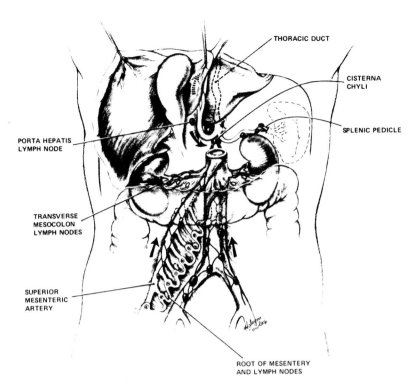

Figure 9.31 Location of major abdominal lymph-node-bearing areas. Arrows show direction of lymphatic flow. The liver and right kidney are retracted superiorly and slightly laterally, respectively. Note location of root of mesentery and transverse mesocolon, which, along with the adjacent bowel, should be included in radiation portals of patients with non-Hodgkin's lymphomas. (Reprinted, by permission of the authors and the Editor of *Cancer,* from the paper by Goffinet et al., 1976.)

whom involvement of the mesenteric lymph nodes occurs much more commonly than in patients with Hodgkin's disease. Nonetheless, where mesenteric adenopathy is known to be present in a patient with Hodgkin's disease, this technique has proven to be extremely useful. Because the lymph nodes of the mesentery and transverse mesocolon extend laterally to lie anterior to both kidneys (Fig. 9.31), it is not ordinarily possible to treat these nodes through opposed anterior and posterior fields without doing irreparable damage to the kidneys. In order to treat the entire abdominal volume anterior to the kidneys to high dose levels and at the

same time protect the kidneys, liver, and intestine from radiation injury, the upper abdomen is treated in three sequential phases through differently shaped and directed fields (Fig. 9.32). In the first phase, the entire upper abdomen, encompassing both kidneys as well as the liver and spleen or splenic pedicle, is included in the field, and the pelvis is usually treated concurrently, through opposed anterior and posterior fields. After a dose of 1,500 rads has been delivered, which is well within kidney tolerance, a new localization procedure is carried out to delineate opposing horizontal decubitus (cross-table) lateral fields with the aid of an

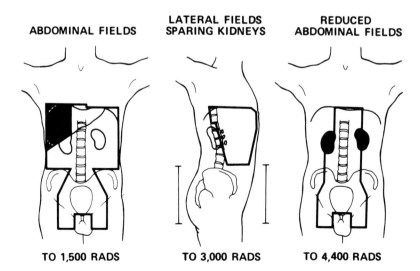

ABDOMINAL FIELDS

LATERAL FIELDS SPARING KIDNEYS

REDUCED ABDOMINAL FIELDS

TO 1,500 RADS

TO 3,000 RADS

TO 4,400 RADS

Figure 9.32 Three-way technique of whole abdomen radiation used at Stanford since 1973. Thick (5 cm.) lead blocks protect the right hepatic lobe for the first 1,500 rads and are also placed over both kidneys and the right lobe of the liver during the final treatment phase, which includes wide para-aortic fields. Note A-P pelvic field and position of pelvic block at level of pubic symphysis. (Reprinted, by permission of the authors and the Editor of *Cancer,* from the paper by Goffinet et al., 1976.)

intravenous urogram to visualize the lateral position of both kidneys. The kidneys usually lie in a plane slightly posterior to that of the lumbar vertebral bodies, whereas the para-aortic lymph nodes lie just anterior to the lumbar vertebrae, and the mesenteric nodes are still further anterior. The lateral radiation portals are delineated in such a way that their posterior margins in the vicinity of the kidneys lie just anterior to the surfaces of both kidneys but far enough posteriorly to encompass the para-aortic lymph nodes, as visualized by lymphangiography (Fig. 9.33); anteriorly, these lateral fields extend to the anterior abdominal wall. Lead blocks 5 cm. in thickness are placed at the posterior margin of the lateral portal, carefully positioned to shield the kidneys. An additional 1,500 rads is delivered in two weeks through these cross-table lateral fields, bringing the total dose to the para-aortic and mesenteric nodes to 3,000 rads. Finally the third phase is undertaken with a modified inverted-Y field, usually widened sufficiently to encompass most of the mesenteric distribution, with

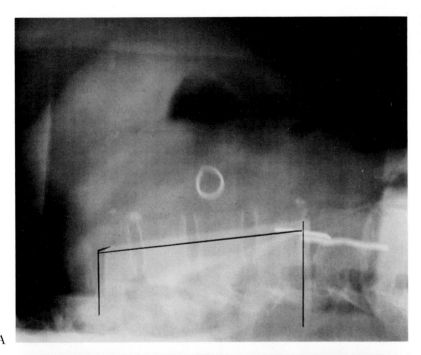

A

Figure 9.33   Horizontal decubitus field of the three-way upper abdomen technique. *A*, localization film taken with the patient supine following intravenous injection of a renal contrast agent, as for intravenous urography. The opacified renal collecting systems may be seen in the plane of the posterior margins of the upper lumbar vertebrae, with the ureters extending obliquely downward and anteriorly to the right of the rectangular area outlined with wax pencil. Two or three small para-aortic lymph nodes containing Ethiodol are seen just anterior to the lumbar vertebrae. The metal circle marks the plane of the isocenter. *B*, port film during treatment of the same patient.

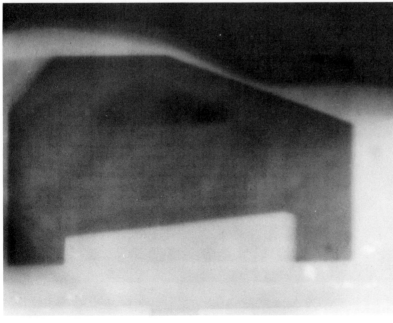

B

LIVER BLOCKED FROM ANTERIOR & POSTERIOR FIELDS

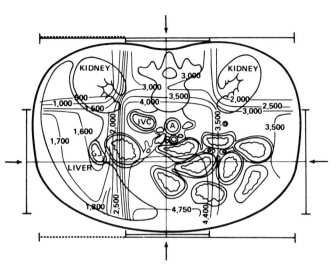

**50% TRANSMISSION LIVER BLOCK —
ANTERIOR + POSTERIOR FIELDS**

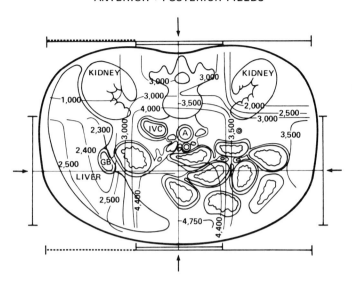

Figure 9.34   Dosimetry for the three-way cross-table lateral technique of whole abdominal irradiation, with initial thick liver block for 1,500 rads. Note radiation doses to right hepatic lobe, intestines, mesenteric and para-aortic lymph nodes, and kidneys. (Reprinted, by permission of the authors and the Editor of *Cancer,* from the paper by Goffinet et al., 1976.)

Figure 9.35   When it is desirable to increase the radiation dose to the right lobe of the liver, one can use a 50 percent transmission block both anteriorly and posteriorly during the initial (1,500 rads) whole abdominal A-P phase of the treatment course. (Reprinted, by permission of the authors and the Editor of *Cancer,* from the paper by Goffinet et al., 1976.)

bilateral 5-cm.-thick lead blocks placed directly over the kidneys during opposed anterior and posterior treatments, which brings the total dose to 4,400 rads to the central abdomen in approximately 50 days. This technique has proven to be safe and effective in our clinical experience to date and provides quite satisfactory dose distributions (Figs. 9.34, 9.35).

The lymphoid tissues of Waldeyer's ring are seldom involved by Hodgkin's disease, but are usually treated prophylactically in patients with high cervical or preauricular lymph node involvement, using small opposed lateral treatment fields shaped as indicated in Figure 9.36.

Dosimetry.   To yield optimal results in the treatment of Hodgkin's disease, megavoltage radiotherapy must be carried out with precise and reproducible beam dosimetry. However, the dosimetry of the irregularly shaped large fields used in such treatment has constituted a complex and difficult problem for radiologic physicists. The dosimetric system utilized must, of course, be matched to the beam energy and type of equipment employed. Dosimetric data for the mantle field has now been developed for 4 and 6 MV linear accelerator X-rays (Page et al., 1970a; Cundiff et al., 1973; Gray and Prosnitz, 1975) and for ^{60}Co gamma rays (An-

derson, D'Angio, and Khan, 1969; Meurk et al., 1968; Svahn-Tapper and Landberg, 1971; Cundiff et al., 1973).

The following simple and practical dosimetry system, devised by Page, Gardner, and Karzmark (1970a) is used at the Stanford University Medical Center for treatment of patients with Hodgkin's disease and other malignant lymphomas with the X-ray beam from our 6 MV linear accelerator. No calculations are required for individual patients; instead, dosimetry is based on the use of tabulated factors which relate to physical measurements of source-skin distances (SSD) and body thicknesses at five anatomic sites. The technique has been planned to give uniformity of total dose within ±5 percent in the midplane throughout the irradiated region within the penumbra. This is achieved very simply by adjusting the number of treatments slightly upward for thicker areas and slightly downward for thinner areas.

A total dose of 4,400 rads in four weeks is routinely given to the midplane of the region covered by anterior and posterior opposing mantle fields. One field is treated per day, and treatments are given on five days per week. It would be desirable to treat *both* the anterior and posterior fields each day in order to deliver half of the prescribed daily

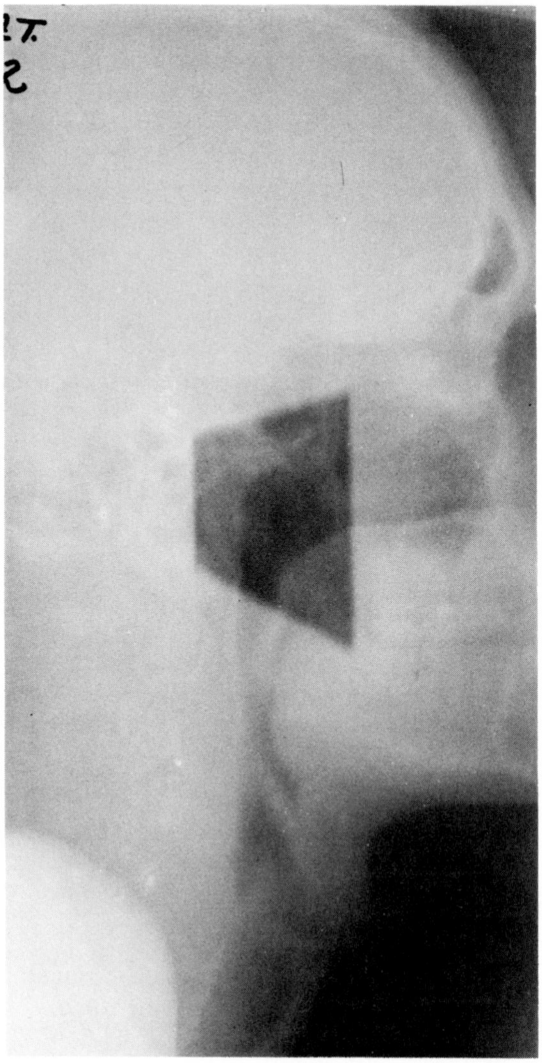

Figure 9.36 Typical port film for a lateral field covering the preauricular nodes as well as the lymphoid structures of Waldeyer's ring.

dose from each direction, thus reducing the potential complication rate (Marks, Agarwal, and Constable, 1973), but logistical considerations do not always permit this refinement of technique in a busy radiotherapy department. All fields are centered at the suprasternal notch (SSN), and the monitor on the accelerator console is set to deliver the prescribed daily dose of 220 rads to the midplane at that point. This midplane dose is designated $D_{1/2\,ssn}$. Doses in the midplane at all other anatomic sites are then related to this dose.

The thickness of the patient's body and the source-skin distance at several specific anatomic sites are measured and recorded at the time of the initial simulator localization procedure in both the prone and the supine position. The anatomic sites

selected for measurement are the mediastinum, the supraclavicular region, the axilla, the neck, and the SSN. Three tables have been prepared, with the aid of which the daily and the total dose in the midplane ($D_{1/2}$) at each of these sites can be determined and the requisite adjustment in numbers of treatments to certain sites derived. Table 9.2 indicates the monitor units required to deliver the prescribed midplane dose at $d_{1/2\,ssn}$. The corresponding subcutaneous dose maxima (D_m) are also tabulated and are recorded during therapy as a check against the possible overirradiation of corpulent patients. Table 9.3 presents the ratios (multiplying factors) of midplane dose at any given anatomic site relative to the reference dose at $d_{1/2\,ssn}$, for different values of SSD and various thicknesses of the anatomic site of interest, recorded as the difference between the thickness to the midplane at that site, and the $d_{1/2\,ssn}(d_{1/2} - d_{1/2\,ssn})$ in centimeters. The third table (Table 9.4) gives the required adjustment in the total number of treatments to be delivered to a particular anatomic site in order to deliver 4,400 rads ± 5 percent at $d_{1/2}$ at that site. Physical measurements of effective field size and of midplane dose throughout the irradiated volume for a number of treatment plans and a variety of field shapes and sizes indicated acceptable agreement with the values given in the tables. The same methods can be adapted to ^{60}Co teletherapy with the tabulated values appropriately recalculated; however, because of the appreciably greater variation in dose with ^{60}Co field size, and the lesser degree of isodose flatness of field, compensatory field flatteners have to be used and certain other minor precautions observed. Such compensating filters have been described by Faw et al. (1971), Svahn-Tapper and Landberg (1971), Walborn-Jorgensen et al. (1972), and Sørensen (1973).

A completed mantle treatment calculation form for a typical patient is shown in Figure 9.37 (top). From the SSD of 130 cm. and the $d_{1/2}$ of 8 cm. at the suprasternal notch for the supine position and the corresponding values of 130 cm. and 8.5 cm. for the prone position, we find from Table 9.2 that, to give a dose at $d_{1/2\,ssn}$ of 275 rads, 572 monitor units would be required with the patient in the supine position and 582 monitor units for the prone position. A total of sixteen such treatments in four weeks will deliver a total of 4,400 rads at $d_{1/2\,ssn}$. As seen from Table 9.3 the multiplying factor (MF) for the neck region is 1.07 for the supine position and 1.05 for the prone position, the average value being 1.06. If all sixteen treatments are delivered to the neck, a total of 4,660 rads would

Table 9.2 Accelerator Monitor Units Required to Deliver a Prescribed Midplane Dose at $d_{1/2ssn}$ during Mantle Treatments

(SSD = 130 cm.; collimator settings[a] = 24 × 24 cm.)

$d_{1/2}$ in cm.	Monitor units required to give a dose at $d_{1/2}$ of:				D_m dose received for a $d_{1/2}$ dose of:			
	100 rads	150 rads	200 rads	275 rads	100 rads	150 rads	200 rads	275 rads
5	187	280	373	513	112	168	223	307
6	194	291	388	533	116	174	232	319
7	204	301	401	552	120	180	240	331
8	208	319	416	572	124	187	249	342
9	215	323	431	592	129	194	258	355
10	224	336	448	615	134	201	268	368
11	234	351	469	644	140	210	281	386
12	246	369	491	676	147	221	294	405
13	256	384	512	705	153	230	307	422
14	268	402	536	737	160	241	321	441
15	281	421	561	772	168	252	336	462

Source: Data obtained at Stanford University Medical Center by Page et al. (1970a).
[a] Field size at 100 cm. SSD assumed to be effectively the same as the true field size at 130 cm. SSD with shielding.
N.B. The monitor units incorporate a 4% factor to allow for absorption by the Lucite shadow tray and the shielding table.

be received in that region; however, by shielding the neck during the last treatment delivered to the patient (-1 treatment) the final dose in the neck at $d_{1/2}$ would be 4,370 rads. The average MF at the axilla is only 1.01, so that no adjustment in total numbers of treatments is required relative to the $d_{1/2\ ssn}$. The supraclavicular region requires an adjustment of -1 treatment to receive a total dose of 4,460 rads, and the mediastinum requires one additional treatment for a total of 4,480 rads. Figure 9.37 (bottom) gives the measurements of midplane dose obtained by the thermoluminescent dosimetry technique, normalized to a prescribed dose of 100 at $d_{1/2\ ssn}$. Note the appreciably lower doses in the shielded regions.

Treatments to the inverted-Y field are also given through large opposing anterior and posterior fields at an increased source-skin distance (usually 120 to 160 cm.) with the 6 MV linear accelerator X-ray beam. Since most patients have relatively uniform body thickness over the entire region treated, the dosimetry is again relatively simple and uniform (Fig. 9.38). The decrease in midplane dose due to an increase in body thickness in a given region is at least partially canceled out by the inverse-square-law increase in incident dose to that region, due to the skin's being nearer to the source. As a rule of thumb, when the thickness of the body over a specified treatment region is within ± 5 cm. of the midpoint thickness, no special calculations are required, and the dose in the midplane throughout the treatment region may then be as-

sumed to be within ± 5 percent of the midpoint dose. When variations in thickness exceed these limits, SSD and thickness measurements are made over the anatomic sites involved, and the requisite dose factors in the midplane can then be found from Table 9.2. When the dose factors differ by more than ± 5 percent from the midplane dose at the midpoint, additional or fewer treatments are given to the specified region as required. Although the tables used for the mantle-field dosimetry apply equally well to the inverted-Y fields, in practice only Table 9.2 is required for most patients (cf. also Page, Gardner, and Karzmark, 1970b).

At the junction of two adjacent fields, it is important to leave an appropriate gap between the fields at the skin surface in order that the diverging edges of the beams can abut perfectly at the midplane (Fig. 9.39) or at other selected treatment depths (Glenn et al., 1968; Page, Gardner, and Karzmark, 1970b). Shifting the position of the junction between fields on a predetermined regular schedule or using a specially shaped filter also helps to obviate inhomogeneity of dose in the region of field junctions.

The required gap per field between the edge of the field illuminated by the light localizer on the skin and the plane projected upward to the skin from the desired junction line at depth may be expressed as:

$$g = 1/2\ Cd \div F$$

for each field, where C is the collimator setting (the

Table 9.3 Mantle Treatments: Multiplying Factor to Find Dose Received at $d_{1/2}$ Normalized to Dose Received at Setting up $d_{1/2ssn}$

(Field sizes = 15 × 15 cm. to max. dial settings; SSD = 130 cm.)

SSD $(d_{1/2} - d_{1/2ssn})$	115	116	117	118	119	120	121	122	123	124	125	126	127	128	129	130	131	132	133	134	135	136	137	138	139	140	SSD $(d_{1/2} - d_{1/2ssn})$
−6	1.57	1.55	1.52	1.50	1.47	1.45	1.42	1.40	1.38	1.35	1.33	1.32	1.30	1.28	1.26	1.24	1.22	1.20	1.18	1.17	1.15	1.14	1.13	1.11	1.09	1.08	−6
−5	1.51	1.49	1.46	1.44	1.41	1.39	1.37	1.35	1.32	1.30	1.28	1.27	1.25	1.23	1.21	1.19	1.18	1.16	1.14	1.12	1.11	1.10	1.08	1.07	1.05	1.04	−5
−4	1.47	1.44	1.42	1.39	1.37	1.35	1.32	1.30	1.28	1.26	1.24	1.22	1.21	1.19	1.18	1.16	1.14	1.12	1.10	1.09	1.07	1.06	1.05	1.04	1.02	.99	−4
−3	1.41	1.39	1.38	1.34	1.32	1.30	1.28	1.26	1.23	1.21	1.20	1.19	1.17	1.15	1.13	1.11	1.10	1.08	1.06	1.05	1.03	1.02	1.01	1.00	.98	.97	−3
−2	1.36	1.34	1.31	1.29	1.27	1.25	1.23	1.21	1.19	1.17	1.16	1.14	1.12	1.11	1.09	1.07	1.06	1.04	1.02	1.01	.99	.98	.97	.96	.95	.93	−2
−1	1.31	1.29	1.27	1.25	1.23	1.21	1.19	1.17	1.15	1.13	1.12	1.10	1.09	1.07	1.05	1.04	1.02	1.00	.99	.97	.96	.95	.94	.93	.92	.90	−1
0 (= $d_{1/2ssn}$)	1.27	1.25	1.22	1.20	1.18	1.16	1.14	1.13	1.11	1.10	1.08	1.06	1.05	1.03	1.02	1.00	.99	.97	.96	.94	.93	.92	.91	.90	.89	.87	0
+1	1.22	1.20	1.18	1.16	1.14	1.12	1.10	1.09	1.07	1.06	1.04	1.03	1.01	1.00	.98	.96	.95	.94	.92	.91	.89	.88	.87	.86	.85	.84	+1
+2	1.18	1.16	1.14	1.12	1.10	1.08	1.06	1.05	1.03	1.02	1.00	.99	.97	.96	.94	.93	.92	.90	.89	.87	.86	.85	.84	.83	.82	.81	+2
+3	1.12	1.11	1.09	1.07	1.05	1.03	1.01	1.00	.98	.97	.96	.94	.93	.92	.90	.89	.87	.86	.85	.84	.83	.82	.81	.80	.79	.78	+3
+4	1.07	1.05	1.04	1.02	1.00	.98	.97	.95	.94	.93	.92	.90	.89	.87	.86	.85	.83	.82	.81	.80	.79	.78	.77	.76	.75	.74	+4
+5	1.03	1.01	.99	.98	.96	.94	.93	.91	.90	.88	.87	.86	.85	.84	.82	.81	.80	.79	.78	.76	.75	.75	.74	.73	.72	.71	+5
+6	.98	.96	.95	.93	.92	.90	.89	.87	.86	.85	.84	.83	.81	.80	.79	.78	.76	.75	.74	.73	.72	.71	.71	.70	.69	.68	+6
+7	.94	.92	.90	.89	.87	.86	.85	.83	.82	.81	.80	.79	.78	.76	.75	.74	.73	.72	.71	.70	.69	.68	.67	.67	.66	.65	+7

Source: Data of Page et al. (1970a).

Table 9.4 Mantle Treatments: Number of Treatments to Be Added or Subtracted to Give 4,400 Rads in the Midplane

(Maximum $d_{1/2}$ dose $\leqq$ 4,500 rads)

Average multiplying factors	Calculated total dose at $d_{1/2}$	Dose at $d_{1/2}$ from one treatment	Incremental no. of treatments	Final total dose at $d_{1/2}$
.90	3,960 rads	248 rads	+2	4,460 rads
.91	4,000	250	+2	4,500
.92	4,050	253	+1	4,300
.93	4,090	256	+1	4,350
.94	4,140	258	+1	4,400
.95	4,180	261	+1	4,440
.96	4,220	264	+1	4,480
.97	4,270	267	0	4,270
.98	4,310	270	0	4,310
.99	4,360	272	0	4,360
1.00	4,400	275	0	4,400
1.01	4,440	278	0	4,440
1.02	4,500	280	0	4,500
1.03	4,540	283	−1	4,260
1.04	4,580	286	−1	4,290
1.05	4,620	289	−1	4,330
1.06	4,660	292	−1	4,370
1.07	4,710	294	−1	4,420
1.08	4,760	297	−1	4,460
1.09	4,800	300	−1	4,500
1.10	4,840	302	−2	4,240
1.11	4,880	305	−2	4,270
1.12	4,920	308	−2	4,300
1.13	4,970	311	−2	4,350
1.14	5,020	314	−2	4,390
1.15	5,060	316	−2	4,430

Source: Data of Page et al. (1970a).

nominal field size at the standard SSD); d is the depth at which the two fields are to abut; and F is the standard SSD. Thus, for a collimator setting of 25 cm. and a standard SSD of 80 cm., the gap at the skin required for that field to match an adjacent field at a depth of 8 cm. is:

$$\frac{25 \times 8}{2} \div 80 = 1.25 \text{ cm.}$$

This gap is then correct for all other values of the actual field size and source-skin distance, including the actual treatment SSD of 120 cm. and measured field size on the skin of 37.5 cm. Accordingly, a simple table (Table 9.5) of gap sizes required for any collimator setting and depth of junction line between adjacent fields has been prepared (Page, Gardner, and Karzmark, 1970b).

However, the data given in the table apply only to situations in which the edge of the field delineated by the light localizer is coincident with the 50 percent decrement line. If this is not the case, sig-

nificant errors in dose can occur when large fields are matched at increased source-skin distances (Hopfan et al., 1977). The relationship of decrement lines to the geometric edge of the light localizer-illuminated field must be carefully measured for large fields, and the possibility of overlap or excessive gap must be checked for all applicable collimator and gantry positions, usually by film dosimetry. An additional table of gap size corrections to be added to or subtracted from the gaps in Table 9.5 must then be calculated for the desired decrement value (Table 9.6). The calculations must be made with particular care for beams with narrow penumbras and for treatments where additional shields are used at one or both of the matching edges. Additional details may be found in the papers by Page, Gardner, and Karzmark (1970b), Cundiff et al. (1973), and Hopfan et al. (1977). Similar calculations of gap requirements for ^{60}Co teletherapy fields at 80 cm. have been presented by Glenn et al. (1968). The serious hazard of radia-

NAME: _____ RANDO _____ DATE: November 1967

| PATIENT SUPINE | PATIENT PRONE |

S.S.D.$_{ssn}$ = 130 $d\frac{1}{2}$ ssn = 8   couch ht = 54

	$d\frac{1}{2}$	S.S.D.	$d\frac{1}{2} - d\frac{1}{2}$ ssn	∴ M.F.
Neck	6	130	-2	1.07
Axilla	$8\frac{1}{4}$	129	$+\frac{1}{4}$	1.00
Sup. Cl.	5	133	-3	1.06
Med.	$10\frac{1}{2}$	127	$+2\frac{1}{2}$	.95

S.S.D.$_{ssn}$ = 130 $d\frac{1}{2}$ ssn = $8\frac{1}{2}$ couch ht = 50

	$d\frac{1}{2}$	S.S.D.	$d\frac{1}{2} - d\frac{1}{2}$ ssn	∴ M.F.
Neck	$5\frac{1}{2}$	134	-3	1.05
Axilla	8	130	$-\frac{1}{2}$	1.02
Sup. Cl.	$4\frac{1}{2}$	$133\frac{1}{2}$	-4	1.095
Med.	10	$128\frac{1}{2}$	$+1\frac{1}{2}$	.97

	Av. M.F.	Expected dose at $d\frac{1}{2}$	Average Dose at $d\frac{1}{2}$ from one treatment	± No. of Treatments	Final dose at $d\frac{1}{2}$
S.S.N.	1.00	4400 RADS	275 RADS	–	4400 RADS
Neck	1.06	4660	292	-1	4370
Axilla	1.01	4440	278	–	4440
Sup. Cl.	1.08	4760	297	-1	4460
Med.	.96	4220	264	+1	4480

N. B. Added treatments with patient supine. Subtracted treatments
with patient prone.

All distances in centimeters.

Definition of points

Mediastinum: thickest part along sternum

Sup. Clav.: mid-clavicular line – just sup. to clavicle

Neck: just below thyroid cartilage

Axilla: intersection of the per- pendicular lines a & b

a) from outer process of clavicle inferiorly parallel to midline
b) from anterior axillary fold medially

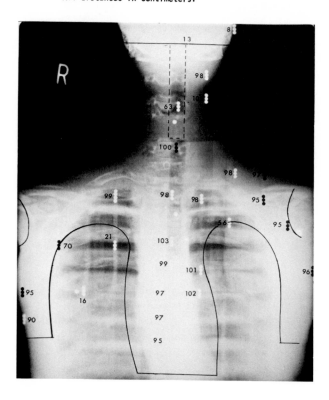

Figure 9.37 *Top,* completed mantle treatment calcula- tion form, indicating typical values for an average adult patient. *Bottom,* Thermoluminescence dosimetry (TLD) measurements of midplane dose for the mantle field in an Alderson RANDO phantom, normalized to the prescribed dose at $d_{1/2\,ssn}$. Note the lower doses under the lung and cervical spine-shielding blocks. (Re- printed by permission from the paper by Page et al., 1970a.)

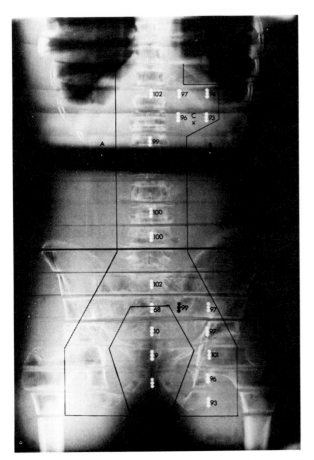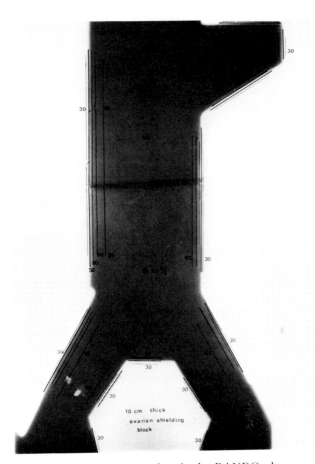

Figure 9.38 Dosimetry of the inverted-Y field. *Left,* TLD measurements of midplane dose in the RANDO phantom, normalized to prescribed dose at $d_{1/2}$. *Right,* isodose curves measured at 10-cm. depth in a Presdwood phantom. (Reprinted by permission from the paper by Page et al., 1970b.)

Table 9.5 Light Gap (g) per Field Required on the Skin when Matching the 50 Percent Decrement Lines of Adjacent Fields at Various Depths (d) and Collimator Settings (C)

Depth	Collimator Setting C (cm.)[a]													
d (cm)	4	6	8	10	12	14	16	18	20	22	24	26	28	30
2	.04[b]	.06	.08	.10	.12	.14	.16	.18	.20	.22	.24	.26	.28	.30
3	.06	.09	.12	.15	.18	.21	.24	.27	.30	.33	.36	.39	.42	.45
4	.08	.12	.16	.20	.24	.28	.32	.36	.40	.44	.48	.52	.56	.60
5	.10	.15	.20	.25	.30	.35	.40	.45	.50	.55	.60	.65	.70	.75
6	.12	.18	.24	.30	.36	.42	.48	.54	.60	.66	.72	.78	.84	.90
7	.14	.21	.28	.35	.42	.49	.56	.63	.70	.77	.84	.91	.98	1.05
8	.16	.24	.32	.40	.48	.56	.64	.72	.80	.88	.96	1.04	1.12	1.20
9	.18	.27	.36	.45	.54	.63	.72	.81	.90	.99	1.08	1.17	1.26	1.35
10	.20	.30	.40	.50	.60	.70	.80	.90	1.00	1.10	1.20	1.30	1.40	1.50
11	.22	.33	.44	.55	.66	.77	.88	.99	1.10	1.21	1.32	1.43	1.54	1.65
12	.24	.36	.48	.60	.72	.84	.96	1.08	1.20	1.32	1.44	1.56	1.68	1.80
13	.26	.39	.52	.65	.78	.91	1.04	1.17	1.30	1.43	1.56	1.69	1.82	1.95
14	.28	.42	.56	.70	.84	.98	1.12	1.26	1.40	1.54	1.68	1.82	1.96	2.10
15	.30	.45	.60	.75	.90	1.05	1.20	1.35	1.50	1.65	1.80	1.95	2.10	2.25

Source: Data of Page et al. (1970b).

[a]The collimator setting is the nominal or geometric field size at the standard source-skin distance, i.e., 100 cm. for the Varian Clinac 6.

[b]Assuming that the 50% decrement line coincides with the geometric edge of the beam as defined by the light field, the gap size per field required $= 1/2 \, Cd/100$.

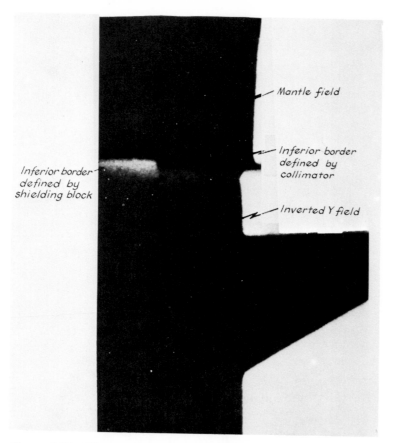

Mantle field

Inferior border defined by collimator

Inverted Y field

Inferior border defined by shielding block

Figure 9.39 Film exposed at 10-cm. depth in a Presdwood phantom, showing the abutment of adjacent fields at the midplane.

tion injury to normal tissues in regions of overlapping dose or of recurrence of disease in regions of inadequate dose due to excessive gap are well illustrated by their cases 1 and 2.

The internal scattering of megavoltage X- or gamma rays after they enter makes it impossible to shield the gonads completely. However, directly incident dose can and should be reduced as much as possible. In male patients we use two 5 cm. thicknesses of lead block cut to trapezoidal shape (Fig. 9.40) to shield the scrotal region; the blocks are placed one above the other on the shielding table or tray and positioned so that their narrower upper edge lies along or slightly above the edge of the symphysis pubis. Alternatively, a scrotal cup may be shaped from a thick lead ingot and positioned to protect the scrotum during treatment (Fig. 9.41). Glenn and Johnson (1972) also used specially fabricated scrotal shielding cups to reduce scattered radiation by about 50 percent. Scattered dose to the scrotum may also be reduced slightly by having patients abduct their legs slightly away

from the midline in both the prone and supine treatment positions. Nonetheless, significant doses, averaging as high as 10 percent of the total dose delivered with 6 MVX-rays to the iliac and inguinal nodes, may reach the testes, as indicated in Table 9.7. Jackson et al. (1970) obtained somewhat lower measured values, averaging 5 to 6 percent, using cobalt teletherapy and specially designed anterior and posterior shielding blocks.

Testicular doses of about 400 rads are sufficient to suppress spermatogenesis for several months or more (Speiser, Rubin, and Casarett, 1973; Slanina et al., 1977), but, except in older patients, permanent suppression of spermatogenesis is not often seen. Recovery of spermatogenesis was documented in 5 of the 11 patients studied by Hahn, Feingold, and Nisce (1976), in three instances to fertile levels. Similar observations were made by Asbjørnsen et al. (1976a), who found azoospermia or severe oligospermia in eight of nine patients, associated with elevated levels of follicle-stimulating hormone (FSH). Seven of these male patients were

Table 9.6 Distance of the 50 Percent Decrement Line from the Light Field Edge at 10 cm. Depth

Field size on the skin, cm.	5	10	15	20	25	30	35	40	45
Added gap/field "a," cm.	0	0.1	0.2	0.3	0.4	0.5	0.6	0.7	0.8

Total light gap required on the skin matching adjacent fields (1) and (2): $G = g_1 + g_2 + a_1 + a_2$

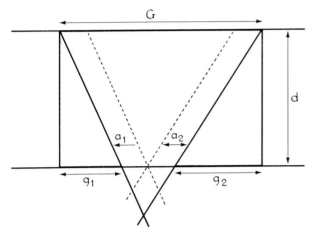

Source: Data of Page et. al. (1970b).

married to women of fertile age, and three of their wives became pregnant and gave birth to healthy children after 18, 40, and 57 months. Our married male patients are usually advised not to try to have children for at least two years after completion of treatment. Several of our male patients have become the fathers of normal offspring after that time; no deformed or otherwise abnormal progeny have been reported to date. In those patients who remain oligospermic, it is possible that restoration of spermatogenesis might be stimulated by treatment with clomiphene, which has been used with some success in the treatment of other types of male infertility (Schellen and Beek, 1974).

In female patients, the problem of gonadal protection is far more difficult, since the ovaries normally lie in immediate proximity to the iliac lymph nodes and thus receive very nearly the same dose during pelvic irradiation. In an attempt to circumvent this difficulty, we have utilized surgical oophoropexy in our young female patients (Trueblood et al., 1970; Ray et al., 1970). When the procedure is carried out as a part of the initial diagnostic laparotomy, it is performed through a long midline vertical incision. However, in other instances where oophoropexy alone is undertaken, a simple Pfannenstiel suprapubic incision suffices. The ovaries are usually quite readily mobile, to-

gether with the intact tube and blood vessels, and can be lifted from their normal lateral position to a position as close to the mid-sagittal plane as possible, either behind or in front of the uterus, where they are sutured in place with a fine metallic wire transfixion suture (cf. Fig. 4.9, Chapter 4). Nahhas et al. (1971) have used a lateral ovarian transposition technique, in which the ovaries are surgically separated from the tubes and broad ligaments but retain their vascular supply along the infundibulopelvic ligament, and are then swung laterally and sutured to the anterior abdominal wall as close as possible to the anterior superior iliac spine. Metallic wire is used to permit radiographic visualization of the location of the ovary on subsequent X-ray films and thus to assist in the placement of lead shields. When the inverted-Y or pelvic field localization procedure is carried out (Figs. 9.42, 9.43), the soft tissues in the midzone of the true pelvis, from the pelvic brim down to the sym-

Table 9.7 Average Gonad Doses Received During Treatment to the Inverted-Y Field, Using a 6 MV. Linear Accelerator

A. *Female*[a]

$d_{1/2}$ (cm.)	Narrow block,[b] (%)	Wide block,[b] (%)
(1) As a percentage of the calibrated dose at $d_{1/2}$:		
5	6.5	5.5
6	7	6
7	8	6.5
8	8.5	7.5
9	9	8.5
10	10	9
11	10.5	9.5
12	10.5	9.5
13	11	9.5
14	11	10
15	11	10
(2) As a percentage of D_m:		
5–15	6.5 ± 1	6 ± 1

B. *Male*[c] = 6–9% of dose at $d_{1/2}$.

Source: Data of Page et al. (1970b) for opposing fields at 150 cm. SSD with 10-cm.-thick gonad-shielding blocks.

[a] Ovaries assumed to be directly below the midpoint of the widest part of the shielding block at a depth of $d_{1/2}$.

[b] Narrow and wide blocks with the shape and dimensions indicated in Figure 9.40B and C, respectively.

[c] Testes assumed to be at 2-cm. depth, 1.5 cm. lateral to the midline, and 6 cm. inferior to the top of a male gonad-shielding block with the shape and dimensions given in Figure 9.40A.

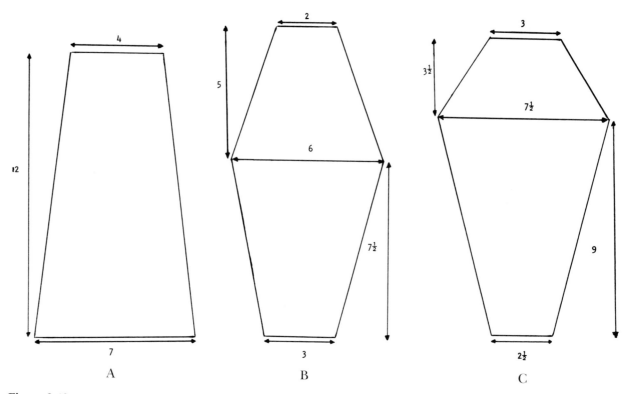

Figure 9.40   Gonad-shielding blocks, with dimensions indicated in centimeters. *A*, male gonad-shielding block. *B*, narrow ovarian shielding block. *C*, wide ovarian shielding block. (Reprinted by permission from the paper by Page et al., 1970b.)

physis pubis, can then be shielded with two 5-cm. thicknesses of lead shield, of appropriate width, precut to the lozenge-like shape and dimensions indicated in Figure 9.40 *B* and *C*. Dose measurements under such double-thickness blocks have been made (Page, Gardner, and Karzmark, 1970b) and are given in Table 9.7. When the ovaries are optimally placed exactly in the midline, the ovarian dose, which is due almost entirely to scattered radiation within the pelvis, is approximately 9 percent of the dose delivered to the iliac lymph nodes along the lateral pelvic walls (Fig. 9.44). With the lateral ovarian transposition technique, the scattered radiation dose to the ovaries has been estimated at 8 percent (Nahhas et al., 1971).

Our first oophoropexy, in a nineteen-year-old patient, was carried out in December 1964. To date, over 150 adolescent and young adult female patients have undergone oophoropexy, without significant morbidity, prior to pelvic radiation therapy with midpelvic shielding. More than 70 percent of the patients thus treated have continued to have normal menstrual periods or have resumed normal menses after a transient interruption of one or a few cycles. In three instances to date, menses have resumed after intervals as long

as twelve to twenty-five months. Thomas et al. (1976b) have used midline oophoropexy and pelvic irradiation with similar results. There is reason to believe that sustained high levels of FSH may contribute to the recovery of ovarian function. Accordingly, we recommend that except when hot flashes and other symptoms attributable to artificial menopause are unusually severe, estrogen therapy for the relief of such symptoms be withheld for at least two years following treatment. The fact that preservation of menstrual function is not achieved in a higher percentage of cases is due in part to the difficulty of placing the ovaries exactly in the midline at the time of surgery; even a 1 cm. shift of the ovary lateral to the midline results in an appreciably larger scatter dose being delivered to the gland.

The first of our patients to become pregnant later delivered a normal full-term infant, though her pregnancy was complicated by an acute glomerulonephritis which later proved fatal. We have now observed a total of 21 pregnancies in female patients who received high-dose pelvic irradiation following laparotomy and oophoropexy. Of these, 9 have been described in some detail by LeFloch, Donaldson, and Kaplan (1976; Fig. 9.45). Of these

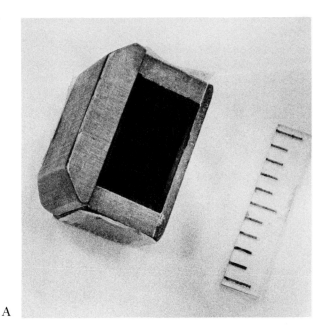

A

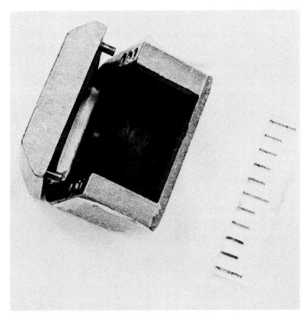

B

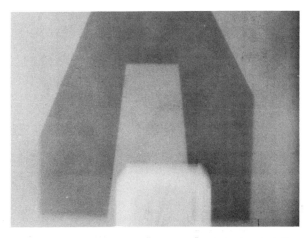

C

Figure 9.41   Scrotal shielding cup used during irradiation of the pelvis. *A*, assembled cup; *B*, cup with cover lifted to show adjustable pin and socket design; *C*, lower end of an inverted-Y posterior port film to show the cup in place below the pelvic midline shield.

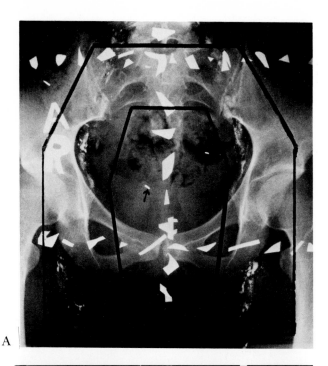

A

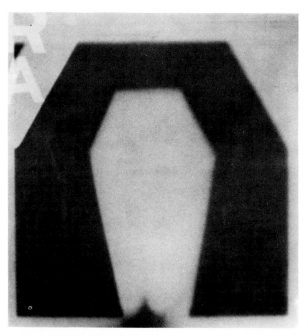

C

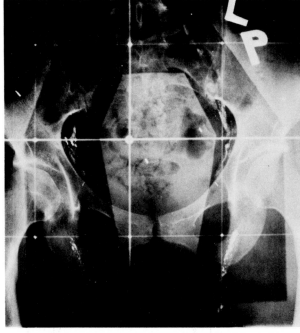

B

Figure 9.42   Pelvic-field localization procedure follow-ing laparotomy and oophoropexy in a 23-year-old fe-male patient with stage III$_S$B Hodgkin's disease. *A*, lo-calization film. The metal clips (arrows) indicate that the right ovary is close to the midsagittal line but the left ovary is undesirably high and lateral in position. For this reason, the radiotherapist has shifted the ovar-ian shielding block slightly to the left in delineating the field contours and dimensions. Note that the field spares most of the iliac wings and the femoral shafts. *B*, simulator verification film. *C*, port film. Note that the wide ovarian shielding block (Fig. 9.40*C*) has been placed eccentrically to the left, with its upper margin at the sacral promontory. (Fig. 9.42*B* is reprinted, by per-mission, from the paper by Trueblood et al., 1970.)

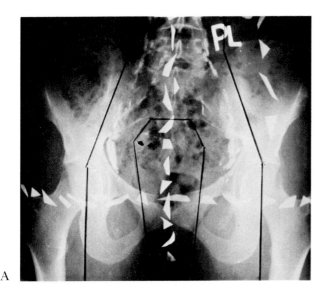

A

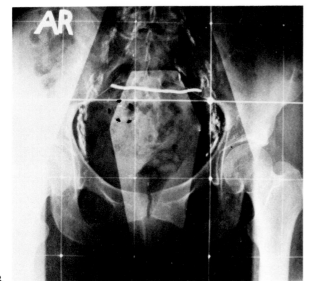

B

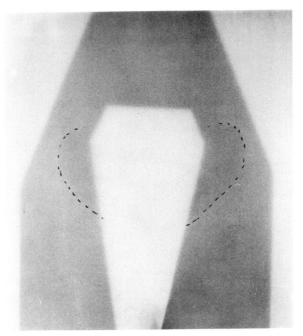

C

Figure 9.43 Positioning of the double-thickness ovarian shield for pelvic irradiation following staging laparotomy and oophoropexy in a nulliparous 31-year-old female with stage III$_S$A Hodgkin's disease. *A*, localization film, revealing the lateral position of the opacified external iliac nodes and the wire transfixion suture through the ovaries (arrows), which lie somewhat to the right of the midline. *B*, simulator verification film with a thin lead sheet cut to the shape of the ovarian shield; note that the wire suture (arrows) lies near and projects beyond the right lateral margin of the shield. *C*, accelerator port film, in which the ovarian shield has been deliberately moved somewhat to the right to improve protection to the transposed ovaries. The patient was treated with total lymphoid and hepatic irradiation, receiving a dose of 4,400 rads to the pelvic lymph nodes. She subsequently resumed normal menstruation and had two successive full-term pregnancies, each resulting in a normal, well-developed child. She remains relapse-free nearly ten years later.

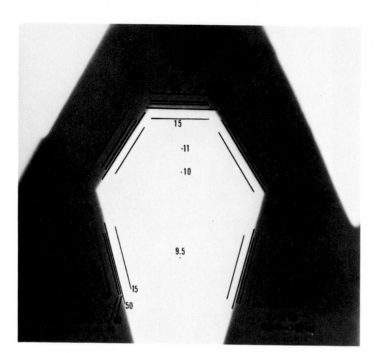

Figure 9.44   Isodose curves in a Presdwood phantom at 10 cm. depth under a wide ovarian shielding block. (Reprinted by permission from the paper by Page et al., 1970b.)

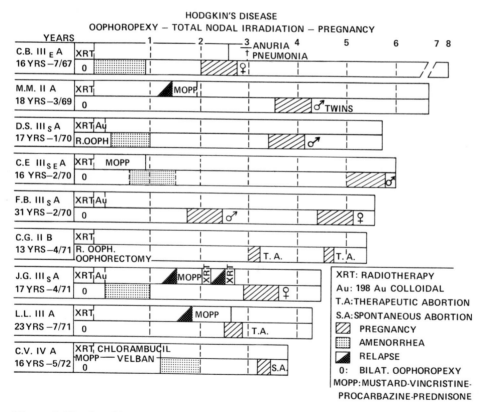

Figure 9.45   Graphic summary of pregnancies in 9 female patients with Hodgkin's disease who received high-dose pelvic irradiation following oophoropexy. Age, date of admission, and pathologic stage are indicated at the left. The upper bar graph for each patient summarizes treatment and disease status; the lower bar graph, gynecologic status and pregnancy data. (Reprinted, by permission of the authors and the Editor of *Cancer,* from the paper by LeFloch, Donaldson, and Kaplan, 1976.)

9 patients, 6 gave birth to a total of 8 normal full-term children (5 boys, 3 girls); one patient, who had also received MOPP combination chemotherapy, had male twins, and another, who had been treated with total lymphoid irradiation plus radioactive colloidal gold, had two successive full-term pregnancies (Fig. 9.43). The remaining 3 patients had abortions, 2 therapeutic and 1 spontaneous. Baker et al. (1972) also reported recovery of menstrual function in a significant proportion of their patients, and one patient who had been amenorrheic for two years, followed by a sustained period of irregular menses, conceived and later gave birth to a normal child six years following high-dose pelvic irradiation. To our knowledge, there have been no reported pregnancies among women who received high-dose pelvic irradiation after oophoropexy by the lateral ovarian transposition technique. Few of the other patients with normal menstrual function have tried to conceive children; some are unmarried, and the married patients have wanted to wait until they have been free of Hodgkin's disease for at least two years after primary treatment before trying to start a family. Most of our amenorrheic patients have developed mild to moderate hot flashes and other menopausal symptoms within two to six months after pelvic radiotherapy. Such symptoms are readily controlled with maintenance estrogen therapy.

The amount of scattered radiation reaching the fetus during a course of 6 MV X-ray therapy to the mantle field has been measured on a phantom by Covington and Baker (1969). They obtained an average value of 0.0026 rads per rad delivered to the tumor, or 7.9 rads for a total dose of 3,500 rads. The 6 MV X-ray beam yielded significantly less scattered radiation than did ^{60}Co-gamma rays or 250 kv. X-rays down to the level of the umbilicus; below this level, the values for the three modalities were about the same. The amount of scattered radiation also depended on the duration of the pregnancy; it was 3.5 to 14 rads in early pregnancy, 31 to 49 rads in midpregnancy, and 129 to 248 rads in late pregnancy, for the same total dose of 3,500 rads.

Radioactive Isotope Therapy for Lymphomatous Adenopathy

Although lymphangiography was developed primarily as a diagnostic procedure, it was not long before its therapeutic potentialities began to be investigated. Of the four beta-ray emitting radioactive isotopes employed to date in endolymphatic

radiotherapy, the two of relatively high beta-ray energy (^{32}P and ^{90}Y) have been used mainly in experimental animals (Edwards et al., 1966), although some of the patients studied by Hennig et al. (1971) received ^{32}P-trioctylphosphate. Radioactive colloidal gold (^{198}Au) has also seen only limited clinical use (Jantet, 1962). Thus, the bulk of present clinical experience pertains to radioactive iodine (^{131}I), incorporated chemically into Lipiodol, the oily contrast medium used for lymphangiography. This material, in the use of which Ratti was a pioneer (1962), has now been used by a number of groups for the treatment of chronic lymphatic leukemia and lymphomas (Chiappa et al., 1966; Ratti and Chiappa, 1966; zum Winkel et al., 1967; Strickstrock et al., 1968; Wolf, 1971; Hennig et al., 1971); and for metastatic melanomas and other solid tumors (Edwards et al., 1967).

The dose employed by Ratti and Chiappa (1966) in Hodgkin's disease was usually 15 to 20 mCi. in 10 ml. of medium injected into the lymphatics of each lower extremity. Although these relatively large volumes were helpful in obtaining more homogenous and complete filling of the femoral, inguinal, iliac, and para-aortic lymph nodes, they were not without potential hazard to the pulmonary parenchyma, since the amount of medium that escaped from the thoracic duct into the subclavian vein and thence into the lungs, and thus the radiation dose to the lungs, was found to be a function of the injection volume (Edwards et al., 1966). Other workers (zum Winkel et al., 1967) have used smaller volumes of higher specific activity material (5 to 10 mCi./ml., total 10 mCi. in each lower extremity). External measurements and calculations of absorbed dose have indicated great variability of the dose delivered to the para-aortic lymph nodes, ranging from 5,020 to 36,140 rads, with a concomitant pulmonary dose of 162 to 916 rads.

In general, remarkably few complications have been observed after endolymphatic ^{131}I-Lipiodol radiotherapy. Fever to 39 C. has occurred in about the same proportion of cases as with nonradioactive, conventional lymphangiography. Hematopoietic depression has not been a problem in patients treated with the limited doses employed for Hodgkin's disease and the malignant lymphomas, although severe and relatively long-sustained lymphopenia has been observed in man after the somewhat larger doses employed for the treatment of metastatic malignant melanoma (Edwards et al., 1967). Strickstrock et al. (1968) have called attention to the serious hazard of endolymphatic radiotherapy in patients who have previously received significant doses of conventional external radiotherapy over one or both lung fields; three of their patients developed fatal pulmonary complications, two of acute exudative form and one with severe chronic diffuse fibrosis. Radiation pneumonitis was also observed by Hennig et al. (1971) in six patients.

Although the method has now been used since 1962, survival data on large numbers of patients with carefully staged Hodgkin's disease are not yet available for analysis. Strickstrock et al. (1968) reported that five of their fifteen patients were apparently free of disease at followup intervals of ten to forty-eight weeks; however, two had recurrence in the retroperitoneal nodes at nine and sixteen weeks, respectively. Hennig et al. (1971) treated 41 patients with Hodgkin's disease and 29 patients with other lymphomas by this technique. They observed no relapses in treated lymph nodes during a two-year followup period. The problem of inhomogeneous and incomplete filling of the retroperitoneal lymph nodes, which is most likely to occur in lymph nodes extensively replaced and partially obstructed by tumor, threatens to limit the usefulness of this method as a form of radiotherapy with curative intent. Zum Winkel et al. (1967) reported that, in their series of thirty-six patients with systemic disease—of which twenty-two had Hodgkin's disease—there were twenty-three instances in which filling of the involved nodes by radioactive Lipiodol was so incomplete or inhomogeneous that external telecobalt radiotherapy had to be administered in any case. They therefore concluded that endolymphatic radiotherapy might be useful as an adjunctive form of treatment but could not be expected to replace external megavoltage radiotherapy as a form of definitive treatment. Bonadonna et al. (1967) suggested that the combination of endolymphatic radiotherapy and chemotherapy, using one of the alkylating agents, might have a place in the palliative treatment of patients with Hodgkin's disease or other malignant lymphomas involving the retroperitoneal lymph nodes.

Radioactive Isotope Therapy for Hodgkin's Disease Involving the Liver

Kaplan and Bagshaw (1968) reported encouraging preliminary results from the use of radioactive colloidal gold (^{198}Au) in an attempt to circumvent the hazard of radiation hepatitis in the definitive radiotherapy of Hodgkin's disease involving the liver. It was once widely believed that the liver was a relatively radioresistant organ. However, the advent of megavoltage radiotherapy beams made it feasible to deliver relatively high radiation doses to the entire liver for the treatment of hepatic metastases due to lymphoma or carcinoma. In a series of forty patients treated to a median dose of 3,900 rads with 5 to 6 MV linear accelerator X-rays, Ingold et al. (1965) observed clinical evidence of hepatic injury in thirteen, of whom three died. The principal histopathologic lesion observed in the liver (Reed and Cox, 1966) was a selective injury of the central veins of the hepatic lobules, with the same sequelae of sinusoidal congestion and secondary atrophy of the liver cords that are observed in veno-occlusive disease of the liver due to other causes. The lowest total radiation dose to the entire liver known to have elicited the clinical syndrome of radiation hepatitis is about 2,500 rads (Kaplan and Bagshaw, 1968) delivered at the rate of approximately 1,000 rads per week. The pathologic changes appear to be reversible; biopsies obtained at later time intervals indicate a diminution of sinusoidal congestion, recanalization of the venous channels, and hyperplasia of hepatic parenchymal cells indicative of repair.

The selective localization of the primary hepatic radiation injury to the central veins of the liver lobules, together with the observation that early foci of Hodgkin's disease of the liver tend to develop in the region of the periportal triad and peripheral sinusoids, suggested that effective irradiation of such foci might be possible with internally deposited radioactive particulate material, providing a dose gradient which would be expected to be maximal in the periportal triads and periphery of the liver lobule, in the region of maximal uptake by the Kupffer cells, and minimal in the central vein region. It seemed possible that the dose gradient thus achieved might be sufficient to afford a significant degree of protection to the radiosensitive elements of the central veins at doses that might be capable of eradicating Hodgkin's disease. To achieve this goal, short-range beta-ray-emitting isotopes were clearly required, and the ready availability and particle size uniformity of radioactive colloidal gold (^{198}Au) made it the isotope of choice for this purpose. However, the short range of the beta rays emitted by this isotope made it essential that foci of Hodgkin's disease first be reduced to microscopic dimensions by either chemotherapy or external radiotherapy. An alternative approach, described by Simon et al. (1971), involves selective catheterization of the hepatic artery and intra-arterial infusion of ^{90}Y microspheres. This method, which is apparently very well tolerated hematologically, has not to our knowledge been used in treatment of Hodgkin's disease involving the liver.

Clinical investigations using intravenous [198]Au were initiated at Stanford University Medical Center early in 1965 (Kaplan and Bagshaw, 1968). Histologic evidence of involvement of the liver by Hodgkin's disease was documented by needle and/or open biopsy. All of the patients also had extensive disease involving the spleen and multiple lymph node chains, usually both above and below the diaphragm. All extrahepatic sites of disease were first treated by extended-field or "total lymphoid" megavoltage radiotherapy, by the techniques described earlier in this chapter.

In addition, radioactive colloidal gold was used as "prophylactic" therapy in a series of patients who were considered to have presumptive evidence of hepatic involvement, despite a negative needle or open biopsy of the liver, on the basis of documented microscopic evidence of Hodgkin's disease in the resected spleen. The evidence linking splenic Hodgkin's disease to the subsequent development of hepatic involvement has been presented in Chapter 7. Among the variables studied were the total dose of radioactive colloidal gold, the use of one or multiple fractionated intravenous injections, the interval between injections, the use of prior external radiotherapy or combination chemotherapy, and the prior occurrence of splenectomy (Kraut, Kaplan, and Bagshaw, 1972).

Hematopoietic depression, of which thrombocytopenia has been the dominant feature, has been a serious problem in several of these patients and has proved fatal in one case additionally complicated by intractable hemorrhagic gastritis. It is of interest that hematologic injury was not a problem in the first patient, despite the large single dose of 60 mCi. of colloidal [198]Au that he received; this patient, unlike most of the subsequent patients, was not subjected to laparotomy and splenectomy, and it is possible that his spleen served as an effective secondary reservoir for much of the radioactive colloidal gold that escaped retention in the liver, thus diminishing the quantity available for deposition in the bone marrow. Although there was some indication that the use of three to four fractionated injections of colloidal gold reduced the hazard of hematopoietic injury, the interval of only one week employed initially was not sufficient to permit decay of all of the radioactive gold deposited in the prior injection. When an interval of at least two weeks was interposed between injections, to permit the radioactive gold to decay through four to five half-lives, three or four successive doses of colloidal gold (total 25–40 mCi.) could be given without significant platelet or white blood cell count depression.

Total lymphoid irradiation combined with colloidal radioactive gold was used in a total of 54 previously untreated patients with PS III$_S$(A + B) disease. Actuarial survival at five years was 76 percent, and 48 percent remained relapse-free (Fig. 9.46). When separately analyzed with respect to constitutional symptoms (Fig. 9.47), the relapse rate in stage III$_S$B patients was clearly unacceptable, since only 20 percent remained relapse-free

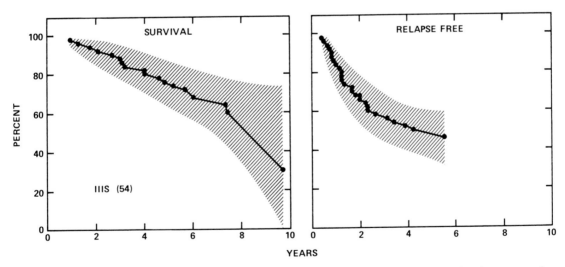

Figure 9.46 Actuarial analysis of survival and freedom from relapse in a series of 54 previously untreated patients with PS III$_S$(A + B) Hodgkin's disease who received total lymphoid irradiation and colloidal radioactive gold ([198]Au). Standard errors are indicated by the striped areas.

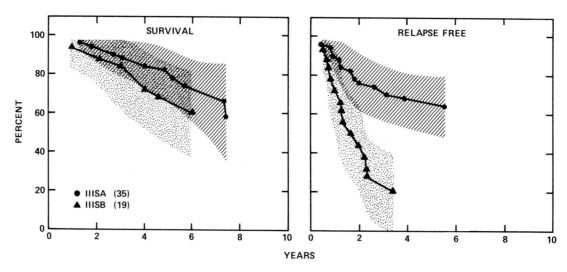

Figure 9.47 Survival and relapse-free data for the same patients, analyzed with respect to constitutional symptoms. Standard errors are indicated by the striped areas for stage III$_S$A, and by the stippled areas for stage III$_S$B.

at 3.5 years, as compared with 64 percent at 5.5 years in stage III$_S$A patients. In 13 patients with biopsy-proven involvement of the liver (PS IV$_H$A + B), five-year survival was 61 percent, and 50 percent were relapse-free at 40 months (Fig. 9.48). However, in both groups a high proportion of the primary relapses occurred in the bone marrow, and many of these patients had poor hematologic tolerance for salvage treatment with MOPP combination chemotherapy, presumably due to the radiation dose delivered to the bone marrow by the small amount of ^{198}Au colloid that was deposited there instead of in the liver. Accordingly, the

use of colloidal radioactive gold was discontinued in 1972, and the technique described earlier of external beam irradiation of the liver through a 50 percent transmission lead block (Figs. 9.29, 9.30) was developed to replace it (Schultz, Glatstein, and Kaplan, 1975).

Radioactive Isotope Therapy of Serous Effusions

Radioactive colloidal ^{198}Au, colloidal ^{32}P-chromic phosphate, and other radioactive substances have been injected intrapleurally and intra-abdominally

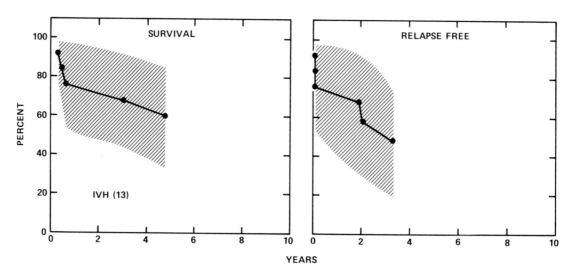

Figure 9.48 Actuarial analysis of survival and freedom from relapse in a series of 13 previously untreated patients with PS IV$_H$(A + B) Hodgkin's disease who received total lymphoid and hepatic irradiation plus radioactive colloidal gold. Standard errors are indicated by the striped area.

for the treatment of serous effusions due to metastatic carcinoma and malignant lymphoma. The usual dose injected into the pleural or peritoneal cavity is 50 mCi. of ^{198}Au or 10 mCi. of ^{32}P-chromic phosphate. It is important that the fluid be freely mobile within the pleural or peritoneal cavity, rather than loculated, to permit uniform distribution of the radioactive material and to obviate the hazard of excessive radiation doses in localized areas.

Although excellent palliation of serous effusions has been obtained in many instances with such treatment, the results of injection of alkylating agents such as nitrogen mustard or triethylene melamine (TEM) have been comparable in efficacy. Moreover, most such patients have other sites of disseminated disease, for which systemic combination chemotherapy is usually indicated.

Palliative Radiotherapy

As the role of radiotherapy in the treatment of Hodgkin's disease with curative intent has grown in importance, its palliative role has become more restricted as a consequence of the introduction of chemotherapeutic agents with a high degree of palliative efficacy. Nonetheless, there are certain clinical situations in which the judicious use of palliative radiotherapy can appropriately be interdigitated with chemotherapy with appreciable benefit to the patient. The wise and judicious use of palliative radiotherapy requires a high degree of clinical judgment and the careful evaluation of each individual patient with respect to the following questions.

Is the Patient's Hodgkin's Disease Really Incurable? It would obviously not be justifiable to use palliative measures in a patient whose Hodgkin's disease is still amenable to definitive treatment with curative intent. Our concepts of the extent of disease that can be eradicated by intensive therapy have undergone appreciable modification in recent years; whereas only stage I and early stage IIA disease might once have been considered appropriate for such treatment, today intensive radiotherapy is the treatment of choice for patients in stages IA and IB, IIA and IIB, and IIIA. Moreover, highly encouraging results have now been obtained with combined modality therapy in stage IIIB and even in selected patients with stage IV disease. Thus, relatively young and vigorous patients with advanced disease deserve definitive

therapy with curative intent and should not be relegated to palliation.

Patients who have been previously treated, with either radiotherapy or chemotherapy, who develop recurrent disease in one or more sites also deserve individualized evaluation, since a significant fraction of them may still be salvageable by additional intensive combination chemotherapy and/or radiotherapy. When the recurrent site of involvement is in a region that has already been subjected to prohibitively high doses of prior radiotherapy or when disseminated disease appears in the bone marrow, both lungs, both pleural cavities, and/or multiple osseous or subcutaneous loci, additional high dose radiotherapy with curative intent is clearly not warranted. However, low to moderate doses of radiotherapy may provide effective relief of pain or other distressing symptoms in patients whose disease has progressed despite prior radiotherapy and/or chemotherapy.

Are Distressing Symptoms Requiring Palliative Intervention Actually Present or Imminent? It is obvious that one cannot offer palliation to a comfortable patient; in some instances, the best treatment for patients with widely disseminated, incurable Hodgkin's disease who are free of distressing symptoms attributable to the disease may be reassurance and careful, continued observation, rather than active therapeutic intervention. However, in certain situations in which the subsequent development of symptoms would probably be particularly distressing or life-threatening, active intervention is indicated, even when symptoms are minimal or absent. Examples include mediastinal disease, which, if left untreated, may progress to tracheobronchial compression or to superior vena cava obstruction, and epidural involvement, which, if left untreated, will progress to paralysis. Extensive lytic destruction of bone is seldom painless, but such infrequent instances should be treated early to prevent pathologic fracture.

Can Palliation Be Most Effectively Managed by Chemotherapy or by Radiotherapy? Chemotherapeutic agents are systemic in their distribution, whereas radiotherapy is an essentially local modality of treatment. Accordingly, it is logical to employ chemotherapy as the principal form of treatment when the palliative problem is attributable to widely-disseminated disease. Examples include patients with severe constitutional symptoms or anemia secondary to bone marrow involvement. Because chemotherapy causes little or no local injury to most normal tissues, whereas radiotherapy may cause significant permanent tissue injury, chemotherapy is also to be preferred in situations in which Hodgkin's disease has recurred after prior radiotherapy carried to doses that would make the hazard of local tissue injury from further radiotherapy prohibitive. Thus, although localized relapsing disease confined to one pulmonary lobe can still be treated intensively with high doses of radiotherapy, such treatment could not be tolerated by the entire volume of both lungs; accordingly, patients with bilateral, multiple foci of pulmonary Hodgkin's disease are obvious candidates for chemotherapeutic management. The same considerations apply in unilateral versus bilateral pleural disease.

Conversely, patients with widely disseminated Hodgkin's disease may be essentially asymptomatic, except for disease in one or two localized sites. For example, a patient with widespread skeletal or marrow infiltration may have local bone pain due to erosion and lytic destruction of some osseous structure. Although chemotherapy employed for the disseminated disease will sometimes also relieve the bone pain and elicit healing of the lytic osseous lesion, a palliative course of local radiotherapy over the affected bone is likely to give relief of pain much more promptly and more reliably and thus constitutes appropriate treatment in addition to whatever chemotherapy may be employed.

Sometimes radiotherapy can fill a gap in the palliative management of patients with Hodgkin's disease when severe hematopoietic depression forces an interruption of drug therapy. When the symptoms presented by such patients are localized to one or a small number of foci of involvement, these may appropriately be treated with localized, palliative radiotherapy and kept under control during an interval of time sufficient for hematopoietic recovery to occur, permitting resumption of effective chemotherapy. Thus, palliative radiotherapy can in effect "buy time" for the patient by stretching out the period during which chemotherapy can be administered prior to the time when hematopoietic or other manifestations of toxicity become so severe as to preclude the continued use of effective agents.

The choice of dose level to be used in palliative radiotherapy requires careful thought. In general, it is desirable to employ relatively high doses only when one desires to obtain relatively long-term control of some particularly distressing or life-threatening manifestation of disease. In all other situations, the smallest dose should be used that will afford substantial relief of symptoms for an interval of time deemed significant in relation to the anticipated survival time of the patient.

We ordinarily employ doses of 2,500 to 4,000 rads, delivered at the rate of 1,000 rads per week, to treat mediastinal lymphadenopathy, epidural disease, or lytic destruction of vertebrae or other weight-bearing skeletal structures in which pathologic fracture could lead to serious disability. The objective of using such high doses is to attempt to eradicate the disease in such sites, or at least to prevent its recurrence during the anticipated residual lifetime of the patient with otherwise incurable disease. Less serious problems, such as local pressure symptoms due to enlarged lymph nodes in the axillae, neck, or groin, or osseous lesions in non-weight-bearing structures are usually treated with doses of 500 to 1,000 rads, which may be repeated at later intervals if necessary.

Acute Morbidity During Radiotherapy

During the course of intensive radiotherapy, a variety of signs and symptoms of acute radiation reaction may occur in the normal tissues traversed by the beam. In almost all instances, these signs and symptoms are transient and promptly reversible when the daily dose is reduced or treatment interrupted for a few days. Such manifestations are appropriately classified under the heading of acute morbidity, rather than as true complications of radiotherapy. This conforms with usage in surgery, where such symptoms and signs as pain along the margins of an incision, gaseous distention and transient adynamic ileus, and mild degrees of basilar pulmonary atelectasis are considered part of the virtually unavoidable acute morbidity following surgery, whereas wound dehiscence, postoperative sepsis, or pulmonary embolism would be appropriately scored as complications.

During intensive megavoltage radiotherapy to the complex irregularly shaped fields described earlier in this chapter, acute morbidity is manifested principally in the gastrointestinal and hematopoietic systems. Anorexia is probably the single most common symptom. Although it is particularly likely to occur when the abdominal and/or pelvic fields are being treated, it is not uncommon during treatment to the "mantle" field as well. Sustained anorexia during much or all of the treatment period is almost invariably accompanied by a significant degree of weight loss. However, loss of more than 10 percent of the pretreatment body weight is unusual, except in patients who develop such additional signs and symptoms of gastrointestinal reaction and irritability as nausea, vomiting, and/or diarrhea. The latter symptoms usually abate readily with symptomatic medication and perhaps a slight, transient diminution of daily radiation dose rate. Occasionally, vomiting or diarrhea may be severe enough to require interruption of treatment for several days; rarely, a brief period of hospitalization for rehydration may be necessary before treatment can be resumed. The association of bleeding with diarrhea is a much more serious symptom, calling for immediate and sometimes permanent interruption of treatment over the abdominal region. Anorexia usually ceases promptly after the completion of treatment, followed by the gradual return of appetite and the restoration of body weight.

Treatment to the supradiaphragmatic lymph node chains through the mantle field produces drying of salivary secretions, loss of taste, sore throat, and/or esophagitis with spasm and dysphagia, none of which are likely to be so severe as to require interruption of treatment (Glicksman and Nickson, 1973). These symptoms also clear within a few weeks after the completion of radiotherapy.

Patients undergoing wide-field radiotherapy often experience a curious fatigue and lassitude, which occurs only on the actual days of treatment, appearing within one or two hours thereafter and lasting for a few hours. Such patients require a great deal more rest and sleep than usual. In striking contrast, other patients may remain buoyant and energetic enough to carry out their full normal workload throughout the course of treatment. Wide individual differences in sensitivity to these and other radiation-induced symptoms are encountered so often that, although radiotherapists should always caution patients prior to treatment about the untoward reactions that may occur, great care should be taken not to convey the impression that such reactions are inevitable.

The peripheral blood cell count must be followed with care during treatment. The complete blood cell count obtained during the initial diagnostic evaluation is an important benchmark against which the radiation-induced hematopoietic changes in individual patients may be measured. Initially, it suffices to obtain white blood cell, platelet, and either hemoglobin or packed red blood cell volume determinations on a weekly basis. When relatively small treatment fields are employed over solitary or contiguous chains of involved peripheral lymph nodes, the white blood cell and/or platelet counts may dip slightly but are unlikely to descend below the normal range at any time during the course of treatment. However, megavoltage radiotherapy to dose levels of approximately 4,000 rads in four weeks through anterior and posterior opposed mantle fields will usually depress these peripheral blood elements to about half of their pretreatment level by the end of the course of treatment to this field. If treatment is immediately resumed over the para-aortic and spleen field, without concomitant treatment of the pelvic region, only a modest further reduction in the white blood cell and platelet counts is likely to occur. However, when irradiation is finally extended to the pelvic field, an additional significant and sometimes sharp drop in the white blood cell and/or platelet counts almost invariably occurs, the average drop again being to about 50 percent of the level reached at the completion of the mantle field (25 percent of the pretreatment level).

When the presence of extensive disease in lymph nodes in each of these treatment fields necessitates uninterrupted treatment from one region to the next without a rest period, leukopenia and/or thrombocytopenia are likely to be severe enough to force one or more interruptions of treatment, each lasting for a few days, or a reduction in the daily dose rate, with a concomitant prolongation of the total treatment time for the last field treated. The same situation obtains when sequential segmental field treatment is carried out in the reverse direction, from below upward: the final field to be treated will then be the "mantle," during the treatment of which a comparable degree of leukopenia and/or thrombocytopenia may be anticipated.

Whenever possible, therefore, a two- to four-week rest period should be permitted between the completion of the initial field, which should always be the region of maximal involvement, either above or below the diaphragm, and the resumption of treatment to the transdiaphragmatic field(s). Patients consistently recover appetite, strength, and a sense of well being during such rest periods. Leukopenia and/or thrombocytopenia may fail to develop, and when present tend to be of significantly reduced severity during the remainder of the course of treatment. Interruptions or delays in completion of the final treatment fields are required much less often, and the total elapsed time from the beginning to the completion of treatment may be the same, or even shorter, despite the rest period.

The most difficult problems of all are those in which actively growing, aggressive disease, both above and below the diaphragm, compels the radiotherapist to use an alternating technique, delivering a "holding" dose of about 1,500 rads in two weeks to either the mantle or the infradiaphragmatic sites of involvement, then a similar dose on the opposite side of the diaphragm to hold the disease in check there, and finally the sequential completion of treatment in each field. Under these circumstances, a great deal of the bone marrow of the entire trunk region is subjected within a very short time to a degree of radiation injury which is sufficient to shut off the production of blood elements. Since most of the active marrow in the adult body is encompassed within these fields, the white blood cell and platelet counts, and sometimes even the hemoglobin values, are usually reduced very quickly to levels that may greatly delay and complicate the completion of treatment.

Blood cell counts should be obtained two to three times a week when the white blood cell level falls below 4,000 or the platelet count below 100,000, and daily prior to treatment when the white blood cell count falls to 2,000 or less or the platelet count to 50,000 or less. At these levels, decisions about continuation or interruption of treatment may have to be made on a day-to-day basis, requiring close personal observation of the patient by the radiotherapist. Often a slight reduction in the daily dose rate is followed by stabilization and partial recovery of the peripheral blood elements levels, whereupon the daily dose rate may once again be cautiously increased.

When we first initiated the "total lymphoid" technique of radiotherapy for stage III Hodgkin's disease in 1962, it was with a great deal of trepidation. A priori, the delivery of tumoricidal doses of about 4,000 rads to virtually every lymphoid structure in the body seemed prohibitively dangerous, since it would entail the intensive irradiation of a large fraction (estimated by Tubiana et al., 1966, at about 55 to 60 percent) of the active bone marrow. The possibility was all too vividly apparent that severe leukopenia and/or thrombocytopenia, complicated by sepsis or hemorrhage, respectively, might occur in a high proportion of cases and might well prove fatal in some. Nonetheless, we decided to proceed with such treatment for stage III cases and for certain stage II cases randomly assigned to extended-field treatment as part of a clinical trial which began at Stanford in June 1962. About eighteen months later, a similar program was initiated by Tubiana and his colleagues at the Institut Gustave Roussy in Paris. By the time of the symposium on Hodgkin's disease held in Paris early in 1965, both groups were able to report that total lymphoid megavoltage radiotherapy for Hodgkin's disease is not at all as dangerous as had been feared (Kaplan and Rosenberg, 1966a and b; Tubiana et al., 1966).

Hematologic data before, during, and after treatment were compiled on sixty-one consecutive patients treated at Stanford University Medical Center with doses of approximately 4,000 rads by the total lymphoid technique (Kaplan, 1970). As may be seen in Table 9.8, the mean white blood cell count prior to treatment was 10,500 per cubic millimeter, with a range from 4,600 to 40,000; it fell during treatment to a mean nadir level of 2,200 (range 1,000 to 5,000) and, within four to eight months after completion of treatment, had climbed again to a mean level of 6,100 (range 3,700 to 12,600). The mean pretreatment platelet count was 350,000 per cubic millimeter (range 184,000 to 890,000); the mean nadir value during treatment was 101,000 with a range of 15,000 to 217,000, recovering within a few months after treatment to a mean level of 269,000 (range 123,000 to 859,000).

Table 9.8 Peripheral Blood Cell Counts on Patients with Hodgkin's Disease before, during, and after "Total Lymphoid" Radiotherapy

	White blood cell count/mm.^{3} ($\times 10^{-3}$)	Platelet count/mm.^{3} ($\times 10^{-3}$)	Packed red cell volume	Hemoglobin (gm.%)
Pretreatment	10.5(4.6–40.0)[a]	350(184–890[b])	40.5(33–50.5)	14.0
Lowest value during treatment	2.2(1.0–5.0)	101(15–217[b])	32.9(26–43.5)	11.4
Typical value 4–8 months posttreatment	6.1(3.7–12.6)	269(123–859)	39.6(32–46)	13.3

Source: Data of Kaplan (1970).
[a] Mean and (range).
[b] After splenectomy.

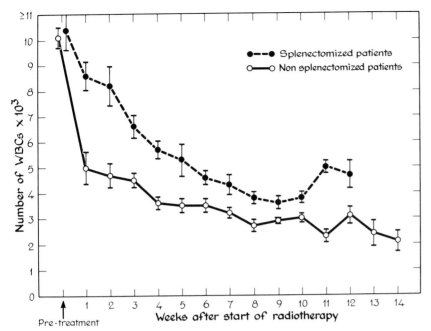

Figure 9.49 Mean white blood cell (WBC) counts before, during, and after total lymphoid radiotherapy in a group of 50 patients subjected to splenectomy prior to treatment, compared with WBC values in a group of 50 patients who did not have splenectomy. (Reprinted, by permission, from Salzman and Kaplan, 1971.)

Higher pretreatment levels for both the white blood cell and platelet count have been consistently observed in patients subjected to splenectomy prior to the initiation of radiotherapy. A detailed analysis (Salzman and Kaplan, 1971) indicates not only that these patients begin radiotherapy with much higher white blood cell and platelet counts, but that their counts are less likely to descend during treatment to levels which require interruption or prolongation of treatment (Figs. 9.49 and 9.50). Similar observations have subsequently been reported by other groups (DiBella, Blom, and Slawson, 1973; Begent and Wiltshaw, 1974).

The hemoglobin concentration and packed red cell volume tend to reach their lowest values near the end of the course of treatment or somewhat thereafter; but the degree of depression is seldom severe, and recovery within a few months is again the rule. Other groups using essentially similar techniques of total lymphoid radiotherapy for patients with Hodgkin's disease have now amply confirmed these hematologic observations (Boutis et al., 1967; Johnson et al., 1969).

Detailed studies have been made of the marrow granulocyte responses to stimulation by etiocholanolone (Vogel et al., 1968) and by preparations

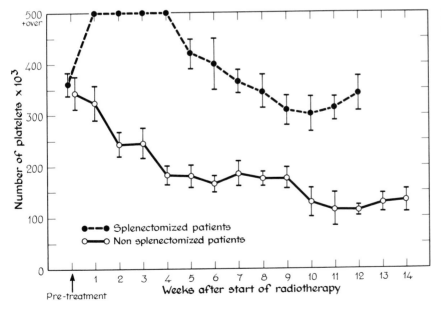

Figure 9.50 Mean platelet counts in the same two groups of patients. (Reprinted, by permission, from Salzman and Kaplan, 1971.)

of bacterial endotoxin (Hellman and Fink, 1965) during mantle field or total lymphoid radiotherapy in patients with previously untreated Hodgkin's disease. In the former study, radiation doses over involved regions were in the range of 3,000 to 4,000 rads, and those over "prophylactic" fields were usually between 2,000 and 3,000 rads delivered at the rate of 1,000 rads per week. Although the impairment of granulocyte mobilization and the reduction of circulating granulocyte and platelet level was somewhat more severe in patients receiving total lymphoid than in those receiving only mantle field irradiation, the return of granulocyte responses to near pretreatment values within five months after therapy was essentially the same in both groups (Fig. 9.51). It was of interest that three patients who failed to respond normally to either etiocholanolone or endotoxin prior to treatment were restored to a state of responsiveness similar to that of other patients after completion of the course of radiotherapy, suggesting that those factors responsible for inhibiting normal granulocyte release mechanisms initially were eliminated or altered by radiotherapy.

Thus, the potential hematopoietic catastrophes which we had anticipated with some dread in 1962 and which have been so much in evidence in chemotherapeutically treated leukemic patients have not materialized. There have been no deaths due to hemorrhage or sepsis in patients with Hodgkin's disease treated at Stanford University Medical Center with total lymphoid megavoltage radiotherapy alone. Indeed, only three of these patients have required hospitalization for transfusion during or subsequent to treatment. Charts of the hematopoietic responses before, during, and after treatment on a number of representative cases treated in that early period are presented in Figures 9.52 to 9.57. Excellent tolerance to subsequently administered chemotherapy may be noted in several of these cases (Figs. 9.58 and 9.59) in which relapses occurred after radiotherapy.

These favorable experiences encouraged us to take the next step and to ascertain whether it was possible to add either fractionated treatment with radioactive gold colloid as described in a preceding section, or six cycles of MOPP combination chemotherapy (De Vita et al., 1970; see Chapter 10) after the completion of total lymphoid radiotherapy. The experimental protocols of these and subsequent clinical trials are described in Chapter 11. It suffices here to state that it has indeed been possible to carry many patients through a complete course of six cycles of chemotherapy, with moder-

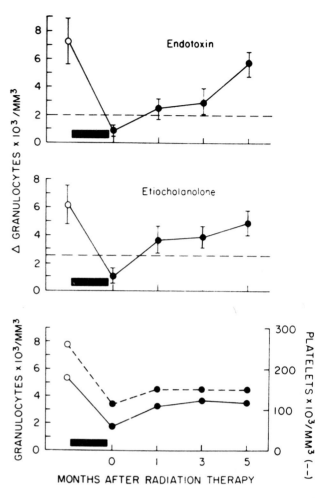

Figure 9.51 Lower panel, peripheral granulocyte (solid line) and platelet (broken line) counts before and after extended field and total lymphoid radiotherapy. The maximum granulocyte increment following administration of etiocholanolone is shown in the middle panel and the response to endotoxin in the upper panel of the figure. The broken lines in the two upper graphs represent the normal responses to each agent; the black bar indicates the duration of radiotherapy; open circles = data before irradiation; closed circles = data after irradiation. (Reprinted, by permission, from the paper by Vogel et al., 1968.)

ate dose reduction of the myelosuppresive drugs in some of the later cycles, after completion of total lymphoid radiotherapy (Bull, DeKiewiet, Rosenberg, and Kaplan, 1970; Moore, Bull, Jones, Rosenberg, and Kaplan, 1972; Rosenberg et al., 1972, 1977).

The administration of four weekly doses of 5 to 10 mCi. each (total 25 to 40 mCi.) of radioactive gold colloid after total lymphoid radiotherapy was also well tolerated by most of our patients, but severe and occasionally long-sustained thrombocyto-

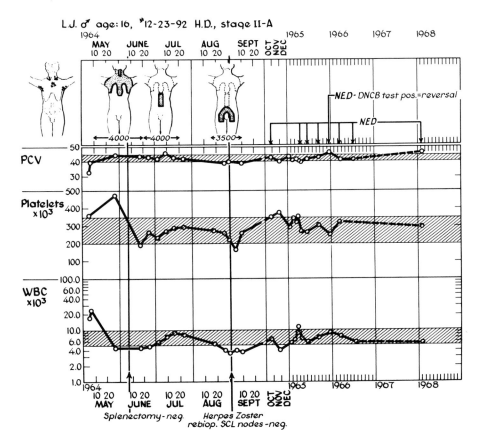

Figure 9.52   L. J., male, age 16, stage IIA. Hematologic responses during and after radiotherapy. The
sites of documented involvement are indicated schematically in this and subsequent examples on the small
manikin at the upper left, followed by diagrams indicating the sequence of fields, time interval, and dose.
PCV = packed red blood cell volume; WBC = white
blood cell count. Note that the time scale has been expanded during periods of active treatment. Repeat
blood cell counts in November 1970 and at irregular
intervals through 1978 were again normal.

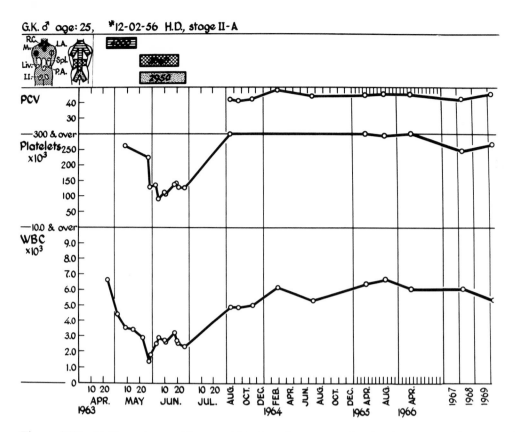

Figure 9.53   G. K., male, age 25, stage IIA. Note how promptly all values returned to normal. He has remained relapse-free and his blood counts have remained normal for more than 15 years.

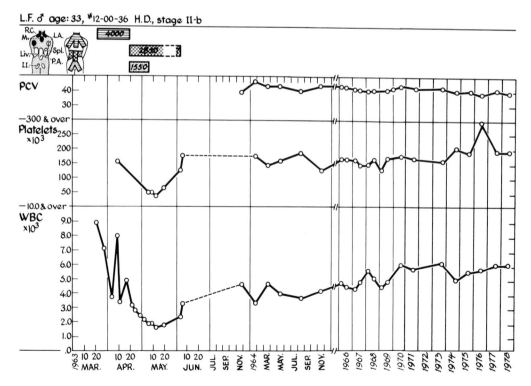

Figure 9.54   L. F., male, age 33, stage IIB. The pelvic field was only carried to 1,500 rads in this early case. Note that his blood counts have remained normal for over 15 years.

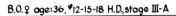

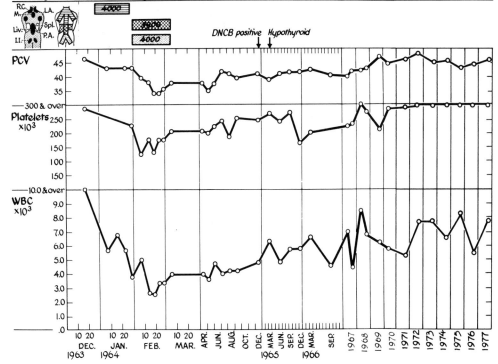

Figure 9.55 B. O., female, age 36, stage IIIA. Note that the delayed hypersensitivity reaction to DNCB, initially anergic, became normal several months after treatment. This patient remained relapse-free for 15 years, and then developed a secondary, non-Hodgkin's (diffuse histiocytic) lymphoma in the thorax.

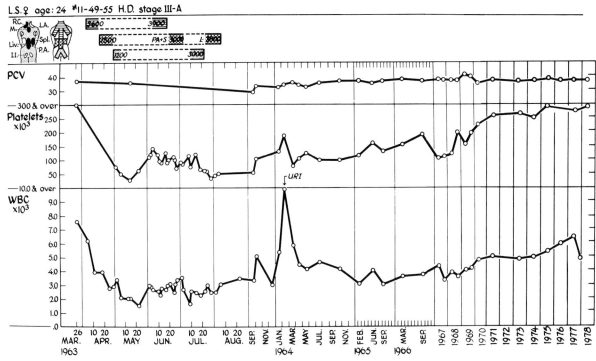

Figure 9.56 L. S., female, age 24, stage III$_s$A. Because of extensive disease both above and below the diaphragm, the mantle, para-aortic, and pelvic fields were not treated to completion in sequence but treated on an alternating schedule, which is less well tolerated hematologically. Nonetheless, the patient was able to respond to an upper respiratory infection (URI) several months later with a sharp increase in white blood cells and in granulocytes. She had mild leukopenia for three years, after which her white blood cell count returned to normal.

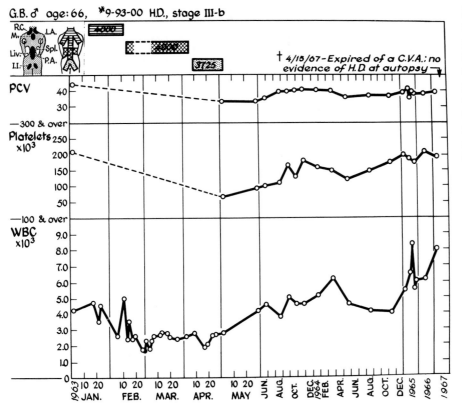

Figure 9.57 G. B., male, age 66, stage IIIB. Despite his age, this patient tolerated total lymphoid radiotherapy reasonably well, except for the slow recovery of his platelet count. He remained free of disease until his death from a cerebrovascular accident 52 months after admission; autopsy revealed no evidence of Hodgkin's disease.

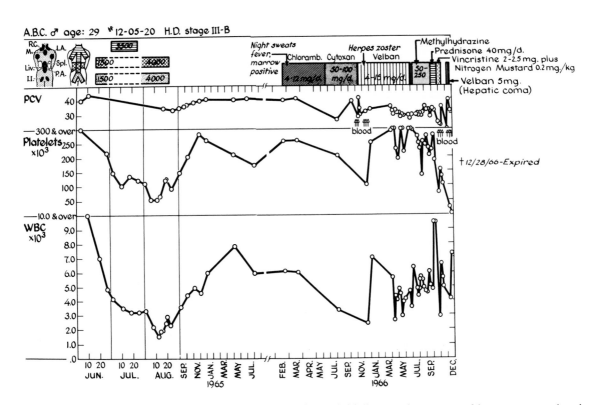

Figure 9.58 A. B. C., male, age 29, stage IIIB. Despite an initially negative marrow biopsy, marrow involvement became clinically evident about 18 months after total lymphoid radiotherapy. Sequential single drug chemotherapy was well tolerated, but the disease progressed despite treatment to a rapidly fatal termination.

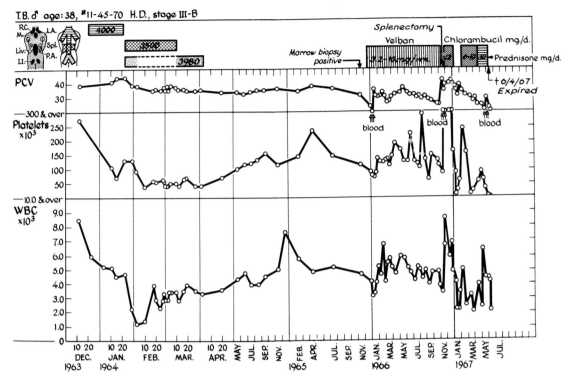

Figure 9.59   T. B., male, age 38, stage IIIB. Occult marrow involvement was also present in this case, with an excellent response to single-drug chemotherapy for nearly 18 months.

penia and moderate leukopenia developed in several others, and in one patient progressed to a fatal termination when further complicated by hemorrhagic gastritis. When the interval between successive doses of radioactive gold colloid was increased to two weeks, the frequency of these serious hematologic reactions was sharply reduced. The possible desirability of direct introduction of radioactive gold colloid or radioactive microspheres into the portal vein, either via intrasplenic injection immediately prior to splenectomy or by percutaneous puncture, or via an intra-arterial catheter into the hepatic artery (Simon et al., 1971), deserves further investigation to ascertain whether a greater percentage of the injected isotope could thus be deposited in the liver and less in the bone marrow.

Complications of Radiotherapy

Complications of radiotherapy, as distinguished from manifestations of acute morbidity described above, are expressed as signs and symptoms of impaired function due to radiation-induced injury of normal tissues, becoming manifest at any time after treatment. Fortunately, only a small proportion of these are major complications, causing severe, permanent disability or even death; the great majority are minor in severity and transient. Complication rates have also been sharply reduced by treatment of both anterior and posterior fields daily (Marks, Agarwal, and Constable, 1973), split course regimens (Landberg, Lidén, and Forslo, 1973; Johnson et al., 1976), and refinements of technique such as the "thin" lung blocks and subcarinal blocks described earlier in this chapter.

Respiratory System. The pathology and clinical features of radiation pneumonitis have been described (Rubin and Casarett, 1968; Gross, 1977). Typically, there is little or no clinical or roentgenographic evidence of pulmonary radiation reaction until two or three months after the completion of treatment to the mantle field, although a small proportion of cases may develop immediately after completion of radiotherapy or as late as five years thereafter (Carmel and Kaplan, 1976). The mediastinal silhouette on conventional chest roentgenograms begins to assume a somewhat less well-defined, shaggy appearance, and irregular strands of density appear in the paramediastinal pulmonary parenchyma in a zone which usually corresponds quite closely to the size and shape of the mediastinal field (Fig. 9.60; Libshitz, Brosof, and

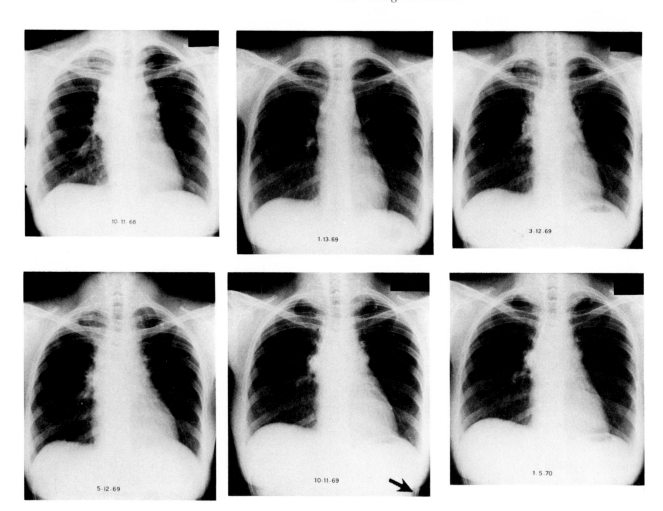

Figure 9.60   Radiographic evolution of paramediastinal postirradiation pulmonary fibrosis. This 32-year-old fe-male patient had severe generalized itching which was ascribed to various dermatoses for two years, until a pre-em-ployment chest X-ray (10/11/68) revealed a large mediastinal mass and supraclavicular node biopsy showed nodular sclerosing Hodgkin's disease. The film of 1/13/69 was made just after a dose of 4,400 rads had been delivered to the mantle field and shows marked regression of the mass, with little or no pulmonary reaction. By 3/12/69, irregu-lar, shaggy infiltrative strands had appeared in the paramediastinal pulmonary parenchyma, and the mediastinal silhouette seemed once again to be growing wider. This process reached its peak on the film of 5/12/69, at which time the mediastinum was almost as wide as it had been before treatment. However, the fibrotic and inflammatory, rather than neoplastic, nature of the process was clearly revealed by the decrease in width and sharper outline of the mediastinum on the films of 10/11/69 and 1/5/70. In March 1969, the patient became short of breath and de-veloped a troublesome cough. After a severe bout of coughing in October 1969, she felt a sharp, persistent pain in the lower left chest, demonstrated on the film of 10/11/69 to be due to a rib fracture (arrow). Her symptoms were relieved by steroids, administration of which was tapered very slowly and carefully until January 1970, since which time she has remained symptom-free.

Southard, 1973). During this time, the patient may have virtually no symptoms; more often, a dry hacking cough is likely to develop and may, in some instances, be accompanied by dyspnea on ex-ertion or, less commonly, at rest.

The frequency with which radiation pneumo-nitis is observed in various centers depends strongly on the sensitivity of the diagnostic criteria by which the condition is defined. In a recent Stan-ford study, Carmel and Kaplan (1976) defined the syndrome of symptomatic pulmonary radiation reaction (SPRR) as: otherwise unexplained cough, shortness of breath, dyspnea on exertion, and/or pleurisy on at least two follow-up clinic visits. The symptoms and signs observed in 75 patients with SPRR are presented in Table 9.9. Physiological studies during this time may reveal some decrease of vital capacity and other parameters of pulmo-

Table 9.9 Symptoms and Signs of Symptomatic
Pulmonary Radiation Reaction in 75 Patients

Symptoms and Signs	Patients
Shortness of breath or dyspnea on exertion	57
Cough	50
Pleurisy	6
Cyanosis	0
Fever	1
Hemoptysis	1
Pleural rub	1
Decreased breath sounds	2
Rales	2
Radiographic signs of pneumonitis	67

Source: Stanford University Medical Center data of Carmel
and Kaplan (1976).

nary function (Høst and Vale, 1973; Lokich, Galvanek, and Moloney, 1973; Evans et al., 1974). In
cases of mild to moderate severity, the cough and
mild dyspnea on exertion will usually last for two
to four months and then gradually disappear, requiring no specific treatment. In our experience,
when this type of mild reaction clears, it clears permanently, leaving behind only slight roentgenographic changes indicative of paramediastinal fibrosis, sometimes accompanied by elevation of the
hila, pulled up by fibrotic strands in the upper pulmonary lobes. The mediastinum tends to become
somewhat wider as a consequence of the blending
of the paramediastinal zone of pulmonary fibrosis
and atelectasis with the previous silhouette of the
mediastinum proper (Fig. 9.60). It is important not
to confuse this widened mediastinal silhouette due
to radiation fibrosis with recrudescence of Hodgkin's disease. We have seen a few tragic instances in
which misinterpretation of the widened mediastinal shadow had led to a second, quite unnecessary course of radiotherapy to the mediastinum,
with serious and even fatal consequences. In such
instances, it is best to wait and to follow the patient
with chest roentgenograms at serial intervals. If
the process involves fibrosis, it will tend to shrink
with time, whereas lymphomatous recurrences will
inevitably grow and cause progressive widening of
the mediastinum.

Severe cases of radiation pneumonitis are much
more likely to occur when very large mediastinal
masses must be irradiated, thus permitting only a
negligible volume of lung to be shielded, or when
the entire lung is treated prophylactically because
of the presence of hilar lymphadenopathy. Such
cases may begin insidiously but increase rapidly in
severity, usually accompanied by the development

of diffuse infiltrating densities of linear and mottled character in the affected segments or lobes of
one or both lungs. Intractable cough, dyspnea,
fever, and air hunger severe enough to require administration of oxygen may develop, and cyanosis
may supervene if both lungs are affected. If such
patients survive, they are likely to have a prolonged convalescence and to manifest significant
impairment of pulmonary ventilatory capacity
long after the acute process has subsided (Slanina
et al., 1977). Extensive distortion of one or both
lungs by fibrotic strands and secondary atelectasis
are seen on the roentgenograms (Fig. 9.61). Such
distorted, scarred lungs are vulnerable to repeated
bouts of pneumonitis, often associated with
progressive bronchiectasis. These patients are
likely ultimately to succumb to a combination of recurrent infection and progressive pulmonary insufficiency.

The risk of significant radiation pneumonitis
depends on total radiation dose and dose rate (Jen-

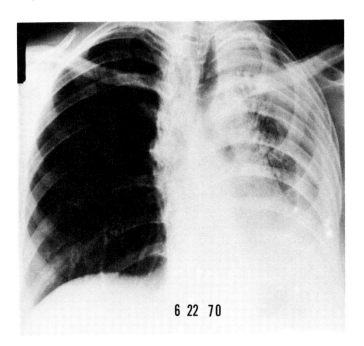

Figure 9.61 Severe unilateral pulmonary radiation fibrosis in a 30-year-old female with Hodgkin's disease
involving the cervical, supraclavicular, mediastinal, and
left hilar nodes and with nodular lesions in the left
mid-lung. In October 1966 she was given a dose of
4,400 rads over a mantle field with the left lung block
omitted for two-thirds of the treatments and a narrow
lung block for the remainder. Though she was severely
dyspneic for several months, she is now asymptomatic
and remains free of disease. Note the shift of the heart
and mediastinum into the left hemithorax and the
compensatory hyperaeration of the right lung.

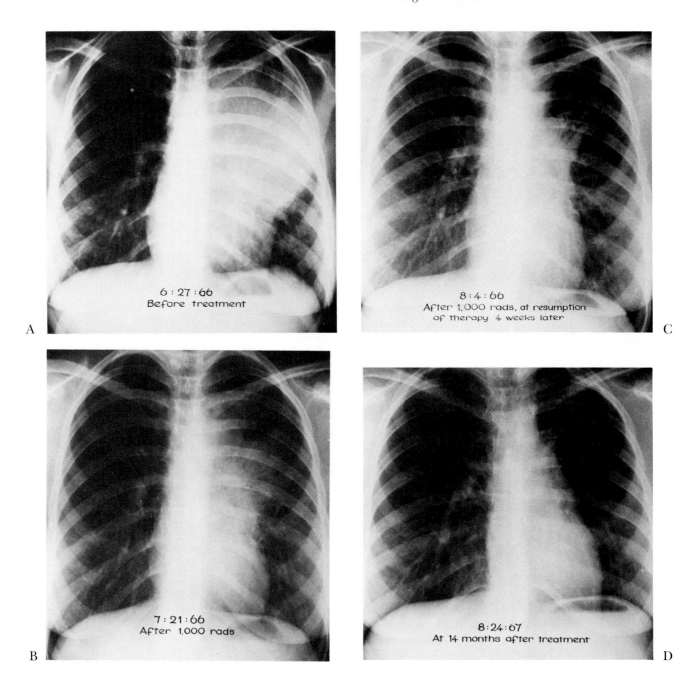

Figure 9.62 Split course technique used for very large mediastinal masses. *A*, pretreatment film, revealing huge mediastinal and left hilar mass invading out into the parenchyma of the left upper lobe. *B*, chest film one week after a midplane dose of 1,000 rads had been given to the mantle field, omitting the left lung block. *C*, chest film four weeks after a dose of 1,000 rads, at which time treatment to the mantle was resumed, using a tightly masked left lung block. *D*, chest film 14 months later, showing minimal fibrosis and distortion of the left hilar and paramediastinal silhouette. The patient had no respiratory symptoms at any time after treatment and remains free of disease, with unimpaired exercise tolerance, to the present time. (Reprinted, by permission, from Kaplan and Rosenberg, 1968.)

nings and Arden, 1962; Phillips and Margolis, 1972; Wara et al., 1973), and on the volume of lung included in the high-dose region. When mediastinal adenopathy is minimal or absent, and the mediastinum can therefore be very tightly masked, permitting most of both lungs to be shielded, the risk of significant pneumonitis is minimal. Lassvik, Rosengren, and Wranne (1977) found no evidence of impairment of pulmonary gas exchange or spirometric function in any of eight patients with Hodgkin's disease who had received mediastinal doses of 4,000–4,600 rads in six weeks. However, when massive mediastinal lymphadenopathy must be treated, the volume of lung that can be shielded is correspondingly smaller, and the risk appreciably greater (Carmel and Kaplan, 1976). In this situation, we have since 1966 made effective use of the split-course technique, in which a small fraction of the anticipated total dose, on the order of 1,000 to 1,500 rads, is delivered over the entire silhouette of the large mediastinal mass, and then treatment is interrupted for one to three weeks, while the regression of the mediastinal mass is followed on serial chest roentgenograms. When regression is dramatic and rapid, as is usually the case, treatment can usually be resumed in one to three weeks, using much larger lung-shielding blocks and masking the much smaller mediastinal mass rather closely. With this variation in technique, even massive mediastinal lesions can be treated effectively with little or no subsequent pulmonary functional impairment (Fig. 9.62; also cf. Fig. 5.1).

An analysis of the incidence of radiation pneumonitis observed in patients treated at Stanford University Medical Center between January 1964 and June 1969 is presented in Table 9.10. A single course of treatment to the mediastinum usually entailed a dose of 4,000 to 4,400 rads in approximately four weeks. It may be noted that 16 (6.4 percent) of 248 patients who received only a single course of treatment to the mediastinum alone developed radiation pneumonitis (Kaplan and Stewart, 1973). Nine of these cases were scored as mild to moderate in severity; of the remaining seven severe cases, one (0.25 percent) was fatal. The risk of significant radiation pneumonitis was appreciably greater when the mediastinum received two or more courses of treatment; in six of forty-one such cases (15 percent) radiation pneumonitis developed, which was severe in five and fatal in one. Finally, the risk was greatest of all when one or both lungs were treated either therapeutically, for demonstrable pulmonary infiltrations due to Hodgkin's disease, or prophylactically in patients with significant hilar lymphadenopathy. Of sixty-nine patients who had treatment to one or both lungs, usually to a dose of approximately

Table 9.10 Incidence of Radiation Pneumonitis after One Course of Radiotherapy for Hodgkin's Disease

Time interval	Area treated	No. of patients at risk	Radiation pneumonitis	
			No.	%
Jan. 1964	Mediastinum Only	248	16[a]	6
to	Mediastinum and One or Both Lungs	69	23[b]	33
June 1969				
	Totals	317	39	12
Jan. 1969	Mediastinum Only	66	0	0
to	Mediastinum and One or Both Lungs[c]	37	0	0
June 1970				
	Totals	103	0	0

Source: Stanford University Medical Center data of Kaplan and Stewart (1973).

[a] One of these was fatal.

[b] Four of these were fatal.

[c] Most of these patients were given a lung dose of 1500 rads in 4 weeks using the "thin lung block" technique.

1,500 rads in ten to twelve days, twenty-three (33 percent) developed radiation pneumonitis. Although most of these cases were only of mild to moderate severity, eight were quite severe and four were fatal (5.8 percent). This relatively high incidence after whole-lung irradiation may be due in part to the fact that the dose transmitted through and scattered around the lung-shielding blocks was not taken into consideration and in part to the use of a relatively high dose rate (1,100 rads per week) in these cases. More recently, we have limited the total lung dose to 1,650 rads, and reduced the dose rate to 75 rads per day, five days per week, using the "thin block" technique described above (Palos, Kaplan, and Karzmark, 1971). A diagrammatic comparison of the old and new mantle techniques (Fig. 9.63) reveals that a marked decrease in the risk of pneumonitis and pericarditis has been achieved. Moreover, the few cases that have been observed have been relatively mild; there have been no instances of severe radiation pneumonitis in patients who had treatment to one or both entire lungs with these reduced dose rates. The risk of SPRR is also a function of total radiation dose. In an analysis of 377 mantle field–treated patients, Carmel and Kaplan (1976) found that SPRR occurred in 45 (16 percent) of 274 pa-

tients whose lungs were shielded throughout, and therefore were exposed only to scattered radiation plus the 6 percent primary transmission through the lead blocks, yielding a whole lung dose ≤ 599 rads (Table 9.11). As lung dose increased above 600 rads, the risk of SPRR increased to 29 percent.

The role of steroids in the treatment of acute radiation pneumonitis remains controversial (Moss et al, 1960). Only 15 of 75 patients with SPRR required steroids, and 55 required no treatment whatever (Carmel and Kaplan, 1976). It has been our policy to use steroids only in those patients whose symptoms of cough and dyspnea are at least moderately severe. Although there is no convincing evidence that steroids play a really important role in such instances, we have observed dramatic and almost catastrophic effects of the sudden interruption of steroid therapy, once started, in patients who have significant radiation reactions in the lung. In most instances, such sudden cessation of steroid therapy has resulted from a misunderstanding on the part of either the patient or the referring physician. Within one to three days after the last dose of steroid, there has been a fulminating onset of severe cough, profound dyspnea, cyanosis, and a diffuse, dense flocculant infiltration in one or more lobes of the lung, depending

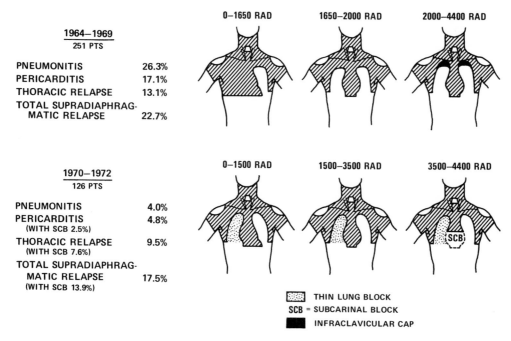

Figure 9.63 Comparative risks of symptomatic radiation pneumonitis and pericarditis, and relative relapse rates with the old high-dose-rate technique of pulmonary irradiation during mantle field irradiation (*upper row*) and the new "thin lung block", low-dose-rate technique (*lower row*). None of the cases of pneumonitis or pericarditis developing in patients treated with the new technique was severe, and there were no fatalities due to these complications in this group. (Reprinted, with slight modifications, from the paper by Carmel and Kaplan, 1976.)

Table 9.11   Symptomatic Pulmonary Radiation Reaction (SPRR) as a Function of Dose to One or Both Lungs in 377 Patients with Hodgkin's Disease

	Radiation dose (rad)			
	≤599	600–1500	1501–3000	>3000
Lung irradiation	274	66	36	1
SPRR[a]	45 (16)	20 (30)	9 (25)	1
SPRR requiring treatment[a]	7 (2.6)	8 (12)	4 (11)	1

Source: Stanford University Medical Center data (Carmel and Kaplan, 1976).

[a] Number of patients in group; percentage of total number in parentheses.

on the previous extent of the radiation treatment fields, and even extending out into segments of lung which were not irradiated (Figs. 9.64, 9.65). Such patients sometimes must be hospitalized, treated with oxygen, and promptly treated with steroids again.

As a consequence of several such cases which have come to our attention (Castellino et al., 1974b), it is now our policy to stress the importance of extremely gradual tapering of steroid therapy if it is once initiated. We usually begin with a dose of about 40 mg. of prednisone daily, which is continued for at least three to four months, after which tapering of the dose is begun at a rate not in excess of 2.5 mg. per week. It is important to explain this carefully, not only to the patient but also to the referring physician, to avoid accidental interruption of steroid therapy due to misunderstanding.

Cardiovascular System. The clinical, pathologic, and radiologic features of a series of cases of radiation-induced heart disease observed at Stanford University Medical Center have been previously described (Cohn et al, 1967; Stewart et al., 1967; Fajardo et al., 1968). Although acute pericarditis developed during the course of radiation therapy in two patients with Hodgkin's disease, these instances were not believed to have been specifically attributable to radiation injury; moreover, in both cases, treatment was continued to a dose of 4,000 rads without further incident. If these two cases are excluded, then all of the other cases observed to date have occurred at doses above 3,500 rads, delivered at the rate of 1,000 to 1,100 rads per week. However, this may not represent a true threshold dose for the induction of radiogenic heart disease, since the sample population of patients treated over the heart and mediastinum at lower dose levels was not sufficiently large to per-

mit detection of a small incidence of such cardiac complications.

Radiation injury to the heart was manifested in a variety of ways. Perhaps the most common was acute pericarditis, often associated with pericardial effusion and sometimes with signs of tamponade. Although most of these cases spontaneously regressed under conservative medical management, a few went on to chronic pericardial effusion or to chronic constrictive pericarditis, sometimes requiring pericardiectomy for relief (Cohn et al., 1967; Masland et al., 1968). Some patients have been reported to respond well to treatment with corticosteroids (Keelan and Rudders, 1974). In some of the more severe instances, there was electrocardiographic, biopsy, or autopsy evidence of myocardial and/or endocardial fibrosis or fibroelastosis. Acute pericarditis developed in thirteen patients within five to forty-eight months after completion of radiotherapy, the great majority of cases appearing within one year. Clinical manifestations usually included fever, pleuritic chest pain, pericardial friction rubs, low voltage and other electrocardiographic abnormalities, radiographic enlargement of the cardiac silhouette, and ultrasound or other evidence of pericardial effusion. The presence of neck-vein engorgement and a paradoxical pulse were noted in several cases, providing evidence of tamponade. These observations have now been confirmed by several other groups (Byhardt et al., 1975; Ruckdeschel et al., 1975; Chebat et al., 1977; Geslin et al., 1977; Markiewicz et al., 1977; Nordman, 1977).

In the first compilation of cases by Stewart et al. (1967) 8 instances of heart disease were encountered among 120 cases of Hodgkin's disease available for assessment, including the 2 above-mentioned cases of acute pericarditis developing during treatment, which were not deemed to be

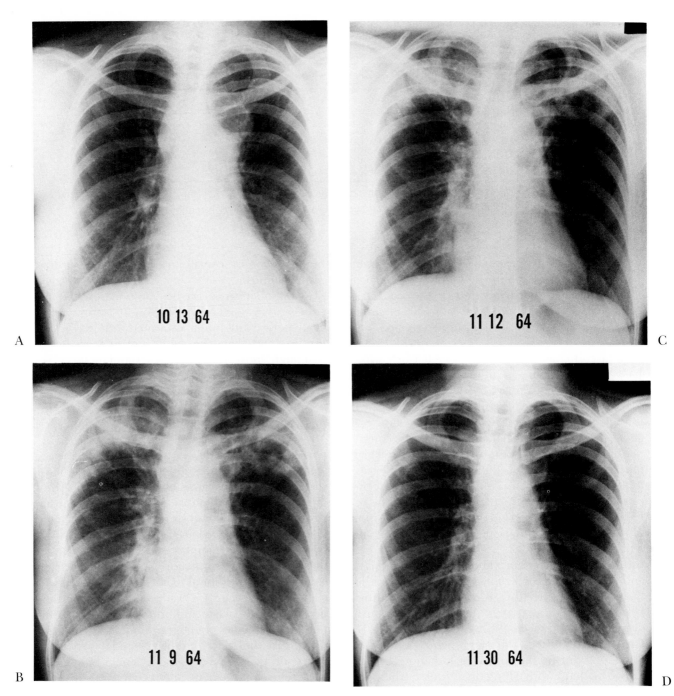

A

B

C

D

10 13 64

11 9 64

11 12 64

11 30 64

Figure 9.64 This young female patient had a biopsy diagnosis of Hodgkin's disease made in Brazil. She was placed on steroids (without any evident indication) and referred to Stanford. *A*, the chest film on admission (10/13/64) revealed a superior mediastinal mass and clear lung fields. Mantle field treatment was started two weeks later, after all staging procedures had been completed, and the steroid therapy was rapidly tapered. *B*, two days after steroid therapy was discontinued (11/9/64) at a radiation dose of only 1,200 rads to the midplane, she was readmitted with severe acute respiratory distress and cyanosis requiring oxygen, and a chest film revealed flocculent, hazy infiltrates in both upper lobes and at the right cardiopulmonary border. Cultures were negative, and there was no leukocytosis. *C*, steroid therapy was reinitiated, with prompt relief of respiratory distress and rapid resolution of the infiltrative process on a repeat film (11/12/64). *D*, the patient was then maintained on steroids without further incident during the rest of her mantle field treatment, at the end of which (11/30/64) there had been almost complete disappearance of the mass, and the lung fields were again clear. Steroid therapy was very slowly and cautiously tapered thereafter without difficulty.

truly radiation-induced cases. In a later analysis by Kaplan and Stewart (1973) of 592 patients who received only one course of treatment of the mediastinum, to a dose of 4,000 to 4,400 rads in approximately four weeks, a total of 32 cases of radiation-induced heart disease were recorded (5.4 percent). Of these, sixteen were clinically asymptomatic and detected only by virtue of roentgenographic evidence of cardiomegaly; in all of these patients the heart has subsequently become normal, either spontaneously or after a brief period of bed rest. Nine other patients had mild to moderate symptoms, but these were also reversible (cf. Fig. 5.38). Only seven cases were classifiable as clinically severe; four of these progressed to chronic constrictive pericarditis requiring surgery, and one case (0.3 percent) proved fatal. Some of these reactions were apparently triggered by acute steroid withdrawal (Castellino et al., 1974). As in the case of radiation-induced pneumonitis, patients requiring repeated courses of irradiation to the mediastinal area had a much higher incidence of radiation-induced heart disease. Of forty-one patients who received two or more courses of treatment over the mediastinum, eight (19.5 percent) developed radiation-induced heart disease, which was scored as mild to moderate in severity in three instances and severe in five, three (7.3 percent) of which later proved fatal. Pericardiectomy for alleviation of constrictive manifestations was required in two of the five severe cases. Defining radiation pericarditis as: significant enlargement of the cardiac silhouette on at least two sequential follow-up chest radiograms, a pericardial effusion on an echocardiogram, pericardial fibrosis on a biopsy, constrictive pericarditis documented by cardiac catheterization, and/or a pericardial friction rub, Carmel and Kaplan (1976) scored a total of 49 patients (13 percent of a series of 377 patients treated with mantle radiotherapy) as having developed radiation pericarditis. The interval between mantle treatment and the development of this complication ranged from 0 to 85 months, with a median of 9 months. When the entire pericardium was included in the radiation field, the incidence was 20 percent, whereas when a portion of the heart was shielded, it was 7 percent. The risk was dose-related (Table 9.12); of 240 patients who received doses to the entire heart of up to 1,500 rads, pericarditis occurred in only 19 (7.9 percent) and required treatment in only 7 (2.9 percent), whereas at doses ranging from 1,501 to over 3,000 rads, this complication developed in 30 (21.9 percent) of 137 patients, and 9.5 percent required treatment. At the National Cancer Institute, a much higher incidence (26 percent) was observed when a single course was delivered entirely via an anterior field, resulting in a significantly higher cardiac dose (Pierce et al., 1969). It is encouraging that only two of more than 400 patients treated at Stanford with the subcarinal block technique (Fig. 9.19) have developed radiation pericarditis, which in both instances was limited to asymptomatic cardiomegaly (Carmel and Kaplan, 1976).

There is also fragmentary evidence that arterial vascular injury may occur following mantle irradiation. The development of coronary arterial disease with precocious myocardial infarction has now been reported several times. The patient described by Ali et al. (1976) was 24 years of age; the two patients described by McReynolds, Gold, and Roberts (1976) were 33 and 42 years old; and the youngest such patient observed by the author (Kaplan, unpublished) was a 14-year-old boy who died of myocardial infarction about two years after mantle treatment. Other such cases have been cited by Prentice (1965), Dollinger, Lavine, and Foye (1966), Rogers (1976), and Carmel and Kap-

Table 9.12 Radiation Pericarditis as a Function of Dose to the Whole Pericardium

	Radiation Dose (rad)			
	≤599	600–1500	1501–3000	>3000
Pericardial irradiation	198	42	123	14
Pericarditis[a]	14 (7)	5 (12)	23 (19)	7 (50)
Pericarditis requiring treatment[a]	3 (1.5)	4 (9.5)	8 (6.5)	5 (36)

Source: Stanford University Medical Center data (Carmel and Kaplan, 1976).

[a] Number of patients in group; percentage of total number in parentheses.

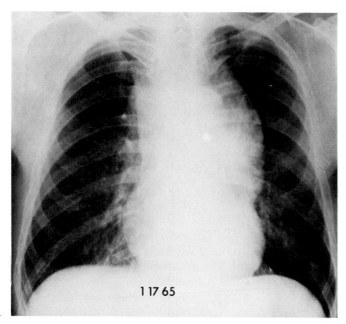

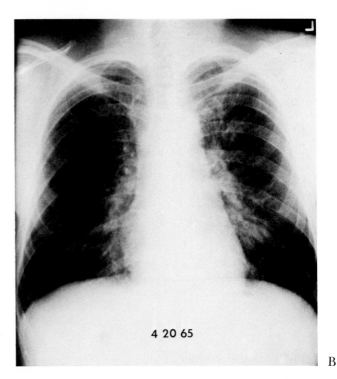

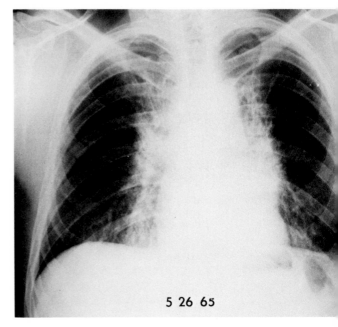

A

B

Figure 9.65   Radiation pneumonitis severely exacerbated by sudden cessation of steroid therapy. *A*, pretreatment chest film (1/17/65). Huge mediastinal and left hilar mass in a 37-year-old male with stage II-B Hodgkin's disease. The entire left lung was treated to 1,500 rads with the mantle. *B*, post-treatment chest film of 4/20/65; marked regression of the mediastinal and hilar masses is apparent, with some paramediastinal pulmonary radiation reaction. Although the patient was asymptomatic, he was placed on steroid therapy prophylactically. *C*, through a misunderstanding, the patient abruptly stopped taking his steroid medication four weeks after it was started, and within 72 hours he was in severe respiratory distress and coughing continuously. Chest film (5/26/65) revealed a shaggy paramediastinal pulmonary infiltrate, roughly corresponding to the mediastinal silhouette of his mantle field. *D*, steroid therapy was immediately reinitiated, with moderately rapid symptomatic relief, though dyspnea on exertion persisted for several months. The chest film of 7/12/65 showed a dense, sharply outlined paramediastinal fibrotic process, with some reaction also appearing along the left diaphragmatic pleura, which was included in the upper margin of the spleen field. *E*, steroid therapy was cautiously tapered over several months without incident, during which time dyspnea gradually disappeared and a surprisingly good degree of exercise tolerance returned. Although his later chest films (11/10/69) remained abnormal due to paramediastinal fibrosis, the patient remained disease-free and had no respiratory symptoms until the time of his death, apparently due to myocardial infarction, in 1977.

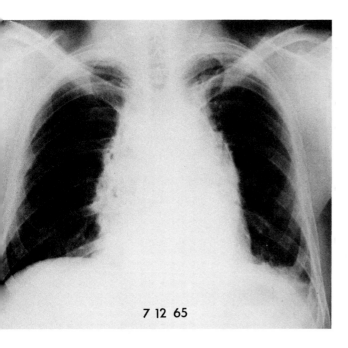

7 12 65

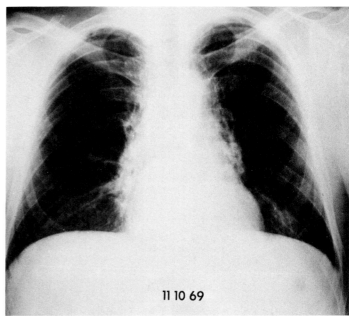

11 10 69

E

lan (1976). Weinstein, Greenwald, and Grossman (1976) described an unusual case of a 27-year-old patient with Hodgkin's disease who was treated with mantle irradiation followed by cycles of MOPP combination chemotherapy, each of which triggered episodes of chest pain, the first of which clinically resembled a myocardial infarction. An isolated instance of fatal aorto-duodenal fistula following abdominal irradiation for Hodgkin's disease has been reported by Zarembok and Brace (1972). Heidenberg, Lupovitch, and Tarr (1966) have reported a case of "pulseless" disease, apparently caused by radiotherapy, in a twenty-one-year-old white female with Hodgkin's disease, who received intensive radiotherapy over the mediastinal and supraclavicular regions in 1953. By February 1962, examination revealed no detectable pulse or blood pressure in either arm. The patient later developed an extradural extension of her Hodgkin's disease and died in March 1965, despite additional radiotherapy.

Nervous System. The neurologic complications of Hodgkin's disease and/or its radiotherapy in a Stanford series of 592 patients are presented in Table 9.13. Ninety-one patients with herpes zoster (17 percent) are listed here, though many of these cases may have been attributable to the enhanced susceptibility associated with Hodgkin's disease or to chemotherapy, rather than to radiotherapy. Although there has been no documented instance of

radiation-induced transverse myelitis in our experience, occasional cases have been reported from other institutions. Castaigne et al. (1970) described the clinical and histopathologic features of four cases occurring after radiotherapy of Hodgkin's disease, and reviewed published information on 274 patients with radiation-induced myelopathy. Two additional cases were recorded by Slanina et al. (1977). It is very likely that most such instances are traceable to errors in technique. For example, the gap left at the skin level to permit matching of the adjacent mantle and subdiaphragmatic fields in the midplane may have been insufficient, thus possibly resulting in a small zone of high-dose overlap. To minimize radiation dose to the spinal cord, we have routinely shielded the cervical cord posteriorly from the beginning of mantle therapy and

Table 9.13 Neurologic Complications of Hodgkin's Disease and Its Treatment in 592 Patients

Complication	No.	%
Lhermitte's syndrome	62	11
Herpes zoster	91	18
Localized peripheral neuropathy	5	0.9
Radiation-induced transverse myelitis	1	0.15
Severe motor disturbance ("chronic Guillain-Barre" syndrome)	3	0.5
Cerebellar dysfunction	1	0.15

Source: Stanford University Medical Center data (Kaplan and Stewart, 1973).

have added a posterior shielding block for the dorsal spinal cord after a dose of 2,000 rads has been delivered. More recently, we have also added an upper lumbar shielding block, extending down to the lower margin of the first lumbar vertebra (Fig. 9.29), after a dose of 2,000 rads has been delivered to an inverted-Y or spade field to provide further protection against any possible hazard of an incorrectly calculated gap. With these precautions and refinements of technique, transverse myelitis should not constitute a significant hazard in patients with Hodgkin's disease treated with a single course of megavoltage radiotherapy to fields above and below the diaphragm to doses in the range of 4,000 rads, delivered at a dose-rate of approximately 1,000 rads per week. When areas that have been previously irradiated develop new manifestations of disease requiring additional radiotherapy traversing the cervical or dorsal spinal cord, the hazard of transverse myelitis becomes a serious consideration, which must be carefully weighed by the radiotherapist against the anticipated benefits of treatment to the patient. Three of our patients developed a complication, designated as "chronic Guillain-Barré syndrome" by our neurologic consultants, characterized by lower extremity paresis or paralysis coupled with lower motor neuron signs, which was probably not due to radiation injury. Two of these three cases resolved spontaneously.

A curious syndrome, originally described by the French neurologist Lhermitte in cases of multiple sclerosis, has now been observed as a transient complication of radiotherapy. Patients complain of numbness, tingling, or "electric" sensations in the upper and/or lower extremities and sometimes also in the lower back, which may be present more or less continuously, but are sharply exacerbated by flexion of the head and neck; more often, patients are asymptomatic except when they sharply flex the head and neck, at which time they immediately experience the sensation of numbness, tingling, or electric shock radiating into the extremities or back. In a series of 592 patients with Hodgkin's disease who received all of their radiotherapy at Stanford University Medical Center, there were sixty-two recorded instances of Lhermitte's syndrome, an incidence of 11 percent (Kaplan and Stewart, 1973). A later analysis of our data revealed an incidence of 15 percent (Carmel and Kaplan, 1976). In no case was there any associated motor weakness or disability, and neurologic examination was not remarkable. Symptoms developed within 1 to 29

months (median 4 months) after the completion of radiotherapy, were sustained for 2 to 8 months (median 5.3 months), and then gradually disappeared, leaving no residual neurologic abnormality or impairment, except for the three above-cited patients who developed Guillain-Barré syndrome.

Although the cause of the Lhermitte syndrome is not established, Jones (1964), in a scholarly analysis, suggested that it may well be due to temporary radiation-induced inhibition of the normal proliferation cycle of spinal cord oligodendrocytes, with ensuing transient demyelination of nerve fibers in the cord, most probably in the posterior columns, lateral spinothalamic tracts, or both. Fortunately, the syndrome is self-limited and reversible and is thus considered a minor complication, though sufficiently alarming that patients should be appropriately cautioned about the possibility of its occurrence.

In some patients with nodular sclerosis treated with a single course, and in others receiving multiple courses of irradiation to the same region for recurrent Hodgkin's disease, intense fibrosis and cicatricial changes in the subcutaneous and deeper tissues may occur, sometimes with compression of peripheral nerves traversing the region, leading to the development of peripheral neuropathy. This complication has occurred in five instances to date (0.9 percent). Several cases of brachial plexus palsy due to radiation injury have been described by Slanina et al. (1977).

Liver. The syndrome of radiation hepatitis has been described by Ingold et al. (1964). Its incidence is dose-dependent, with an apparent threshold at 2,500 to 3,000 rads to the entire liver. It develops within a few weeks to a few months after completion of radiotherapy; the liver becomes enlarged and frequently somewhat tender, and ascites of variable severity commonly appears, usually unaccompanied by jaundice. The serum alkaline phosphatase level becomes elevated, and the bromsulphalein retention test becomes abnormal. Other liver function tests are more variable in response but may also exhibit abnormality. In reversible cases, these manifestations are sustained for several weeks or months and then gradually disappear. In the severe cases intractable ascites and electrolyte disturbances develop and may progress to a fatal termination.

In many respects, the hazard of radiation hepatitis can be said to have vanished with the recognition of the fact that a hazard existed. The liver was formerly thought to be quite radioresistant, and it was not until the advent of megavoltage radiotherapy encouraged efforts to control disease in the liver by whole-liver irradiation to relatively high doses that this was shown to be a misconception. It is now clear that the hazard of radiation hepatitis can be obviated if either of two conditions can be satisfied: some substantial fraction of the liver must be left unirradiated or, if the entire liver must be irradiated, the radiation dose should be kept under 2,500 rads, delivered at the rate of approximately 1,000 rads per week. Although the chance of clinically significant radiation hepatitis occurring at doses less than 3,000 rads is small, it is not zero. We have seen two documented instances of clinically apparent radiation hepatitis at doses of 2,500 and 2,750 rads, respectively. In one other instance, in a patient coming to autopsy three years after a dose of 2,000 rads to the entire liver, mild radiation changes were detectable at postmortem examination. In a series of 23 patients with stage III Hodgkin's disease treated by Poussin-Rosillo, Nisce, and D'Angio (1976) with a modified "3 and 2" technique which delivered a dose of 2,000 rads in ten days to the entire liver, and an additional 1,800–2,000 rads to the left lobe, elevated levels of serum alkaline phosphatase were observed in 18 (78 percent) and of glutamic-oxaloacetic transaminase in 8 (35 percent). The abnormal serum enzyme levels appeared within 3 to 12 months (median 5 months) after radiotherapy and persisted for 3 to 23 months (median 10 months). However, none of these patients had clinically overt radiation hepatitis.

We have investigated the possibility of using radioactive colloidal gold to replace part or all of the external radiotherapy required for the treatment of established or suspected Hodgkin's disease of the liver, as described earlier in this chapter (Kaplan and Bagshaw, 1968). However, two of the long-term survivors who received massive single doses of radioactive gold colloid for proved Hodgkin's disease of the liver subsequently developed hepatic fibrosis with ascites, which was readily controlled with diuretics. We therefore tried split-course combined external and internal radiotherapy, giving 1,000 rads in one week, then a rest period of two weeks, and then another 1,000 rads, followed by three or four doses of [198]Au of 5–10 mCi each at two-week intervals (Kraut, Kaplan, and Bagshaw, 1972). However, as indicated earlier in this chapter, enough of the radioactive gold colloid reached the bone marrow in these patients to interfere with

subsequent MOPP combination chemotherapy in those patients who later relapsed. Accordingly, it is our current policy to use external radiotherapy alone over the entire liver in patients with laparotomy-documented involvement of the liver or spleen and to deliver a dose of 2,200 rads in four to five weeks through a 50 percent transmission lead block (Schultz, Glatstein, and Kaplan, 1975). This is supplemented by adjuvant combination chemotherapy in those instances in which stage IV disease involving the liver is known to be present. We have observed moderate transient elevations of serum alkaline phosphatase levels in patients treated by this technique, with or without supplementary chemotherapy, but there have been no instances to date of clinically overt radiation hepatitis.

Gastrointestinal Tract. Our experience in the radiotherapy of a large number of patients with Hodgkin's disease to fields below the diaphragm, though undertaken with considerable trepidation, has been remarkable for the almost complete absence of significant gastrointestinal complications. Two patients have developed clinical and roentgenographic evidence of gastric ulcer, and two other patients had rather severe episodes of gastrointestinal bleeding, the site of which could not be established. However, one other patient had an even more massive gastrointestinal bleeding episode just *before* the initiation of radiotherapy to the abdomen. One other patient, who had a long-established gastric ulcer, was symptomatically greatly relieved after radiotherapy. Kellum et al. (1977) have described radiation gastritis and gastric fibrosis requiring surgical correction in six patients (three with Hodgkin's disease and three with other lymphomas) who received appreciably higher doses to the stomach. We have seen one patient, treated with a mantle field at another institution, who developed a tracheoesophageal fistula about one year later (Fig. 9.66). There was some evidence of dosimetric error which may have resulted in an excessive dose to the mediastinum.

Although nausea, vomiting, and/or diarrhea are often noted during radiotherapy, sustained subacute or chronic radiation enteritis with stenosis has been observed in only one instance in our experience; that this patient, a twenty-five-year-old female, may have had a truly idiosyncratic sensitivity to radiation injury is suggested by the fact that she also developed hypothyroidism and radiation pericarditis with constriction.

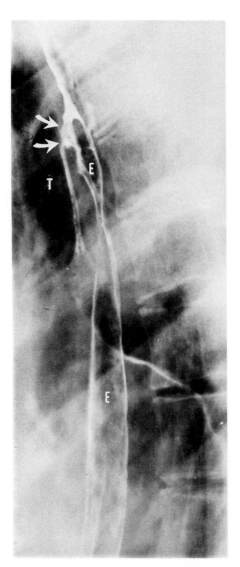

Figure 9.66 Tracheoesophageal fistula, proved at autopsy, developing in a young female patient treated with mantle field radiotherapy at another institution. It appears likely that an overdose of radiation was delivered to the mediastinum in this case. T, trachea; E, esophagus; arrows indicate site of fistula.

Genitourinary Tract. Radiation nephritis is a well-established hazard when radiation doses to both kidneys exceed 2,300 to 2,500 rads, delivered at the rate of approximately 1,000 rads per week (Luxton, 1953). However, with megavoltage radiotherapy, it is readily possible to encompass minimal to moderate degrees of para-aortic lymphadenopathy, as demonstrated by the lymphangiogram, with sharply collimated beams which can be shaped to spare all of the right kidney and all but the upper pole of the left kidney. When lymphadenopathy in the upper abdomen is more massive

and spreads farther laterally to overlie the kidneys, it is sometimes possible to use the split-course technique, delivering approximately 1,500 rads in two weeks and then interrupting treatment for one to two weeks to permit regression of the lymphangiographically opacified nodes. When these shrink medially far enough to permit resumption of treatment with the kidneys shielded, the dose to the lymph nodes can then be carried to approximately 4,000 rads with impunity. When the lymph node mass remains too wide to permit shielding the kidneys while continuing treatment through anterior and posterior opposed fields, it is usually possible to continue treatment with opposing horizontal decubitus fields, with the patient in the supine position (Fig. 9.33), using lead blocks laterally to shield the kidneys (Goffinet et al., 1976). There have been no instances of radiation nephritis in our series of over 1,200 patients with Hodgkin's disease treated since 1961. This favorable experience suggests that the case of total unilateral renal destruction described by Danforth and Javadpour (1975) was almost certainly due to an error in dosimetry, radiation field delineation, or beam alignment, although no details of radiation technique are given.

As mentioned earlier, radiation injury to the gonads occurs in virtually all instances in which the pelvic field is irradiated (Speiser, Rubin, and Casarett, 1973; Asbjørnsen et al., 1976a; Dana et al., 1976; Slanina et al., 1977). In male patients, transient aspermia or oligospermia is the rule, but recovery of spermatogenesis has been documented in several of our younger male patients who have become fathers of normal offspring within a few years after completion of radiotherapy, as well as in 3 of 7 patients studied by Asbjørnsen et al. (1976a), and 5 of 11 patients studied by Hahn, Feingold, and Nisce (1976). In other instances, no specific testing of spermatogenic function has been performed. Gradual regeneration of testicular stem cells has been well documented in irradiated mice (Meistrich et al., 1978). However, there are documented instances of chronic aspermia or hypospermia persisting long after completion of treatment of male patients with Hodgkin's disease. In female patients, ovarian function is usually permanently abolished if doses in excess of 500 to 800 rads are delivered to the ovaries on both sides. As mentioned above, we have investigated the possibility of sparing the ovaries while treating the iliac and other pelvic nodes by moving the ovaries, together with the intact pedicle and tubes, toward the midline of the pelvis and then using double-thickness lead blocks shaped to provide maximal protection to the midsagittal point (Figs. 9.42, 9.43; Ray et al., 1970). More than 70 percent of the young female patients subjected to oophoropexy and radiotherapy to the pelvis by this technique have continued to have or have later resumed normal menstrual function. Twenty-one of these patients later proved fertile and fifteen were able to carry one or more pregnancies to term, yielding a total of 20 children, all of whom were normal. Several of these cases have been described in detail by LeFloch, Donaldson, and Kaplan (1976). Baker et al. (1972) have also reported a normal full-term pregnancy in a patient with Hodgkin's disease who received high-dose pelvic irradiation after ovarian transposition.

Skin and Subcutaneous Tissues. The skin surface usually receives only a small fraction of the dose delivered by a megavoltage X-ray beam of any given energy. Accordingly, severe skin reactions, once the principal limiting factor in kilovoltage X-ray therapy, have been virtually eliminated. When megavoltage X-ray beams are directed perpendicularly at relatively flat skin surfaces, there is little or no discernible cutaneous reaction at the completion of a course of treatment which delivers a dose of approximately 4,000 rads to the depth of the midplane of the body, and the late cosmetic appearance is often indistinguishable from that of adjacent unirradiated skin. Where skin contours are curved in such a way that some of the entering rays strike the skin tangentially, particularly in individuals with fair skin who are known to be sensitive to sunlight, significant acute reactions may occur, particularly when low-energy scattered radiation from beam-shaping lead blocks contributes to the entrance dose. We have successfully circumvented this problem by using curved shielding blocks which follow the contours of the axilla and shield the skin along the axillary silhouette from the tangential rays of the mantle field (Fig. 9.12).

In certain sites, the hair follicles are placed sufficiently deeply to lie in or near the plane of maximal ionization. One such site is the suboccipital area and the nape of the neck. Accordingly, patients receiving megavoltage radiotherapy to the mantle field through both anterior and posterior opposing matched fields should be cautioned to anticipate epilation in suboccipital areas on either side of the shielded midline. Under the dosimetric conditions described previously, in which the anterior and posterior fields jointly contribute a mid-cervical dose of approximately 4,400 rads in four weeks, this epilation has been transient in almost all cases to date, although we have recorded a few among the hundreds treated in which the hair returning in the treated region remained sparse, indicating a partial permanent epilation.

There have been no instances to date of significant subcutaneous fibrosis in patients receiving only a single course of radiotherapy to a dose of 4,400 rads over any one treatment region. However, two obese patients subsequently developed a brawny edema believed due to subcutaneous fat necrosis, followed by a deep cicatricial fibrosis in the lower abdominal and suprapubic region, unaccompanied by significant disability.

The problem of subcutaneous fibrosis may be much more serious, however, in patients who require a second course of radiotherapy for recurrent disease in a previously treated field. We have been particularly impressed with this hazard in patients whose original course of treatment was given at other institutions with kilovoltage X-rays and who had moderate to severe degrees of cutaneous atrophy, deep pigmentation, and telangiectasia, as well as some degree of subcutaneous scarring as a consequence of the original course of treatment (Fig. 9.5). In such patients, fibrosis after retreatment may progress to an almost boardlike rigidity, sometimes associated with impairment of mobility, particularly in the neck. In the low posterior cervical region traversed by the branches of the brachial plexus, scarring of such severity may cause severe and debilitating pain due to compression of peripheral nerves, sometimes with associated motor weakness or paralysis (Slanina et al., 1977). Comment has already been made about a case report in which subcutaneous fibrosis induced by radiotherapy apparently also caused obliteration of the pulse in the upper extremities (Heidenberg et al., 1966).

Skeletal System. There is no discernible acute radiation reaction in bone or cartilage. Although late pathologic fractures are known to occur after higher doses of radiation, there has been only one such instance to date among our patients with Hodgkin's disease treated with a single course of megavoltage radiotherapy to a dose of approximately 4,400 rads in four weeks. There has been no evidence of late cartilaginous injury. Two others have had painless atrophy and resorption of part of the clavicle without fracture.

In young children with Hodgkin's disease, radiation is known to impair growth and development of the sternum (Morris et al., 1975), clavicles, rib cage, and vertebral column (Ďurkovský and Krajči, 1972; Probert, Parker, and Kaplan, 1973; Probert and Parker, 1975). When lesions on one side of the vertebral column have been treated, severe deformities of the spine have later developed as a consequence of unilateral asymmetrical growth retardation. However, unilateral paravertebral treatment is rarely, if ever, appropriate in patients with Hodgkin's disease and other malignant lymphomas; instead, the tendency of lymph nodes to become involved more or less symmetrically along the spinal axis usually constitutes a strong argument for treating a field which encompasses the entire width of the vertebrae. Accordingly, whatever growth inhibition may be induced is symmetrical and not subsequently conducive to the development of kyphoscoliosis. We have observed one instance of growth inhibition in a female patient treated successfully at the age of five years for stage III-B Hodgkin's disease. In this patient, there has been appreciable reduction of the rate of growth in height of the trunk relative to that of the extremities. Deformity of the vertebral bodies, with flattening, and a failure to attain normal vertical height have been noted in several other patients (Probert and Parker, 1975). Similar observations have been reported by Gutjahr, Greinbacher, and Kutzner (1976). Accordingly, when confronted almost simultaneously in 1970 with two children, aged 21 months and four and a half years, both with stage III$_S$B Hodgkin's disease, the author decided to limit the radiation dose during total lymphoid irradiation to 1,500 rads in the infant and 2,000 rads in the older child and then to administer adjuvant MOPP chemotherapy. Both children are alive and free of relapse more than nine years later and are within one standard deviation of normal growth in sitting and standing height. Encouraged by this experience, we have developed a combined modality protocol using low-dose irradiation plus adjuvant MOPP chemotherapy for young children with Hodgkin's disease, as described in greater detail in Chapter 11.

Endocrine System. The development of overt hypothyroidism has been documented in 47 (20 percent) of 235 patients who received their primary radiotherapy for Hodgkin's disease at Stanford University Medical Center (Fuks et al., 1976a); one other patient developed signs of hyperthyroidism with exophthalmos, and an increased blood level of the long-acting thyroid stimulator. Several additional patients have had symptoms strongly suggestive of hypothyroidism, but clearcut confirma-

tion via the usual laboratory tests has not been forthcoming. Prager, Sembrot, and Southard (1972) detected hypothyroidism in 5 of 23 patients within one year following completion of mantle irradiation. Similar observations have been reported by Shalet et al. (1977) and by Schimpff et al. (1978). Moreover, 103 (44 percent) of 235 of our patients who completed mantle therapy for Hodgkin's disease have developed "compensated hypothyroidism," as revealed by significant and long-sustained elevations of the level of pituitary thyroid-stimulating hormone (TSH) in the presence of normal thyroxine levels (Glatstein et al., 1971; Fuks et al., 1976a). The fact that these patients are euthyroid, rather than hyperthyroid, in response to the elevated TSH level, indicates that a subclinical degree of radiation injury to the thyroid gland has occurred, but that sufficient thyroid tissue has persisted to permit the thyroid to function at normal levels in response to an increased TSH stimulus. There is evidence that the iodine load contributed by lymphangiography may be a co-factor in the genesis of hypothyroidism in these patients (Glatstein et al., 1971). Of particular interest is the observation that nine of nineteen patients in whom radiation pericarditis or pancarditis developed were also overtly hypothyroid, and sixteen had elevated TSH levels (Glatstein et al., 1971), suggesting that the hormonal disturbance may well have been a contributing factor in the genesis of the cardiac complication.

The pituitary gland is relatively insensitive to radiation. We have observed one serious disturbance of skeletal growth in a boy treated to a dose of about 7,000 rads in six and one-half weeks over the sphenoid region for a malignant rhabdomyosarcoma of the sphenoid; in this instance, it is presumed that radiation injury to the hypophysis led to impaired secretion of pituitary growth hormone (Fuks et al. 1976a). However, no such instance has been observed in any of the children treated to date to significantly lower doses for Hodgkin's disease or other malignant lymphomas, even when the structures of Waldeyer's ring have been irradiated. Nonetheless, it is desirable to shield the pituitary fossa as much as possible during treatment of the Waldeyer field in young children.

We have not made serial laboratory observations of adrenal gland function after radiotherapy. There have been no instances in which the clinical syndrome of Addison's disease has appeared. Moreover, the likelihood of significant radiation-induced adrenal dysfunction is small a priori, since the right adrenal gland is ordinarily outside the para-aortic treatment field, and only the left adrenal is usually included in the extension of the para-aortic field shaped to encompass the spleen or splenic pedicle.

Several of our patients had known diabetes mellitus at the time when their Hodgkin's disease was diagnosed. There has been no discernible exacerbation of their diabetes as a consequence of the course of radiotherapy, which in several instances has of necessity included virtually the entire volume of the pancreas in the para-aortic field. This is consistent with the prevailing impression that the pancreatic islets are relatively radioresistant.

Hematopoietic System. The changes in peripheral blood element levels during and soon after total-lymphoid radiotherapy have been described in a preceding section (cf. Table 9.8). The white blood cell count has returned to normal within a few months after completion of radiotherapy and remained in that range permanently thereafter in all but a few of our patients (Figs. 9.52 to 9.57). These few have shown sustained leukopenia of mild degree, usually in the range of 3,500 to 4,500 white blood cells per cubic millimeter for some years after completion of radiotherapy, with no untoward effects and no obvious enhancement of susceptibility to infection. Similar observations have been made by Kun and Johnson (1975). The profound effects of total lymphoid irradiation on T-lymphocytes and the prolonged impairment of several parameters of cell-mediated immunologic function (Fuks et al., 1976b) have been fully detailed in Chapter 6. Progressive restoration to normal of the marrow granulocyte reserves over a period of five months after completion of extended-field radiotherapy has been documented by Vogel et al. (1968), using the marrow response to etiocholanolone and to bacterial endotoxin as a measure of the capacity for marrow granulocyte response. There have been only a few instances in our experience in which the platelet count after completion of radiotherapy has not returned to a level of 200,000 per cubic millimeter or more; in these, the platelet count has exceeded 100,000, and there have been no bleeding episodes. Thus, the incidence of incomplete hematopoietic recovery after total lymphoid radiotherapy alone has been approximately 1 percent, and there have been no instances of aplastic anemia or pancytopenia.

Moreover, there has now been unequivocal histopathologic and radioisotopic evidence of bone marrow regeneration in the irradiated fields in pa-

tients who have received total lymphoid radiotherapy for Hodgkin's disease. This was a pleasant surprise, inasmuch as earlier studies had suggested that the marrow is incapable of regeneration after localized irradiation to doses of 4,000 rads or more (Sykes et al., 1964; Bell, McAfee, and Constable, 1969). Rubin and co-workers (1973, 1978) used ^{99m}Tc sulfur colloid scans to study the bone marrow of 27 patients, of whom 10 were reexamined at serial intervals. They observed profound impairment of uptake in the irradiated regions of bone marrow following total lymphoid irradiation which persisted for one to two years. Thereafter, there was partial to complete regeneration of bone marrow in approximately 85 percent of bone marrow sites. Morardet, Parmentier, and Flamant (1973), Cionini (1973), and DeGowin et al. (1974) used ^{59}Fe uptake by erythropoietically active bone marrow to study the response to radiotherapy in patients with Hodgkin's disease, at least one of whom had also received MOPP combination chemotherapy. The latter authors observed little or no uptake in irradiated bone marrow areas for periods of one to three years and compensatory hyperplasia of erythropoietic tissue in the unirradiated portions of ribs and axial skeleton in several patients. Since the highly energetic gamma emission of ^{59}Fe impairs the quality of scans obtained with this isotope, Knospe et al. (1976) used another iron radionuclide, ^{52}Fe, to study 25 patients with malignant lymphomas at various intervals after radiotherapy. They found a significant inhibition of erythropoiesis in irradiated zones in all patients at intervals less than one year following completion of radiotherapy. However, between 12 and 24 months after treatment, at least moderate recovery was observed in one or more radiation fields in 7 of 8 patients. The degree of recovery was not uniform in all treated fields, and the last field treated often showed a lesser degree of regeneration.

Bone marrow regeneration was also observed by Sacks et al. (1978b) using ^{111}InCl$_3$ as a bone marrow scanning agent (Fig. 9.67). The ability of the irradiated marrow to regenerate, as scored by relative uptake on a scale of 0 to 4, was a function of radiation dose, and decreased sharply at doses over 4,000 rads (Table 9.14) in patients receiving total lymphoid irradiation. There was an apparently inverse correlation between the volume of central marrow irradiated and the subsequent occurrence of marrow regeneration (Fig. 9.68). The mean extent of regeneration for any given dose level was appreciably less in patients who had only limited field irradiation than in those who had received

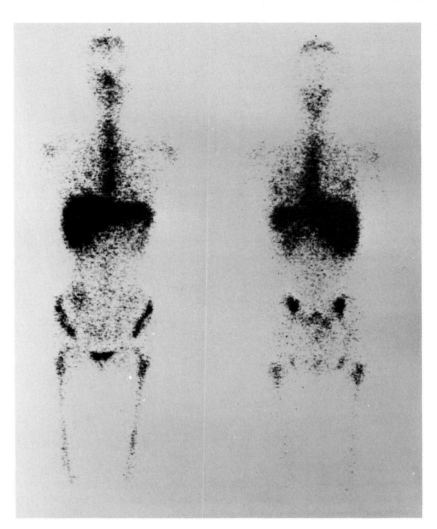

Figure 9.67   A 17-year-old female with pathological stage III$_S$A nodular sclerosing Hodgkin's disease treated with total lymphoid irradiation and colloidal gold (^{198}Au), scanned 55 months after radiation therapy, demonstrating complete bone marrow regeneration in the thorax, modest regeneration in the pelvis, no regeneration in the para-aortic region, and extension of marrow activity to the femurs and calvarium. Left, anterior view; right, posterior. (Reprinted, by permission of the authors and the Editor of *Cancer*, from the paper by Sacks et al., 1978b.)

total lymphoid irradiation. For example, isotope uptake was poor to absent in the irradiated region in 10 of 11 patients treated with either a mantle or an inverted-Y field alone, whereas failure of regeneration in the irradiated regions was observed in only 6 of 31 patients who received treatment on both sides of the diaphragm to a dose of approximately 4,400 rads. Regeneration was markedly greater in patients under 20 years of age and was poor in patients over 40 years of age at the time of treatment (Table 9.15). Most of the observed regeneration occurred within 12 to 36 months, and there was little further regeneration in patients examined more than 5 years after completion of radiotherapy. The occurrence of marrow regeneration following total lymphoid radiotherapy in patients with Hodgkin's disease has also been confirmed histopathologically. Active, essentially normocellular marrow was observed at autopsy in irradiated skeletal regions in five of our patients who

died of intercurrent disease some years after total-lymphoid radiotherapy.

Collectively, these observations are consistent with the view that the intensity of the stimulus for regeneration is directly related to the volume of marrow irradiated. This would explain the paradox that there is little or no regeneration after high-dose irradiation of small, localized volumes of marrow (Sykes et al., 1964; Bell et al., 1969), whereas substantial regeneration occurs after total lymphoid irradiation, particularly in adolescent and young adult patients. Sacks et al. (1978b) also found that regeneration was more active in regions of marrow that had received reduced doses as a consequence of the use of lead shielding blocks, as for example in the lower thoracic spine regions partially protected by the subcarinal blocks used in mantle field irradiation (Fig. 9.69). This suggests that shielding blocks might be selectively used over other areas of the body, such as the lumbar spine,

Table 9.14   Effect of Radiation Dose and Fields on Bone Marrow Activity Assessed by Uptake of [111]Indium

Extent of radiation fields	Radiation Dose (rad)		
	<3,000	3–4,000	>4,000
TLI[a]	2.8 ± 0.8 (20)	2.5 ± 1.1 (45)	1.3 ± 1.3 (59)
IF, EF, or subtotal[b]	1.0 ± 1.2 (4)	1.2 ± 1.5 (8)	0.8 ± 1.0 (16)

Source: Stanford University Medical Center data (Sacks et al., 1978b)

[a] TLI: total lymphoid irradiation; IF: involved field irradiation; EF: extended field irradiation.

[b] Uptake in irradiated marrow regions was graded on a relative scale from 0 to 4; numbers indicate the mean grade ± square root of the mean square difference, with numbers of observations given in parentheses.

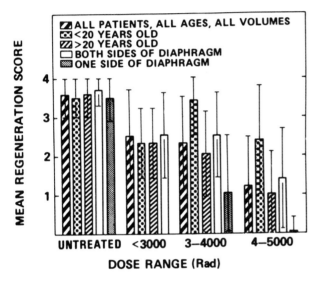

Figure 9.68   Bar graph representation of bone marrow regeneration in evaluated sites versus dose range. The effects of age, dose, and volume treated are seen in the dose ranges 3–4,000 rads and 4–5,000 rads. (Reprinted, by permission of the authors and the Editor of *Cancer,* from the paper by Sacks et al., 1978b.)

to enhance the probability of marrow regeneration, particularly in older patients.

The risk of late radiation-induced leukemia after extensive high-dose irradiation of the bone marrow is one that must be taken seriously in the light of the evidence from survivors of the atomic bombings in Japan (Bizzozero et al., 1966) and from patients treated over the vertebral column for ankylosing spondylitis (Court Brown and Doll, 1957; Court Brown, 1958). However, it may prove to be of importance that the conditions of radiation exposure of our patients with Hodgkin's disease were significantly different from those of the other groups mentioned. The atomic bomb survivors obviously received a single, relatively massive, total-body exposure; the British patients treated for ankylosing spondylitis received, as a rule, multiple courses of treatment spaced over appreciable intervals of time, to the spinal marrow, with aggregate total doses estimated in some instances to have been quite high. In contrast, the patients with Hodgkin's disease have been treated, for the most part, with a single fractionated course of treat-

Table 9.15   Effect of Age on Bone Marrow Activity in Patients Treated with Total Lymphoid Irradiation, as Assessed by Uptake of [111]Indium

Age in years at irradiation	Radiation Dose (rad)		
	<3,000	3–4,000	>4,000
0–20	3.0 (1)[a]	3.7 ± 0.6 (11)	2.6 ± 1.4 (12)
20–40	3.1 ± 0.6 (7)	2.3 ± 0.6 (16)	1.2 ± 1.2 (25)
40–70	2.6 ± 0.9 (12)	1.9 ± 1.1 (18)	0.8 ± 0.9 (22)

Source: Stanford University Medical Center data (Sacks et al., 1978b).

[a] Uptake in irradiated marrow regions graded on a relative scale from 0 to 4; numbers indicate the mean grade ± square root of the mean square difference, with numbers of observations given in parentheses.

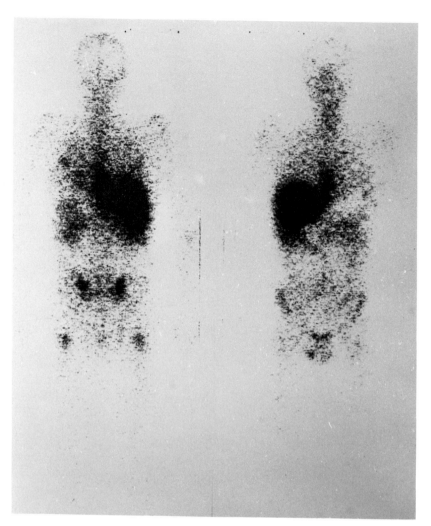

Figure 9.69 A 39-year-old male with pathologic stage IA nodular sclerosing Hodgkin's disease scanned 76 months following treatment with total lymphoid irradiation (subcarinal block inserted at 2,000 rads). There is modest regeneration in the upper thoracic spine and pelvis, normal uptake in the lower thoracic spine, and no uptake in the para-aortic area. Anterior view is on the right. (Reprinted, by permission of the authors and the Editor of *Cancer*, from the paper by Sacks et al., 1978b.)

ment, receiving about 4,400 rads in four weeks to all of the lumbar and part of the upper sacral marrow, and a somewhat lower dose, due to the use of lead shields for the spinal cord, to the cervical and dorsal spinal marrow. On the basis of published data on the latent period of leukemias induced in the other series of patients mentioned, we would expect that the peak incidence of leukemia induced in survivors treated for Hodgkin's disease or other malignant lymphomas would occur within five to ten years after completion of treatment. Some of our patients treated with total-lymphoid radiotherapy alone for advanced stage II and stage III Hodgkin's disease are now in their seventeenth year of followup observation, and many others have passed the ten-year mark. To date, there has not been a single instance of leukemia among them. In a more recent analysis of 680 previously untreated patients with Hodgkin's disease treated at Stanford University Medical Center from 1968 through 1975, Coleman et al. (1977) encountered

a total of 8 cases of acute and 1 of subacute leukemia, all in patients who had received both radiotherapy and chemotherapy. There were no leukemias among 320 patients treated with external radiotherapy alone, but acute leukemia did occur in one patient treated with both total lymphoid irradiation and intravenous ^{198}Au. Several case reports of acute leukemia following treatment with radiotherapy alone have appeared in the literature during the past decade (Ezdinli et al., 1969; Newman et al., 1970; Roozendaal and Schreuder-Van Gelder, 1971; Chan and McBride, 1972; Kim and Harley, 1972; Weiden et al., 1973; Zwaan and Speck, 1973; Raich et al., 1975; Stenfert-Kroese, Sizoo, and Somers, 1976; Cadman, Capizzi, and Bertino, 1977; Larsen and Brincker, 1977; Saxe and Mandel, 1978; A. M. Nordentoft et al., personal communication, 1978).

In the case described by Osta et al. (1970) the interval between the start of localized radiotherapy and the onset of acute myeloid leukemia was only nine months, casting serious doubt on the etiologic role of radiation exposure. Several cases of acute leukemia have occurred in patients treated with chemotherapy alone, and a much greater number in patients treated with both radiotherapy and chemotherapy, in either sequence. Accordingly, the hazard of developing acute leukemia is discussed again in Chapters 10 and 11. Since even the highest risk group among the ankylosing spondylitis patients had a leukemia incidence of less than 0.1 percent per year (Court Brown and Doll, 1957), a longer period of observation of a greater number of patients will be required before we can conclude with confidence that the leukemia risk after treatment of Hodgkin's disease with these techniques is really within acceptable limits, relative to the profound therapeutic benefit which such treatment obviously confers on these patients.

Leukemia is not the only form of malignant disease developing secondarily in patients treated for Hodgkin's disease. Krikorian et al. (1979a) have reported the development of six cases of non-Hodgkin's lymphoma, predominantly involving the gastrointestinal tract or abdomen. The actuarial risk of developing such a secondary non-Hodgkin's lymphoma at ten years after primary treatment of Hodgkin's disease was approximately 4.4 percent, comparable to or slightly greater than that for developing acute leukemia. All of these patients had received both radiation therapy and chemotherapy. However, we have now seen one adult female patient who developed a new, non-Hodgkin's (diffuse histiocytic) lymphoma in the thorax 15 years after treatment with total lymphoid radiotherapy alone for stage IIIA Hodgkin's disease. McDougall et al. (1979) have described three cases of thyroid carcinoma arising in patients with Hodgkin's disease following radiotherapy to the mantle field. Another such case has been reported by Weshler et al. (1978). It is probable that these instances developed on a background of "compensated hypothyroidism" which was clinically unrecognized and thus that the development of malignant change in the thyroid might have been prevented by replacement therapy. A number of miscellaneous secondary neoplasms in epithelial and connective tissues have also been reported following radiotherapy for Hodgkin's disease, but the anecdotal nature of these reports makes it difficult to assess the extent to which these secondary neoplasms can indeed be attributed to radiation therapy and not merely to chance.

Chapter 10   Chemotherapy

Historical Aspects

Around the turn of the century, before radiotherapy equipment became widely available, physicians attempted with discouragingly little success to stem the progress of Hodgkin's disease and to alleviate its distressing symptoms with arsenicals, iodides, and other medications, as well as with a variety of serums, vaccines, and other biologic preparations. Of these, only the arsenicals appear to have elicited objective responses. Senn (1903), in one of the first published papers on X-ray therapy for the treatment of "pseudoleucemia" (one of many synonyms then in vogue for Hodgkin's disease), undoubtedly reflected the widely prevailing view at the time: "The writer has seen many cases of pseudoleucemia and has never known one to be permanently benefited by either medical or surgical treatment." Gilbert (1939) also refers to the use of arsenicals as an adjunct in the maintenance therapy of patients who had been brought into remission with radiotherapy; this practice was apparently continued into the 1930's.

The modern era of chemotherapy for the leukemias and lymphomas is only slightly over thirty years old (Karnofsky, 1968). Gilman, Goodman, Lindskog, and Dougherty, in studies initiated in 1942–1943 but not published because of wartime military security considerations, first administered a derivative of mustard gas, tris-β-chloroethylamine hydrochloride (HN$_3$), to patients with leukemias and lymphomas and noted significant though transient regressions of disease. Soon thereafter, Jacobson et al. (1946) and Goodman et al. (1946) used the closely related compound, methyl-bis-β-chloroethylamine hydrochloride (nitrogen mustard, HN$_2$), which elicited dramatic clinical responses in patients with Hodgkin's disease. These early studies were confirmed and extended by Karnofsky et al. (1947) and Zanes et al. (1948). Since that time a host of polyfunctional alkylating agents have been synthesized and tested clinically against a spectrum of malignant neoplasms, including the leukemias and lymphomas, in a search for more specific antitumor activity, reduced hematopoietic toxicity, and/or diminished acute gastrointestinal intolerance. Karnofsky (1968) has summarized the current status of these efforts: "Occasional reports have suggested that one alkylating agent is more beneficial than another in specific clinical situations, but a more acceptable generalization is that the polyfunctional alkylating agents have a similar spectrum of therapeutic activity in the lymphomas, when given at equivalent doses in relation to the individual patient's tolerance to the drug."

Interestingly enough, the experimental foundations for the use of the adrenal steroids in the treatment of leukemias and lymphomas were also laid at about the same time that the nitrogen mustards were being explored. In 1943, Dougherty and White demonstrated that the adrenocorticotrophic hormone (ACTH) caused lymphoid atrophy in mice, and in the following year, Heilman and Kendall (1944) reported that compound E (11-dehydro-17-hydroxycorticosterone, cortisone) caused regression of transplanted lymphosarcomas in mice. ACTH and cortisone did not become available for clinical use until 1949–50 and were almost immediately tried in patients with lymphomas. ACTH appeared to act indirectly through stimulation of the adrenal cortex and was ultimately discarded, and a series of more active derivatives of cortisone were gradually introduced, of which prednisone is today perhaps the most widely used.

These two discoveries may appropriately be credited with having ushered in modern cancer chemotherapy. In the 1950's, the scale of research in this field was rapidly and vastly expanded in a search for new classes of compounds with antitumor activity. Although some such compounds were brought to light as a consequence of massive screening programs undertaken both in this country and abroad, a number of the more effective anticancer compounds in use today were synthesized deliberately on the basis of rational considerations, stemming from newer knowledge of the metabolic pathways for the synthesis of DNA precursors. Of these, the antifolic agents (Farber et al., 1948; Farber, 1949) and 5-fluorouracil are perhaps the most outstanding examples. Other active anticancer agents include the *Vinca* alkaloids, vinblastine and vincristine; procarbazine, a methylhydrazine; the nitrosoureas (BCNU, CCNU); and the antibiotics, such as actinomycin D, daunomycin, adriamycin, and bleomycin. The availability of an ever-broadening spectrum of potentially clinically useful drugs (Hall, 1966; Carter and Livingston, 1973; Desser and Ultmann, 1973) has in turn led to the development of quantitative studies of their mechanisms of action in model tumor systems in experimental animals (Chabner et al., 1975) as well as to the development of criteria for the objective analysis of clinical responses and for the comparative assessment of the efficacy of different types of drugs through the device of the randomized clinical trial.

General Considerations

Mechanisms of Drug Action in the Lymphomas. The mechanisms of action of some of the antilymphoma drugs are now reasonably well established, whereas others remain to be elucidated. As their name implies, the polyfunctional alkylating agents, of which nitrogen mustard is the prototype, are highly reactive compounds capable of attacking certain chemical groups to which they become firmly bound by alkylation reactions. In contrast to the other alkylating agents, cyclophosphamide is inert and requires activation by hepatic microsomal enzymes to active metabolites, which are then distributed to target sites via the systemic circulation. The alkylating agents have been shown to act preferentially on the guanine bases of DNA. Since they can simultaneously attack different molecules, one possible consequence of alkylation is the formation of a cross-link between the two strands of DNA (Brookes and Lawley, 1961). Unless such a lesion can be repaired soon enough, it may be expected to be lethal for any cell which is still actively replicating. A number of the antibiotic compounds, such as mitomycin C, resemble the alkylating agents in their capacity to cause cross-links in DNA (Iyer and Szybalski, 1963). A somewhat more selective type of alteration of DNA structure is brought about by actinomycin D, which becomes attached to DNA in such a way as to prevent the attachment of the enzyme RNA polymerase, thus interfering with DNA-dependent RNA synthesis

and, in particular, with the synthesis of messenger RNA (Goldberg and Rabinowitz, 1962; Goldberg and Reich, 1964). The anthracycline antibiotics, daunomycin and adriamycin, bind to DNA by intercalation between adjacent base pairs along the DNA strand, distorting the helical structure of the molecule and interfering with the activity of both DNA and RNA polymerases (Chabner et al., 1975). The mechanisms of action of procarbazine and of the nitrosoureas are not well understood, but appear to involve inhibition of DNA synthesis. The action of the nitrosoureas resembles that of alkylating agents in some respects, but the fact that patients who have become refractory to the alkylating agents are often still responsive to the nitrosoureas suggests that there must be significant differences. Bleomycin may cause strand breakage in DNA; it also interferes with DNA synthesis and with the progression of cells through the premitotic (G_2) and mitotic (M) phases of the cell cycle (Chabner et al., 1975).

A variety of antimetabolites have now been developed for clinical use. These are compounds which closely simulate naturally occurring metabolic intermediates and precursor compounds. They are able to bind to certain key enzymes in the biosynthetic pathway utilized by the normal compound to which they are related and thus to block either its synthesis or its utilization. Most of the antimetabolites currently in wide clinical use are those which block purine and pyrimidine metabolic pathways and thus interfere with the synthesis of DNA and RNA. The folic acid antagonists, such as methotrexate, and the fluorinated pyrimidines, such as 5-fluorouracil and its derivatives, interfere with the action of the enzyme thymidylate synthetase, thus preventing the synthesis of thymidylate, an essential precursor of DNA synthesis. Cytosine arabinoside (ara-C) is believed to interfere with the reduction of cytidine diphosphate to deoxycytidine diphosphate, another essential precursor in the pathway leading to DNA synthesis (cf. Karnofsky and Clarkson, 1963; Chabner et al., 1975).

The *Vinca* alkaloids share with colchicine and its derivatives the property of acting as mitotic spindle poisons, thus interfering with mitosis (Palmer et al., 1960). For this reason, their activity is highly cell-cycle-dependent. However, there is also evidence that they may interfere with the metabolism of certain amino acids and with the synthesis of DNA (Desser and Ultmann, 1973). The mechanism whereby the adrenal steroids exert their remarkable lymphocytolytic effects is not yet well understood. Cellular susceptibility is clearly related to the extent of differentiation; the small lymphocyte is exquisitely sensitive, the immature lymphocyte or lymphoblast appreciably less so, and the histiocyte apparently unaffected, even by large doses. It is also established that the adrenal steroids inhibit protein synthesis in connective tissue and interfere with growth in the mesenchymal tissues generally.

Kinetics of Antitumor Drug Action. The end result common to the diverse biochemical mechanisms of action of these drugs is the killing of cells. It must be stressed that all of the chemotherapeutic agents currently used in the treatment of Hodgkin's disease have the capacity to kill certain classes of normal cells and are thus not highly selective for tumor cells. Yet, they may, under certain circumstances, cause dramatic regression and even apparently complete disappearance of lymphomatous masses and alleviate systemic symptoms at dose levels which elicit only moderate and readily tolerable degrees of host toxicity. Even the most dramatic and apparently complete regressions after single-drug administration have not been permanent, however. There is no well-documented instance of cure of a patient with Hodgkin's disease by treatment with any single drug alone. When efforts were made to achieve tumor eradication by increase in drug dose, normal tissue toxicity escalated to prohibitive levels.

Experimental systems have been developed, due in large measure to the work of Goldin et al. (1956, 1958), Skipper et al. (1964, 1970), and Bruce et al. (1966, 1967, 1969), for the quantitative analysis of the kinetics of tumor-cell killing as a function of drug dose and timing of administration. Many of these studies have been done with transplantable lymphoblastic leukemias of mice, such as the L1210 leukemia. It has been possible to demonstrate that the killing of these tumor cells by a variety of chemotherapeutic agents, just as in the case of radiation, is essentially an exponential function of dose. This implies that the proportion of cells killed by a given dose of drug is constant, regardless of the number of cells present at the time of treatment (Goldin et al., 1956, 1958). Skipper (1964, 1968) has pointed out that the effect of a drug depends not only on dose but also on the spacing of successive doses and on the rate of proliferation of the surviving tumor cell population during that time interval. Thus, in the experimental treatment of leukemia in mice with a rate of proliferation such that the population doubles

every twelve hours, the administration of a daily dose of a drug that kills less than 75 percent of the tumor cell population is doomed to failure simply because the cell population increases faster than the rate at which cells are being killed. Goldin et al. (1958) reported that this was partly due to the adherence to a daily schedule of drug administration. By going to a schedule in which maximally tolerated doses of drug were given every fourth day, they found that very significant increases in life span in mice bearing the L1210 leukemia could be obtained with the folic acid antagonist amethopterin. The therapeutic gain achieved with this more optimal treatment interval was presumably due to the fact that the critically sensitive normal stem-cell populations of the bone marrow and intestinal crypts of the host could renew themselves more effectively on a four-day cycle than on a daily treatment basis.

Bruce and his associates (1967, 1969; Valeriote, Bruce, and Meeker, 1968) demonstrated that certain classes of chemotherapeutic agents possess an appreciable degree of selectivity for the killing of leukemic cells, relative to their ability to kill normal colony-forming stem cells. They attributed this selectivity to the fact that these drugs are mitotic cycle-dependent and to the differences in proliferative state of normal and leukemic cells. Whereas the leukemic cell population is continuously proliferating and thus continuously susceptible to the lethal action of these chemical agents, an appreciable fraction of the normal stem-cell population is temporarily in a resting state, out of the mitotic cycle, and thus relatively insensitive to the same drug. A detailed analysis of these concepts has been presented by Valeriote and van Putten (1975).

These studies also suggested the rationale of using two or more different classes of chemotherapeutic agents in combination. Such combinations would be expected to be effective if the drugs all had the ability to kill some proportion of the tumor cell population, but exhibited differential, nonoverlapping toxicities for the normal host tissues. Animals treated with such combinations would exhibit a greater spectrum of host-tissue toxicities, but each of these could be maintained in the tolerable range under circumstances in which the doses of the various drugs would have additive effects upon the tumor cell population (Valeriote et al., 1968; De Vita, Young, and Canellos, 1975). This has proved to be a powerful concept which, as described later in this chapter, has now been very successfully applied to the treatment of patients with advanced Hodgkin's disease.

Criteria of Clinical Response. As time went on, chemotherapists became aware of the need to develop measurable and reproducible criteria of response to treatment with the various cancer chemotherapeutic agents. Karnofsky (1968) has fully described one long-established system for the evaluation of chemotherapeutic efficacy. In addition to recording a number of parameters of response in considerable detail, a simplified system has been devised to score the *category of response,* which relates not only to the production of symptomatic or objective improvement but also to the degree of practical benefit experienced by the patient. Karnofsky has also developed a practical and useful index of the performance status of the patient (Table 10.1).

The terms "complete remission" and "partial remission" are frequently used in publications on the chemotherapy of the lymphomas, although it has been pointed out (Karnofsky, 1968) that these terms are misnomers, since what is really being observed is the "complete or partial suppression of manifestations of disease." In another clinical trial (Jacobs et al., 1968), an objective response was defined as "a reduction of more than 50 percent in the diameter of a measurable tumor, or a decrease of 50 percent in the vertical distance of the spleen tip and the liver edge, or both, when measured below the costal margin, for one month or longer." A partial response was defined as a reduction of 25 to 50 percent in the diameter of the measurable tumor for one month or longer.

In another study (Carbone and Spurr, 1968), several categories of response were defined as follows: *complete remission* (CR) = complete disappearance of all measured lesions; *partial remission* (PR) = decrease in the sum of the product of tumor diameters by equal to or greater than 50 percent over two consecutive measurement periods; *minimal or no remission* (NR) = decrease of less than 50 percent of the sum of the product of diameters or an increase of less than 125 percent over the original measurements; *progression* = increase equal to or greater than 125 percent over the original measurements; *relapse* = either the appearance of a new lesion (at least 2 cm.^{2}) persisting for two weeks or an increase of the product of diameters of any lesion by 50 percent over the size recorded at the time of maximum regression over two consecutive weekly measurement periods.

Karnofsky (1968) has challenged the relevance of such comparative response data to the practical management of the patient with a malignant lymphoma. He pointed out that the purportedly less effective drugs will be tried in any case when the more effective drugs have lost their effectiveness in a given patient and that individual variations in patient response may well be manifested in a reversal of the relative efficacies of different drugs. However, some of the clinical trials have been

Table 10.1 Karnofsky Performance Status Index

General category	Index	Specific criteria
Able to carry on normal activity; no special care needed	100	Normally no evidence of disease
	90	Normal activity; minor signs or symptoms of disease
	80	Normal activity with effort; some signs or symptoms of disease
Unable to work; able to live at home and care for most personal needs; varying amount of assistance needed	70	Cares for self; unable to carry on normal activity or to do work
	60	Requires occasional assistance from others
	50	Requires considerable assistance from others and frequent medical care
Unable to care for self: requires institutional or hospital care or equivalent; disease may be rapidly progressing	40	Disabled; requires special care
	30	Severely disabled; hospitalization indicated; death not imminent
	20	Very sick; hospitalization necessary; active supportive treatment necessary
	10	Moribund
	0	Dead

aimed at resolving more meaningful questions. In two such studies cited by Frei and Gamble (1966), patients with Hodgkin's disease and lymphosarcoma were randomly assigned to two different dose levels of the alkylating agent Thio-TEPA, or to two different dose levels of certain folic acid antagonists. It was demonstrated that a sharp increase in the frequency of objective responses as well as a concomitant increase in significant toxicity resulted from a doubling of dose in each study. Lethality studies in rats were then undertaken which provided support for the postulate that combinations of agents whose toxicities are independent and nonoverlapping could be given safely at dose levels close to the maximally tolerated dose for each drug. Conversely, when the toxicities of two or more drugs overlapped, combinations of those drugs given at much lower dose levels proved highly toxic, due to additivity of their toxic effects.

In other studies, it has been demonstrated that maintenance chemotherapy during complete remission can prolong the duration of remission after single-drug treatment to a very significant degree in patients with Hodgkin's disease (Scott, 1963). Remission was induced with nitrogen mustard, after which half of the patients were assigned at random to maintenance daily treatment with the alkylating agent, chlorambucil, the other half remaining untreated during remission. The median duration of the unmaintained remissions was only ten weeks; that for the patients receiving maintenance chlorambucil was thirty-two weeks, a highly significant increase. Thus, despite the far greater difficulty of quantifying palliative, rather than curative, responses, meaningful questions about drug therapy can indeed be answered by appropriately designed clinical trials.

It is perhaps relevant to point out that the radiotherapist does not tend to think in terms of complete and partial remissions. The occurrence of a complete remission in patients with Hodgkin's disease, after radiotherapy to adequate dose levels, may ordinarily be taken for granted, since remission rates (1.0 − recurrence rates) in excess of 90 percent have regularly been recorded (Musshoff et al., 1968; Kaplan, 1966a, 1970). Instead, the radiotherapist is concerned with the *permanence* of the complete regressions which he induces and thus scores recurrences per treated field as a significant criterion of therapeutic failure (cf. Fig. 9.3). It is important to bear these differences in terminology and emphasis in mind in evaluating published reports about the treatment of Hodgkin's disease and the other malignant lymphomas by radiotherapists and chemotherapists, respectively.

Conventional Chemotherapy of Hodgkin's Disease

The Established Drugs (Table 10.2).

Alkylating Agents. The alkylating agents are best thought of as a group, despite the fact that individual differences in mode of administration and nature of toxicity distinguish some of the available drugs in this category. There is, however, a considerable degree of cross-resistance among them, with the consequence that a patient who has become refractory to any one of the alkylating agents is likely to respond poorly, if at all, to others in the same group.

The prototype drug among the alkylating agents was the first to be extensively used clinically, *nitrogen mustard* (methyl-bis-β-chloroethylamine hydrochloride, mechlorethamine, HN_2). This drug must be given by intravenous injection; it is highly reactive and decays rapidly in solution, hence must be injected promptly after being dissolved. The usual dose is 0.4 mg per kilogram, which may be given either as a single injection or in divided doses spaced over a few days. Objective responses may be expected in approximately 65 percent of patients with Hodgkin's disease (Jacobs et al., 1968; Carter and Livingston, 1973). They usually occur quite rapidly, within a few days after the first injection. Partial responses are likely to occur in an additional 20 percent of cases. Because of its rapid action, nitrogen mustard is the preferred alkylating agent in patients who are quite ill and present relatively urgent problems, such as high fever, respiratory or superior vena caval obstruction by mediastinal lymphadenopathy, or the spinal cord compression syndrome.

The drug almost invariably induces nausea, vomiting, and anorexia, which usually develop within a few hours after injection and are ordinarily of brief duration and moderate severity. These symptoms may be lessened or prevented if the patient is concurrently sedated with phenothiazine or barbiturate medications. Although its gastrointestinal toxicity is essentially just a minor nuisance, the hematopoietic toxicity of nitrogen mustard is a potentially serious hazard. The white blood cell and platelet counts fall rapidly within a few days after injection and remain depressed for two to four weeks thereafter. Additional full doses of nitrogen mustard can ordinarily not be given safely in less than one month after a prior injection, and serial monthly injections of the drug soon elicit a degree of leukopenia and/or thrombocytopenia that contraindicates its further use.

It was therefore a considerable advantage when

it was discovered (Scott, 1963) that remissions induced by nitrogen mustard, which have an average duration of only ten weeks, can be prolonged to an average of thirty-two weeks if maintenance therapy with chlorambucil is instituted, beginning about two to four weeks after the nitrogen mustard infusion, as soon as the white blood cell and platelet counts begin to rise. It is not desirable for the blood counts to return completely to normal levels, since relapse of the Hodgkin's disease is then often also observed, and more intensive chemotherapy is then required to induce a new remission. *Chlorambucil* is administered orally, usually starting at a dose of 0.1 to 0.2 mg. per kilogram per day (usually 6 to 12 mg. per day in adults). After two to four weeks, the blood picture and the therapeutic response of the patient may be used as guides to titrate the dose individually to the lowest effective maintenance level. The skillful use of chlorambucil to maintain remissions induced by nitrogen mustard can obviate the need for repeated courses of the intravenous drug.

Cyclophosphamide has the advantage that it may be given either intravenously or orally. Because its gastrointestinal toxicity is relatively mild, successive daily intravenous injections induce little discomfort. Accordingly, the intravenous use of cyclophosphamide instead of nitrogen mustard is advantageous in patients whose symptoms are of intermediate severity and do not require immediate relief. It is usually given at a dose level of 40 mg./kg. in either single or divided doses intravenously; when given orally, the usual induction dose is 3 to 5 mg./kg. (200 to 300 mg. per day), followed by maintenance at a level of 50 to 100 mg. per day orally in patients who exhibit a favorable response. The response rate in Hodgkin's disease when intravenous cyclophosphamide is used for induction and oral cyclophosphamide is used for maintenance is about 60 percent (Jacobs et al., 1968; Carter and Livingston, 1973).

Cyclophosphamide is believed to produce less severe platelet depression than the other alkylating agents at therapeutically equivalent doses and is therefore often preferred in patients with impaired marrow function. It does, however, produce significant leukopenia, and at dose levels which elicit significant marrow toxicity, alopecia is also likely to occur, with concomitant emotional distress, particularly in women and children. A more serious toxic manifestation is cystitis, which, if the physician is not alert to its early manifestations, may progress to a serious hemorrhagic form, requiring fulguration, multiple transfusions, and sometimes even cystectomy for its control. The hazard of cyclophosphamide-induced cystitis can be minimized by stressing the importance of a high fluid intake and the maintenance of a high urine volume (Philips et al., 1961). Whenever the symptoms of cystitis appear, consideration should promptly be given to reducing the dose or discontinuing the use of the drug.

Thiotriethylene phosphoramide (Thio-TEPA) closely resembles nitrogen mustard in its action but seems to be somewhat less therapeutically reliable at equivalent doses on a weight basis. It is less likely to induce nausea and vomiting after intravenous injection than nitrogen mustard. The usual dose is 0.6 to 1.0 mg./kg., given intravenously in a single injection or in divided doses. This drug is now less often used systemically; nitrogen mustard is preferred in the most urgent cases, and intravenous cyclophosphamide in patients with symptoms of intermediate severity. However, Thio-TEPA may be given by direct injection into serous effusions and is still a widely used drug for this purpose, particularly for intrapleural injection, the usual dose being 0.8 mg./kg.

Many other alkylating agents have been synthesized and introduced into clinical use. While some of these have apparent advantages in other types of neoplastic disease, none has established a place for itself in the treatment of patients with Hodgkin's disease comparable to that of the tried and proved agents discussed above (cf. Hall, 1966, table I).

Vinca Alkaloids. Stimulated by his observation that extracts of the periwinkle plant, *Vinca rosea Linn.*, had leukopenic activity, Noble and his associates (Noble et al., 1958a,b) purified and chemically characterized one of its alkaloids, vincaleukoblastine (Vinblastine, Velban, Velbe). Soon thereafter, a second alkaloid, leurosine (Vincristine, Oncovin), was also isolated. These alkaloids are entirely unrelated to the polyfunctional alkylating agents; they represent a different class of chemotherapeutic compound, characterized by the presence of indole and dihydroindole moieties. Laboratory studies utilizing mammalian cells in culture revealed that these compounds exert a powerful inhibitory action on mitosis, apparently by acting as mitotic spindle poisons in much the same manner as colchicine (Palmer et al., 1960). Clinical studies soon demonstrated that these drugs had significant chemotherapeutic efficacy in Hodgkin's disease and, less consistently, in the other malignant lymphomas. Vinblastine is generally preferred to vincristine in the treatment of patients with Hodgkin's disease, since it causes significantly less neurotoxi-

Table 10.2 Chemotherapeutic Agents Active in Hodgkin's Disease

Drug	Abbrev.	Dose	Route[a]			
			IV	IM	SC	PO
Nitrogen mustard	HN_2	0.2–0.4 mg./kg.	√			
Cyclophosphamide (Cytoxan)	CTX	100–200 mg./day				√
		30–40 mg./kg.	√			
Chlorambucil	CLB	0.1–0.2 mg./kg./day				√
ThioTEPA	TTPA	0.2–0.4 mg./kg./day				√
Vinblastine	VLB	0.15–0.30 mg./kg./ week	√			
Vincristine	VCR	0.1–0.2 mg./kg./ week	√			
Procarbazine (Natulan, Matulane)	PCB	50–150 mg./day				√
Carmustine	BCNU	100–200 mg./m² q. 6 weeks	√			
Lomustine	CCNU	100–130 mg./m² q. 6 weeks				√
Prednisone	PRD	40–60 mg./day				√
Adriamycin	ADM	25–60 mg./m²	√			
Epipodophyllotoxin	VM26	50 mg./m²/ 2×/week	√			
Bleomycin	BLM	5 mg./m²	√	√	√	
Streptozotocin	STZN	500 mg./m²/5 days q. 2 weeks	√			
Piperazinedione	PPZD	9–12 mg./m²/ q. 3–4 weeks	√			
Dimethyltria-zeno-imidazole carboxamide	DTIC	200 mg./m²/5 days	√			
Trimethylcol-chicinic acid methyl ether d-tartrate	TMCA	0.025–0.075 mg./ kg./day				√
Rubidazone	RBZN	200 mg./m² q. 3 weeks	√			

[a] IV, intravenous; PO, orally; IM, intramuscular; SC, subcutaneous.

| Remission Rate (%) | | | | |
Complete	Partial	Total	Toxicity	Reference
13	52	65	Acute nausea and vomiting; myelo-toxicity	Huguley et al., 1975; Carter and Livingston, 1973
12	42	54	Myelotoxicity; hemorrhagic cystitis	Desser and Ultmann, 1973; Carter and Livingston, 1973
16	44	60	Myelotoxicity	Desser and Ultmann, 1973; Carter and Livingston, 1973
—	—	41	Myelotoxicity	Desser and Ultmann, 1973; Carter and Livingston, 1973
30	38	68	Myelotoxicity; occasional neurotoxicity	Desser and Ultmann, 1973; Carter and Livingston, 1973
36	22	58	Neurotoxicity, occasionally severe	Desser and Ultmann, 1973; Carter and Livingston, 1973
38	31	69	Myelotoxicity; nausea	Desser and Ultmann, 1973; Carter and Livingston, 1973
4	43	47	Delayed, often severe myelotoxicity	Young et al., 1971; Marsh et al., 1971
3	31	34	Delayed, often severe myelotoxicity	Hoogstraten et al., 1973; Stolinsky et al., 1976b
0	61	61	Cushing's syndrome, peptic ulcer, sepsis, mental aberrations	Carter and Livingston, 1973; Desser and Ultmann, 1973
8	33	41	Nausea and vomiting; alopecia; myelotoxi-city; cardio-myopathy; recall radiation reactions	Blum and Carter, 1974; Chabner et al., 1975
12	56	68	Nausea and vomiting; myelotoxicity	Sonntag et al., 1974
6	31	37	Nausea and vomiting; febrile reactions; pulmonary fibrosis	Yagoda et al., 1972
6	38	44	Renal tubular injury, tubular acidosis	Schein et al., 1974
0	72	72	Myelotoxicity	Jones et al., 1977
6	50	56	Nausea, vomiting; occasional myelo-toxicity	Frei et al., 1972
0	33	33	Nausea, diarrhea, stomatitis; alopecia, dermatitis; myelo-toxicity	Stolinsky et al., 1976a
0	83	83	Nausea, vomiting; cardiomyopathy, myelotoxicity	Chauvergne et al., 1978

city. Both agents have the advantage that they tend to be platelet-sparing; indeed, thrombocytopenic patients may show an increase in the platelet count during vinblastine treatment. Both compounds tend to induce myelopoietic suppression with peripheral granulocytopenia.

These alkaloids must be given by intravenous injection, though oral derivatives have been introduced for investigational use (MacDonald and Lacher, 1966; Armstrong et al., 1967; Wilson and Louis, 1967). Injections of vinblastine are usually given weekly, at a dose of 0.05 to 0.20 mg./kg. and occasionally as high as 0.30 mg./kg. The weekly dose must be carefully titrated in relation to the white blood cell count. When granulocytopenia is present, it is usually reversible simply by a reduction in the weekly dose or an increase in the interval between injections. Patients can occasionally be maintained in complete remission with injections given every two weeks or even once per month. Responses to vinblastine usually occur less rapidly than those after nitrogen mustard or cyclophosphamide therapy. Some degree of response is ordinarily apparent after the second or third injection; occasionally, four to six weekly injections are required before a response is observed.

In a clinical trial described by Carbone and Spurr (1968), 15 of 56 previously untreated patients with Hodgkin's disease assigned at random to treatment with vinblastine experienced a complete remission and 27 others a partial remission for a total response rate of 75 percent, compared with a 54 percent remission rate in those treated with cyclophosphamide. There was, however, no significant difference in survival of the two groups of patients that could be attributed to either drug. In another clinical trial, the relative efficacies of vinblastine and nitrogen mustard in the treatment of Hodgkin's disease were compared (Ezdinli and Stutzman, 1968). Nitrogen mustard yielded objective responses in 80 percent of cases, as compared with 73 percent with vinblastine, in a series of 27 patients with stage III or IV Hodgkin's disease given full courses of both drugs. Of interest in this study was the finding that the sequence of administration of the two drugs may be an important consideration. When nitrogen mustard was given first and vinblastine treatment initiated after relapse or progression of disease had become apparent, there was an 80 percent overall response rate, whereas the reverse sequence yielded only a 65 percent response rate. The median duration of remission was 2.5 months for each drug. When vinblastine is used both for remission induction

and for maintenance therapy, Hodgkin's disease may be kept in sustained remission for many months and occasionally for years.

Vincristine is less often used in Hodgkin's disease than it is in the other malignant lymphomas, particularly in the diffuse histiocytic lymphomas, where it is sometimes dramatically effective. Although it causes somewhat less marrow toxicity, its use may be severely limited by its much greater tendency to elicit significant peripheral neuropathy, which can progress to become severe and disabling, if relatively high doses of drug are maintained for long periods of time (Watkins and Griffin, 1978). Sensory changes usually develop first, after several weekly intravenous injections have been given; if the drug is continued, motor changes soon supervene. The initial intravenous dose is usually 0.015 to 0.050 mg./kg. and the weekly maintenance dose is held to 0.01 to 0.015 mg./kg., if possible, to minimize the hazard of neurotoxicity. Refractoriness to vincristine appears to develop earlier than with vinblastine, and this, coupled with the limitation of its use imposed by neurotoxicity, seldom makes it possible to use vincristine for more than a few months at most.

Procarbazine. A third class of compound is represented by N-methylhydrazine (procarbazine, Natulan, Matulane), which was introduced for the treatment of Hodgkin's disease in 1963 by Mathé and his colleagues. An important advantage is that patients exhibit no cross-resistance to this drug relative to the alkylating agents or the periwinkle alkaloids. Thus it may be therapeutically active in patients who have become refractory to the other agents, as well as in previously untreated patients with Hodgkin's disease (Brunner and Young, 1965).

It is usually given orally, although intravenous administration is also possible. The starting dose is 50 mg. per day, increased gradually during the first week to 200 to 300 mg. per day (3 to 5 mg./kg.), after which the daily dose is carefully adjusted in relation to the therapeutic response and the white blood cell and platelet counts. The usual maintenance dose is in the range of 50 to 100 mg. per day. Patients often experience nausea and vomiting, particularly during the initiation of therapy, which can be minimized by careful adjustment of dose. Procarbazine may also cause mental depression or enhance the depressant effects of the phenothiazine drugs, which should therefore be avoided during its administration (Karnofsky, 1968). "Procarbazine lung," manifested as a pulmonary infiltrate resembling that seen in certain collagen diseases, and often associated with pleural effusion, is another reported complication (Ecker, Jay, and Keshane, 1978).

Most of the patients with Hodgkin's disease selected for phase II treatment with this drug had been previously treated with the alkylating agents and with vinblastine until they became refractory to these drugs. Perhaps because the marrow reserve of these patients had already been depleted before therapy with procarbazine was started, the marrow toxicity which it has elicited has often been remarkable for its prolonged and unremitting character. The early development of marrow toxicity under these circumstances has often limited the duration of benefit conferred by the drug. However, when procarbazine was administered earlier in the course of disease, it appeared to be about as effective as the alkylating agents or the periwinkle alkaloids (Table 10.2).

Nitrosourea Compounds. The first representative of this class of compounds which was tested clinically in patients with Hodgkin's disease was 1,3,bis-(β-chloroethyl)-1-nitrosourea (BCNU), which is administered intravenously. An orally administered derivative, 1-(2-chloroethyl)-3-cyclohexyl-1-nitrosourea (CCNU), was subsequently introduced. Dramatic and rapid objective responses were obtained with BCNU in 17 of 31 patients with advanced Hodgkin's disease who had become refractory to the standard chemotherapeutic agents; the median duration of maintained remission was in excess of 120 days (Lessner, 1968). An important advantage of these drugs is their ability to cross the blood-brain barrier (Rall and Zubrod, 1962; De Vita et al., 1967), because of their high degree of solubility in lipids and aqueous media.

Dispensed as a lyophilized powder, BCNU is dissolved in absolute ethanol, then diluted with distilled water, and further diluted in 200 to 500 ml. of saline prior to its slow intravenous infusion over a period of 30 to 60 minutes. The drug was initially recommended for use at 100 mg. per square meter per day for three consecutive days. When it was discovered that this dose causes excessively severe marrow toxicity, the dose was reduced to 100 mg. per square meter per day on two consecutive days. The dose of CCNU used in patients with good marrow tolerance is 130 mg. per square meter; when leukopenia or thrombocytopenia are present due to prior chemotherapy or radiotherapy, the dose of CCNU is ordinarily reduced to 100 mg. per square meter. No additional drug is given for

at least six weeks because the marrow toxicity associated with BCNU or CCNU is characteristically delayed in onset, and the premature resumption of treatment may have serious consequences if the nadir response to prior doses has not been passed. Maintenance therapy with CCNU, when instituted, is at a dose of 100 mg. per square meter every six weeks, while carefully monitoring the peripheral white blood cell and platelet counts. The mechanism of action of these drugs is not yet well established, though their major mode of action is similar to that of the alkylating agents (Schabel et al., 1965).

Bleomycin. Bleomycin is a mixture of several polypeptide antibiotics isolated from *Streptomyces verticillus*. It is usually given by slow intravenous injection but may also be injected intramuscularly or subcutaneously. In preliminary studies in which it was administered at a dose level of 0.25 mg./kg. daily, severe mucocutaneous reactions were observed after seven to ten days (Yagoda et al., 1972). Subsequent studies have suggested that twice-weekly administration of bleomycin at a dose of 15 mg. per square meter is generally well tolerated. However, fever and chills may follow the injection of bleomycin within a few hours and are occasionally of sufficient severity to require dose reduction. Of greater concern is the occasional occurrence of anaphylactoid reactions, which may be acutely fatal; we have seen one such case. However, bleomycin has the great advantage that it has no bone marrow toxicity and thus may be given with impunity to patients whose hematologic tolerance has been severely impaired by prior chemotherapy or radiotherapy. For this reason it has also recently been introduced in certain drug combinations as an agent that can safely be given during the recovery period between successive cycles of myelotoxic drugs.

The major limiting factor in the use of bleomycin has been the unpredictable and occasionally fatal development of pulmonary fibrosis, which was observed in as many as 10 percent of patients in early studies. The clinical manifestations of this complication may be abrupt in onset and are manifested by dyspnea, cough, rales at the pulmonary bases, evidence of a bilateral interstitial infiltrate on chest radiograms, and laboratory evidence of decreased arterial oxygen saturation, pulmonary vital capacity, and diffusion capacity. Histopathologic studies have revealed interstitial edema, intra-alveolar hyaline membrane formation, increased numbers of alveolar macrophages, and the deposition of collagen in the alveolar walls (De Lena et al., 1972). Although there is some evidence that the risk of serious pulmonary fibrosis increases at cumulative total doses exceeding 400 mg., cases have been reported at total doses of as little as 50 mg. (Iacovino et al., 1976). There is believed to be a greater risk of this complication in elderly individuals, in whom the use of this drug is therefore to be undertaken with great caution. The drug is also contraindicated for these reasons in patients who have other forms of significant pulmonary disease. There have been anecdotal reports that corticosteroid treatment may alleviate the symptoms associated with bleomycin-induced pulmonary fibrosis (Blum, Carter, and Agre, 1973).

Adriamycin. Adriamycin (14-hydroxy-daunomycin) is a member of the anthracycline antibiotics obtained as fermentation products of the fungus *Streptomyces peucetius* var. *caesius.* It has been shown to have significant clinical activity against a broad spectrum of malignant neoplasms, including the soft tissue sarcomas, carcinoma of the breast and lung, and the lymphomas (Blum and Carter, 1974). After intravenous administration, the drug is rapidly cleared from plasma and widely distributed in tissues throughout the body. It is metabolized in the liver and excreted primarily via the biliary tract. Severe toxic reactions associated with the delayed excretion of the drug have been observed in patients with impaired hepatic function, in whom dose reduction is usually necessary (Chabner et al., 1975). Small amounts of the drug or its metabolites are also excreted in the urine. Adriamycin, unlike the nitrosoureas, has little ability to cross the blood-brain barrier and to enter the central nervous system.

The drug is usually given at a dose level of 25–50 mg. per square meter by rapid intravenous infusion. Alternatively, it may be given at a dose of 60–75 mg. per square meter every three weeks. Its administration may be attended by nausea and vomiting and is consistently associated with the development of severe or complete alopecia. It also has very significant myelotoxicity, and must therefore be used with caution in leukopenic or thrombocytopenic patients. An interesting and potentially serious aspect of adriamycin toxicity is its interaction with ionizing radiation effects on tissues. Typical radiation reactions, sometimes of considerable severity, have reappeared during adriamycin treatment in tissues treated months or even years earlier with X-irradiation (Cassady et

al., 1975; Phillips and Fu, 1976). However, the most serious complication associated with adriamycin administration is cardiomyopathy, sometimes of sufficient severity to lead to congestive heart failure and death. At autopsy, fragmentation of myocardial myofibrils, mitochondrial swelling, intracellular inclusions, and loss of myocardial muscle cells, with replacement by fibrous tissue, have been observed (Bristow et al., 1978). The risk of clinically manifest cardiomyopathy increases rapidly at cumulative total doses exceeding 550 mg. per square meter. However, serial transcatheter endomyocardial biopsies have revealed that destruction of cardiac muscle may appear focally even after a single dose of adriamycin (Billingham et al., 1977). Thus cardiac damage probably occurs in all instances, though clinically silent in most. This is of importance in patients who have previously received mantle field irradiation, in whom adriamycin cardiac toxicity may be superimposed on a recall radiation reaction triggered by adriamycin administration.

Adrenal Corticosteroids. Prednisone and other adrenal steroids have for the most part been used in patients with Hodgkin's disease who develop severe hemolytic anemias or who are in the near-terminal stages of the disease, when bone marrow reserves have been so severely depleted by other chemotherapeutic agents as to preclude their continued use. Perhaps because they have been used almost entirely under such extremely adverse circumstances, steroids have reportedly yielded disappointing results in terms of objective response (Fadem et al., 1951; Ranney and Gellhorn, 1957; Rosenberg et al., 1961). However, massive doses of prednisone or prednisolone (200 mg. to 5 gm. per day for 9 to 68 days) were used by Hill, Marshall, and Falco (1956) in 16 patients with leukemia and 3 with lymphoma, with reportedly good results. Moloney et al. (1961) were not able to obtain similar responses in patients with Hodgkin's disease, but Hall et al. (1967) reported objective remissions in 16 of 24 patients with Hodgkin's disease and in 5 of 12 patients with other types of malignant lymphoma, all of whom had advanced disease refractory to radiation therapy and alkylating agents prior to the initiation of corticosteroid therapy. Most of their patients received either prednisone at doses ranging from 45 to 300 mg. per day for periods of 3.5 to 75 weeks or methyl prednisolone (Medrol) at 60 to 600 mg. per day for 4 to 42 weeks. Several criteria of objective response were scored: regression of lymphadenopathy in 20 of 29 patients, lasting for 3 to 104 weeks; diminution of hepatosplenomegaly in 8 of 14; clearance of peripheral edema in 4; relief of recurrent pleural effusion in 4 of 6 instances; significant increases in hemoglobin levels in 19, and in white blood cell levels in 11 of 19 patients. Hall et al. concluded: "The use of high-dose corticoids seems justified in those patients who have progressive disease and drug- or radiation-induced myelosuppression and in whom the risk of gastrointestinal and infectious complications is justified in comparison with further myelosuppressive therapy."

However, prolonged maintenance on corticosteroids is likely to be both dangerous and difficult. Virtually all patients who receive significant doses of steroids over several weeks develop Cushingoid manifestations, which are sometimes quite disagreeable, particularly in female patients. More serious, however, is the induction of susceptibility to bacterial, viral, and fungal infections and the hazard of gastrointestinal bleeding and ulceration. The adrenal steroids may also induce severe psychiatric disturbances requiring discontinuation of treatment.

Miscellaneous. Reviews of the literature concerning other drugs tested in patients with Hodgkin's disease have been presented by Hall (1966), Carter and Livingston (1973), and Desser and Ultmann (1973). In general, the antimetabolite drugs (6-mercaptopurine, cytosine arabinoside, 5-fluorouracil, and methotrexate) have been surprisingly ineffectual, in view of their demonstrated therapeutic activity in other types of neoplastic disease. In four clinical studies cited by Hall, actinomycin C (Sanamycin) elicited responses in 9 of 14, 13 of 19, 41 of 92, and 26 of 44 cases of Hodgkin's disease, respectively. The methyl ester of streptonigrin, another antibiotic, was effective in 6 of 9 and 9 of 15 patients, respectively, in two additional studies. Aurantin, a complex antibiotic of the actinomycin group, was reportedly effective in 26 of 40 instances. Conversely, the antibiotics mitomycin C and mithramycin were relatively unimpressive (cf. Hall, 1966, table 3).

Among the miscellaneous drugs, desacetyl methylcolchicine was reported by Santos Silva (1963) to elicit responses in six of six patients with advanced Hodgkin's disease. Another analog of colchicine, trimethylcolchicinic acid methyl ether d-tartrate (TMCA), yielded partial remissions in one-third of the patients studied by Stolinsky et al. (1976a). Another agent which has shown useful levels of clinical activity in the treatment of patients with Hodg-

kin's disease and other lymphomas, and has therefore found its way into some of the recent multiple drug combinations, is 5-(3,3-dimethyl-1-triazeno) imidazole-4-carboxamide (DTIC; Frei et al., 1972). Methylglyoxal-bis-guanylhydrazone elicited responses in two of four and four of four patients, respectively, in two brief clinical trials. Hydroxyurea was relatively ineffectual in reported studies to date. Cycloheximide has been shown by Young, MacDonald, and Karnofsky (1964) to have useful antipyretic effects in patients with Hodgkin's disease, without observable effects on the growth of lymph node or other tumor masses.

Multiple-Drug Chemotherapy

Theoretical and Experimental Background. As each new class of chemotherapeutic compound emerged, it reawakened the hope that a chemical cure for Hodgkin's disease and other malignant lymphomas might at last have been found; and as the inevitable relapses have developed after initially favorable responses to each of the new chemotherapeutic agents, hope has given way to disillusionment and even to despair about the curative potential of chemotherapy for the lymphomas. The emergence of a new conceptual approach has rekindled that hope. As discussed above, it was the experimental work of Goldin et al. (1956,1958), Skipper et al. (1964), and Bruce et al. (1966,1967, 1969) that laid the conceptual framework for the new approach. Their studies, using transplantable leukemias of mice as model systems, yielded the following conclusions.

1. For practical purposes, it is necessary to kill every tumor cell in order to effect a cure. It is not sufficient to kill 99 percent of the tumor cells; the surviving 1 percent will inevitably repopulate the tumor. (There are, however, certain apparent exceptions to this view, in which immunologic defenses against the tumor may be sufficiently strong to eradicate a small residual tumor cell population; examples are the choriocarcinoma of females and the African Burkitt lymphoma.)

2. The killing of tumor cells (and of normal cells) by chemotherapeutic agents, as had previously been established for radiation, is exponential relative to dose. That is, a certain proportion, rather than a fixed number, of the tumor cells present at the beginning of treatment will be killed by any given dose of an agent.

3. Since any systemic agent will also kill normal proliferating cell populations and since no drug developed to date has a high degree of selectivity

for the killing of tumor cells, even near-lethal doses of any single drug will still fall far short of the dose levels needed to eradicate all of the cells in a tumor population. Thus, unless some as yet unknown, qualitative biochemical difference between tumor cells and normal cells can be discovered and chemically exploited, it would appear that single-drug chemotherapy is a priori doomed to failure in most tumors.

4. However, experiment confirmed the expectation that *combinations* of two or more agents, each of which was independently active against a tumor, would act additively to kill a much greater fraction of the initial tumor cell population than could have been achieved with maximally tolerable doses of any one agent alone, *provided* that the major toxicity of each agent employed acts on a different normal cell population (Valeriote et al., 1968). Only when their toxicities are independent and non-overlapping can it be anticipated that there will be any therapeutic gain by combining two or more agents.

These experimental concepts were then tested and substantially confirmed in patients with acute leukemia by Frei and his colleagues (1965). Encouraged by their results with combination chemotherapy in acute leukemia, these investigators then initiated a search for effective combinations of agents in the treatment of patients with Hodgkin's disease. In addition, a number of workers had, for nearly thirty years, explored the potentialities of chemotherapy combined with radiotherapy in the management of Hodgkin's disease. Although the results of combining single drugs with radiotherapy were, for the most part, unimpressive, clinical trials in which multiple drugs were used in addition to total lymphoid radiotherapy (combined modality therapy) have yielded highly significant gains. The experience to date with combined modality therapy is presented in Chapter 11.

Combination Chemotherapy for Hodgkin's Disease. An alkylating agent, chlorambucil, and the periwinkle alkaloid, vinblastine, were selected by Lacher and Durant (1965) as a two-drug combination for the treatment of patients with advanced Hodgkin's disease. They observed complete remissions in 10 of 16 patients (63 percent) and partial responses in 3 others, for a total remission rate of 81 percent. No simultaneous randomized controls were included in their study.

Quadruple-drug combinations were first used by the National Cancer Institute group. Moxley et al. (1967) reported preliminary results of a study in which one patient with stage IIIA and four others with stage IIIB Hodgkin's disease were treated with three two-week cycles of combination chemotherapy, separated by rest periods of ten days or more. The drugs employed were cyclophosphamide, vincristine, methotrexate, and prednisone. Nine other patients with more localized disease who received this combination of drugs in conjunction with radiotherapy to all involved sites are discussed separately in Chapter 11.

The results in the patients treated with this drug combination were not particularly impressive. Two of the four patients with stage IIIB disease failed to enter a remission; remissions were induced in the other two, but they developed relapses at two and twelve months, and all four patients with stage IIIB disease died of uncontrolled disease. The lone patient with stage IIIA disease treated with this four-drug combination alone entered a remission which persisted without maintenance therapy for more than thirty-two months. The mean nadir white blood cell count in the five patients treated with chemotherapy alone was 5,700 per cubic millimeter, with a range of 1,500 to 9,400 during the first cycle of treatment; 4,980 (range 800 to 7,600) during the second cycle; and 3,360 (range 600 to 5,600) during the third cycle. There were no deaths attributable to drug toxicity. Aside from hematopoietic depression, other toxic manifestations included paresthesias and foot drop, attributable to vincristine; buccal and other gastrointestinal mucosal ulcerations, attributable to methotrexate, with gross bleeding in one instance; Cushingoid changes attributable to prednisone; and hair loss, probably due to the combined action of methotrexate and cyclophosphamide.

The National Cancer Institute group then went on to study a different quadruple drug combination, essentially similar to the first, with the following exceptions: (1) six rather than three two-week cycles were utilized; (2) methotrexate, the drug with the least well-established activity against Hodgkin's disease, was replaced by procarbazine; and (3) nitrogen mustard was substituted for cyclophosphamide as the alkylating agent (Carbone, 1967). This so-called MOPP program derives its acronym from M for mustard, O for Oncovin (vincristine), P for procarbazine, and P for prednisone. The doses, routes of administration, and schedules are summarized in Table 10.3. It may be seen that two of the drugs, nitrogen mustard and vincristine, were given intravenously on days 1 and 8 of each cycle, whereas the other two, procarbazine and prednisone, were given orally throughout a 14-day period of treatment, which was then followed by a 14-day rest interval before the initiation of the next cycle. Prednisone was administered only in cycles 1 and 4 of a sequence which usually involved six cycles of treatment. Maintenance therapy was not given at the completion of the six cycles of quadruple chemotherapy, but additional chemotherapy was administered in those cases in which relapses developed.

DeVita, Serpick, and Carbone (1970) reported that 43 patients with advanced Hodgkin's disease completed six cycles of MOPP quadruple chemotherapy during the interval from 1964 to July 1, 1967. Thirty-five of these (81 percent) entered complete remission, the median duration of which, calculated from the end of the sixth cycle, was 29 to 42 months as of March 1970 (Tables 10.4 and 10.5). Eighteen of these patients had relapsed at the time of their report, with a median time to relapse of eleven months. Relapse intervals ranged from 2 to 42 months. The remaining seventeen patients were still in unmaintained remission at the time of the report, the longest continuing remission being 52 months. Particularly encouraging was the fact that of the twenty patients with unmaintained remission lasting longer than two years, only three had exhibited relapses to the date of reporting. Several other groups were subsequently able to obtain essentially identical complete remission rates with the MOPP regimen (Table 10.3). Moreover, a ten-year followup report on 194 patients with stage III or IV disease treated with MOPP at the National Cancer Institute revealed an 80 percent complete remission rate; of those achieving complete remission, 66 percent remained relapse-free at five and ten years after all treatment had been discontinued. The five- and 10-year survival rates of all patients in the series were 65 and 58 percent, respectively; corresponding survival figures for patients who achieved complete remissions were 82 and 72 percent, respectively (De Vita et al., 1976).

The first modification of the MOPP program was MVPP (Table 10.3), which was initiated at St. Bartholomew's Hospital, London, by Nicholson et al. (1970). In this regimen, vinblastine was substituted for vincristine, prednisone was used in all six cycles at lower dosage, and the interval between cycles was lengthened to four weeks. The long-term results of the MVPP combination appear to be quite comparable to those achieved with MOPP (McElwain et al., 1973; Sutcliffe et al., 1978). In the several years that have elapsed since the MOPP program was first reported, a number of other

combination chemotherapy regimens have been investigated. Some of these were initially developed for the treatment of patients who failed to respond to MOPP, or who relapsed after obtaining complete or partial remissions, and were then utilized as primary chemotherapeutic programs after initial experience with their use proved favorable. The drug combinations, dose levels, and schedules of administration, as well as remission rates obtained with each of these regimens are summarized in Table 10.3. It is evident that the results obtained with most of these multiple drug programs have been remarkably similar. However, none of the newer combinations has proven to be significantly better than MOPP, as measured by complete remission rate, though some, such as MVPP, appear to be advantageous with respect to acute toxicity and hematologic tolerance.

The degree of leukopenia (Table 10.6) and neurotoxicity observed by DeVita et al. (1970) were generally within tolerable limits and readily reversible after the completion of individual cycles. Thrombocytopenia was not a major problem. Two patients died during the initial cycle of chemotherapy, as a consequence both of rapid necrosis in lymphoid tumor masses and sepsis. One other patient developed staphylococcal septicemia but responded well to antibiotics. MOPP combination chemotherapy was also well tolerated by and efficacious in patients relapsing after prior limited field radiotherapy, but hematologic tolerance was often poor, and complete remission rates significantly lower, in patients who were treated with MOPP after prior single-drug chemotherapy (Lowenbraun et al., 1970).

Although the experience reported by the Bethesda group in previously untreated patients with stage IIIB and stage IV Hodgkin's disease was highly impressive, the lack of a concurrent control group treated with comparably intensive single-drug chemotherapy made it difficult to draw firm conclusions concerning the superiority of MOPP or other multiple-drug combinations. Convincing evidence for this view was later provided in a prospective randomized clinical trial conducted by Huguley et al. (1975), the design and results of which are presented in Chapter 11.

Our experience at Stanford University Medical Center (Moore et al., 1973; Portlock et al., 1976) with the MOPP quadruple chemotherapy program, used as primary treatment in patients with disseminated (stage IV) disease and as secondary treatment in patients relapsing after prior radiotherapy or single-drug chemotherapy, has been

Table 10.3 Combination Chemotherapy Regimens in Advanced Hodgkin's Disease

Acronym	Drug[a]	Dose	Route	Schedule (days)	Interval between cycles (days)	Remission rate (%) Complete	Remission rate (%) Partial	Reference
MOPP	HN₂	6 mg./m²	IV	1, 8	28	81	—	De Vita et al., 1970
	VCR	1.4 mg./m²	IV	1, 8		83	—	Cooper et al., 1972
	PCB	100 mg./m²	PO	1–14		80	—	Jacobs et al., 1976
	PRD	40 mg./m²	PO	1–14		62	17	Bonadonna et al., 1977
				(cycles 1 and 4 only)				
MVPP	HN₂	6 mg./m²	IV	1, 8	42	82	—	Nicholson et al., 1970; McElwain et al., 1973; Sutcliffe et al., 1978
	VLB	6 mg./m²	IV	1, 8				
	PCB	100 mg./m²	PO	1–14				
	PRD	40 mg.	PO	1–14				
MVVPP	HN₂	0.4 mg./kg.	IV	1	57	78	22	Levitt et al., 1970
	VCR	1.4 mg./m²	IV	1, 8, 15				
	VLB	6 mg./m²	IV	22, 29, 36				
	PCB	100 mg./day	PO	22–43				
	PRD	40 mg./m²	PO	2–22				
				(tapered days 23–36, cycle 1 only)				
MABOP	HN₂	6 mg./m²	IV	1, 8	28	72	16	Bonadonna et al., 1972
	ADM	25 mg./m²	IV	1, 8				
	BLM	30 mg./m²	IV	1, 8				
	VCR	1.2 mg./m²	IV	1, 8				
	PRD	40 mg./m²	PO	1–14				
—	VM-26	40 mg./m²	IV	1, 4, 8, 11, 14	28	40	44	Eckhardt et al., 1975
	PCB	100 mg./day	PO	1–14				
	PRD	40 mg./day	PO	1–14				
B-DOPA	BLM	4 mg./m²	IM	2, 5	28–35	60	20	Lokich et al., 1976
	DTIC	150 mg./m²	IV	1–5				
	VCR	1.5 mg./m²	IV	1, 5				
	PRD	40 mg./m²	PO	1–6				
	ADM	60 mg./m²	IV	1				
ABCD	ADM	25–30 mg./m²	IV	1	42	33	33	Abele et al., 1976
	BLM	15 mg./m²	IV, IM or SC	1–5				
	CCNU	60 mg./m²	PO	1				
	DTIC	90–100 mg./m²	IV	1–5				

(continued)

Regimen	Drug	Dose	Route	Days				Reference
CVPP (1)	CTX	300 mg/m²	IV	1, 8	42	74	—	Bloomfield et al., 1976
	VLB	10 mg,	IV	1, 8, 15				
	PCB	100 mg/m²	PO	1–15				
	PRD	40 mg/m²	PO	1–15 (cycles 1 and 4 only)				
CVPP (2)	CTX	1,000 mg/m²	IV	1	28	62	—	Diggs et al., 1977
	VLB	0.1 mg./kg.	IV	1, 8				
	PCB	100 mg/m²	PO	1–7				
	PRD	40 mg/m²	PO	1–7				
BVPP	BCNU	100 mg/m²	IV	1–3	42	83	17	Harrison and Neiman, 1977
	VCR	1.4 mg./m²	IV	1, 8, 15				
	PCB	100 mg/m²	PO	1–10				
	PRD	40 mg/m²	PO	1–14				
ABVD	ADM	25 mg/m²	IV	1, 15	28	70	11	Bonadonna et al., 1977
	BLM	10 mg/m²	IV	1, 15				
	VLB	10 mg/m²	IV	1, 15				
	DTIC	375 mg/m²	IV	1, 15				
CLVPP	CLB	6 mg/m²	PO	1–14	28	76	17	McElwain et al., 1977
	VLB	6 mg/m²	IV	1, 8				
	PCB	100 mg/m²	PO	1–14				
	PRD	40 mg.	PO	1–14				
B-MOPP	MOPP, as above, plus				28	84	14	Coltman and Jones, 1978
	BLM	2 mg./m²	IV	1, 8				
SCAB	STZN	500 mg/m²	IV	1–5	42	80	10	Diggs et al., 1978
	CCNU	100 mg/m²	PO	1				
	ADM	45 mg/m²	IV	1				
	BLM	15 mg/m²	IM	1, 8				
PAVe	ALK	7.5 mg./m²	PO	1, 2, 8, 9	28	—	—	Rosenberg et al., 1978
	VLB	6 mg/m²	IV	1, 8				
	PCB	100 mg/m²	PO	1–14				
VAPP	VCR or	0.03 mg./kg.	IV	1	28	75	19	Marinone et al., 1978
	VLB	0.6 mg./kg.	IV	1, 3, 5				
	ADM	0.4 mg./kg.	IV	1–14				
	PCB	3 mg./kg.	PO	1–14				
	PRD	1–1.5 mg./kg.	PO	1–21				

[a] Abbreviations as in Table 10.2.

Table 10.4 Results of MOPP Combination Chemotherapy in Forty-Three Patients with Advanced Hodgkin's Disease

Mean duration of treatment	5.8 months
Deaths during treatment	2
Responded but failed to achieve a complete remission	6
Achieved a complete remission	35 (81%)
Mean time to complete remission	3 months
Median duration of complete remission (from the cessation of all therapy)	29–42 months
Number who have relapsed	18 (51%)
Median time to relapse	11 months

Source: Data of DeVita, Serpick, and Carbone (1970). Reproduced with permission.

generally consistent with that reported by De Vita et al. (1970,1976). Dramatic regression of advanced disease and prompt lysis of cyclic fever, even after a single cycle of drugs, has been observed in several instances (Figs. 4.3, 10.1, 10.2, and 10.3). However, a much higher primary relapse rate has been observed in the Stanford series in stage IV patients presenting with bone marrow involvement. Patients over 45 years of age also had a very significantly higher relapse rate than patients less than 20 years of age (Moore et al., 1973). Our experience with MOPP treatment in the salvage of patients relapsing after prior radiotherapy

or combined modality therapy, which is detailed in Chapter 12, has also been highly encouraging (Weller et al., 1976; Portlock et al., 1978).

Thus, the advent of multiple-drug combination chemotherapy has dramatically changed the prognosis of patients with previously untreated stage III or IV Hodgkin's disease, as well as that of patients with regionally localized disease relapsing after prior radiotherapy. Combination chemotherapy appears to have significant curative potential even in some patients with stage IVB disease. Accordingly, except for elderly or medically infirm individuals, patients with advanced Hodgkin's disease, who were formerly deemed to have no significant chance for cure and were therefore relegated to palliative treatment with single-drug chemotherapy, are now candidates for possible curative treatment with combination chemotherapy or, as described in Chapter 11, with combined modality therapy. Moreover, the success of combination chemotherapy, used as primary treatment for advanced disease and as salvage treatment for relapsing disease, has prompted clinical investigations in which MOPP and other multiple-drug combinations have been used as adjuvant treatment following or associated with radiotherapy in an effort to eradicate occult sites of microscopic disease. The design and the results of clinical trials involving adjuvant chemotherapy are detailed in Chapter 11.

Table 10.5 Results of Combination Chemotherapy: Response and Status by Stage of Disease

Stage[a]	Number	Induction failures	Complete remissions	First remission continuing	Deaths
IV-B	31	8[b]	23	9	13[b]
IV-A	4	0	4	4	0
III-B	5	0	5	2	0
III-A	3	0	3	2	1

Source: Data of DeVita, Serpick, and Carbone (1970). Reproduced with permission.
[a] Rye classification.
[b] Includes both deaths following initial cycle of treatment.

Table 10.6 White Blood Cell Count Suppression During Successive Cycles of MOPP Combination Chemotherapy

Cycle	Mean nadir WBC count	Percentage of patients with WBC counts			
		$<1000/mm.^3$	$<2000/mm.^3$	$<3000/mm.^3$	$<5000/mm.^3$
1	7,800	2	20	37	63
2	3,300	0	27	46	88
3	3,900	3	18	49	82
4	4,000	0	9	49	77
5	3,000	3	26	62	97
6	3,000	3	21	53	91

Source: Data of DeVita, Serpick, and Carbone (1970). Reproduced with permission.

Combination Chemotherapy for MOPP Relapses. Despite the very impressive results obtained with MOPP combination chemotherapy, as detailed in the preceding section, approximately 20 to 30 percent of previously untreated patients with advanced disease fail to achieve complete remission with MOPP, and a significant proportion of those who enter complete remission subsequently relapse with recurrent disease (Figs. 10.3, 10.4, 10.5). In the National Cancer Institute experience, 52 (32 percent) of 161 patients with advanced Hodgkin's disease who achieved complete remission with MOPP chemotherapy subsequently relapsed (Young et al., 1978). Relapses occurred principally in sites of previous disease (92 percent), especially in previously involved lymph nodes (75 percent).

For patients relapsing more than one year after the completion of six cycles of MOPP chemotherapy, reinitiation of the MOPP regimen was often successful in inducing a second complete remission (De Vita et al., 1970; Fisher et al., 1977). In our ex-perience, however, such second remissions have not been sustained; indeed, we have not succeeded in a single such patient to date in preventing the ultimate progression of disease by retreatment with MOPP (S. A. Rosenberg, personal communication).

When relapse occurs earlier, or when patients fail to enter complete remission, the MOPP program must be abandoned. At one time, the only available treatment for such patients was single-drug palliative chemotherapy, a situation in which vinblastine was perhaps the single most effective agent, inducing complete remissions in about 7 percent and partial remissions in about 55 percent (Warren et al., 1978).

In the past decade, medical oncologists have sought to develop other multiple-drug programs utilizing agents to which the MOPP combination would not have been expected to induce cross-resistance. Several such "cross-over regimens" have been developed and tested in patients with MOPP-

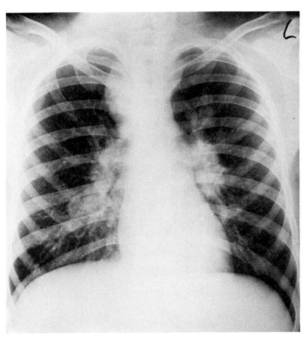

A

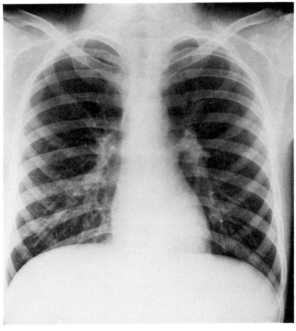

B

Figure 10.1 Dramatic regression of advanced (stage IVB) Hodgkin's disease after only one cycle of MOPP quadruple chemotherapy. The patient, a 12-year-old male, was admitted with generalized lymphadenopathy, a palpably enlarged spleen, drenching night sweats and fever, and radiographic evidence (*A*, 12/5/69) of mediastinal, bilateral hilar and bilateral pulmonary parenchymal disease (cf. also Fig. 5.18). An abdominal film (*C*) confirmed the presence of splenomegaly (arrows); lymphangiogram on 12/9/69 (*D*) revealed multiple grossly enlarged, foamy para-aortic and splenic hilar nodes; and a splenic arteriogram and splenogram (*E*) revealed diffuse mottling due to the presence of multiple filling defects. Because his constitutional symptoms were so severe and his bilateral pulmonary disease placed him in stage IV, MOPP chemotherapy was instituted, with prompt lysis of fever (Fig. 4.3, Chapter 4), cessation of night sweats, and increase in appetite and vigor. At the completion of the first two-week cycle on 12/17/69, repeat films of the chest (*B*) and abdomen (*F*) revealed dramatic diminution in size of the involved lymph nodes and spleen. At laparotomy two weeks later, the spleen revealed large areas of hypocellularity, largely filled with red blood cells, but no histologic evidence of viable residual Hodgkin's disease.

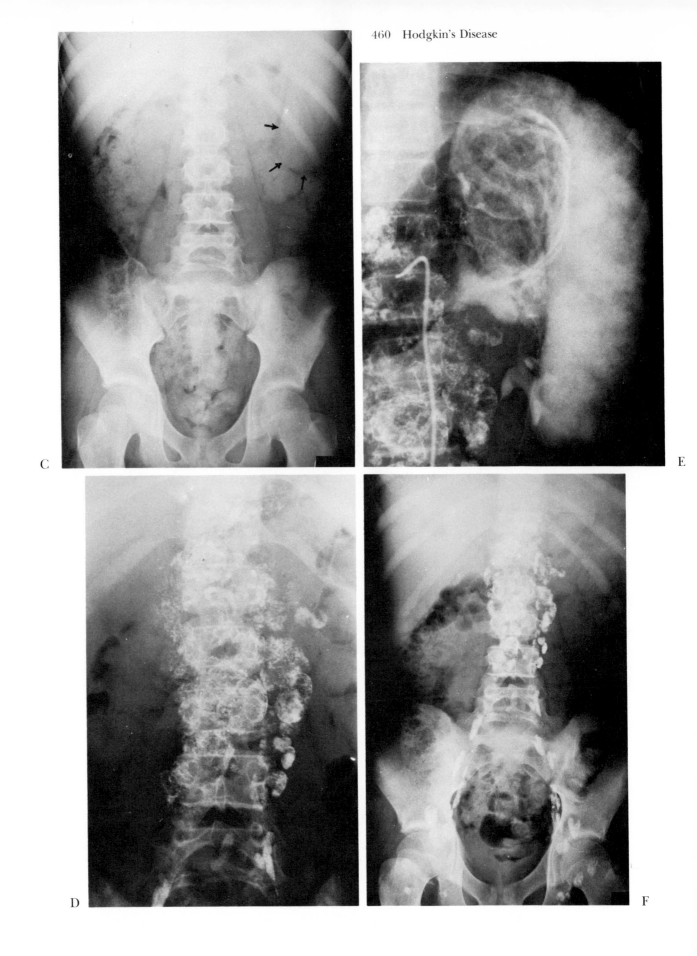

C

D

E

F

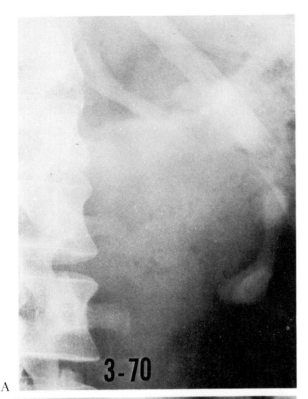

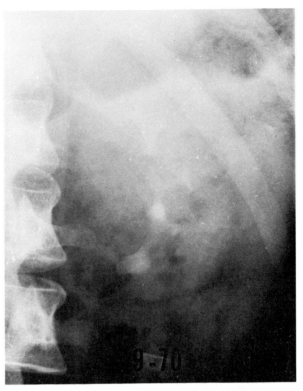

A

C

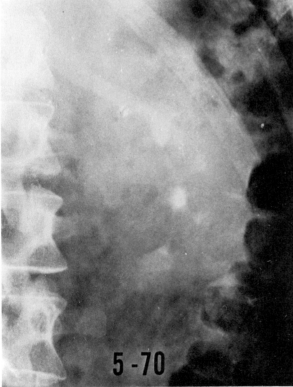

B

Figure 10.2 Response of renal involvement to MOPP quadruple chemotherapy. This 23-year-old male was initially treated at Stanford with total lymphoid radiotherapy in 1965 for stage IIIA Hodgkin's disease. Unfortunately, at that time the importance of the nodes along the splenic pedicle was not appreciated, and his spleen field was therefore separated from his para-aortic field by a gap of 3 to 4 cm. He was apparently well for four and one-half years, but then returned in March 1970 with low back and left costovertebral angle pain and weakness and paralysis of the lower extremities. Diagnostic studies revealed a large mass in the left upper lumbar region, displacing the left kidney laterally, directly invading the renal pelvis and medulla and producing marked caliectasis (*A*). It was felt that he could not be reirradiated safely; instead, treatment with MOPP quadruple chemotherapy was started, with progressive improvement in the appearance of the left kidney on serial intravenous urograms in May and September 1970 (*B* and *C*).

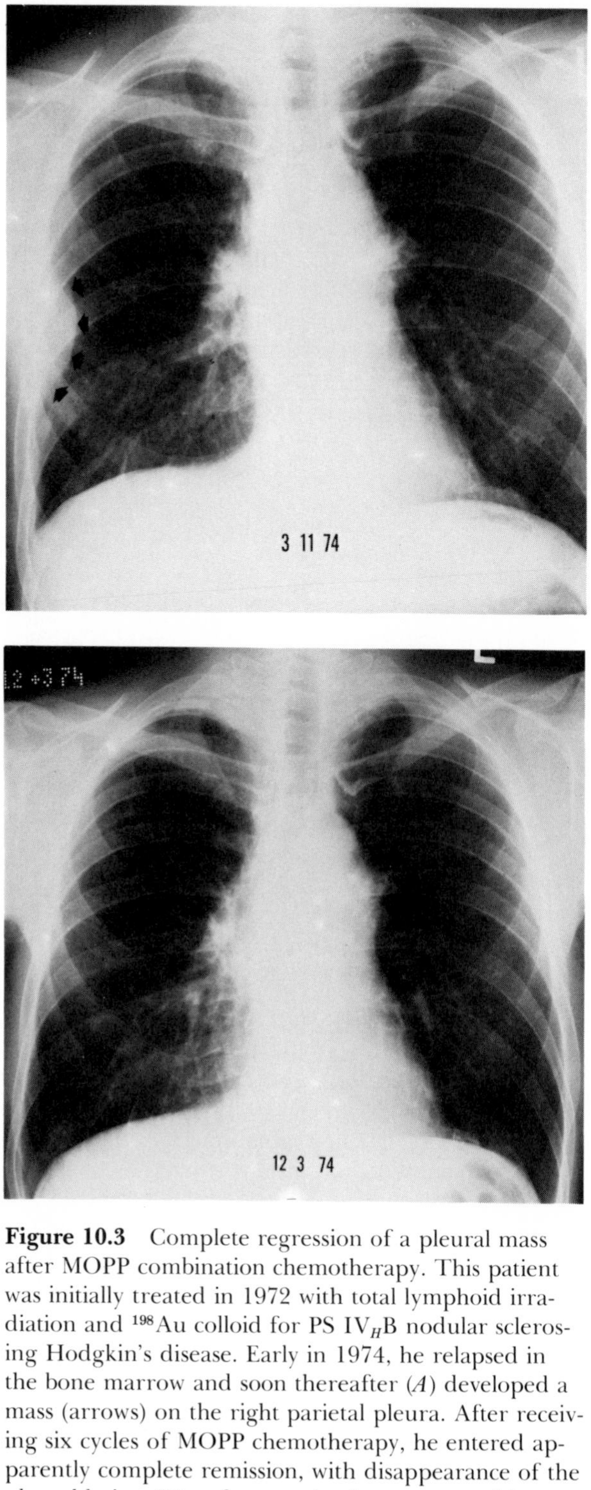

Figure 10.3 Complete regression of a pleural mass after MOPP combination chemotherapy. This patient was initially treated in 1972 with total lymphoid irradiation and ^{198}Au colloid for PS IV$_H$B nodular sclerosing Hodgkin's disease. Early in 1974, he relapsed in the bone marrow and soon thereafter (A) developed a mass (arrows) on the right parietal pleura. After receiving six cycles of MOPP chemotherapy, he entered apparently complete remission, with disappearance of the pleural lesion (B) and a negative bone marrow biopsy. His response was of brief duration, however, perhaps because his drug doses were suboptimal due to poor hematologic tolerance. Subsequent relapses could not be controlled by various crossover regimens or by palliative single-drug chemotherapy, and he died with active disease in 1976.

resistant Hodgkin's disease. The drugs, dose levels, and schedules of administration, as well as the remission rates achieved with each of these combinations, are detailed in Table 10.7. It is evident that a significant complete remission rate has been obtained with a number of these combinations. In most instances, however, the duration of such remissions has been discouragingly brief, and it would appear that few patients have been permanently salvaged by any of the cross-over regimens available to date.

Maintenance Therapy. The value of maintenance therapy in single-agent chemotherapy with the alkylating agents was well documented years ago by Scott (1963). Accordingly, several groups of investigators have used either single drugs or combinations of drugs, given on a less intensive schedule, every two or three months, following the induction of complete remission with MOPP or other combination chemotherapy regimens. Although short-term observations have suggested a decrease in relapse rates in some of the reported studies, there has been no convincing evidence that long-term survival is significantly improved by maintenance chemotherapy.

Luce et al. (1973) randomly allocated patients who had achieved complete remission after six or more courses of MOPP combination chemotherapy either to no maintenance therapy or to a maintenance regimen which consisted of two more cycles of MOPP at four-week intervals, followed by additional cycles of MOPP at eight-week intervals for at least two years, omitting prednisone. The early results were quite encouraging. At the time of their analysis, Luce et al. reported that only 8 (23 percent) of 35 patients on the maintenance regimen had relapsed, as compared with 14 (42 percent) of 33 patients allocated to no maintenance therapy. The median duration of maintained remission was estimated by extrapolation to be 180 weeks in the maintained group, almost twice as long as that in the unmaintained group (95 weeks). The additional toxicity attributable to maintenance therapy was considered to be well within acceptable limits. However, a later analysis by the same group (Coltman, Frei, and Moon, 1976) revealed that relapses were postponed, rather than permanently prevented, in the patients who had received maintenance treatment; within a few years after the cessation of maintenance therapy, the relapse rates in both groups were no longer significantly different, nor was long-term survival differentially affected.

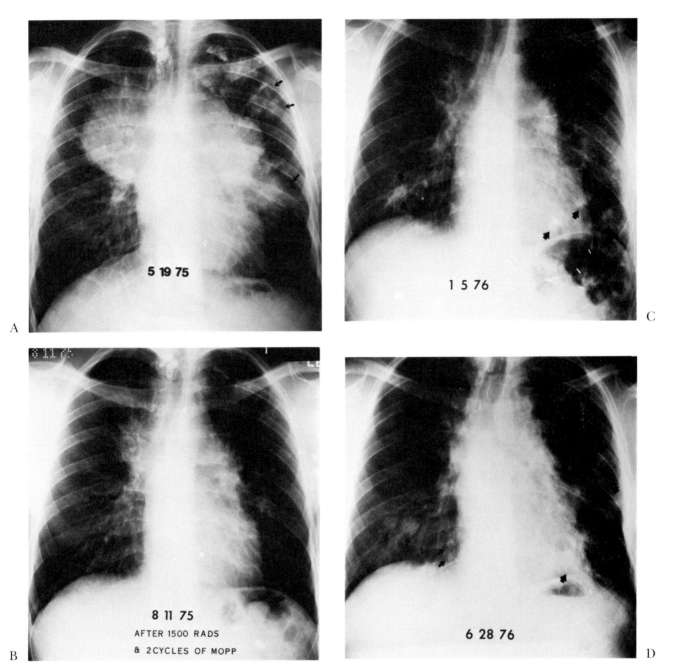

Figure 10.4 Relapse of Hodgkin's disease in the lung after MOPP chemotherapy. *A*, this patient presented in May 1975 with massive mediastinal and bilateral hilar adenopathy and multiple pulmonary parenchymal nodules (arrows) and was classified as having stage IV_LB disease. He received 1,500 rads in two weeks to the entire thorax and then was started on MOPP, with an excellent, though incomplete, response after two cycles (*B*). However, a repeat chest film (*C*) in January 1976, shortly after the sixth cycle, revealed unequivocal evidence of new pulmonary parenchymal disease bilaterally. Attempted salvage with ABVD combination chemotherapy was unsuccessful (*D*), and he died in January 1977 with uncontrolled disease.

In a study at the National Cancer Institute, 57 patients with advanced Hodgkin's disease who attained a complete remission after MOPP chemotherapy were randomly allocated to one of three regimens: (1) no additional therapy; (2) intermit- tent therapy with two consecutive monthly cycles of MOPP chemotherapy at 3-month intervals for 15 months following the completion of remission induction; or (3) intermittent BCNU maintenance at doses of 200 mg. per square meter intrave-

Table 10.7 Cross-over Combination Chemotherapy Regimens in MOPP-Resistant Hodgkin's Disease

Acronym	Drug[a]	Dose	Route	Schedule (days)	Interval between cycles (days)	Remission rate (%) Complete	Partial	Reference
ABVD	ADM	25 mg./m²	IV	1, 15	28	60	—	Bonadonna et al., 1975, 1977
	BLM	10 mg./m²	IV	1, 15		33	53	Vicente and Cortès-Funes, 1976
	VLB	6 mg./m²	IV	1, 15		22	15	Krikorian et al., 1978
	DTIC	375 mg./m²	IV	1, 15		0	11	Clamon and Corder, 1978
—	BLM	0.25 units/kg. then, 0.75 units/kg.	IV	2×/week for 3 weeks, 2×/week for 2 weeks	42	9	50	Kurnick et al., 1975
	CCNU	130 mg./m²	PO	1				
B-DOPA	BLM	4 mg./m²	IV	2, 5	28–35	60	20	Lokich et al., 1976
	DTIC	150 mg./m²	IV	1–5				
	VCR	1.5 mg./m²	IV	1, 5				
	PRD	40 mg./m²	PO	1–6				
	ADM	60 mg./m²	IV	1				
CVB	CCNU	100 mg./m²	PO	1	42	26	59	Goldman & Dawson, 1975
	VLB	6 mg./m²	IV	1, 8				
	BLM	15 mg.	IM	1, 8				

Regimen	Drug	Dose	Route	Days				Reference
B-CAVe	BLM	5 mg./m²	IV	1, 28, 35	42	50	27	Porzig et al., 1978
	CCNU	100 mg./m²	PO	1				
	ADM	60 mg./m²	IV	1				
	VLB	5 mg./m²	IV	1				
BVDS	BLM	5 mg./m²	IV	1, 15	28	30	20	Vinciguerra et al., 1977
	VLB	6 mg./m²	IV	1, 15				
	ADM	30 mg./m²	IV	1				
	STZN	1,500 mg./m²	IV	1, 15				
SCAB	STZN	500 mg./m²	IV	1-5	42	35	24	Levi et al., 1977
	CCNU	100 mg./m²	PO	1				
	ADM	45 mg./m²	IV	1				
	BLM	15 mg./m²	IM	1, 8				
ABDIC	ADM	45 mg./m²	IV	1	42	23	45	Loh et al., 1977
	BLM	5 mg./m²	IV	1, 5				
	DTIC	200 mg./m²	IV	1-5				
	CCNU	50 mg./m²	PO	1				
	PRD	40 mg./m²	PO	1-5				
——	ADM	60 mg./m²	IV	1	42	50	30	Williams & Einhorn, 1977
	ADM	45 mg./m²	IV	22				
	CCNU	100 mg./m²	PO	1				
ABDV	ADM	25 mg./m²	IV	1, 15, 18-26	28	4	57	Case et al., 1977b
	BLM	2 mg.	SC	4-12				
	DTIC	250 mg./m²	IV	1, 15				
	VLB	6 mg./m²	IV	1, 15				

[a] Abbreviations as in Table 10.2.

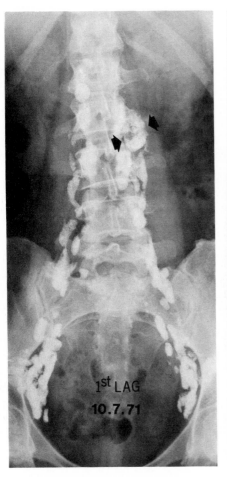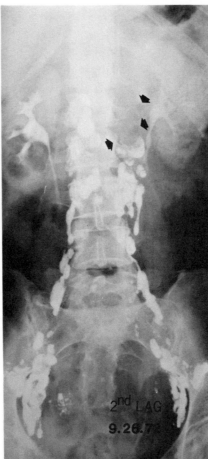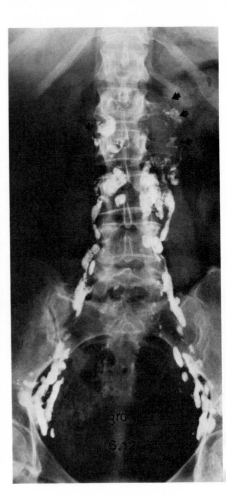

Figure 10.5   Relapse in the upper para-aortic nodes following MOPP chemotherapy for stage IV$_{M+}$ disease, as visualized on three successive lymphangiograms in 1971, 1972, and 1975.

nously every 3 months for 15 months. The results after a median followup interval of 33 months are presented in Table 10.8. Maintenance therapy had no significant influence on relapse rates, although the mean interval to relapse was significantly shorter for patients who received no maintenance therapy. The median duration of initial remission for patients who received no maintenance therapy was projected by extrapolation to be greater than 48 months, essentially identical to the 48.2-month estimate for patients receiving maintenance therapy. Only one patient in each group had died of Hodgkin's disease at the time of the report, and the survival curves were not significantly different for the three groups (Young et al., 1973a).

A third study of the effect of maintenance therapy was carried out by Diggs et al. (1977) in patients achieving complete remission on the 21-day CVPP combination chemotherapy regimen. Such patients were randomly allocated to no mainte-

nance therapy or to treatment with alternating monthly doses of vinblastine (0.2 mg./kg. iv) or CCNU (110 mg./m² po) for one year or until relapse. Actuarial analysis of remission duration revealed no significant difference between the group that received maintenance and the group that received no additional treatment following remission induction, nor was there any significant difference in survival between the two groups.

Palliative Single-Drug Chemotherapy. Combination chemotherapy is indicated as primary treatment for patients with disseminated stage IV Hodgkin's disease, particularly those with demonstrable involvement of the bone marrow, and, in conjunction with radiotherapy, for patients with stage IIIB disease. Together, such cases account for about 25 to 30 percent of all previously untreated cases of Hodgkin's disease in the United States. Combination chemotherapy is also under

Table 10.8 Influence of Maintenance Chemotherapy on the Duration of Complete Remissions Induced by MOPP Combination Chemotherapy

	No maintenance	Intermittent MOPP	Intermittent BCNU
No. of patients	21	20	16
No. of relapses	5 (24%)	5 (25%)	2[a] (13%)
Mean time to relapse (mos.)	6[b]	25.8	25.5
No. dead of Hodgkin's disease	1	1	1
Time to death (mos.)	11	35	52
Median duration of remission (mos.)	>48	48.2	—

Source: National Cancer Institute data of Young et al. (1973a), reported after a median followup interval of 33 months.

[a] Difference not significant.

[b] Difference significant ($p < 0.05$).

investigation as an adjuvant treatment in certain patients with stage I, II, or IIIA disease, in which its use is intended to eradicate occult microscopic disease. This is still a controversial topic which is discussed in greater detail in Chapter 11. Finally, chemotherapy has an important place in the palliative treatment of patients who have relapsed one or more times after radiotherapy and/or combination chemotherapy and who are no longer candidates for intensive chemotherapy or radiotherapy. Moreover, palliative single-drug chemotherapy may be indicated for patients who are aged and infirm or who suffer from other life-threatening medical disabilities which preclude the use of intensive combination chemotherapy or radiotherapy. Chemotherapy is sometimes the only option available when disease recurs in areas that can no longer be safely reirradiated. Chemotherapy with palliative intent should be initiated in patients who present with local or significant constitutional symptoms, such as fever, night sweats, generalized pruritus, anemia, and debility. In patients with advanced disease who are essentially asymptomatic, it is usually best to defer chemotherapy and to observe such patients at periodic intervals until some clear-cut indication for treatment develops; the exceptions to this rule are those cases in which the tempo of the disease is so rapid as to indicate that distressing symptoms will supervene in a relatively short time.

As Rosenberg (1970) has pointed out, "The choice among agents, and their sequential usage, depends more on the experience of the physician and the individual patient situation than on any major superiority of one drug over another." The regimen described here is the one we have employed for several years, with generally good and sometimes remarkably gratifying results. Although it is recommended for general use in those cases of Hodgkin's disease in which a valid indication for single-drug chemotherapy exists, physicians should be prepared to alter the sequence of drug utilization from that described here to meet specific clinical situations.

In previously untreated patients with advanced disease who are not deemed candidates for combination chemotherapy due to medical contraindications or old age, we prefer to initiate chemotherapy with the alkylating agents. Conversely, when single-drug palliative chemotherapy is required for patients who have relapsed after multiple regimens of combination chemotherapy and who are no longer candidates for intensive treatment, bone marrow reserve is often seriously eroded. It is then preferable to start with one of the *Vinca* alkaloids; vinblastine is usually preferred if leukopenia is not a major problem. When either constitutional or distressing local symptoms are present, it is desirable to achieve a rapid response by the administration of an intravenous agent. The alkylating agent most often employed for this purpose is nitrogen mustard, given in a single injection of 0.4 mg./kg.; cyclophosphamide given intravenously in fractionated doses over several days may be better tolerated in less urgent situations. If objective response is induced with either of these alkylating agents, maintenance therapy with an oral alkylating agent is indicated thereafter. When nitrogen mustard is used initially, we usually prefer to start maintenance therapy with chlorambucil; comparable results, however, are obtained when maintenance therapy with cyclophosphamide is used after initial intravenous use of cyclophosphamide (Jacobs et al., 1968). In either case, oral maintenance therapy should be initiated as soon as the white blood cell and platelet counts begin to recover after the intravenous induction course. Regardless of whether chlorambucil or cyclophosphamide is used for oral maintenance therapy, it is important to adjust the dose carefully, obtaining white blood cell and platelet counts at weekly intervals and seeing patients at weekly or biweekly intervals for clinical evaluation and adjustment of dosage.

It has been our policy to continue maintenance therapy with a given alkylating agent until it becomes evident that maximally tolerated doses of the drug no longer prevent progression of the disease, or until bone marrow toxicity no longer makes it possible to use therapeutically effective doses. Significant benefit is seldom obtained by shifting from one maintenance alkylating agent to another at this point, and it is generally preferable to shift to the periwinkle alkaloid drugs instead. In most instances, vinblastine is preferred to vincristine in the treatment of patients with Hodgkin's disease. Patients are initially treated with weekly intravenous injections, adjusting the dose to the therapeutic response and to the white blood cell count. In those patients who respond unusually well, it is sometimes possible, once an initial therapeutic response has been obtained with vinblastine, to lengthen the interval between injections to two weeks or even one month. Such patients can often be maintained for remarkably long periods of time in excellent health and with minimal deterioration of the white blood cell count. Although initiation of vinblastine therapy in patients who have previously developed severe leukopenia with alkylating agent therapy must be deferred until the white blood cell count has recovered, those patients whose marrow toxicity has been primarily expressed as thrombocytopenia can safely be transferred to vinblastine treatment without delay and may actually have an increase in platelet counts during the induction phase.

Once again, the policy has been to continue with maintenance therapy for as long as the drug continues to keep the disease under control. When progression of the disease occurs despite weekly doses of vinblastine sufficient to induce significant leukopenia, use of the drug should be discontinued. Since cross-resistance may be anticipated, there is no valid indication for using vincristine at this point. Instead, we have next moved to procar-

bazine, after a long enough interval to permit white blood cell counts to return to safe levels. When patients are suffering from high fever, advantage may be taken of the antipyretic efficacy of indomethacin to provide symptomatic relief during this rest period until procarbazine therapy can be started. One may also use bleomycin or prednisone during this interval, in a course of limited duration, to permit bone marrow recovery and to elicit occasional objective regressions of growing lymph node masses or to hold these in check until procarbazine treatment can be safely begun.

When intractable bone marrow toxicity or progression of the disease once again supervenes, procarbazine in its turn must be abandoned. Since myelosuppression is usually severe at this stage in the course of the disease, it may not be possible to use one of the nitrosoureas, unless the patient's condition permits a relatively prolonged rest period between drugs. However, whenever the condition of the bone marrow permits, the use of CCNU (or BCNU, if an intravenous agent is preferred) may be indicated. Because bone marrow reserves are often seriously depleted by this time, very careful observation of these patients is required, since the hematopoietic toxicity of the nitrosoureas is typically delayed and thus particularly treacherous in patients who are already leukopenic and/or thrombocytopenic. When BCNU or CCNU cannot safely be utilized, remissions can sometimes again be obtained with the marrow-sparing antibiotic bleomycin. However, sustained use of bleomycin is associated with the hazard of severe pulmonary reactions. Partly for this reason, remissions induced by this drug usually cannot be maintained very long. Finally, when all of these categories of drugs have been used up, the adrenal steroids constitute the last resort in the chemotherapeutic armamentarium. Although symptomatic and subjective improvement is often noted, objective regressions of the disease at this stage have not occurred frequently in our experience and, when observed, have seldom been long-lasting. Accordingly, it is likely that physiologic disturbance due to the unrelenting growth of the neoplastic process at this advanced stage (Fig. 10.6) or the development of serious infections or other complications of sustained steroid therapy will usher in the terminal episode of the disease.

Comment is indicated here concerning the still distressingly widespread practice of initiating chemotherapy in patients who have not been fully staged. This practice is sometimes defended on the ground that patients present with fever or other constitutional symptoms requiring alleviation. However, fever and other constitutional symptoms are usually controllable, at least for the relatively short interval during which staging procedures are underway, by nonspecific agents such as aspirin or indomethacin. It cannot be too strongly stressed that when chemotherapy is instituted prior to the completion of the diagnostic evaluation, it may prevent the detection of disease in the bone marrow or in intra-abdominal sites and thus introduces serious errors into clinical staging (Fig. 10.7). Moreover, when such ill-advised primary chemotherapy is carried to the point of marrow toxicity, it can seriously interfere with the administration of curative doses of radiotherapy to the extensive fields which may be required. Finally, as reported by Johnson and Brace (1966), prior chemotherapy may render recurrent sites of lymphadenopathy appreciably more radioresistant than they would have been if treated primarily with radiotherapy.

Complications of Chemotherapy

The complications of chemotherapy, like those of radiotherapy, are expressed as signs and symptoms of impaired function due to drug-induced injury to normal tissues. In some instances, acute toxic manifestations occurring during chemotherapy may persist and become irreversible even after drug treatment is stopped, sometimes progressing to a fatal outcome. In other instances, however, complications appear at a later time, sometimes long after patients have entered remission and no longer require active chemotherapy. Fortunately, again as in the case of radiotherapy, only a small proportion are major complications causing severe permanent disability or death. Complications may also arise as the consequence of an interaction of drug and radiation effects on specific tissues (Phillips and Fu, 1976). Such interactions have been particularly notable with actinomycin D, which sensitizes or enhances radiation effects in the lung, intestine, skin, and mucous membranes; adriamycin, which interacts with radiation injury in the myocardium and lung and may also induce "recall" reactions in skin or mucous membranes; methotrexate, which may potentiate central nervous system injury in previously or concurrently irradiated patients with acute leukemias; and bleomycin, which may enhance radiation injury to the lung or mucous membranes. It has therefore been suggested that, in patients who are scheduled to receive both radiotherapy and combination chemotherapy, careful consideration be given to the reduction of radiation dose in anticipation of additive or sensitizing effects of these chemotherapeutic agents.

Respiratory System. Although acute pulmonary interstitial reactions, sometimes progressing to chronic interstitial pulmonary fibrosis, have most often been associated with the chronic administration of bleomycin, this complication has also been described in occasional patients receiving MOPP chemotherapy (Farney et al., 1977), and acute pulmonary reactions thought to be due to drug hypersensitivity reactions have been observed with procarbazine (Jones et al., 1972; Ecker, Jay, and Keshane, 1978). The cyclic administration of prednisone in combination chemotherapy regimens, followed by its abrupt cessation, as well as the administration of adriamycin, either alone or in conjunction with other drugs, may trigger "recall" radiation reactions in the lung (Castellino et al., 1974; Phillips and Fu, 1976).

The clinical manifestations of the pulmonary reactions induced by bleomycin have been fully described by De Lena et al. (1972). Early symptoms may include pleuritic pain, cough, and dyspnea. Physical examination may reveal rales in one or both lungs. A reticular interstitial infiltrate becomes manifest on chest roentgenograms either prior to or concomitant with development of overt symptoms. The infiltrate usually progresses, at a variable rate, to alveolar consolidation. Alterations in pulmonary function are usually manifested as a simultaneous decrease in vital capacity and diffusing capacity. Even when bleomycin administration is promptly discontinued, the pulmonary process may progress inexorably, sometimes to a fatal outcome, and in other instances to severe chronic pulmonary insufficiency. Although there have been occasional reports of successful treatment of this complication with corticosteroids (Yagoda et al., 1972), the general experience has been that steroids offer little or no benefit in most instances. If all manifestations of this toxic effect are counted, ranging from asymptomatic individuals with abnormalities confined to roentgenograms or physical examination through severe crippling pulmonary insufficiency, the total hazard may be in excess of 40 percent of patients receiving chronic bleomycin treatment. However, significant clinical abnormality is encountered in less than 15 percent, and fewer than 5 percent of these reactions have been fatal. The hazard of bleomycin-induced pulmonary reactions is thought to be dose-dependent, increasing at cumulative doses exceed-

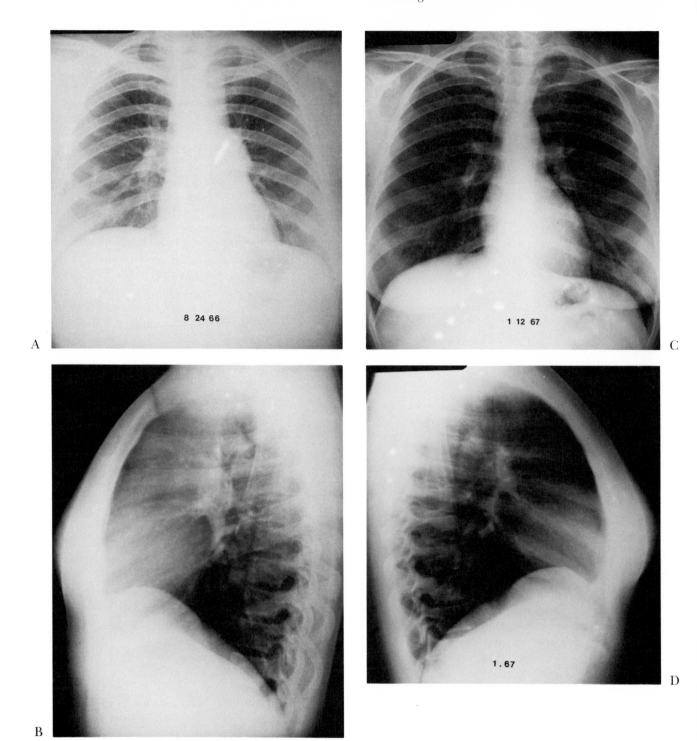

Figure 10.6 An example of inexorable relapse and progression of Hodgkin's disease during single-drug chemotherapy. *A,B,* this young woman was treated with nitrogen mustard in August 1966 in Central America for clinical stage IIA disease involving the cervical, mediastinal, and hilar lymph nodes. *C, D,* there was an apparently complete response on subsequent chest roentgenograms in January 1967. However, by May 1971 (*E*), recurrent adenopathy was evident in the right hilum and in the azygos vein region of the right superior mediastinum, and suspicious pulmonary infiltrates were present in the right mid lung and at the left base; additional pulmonary nodules appeared and progressed to massive involvement, despite renewed chemotherapy with a series of other drugs, as seen in the films of October 1971 (*F*), December 1972 (*G*), and April 1973 (*H*).

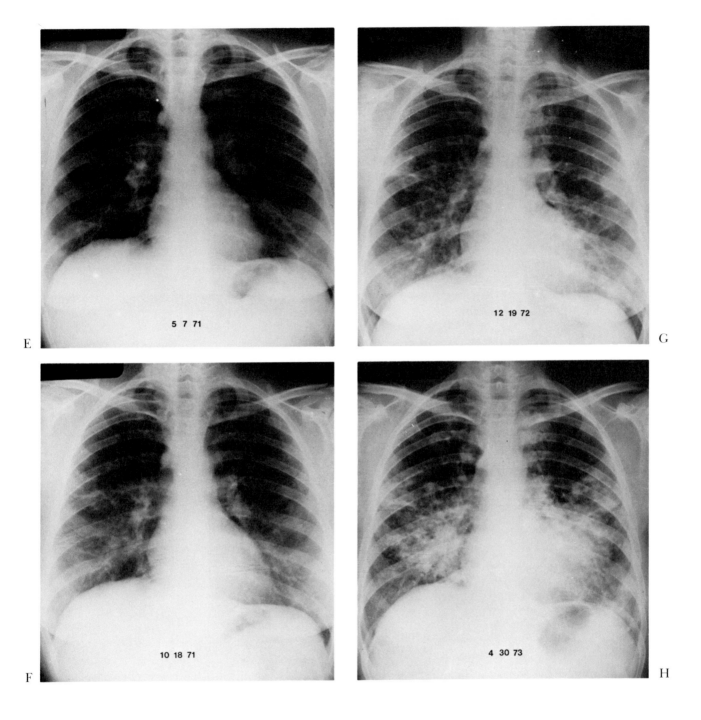

E

5 7 71

G

12 19 72

F

10 18 71

H

4 30 73

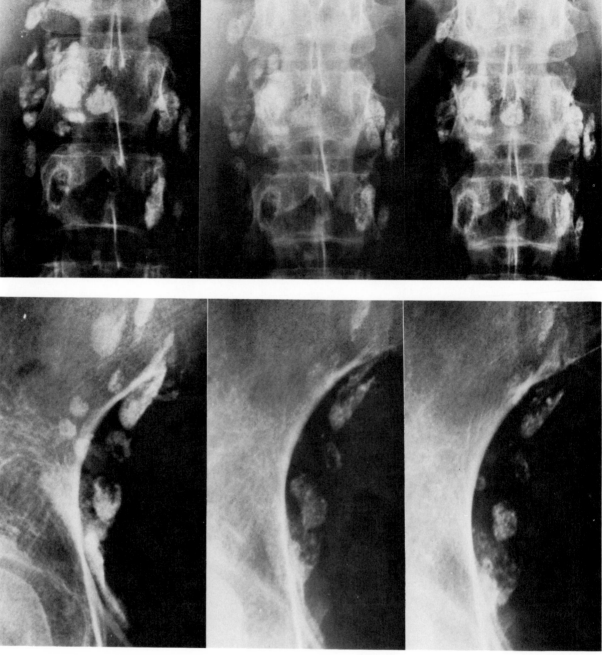

Figure 10.7 An example of staging error induced by premature and ill-advised chemotherapy. *Top,* mid-lumbar para-aortic nodes. *Bottom,* detail of right iliac nodes. The left panel is from the initial 24-hour lymphangiogram of 8/3/67; the middle panel, a surveillance film of 10/6/67; and the right panel, a surveillance film of 11/9/67. This 25-year-old female patient had a cervical node biopsy diagnosis of Hodgkin's disease made at another hospital after the discovery of mediastinal lymphadenopathy on a chest radiograph. No lymphangiogram or other staging procedures were performed. Instead, she was treated with Velban, receiving three weekly injections of 10 mg. each. She was referred to Stanford University Medical Center slightly more than two months after the biopsy. A lymphangiogram on 8/3/67 was apparently normal, and her disease was tentatively classified in stage IIA. However, in view of the prior chemotherapy, for which no valid indication had existed, it was recognized that the staging might be erroneous. To gain time for later reevaluation of her status, we decided to proceed on a step-by-step treatment plan. Accordingly, she was treated first to a mantle field, receiving 4,400 rads to the midplane in four weeks, at the end of which (10/6/67) a surveillance film of the abdomen was obtained. This revealed unequivocal interval enlargement of the mid-lumbar para-aortic nodes (*top,* middle panel). Treatment to the para-aortic-spleen field was thus clearly indicated and was carried out to the same dose. A second surveillance film, of 11/9/67, showed regression of the mid-lumbar nodes (*top,* right panel) but definite interval enlargement of the right iliac nodes (*bottom,* right panel), whereupon an oophoropexy was performed, followed by radiotherapy to the pelvic nodes. Thus, in retrospect, this patient must have had occult stage IIIA disease, the infradiaphragmatic component of which had been rendered clinically inapparent by Velban therapy. She is alive and free of disease to date and regained normal menstrual function after an interruption of several months.

ing 200 units per square meter. However, there have been several reports of fatal bleomycin-induced pulmonary toxic reactions in patients who received much lower doses, ranging from 50 to 165 units (Bonadonna et al., 1972b; Krakoff, 1974; Iacovino et al., 1976). In some of these instances, patients had received prior radiation to the lungs. Accordingly, it is suggested that patients receiving bleomycin should be monitored very closely with respect to pulmonary symptoms and physical examination of the lungs prior to each treatment. Chest roentgenograms and tests of pulmonary vital capacity and diffusing capacity should be performed at regular intervals. It is essential that administration of the drug be discontinued promptly at the appearance of any unexplained sign or symptom referable to the lungs or at the development of suspicious changes in either the chest roentgenogram or pulmonary function tests.

Cardiovascular System. Cardiomyopathy is the single most important complication induced by the anthracycline antibiotics, adriamycin (doxorubicin) and daunomycin. In a series of 399 patients with various types of neoplastic disease in whom adriamycin was used as a phase II agent, Lefrak et al. (1973) noted transient electrocardiographic changes in 45 (11 percent). In 11 other patients (2.8 percent), severe congestive heart failure developed, and 8 of these individuals died within three weeks. Adriamycin-induced diffuse cardiomyopathy is usually manifested as congestive heart failure which develops suddenly, with the classical signs of tachycardia, frequently a gallop rhythm, tachypnea, hepatomegaly, cardiomegaly, peripheral or pulmonary edema, venous congestion, and pleural effusion. Some patients may complain of weakness or dyspnea on exercise associated with cough for a few days before the onset of overt congestive failure. The syndrome may occur at any time up to six months after the last dose of the drug. There is some evidence that congestive heart failure is more severe when the interval from the last dose of drug is relatively short (one to seven weeks). After the onset of severe congestive heart failure, death supervenes rapidly, usually within one to ten days, with a median of two days. The most frequent electrocardiographic alterations are decreased QRS voltage, abnormalities of cardiac rhythm, premature ventricular and supraventricular contractions, abnormalities of conduction, such as left axis deviation, and various nonspecific S-T wave abnormalities. Most of these are transient, but decreased voltage of the QRS complex is

usually persistent and a more ominous sign. At autopsy, the heart is enlarged, pale, and flabby, with ventricular dilatation and hypertrophy. Pericardial effusions may be noted, and mural thrombi are occasionally seen. The coronary arteries and cardiac valves are unaffected. Histologic examination of the myocardium reveals a profound decrease in number of myocytes and degenerative changes in the remaining cardiac muscle cells. Interstitial edema and/or interstitial fibrosis are usually prominent. Electron microscopy reveals extensive loss of myofibrils, swelling and degenerative changes in the mitochondria, and the presence of dense intramitochondrial inclusion bodies.

Initial studies suggested that there was a dose-related threshold for the occurrence of cardiomyopathy following adriamycin administration. Lefrak et al. (1973) reported that only 1 of 366 patients given a cumulative dose less than 550 mg. per square meter (0.27 percent) developed cardiomyopathy, as contrasted with 10 of 33 patients (30 percent) given doses exceeding this level. A later tabulation by Minow, Benjamin, and Gottlieb (1975) revealed no cases among 764 patients receiving cumulative doses up to 500 mg. per square meter, 3 cases among 32 patients receiving 501–550 mg. per square meter (9 percent), 3 among 15 receiving 551–600 mg. per square meter (20 percent), and 15 among 37 patients receiving more than 600 mg. per square meter (41 percent). Overall, 52 patients received more than 550 mg. per square meter, of whom 18 (32 percent) developed cardiomyopathy. However, in a series of 33 adult patients studied at serial intervals during adriamycin treatment by a battery of methods, including phonocardiography, endomyocardial biopsy, and cardiac catheterization, Bristow et al. (1978) found clear-cut evidence of damage to myocytes at much lower dose levels. Endomyocardial biopsies revealed degenerative changes and loss of myocytes in 27 of 29 patients at doses of 240 mg. per square meter or greater. These investigators found that another widely used index of impending cardiomyopathy, the ratio of the preejection period to the left ventricular ejection time (PEP/LVET) was not as sensitive a criterion as endomyocardial biopsy and did not begin to increase significantly until doses of 400 mg. per square meter or more had been administered. They found that seven patients with catheter-proven heart failure had a significantly greater extent of myocyte injury on endomyocardial biopsy than dose-matched patients who were not in heart failure. Two types of myocyte damage were observed: (1) cells totally devoid of myofibrillar content, though their nucleus and mitochondria were often intact, and (2) cells exhibiting vacuolar degeneration of the sarcoplasmic reticulum. In severe cases, there was evidence of cell necrosis and of replacement fibrosis.

Bristow et al. (1978) noted that prior mediastinal irradiation and age over 70 years were factors apparently associated with an increased risk of adriamycin-induced cardiomyopathy. This is consistent with the reported observation of cardiomyopathy at significantly lower doses of adriamycin in several previously or concurrently irradiated patients in a series of case reports collated by Phillips and Fu (1976). In an experimental study, Eltringham, Fajardo, and Stewart (1975) demonstrated that rabbits treated with a single dose of 1,600 rads and a low dose of adriamycin (167 mg./m^2) developed cardiac damage comparable to that of animals receiving a significantly higher dose (255 mg./m^2) of adriamycin alone. There is also some evidence that little or no cardiac repair occurs during intervals as long as one year following adriamycin therapy, and thus resumption of adriamycin therapy in patients who have had significant prior cumulative doses is particularly hazardous (Lenaz and Page, 1976). An encouraging development is the recent report by Bristow et al. (1979) indicating that adriamycin cardiotoxicity is mediated by the release of histamine and catecholamines, and may be prevented or minimized by the administration of histamine and catecholamine blocking agents.

Gonadal Injury. Sherins and De Vita (1973) studied reproductive functions in 16 male patients who had been in complete remission for two months to seven years from the completion of combination chemotherapy for Hodgkin's disease and other types of lymphomas. Nine of these patients had been treated with six cycles of MOPP chemotherapy, and the others had had a variety of other multiple drug regimens. Ten of these 16 patients were azoospermic or virtually so, and showed total aplasia of spermatogenic elements on testicular biopsy; in two other patients who were also azoospermic, the seminiferous tubules still contained a few scattered germ cells, despite the widespread presence of germinal aplasia. In a similar study, Asbjørnsen et al. (1976b) noted azoospermia in seven of eight patients who received at least six courses of MOPP, MVPP, or CVPP chemotherapy. Serum follicle-stimulating hormone (FSH) levels were increased in all but one of these patients, whereas testosterone and luteinizing hormone (LH) were generally within normal limits. Sexual function and libido

were unaffected in both of these groups of patients. Roeser, Stocks, and Smith (1978) noted azoospermia in all of 15 patients in whom sperm counts were performed and evidence of testicular damage in 31 of 32 patients studied. Elevated levels of FSH have also been observed by Jacobson et al. (1978) in eight male patients treated with alkylating agents. Experimental studies have incriminated the alkylating agents and procarbazine; adult male rhesus monkeys chronically treated with procarbazine developed testicular atrophy with complete aplasia of the germinal epithelium (Sieber et al., 1978).

Although azoospermia persisted for as long as four years after cessation of all drug treatment in some of the patients studied by Sherins and De Vita (1973), there was some indication, both in their study and in that of Asbjørnsen et al. (1976b), that recovery may occur in an as yet undetermined but probably rather small proportion of patients who receive six or more cycles of MOPP or similar combination regimens. Two of the patients studied by Sherins and De Vita who had been off all drug treatment for four and seven years, respectively, had essentially normal sperm counts and normal testicular biopsies. One other adolescent male who had been treated with cyclophosphamide alone was initially oligospermic and when retested one year later was found to have a significant increase in sperm concentration to 15 million/ml. Concurrently with this improvement in the quality of his semen, his wife became pregnant. One of the patients studied by Asbjørnsen et al. was azoospermic at 13 months after the completion of his eighth cycle of MVPP treatment. However, on reexamination at 17 months (4 months later), he had a sperm count of <1 million/ml., and at 21 months after completion of treatment, his sperm count had risen to 5 million/ml. We have also seen one patient whose wife became pregnant about four years after completion of MOPP chemotherapy for Hodgkin's disease. However, only one of six patients studied by Roeser, Stocks, and Smith (1978) had any increase in sperm count within 52 months. Accordingly, it is probably wise to inform patients that the probability of recovery of spermatogenic function and fertility is low. Those patients who are deeply concerned about loss of fertility should be advised to store sperm in a frozen-sperm bank prior to the initiation of drug treatment.

Adolescent males may develop hormonal abnormalities in addition to germinal aplasia. Of 21 Ugandan boys with Hodgkin's disease who achieved complete remission after three to six cycles of MOPP chemotherapy, Sherins, Olweny, and Ziegler (1978) selected for study 19 who survived more than two years. Thirteen of these patients were 11 to 16 years old at the time of treatment; the remaining six were prepubertal (less than 10 years of age) at the time of treatment. Nine of the 13 pubertal boys developed moderate to severe gynecomastia, complete germinal aplasia, a tenfold increase in their mean serum FSH levels, a threefold increase in their mean LH levels, and reduced serum testosterone levels. In contrast, the prepubertal boys showed no change in serum gonadotropin levels and did not develop gynecomastia.

Gonadal injury also occurs in women following combination chemotherapy. Morgenfeld et al. (1972) noted amenorrhea in 6 of 13 adult female patients treated with chlorambucil, vinblastine, and procarbazine, either simultaneously or sequentially. Ovarian biopsies performed in the amenorrheic individuals by posterior colpotomy revealed fibrohyalinization, absence of primordial follicles, vascular injury, and hemorrhage. Urinary gonadotrophin levels were elevated. Similar observations were made by Sobrinho, Levine, and DeConti (1971), who found that ten young women with advanced Hodgkin's disease, who had had no prior pelvic or para-aortic radiotherapy and all of whom had had a normal menstrual history prior to treatment, developed menstrual abnormalities and amenorrhea after the initiation of chemotherapy. Three of these patients received vinblastine alone, five received alkylating agents alone, and two received combinations containing both alkylating agents and one or both of the *Vinca* alkaloids. The onset of amenorrhea was appreciably earlier in patients treated with alkylating agents than in those treated with vinblastine alone, and one of the latter patients began to have normal periods again within two months after discontinuation of the drug. One other patient became pregnant while on vinblastine, despite the fact that she was apparently amenorrheic during this time. FSH and LH levels were significantly elevated in six of eight patients. Postmortem histologic examination of the ovaries was performed in two patients. In one of these patients, who had been amenorrheic for more than two years, the ovaries were markedly atrophic, highly vascularized, and showed no signs of follicle activity or primordial follicles. The other patient, whose amenorrhea was of much shorter duration, had ovaries which contained several small cysts, but no oocytes were seen. In our experience at Stanford University Medical Center, amenorrhea

has been a frequent but by no means a consistent manifestation in young adult female patients during MOPP chemotherapy, and at least one patient became pregnant after two cycles of MOPP and required a therapeutic abortion. Additional studies of the effect of combination chemotherapy on the ovary will be needed to provide realistic estimates of the extent of this risk and its relationship to specific drugs, drug doses, and other therapeutic parameters.

Teratogenic effects on the fetus have also been noted after combination chemotherapy (Chauvergne, 1971). Garrett (1974) has reported the case of a 27-year-old woman with stage IIB Hodgkin's disease, who received six cycles of MOPP chemotherapy at monthly intervals and a seventh cycle three months thereafter, at which time she was found to be two months pregnant. At the twenty-fourth week, she was delivered of a male child who had only four toes on each foot, with webbing of the third and fourth toes of the right foot, four metatarsals on the left side but only three on the right, and bowing of the right tibia. Mennuti, Shepard, and Mellman (1975) described the case of a 20-year-old female patient with stage IIIB Hodgkin's disease who was treated with four cycles of MOPP combination chemotherapy for relapsing disease after prior supradiaphragmatic radiotherapy and subsequent single-agent treatment with vinblastine. She apparently became pregnant shortly after her last normal menstrual period on August 9, 1972. Before it was recognized that she was pregnant, she received a partial additional cycle of MOPP treatment on September 21, 1972. Pregnancy was diagnosed in November and shortly thereafter was terminated by hysterotomy. The fetus was an externally normal male in whom both kidneys were located just above the pelvic inlet, below the bifurcation of the aorta. The kidneys were also of markedly reduced size. All other internal organs were normal in size and location. Although no precise data are available concerning the risk of teratogenic effects in fetuses exposed to MOPP combination chemotherapy, it has generally been assumed that the risk is sufficiently high to warrant the general recommendation of therapeutic abortion in patients who become pregnant during such treatment.

Miscellaneous Complications. Hemorrhagic cystitis is a well-recognized hazard of cyclophosphamide treatment. Patients receiving this drug should be cautioned to maintain a high fluid intake and to report promptly the occurrence of frequency, dysuria, or hematuria. When symptoms are mild, the dose of drug may be reduced and the patient closely observed for a short time, but if symptoms persist or hematuria develops, discontinuation of the drug is mandatory. In severe cases, surgical intervention has been necessary to control bleeding. One case of hemorrhagic cystitis has been described following twelve cycles of MOPP chemotherapy for Hodgkin's disease (Royal and Seller, 1978).

Several groups have described the development of avascular necrosis of the femoral head in patients with Hodgkin's disease or other malignant lymphomas treated with multiple courses of combination chemotherapy (Ihde and De Vita, 1975; Sweet et al., 1976; Timothy et al., 1978). The lesions may be either unilateral or bilateral. Clinically, the condition is manifested by pain and limitation of motion in one or both hips, with evidence of flattening and progressive collapse and osteoblastic change in the femoral heads on roentgenograms. These changes are essentially identical to those observed when patients with a variety of non-neoplastic diseases have been treated with steroids. Accordingly suspicion has focused on prednisone in the MOPP or other combination chemotherapy regimens which these patients have received. However, since the total dose of steroid received by these lymphoma patients was much smaller than that usually associated with the development of avascular necrosis, it is possible that the use of other drugs with known cytotoxic effects in conjunction with prednisone may have contributed to the development of this complication.

Local skin necrosis is an infrequent but potentially serious complication which may occur at the site of intravenous or intra-arterial infusion of adriamycin (Rudolph, Stein, and Pattillo, 1976). When extravasation occurs during drug injection, progressive slough of skin may develop in the adjacent area. Such sloughs are initially quite superficial but slowly progress to become quite deep and painful indolent ulcers, sometimes with exposure of underlying structures such as tendon or bone. The risk is particularly great on the dorsum of the hand, where the tendons are covered by only a thin layer of subcutaneous tissue and surgical reconstruction is difficult. Adriamycin administration following radiotherapy may also elicit "recall" radiation-like reactions in skin, subcutaneous tissues, and mucous membranes in the previously irradiated regions. In some instances, these may be severe, progressing to moist desquamation and local necrosis (Cassady et al., 1975).

Secondary Neoplasia

There is increasing evidence that several of the chemotherapeutic agents commonly used in the treatment of Hodgkin's disease and other malignant lymphomas are carcinogenic and/or leukemogenic when administered to experimental animals (O'Gara et al., 1971; Croft, Skibba, and Bryan, 1975; Price et al., 1975; Sieber and Adamson, 1975; Marquardt and Marquardt, 1977; Sieber et al., 1978). Evidence presented in Chapter 11 suggests that patients with Hodgkin's disease who receive intensive treatment with both radiotherapy and chemotherapy have a very significantly increased risk of developing secondary malignant tumors, particularly acute myeloblastic or myelomonocytic leukemias and non-Hodgkin's undifferentiated lymphomas. However, the increased risk is not confined solely to patients who receive combined modality therapy. Arseneau et al. (1972) noted 3 cases of secondary malignant tumors among 110 patients treated with intensive chemotherapy alone after a total of 371 man-years of observation. Only 0.94 cases would have been expected, indicating a 3.2-fold increased risk in this group of patients. A review of the literature reveals several published cases of acute leukemia developing after chemotherapy alone in patients with Hodgkin's disease, to which we can now add one patient with stage IVB disease from the Stanford University Medical Center series who was treated with multiple cycles of MOPP chemotherapy alone and developed acute myeloblastic leukemia approximately four years after the initiation of treatment. A tabulation of the 15 cases recorded to date is presented in Table 10.9. Unfortunately, the numbers of individuals at risk in each of the institutions from which these cases were reported are unknown, with the exception of the Stanford series, in which 30 patients treated with MOPP chemotherapy alone were among the group analyzed by Coleman et al. (1977). At the time of that report, none of these patients had yet developed acute leukemia, but the stage IVB patient cited above, who was among that group of 30 patients, has now developed overt clinical evidence of acute myeloblastic leukemia. Since the total number of patients is small, the risk estimate of 3 percent derived from these data cannot be considered reliable.

The drugs which have been most clearly incriminated as carcinogenic or leukemogenic agents in experimental studies include the alkylating agents (Sieber and Adamson, 1975), adriamycin (Price et

Table 10.9 Secondary Leukemias in Patients with Hodgkin's Disease Treated with Chemotherapy Alone

Age, Sex	Clinical stage	Chemotherapy	Interval[a] (months)	Type of leukemia[b]	Reference
43, F	IIIA	HN$_2$, PRD, CLB	12	AML	Bignotti et al., 1970
56, M	IVA	COPP	14	AML	Castro et al., 1973
N.A.[c]	IV	MABOP	38	AML	Bonadonna et al., 1973
44, M	IIIA	MOPP	21	AML	Cuny et al., 1973
49, M	IVB	MOPP + BCNU	9	AMML	Sahakian et al., 1974
N.A.	IV	MOPP	22	AMML	Parmley et al., 1975
N.A.	IV	MOPP	54	AML	Huguley et al., 1975
N.A.	N.A.	PCB, VLB; VLB, CLB, PRD	95	ALL	Falkson et al., 1976
N.A.	N.A.	MOPP, CLB	78	AEL	Falkson et al., 1976
N.A.	N.A.	—	N.A.	AML	Garrett et al., 1977
N.A.	N.A.	—	N.A.	AML	Garrett et al., 1977
35, F	IIIB	Multiple → MOPP	75	AML	Rowley et al., 1977
51, F	IVA	VCR, PRD, COPP, CTX	51	BL-MPD	Rowley et al., 1977
53, M	IVB	MOPP	52	AML	Stanford University Medical Center, 1978 (unpublished)
49, F	IIIA	MOPP, VLB, CLB	62	AML	Danish LYGRA Project (A. M. Nordentoft and S. Kaae, personal communication).

[a] Interval from initiation of treatment to diagnosis of leukemia.

[b] AML, acute myelogenous leukemia; AMML, acute myelomonoblastic leukemia; ALL, acute lymphoblastic leukemia; AEL, acute eosinophilic leukemia; BL-MPD, blastic phase of myeloproliferative disease.

[c] N.A., not available.

al., 1975), and procarbazine (Sieber et al., 1978). Of 42 monkeys autopsied after chronic treatment with procarbazine alone, 11 (26 percent) were found to have a malignant neoplasm, as compared with 2 (3.1 percent) of 66 control animals that died during the same time interval. Six of the 11 malignant neoplasms were acute leukemias, of which 5 were acute myelogenous and one was undifferentiated. One animal developed a poorly differentiated lymphocytic lymphoma. Two others developed osteogenic sarcomas, and the remaining two developed hemangioendothelial sarcomas. The induction times ranged from 16 to 73 months. A similar spread of induction intervals is evident in the human data summarized in Table 10.9; the shortest interval from the initiation of treatment to the development of leukemia was 9 months and the longest was 95 months. Since many centers did not actively adopt combination chemotherapy with drug regimens containing procarbazine and alkylating agents until approximately 1970, an increasing number of patients who entered complete remission and have remained relapse-free for several years are now entering the time interval in which they may be at significantly increased risk of developing leukemia. It is to be hoped that as additional cases are reported, the total numbers of patients with Hodgkin's disease similarly treated during the interval will be stated in published reports so that estimates of risk can be based on substantially larger denominators than are currently available.

Chapter 11

Selection of Optimal Treatment

Introduction: Changing Therapeutic Perspectives

Therapeutic advances have evolved so dramatically during the past several years as to render obsolete much of the discussion presented in the chapter on general therapeutic considerations in the first edition of this book. At that time, many previously untreated patients with advanced disease appeared to have little or no chance for cure, and it was thus appropriate to devote a significant amount of space to a discussion of the indications for treatment with curative rather than palliative intent. Today, an appreciable chance for cure can be offered to virtually all previously untreated patients, even those with stage IV disease involving the bone marrow or the liver, the only exceptions being those patients who, by virtue of advanced age or other life-threatening disease, cannot withstand intensive radiotherapy and/or combination chemotherapy. All other previously untreated patients must now be considered appropriate candidates for treatment with curative intent. Thus, the arena for therapeutic decisions shifts to a consideration of which form of treatment offers the best chance for cure. Where the probabilities of cure are similar for different treatments, which treatment can be administered with the least morbidity and the lowest risk of late complications? The selection of optimal treatment may now appropriately take into consideration factors which were formerly of secondary importance, such as the preservation of normal bone growth in children; preservation of fertility; and minimization of the hazard of pulmonary, cardiac, or bone marrow injury. These advances are due to technical refinements which have increased the scope and decreased the morbidity of radiotherapy; to the fact that the curative potential of combination chemotherapy in advanced disease has now been firmly established; and to the advent of combined modality therapy, employing both irradiation and chemotherapy. However, as is detailed in a later

section of this chapter, the gains achieved by combined modality therapy have exacted a sobering price in terms of increased complication rates and a greatly increased hazard of late secondary neoplasia. Accordingly, combined modality therapy must not be regarded as a panacea for Hodgkin's disease; instead, it must be used judiciously and selectively in patients who present the appropriate indications.

The advent of combination chemotherapy has brought about an even greater change in our views concerning the prognostic import of relapsing disease. When the first edition of this book appeared, the mainstay of treatment for relapsing disease was single-agent chemotherapy, which offered excellent palliation but no significant chance for cure. The use of high-dose radiotherapy was limited to patients whose relapses appeared in previously untreated nodal sites. Even in this relatively favorable group, the long-term salvage rate was only about 15 to 25 percent. Combination chemotherapy, supplemented in selected situations by radiotherapy, now offers patients with initial relapses a chance for long-term survival, free of secondary relapse, of approximately 40 to 50 percent. However, as is detailed in a later section of this chapter, the chance for salvage depends in considerable degree on the type of previous treatment which the patient has received, the site of relapse, and on other factors such as the age and general condition of the patient. Although relapsing disease is far more effectively managed today than formerly, the patient with an initial relapse still has a distinctly less favorable prognosis than the relapse-free patient. Accordingly, each previously untreated patient deserves the thoughtful and informed selection and skilled administration of optimal treatment for the specific clinical situation which he or she presents. There is no justification whatever for the initial use of suboptimal radiation or drug regimens in anticipation that later intensive treatment can readily salvage those who relapse. Such a policy clearly deprives patients of a very substantial measure of their initial chance for cure, and is thus indefensible.

This chapter presents a detailed review of the results of different forms of treatment for a broad spectrum of clinical situations. In some instances, data from randomized clinical trials are available to provide definitive and unambiguous answers to therapeutic questions. In other instances, however, comparisons must be made between results achieved with one form of treatment administered in a nonrandomized study in one institution and those of a contrasting treatment approach in some other institution. Such comparisons are clearly of doubtful validity and cannot fully resolve therapeutic controversies. Near the end of the chapter, on the basis of the broad mass of evidence currently available, a series of general therapeutic recommendations are set forth for the management of patients with previously untreated disease and for patients with relapsing disease.

Therapeutic Options in Previously Untreated Patients

Different Techniques of Radiotherapy Alone. Controversy has raged for at least forty years as to the desirability of irradiating lymph node regions that appear clinically to be uninvolved but which are so located as to be deemed probable sites of subsequent spread of the disease ("prophylactic" irradiation). As has been mentioned earlier, Gilbert (1939) strongly advocated such treatment, while Voorhoeve (1925), Kruchen (1929), Merner and Stenstrom (1947), and others were just as firmly opposed to the concept and considered it important to preserve the normal tissues of the lymphatic system as far as possible. Peters (1966) has pointed out that the term "prophylactic" is in any case inappropriate, since the treatment is not intended to prevent the *de novo* development of tumor in disease-free lymph nodes but rather to eradicate microscopic, clinically undetectable foci of disease already present in lymph node chains beyond those in which the disease is clinically evident. Accordingly, she suggested the term "complementary" to refer to such treatment, since its intent is to complete the therapeutic effort. We have preferred to use the term "involved field" (IF) to refer to fields confined to areas of clinically evident disease and the term "extended field" (EF) to refer to the increased numbers or sizes of fields needed to encompass all contiguous lymphatic structures to which microscopic spread of disease is likely to have occurred. When the initial extent of

clinically evident disease, either above or below the diaphragm, involves several lymph node chains, EF treatment may entail the irradiation of virtually all lymph node chains and even of other lymphatic structures, such as the spleen and Waldeyer's ring, in which case it becomes synonymous with "total nodal" or "total lymphoid" irradiation (TLI), respectively.

The doses delivered to clinically uninvolved lymph node chains have gradually increased. In Toronto, where such treatment has long been in use, the usual dose to uninvolved regions in the years 1928 to 1935 was 600 to 800 rads of 200 kv. X-rays (Peters, 1950, 1966). After the advent of ^{60}Co teletherapy apparatus, the dose was increased to 1,500 to 2,000 rads in two weeks (Peters, 1966). I have argued (1962) that microscopic tumor might require virtually the same dose for its eradication as clinically apparent disease and have therefore advocated the use of doses in the range of the optimal tumoricidal dose (3,500 to 4,000 rads of 6 MV X-rays in three and one-half to four weeks).

Peters (1966) has presented a detailed retrospective analysis of survival in groups of patients with Hodgkin's disease of various stages, treated to clinically involved areas with relatively high doses (approximately 3,500 rads in three weeks) versus low doses (less than 2,500 rads). In each dose range, some patients had received "prophylactic" radiation to clinically uninvolved lymph node regions, and other patients had not. Her data for five- and ten-year survival rates in these various treatment groups are summarized in Tables 11.1 and 11.2. In general, it will be seen that the best survival rates were those achieved in the high tumor dose group who received "prophylactic" radiation in addition. In several instances, the difference between the survival in this group and that in the high-dose group without "prophylactic" irradiation was statistically significant, provided that the cases assigned to these different forms of treatment were really comparable and not selected in some subtle manner. It is around this specific point that the difficulty of evaluation of her data turns; since this was a retrospective analysis, it was not possible to eliminate the possibility that some subtle bias had entered into the decision to use or not to use "prophylactic" irradiation in specific cases. The only way to eliminate such bias is to allocate cases to treatment groups *at random* after they have been ascertained to be eligible for admission into clinical trial and to be of comparable clinical extent. The lack of a fully acceptable animal counterpart of Hodgkin's disease has also forestalled attempts to

Table 11.1 Hodgkin's Disease, 1928–1954; Complementary Radiation Study at Five Years (Percentage of Total Number Surviving)[a]

Stage	$H\bar{c}$	$H\bar{s}$	$L\bar{c}$	$L\bar{s}$	Total/stage
I	39	13	13	5	70
	72%	69%	77%	(60%)	71%
IIA	32	12	4	3	51
	91%	100%	(75%)	(33%)	88%
IIB	25	22	6	10	63
	28%	18%	(17%)	(20%)	22%
III	28	16	60	31	135
	32%	19%	13%	0%	15%
All cases	124	63	83	49	319
	59%	44%	27%	12%	40%

Source: Data from the paper by Peters (1966).

[a]Code: $H\bar{c}$, high tumor dose to involvement with radiation of adjacent areas; $H\bar{s}$, high tumor dose to involvement without radiation of adjacent areas; $L\bar{c}$, low tumor dose to involvement with radiation of adjacent areas; $L\bar{s}$, low tumor dose to involvement without radiation of adjacent areas. The survival rate comparisons which are underlined demonstrate significant differences.

resolve the question by controlled experimental studies in mice (Rubin and Haluska, 1969).

In 1962, one of the first randomized clinical trials ever undertaken in patients with Hodgkin's disease was initiated at Stanford University Medical Center to assess the relative merits of two different techniques of radiotherapy in patients with clinical stage I and II disease (Fig. 11.1). All patients received intensive radiotherapy with linear accelerator X-rays to a dose of approximately 4,000 rads. However, in half of the patients, the treatment field was confined to the specific chains of lymph nodes in which macroscopic involvement had been documented by biopsy, physical examination, and/or radiography (involved field or IF radiotherapy), whereas patients allocated to the other treatment arm received, in addition, treatment to the contiguous lymph nodes believed at that time to be at risk of containing microscopic disease ("extended field" or EF radiotherapy). Criteria for patient eligibility and other details of protocol design have been previously described (Kaplan, Bagshaw, and Rosenberg, 1964; Kaplan and Rosenberg, 1966b, 1973). A large-scale randomized clinical trial of essentially similar design was initiated a few years later by a national collaborative group (Nickson, 1966; Nickson and Hutchison, 1972; Hutchison, 1973).

The only really valid criterion in such a clinical trial is survival; if survival proved to be insignificantly different between the two types of treatment, then such subsidiary considerations as morbidity and complication rates could appropriately be taken into consideration to help decide the issue. Since many more lymph node chains are left untreated in IF than EF treatments, it would be expected that a greater proportion of patients receiving IF treatment would have relapses after the initial course of radiotherapy, owing to the appearance of clinical extensions of disease in previously untreated lymph node chains. In the course of time, therefore, the IF group of cases would gradually segregate into two groups of patients: those without any subsequent extension of the disease, who would have benefited from IF treatment because their treatment fields were initially smaller and the total time required for their treatment less, and those who developed later relapses, who would once again be at risk of dying of Hodgkin's disease unless all of their new sites of disease could be successfully eradicated by a second course of radiotherapy or by combination chemotherapy. Conversely, the success of EF treatments would depend critically on two factors: the validity of the delineation of EF treatment fields in relation to the actual patterns of spread of the disease, and the

Table 11.2 Hodgkin's Disease, 1928–1954; Complementary Radiation Study at Ten Years (Percentage of Total Number Surviving)[a]

Stage	Hc	$H\bar{s}$	$L\bar{c}$	$L\bar{s}$	Total/stage
I	39	13	13	5	70
	59%	62%	31%	(0%)	50%
IIA	32	12	4	3	51
	78%	75%	(0%)	(0%)	67%
IIB	25	22	6	10	63
	8%	9%	(17%)	(10%)	(10%)
III	28	16	60	31	135
	18%	6%	2%	0%	5%
All cases	124	63	83	49	319
	44%	32%	7%	2%	26%

Source: Data from the paper by Peters (1966).

[a]Code: $H\bar{c}$, high tumor dose to involvement with radiation of adjacent areas; $H\bar{s}$, high tumor dose to involvement without radiation of adjacent areas; $L\bar{c}$, low tumor dose to involvement with radiation of adjacent areas; $L\bar{s}$, low tumor dose to involvement without radiation of adjacent areas. The survival rate comparisons which are underlined demonstrate significant differences.

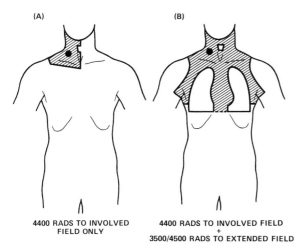

(A)   (B)

4400 RADS TO INVOLVED   4400 RADS TO INVOLVED FIELD
FIELD ONLY   +
                                   3500/4500 RADS TO EXTENDED FIELD

L₁ PROTOCOL (1962)

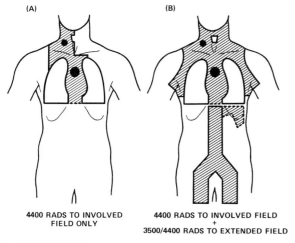

(A)   (B)

4400 RADS TO INVOLVED   4400 RADS TO INVOLVED FIELD
FIELD ONLY   +
                                   3500/4400 RADS TO EXTENDED FIELD

L₁ PROTOCOL (1962)

Figure 11.1 Diagram of the L-1 randomized clinical trial initiated at Stanford University Medical Center in May 1962 to compare local-field (IF) versus extended-field (EF) radiotherapy in the treatment of clinical stage I and II Hodgkin's disease. Two different examples are presented. As explained in the text, prior to July 1967 extended-field treatment would not have extended below the diaphragm in patients with involvement limited to the cervical-supraclavicular and/or axillary nodes. Note also that the inverted-Y field in that era did not include the spleen.

morbidity and complication rate associated with such extensive treatment. Similar considerations clearly apply also to clinical trials testing the relative merits of radiotherapy alone, for limited disease, or of multiple-drug chemotherapy alone, for advanced disease, and combined modality therapy. It is to be expected that the latter would be followed by fewer relapses; however, the relative salvage rates among those relapsing patients who initially received only single modality therapy might well be enough better than those among the combined modality-treated relapsers to tip the balance in favor of the former group with respect to the crucial endpoint, survival.

Unfortunately, these trials were conducted at a time when our knowledge concerning the patterns of spread of Hodgkin's disease was both erroneous and incomplete. For example, it was assumed that the disease had to progress from the neck to the mediastinal lymph nodes before reaching lymphatic sites below the diaphragm. Accordingly, EF treatment for patients with lymphadenopathy confined to the neck and/or the axillae was limited to a mantle field, without any subdiaphragmatic treatment. Moreover, these studies antedated by several years the routine adoption at Stanford University Medical Center of staging laparotomy with splenectomy, which revealed for the first time the hitherto unappreciated frequency with which silent disease is present in the spleen in patients with involvement in the cervical-supraclavicular regions, with or without associated mediastinal or axillary involvement. In retrospect, the delineation of EF treatment fields in these early studies was clearly inadequate and failed in many instances to provide protection against the growth of microscopic disease in the upper para-aortic lymph nodes and/or the spleen. Accordingly, it is not surprising that the long-term results of the Stanford L-1 trial revealed no significant differences between IF and EF radiotherapy with respect to either survival or freedom from relapse (Fig. 11.2).

The national cooperative clinical trial (Collaborative Study, 1976) also failed to reveal any significant difference in survival between the involved and extended field regimens for the total patient group and for most subgroups defined by age, sex, histology, stage, and constitutional symptoms. There were fewer local or distant extensions of disease in the extended field treatment group, but this advantage was offset by an increased incidence of complications. One important difference between the two studies was that the Stanford L-1 protocol for several years revealed a significant advantage of extended field radiotherapy with respect to both survival and freedom from relapse in patients with constitutional symptoms (CS IB and IIB; Fig. 11.3). Many patients with constitutional symptoms assigned to the EF treatment arm had mediastinal involvement and thus received supplementary treatment below the diaphragm (cf. Fig. 11.1, lower panel) which rendered their treatment tantamount to total lymphoid irradiation (TLI).

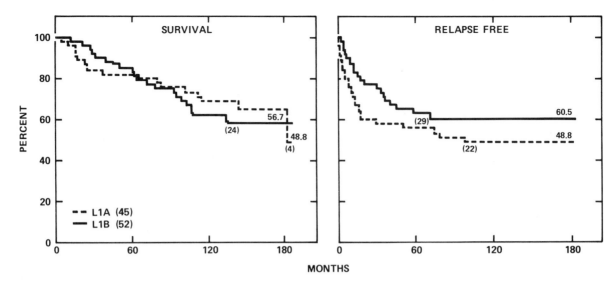

Figure 11.2   Actuarial analysis (by the method of Kaplan and Meier, 1958) of survival and freedom from relapse during the first 15 years for patients with CS I and II Hodgkin's disease treated in the Stanford L-1 randomized trial. Those allocated to the L-1A group received involved field (IF) radiotherapy to a dose of 4,400 rads in four weeks; those allocated to the L-1B group received, in addition, treatment to extended fields, as indicated in the examples in Figure 11.1, to a dose of 3,500–4,400 rads in four weeks. It is evident from the curves that there is no significant difference between the two groups with respect to either survival or freedom from relapse, perhaps in part due to faulty definition of extended fields, as explained in the text. Numerals in parentheses: numbers of patients (a) randomized to each treatment area; and (b) at risk after the indicated interval (below the corresponding curve).

Thus, it seemed more appropriate to ascribe the improved survival and freedom from relapse seen in these patients to TLI rather than to EF treatment. Despite the fact that late deaths in the L-1B treatment group subsequently reduced the survi-val difference, we concluded that TLI treatment is superior to IF treatment in patients with stage IB and IIB disease and, in July 1968, adopted this as our standard treatment for such patients.

In July 1967, we initiated a new clinical trial,

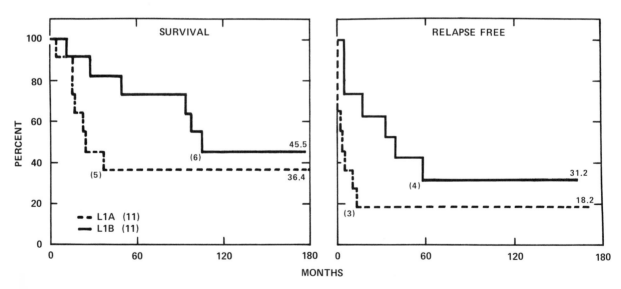

Figure 11.3   Survival and freedom from relapse in the subset of patients in the L-1 protocol who had constitutional symptoms (defined at that time as fever, night sweats, and/or generalized pruritus) and were thus classified in stage IB or IIB. The treatment options were those described in the legend to Figure 11.2 and illustrated schematically in Figure 11.1. The difference in survival was statistically significant from five through eight years, but late deaths in the L-1B group have almost eliminated this difference. However, relapse-free survival in the L-1B group remains significantly better ($p = .02$).

H-1, in which the treatment options in patients with stage IA and IIA disease were sharply polarized between IF and TLI radiotherapy. One year later, this clinical trial was modified by the routine introduction of staging laparotomy with splenectomy, with the result that all patients allocated after that time were pathologically staged. It may be seen in Figure 11.4 that although there is a highly significant difference in relapse rates, in favor of total lymphoid irradiation, there is little or no difference in survival at approximately ten years. In all probability, this was due to the effective salvage of relapsing patients with MOPP combination chemotherapy. However, there has been a sharp drop in survival of the H-1A (IF) group during the eleventh year; it is therefore not unlikely that a significant difference in survival, in favor of TLI, will emerge as the remaining patients continue to be followed out to fifteen or more years.

The TLI treatment requires several weeks longer to complete than IF treatment, and there is usually somewhat more severe hematopoietic depression and weight loss during treatment. However, there have been remarkably few significant complications due to treatment below the diaphragm; instead, the most significant complications have been those associated with treatment in the vicinity of the mediastinum: radiation pericarditis and radiation pneumonitis (Carmel and Kaplan, 1976). Whatever additional complication hazard may have been entailed in EF or TLI treatment was offset by the fact that patients receiving IF treatment initially who suffered a relapse of disease in close proximity to the initial treatment fields were at serious risk of suffering injury to normal tissues from a second course of radiotherapy. One such example occurred in a patient with cervical and mediastinal disease, treated by the IF technique initially, who developed extensions of disease in the pericardium and in the para-aortic lymph nodes. The second course of radiotherapy necessarily overlapped parts of the heart and mediastinum that had been included in the original mediastinal field, with the consequence that an intractable radiation pericarditis developed which failed to respond to surgical pericardiectomy and ultimately proved fatal. Thus, the risk of complications is not entirely on the side of TLI treatment.

Another randomized clinical trial, the L-2 protocol, which is now largely of historical interest, was also initiated at Stanford University Medical Center in 1962. It involved an unprecedented attempt to offer curative radiotherapy to patients with clinical stage III disease, using the total lymphoid irradiation technique; the results of such treatment were compared with those in a group of patients randomized to conventional palliative treatment with low-dose radiotherapy (1,500 rads in two weeks) to all involved lymph node chains above

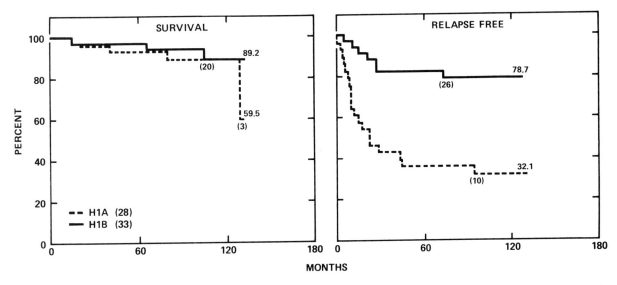

Figure 11.4 Survival and freedom from relapse in the H-1 protocol, in which patients with CS (later PS) IA and IIA disease were randomized to H-1A, IF radiotherapy (4,400 rads/4 weeks) or H-1B, TLI radiotherapy (4,400 rads/4 weeks to involved regions, 3,500–4,400 rads to all other regions). Although there is a highly significant difference in relapse rates in favor of TLI treatment, there was no difference in survival until the eleventh year, when a sharp decrease in survival occurred in the H-1A group. However, the numbers of patients at risk for more than ten years are too few for this result to be statistically significant.

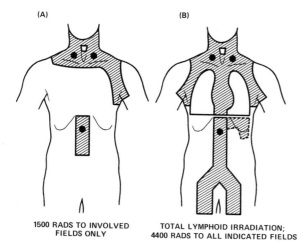

1500 RADS TO INVOLVED FIELDS ONLY

TOTAL LYMPHOID IRRADIATION; 4400 RADS TO ALL INDICATED FIELDS

L₂ PROTOCOL (1962)

Figure 11.5 Diagram of the L-2 randomized clinical trial initiated at Stanford University Medical Center in 1962. Previously untreated patients with CS III (A + B) Hodgkin's disease were allocated at random either to L-2A, palliative treatment with low-dose (1,500 rads/2 weeks) involved field irradiation, or to L-2B, treatment with curative intent, involving high-dose (4,400 rads/4 weeks) total lymphoid irradiation (TLI).

and below the diaphragm (Fig. 11.5). Accessions into this protocol were stopped after five years, at which time there was a highly significant difference in relapse rate and a near-significant difference in survival in favor of the intensive TLI treatment regimen. Patients who had initially received only palliative low-dose radiotherapy were treated with intensive TLI radiotherapy if they relapsed in lymph node sites, and, beginning in 1968, with MOPP combination chemotherapy if they relapsed in extralymphatic sites. Perhaps as a consequence of the efficacy of these salvage treatments, the ultimate survival in the L-2A group, initially treated with low-dose palliative radiotherapy, was 43 percent at 10 years and 28.6 percent at 12 years. Survival in the group treated initially with intensive TLI radiotherapy was 64 percent at 5 years, 50 percent at 10 years, and 45.5 percent at 12 years (Fig. 11.6). Though survival was appreciably higher in this group at 5 years, the differences in survival are not significantly different at 10 or 15 years, even when patients with and without constitutional symptoms are considered separately (Figs. 11.7, 11.8). Nonetheless, it will be noted that 41 percent of the patients with clinical stage III disease who were

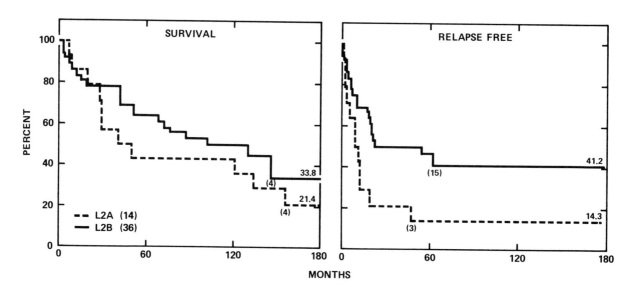

Figure 11.6 Survival and freedom from relapse during the first 15 years in the Stanford L-2 clinical trial. Relapses occurred earlier and significantly more frequently among the palliatively treated group. However, their ultimate survival, though less than that of the L-2B group, was not significantly less, due to the success of salvage treatment with TLI and, after 1968, with MOPP combination chemotherapy. Note that one-third of the L-2B group, treated initially with TLI, survived 15 years or more, and that 41.2 percent of this group remained relapse-free, with no primary relapses beyond the sixth year. Thus an appreciable number of patients with stage III Hodgkin's disease had been cured for the first time in history. Deaths due to intercurrent disease account for the fact that survival is lower than freedom from relapse in the L-2B group.

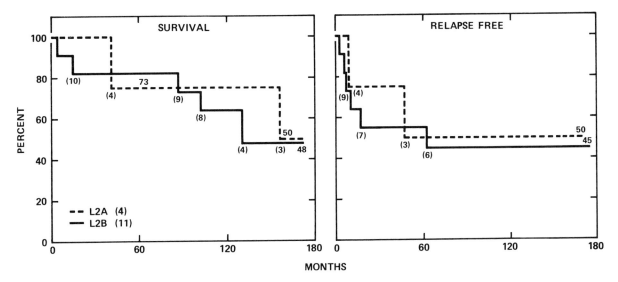

Figure 11.7   Stanford L-2 clinical trial results for patients without constitutional symptoms (CS IIIA).

treated with TLI radiotherapy have remained re-lapse-free for 15 years or more, and essentially all of these patients can be considered permanently cured. Thus, the L-2 protocol has indeed proved to be of great historical significance, since it was the first systematic study in which the curability of stage III Hodgkin's disease by any method of treatment was conclusively demonstrated. Moreover, since this clinical trial antedated our routine use of staging laparotomy by several years, essentially all of these patients were classified as having stage III disease by virtue of a positive lymphangiogram; thus their extent of involvement was generally greater than that of many patients today who are assigned to stage III on the basis of histopathologic

evidence obtained at laparotomy. As is discussed in later sections of this chapter, these long-term survi-val and relapse-free results, though remarkable for their time, have now been superseded by the greatly improved results of combined modality therapy in patients with stage III disease.

Different Forms of Chemotherapy Alone. The re-markable complete remission and long-term survi-val rates achieved with MOPP combination chemo-therapy in advanced Hodgkin's disease have been detailed in Chapter 10. The complete remission rates reported by several clinical groups appeared to be far superior to those achieved in earlier stud-ies utilizing single-agent chemotherapy. However,

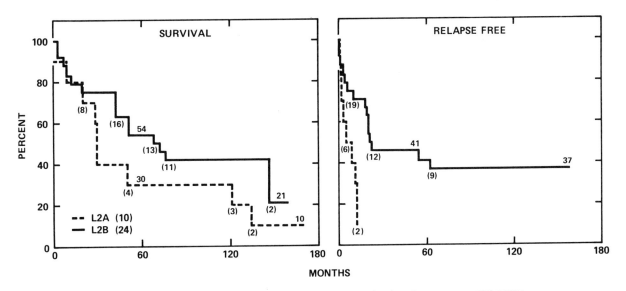

Figure 11.8   Stanford L-2 clinical trial results for patients with constitutional symptoms (CS IIIB).

single-agent chemotherapy had been employed with palliative intent, with the result that neither the dose nor the duration of treatment had been carried to tolerance levels, whereas MOPP combination chemotherapy was, from the beginning, employed as an aggressive regimen aimed at treatment with possibly curative potential. The Southeastern Cancer Study Group concluded that it was of critical importance to establish whether the apparently superior results of combination chemotherapy were due to the use of a combination of multiple drugs or to the intensity and long duration of treatment.

Accordingly, in April 1967 this group initiated a randomized control study to test the difference in efficacy of six cycles of MOPP chemotherapy versus treatment for an equal period of time with a single agent, nitrogen mustard, administered at tolerance dose levels. Eligibility for the clinical trial was confined to patients with Rye stage III or IV Hodgkin's disease, staged with the aid of lymphangiography; staging laparotomy and splenectomy were not performed. Patients were further stratified according to whether they had had no prior therapy (group A); minimal prior IF radiotherapy (no more than 3,000 rads to no more than three lymph-node-bearing areas, and in any case less than a full mantle field; group B-1); patients who had received single-agent chemotherapy with alkylating agents, vincristine, or procarbazine, except for those who had failed to respond or had relapsed while still on treatment (group B-2); and a poor-risk category (group C) which included patients who had had radiotherapy exceeding the doses or field distributions described for group B-1 or who had had a positive bone marrow biopsy. Randomization to MOPP or intensive nitrogen mustard therapy was separately performed within each of the stratification groups.

A total of 179 patients was entered into this clinical trial, of whom 108 were considered evaluable. The characteristics of the evaluable patients in each treatment group have been detailed by Huguley et al. (1975). Patients treated by the two chemotherapeutic regimens were identically distributed with respect to sex, histopathologic classification, and age at onset of treatment. Six (12.8 percent) of 47 patients treated with nitrogen mustard alone achieved a complete remission, and an additional 6 patients had a partial response, for a total response rate of 25.5 percent. Complete remissions were achieved in 29 (47.5 percent) of 61 patients treated with MOPP, and an additional 11 patients had a partial remission, for a total re-

sponse rate of 65.6 percent. Both the complete and the total remission rates with MOPP were significantly better than those with nitrogen mustard ($p < .001$). The differences in complete remission rates were also significant within the individual stratification groups. In group A patients with no prior therapy, complete remissions were obtained in 5 (20 percent) of 25 patients treated with nitrogen mustard alone versus 16 (46 percent) of 35 treated with MOPP; in group B, the corresponding figures were 0 of 6 versus 6 of 12; and in group C, they were 1 of 16 versus 7 of 14. Complete remission rates were also significantly different, again in favor of MOPP chemotherapy, for patients with stage IIIB or IVB, for all patients with constitutional symptoms, and for all patients with mixed cellularity histologic type.

Of the six patients who achieved a complete remission with nitrogen mustard alone, two remained in complete remission at 22 and 48 months after completion of therapy, the others having relapsed at 3, 8, 11, and 31 months, yielding a median duration of unmaintained remission of 12 months. Of the 29 patients who achieved a complete remission during MOPP chemotherapy, 11 remained in complete remission at from 19 to 56 months. It is of interest that 1 of the remaining 18 died of acute myelocytic leukemia without evidence of recurrent Hodgkin's disease 48 months after the completion of treatment. The remaining 17 patients relapsed at from 1 to 24 months after the completion of treatment, yielding a median duration of unmaintained complete remission of 15 months. The curves for duration of remission in patients treated with MOPP and those treated with nitrogen mustard who achieved complete remission were not significantly different. However, the overall survival curves, plotted from the time of initiation of treatment, revealed a median survival for all patients treated with nitrogen mustard alone of 13 months, as compared with a median survival in those treated with MOPP of 38 months, a difference which is statistically significant ($p = .04$). The difference in survival was due almost entirely to the fact that a much smaller percentage of patients treated with nitrogen mustard alone achieved a complete remission. There was little or no difference in survival among those achieving complete remission with either treatment regimen, nor was there an appreciable difference in survival of those failing to achieve complete remission with either technique of treatment. It was concluded that the complete remission rate attainable with MOPP chemotherapy is significantly better than that attainable with intensive use of nitrogen mustard alone and that this superiority is indeed attributable to the use of multiple chemotherapeutic agents, rather than to the intensiveness of the MOPP regimen. Despite the fact that the results obtained with intensive nitrogen mustard therapy alone were less satisfactory than those with MOPP, they were nonetheless of considerable interest in comparison to those previously observed when nitrogen mustard was used with palliative intent. One of the patients induced into complete remission by nitrogen mustard remained in complete remission four years after cessation of therapy. Huguley et al. (1975) were able to find only one other report of a patient who remained in complete remission for more than five years after only two courses of nitrogen mustard; in virtually all other patients, the remissions induced by a brief course of single-agent chemotherapy had been of short duration. Accordingly, they concluded that long unmaintained remissions are related to the duration of intensive induction therapy and that a long duration of intensive induction is more effective than a continuous low-dose maintenance regimen.

The fact that radiotherapy is not available in Uganda permitted a study of the efficacy of MOPP combination chemotherapy alone in a series of 48 children with Hodgkin's disease of all stages, including those with localized disease in clinical stages I and II, who were treated at the Uganda Cancer Institute between 1967 and 1977 (Ziegler et al., 1972; Olweny et al., 1978). Complete remissions were achieved in all of 11 patients with clinical stage I or II disease, in 21 of 23 (91 percent) of those with clinical stage III disease, and in 10 of 14 (72 percent) of those with clinical stage IV disease, for an overall complete remission rate of 88 percent. Eleven (36 percent) of the patients who entered complete remission later relapsed. Three patients were lost to followup, and 15 died, 12 due to advancing Hodgkin's disease, 1 due to a Burkitt's lymphoma, and 2 of other causes. Actuarial survival in stages I and II was 75 percent; that in stages III and IV, 60 percent. Comment has already been made in Chapter 10 about the unexpected complication of gonadal dysfunction and gynecomastia in the adolescent boys in this study. Although the authors concluded that childhood Hodgkin's disease of all stages can be successfully managed with MOPP chemotherapy alone, a comparison of the survival obtained in clinical stages I and II with MOPP chemotherapy alone, as contrasted with that achievable with TLI radiotherapy, clearly indicates the superiority of radiotherapy. For example, in patients with stage I and stage II (A + B) disease treated with TLI radiotherapy alone in the H-1 and H-2 protocols at Stanford University Medical Center, survival at ten years ranged from 79.2 to 89.4 percent, and freedom from relapse from 78.2 to 84.2 percent. Since the initial complete remission rate achieved with MOPP combination chemotherapy at various major medical institutions is only about 80 percent, and approximately 40 to 50 percent of such patients later relapse, it seems difficult to defend the use of MOPP chemotherapy alone as definitive treatment for patients with stage I or II Hodgkin's disease.

Finally, a number of clinical studies have compared the relative efficacy of the MOPP regimen versus other combination chemotherapy regimens in patients with advanced (stage III and IV) disease. Representative data on complete remissions achieved with various drug combinations have been presented in Chapter 10. No other combination chemotherapy regimen has yet been shown to have any appreciable advantage over the MOPP regimen. This conclusion is further supported by the results of a randomized clinical trial reported by Bonadonna et al. (1977). In a comparison of MOPP versus ABVD in patients with pathologic stage IIB, IIIB, III$_S$, and IV disease, the complete remission rate observed with MOPP was 62 percent, that with ABVD was 70 percent, increasing to 95 percent and 89 percent, respectively, after supplementary radiotherapy. Of the complete responders at risk for 30 months after the termination of all treatment, 88.9 percent of those treated with MOPP and 93.4 percent of those treated with ABVD remained relapse-free. Three-year survival from the initiation of treatment was 65.7 percent in the MOPP group, as compared with 73 percent in the ABVD group; the differences were not statistically significant.

Since the studies of Bonadonna et al. (1975, 1977) had indicated that there was little or no cross-resistance between the MOPP and the ABVD regimens, it was logical for investigators to raise the question whether the sequential or alternating use of these two different combination chemotherapy regimens would be attended by a lower relapse rate than the use of either regimen alone. Case et al. (1976b) treated 37 patients with advanced Hodgkin's disease for three or more months with a protocol involving alternate monthly courses of MOPP and ABVD, supplemented by local radiotherapy to areas of originally bulky disease. Such treatment produced complete remission in 19 (100 percent) of 19 previously untreated patients, in 8 (89 percent) of 9 previously treated with radiotherapy alone, and in 6 (67 percent) of 9 previously treated with both radiotherapy and MOPP. After an induction period of eight cycles of chemotherapy, the patients were started on alternate-month maintenance treatment using the same drug combinations in alternating sequence. During the maintenance phase, two patients developed relapses, and one a probable second primary lymphoma. A later report on this study (Straus et al., 1978) reveals that a total of five relapses occurred within 7–24 months after the start of treatment, four of which occurred in patients who had entered complete remission, and that three patients died, two of progressive Hodgkin's disease and one of sepsis. A number of other clinical investigations employing alternating combination chemotherapy regimens are currently in progress (Bonadonna et al., 1978), but results to date are too preliminary to permit evaluation. In principle, the use of two different combination chemotherapy regimens which are known not to induce cross-resistance appears to be eminently logical, but a prolonged period of observation of adequate numbers of patients will be required before it can be ascertained that such treatment actually yields significantly improved long-term survival and acceptable risks of late complications and secondarily induced neoplasms.

Radiotherapy Versus Chemotherapy. The Stanford L-2 protocol described earlier established for the first time that patients with clinical stage III Hodgkin's disease could be permanently cured with total lymphoid radiotherapy alone. Subsequently, excellent results were obtained with MOPP combination chemotherapy alone in a very small number of patients with stage IIIA Hodgkin's disease who were included in the original NCI study reported by De Vita, Serpick, and Carbone (1970). In another study, eight patients with stage IIIA disease all entered complete remission after MOPP chemotherapy and remained relapse-free for 8 to 32 months (Nixon and Aisenberg, 1974). However, neither of these studies was a randomized clinical trial. Thus, no concurrent group treated with total lymphoid irradiation alone was available for comparison.

This deficiency was remedied in a randomized clinical trial initiated in 1970 by the British National Lymphoma Investigation group. Patients with stage IIIA Hodgkin's disease were randomly allocated to either TLI alone or MOPP chemotherapy alone. The results of this study (British Na-

tional Lymphoma Investigation, 1976) were separately analyzed for the 81 patients staged by laparotomy and for 36 others in whom staging laparotomy was not performed. In the former group, complete remission was achieved in 40 of the 42 patients treated by TLI alone (95 percent); the remaining 2 patients entered partial remission. Complete remission was maintained in 31; 9 other patients relapsed, and 3 had died at the time of reporting. In contrast, only 29 of 39 patients treated with MOPP alone (74 percent) entered complete remission; partial remission was achieved in the remaining 10 patients. Remission was maintained in 18 of the 29 patients who entered complete remission. Of the 11 patients who relapsed, 1 had died at the time of reporting. Three of the 10 patients who entered partial remission on MOPP had also died. The curve for freedom from relapse of patients treated with TLI alone is very significantly better ($p < .01$) than that for patients treated with MOPP alone (Fig. 11.9). However, the overall survival curves for these two groups of patients were not significantly different at the time of reporting (Fig. 11.10).

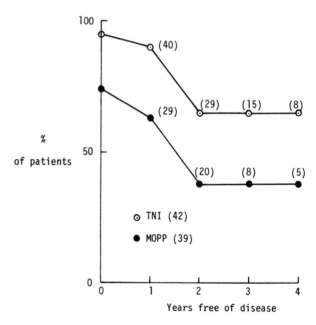

Figure 11.9 Actuarial analysis of disease-free survival up to four years for patients with stage IIIA Hodgkin's disease treated by total node irradiation (TNI) versus MOPP chemotherapy in the British National Lymphoma Investigation (1976). The number of patients entering each yearly interval is given in parentheses. The curves do not start at 100 percent at zero time, because some patients in each group did not have a complete remission. (Reprinted by permission of Dr. A. M. Jelliffe and the Editor of *Lancet*.)

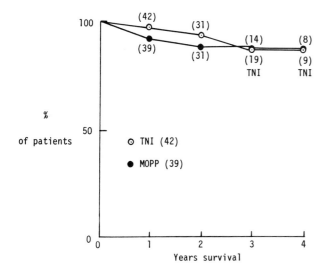

Figure 11.10 Actuarial analysis of survival up to four years for laparotomy-staged patients with PS IIIA Hodgkin's disease treated by total nodal irradiation (TNI) versus MOPP chemotherapy in the British National Lymphoma Investigation (1976). The number of patients entering each yearly interval is given in parentheses. (Reprinted by permission of Dr. A. M. Jelliffe and the Editor of *Lancet*.)

In the 36 patients staged without laparotomy, there were no significant differences in the incidence of complete remission or in relapse-free or overall survival during the first four years after treatment with either TLI or MOPP. It was pointed out that these findings may differ from those observed in the laparotomy-staged group of patients because of the inclusion of patients with more advanced occult disease in both treatment arms of the nonlaparotomized group. Such occult stage IV sites of disease would remain untreated in the TLI group but would be effectively treated by systemic combination chemotherapy. Thus, this randomized study carried a built-in bias in favor of MOPP chemotherapy in patients staged without the aid of laparotomy and splenectomy. This suggests that the results obtained in the laparotomy-staged patients are of greater validity; if so, they clearly speak in favor of total lymphoid radiotherapy alone, as compared with MOPP alone, in the management of patients with stage IIIA disease. Whether a further significant improvement in long-term results can be achieved by combined modality therapy, employing both total lymphoid irradiation and MOPP, is discussed in the next section of this chapter. However, it is appropriate to note here that in randomized clinical trials in which TLI alone was compared with TLI followed

by adjuvant MOPP chemotherapy in patients with pathologic stage IIIA Hodgkin's disease, confirmation of the excellent results observed by the British group with TLI alone has been obtained (Rosenberg et al., 1978). In patients with pathologic stage IIIA disease treated with TLI alone, survival at nine years was 81 percent, and 67 percent of this group was relapse-free.

Appreciably less satisfactory relapse-free survival has been obtained by the Yale group (Prosnitz et al., 1978) in PS IIIA disease with total lymphoid radiotherapy alone. In a series of 48 such patients, 46 (96 percent) entered complete remission after irradiation, but 26 (57 percent) of these later relapsed, and the relapse-free survival rate at five years was only 35 percent. Examination of the reported sites of extranodal relapse was revealing; four were in the liver, three in the lung, two each in the marrow and skin, and one each in the heart and in bone. These patients had been treated routinely with mantle and inverted-Y fields; irradiation of the liver through a 50 percent transmission block was not used in those with involved spleens, nor was irradiation of one or both lungs through 37 percent transmission blocks used in those with ipsilateral or bilateral hilar adenopathy, and there is no indication that the entire cardiac silhouette was irradiated during mantle treatment in those with massive mediastinal disease. These refinements of radiotherapeutic technique, which have been fully described in Chapter 9, might well have been able to prevent 8 (4 liver, 3 lung, 1 heart) of these 13 extranodal relapses. On the basis of their discouraging experience, Prosnitz et al. (1978) concluded that TLI alone is not adequate treatment for PS IIIA disease and recommended the routine addition of adjuvant combination chemotherapy. Glick (1978), in a thoughtful analysis of this recommendation, pointed out that better results have been obtained with TLI alone by other groups, that the routine use of combined modality therapy carries a greatly increased risk of late secondary neoplasia, especially acute myeloblastic leukemia (a subject discussed in detail in a later section of this chapter), and that salvage therapy with MOPP affords an excellent chance for long-term survival to the relapsers. Glick suggested that combined modality therapy, if used at all in this situation, may be indicated in the subset of patients with CS IIIA/PS IIIA or with PS III$_2$A disease, rather than in the more favorable group with CS IA or IIA/PS IIIA disease or those with disease of PS III$_1$A extent. This point is addressed in more detail in the next section.

The results of TLI alone and of MOPP alone in stage IIIB Hodgkin's disease both leave much to be desired. Although all 13 of the stage IIIB patients treated with MOPP alone by Nixon and Aisenberg (1974) entered complete remission, only 6 remained relapse-free at intervals ranging from 6 to 63 months. The remaining 7 patients relapsed at 4 to 40 months after completion of treatment, and 1 of these was dead at 20 months. The data of the National Cancer Institute group also suggest that patients with stage IIIB disease treated with MOPP alone are likely to experience a long-sustained complete remission in less than half of all instances. The Stanford clinical trials (Rosenberg et al., 1978) indicate that the results of TLI radiotherapy alone in stage IIIB are somewhat worse. Although 44 percent of such patients were alive at nine years, only 7.2 percent were relapse-free. To the author's knowledge, no randomized clinical trial directly comparing MOPP alone versus TLI alone in stage IIIB has been reported. The poor results obtained with either of these treatments makes it pointless to debate which of them is superior to the other. Instead, our energies should be directed toward the investigation of combined modality therapy or other innovative approaches which offer promise of improving the situation.

Finally, although combination chemotherapy appears to be the treatment of choice for most patients with stage IV disease, a possible exception to this generalization is worthy of note in the case of patients whose stage IV site of involvement is the liver (stage IV_H). In early 1965, we began to treat such patients with total lymphoid irradiation supplemented with external low-dose irradiation of the liver and, in some instances, single or fractionated doses of intravenous colloidal radioactive gold (^{198}Au). This treatment regimen was generally well tolerated (though serious complications were observed in a small number of early patients), and the initial complete remission rate was highly encouraging (Kaplan and Bagshaw, 1968; Kraut, Kaplan, and Bagshaw, 1972). In a subsequent update of the results achieved in 22 patients with biopsy-proved stage IV_H Hodgkin's disease treated at Stanford University Medical Center by this combined radiotherapeutic technique, Glatstein (1977) reported an actuarial survival of 63 percent at seven years, with 50 percent of the group relapse-free (Fig. 11.11). These results of radiation therapy alone in this specific subtype of stage IV Hodgkin's disease are surprisingly good. Unfortunately, there has been no reported randomized clinical trial directly comparing radiotherapy alone, in-

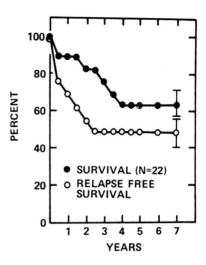

Figure 11.11 Actuarial analysis of survival and relapse-free survival of 22 patients with biopsy-proved stage IV_H Hodgkin's disease involving the liver at presentation. Patients were treated from 1965–1974 with total lymphoid irradiation to doses of approximately 4,000 rads plus 2,000 rads to the entire liver and 25–40 mCi of colloidal ^{198}Au. (Reprinted by permission of the author and the Editor of *Cancer,* from the paper by Glatstein, 1977.)

cluding irradiation of the liver, with combination chemotherapy. Although these results may well be surpassed by combined modality therapy, currently they provide ample justification for the use of total lymphoid radiotherapy, supplemented by hepatic irradiation, as an acceptable alternative to MOPP in the primary treatment of patients with stage IV_H disease.

Radiotherapy Plus Chemotherapy (Combined Modality Therapy). The idea of using chemotherapeutic agents in conjunction with radiotherapy in the treatment of Hodgkin's disease is not new. Soon after nitrogen mustard was first demonstrated to have therapeutic activity in Hodgkin's disease, several groups of investigators began to use this drug together with radiotherapy in the treatment of selected cases, with somewhat discordant results. As early as 1951, Gellhorn and Collins were able to report on a series of 67 patients treated from 1946 through 1950 with nitrogen mustard plus radiotherapy and to compare their responses with those of 65 consecutive patients treated by radiotherapy alone prior to 1946. Although the dose of nitrogen mustard they used (0.2 mg. per kilogram on each of two successive days) is the dose level still employed today, their radiation doses appear to have been, for the most part, in what would now be considered the palliative dose range. Actuarial analysis yielded a four-year survival rate of 48.2 percent in their patients receiving radiation therapy together with nitrogen mustard and 47.6 percent in those receiving radiotherapy alone. They concluded that nitrogen mustard did not contribute significant prolongation of life, beyond that afforded by radiotherapy alone, to patients with Hodgkin's disease. Essentially similar conclusions were reached by Dameshek et al. (1949), Heilmeyer et al. (1957), Paterson (1958), and Papillon et al. (1966).

However, a slightly different result was reported by Cook, Krabbenhoft, and Leucutia (1959) in an analysis of 347 patients with Hodgkin's disease treated from 1922 through 1952, of which 102 of those treated between 1944 and 1952 had received combined roentgen therapy and nitrogen mustard. They observed five-year survival in 40 of these 102 cases (39.2 percent), compared with 41 of 110 patients receiving roentgen therapy alone (37.2 percent). They interpreted these virtually identical five-year survival rates as "indicating an advantage of the combined method, since this was used only in cases of generalized involvement." It is clear, however, that a randomized clinical trial, in which patients with disease of comparable extent and severity are assigned to the two different forms of treatment, would be required for a valid conclusion on this point.

Whereas both radiotherapy and nitrogen mustard were used with essentially palliative intent in the studies just described, three groups of investigators have conducted limited clinical trials in which the same two agents, nitrogen mustard and radiotherapy, have been used with curative intent. Their rationale was to use significantly greater doses of radiation to eradicate all detectable macroscopic foci of disease and to use nitrogen mustard primarily for the purpose of eradicating whatever additional microscopic foci of disease might also be present. I initiated such a study in 1951 but abandoned it several years later after observing the development of new disease in contiguous lymph node chains just beyond the field of radiotherapy in three of the first six patients thus treated, suggesting that nitrogen mustard had failed to eradicate microscopic disease in these adjacent lymph node chains. In place of the nitrogen mustard, I substituted additional radiotherapy carried to high dose levels over the clinically uninvolved contiguous lymph node chains, a procedure which the advent of megavoltage radiotherapy beams had made technically feasible (Kaplan, 1962).

Karnofsky, Miller, and Phillips (1963) began a similar study with stage I and II Hodgkin's disease in 1949. Of the 22 patients whom they treated by this method, 13 remained continuously free of disease, 8 for more than five years. This is a result not substantially different from that reported by Peters (1961) with roentgen therapy alone. Moreover, confirming my observations (1962), 9 of their 22 patients had developed extensions of disease in unirradiated areas, indicating the inability of nitrogen mustard alone to eradicate microscopic foci of disease. Five of the nine patients with relapsing disease had died; the other four were alive with disease.

A third clinical trial, reported by Thompson Hancock and Ledlie (1967), was initiated in England in 1959. It was concerned with apparently early, previously untreated cases, subject to the limitation that lymphangiography was not utilized for staging of patients admitted prior to 1965. Both groups received radiotherapy (2,500 rads minimal tumor dose to the involved area and 1,000 rads minimal dose to adjacent regions), and the experimental group alone was subsequently treated with nitrogen mustard in a single dose of 0.3 mg./kg. Survival in the control group was 41/45 (92 percent) at one year; 19/27 (72 percent) at three years; and 7/16 (45 percent) at five years. The corresponding figures in the experimental group were 46/46 (100 percent); 30/36 (85 percent); and 12/17 (73 percent). The actuarial survival curves derived from these data were analyzed by Pike, Thompson Hancock, and Ledlie (1967), using the modified Wilcoxon rank test, which revealed that the curves were significantly different ($p = .02$). However, when ten-year followup data became available on the same two groups of patients, the difference in survival that was apparent after four years was no longer discernible, and the difference between the two curves was not statistically significant. The estimated ten-year survival rate was about 40 percent in both groups, and about 25 percent of patients remained relapse-free at ten years (Thompson Hancock, Austin, and Smith, 1973).

Two other reports of the combination of a single drug with radiotherapy deserve mention. Linke (1960) reported a very appreciable improvement in survival rates over those that he obtained with roentgen therapy alone when another alkylating agent, Trenimon (2,3,5-tris-ethyleniminobenzoquinone, 1,4, a soluble form of E-39) was added to the treatment regimen. However, his results with radiotherapy alone were far inferior to those obtained by Peters (1961), suggesting that the alkylating agent may merely have compensated for his less aggressive radiotherapy. Karnofsky et al. (1963) have pointed out that Linke's results with combined treatment were not significantly better than those of Peters with more intensive radiotherapy alone.

From 1964 to 1971, the European Oncology-Radiation Therapy Cooperative Group (EORTC) conducted a randomized clinical trial in several European medical centers which compared the results in clinical stage I and II patients of radiation therapy alone versus radiation therapy followed by weekly injections of vinblastine for a period of two years. The trial therefore constituted a test of the usefulness of maintenance single-drug chemotherapy following radiotherapy for regionally localized disease. The early results, after a followup interval of four to five years, revealed differences in survival in certain specific histopathologic subgroups in favor of the use of supplementary vinblastine (EORTC Group, 1972; Tubiana and Mathé, 1973), but after a followup interval of seven to eight years, the favorable influence of supplementary vinblastine on survival had disappeared (Burgers et al., 1976; Tubiana et al., 1977).

More recently, multiple-drug chemotherapy has been used in conjunction with radiotherapy in limited clinical trials. Moxley et al. (1967) used megavoltage radiotherapy to tumor doses of 3,600 to 4,000 rads given at the rate of 1,000 rads per week to supradiaphragmatic sites of involvement, in conjunction with a quadruple chemotherapy program consisting of cyclophosphamide, vincristine, methotrexate, and prednisone, in seven patients with stages I and II and in two patients with stage IIIA Hodgkin's disease. The latter two patients received no radiation treatment below the diaphragm. All nine patients entered remission, and all but one were still in unmaintained remission for intervals exceeding thirty months at the time of reporting. The one exception suffered a relapse at two months and died soon thereafter.

It is extremely difficult to evaluate these results, since there was no concurrent randomized control group receiving radiotherapy alone for disease of comparable extent and severity. Other groups treating patients with stage I and stage IIA and B Hodgkin's disease to comparable dose levels with radiotherapy alone have now achieved comparable results, suggesting that this particular combination of four drugs may not really have added significantly to the degree of tumor control achieved by radiotherapy in the small series of patients studied by Moxley et al. The many pitfalls in the assessment of results of nonrandomized therapeutic studies have been carefully considered by Rosenberg (1977).

From 1967 through 1974, Lagarde et al. (1976) conducted a nonrandomized study on a series of 100 patients with clinical stage I or II Hodgkin's disease. All patients received one three-week cycle of a modified CVPP regimen, followed immediately by extended field radiotherapy. Most of those patients who had entered complete remission by the end of radiotherapy then received one additional consolidation cycle of chemotherapy. Complete remissions were obtained in 93 of 98 evaluable patients (95 percent). Nearly 90 percent of those who received both the initial and the subsequent consolidation cycle of chemotherapy remained relapse-free at four years, whereas only 70 percent of those who received the first cycle of chemotherapy alone remained relapse-free after two to five years. Overall survival for the entire group was approximately 75 percent at five years. Once again, the absence of a concurrent group randomized to radiotherapy alone makes it difficult to assess the significance of these observations. However, since comparable or superior five-year survival rates with total lymphoid radiotherapy alone have been reported from several other medical centers, the benefit conferred by the administration of one or two cycles of combination chemotherapy does not seem impressive.

The first randomized clinical trial in which multiple cycles of MOPP combination chemotherapy were administered following total lymphoid radiotherapy was initiated at Stanford University Medical Center in 1968 (Bull et al., 1970; Moore et al., 1972; Rosenberg et al., 1972). It proved technically possible to deliver total lymphoid radiotherapy to doses of approximately 4,400 rads, given to each of two to three large fields at the rate of 1,100 rads per week, followed by a complete course of six cycles of MOPP chemotherapy. The use of a rest period of approximately six to eight weeks between the completion of radiotherapy and the initiation of chemotherapy permitted successful completion of this formidable program in about 90 percent of our patients in whom it was attempted. Since 1973, prednisone has been eliminated from the MOPP combination in patients who had received radiotherapy to the mediastinal region, to avoid the anamnestic reactivation of pulmonary and cardiac radiation reactions which we had previously observed following steroid withdrawal (Castellino et al., 1974b).

Leukopenia usually reached nadir values during or after the fourth drug cycle. Although white blood cell counts less than 500 per cubic millimeter have occasionally been observed, there have been no serious bacterial infections or bleeding episodes to date in the combined therapy group. There has been a remarkably high incidence (over 30 percent) of herpes zoster infection among the MOPP-treated patients, with nonfatal dissemination in several instances. Neuropathy attributable to vincristine has been a significant problem in many cases. Foot drop has occasionally been a troublesome manifestation; although it has usually been reversible, one patient showed no recovery 18 months after completion of treatment. Alopecia and constipation attributable to vincristine have also been noted with some regularity. The prolonged duration (nine to twelve months) of the combined therapy, and the recurrent discomfort of drug-induced vomiting and malaise have also made the treatment psychologically difficult for patients to tolerate. Finally, it must be presumed, in view of the data presented in Chapter 10, that virtually all of the male patients have been sterilized by the MOPP chemotherapy, most of them permanently.

The favorable early results observed in the series of randomized clinical trials (H-2 through H-7) established in 1968 led to the initiation of two new trials, R-1 and K-1, for patients with regionally localized disease in what were then considered "favorable" versus "unfavorable" sites above the diaphragm. In 1974 a new (S) series of randomized trials was initiated. The stages of disease and the treatment options tested in each of the Stanford clinical trials to date are summarized in Table 11.3. Schematic diagrams illustrating the fundamental aspects of design of each of these protocols are presented in Figures 11.1, 11.5, and 11.12 through 11.21. It will be apparent that the H-2 through H-5 protocols tested essentially the same question, the value of adding six cycles of adjuvant MOPP chemotherapy to total lymphoid irradiation, in different clinical settings ranging from patients with pathological stage IB and IIB disease in the H-2 protocol through pathological stage II_S (A + B) and III_S (A + B) disease in the H-5 protocol. The H-6 protocol tested the relative merits of radiotherapy alone versus split course MOPP chemotherapy plus radiotherapy in patients with stage IV_H (A + B) disease involving the liver, and the H-7 protocol tested the value of adding high-dose total lymphoid radiotherapy between the second and the third cycles of a split course program of MOPP chemotherapy, as compared with six cycles of MOPP chemotherapy alone.

An entirely new concept was introduced in the R-1 and K-1 protocols (Rosenberg and Kaplan,

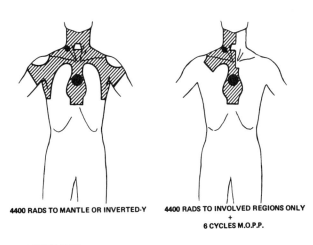

**HODGKIN'S DISEASE
STANFORD RANDOMIZED CLINICAL TRIAL
STAGES IA, IIA, II$_E$A – "FAVORABLE"**

4400 RADS TO MANTLE OR INVERTED-Y   4400 RADS TO INVOLVED REGIONS ONLY
+
6 CYCLES M.O.P.P.

R$_1$ PROTOCOL (1970)

Figure 11.12 Schematic diagram of the Stanford R-1 clinical trial for patients with PS IA, IIA, and II$_E$A Hodgkin's disease involving "favorable" sites. (Reprinted by permission of the Editor of *Cancer,* from the paper by Rosenberg and Kaplan, 1975.)

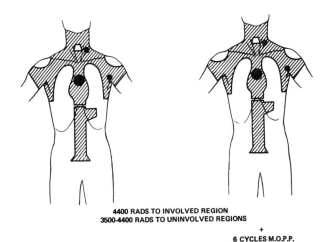

**HODGKIN'S DISEASE
STANFORD RANDOMIZED CLINICAL TRIAL
STAGES IA, IIA, II$_E$A – "UNFAVORABLE"**

4400 RADS TO INVOLVED REGION
3500-4400 RADS TO UNINVOLVED REGIONS
+
6 CYCLES M.O.P.P.

K$_1$ PROTOCOL (1970)

Figure 11.13 Schematic diagram of the Stanford K-1 clinical trial for patients with PS IA, IIA, and II$_E$A Hodgkin's disease involving "unfavorable" sites. (Reprinted by permission of the Editor of *Cancer,* from the paper by Rosenberg and Kaplan, 1975.)

Table 11.3 Stanford Randomized Clinical Trials in Hodgkin's Disease

Protocol	Year initiated	Stage(s) represented	Treatment option[a]	
			A	B
L-1	1962	I and II (A + B)	IF radiotherapy (4,400 rads/4 wk.)	Limited EF radiotherapy (4,400 rads/4 wk.)
L-2	1962	III (A + B)	Low-dose (1,500 rads/2 wk.) IF radiotherapy	High-dose (>3,500 rads/4 wk.) TLI radiotherapy
H-1	1967	IA and IIA	IF radiotherapy (4,400 rads/4 wk.)	TLI radiotherapy (4,400 rads/4 wk.)
H-2	1968	IB and IIB	TLI radiotherapy only (4,400 rads/4 wk. to involved sites, 3,500–4,400 to uninvolved)	TLI radiotherapy, then MOPP (6 cycles)
H-3	1968	III (A + B)	TLI radiotherapy only (4,400 rads/4 wk. to involved sites, 3,500–4,400 to uninvolved)	TLI radiotherapy, then MOPP (6 cycles)
H-4	1968	I_EB, II_EB, III_E (A + B)	TLI radiotherapy only (4,400 rads/4 wk. to involved sites, 3,500–4,400 to uninvolved)	TLI radiotherapy, then MOPP (6 cycles)
H-5	1968	II_S (A + B), III_S (A + B)	TLI radiotherapy and liver irradiation (combined external and ^{198}Au gold colloid)	TLI radiotherapy, then MOPP (6 cycles)
H-6	1968	IV_H (A + B)	TLI radiotherapy + liver irradiation	Split course MOPP (3 cycles before, 3 cycles after TLI radiotherapy)
H-7	1968	IV_M, IV_L, etc.	Split course MOPP (2 cycles before, 4 cycles after TLI radiotherapy)	MOPP alone (6 cycles)
R-1	1970	IA, I_EA, IIA, II_EA ("favorable" sites)	Mantle or inverted-Y field radiotherapy only (4,400 rads/4 wk.)	IF radiotherapy (4,400 rads/4 wk.) + MOPP (6 cycles)
K-1	1970	IA, I_EA, IIA, II_EA ("unfavorable" sites)	Subtotal radiotherapy (STLI) (pelvis omitted for supradiaphragmatic involved sites; 4,400 rads/4 wk.)	Subtotal radiotherapy (STLI) + MOPP (6 cycles)

S-1	1974	IA, IIA	STLI radiotherapy	IF radiotherapy followed by MOPP (6 cycles)
S-2	1974	$I_{E}A$, $II_{E}A$	STLI radiotherapy + MOPP (6 cycles)	STLI radiotherapy + PAVe (6 cycles)
S-3	1974	$I_{E}B$, $II_{E}B$	TLI radiotherapy + MOPP (6 cycles)	TLI radiotherapy + PAVe (6 cycles)
S-4	1974	$II_{S}A$, IIIA, $III_{S}A$	TLI (only 3,000 rads to uninvolved mediastinum and/or pelvis) + MOPP (6 cycles)	TLI as in option A, + PAVe (6 cycles)
S-5	1974	$II_{S}B$, IIIB, $III_{S}B$	Split course MOPP with TLI radiotherapy, including 2,200 rads to liver, between 2nd and 3rd cycles of MOPP	Split course PAVe, with TLI radiotherapy as in option A
S-6	1974	IV_{L}	Split course MOPP with TLI radiotherapy between 2nd and 3rd cycles of MOPP. Radiation dose reduced to 3,000 rads to uninvolved pelvis. At completion of treatment, patients randomized to no maintenance versus maintenance PAVe chemotherapy	Split course PAVe with TLI radiotherapy between 2nd and 3rd cycles
S-7	1974	IV_{H}	TLI radiotherapy including 2,200 rads to liver followed by MOPP (6 cycles). At completion of treatment, patients randomly allocated to no maintenance treatment versus maintenance PAVe chemotherapy	MOPP (6 cycles) followed by TLI radiotherapy with 2,200 rads to liver and 3,000 rads to nodal areas
S-8	1974	IV_{M} and other stage IV sites	Split course MOPP with TLI radiotherapy between 3rd and 4th cycles (3,000 rads to uninvolved nodes). At completion of treatment, patients randomized to no maintenance treatment versus maintenance PAVe chemotherapy	MOPP alone (8 cycles)

[a] IF, involved field; EF, extended field; TLI, total lymphoid irradiation; STLI, subtotal lymphoid irradiation; MOPP, combination of mechlorethamine, vincristine, procarbazine, and prednisone; PAVe, combination of procarbazine, alkeran (L-phenylalanine mustard), and vinblastine (cf. Table 10.3, Chapter 10).

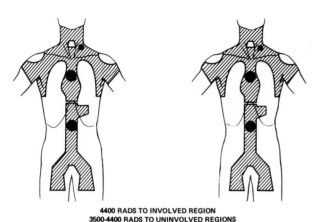

HODGKIN'S DISEASE
STANFORD RANDOMIZED CLINICAL TRIAL
STAGES IB, IIB, II$_E$B, IIIA, IIIB

4400 RADS TO INVOLVED REGION
3500-4400 RADS TO UNINVOLVED REGIONS
+
6 CYCLES M.O.P.P.

H$_2$, H$_3$, H$_4$ PROTOCOLS (1968)

Figure 11.14 Schematic diagram of the Stanford H-2, H-3, and H-4 clinical trials for patients with PS IB, IIB, II$_E$B, IIIA, IIIB, III$_E$A, and III$_E$B Hodgkin's disease. (Reprinted by permission of the Editor of *Cancer,* from the paper by Rosenberg and Kaplan, 1975).

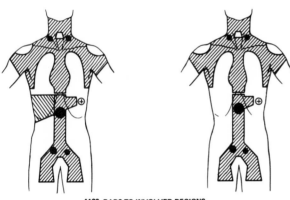

HODGKIN'S DISEASE
STANFORD RANDOMIZED CLINICAL TRIAL
STAGES II$_S$, III$_S$ A OR B

4400 RADS TO INVOLVED REGIONS
3500-4400 RADS TO UNINVOLVED REGIONS
+   +
2500 RADS TO LIVER (EXTERNAL   6 CYCLES M.O.P.P.
AND COLLOIDAL Au^{198})

H$_5$ PROTOCOL (1968)
⊕ *INVOLVED SPLEEN, REMOVED AT SURGERY*

Figure 11.15 Schematic diagram of the Stanford H-5 clinical trial for patients with PS II$_S$A, II$_S$B, III$_S$A, III$_S$B Hodgkin's disease. (Reprinted by permission of the Editor of *Cancer,* from the paper by Rosenberg and Kaplan, 1975.)

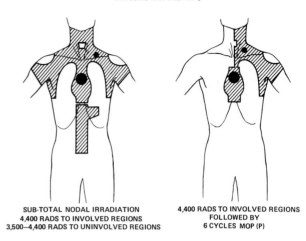

HODGKIN'S DISEASE
STANFORD RANDOMIZED CLINICAL TRIAL
STAGES IA AND IIA

SUB-TOTAL NODAL IRRADIATION   4,400 RADS TO INVOLVED REGIONS
4,400 RADS TO INVOLVED REGIONS   FOLLOWED BY
3,500–4,400 RADS TO UNINVOLVED REGIONS   6 CYCLES MOP (P)

S$_1$ PROTOCOL (1974)

Figure 11.16 Schematic diagram of the Stanford S-1 clinical trial for patients with PS IA and IIA Hodgkin's disease.

1975), which asked whether MOPP chemotherapy could act effectively as an adjuvant treatment to eradicate microscopic sites of disease beyond the margins of involved field radiotherapy for patients with localized (stage IA and IIA) disease, as compared with extended field or subtotal lymphoid (STLI) radiotherapy alone. The S-1 protocol was

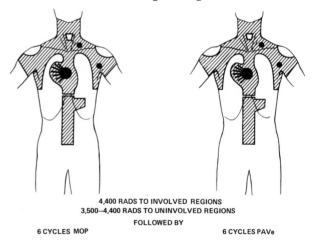

HODGKIN'S DISEASE
STANFORD RANDOMIZED CLINICAL TRIAL
STAGES I$_E$A AND II$_E$A

4,400 RADS TO INVOLVED REGIONS
3,500–4,400 RADS TO UNINVOLVED REGIONS
FOLLOWED BY
6 CYCLES MOP   6 CYCLES PAVe

S$_2$ PROTOCOL (1974)

Figure 11.17 Schematic diagram of the Stanford S-2 clinical trial for patients with PS I$_E$A and II$_E$A Hodgkin's disease.

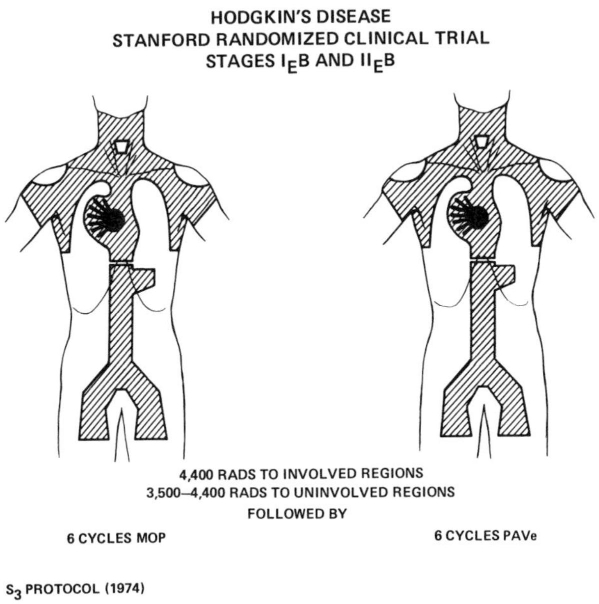

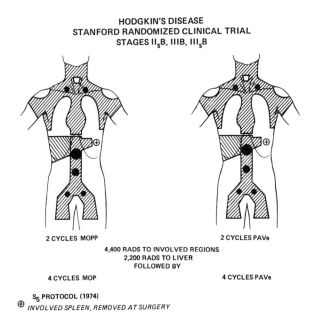

Figure 11.18 Schematic diagram of the Stanford S-3 clinical trial for patients with PS I$_E$B and II$_E$B Hodgkin's disease.

Figure 11.20 Schematic diagram of the Stanford S-5 clinical trial for patients with PS II$_S$B, IIIB, and III$_S$B Hodgkin's disease.

essentially an extension of the combined R-1 and K-1 protocols, comparing the relative efficacy of STLI radiotherapy alone versus involved field radiotherapy plus six cycles of MOPP in stage IA and IIA disease. In the S-2 through S-6 protocols, the radiotherapy employed in each treatment arm remained constant and the MOPP and PAVe chemotherapy regimens were compared with respect to

their value as adjuvants. The details of the PAVe regimen are presented in Table 10.3, Chapter 10. In the S-7 protocol, which dealt with stage IV$_H$ disease involving the liver, both radiotherapy and MOPP chemotherapy were used, but in opposite sequences, beginning with radiotherapy in the A treatment arm and with chemotherapy in the B treatment arm. Finally, in the S-8 protocol, which

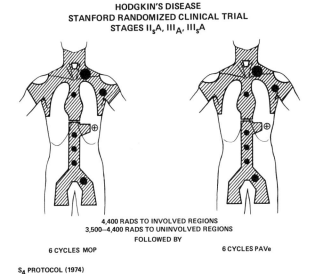

Figure 11.19 Schematic diagram of the Stanford S-4 clinical trial for patients with PS II$_S$A, IIIA, and III$_S$A Hodgkin's disease.

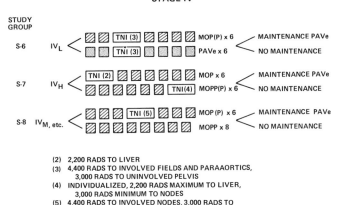

Figure 11.21 Schematic diagram of the Stanford S-6, S-7, and S-8 clinical trials for patients with PS IV Hodgkin's disease. (Reprinted by permission of the Editor of *Cancer,* from the paper by Rosenberg et al., 1978.)

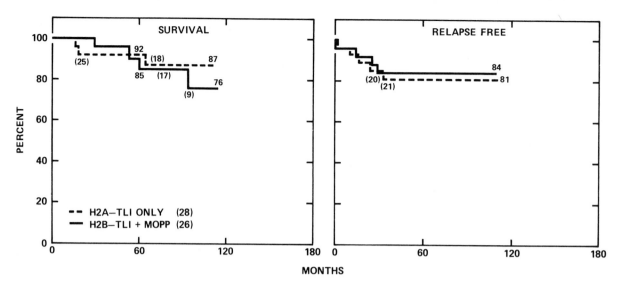

Figure 11.22   Actuarial analysis (by the method of Kaplan and Meier, 1958) of survival and freedom from relapse in the Stanford H-2 clinical trial, the design of which is indicated in Table 11.3 and Figure 11.14. The numbers of patients entered in each treatment arm are given in parentheses.

was concerned primarily with patients with stage IV$_M$ disease involving the bone marrow, the comparison was between split course MOPP plus moderate dose (3,000 rads) involved field radiotherapy (inserted between the third and fourth cycles of chemotherapy) versus eight cycles of MOPP chemotherapy alone.

Actuarial curves for survival and freedom from relapse in these randomized clinical trials are presented in Figures 11.22 through 11.33. In some of the clinical trials (K-1, H-5), but not in others (H-2), there has been a considerable decrease in relapse rate as a consequence of the use of adjuvant

combination chemotherapy (Fig. 11.22 vs. Figs. 11.24, 11.25). After a followup interval of about four years, no significant differences in the adjuvant value of the MOPP versus the PAVe regimens are apparent in the relapse-free survival curves of the S-4 or S-5 protocols (Figs. 11.31, 11.32); there has been only one death to date, in the S-5B group. There is as yet no significant improvement in survival as a consequence of adding adjuvant chemotherapy to radiotherapy, with the probable exception of the H-5 protocol, in which there appears to be a growing difference in survival, approaching significance at the 5 percent level, in patients with

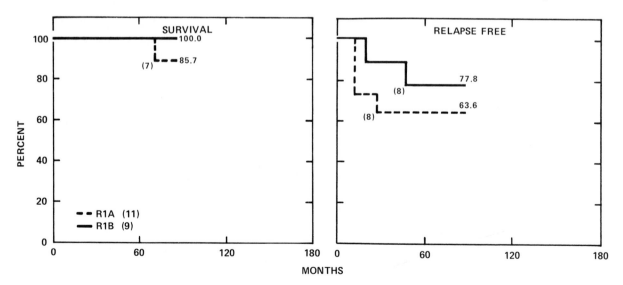

Figure 11.23   Survival and freedom from relapse in the Stanford R-1 protocol, the design of which is schematized in Figure 11.12. The numbers of patients entered in each treatment arm are given in parentheses.

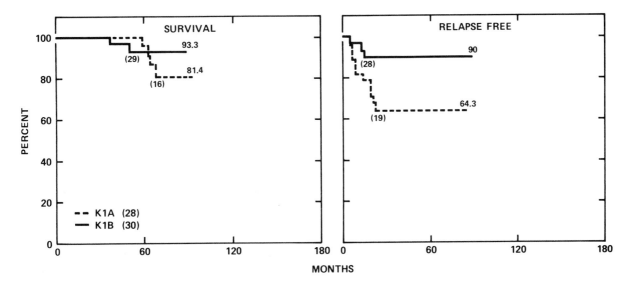

Figure 11.24 Survival and freedom from relapse in the Stanford K-1 protocol, the design of which is schematized in Figure 11.13. The numbers of patients entered in each treatment arm are given in parentheses.

stage III$_S$A disease treated with combined modality therapy, as compared to results with TLI and liver irradiation alone (Fig. 11.26). Thus, if one were to ask whether adjuvant chemotherapy should be used for all patients following radiation therapy for Hodgkin's disease, the answer must clearly be *no* at the present time. However, in stage IIIA, its use in selected patients with multiple (> 4) sites of involvement, or with massive node or spleen involvement, appears to be indicated on the basis of a recent analysis of data from the H-5 and S-4 protocols (Hoppe et al., 1979a). In patients

with stage IIIB disease, MOPP chemotherapy plays a therapeutic rather than an adjuvant role; combined modality therapy appears to be yielding results superior to those of MOPP alone and has now been adopted as our standard treatment for all such patients.

Can adjuvant combination chemotherapy effectively substitute for "prophylactic" radiotherapy of apparently uninvolved regions in patients with localized disease? The results of the R-1 and S-1 protocols appear to answer the question in the affirmative (Figs. 11.23, 11.30). Survival and relapse

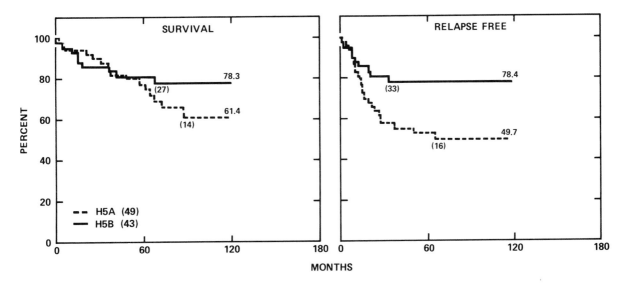

Figure 11.25 Survival and freedom from relapse in the Stanford H-5 protocol, the design of which is schematized in Figure 11.15. These data are for patients with and without constitutional symptoms. The numbers of patients entered in each treatment arm are given in parentheses.

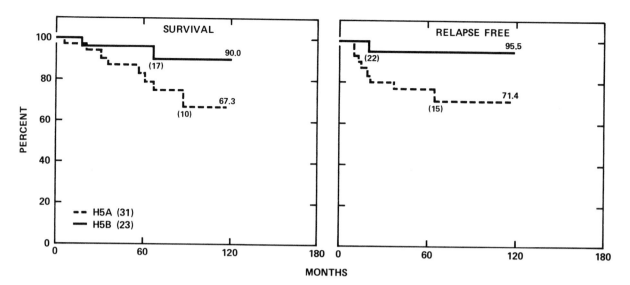

Figure 11.26 Survival and freedom from relapse in the Stanford H-5 protocol, the design of which is schematized in Figure 11.15. These data are for patients without constitutional symptoms (PS II$_S$A, III$_S$A). The numbers of patients entered in each treatment arm are given in parentheses.

rates are at least comparable to those of EF or TLI radiotherapy alone after several years. However, it is important to recognize that this has been achieved at a cost which is not insignificant: virtually all of the male patients (and probably also some of the females) randomized to the limited field radiotherapy plus MOPP program have undoubtedly been sterilized, many of them permanently. In addition, patients have been exposed to an increased hazard of late acute myelogenous leukemia and other secondary neoplasms, a topic which is developed in greater detail later in this section.

Another randomized clinical trial designed to test this question was the LYGRA project, initiated in September 1971, by several oncology centers in Denmark.[1] A total of 202 patients with stage I and II (A + B) Hodgkin's disease (most laparotomy-staged) were entered into the study. Half were allocated to total nodal irradiation (TNI) alone, the other half to mantle field irradiation followed by six cycles of MOPP chemotherapy. Freedom from relapse was slightly greater in the group treated with adjuvant chemotherapy (89 percent) than in those treated with radiation alone (78 percent), but at seven years, survival in both groups was identical (92 percent; Fig. 11.34).

We may also ask whether the use of adjuvant combination chemotherapy can eliminate or reduce the need for staging laparotomy and splenectomy in patients with Hodgkin's disease. At present, it would appear that the answer to this question is negative, since patients with PS IB and IIB disease have not yet manifested any significant benefit from the use of adjuvant chemotherapy (Fig. 11.22), whereas both combination chemotherapy and radiotherapy appear to be essential in the management of patients with PS IIIB disease. In many instances, staging laparotomy is the most reliable way to distinguish between these two groups of patients. In asymptomatic patients, staging laparotomy remains important because the radiotherapy fields appropriate for patients with PS IA and IIA disease are of lesser extent than those used in patients with PS IIIA disease.

Is adjuvant radiation therapy indicated in addition to combination chemotherapy in patients with PS IV disease? The answer to this question is complex, in part because stage IV is a heterogeneous category. It has already been noted in the previous section that our results of total lymphoid plus liver irradiation alone for patients with stage IV$_H$ disease involving the liver were surprisingly good, though no better than those with MOPP alone (Fig. 11.28). At present, there is no clear evidence that high-dose total lymphoid radiotherapy signifi-

1. I am greatly indebted to Prof. S. A. Kaae and Dr. A. M. Nordentoft of the Radiumcentre, Århus, for permission to cite these data prior to their publication. The participants in the LYGRA project were: S. Kaae, A. M. Nordentoft, K. Bjørn Jensen, K. Thorling, A. Sell, and Niels Ulsø from Radiumcentre, Århus; M. Pedersen, Jens Hvolby, and M. Krogh-Jensen from Radiumcentre, Alborg; T. Skov Jensen, H. Brincker, and J. Munk from Radiumcentre, Odense; S. Walbom, H. Sand Hansen, A. Nybo-Rasmussen, N. Nissen, S. Pedersen-Bjergaard, A. Videbaek, E. Anderson, S. Aa. Killmann, J. Boye-Nielsen, J. Ipsen, N. Kjaergard, M. Petersen, J. Clemmesen, J. Hastrup, N. K. Jensen from Radiumcentre, Copenhagen.

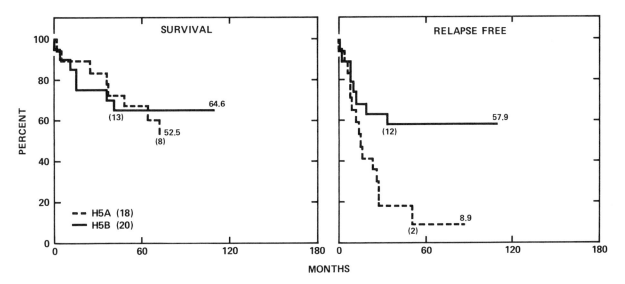

Figure 11.27 Survival and freedom from relapse in the Stanford H-5 protocol, the design of which is schematized in Figure 11.15. These data are for patients with constitutional symptoms (PS II_SB, III_SB). The numbers of patients entered in each treatment arm are given in parentheses.

cantly improves survival or freedom from relapse in patients with stage IV_M disease involving the bone marrow, or in other miscellaneous stage IV sites such as the lungs or bones (Fig. 11.29). However, the numbers of patients in these clinical studies are relatively small, and additional periods of observation on larger numbers of patients will be required before a clear-cut answer is obtained.

The fact that the sites of relapse with MOPP combination chemotherapy alone show a marked predilection for initial sites of bulky lymphadenopathy (Frei et al., 1973; Young et al., 1978) provides a plausible rationale for the use of at least low-dose radiotherapy to all sites of initial lymphadenopathy (Prosnitz et al., 1973, 1976) in patients receiving MOPP or other forms of combination chemother-

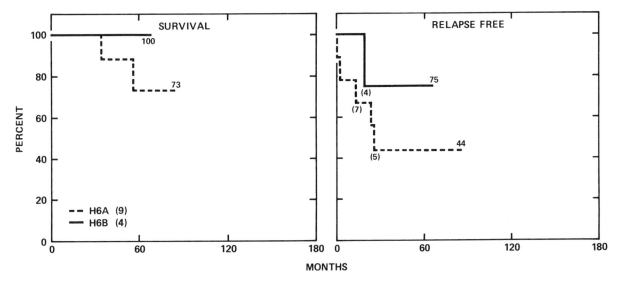

Figure 11.28 Survival and freedom from relapse in the Stanford H-6 protocol, in which patients with PS IV_H (A + B) disease involving the liver were randomized to total lymphoid irradiation, hepatic irradiation, and colloidal [198]Au (H-6A) versus MOPP combination chemotherapy alone (H-6B). It is noteworthy that all four of the patients treated with MOPP alone are alive, and only one has had a relapse. However, the numbers of patients entered into the study are too small for the apparent differences to be significant.

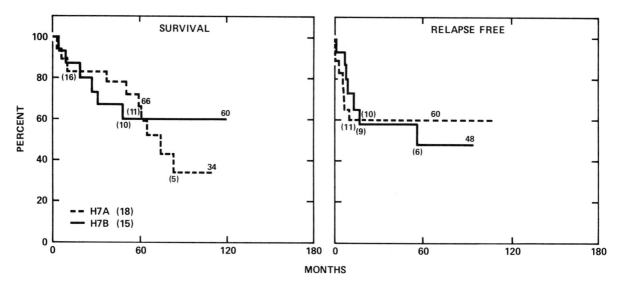

Figure 11.29 Survival and freedom from relapse in the Stanford H-7 protocol, in which patients with stage IV disease involving the bone marrow, lungs, or other extralymphatic sites (excluding the liver) were randomized to treatment with eight cycles of MOPP combination chemotherapy alone (H-7B) versus split course MOPP plus total lymphoid irradiation (two cycles before, four after TLI; H-7A). The numbers of patients (indicated in parentheses) are too small for the apparent differences to be significant.

apy for stage IV disease. The issue of radiation dose in combined modality therapy is discussed further in a later section of this chapter.

Scheduling of Combined Modality Therapy. The scheduling of radiotherapy and chemotherapy in combined modality treatment programs is a complex problem which has undergone an interesting evolution. As has already been mentioned, in the Stanford clinical trials which ushered in the modern era of combined modality therapy in July 1968, we elected to use total lymphoid irradiation first and to carry the radiotherapy to completion, after which a rest interval of six to eight weeks intervened before the first of six cycles of MOPP combination chemotherapy was started. Although

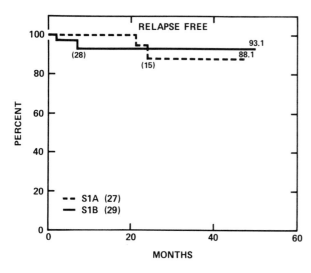

Figure 11.30 Freedom from relapse during the first four years of the Stanford S-1 clinical trial, the design of which is schematized in Figure 11.16. The numbers of patients entered into each treatment arm are indicated in parentheses. There has been one death to date, in the S-1A group.

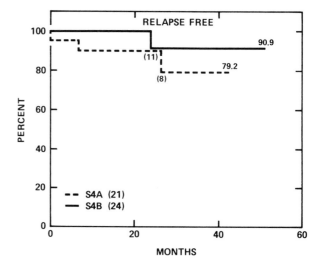

Figure 11.31 Freedom from relapse during the first four years of the Stanford S-4 clinical trial, the design of which is schematized in Figure 11.19. The numbers of patients entered into each treatment arm are indicated in parentheses. There has been one death to date, in the S-4A group.

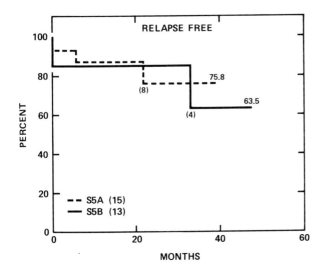

Figure 11.32 Freedom from relapse during the first four years of the Stanford S-5 clinical trial, the design of which is schematized in Figure 11.20. There has been one death to date (in the S-5B treatment group). The numbers of patients entered into each treatment arm are indicated in parentheses.

we had had very serious misgivings as to whether these two formidable treatment regimens could be tolerated, we were pleased to observe that both TLI and MOPP chemotherapy could be completed essentially on schedule in 50 of the first 54 patients thus treated (Moore et al., 1972; Rosenberg et al., 1972). However, some patients required significant reductions of drug dosage, particularly after the first MOPP cycle, and an appreciable percent-

age of patients required delays in the time of initiation of the later cycles of the MOPP program, due to prolonged leukopenia or thrombocytopenia. Thus by 1974 we began to experiment with modifications of radiation and drug treatment schedules in the hope of improving overall tolerance.

Meanwhile in 1969 the National Cancer Institute group had initiated their combined modality studies in patients with stage IIB and IIIB disease, using a scheduling sequence which was the reverse of that employed at Stanford (Kun et al., 1976). By beginning treatment with six cycles of combination chemotherapy, they hoped to alleviate systemic symptoms rapidly, reduce the volume of normal tissue requiring irradiation by inducing regression of tumor masses, and use the chemotherapy at the time when the extent of occult disseminated disease would be minimal. They also anticipated that hematologic depression would be more transient after chemotherapy than after total lymphoid irradiation and thus would favor the use of maximal doses of both modalities. In a series of 28 patients, they achieved complete remissions with the chemotherapy in 27, of whom 5 had relapses during the interval between the completion of chemotherapy and the initiation of radiotherapy. Thus 22 (79 percent) of 28 patients were clinically free of disease at the time when radiotherapy was commenced. By the time of completion of radiotherapy, 26 patients were in complete remission. After a median followup interval of 48 months, 17 patients (61 percent) remained continuously free of

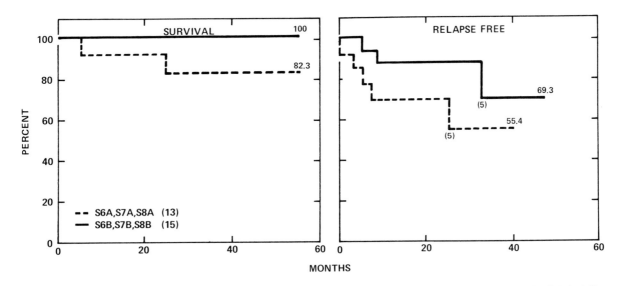

Figure 11.33 Survival and freedom from relapse during the first four years in the combined Stanford S-6, S-7, and S-8 clinical trials involving patients with stage IV disease, as schematized in Figure 11.21. There have been 2 deaths among the 13 patients entered into the A treatment arms and none among the 15 in the B treatment arms. The differences are not statistically significant.

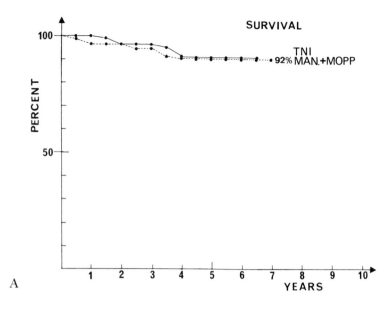

A

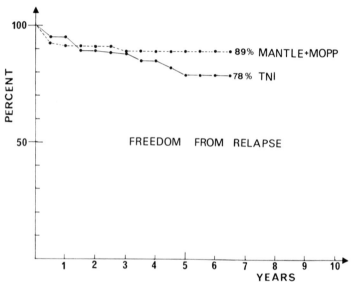

B

Figure 11.34   Results of a multicenter randomized clinical trial conducted by the Danish LYGRA group to compare total nodal irradiation (TNI) with mantle field irradiation plus six cycles of MOPP combination chemotherapy in patients with stages I and II (A + B) Hodgkin's disease. *A,* survival; *B,* freedom from relapse. (Reprinted by permission of the Danish LYGRA group through the courtesy of S. Kaae and A. M. Nordentoft.)

disease, 4 were alive with active Hodgkin's disease, and 7 had died, one from acute myelocytic leukemia at 31 months after combined therapy, 2 from Hodgkin's disease, and 4 from complications of treatment. Four patients developed a local or marginal recurrence of Hodgkin's disease within an irradiated field as the first evidence of relapse.

The initial cycles of chemotherapy were generally well tolerated, and no serious complications secondary to hematologic depression were encountered during this part of the treatment program. However, the subsequent radiotherapy was associated with far more severe hematologic depression than is ordinarily encountered with radiotherapy alone. The most serious problem was prolonged thrombocytopenia; 12 patients had

platelet counts below 50,000/mm³ for many weeks or months, and 8 were below 30,000/mm³. The mean nadir white blood cell count was 2,600/mm³, and values below 2,000 were encountered in 6 cases. It was stated that the nadir values would have been significantly lower if planned segments of the radiotherapy program had not been either delayed or interrupted. The median time for completion of radiotherapy was seven months, and in 11 patients, delays of more than eight weeks between the irradiation of successive lymphatic regions were required because of serious hematologic depression. The overall median time for the combined chemotherapy-radiotherapy treatment program was 15 months, with a range of 11 to 25 months. Thus, it would appear that tolerance for combined modality treatment was significantly less favorable when six cycles of MOPP chemotherapy were used first, followed by total lymphoid irradiation, than was observed with the reverse sequence in the Stanford experience.

The possibility that a more flexible scheduling sequence might yield appreciably better results remained to be explored. In 1974, we initiated such studies in patients with stage IIIB and stage IV (A + B) disease. Emphasis was placed on close cooperation between the radiation therapists and medical oncologists in order to interdigitate successive segments of the radiotherapy and the MOPP or PAVe combination chemotherapy programs. A number of variations of the scheduling sequence have been employed in an effort to individualize treatment wherever possible (Hoppe et al., 1979b). In general, two scheduling patterns have emerged.

The split course pattern (Fig. 11.35), used most often in patients with stage IIIB and IV disease, typically employed two or three cycles of MOPP combination chemotherapy followed by high-dose radiotherapy to areas of initially bulky lymphadenopathy, after which three or four additional cycles of MOPP chemotherapy were delivered, sometimes followed by reduced-dose (3,000 rads) radiotherapy to apparently uninvolved lymph node regions. In patients with bone marrow involvement, this program was followed by consolidation cycles of MOPP chemotherapy, and in some patients by maintenance chemotherapy with monthly vinblastine and chlorambucil or with CCNU given at six-week intervals.

The second pattern, which has been termed the "alternating" technique, was also used principally in patients with stage IIIB and IV disease. The timing of successive components of such treatment programs varied somewhat from case to case; representative examples are diagrammed in Figures 11.36 and 11.37. It will be seen that treatment usually started with two or three cycles of MOPP chemotherapy, after which high-dose irradiation was administered to the region (usually the mantle or the upper abdomen) in which lymphadenopathy was initially most pronounced. After a short rest period, two or three more cycles of MOPP were delivered, following which the patient returned to the radiation therapy department for treatment of the next most impressive region of involvement. In the most typical sequence (Fig. 11.36), this was again followed after a short rest period by two more cycles of MOPP, and the patient was then returned to radiation therapy for

treatment of the final segment of the total lymphoid irradiation sequence (usually the pelvis), which was treated to reduced dose levels (3,000 rads) if the lymph nodes in this region were deemed to have been uninvolved initially.

The alternating and split course programs were associated with an appreciable improvement in the percentage of planned drug dose that could be delivered in each cycle (Fig. 11.38). Overall, 78 percent of the planned alkylating agent dose and 75 percent of the procarbazine dose were successfully delivered in the alternating technique, figures which are comparable with the 82 percent and 76 percent, respectively, reported by De Vita, Serpick, and Carbone (1970), using MOPP chemotherapy alone. The corresponding figures for the split course sequence were somewhat less favorable: 68 percent and 62 percent, respectively. It will be seen in Figures 11.35 and 11.36 that hematologic tolerance was remarkably good throughout the entire treatment program. The mean nadir white blood cell count was 2,200/mm^3, with a range of 1,200–2,600. The mean nadir platelet count was 101,000/mm^3, although 53 percent of the patients had platelet counts less than 100,000/mm^3 on at least one occasion. There was only one episode of sepsis and two of bleeding during treatment. White blood cell or platelet transfusions were not required in any of 25 patients treated with the alternating or split course schedules. One patient developed hypersensitivity to procarbazine, for which CCNU (100 mg PO on day 1 of each cycle) was substituted. Seven patients developed evidence of significant motor neuropathy attributable to vincristine, requiring substitution by vinblastine (6 mg/m^2 IV, days 1 and 8).

The duration of therapy ranged from 9 to 18 months with a median of 13 months (Hoppe et al., 1979b). After approximately four years of followup, the alternating irradiation-chemotherapy program appears to be yielding a significant improvement in both survival and freedom from relapse as compared with previous experience with irradiation alone or sequential irradiation followed by MOPP chemotherapy in patients with stage IIIB disease (Figs. 11.39 and 11.40). There have been only 2 relapses among the 22 patients who achieved complete remission with either the split course or alternating sequences of combined modality treatment. It may be noted that 84 percent of these patients are alive at approximately four years, and 79 percent are relapse-free, as compared with 62 percent survival and 50 percent freedom from relapse in the earlier group that

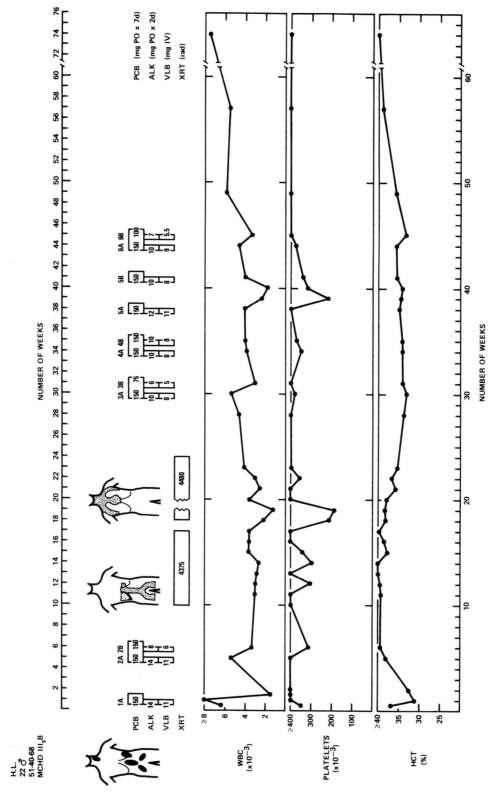

Figure 11.35   Split course combined modality therapy in a 22-year-old male patient with PS III$_s$B mixed cellularity Hodgkin's disease. The sites of documented involvement are indicated on the manikin at upper left. The patient received one and a half cycles of PAVe chemotherapy first, followed by high-dose total lymphoid irradiation which began with an inverted-Y field because he had massive subdiaphragmatic adenopathy. About seven weeks after the completion of his radiotherapy, PAVe chemotherapy was resumed and carried to completion (six cycles) on schedule. Note that his nadir platelet counts were close to 200,000/mm³; however, nadir white blood cell counts less than 2,000/mm.³ were observed on three occasions. All values returned to normal levels within a few weeks after the last drug cycle, and the patient remains relapse-free three years after admission.

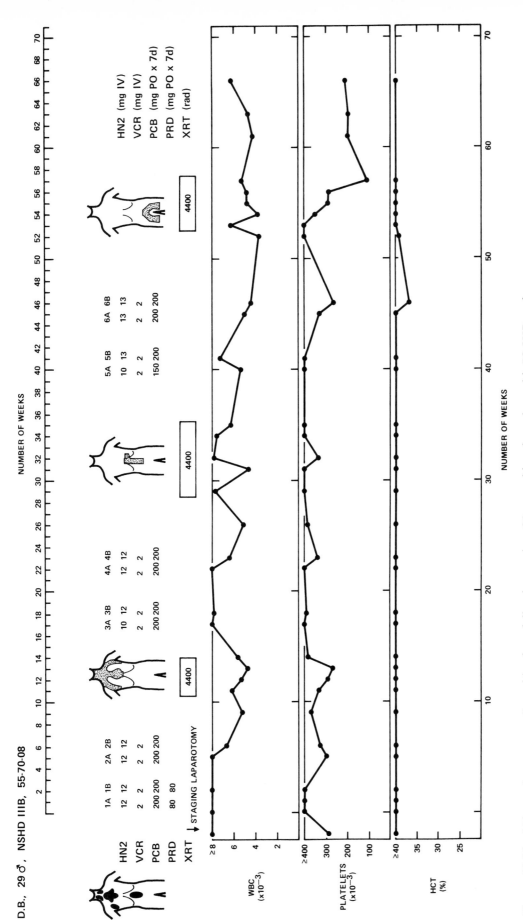

Figure 11.36 "Alternating sequence" combined modality therapy in a 29-year-old male patient with PS IIIB nodular sclerosing Hodgkin's disease. The sites of documented involvement are shown on the manikin. After two cycles of MOPP, chemotherapy was interrupted for several weeks while the mantle field was irradiated to 4,400 rads. Two more cycles of MOPP were then given, followed by irradiation of the para-aortic and splenic pedicle regions to 4,400 rads, cycles 5 and 6 of MOPP, and pelvic irradiation to 4,400 rads. The white blood cell count fell slightly below 4,000/mm.³, and the platelet count decreased to about 100,000/mm.³ when the pelvis was irradiated. All values returned to normal within a few weeks thereafter. At 28 months, the patient is relapse-free.

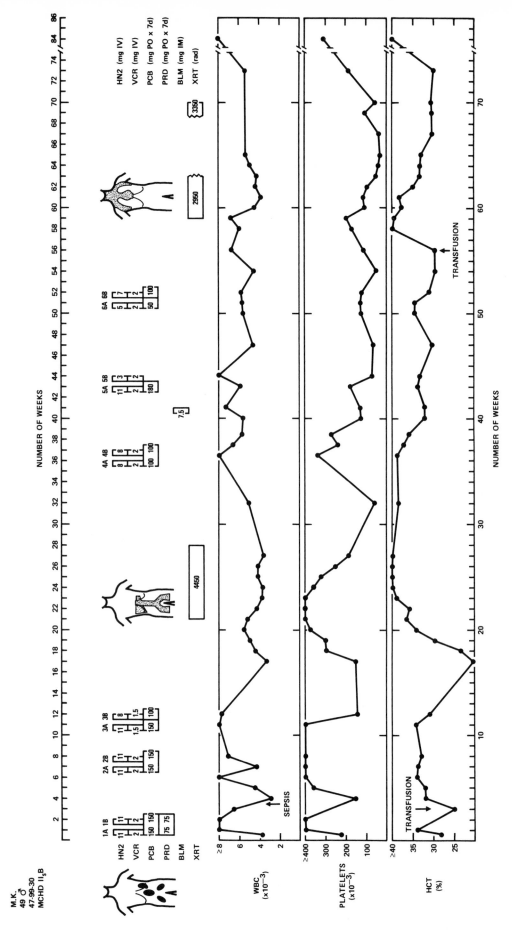

Figure 11.37 Another variation of alternating sequence combined modality therapy in a 49-year-old male with PS II$_S$B mixed cellularity Hodgkin's disease. Because of the severity of his constitutional symptoms (high fevers, drenching night sweats, 80-pound weight loss, anemia), we elected to start with three cycles of MOPP, which caused all of these symptoms to disappear. After hematologic recovery, he received 4,450 rads to an inverted-Y field (plus 2,225 rads to the liver through a 50 percent transmission lead block). A few weeks later, MOPP chemotherapy was resumed, and cycles 4, 5, and 6 were given on schedule, followed by reduced dose (2,950 rads) irradiation of the mantle field. Hematologic values returned promptly to normal, and the patient gained 60 pounds and is relapse-free more than four years later.

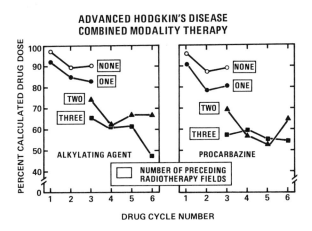

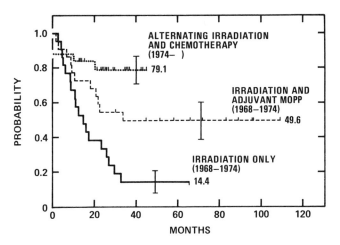

Figure 11.38 Percentage of planned drug doses delivered during combined modality treatment by the split course and alternating schedules. (Reprinted, by permission of the authors and the Editor of *Cancer,* from the paper by Hoppe et al., 1979b.)

Figure 11.40 Actuarial analysis of freedom from relapse in patients with stage IIIB disease treated with an alternating sequence of combined modality therapy, compared with prior relapse-free survival data in such patients treated with total lymphoid irradiation (TLI) alone or followed by six cycles of MOPP chemotherapy. (Reprinted, by permission of the authors and the Editor of *Cancer,* from the paper by Hoppe et al., 1979b.)

received sequential total lymphoid irradiation and MOPP chemotherapy. Both combined modality results are appreciably better than those with total lymphoid irradiation alone, which yielded a survival rate of 44 percent at about nine years, with only 14.4 percent of patients remaining relapse-free at five years. On the basis of this highly favorable experience, the alternating technique appears to be the new standard of comparison in future thera-

peutic investigations in patients with stage IIIB disease and is recommended for general use whenever combined modality therapy is indicated.

Modification of Dose in Combined Modality Therapy. Improved hematologic tolerance during combined modality therapy can also be achieved by reductions of radiation dose, decreases in the extent of radiation fields, planned reductions of drug doses, and/or decreased numbers of planned drug cycles. Some of these parameters have not yet been manipulated experimentally. However, the data presented in this section indicate that reduction of radiation dose and of field extent has been associated with highly favorable initial responses.

The first clinical study in which low-dose radiotherapy was used in conjunction with combination chemotherapy was initiated in 1969 at Yale University School of Medicine in adult patients with stage IIIB and IV Hodgkin's disease (Prosnitz et al., 1973). The chemotherapy regimen employed was a modified version of MOPP, which included five drugs: nitrogen mustard, vinblastine, vincristine, procarbazine, and prednisone, given in a 43-day cycle with a 14-day rest interval. Radiotherapy was initiated one month following completion of the third cycle and was delivered to each of the anatomic areas known to be involved with Hodgkin's disease prior to the institution of chemotherapy. The radiation dose was 1,500–2,500 rads, given at

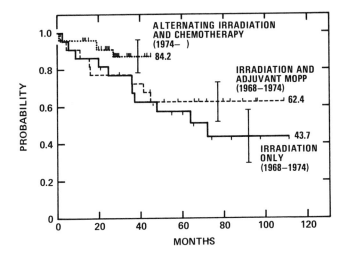

Figure 11.39 Actuarial analysis of survival in patients with stage IIIB disease treated with an alternating sequence of combined modality therapy, compared with prior survival data in such patients treated with total lymphoid irradiation (TLI) alone or followed by six cycles of MOPP chemotherapy. (Reprinted, by permission of the authors and the Editor of *Cancer,* from the paper by Hoppe et al., 1979b.)

a rate of 800–1,000 rads per week. When more than one radiation field was treated, a three-week interval was interposed between successive fields to permit hematologic recovery. Following the completion of radiotherapy, a rest interval of three to four weeks intervened before the delivery of a fourth and fifth cycle of combination chemotherapy.

In a subsequent report, Prosnitz et al. (1976) analyzed the long-term results of this treatment program. A total of 80 patients had been treated, and the followup interval in those entering complete remission was one year or more in all instances. There were 18 induction failures, only 1 of whom remained alive. One other patient, who failed to achieve a complete remission during the induction chemotherapy because of relapsing disease in an axillary node, entered complete remission following radiotherapy and remained apparently disease-free thereafter. Two deaths occurred due to infection during the induction phase of chemotherapy, one from cryptococcal meningitis, the other from pneumococcal sepsis. A total of 60 patients (75 percent) entered complete remission, of whom 54 (68 percent) remained in complete remission for intervals ranging from one to six years. At the time of reporting, only 5 of 60 patients had developed relapses, of whom 3 were dead of Hodgkin's disease. One other patient developed acute myelogenous leukemia three years after completion of combined modality treatment. Overall survival for the entire series of patients was 68 percent at five years; those who had entered complete remission had a 92 percent 5-year survival, whereas survival in the group of induction failures was only 19 percent at two years. Forty-four of the 80 patients were previously untreated patients with stage IIIB and stage IV disease, of whom 32 (73 percent) achieved complete remission. There was no obvious relationship between stage of disease and the probability of achieving complete remission. However, patients with constitutional symptoms had a 69 percent complete remission rate, as compared with 86 percent in patients who were asymptomatic. Age was also a factor in response: complete remissions were obtained in 13 of 14 patients less than 20 years of age (93 percent), 40 of 49 (82 percent) who were 20–39 years of age, and only 7 (41 percent) of 17 who were 40 years of age or older. In a later update encompassing 135 patients at risk for one year or more, Farber et al., (1978) reported that the complete remission rate remained stable at 75 percent, and that only 9 (15 percent) of the 60 patients who had attained complete remission at the time of the 1976 report had relapsed.

The Yale combined modality treatment regimen was generally well tolerated. However, even at these low dose levels, the addition of radiotherapy following three cycles of combination chemotherapy adversely affected bone marrow tolerance, with the result that the fourth drug cycle had to be delayed for one to two months following radiation treatment, and drug doses often had to be reduced. Moreover, the mean nadir white blood cell counts and platelet counts observed after the fourth cycle (1,900/mm³ and 78,000/mm³, respectively) were the lowest observed after any of the five drug cycles. However, it was possible to deliver these radiation doses not only to involved lymph node chains but also to extranodal tissues such as the lungs and liver. Whole lung irradiation was given to nine patients to a dose of 1,500 rads in ten fractions without complications. In ten patients, the entire liver was irradiated to a dose of 2,000 rads, given at a rate of 150 rads per day, with a transient rise in serum alkaline phosphatase and transaminase levels but no other indications of significant hepatic dysfunction.

Our first use of low-dose radiotherapy in combination with six cycles of MOPP combination chemotherapy occurred in two young male children, aged 21 months and 50 months, who were admitted to Stanford University Medical Center in March and April 1970. Following a diagnostic investigation which included staging laparotomy with splenectomy, both were found to have stage III$_S$B Hodgkin's disease. Prompted by concern about the profound impairment of bone growth that could be anticipated in these young children if high-dose total lymphoid irradiation were employed, I decided to ascertain whether multiple cycles of MOPP combination chemotherapy could replace part of the radiation dose. It was elected to give a total of 1,500 rads to each of the total lymphoid irradiation fields in the smaller child, and 2,000 rads to each field in the four-year-old child. Both children tolerated all six cycles of MOPP chemotherapy extremely well after completion of the low-dose total lymphoid irradiation. Both entered complete remission and have remained relapse-free for more than nine years. Moreover, they have continued to grow normally with respect to body weight and standing height and have only a modest decrease in sitting height, presumably due to transient impairment of dorsolumbar vertebral growth (Fig. 11.41).

Encouraged by this favorable preliminary expe-

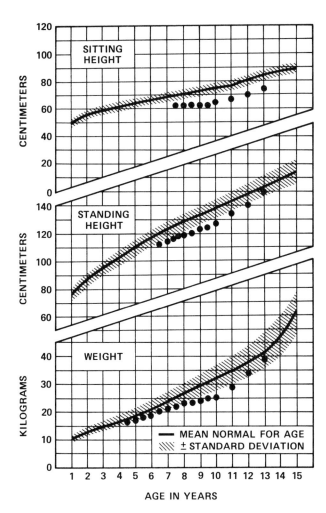

Figure 11.41 Sitting height, standing height, and body weight measurements of a boy who was admitted in May 1970 with PS III$_S$B Hodgkin's disease and was treated with low-dose (2,000 rads) total lymphoid irradiation followed by six cycles of MOPP chemotherapy. The solid lines and striped areas are the mean ± standard deviation for age. The patient's body weight and standing height, after being slightly subnormal for a few years, are again within less than one standard deviation from the mean; sitting height remained static for about three years but is now increasing parallel to the normal curve.

rience, a formalized protocol for treatment of pediatric Hodgkin's disease with low-dose, involved field radiotherapy and MOPP combination chemotherapy was initiated at Stanford. Radiation dose was graduated in relation to bone age, as determined from radiographs of the wrist. Children with a bone age of less than 6 years received 1,500 rads; 6–9 years, 2,000 rads; and 10–14 years, 2,500 rads. When necessary, massive lymphadenopathy was locally supplemented to 3,000 rads

through reduced fields. All children received six cycles of MOPP chemotherapy, which was initiated six to eight weeks after completion of the radiotherapy in all but the stage IV cases, in which two or three cycles preceded radiotherapy, and the stage I cases, in which the first drug cycle was administered concomitantly with radiotherapy. To date, 28 children with Hodgkin's disease of all stages (4 PS I, 12 PS II, 10 PS III, 2 PS IV) have completed treatment. The results of this pediatric protocol (Fig. 11.42) are indeed excellent; actuarial survival for the entire group is currently 96 percent at eight years, and 90 percent are relapse-free (S. S. Donaldson and H. S. Kaplan, previously unpublished data). Growth impairment has generally been minimal, and there have been no major complications.

The Milan group has also explored the use of reduced dose radiotherapy in conjunction with either MOPP or ABVD combination chemotherapy (Bonadonna et al., 1977). All six cycles of combination chemotherapy were given first, following

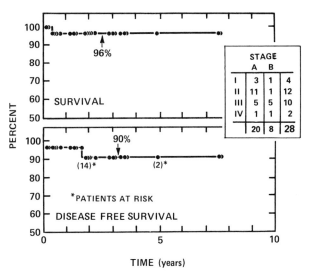

Figure 11.42 Actuarial analysis of survival and freedom from relapse of 28 pediatric patients with Hodgkin's disease, pathologically staged as shown in the insert, who were treated in the Stanford pediatric Hodgkin's disease protocol with low-dose (1,500–2,500 rads, depending on bone age) involved field radiotherapy followed by six cycles of MOPP. The only death was that of a boy with stage IV$_B$ disease who failed to enter remission. Data of S. S. Donaldson and H. S. Kaplan, from S. Murphy and S. S. Donaldson, "Pediatric Lymphoma," in *Principles of Cancer Treatment*, eds. S. K. Carter, E. Glatstein, and R. B. Livingston (New York: McGraw-Hill, in press). Used with permission of McGraw-Hill Book Company.

which patients who had entered either complete or partial remission were started on radiotherapy after an interval of four to six weeks from the end of the induction chemotherapy phase. Radiotherapy was administered to total doses of 3,000–3,500 rads at a rate of 750–800 rads per week, with rest intervals between successive segments when severe and prolonged bone marrow suppression was observed. Patients who initially had involvement of para-aortic and/or iliac chains received total lymphoid irradiation, whereas only the mantle and para-aortic fields were treated in those who had no evident subdiaphragmatic disease. Patients with extranodal involvement initially received low-dose radiotherapy (2,000–2,500 rads) to all nodal and extranodal sites of pretreatment involvement except the bone marrow.

One patient in the ABVD group who received radiotherapy to both lungs developed fatal radiation pneumonitis about two months later, and another, also in the ABVD group, developed cardiomegaly with repeated episodes of congestive heart failure, probably due to exacerbation by radiotherapy by an adriamycin-induced cardiomyopathy. In other respects, however, the radiotherapy was apparently better tolerated by patients who received ABVD than by those who had been treated with MOPP. Prolonged bone marrow suppression, particularly thrombocytopenia, was observed more often after MOPP than after ABVD, and radiotherapy in one patient previously treated with MOPP had to be discontinued because of persistent low blood cell counts. However, no patient in either group showed a white blood cell count less than 1,500/mm³ and/or a platelet count less than 50,000/mm³, nor was there an apparently increased incidence of viral or bacterial infection. One patient in the MOPP group developed an acute myelomonocytic leukemia 22 months after the completion of radiotherapy and died six weeks later. The supplementary radiotherapy clearly had a very favorable influence on complete remission rates in this study. After six cycles of combination chemotherapy alone, complete remissions were observed in 62 percent of those treated with MOPP and 70 percent of those treated with ABVD. After completion of radiotherapy to the patients who experienced either a complete remission or a >75 percent partial response, the complete remission rates had increased to 95 percent in the MOPP group and 89 percent in the ABVD group. Of the complete responders at risk for 30 months or more from the completion of both chemotherapy and radiotherapy, 88.9 percent of those in the MOPP

group and 93.4 percent of those in the ABVD group remained continuously free of disease. Overall survival at three years was 65.7 percent in the MOPP group and 73 percent in the ABVD group; these differences were not statistically significant.

Reduction of radiation field size and extent, rather than reduction of radiation dose, was used in conjunction with MOPP combination chemotherapy in patients with stage IA, IIA or B, and IIIA Hodgkin's disease in a clinical trial initiated at the Baltimore Cancer Research Center in 1970 (O'Connell et al., 1975b; Wiernik and Lichtenfeld, 1975). Half of the patients admitted to the clinical trial were randomized to megavoltage extended field radiotherapy alone, and half to combined modality treatment. The combined modality program involved high-dose radiotherapy (4,000 rads) to involved fields only (at least a mantle field in those with stage I or stage II disease) followed by six cycles of MOPP chemotherapy. Four patients (4.6 percent) failed to achieve remission with the initial radiation therapy. Of 41 patients who achieved complete remission after extended field radiation therapy alone, 10 later relapsed, as compared to only 1 of 31 achieving complete remission following involved field radiation plus chemotherapy. There were only 4 deaths among patients who initially achieved complete remission, all in the group treated with extended field irradiation alone. At the time of reporting, however, survival rates were not significantly different in the two treatment arms.

Fatal radiation pneumonitis occurred in one patient with massive mediastinal involvement whose radiation fields encompassed large volumes of normal lung tissue. Four other patients, two in each randomization category, developed radiation pericarditis requiring pericardiectomy. The subsequent combination chemotherapy was reasonably well tolerated. All 31 patients were able to complete three cycles; 29 completed four cycles; 26, five cycles; and 23 (74 percent) completed all six cycles. Tolerance for subsequent chemotherapy was perhaps somewhat better among the patients whose radiation treatment was confined to the mantle field alone. Fifteen of 18 such patients (83 percent) were able to complete six courses of chemotherapy, as compared with 8 of 13 (62 percent) receiving treatment both above and below the diaphragm prior to chemotherapy. No severe infections or complications due to bleeding occurred during the course of chemotherapy administration, although platelet transfusions were given prophylactically in three instances when platelet counts fell below 20,000/mm³.

In the S-1 protocol initiated at Stanford University Medical Center in 1974, patients with stage IA or IIA Hodgkin's disease were randomized to high-dose IF radiotherapy plus six cycles of MOPP versus subtotal lymphoid (STLI) irradiation alone (Fig. 11.16). This type of combined modality therapy was quite well tolerated; indeed, it was often possible to initiate MOPP chemotherapy concurrently with the IF radiotherapy. Twenty-eight patients have been randomized to subtotal lymphoid irradiation alone, and 29 patients to involved field radiation plus MOPP. Survival in both treatment arms was nearly 100 percent at four years, at which time the proportion of relapse-free patients was slightly, but not significantly, higher in the group treated with involved field radiation plus MOPP (95.8 percent) than in those treated with radiation alone (86.7 percent; Fig. 11.30).

A clinical trial of interesting design was conducted at the Baltimore Cancer Research Center from July 1967 to July 1969 (Brace et al., 1973). Previously untreated patients with clinical stage I or stage II Hodgkin's disease (excluding those with E lesions) were randomly allocated to one of three treatment options: group A received EF radiation therapy alone to all involved and adjacent lymph-node-bearing areas to a tumor dose of 4,000 rads; group B, IF radiation therapy to a tumor dose of 4,000 rads, followed one month later by three cycles of MOPP combination chemotherapy; and group C, three cycles of MOPP combination chemotherapy followed one month later by IF radiation therapy. This was apparently the first study of the efficacy of a reduced number of cycles with MOPP combination chemotherapy as adjuvant treatment in association with involved field radiotherapy and the first to allocate patients receiving such combined modality treatment to reciprocal sequences of radiotherapy and chemotherapy.

Unfortunately, the fact that only 22 patients were entered into this small-scale study precludes any definitive answers to the questions underlying the study design. However, in an analysis of the results after seven years of followup, Wiernik and Lichtenfeld (1975) reported that all patients tolerated their respective treatment regimens well and that there had been no treatment deaths. All patients achieved complete remission by the completion of the initial mode of treatment (radiation in groups A and B, chemotherapy in group C). In group A four of the seven patients treated with EF radiation therapy alone relapsed at 3, 21, 42, and 47 months. All of the relapsing patients have apparently been salvaged by subsequent chemotherapy and/or radiation therapy, and all patients in group A were alive and apparently free of disease at the time of reporting, with a median survival of 87 + months. In group B, two of eight patients relapsed at 63 and 67 months following completion of treatment; one of these failed to respond to further treatment and died six months later. A third patient in this group developed acute nonlymphocytic leukemia 34 months following completion of treatment and died shortly thereafter. Median survival in group B, calculated from the time of completion of treatment, was 74.5 + months. In group C, four of seven patients relapsed at 6, 6, 15, and 20 months following completion of IF radiation therapy, one in a previously unirradiated lymph node and three in parenchymal sites. Two of the latter patients failed to respond to further treatment and died, whereas the other two relapsing patients were apparently salvaged. Median survival in group C from the time of completion of treatment was 75 + months. The authors expressed concern that the decreased relapse rates following adjuvant treatment with three cycles of MOPP may have been obtained at the expense of decreased salvage rates among those patients who subsequently did relapse and a decreased absolute survival among the groups receiving both radiotherapy and chemotherapy, in either sequence.

Coltman, Montague, and Moon (1977) described a study in which patients with pathological stage IIB, IIIA, and IIIB Hodgkin's disease were given three cycles of MOPP followed after four weeks by total lymphoid irradiation, giving a dose of 4,000 rads to all initially involved lymph node chains. After eleven months, when this program appeared to be well tolerated, the induction chemotherapy phase was increased to four, and later to five and six cycles. Of 144 evaluable patients, 125 (87 percent) entered complete remission. There were no complete remissions in 6 patients who received only two cycles of MOPP. However, the complete remission rate among those who received three cycles of MOPP (62 of 68, or 91 percent) was almost identical with that in patients who received four, five, or six cycles (63 of 70, or 90 percent). Treatment complications included three deaths due to thrombocytopenia, three instances in which platelet counts fell below 50,000/mm³, and four with white blood cell counts less than 500/mm³. Overall survival was 86 percent at six years, with flattening of the relapse-free survival curve at 70 percent. It was concluded that three cycles of

MOPP are just as effective as longer courses when given as adjuvant treatment in association with radiation therapy.

There have apparently been no attempts to date to investigate the use of reduced doses of the component drugs of the MOPP regimen in combined modality therapy. However, another approach to the improvement of drug tolerance involves the deletion of one of the drugs from the MOPP regimen. A prospective randomized multicenter trial was initiated in 1969 by the Cancer and Leukemia Group B (Nissen et al., 1979) in which 537 evaluable patients with stage IIIB or IV Hodgkin's disease were allocated to one of four drug treatment regimens, all involving a six-cycle induction phase: group 1, MOPP; group 2, BOPP, in which BCNU (80 mg/m² IV on day 1) was substituted for nitrogen mustard in the MOPP regimen; group 3, BOP, in which the procarbazine of the BOPP regimen was deleted; and Group 4, OPP, in which the alkylating agent of either regimen was deleted. In previously untreated patients, the four-drug combinations yielded significantly higher complete remission rates than either of the three-drug regimens. Complete remissions were achieved in 23 (66 percent) of 35 patients treated with MOPP, 32 (74 percent) of 43 treated with BOPP, 17 (49 percent) of 35 treated with BOP, and 15 (41 percent) of 37 treated with OPP. The median survival of all patients randomized to either of the four-drug regimens was approximately five years, whereas that among patients randomized to the three-drug regimens was only two years. There was essentially no difference in the efficacy of BOPP as compared to MOPP, and the use of this modified four-drug combination was attended by a significantly lower frequency of severe leukopenia and thrombocytopenia. There were three definite and two probable cases of acute myelocytic leukemia, three in patients who had received prior radiotherapy, and two who had received no treatment other than combination chemotherapy. The results of this interesting study suggest that the efficacy of the MOPP and BOPP combinations depends on the presence of both the alkylating agent (nitrogen mustard or BCNU) and procarbazine. Although these results suggest that currently available three-drug regimens are not as effective as four-drug regimens, it should be remembered that the combination chemotherapy programs in this study were used therapeutically, rather than as the adjuvant component of a planned combined modality therapy program. The possibility has thus not been excluded that three-drug regimens of significantly reduced toxicity might be used effectively in conjunction with low-dose total lymphoid irradiation in the combined modality therapy of patients with localized (stage I, II, or IIIA) Hodgkin's disease.

Complications and Secondary Neoplasms. It is well established that the effects of radiation therapy and of various chemotherapeutic agents may interact to yield an augmented frequency or extent of normal tissue injury (Phillips and Fu, 1976). Actinomycin D, which is the best-known chemotherapeutic radiosensitizer, has been reported to enhance radiation damage in the lung, intestine, and other tissues. Fortunately, it is not a component of any of the currently used combination chemotherapy regimens in patients with Hodgkin's disease. Enhanced or anamnestic cutaneous radiation reactions have been well documented following the administration of adriamycin to previously irradiated patients, and there is also some evidence of an increased severity of cutaneous or mucous membrane reactions following treatment with bleomycin and radiation therapy. However, the reactions observed in critical tissues such as the lung and heart are of much greater importance. There is now clear-cut evidence in experimental studies in rabbits (Eltringham, Fajardo, and Stewart, 1975), as well as in patients, that the use of adriamycin and radiotherapy over the heart is associated with an increased risk of cardiomyopathy and heart failure. Fatal cardiac injury has been reported at adriamycin doses substantially lower than those ordinarily causing such injury when adriamycin is used alone. There is also some evidence of an increased risk of radiation pneumonitis in patients receiving drug combinations containing bleomycin and/or adriamycin (cf. Phillips and Fu, 1976). Finally, since many of the drugs used alone or in various combinations in the treatment of Hodgkin's disease have systemic myelotoxic effects, and radiation therapy causes severe injury to bone marrow within the irradiated fields, it is not surprising that the frequency and severity of leukopenia and thrombocytopenia observed after combined modality therapy are generally greater than those seen with either radiotherapy or combination chemotherapy alone. However, as has been indicated in the section above on the scheduling of combined modality treatment, the use of more flexible alternating or split course schedules has permitted combined modality therapy to be carried to completion with minimal bone marrow suppression in substantial numbers of patients with advanced Hodgkin's disease.

Acute leukemias are the most commonly observed secondary neoplasm developing in patients with Hodgkin's disease treated either with radiation therapy alone (Chapter 9) or chemotherapy alone (Chapter 10). A survey of the published literature to late 1978 reveals a total of 93 patients who developed acute leukemia after treatment with both radiation and chemotherapy (Table 11.4). The earlier cases were treated primarily with IF radiotherapy, often to multiple fields as new relapses appeared, and subsequently with various single chemotherapeutic agents. Subsequently, acute leukemias appeared among patients who were treated with MOPP chemotherapy for relapsing disease following extended field or total lymphoid irradiation. Finally, cases have recently been reported in which both radiotherapy and combination chemotherapy were used, in either sequence, as part of a planned combined modality regimen. The interval between initiation of treatment for Hodgkin's disease and the diagnosis of acute leukemia has varied widely from as little as 4 months to as long as 223 months (18.6 years). As will be noted in Table 11.4, most of the cases have been of the acute myeloblastic type, but there have also been several instances of acute myelomonoblastic, acute monocytic, and acute erythroid leukemia.

Most of the reported cases are essentially anecdotal in nature, and little or no information is given concerning the total numbers of patients similarly treated within the same institution who did not develop leukemia during a comparable time interval. Arseneau et al. (1972) were the first to draw attention to the significantly increased risk of development of secondary malignant tumors in patients with Hodgkin's disease who had received both radiotherapy and chemotherapy. Their data, which are summarized in Table 11.5, reveal a ratio of observed to expected secondary neoplasms of 3.8 among 149 patients receiving intensive radiotherapy alone, 3.2 among 110 patients receiving intensive chemotherapy alone, and 29.0 among 35 patients receiving both intensive radiotherapy and intensive chemotherapy. Of six secondary neoplasms observed in patients receiving both intensive radiotherapy and intensive chemotherapy, two were acute leukemias, one myeloblastic, the other myelomonocytic. In a later study which included a larger number of patients (48) treated with combined modality therapy, Arseneau et al. (1977) found a total of 5 neoplasms in 171 person-years, for an observed to expected ratio of 23.0, which was still very significantly greater than that observed with either intensive chemotherapy alone,

intensive radiotherapy alone, or no intensive treatment. Stenfert-Kroese, Sizoo, and Somers (1976) surveyed cases of leukemia developing in patients with Hodgkin's disease treated at various hematologic centers in the Netherlands. They were able to discover a total of 21 such cases (2 of which had been previously published). In 3 of these, the Hodgkin's disease had been treated with radiotherapy alone; in 4, with chemotherapy alone; and in 14, with both radiotherapy and intensive chemotherapy. The interval from the initiation of treatment of Hodgkin's disease to the time of development of leukemia varied from 11 to 168 months, with an average of 66 months. Cavallin-Ståhl et al. (1977) encountered 3 cases of leukemia among 153 patients with Hodgkin's disease between 1971 and 1977; all 3 had been treated with both irradiation and chemotherapy. Larsen and Brincker (1977) reported the later development of acute leukemia in 3 of 201 consecutive patients with Hodgkin's disease treated between 1964 and 1975; of these, two had received both radiotherapy and MOPP combination chemotherapy; the third, radiotherapy alone.

Coleman et al. (1977) studied the risk of development of a secondary hematologic malignancy among 680 previously untreated patients with Hodgkin's disease who were treated at Stanford University Medical Center from July 1, 1968 through December 31, 1975. They encountered 6 cases of leukemia among patients in clinical remission and 2 additional cases in patients with active Hodgkin's disease. All 8 of these cases of leukemia occurred among the 330 patients who had been treated with both radiation therapy and chemotherapy. There were no cases of leukemia among 320 patients treated with external radiotherapy alone. One case of subacute leukemia occurred in a patient treated with radiation therapy and intravenous radioactive colloidal gold. At the time of reporting, there were no cases of leukemia among 30 patients treated with MOPP combination chemotherapy alone. During the first year following publication of this paper, one patient with stage IVB Hodgkin's disease, treated with MOPP chemotherapy alone, has developed acute myeloblastic leukemia, and there has been one additional case of leukemia, also of acute myeloblastic type, in the combined modality group. The actuarial risk of developing leukemia after treatment of Hodgkin's disease with combined radiation therapy and chemotherapy was 2.9 percent at five years, increasing to 3.9 percent at seven years (Fig. 11.43). The median survival among the patients de-

Table 11.4 Acute Leukemia Developing in Patients with Hodgkin's Disease Treated with Both Radiotherapy and Chemotherapy

Case No.	Age	Sex	Radiotherapy[a]	Chemotherapy[b]	Interval, months[c]	Type of Leukemia[d]	Reference
1	44	M	IF (2,280)	HN_2	89	AMoL	Greenberg & Cohen, 1962
2	17	F	IF (2,000)	HN_2, CLB	30	AL	Lacher & Sussman, 1963
3	37	M	Mult. IF (200–2,016)	HN_2, CLB, CTX, VLB, PCB	130	AEL	Durant & Tassoni, 1967
4	33	F	Mult. IF (1,485–3,034)	HN_2, CLB	88	AML	Ezdinli et al., 1969
5	36	F	Mult. IF	CLB, VLB, HN_2	~180	AEL	Steinberg et al., 1970
6	30	M	Mult. IF	CLB, HN_2	108	AML	Steinberg et al., 1970
7	38	F	Mult. IF	HN_2, CLB	65	AMML	Newman et al., 1970
8	9	M	Mult. IF	HN_2	223	AMML	Newman et al., 1970
9	60	M	Mult. IF	VLB	9	AML	Osta et al., 1970
10	34	F	Mult. IF	HN_2, CLB, 5-FU, VLB, PCB	43	ALL	Burns et al., 1971
11	13	F	Mult. IF (later)	HN_2, CLB, PCB	80	AMML	Wakem & Bennett, 1972
12	29	F	Mult. IF	CLB	~72	AL	Chan & McBride, 1972
13	28	F	IF	CLB, VLB	~60	AMML	Chan & McBride, 1972
14	23	M	Mult. IF	HN_2, CLB, CTX, VLB	~96	AEL	Bergevin & Blom, 1972
15	16	M	Mult. IF	CLB, VCR, VLB, PCB	~100	AMML	Weiden et al., 1973
16	22	F	Mult. IF	CLB, other SA	~96	AML	Jacquillat et al., 1973
17	26	F	Mult. IF	HN_2, CLB, other SA	~96	AML	Jacquillat et al., 1973
18	23	F	Mult. IF	CLB, other SA	~84	AML	Jacquillat et al., 1973
19	42	F	Mult. IF	CLB, other SA	~84	AML	Jacquillat et al., 1973
20	60	F	IF	HN_2	~132	AML	Jacquillat et al., 1973
21	31	F	IF	CLB, other SA	~96	AML	Jacquillat et al., 1973
22	8	M	Mult. IF	CLB, VLB, PCB, HN_2	~168	AML	Veenhof et al., 1973
23	—	M	TLI	MOPP	~36	AML	Arseneau et al., 1974
24	—	—	TLI	MOPP	~30	AMML	Arseneau et al., 1974
25	34	M	TLI	MOPP	32	AML	Focan et al., 1974
26	32	F	Mult. IF (later)	CLB, VLB, PCB, BLM	102	AMML	Sahakian et al., 1974
27	21	F	Mantle (3,100)	CLB, PCB, VCR, BLM	89	AMoL	Sahakian et al., 1974
28	12	M	Mult. IF	MOPP, MABOP, VLB, CLB, CTX	~120	AML	Mauri & Quaglino, 1974
29	22	F	Mult. IF	MOPP	44	AEL	Moloney & Long, 1974
30	27	F	IF (4,000)	MOPP, CTX, PCB	56	AML	Kardinal et al., 1974
31	37	M	Mantle (4,000)	MOPP (adj.)	39	AMML	Rosner & Grünwald, 1975
32	74	M	Mult. IF	VLB	~60	AML	Rosner & Grünwald, 1975
33	49	M	Mult. IF	VLB, UrN_2	70	AML	Rosner & Grünwald, 1975
34	40	M	Mult. IF (later)	CTX, VCR, VLB, PCB, BLM, CLB	88	AMML	Rosner & Grünwald, 1975
35	30	F	Mantle (4,500), PA (3,000)	TEM, TTPA, CLB, other SA	~144	AMoL	Rosner & Grünwald, 1975

No.	Age	Sex	Radiation	Chemotherapy	Number	Diagnosis	Reference
36	19	F	Mult. IF	PCB	120	AMML	Rosner & Grünwald, 1975
37	33	F	Mult. IF	MVPP	79	AMML	Rosner & Grünwald, 1975
38	13	M	Mult. IF (900–4,650)	VLB, VCR, PCB, HN$_2$, CLB, BLM	116	AML	Quaglino et al., 1975
39	38	M	TLI (4,050)	VLB, MOPP	26	AML	Lundh et al., 1975
40	39	F	Mult. IF	MOPP, BLM	83	AML	Armenta et al., 1975
41	54	M	Mult. IF	HN$_2$, CLB, MOPP	59	AML	Armenta et al., 1975
42	23	F	Mult. IF (later)	VLB, CLB, PCB, BLM	98	AMoL	Connolly, 1975
43	57	F	Mantle (4,000)	CTX	56	AML	Raich et al., 1975
44	45	M	Mult. IF	VLB, CTX, PCB	~80	AMoL	Tittor et al., 1975
45	—	—	TLI	MOPP (adj.)	—	AL	Toland & Coltman, 1975
46	—	—	TLI	MOPP (adj.)	—	AL	Toland & Coltman, 1975
47	—	—	TLI	MOPP (adj.)	—	AL	Toland & Coltman, 1975
48	37	M	IF	MOPP × 3 (adj.)	~40	ANLL	Wiernik & Lichtenfeld, 1975
49	—	—	TLI	MOPP × 6	~34	AML	Kun et al., 1976
50	47	F	Mantle	CTX, MOPP × 2, VLB	94	AML	Stenfert Kroese et al., 1976
51	66	F	Mult. IF	MOPP × 9	50	AML	Stenfert Kroese et al., 1976
52	43	M	TLI	HN$_2$, CTX, PCB, VLB	72	AML	Stenfert Kroese et al., 1976
53	16	M	TLI	MOPP × 6, VLB, CCNU	59	AMML	Stenfert Kroese et al., 1976
54	25	F	Mult. IF	MOPP × 12	141	AMML	Stenfert Kroese et al., 1976
55	27	M	TLI	MOPP × 6, CLB	60	AMML	Stenfert Kroese et al., 1976
56	25	F	IF	HN$_2$	80	AMoL	Stenfert Kroese et al., 1976
57	57	M	Mantle	HN$_2$, PCB, VLB, CTX	72	AEL	Stenfert Kroese et al., 1976
58	44	M	Mantle, PA, Spl.	MOPP × 6, CTX	44	AEL	Stenfert Kroese et al., 1976
59	39	F	IF	MOPP × 8, CCNU	45	AL	Stenfert Kroese et al., 1976
60	26	F	IF	CLB, VLB	132	AL	Stenfert Kroese et al., 1976
61	42	F	Mantle	MOPP × 8	28	AL	Stenfert Kroese et al., 1976
62	28	F	Mult. IF	HN$_2$, CLB, VLB, PCB	106	ANLL	Cadman et al., 1977
63	44	F	Abd. (3,000)	Modif. MOPP	69	ANLL	Cadman et al., 1977
64	27	M	Mult. IF (1,700–2,000)	Modif. MOPP	43	ANLL	Cadman et al., 1977
65	28	M	Mantle	MOPP × 8	39	AML	Cavallin-Ståhl et al., 1977
66	52	M	Inv-Y	MOPP × 6	79	AML	Cavallin-Ståhl et al., 1977
67	27	M	TLI	VLB; MOPP × 2	26	AML	Cavallin-Ståhl et al., 1977
68	43	M	IF (3,600)	CTX; MOPP × 11	100	AEL	Larsen and Brincker, 1977
69	23	M	Mantle (3,700); Inv-Y (3,700)	MOPP × 6	79	AMML	Larsen and Brincker, 1977
70	37	F	Mult. IF (4,000–5,500)	CLB	132	AML	Rowley et al., 1977
71	37	M	TLI (4,000)	COPP (adj.)	41	AML	Rowley et al., 1977
72	27	F	TLI (4,000)	COPP	76	BL-MPD	Rowley et al., 1977
73	50	F	Mult. IF	COPP × 9	74	APL	Rowley et al., 1977
74	31	M	TLI (4,000)	MOPP × 3, COPP × 3	51	AML	Rowley et al., 1977

Table 11.4 (*Continued*)

Case No.	Age	Sex	Radiotherapy[a]	Chemotherapy[b]	Interval, months[c]	Type of Leukemia[d]	Reference
75	26	M	TLI (4,000)	MOPP × 6 (adj.)	34	AML	Coleman et al., 1977
76	29	M	TLI (4,000)	MOPP × 5 (adj.)	54	AML	Coleman et al., 1977
77	19	F	TLI (4,000)	MOPP × 3 (adj.)	17	AML	Coleman et al., 1977
78	27	F	TLI (4,000)	MOPP × 6 (adj.)	91	AML	Coleman et al., 1977
79	32	M	TLI (4,000)	MOPP × 6 (adj.)	32	AML	Coleman et al., 1977
80	41	M	Mantle, later inv-Y	MOPP × 6	66	AML	Coleman et al., 1977
81	56	M	TLI + ^{198}Au	Mult. SA	50	AML	Coleman et al., 1977
82	39	M	Mantle (800)	MOPP × 6, SA	58	AML	Coleman et al., 1977
83	12	F	TLI	Mult. SA	44	AML	Coleman et al., 1977
84	—	—	TLI	MOPP	~33	AMML	Bonadonna et al., 1977
85	23	M	IF	TTPA, VCR, PCB	4	AML	Cavalli et al., 1977
86	35	F	Mult. IF	CLB, TTPA, VLB	212	AML	Cavalli et al., 1977
87	33	M	Mantle	COPP, VLB, PCB	90	AML	Cavalli et al., 1977
88	35	F	Mult. IF	VLB, CLB, VCR, PCB, TTPA, BLM, ADM	92	AML	Cavalli et al., 1977
89	29	F	Mantle, PA	VCR	52	AML	Cavalli et al., 1977
90	18	F	TLI, mult. IF	MOPP, VLB, ADM, BLM, VP-16-213	90	AMML	Cavalli et al., 1977
91	57	M	TLI	MOPP	48	AMML	Neufeld et al., 1978
92	51	M	Mantle	COPP	37	AML	Neufeld et al., 1978
93	—	—	TLI	MOPP	60	AML	Saxe and Mandel, 1978

[a] Fields abbreviated as in Table 11.3; total dose in parentheses.

[b] Abbreviations for drugs and drug combinations as in Tables 10.2 and 10.3, respectively; SA, single agents; UrN$_2$, uracil mustard.

[c] Interval from initiation of treatment for Hodgkin's disease to diagnosis of leukemia.

[d] AML: acute myelogenous leukemia; AMML: acute myelomonocytic leukemia; AMOL: acute monocytic leukemia; AEL: acute erythrobiastic leukemia; AMOL: acute monocytic leukemia; AL: acute leukemia, type unspecified; ANLL: acute non-lymphocytic leukemia; BL-MPD: blastic phase of mycloproliferative disease.

Table 11.5 Risk of Secondary Malignant Tumor, According to Treatment Group

Group	No. of cases	Man years of observation	Secondary neoplasms Observed	Secondary neoplasms Expected	Ratio of observed to expected
Intensive radiotherapy (IR) alone	149	562	4	1.05	3.8[a]
Intensive chemotherapy (IC) alone	110	371	3	0.94	3.2
IR plus IC	35	108	3	0.10	29.0[a]
No intensive therapy	131	543	2	1.28	1.6
Total cases studied	425	1584	12	3.38	3.5[a]

Source: Data of Arseneau et al. (1972).

[a] Significant at $p < 0.05$.

veloping secondary leukemias was four months. Four of the six patients who developed leukemia while in complete remission had a prolonged period of pancytopenia, which persisted for 3 to 11 months (median 6 months) before frank AML became evident.

The clinical course of the leukemic patients studied by Coleman et al. (1977) is presented in Figure 11.44. The first five patients all received total lymphoid irradiation and multiple cycles of adjuvant MOPP chemotherapy in a planned combined modality program. The sixth patient received mantle field irradiation alone, developed a subdiaphragmatic relapse more than two years later, and was then treated with an inverted-Y field, followed by six cycles of MOPP chemotherapy. He entered complete remission but then developed a myeloproliferative syndrome; although acute leukemia could not be diagnosed during life, a diagnosis of

probable AML was made after the examination of bone marrow at autopsy. Among these six patients, the median interval from the diagnosis of Hodgkin's disease to the diagnosis of leukemia was 41 months, with a range of 17 to 91 months.

A further analysis of this same series of patients with Hodgkin's disease who were treated at Stanford University Medical Center brought to light six cases of non-Hodgkin's lymphoma, four of which were of diffuse undifferentiated type and two of diffuse histiocytic type (Krikorian et al., 1979a). A seventh case, of undifferentiated type, has now been diagnosed. All of these patients had received both radiation therapy and chemotherapy, and none had evidence of active Hodgkin's disease when the diagnosis of non-Hodgkin's lymphoma was made. The histopathologic features of the initial biopsy on which the diagnosis of Hodgkin's disease was based and of the subsequent biopsy documenting the development of a non-Hodgkin's lymphoma in one such case are illustrated in Figures 11.45 and 11.46. The diffuse undifferentiated lymphomas were composed of relatively uniform cells with ovoid nuclei, finely dispersed chromatin, small nucleoli, and rims of well-defined cytoplasm which were pyroninophilic with the methyl green–pyronin stain. Mitotic figures were frequent and, in most instances, karyorrhexis was pronounced, usually associated with a starry sky appearance similar to that seen in African Burkitt's lymphoma. The gastrointestinal tract or abdomen was involved in four of these five patients. Two patients were diagnosed as having diffuse histiocytic lymphomas at autopsy. In both, the tumor was widely disseminated, involving the gastrointestinal tract as well as multiple lymph nodes. The histiocytic lymphomas were composed of larger and more pleomorphic cells than those diagnosed as diffuse undifferentiated lymphomas; mitoses were less frequent and starry sky patterns absent. Cells

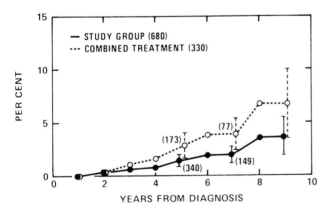

Figure 11.43 Actuarial analysis of the risk (mean ± S. E.) of developing leukemia among a series of 680 patients with Hodgkin's disease, of whom 330 were treated with combined modality therapy. (Reprinted, by permission of the authors and the *New England Journal of Medicine,* from the paper by Coleman et al., 1977.)

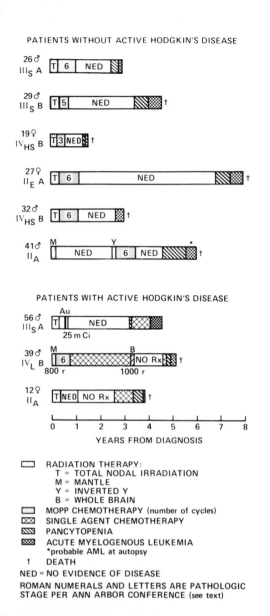

Figure 11.44 Clinical course of patients with Hodgkin's disease who developed AML and related hematologic malignancies following treatment with irradiation and chemotherapy. (Reprinted, by permission of the authors and the *New England Journal of Medicine,* from the paper by Coleman et al., 1977.)

resembling Reed-Sternberg cells were not observed in these cases. Thus, possible diagnostic confusion with lymphocyte depletion type Hodgkin's disease could be eliminated. In one of these two cases, the large cells had plasmacytoid features which would have resulted in classification of this tumor as an "immunoblastic sarcoma" in the classification of Lukes and Collins (1974). This lymphoma also involved the perivascular region of the brain. There was no evidence of residual Hodg-

kin's disease in either of these cases of diffuse histiocytic lymphoma at postmortem examination. At ten years, the actuarial risk of developing a non-Hodgkin's lymphoma in patients receiving combined modality therapy was approximately 15 percent, as compared to approximately 4 percent for the risk of developing acute leukemia in the same group.

A variety of nonhematologic malignancies has also been reported in patients with Hodgkin's disease treated with combined modality therapy; however, there is no conclusive evidence to date that any specific type of neoplasm occurs with a frequency significantly exceeding expectation. Among the secondary tumors observed by the NCI group were a carcinoma of the colon, a fibrosarcoma of the chest wall, an undifferentiated mucin-secreting carcinoma of the lung, and a squamous cell carcinoma of the skin (Canellos et al., 1975). Neufeld, Weinerman, and Kemel (1978) encountered 5 cases of secondary malignant neoplasms among 232 patients with Hodgkin's disease treated at the University of Manitoba from January 1965 through December 1973. These included two cases of acute leukemia, one squamous cancer of the lip, a cancer of the prostate, and a glioblastoma. Brody, Schottenfeld, and Reid (1977) noted a highly significant 18-fold increase in the frequency of multiple primary cancers among adolescent and young adult patients who survived six to ten years following treatment with radiation and single-agent chemotherapy at Memorial Sloan-Kettering Cancer Center during the years 1960–1964. They also noted the occurrence of two multiple primary cancers in a relatively small group of patients treated with chemotherapy alone during the period 1968–1972.

It is clear that these secondary malignancies constitute a problem of major concern to both radiation therapists and chemotherapists. Although the risk of such neoplasms is relatively small when compared to the marked improvement in survival resulting from combined modality therapy in stage IIIB and IV Hodgkin's disease, the same risk would be unacceptable in patients with regionally localized (stage I and II) Hodgkin's disease, whose long-term relapse-free survival with radiation therapy alone is excellent. In such patients, unless current randomized clinical trials convincingly demonstrate a highly significant improvement in absolute survival, it may well be preferable to hold MOPP combination chemotherapy in reserve for the small subgroup of patients who relapse following initial radiation therapy.

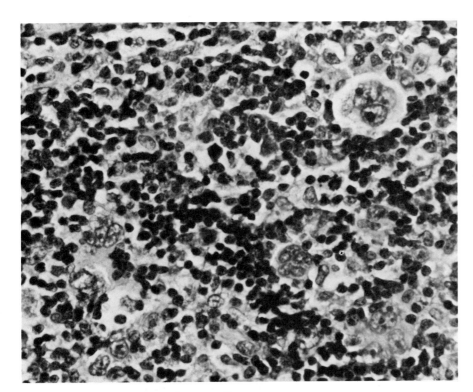

Figure 11.45 Polymorphous infiltrate of lymphocytes, transformed lymphocytes, histiocytes, lacunar cells, and Sternberg-Reed cells in the original biopsy of case 5 of Krikorian et al. (1979a). Hematoxylin and eosin, ×480. (Photomicrograph courtesy of Dr. Jerome Burke, Department of Pathology, Stanford University Medical Center.)

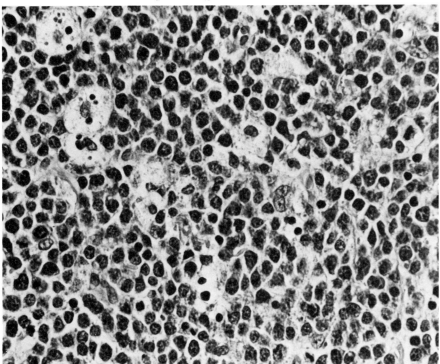

Figure 11.46 Relatively monomorphous cell population with starry sky pattern of undifferentiated lymphoma in a biopsy of an upper abdominal lymph node mass which developed six years after the initial diagnosis of Hodgkin's disease in case 5 of Krikorian et al. (1979a). Hematoxylin and eosin, ×480. (Photomicrograph courtesy of Dr. Jerome Burke, Department of Pathology, Stanford University Medical Center.)

Salvage Therapy for Patients with Relapsing Disease

Although any relapse must be considered a prognostically unfavorable event, several different subtypes of relapse can be distinguished which differ significantly in prognosis. The many factors which influence the prognosis of an initial relapse are discussed in greater detail in Chapter 12. For the purposes of this section, it suffices to distinguish those initial relapses which occur after primary radiotherapy alone, after MOPP chemotherapy alone, and after combined modality treatment; nodal versus extranodal relapses; relapses within high-dose radiation therapy fields versus those at the field margins or in lymph nodes which have received no prior irradiation. These categories are of importance because they relate to the kinds of salvage treatment which can be employed. Relapses occurring in lymph nodes within a region previously irradiated to high dose obviously cannot be reirradiated to high dose with impunity. In such instances, MOPP or other combination chemotherapy, sometimes supplemented by low-dose irradiation (approximately 1,500 rads), is the only therapeutic choice available. Conversely, nodal relapses in regions which have never previously been irradiated can be treated safely with high-dose radiation therapy with an excellent probability of achieving complete remission. Patients who relapse after previous MOPP chemotherapy, particularly within the first year after the completion of treatment, are commonly refractory to retreatment with MOPP and may require some type of crossover regimen, usually of sharply reduced efficacy. Patients who relapse after combined modality therapy often have markedly reduced hematologic tolerance for retreatment with MOPP or any other combination chemotherapy regimen. It is also important to distinguish different types of extranodal relapses. Solitary relapses in an osseous site, such as a lumbar vertebra or the sternum, can be effectively treated with high-dose irradiation, provided that the region has not previously been heavily irradiated. Relapses in the liver, as well as solitary relapses in the lung, can be treated with a combination of low-dose irradiation and MOPP chemotherapy. In contrast, multiple bilateral pulmonary lesions, as well as relapses in the bone marrow, are obviously beyond the scope of high-dose radiotherapy; in such instances, the sole therapeutic option is MOPP or some other combination chemotherapeutic regimen. Finally, in patients who have failed on MOPP as well as the major cross-

over combination regimens, palliative single-drug chemotherapy, sometimes supplemented by palliative low-dose involved field radiotherapy for the relief of localized symptoms, is the only form of treatment which remains available.

There has apparently been a significant improvement in the prognosis of patients with Hodgkin's disease who develop initial relapses. In an earlier study, the after-survival, calculated from the time of initial relapse, of 87 patients who relapsed after IF or EF radiotherapy for stage I or II Hodgkin's disease was only about 25 percent at five years (Fig. 11.47). Second complete remissions of long duration could be induced in about one-third to one-half of patients with local or regional relapses, in about 25 percent of those with trans-diaphragmatic relapses, and in only 15 percent of those with extralymphatic relapses (Spittle et al., 1973). During that era, all patients with relapses occurring in bone marrow and virtually all of those with relapses occurring in the liver were destined to die of Hodgkin's disease. Somewhat more favorable results were reported by Musshoff et al. (1976), who obtained complete remissions after a second course of radiotherapy in 86 percent of 32 patients who developed an initial relapse after having entered a primary complete remission. Of those who achieved a second complete remission,

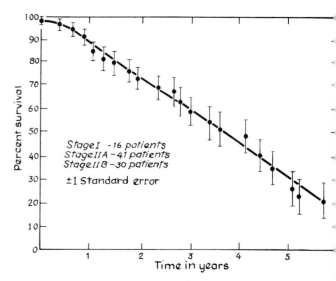

Figure 11.47 Survival, calculated from the time of initial relapse, of 87 patients with stage I and II Hodgkin's disease who developed relapses after radiation therapy and whose relapses were treated in the pre-MOPP era with additional local radiotherapy and/or single drug chemotherapy. (Reprinted by permission from the paper by Spittle et al., 1973.)

57 percent survived relapse-free for five years or more. In contrast, all of 34 patients who had an initial partial remission relapsed, and only 24 percent of these entered a second complete remission after retreatment. However, it is noteworthy that all of those who did enter a second complete remission remained relapse-free for five years. These two studies, which date back to the period in which the only form of intensive treatment for relapsing disease was radiotherapy, clearly document that intensive radiotherapy alone was able to offer an appreciable, though clearly suboptimal, probability of salvage.

More recent analyses reveal the impact of MOPP combination chemotherapy on the prognosis of relapsing disease. Two extensive studies have been made of patients with Hodgkin's disease who developed initial relapses following primary treatment at Stanford University Medical Center during two different, though overlapping, time intervals. The study by Weller et al. (1976) was concerned with 243 initial relapses occuring among 701 consecutive patients treated with curative intent between 1961 and the end of 1972. All patients had completed a minimum followup period of two years, and all had been staged initially with the aid of lymphangiography and bone marrow biopsy. Approximately 400 of the 701 patients had also undergone staging laparotomy with splenectomy. Only those aspects of this report which relate specifically to the efficacy of different forms of salvage therapy are discussed here; the remainder of the data are presented in Chapter 12. Since MOPP combination chemotherapy was not employed at Stanford University Medical Center until August 1968, it was possible to compare survival and freedom from second relapse in patients who received treatment for initial relapses between 1961 and August 1968 and a second group who were treated for initial relapses between August 1968 and the end of 1972. The earlier group comprised 83 patients; the later group, 126 patients, of whom 88 were treated with MOPP, alone or in conjunction with radiotherapy. As may be seen in Figure 11.48, there was a significant improvement in freedom from second relapse at five years after the completion of second therapy in the post-MOPP era. Only 14 percent of patients remained free of second relapse in the earlier group, as compared to 39 percent who were alive and relapse-free in the latter. However, survival in the post-MOPP period, though apparently improved up to four years after second treatment, showed no significant difference at five years.

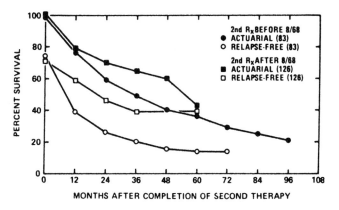

Figure 11.48 Historical comparison of survival and freedom from second relapse in patients retreated for an initial relapse before and after August 1968, when MOPP combination chemotherapy was adopted for use at Stanford University Medical Center. (Reprinted, by permission of the authors and the Editor of *Cancer,* from the paper by Weller et al., 1976.)

Of 33 patients treated with single-agent chemotherapy for initial relapsing disease prior to August 1968, only 14 percent survived at four years (Fig. 11.49). Patients with localized initial relapses prior to August 1968 were treated with high-dose radiation therapy with curative intent, whereas those relapsing after August 1968 were treated either with MOPP chemotherapy alone or with MOPP plus involved field radiation therapy to doses of 2,000 rads or more to areas of clinically evident disease. Curves for survival and freedom from second relapse of these various treatment

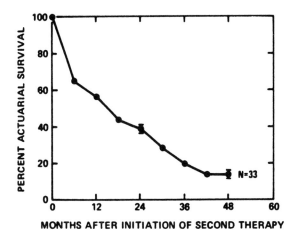

Figure 11.49 Survival following retreatment of patients with initial relapses with single-drug chemotherapy. (Reprinted, by permission of the authors and the Editor of *Cancer,* from the paper by Weller et al., 1976.)

groups are presented in Figure 11.50. At three years, 50 percent of patients who received MOPP alone and 44 percent of those who received MOPP plus local radiotherapy remained free of second relapses, whereas only about 25 percent of patients treated with radiotherapy alone in the earlier era remained relapse-free for a corresponding interval. Survival among those treated with MOPP alone was about 60 percent at four years, and of those treated with radiotherapy alone about 55 percent at four years, a difference which was not statistically significant. Survival at three years in those treated with MOPP plus radiotherapy was 81 percent. However, this difference may have been more apparent than real, since patients who relapsed in bone marrow, and thus had a much less favorable prognosis, were necessarily treated with MOPP alone. The influence of the site of initial relapse on after-survival and on the probability of freedom from second relapse are indicated in Figure 11.51. It is readily apparent that relapses in the

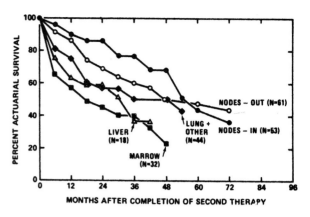

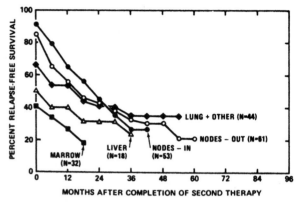

Figure 11.51 Influence of anatomic site of relapse on survival (*top*) and freedom from second relapse (*bottom*) of patients who developed an initial relapse. Nodal relapses are separately analyzed according to whether they were in the field(s) of prior radiotherapy ("nodes in") or outside those fields ("nodes out"). Extralymphatic relapses are divided into three subcategories: those in bone marrow, those in the liver, and those in the lung and/or other sites. (Reprinted, by permission of the authors and the Editor of *Cancer,* from the paper by Weller et al., 1976.)

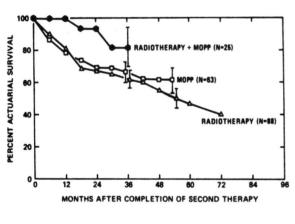

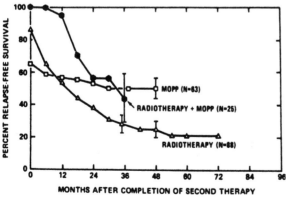

Figure 11.50 Influence of mode of relapse treatment on survival (*top*) and freedom from second relapse (*bottom*) of patients who developed an initial relapse. (Reprinted, by permission of the authors and the Editor of *Cancer,* from the paper by Weller et al., 1976.)

bone marrow and liver had a more unfavorable prognosis than relapses in lymph nodes and lung. In a subsidiary study, Weller et al. (1977) presented evidence indicating that MOPP chemotherapy in addition to radiotherapy had improved the prognosis of patients whose initial relapses were retrograde transdiaphragmatic extensions from supradiaphragmatic stage I or stage II Hodgkin's disease. Improved salvage rates with MOPP chemotherapy have also been documented in our experience with relapsing Hodgkin's disease in childhood (S. S. Donaldson and H. S. Kaplan, unpublished).

Another Stanford study of the impact of salvage treatment (Portlock et al., 1978) was concerned exclusively with initial relapses among 244 patients with previously untreated Hodgkin's disease, stage I–III, who had participated in clinical trials in which they were prospectively randomized to treatment with radiation therapy alone versus radiation therapy plus adjuvant MOPP. Of the 64 evaluable patients with initial relapses, 46 had received radiation therapy alone, and 18, radiation therapy plus MOPP. At the time of reporting, 29 patients appeared to have been salvaged by retreatment; these included 23 (50 percent) of the 46 postradiotherapy relapses and 6 (33 percent) of the 18 relapses following radiotherapy plus MOPP. The former group were treated with MOPP and/or additional radiotherapy, the latter with either chemotherapy or radiotherapy. Although the actuarial probability of remaining free of second relapse was similar for both groups, the median survival of those relapsing after radiotherapy plus MOPP was only 33 months, whereas 58 percent of those relapsing after radiotherapy alone were alive at five years (Fig. 11.52). Complete remissions were obtained with second treatment in 78 percent of the patients relapsing after radiotherapy alone and in 53 percent of those relapsing after radiotherapy plus MOPP. Among those achieving complete second remission, freedom from second relapse was 60 percent at 50 months for both groups, and more than 70 percent of both groups were alive at 40 months.

Salvage treatment was significantly less effective in patients with initial relapses involving the bone marrow. Only 2 of 15 such patients were salvaged, as compared to 40 percent of those with relapses in lymph nodes or extranodal sites other than the bone marrow (Table 11.6). Among patients with relapses in lymph nodes, 58 percent remained free of second relapses at five years, as compared to a median interval to second relapse of only five months for those with initial relapses in bone marrow, a highly significant difference. The probability of second relapse in patients with initial relapses in extranodal sites other than bone marrow was intermediate, with a median of 20 months (Fig. 11.53). Five-year survival was 78 percent among those with initial relapses in lymph nodes, in contrast to less than 20 percent among patients whose initial relapses were in the bone marrow.

Thus salvage therapy was rather effective in patients developing initial relapses after radiotherapy alone and also effective, though less so, among patients developing initial relapses after radiotherapy plus MOPP. The duration of remission prior to initial relapse was found to have an important influence on the effectiveness of salvage therapy in patients relapsing after radiotherapy plus MOPP, but not in those who relapsed after radiotherapy alone. All five of the patients who relapsed less than 12 months after completion of radiotherapy plus MOPP developed progressive disease again within 6 months after the initiation of salvage therapy and had a survival at three years of only 20 percent, as compared to a survival of 54 percent among those patients who relapsed more than 12 months after completion of radiotherapy plus MOPP. In contrast, there was no significant difference in either freedom from second relapse or survival in the patients treated with radiotherapy alone who relapsed less than or more than 12 months later. The overall survival rate of 50 percent at seven years in these 64 patients with relaps-

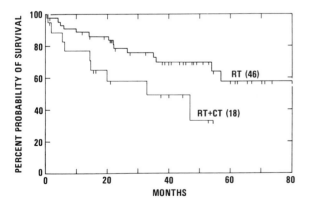 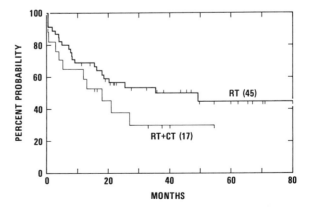

Figure 11.52 Actuarial analysis of survival (*left*) and of freedom from second relapse (*right*), calculated from the date of first relapse, in patients treated with various types of salvage therapy for relapses developing after radiotherapy alone (RT) or after combined modality therapy (RT + CT). The probability that these curves differ significantly, calculated by the Gehan (1965) test, was: $p = 0.06$ for survival and $p = 0.24$ for freedom from second relapse. (Reprinted, by permission of the authors and the Editor of *Blood,* from the paper by Portlock et al., 1978.)

Table 11.6 Salvage Treatments of 64 Relapsing Patients According to Sites of Relapse

Salvage Treatment[b]	Sites of Relapse[a]			
	Nodes	Lung	Marrow	Other Extranodal
MOPP	19 (12)	8 (4)	8 (2)	6 (3)
Re-MOPP	3 (1)	—	4 (0)	2 (0)
MOPP + RT	1 (1)	—	—	—
RT	4 (3)	—	—	—
B-CAVe	1 (1)	1 (1)	—	1 (0)
SA	1 (0)	—	3 (0)	1 (1)
Other	—	1 (0)	—	—

[a] Numbers in parentheses refer to patients disease-free.

[b] MOPP regimen as in Table 10.3; B-CAVe as in Table 10.7; RT: radiation therapy; SA: single agent chemotherapy.

ing Hodgkin's disease, of whom 40 percent remained free of second relapse, constitutes a highly encouraging advance relative to the earlier era in which only single-agent chemotherapy was available for the treatment of disseminated relapsing disease. Moreover, the high salvage rates with MOPP chemotherapy in patients previously treated with radiotherapy alone clearly have important implications with respect to ultimate survival in clinical trials comparing radiotherapy alone versus radiotherapy plus MOPP. Nonetheless, it must not be forgotten that 50 percent of these patients with initial relapses died of Hodgkin's disease despite salvage treatment. Thus an initial relapse remains a prognostically unfavorable event, the probability of which must continue to be minimized by meticulously thorough staging and optimal initial treatment of all patients.

Finally, comment is in order here concerning the efficacy of salvage treatment with "cross-over" combination chemotherapy regimens in MOPP-resistant patients. The probability of achieving complete remissions with cross-over chemotherapy in such patients has been discussed in Chapter 10. Selected data on complete and partial remission rates induced with certain of the more promising cross-over regimens are summarized in Table 11.7. It will be noted that there is an appreciable discrepancy in the experience of the Milan and the Stanford groups with respect to the efficacy of ABVD as a cross-over regimen. Bonadonna et al. (1977) observed complete remissions in 9 (60 percent) of 15 evaluable MOPP-resistant patients, with a remission duration ranging from 3 to 24 + months, whereas Krikorian et al. (1978) observed complete remissions in only 6 (22 percent) of 27 such patients, 2 of whom relapsed again within less than ten months. The Stanford group concluded that ABVD was not an effective curative regimen for patients with Hodgkin's disease who had failed MOPP. Clamon and Corder (1978) reached the same conclusion after obtaining no complete remissions and only one partial remission among nine MOPP-resistant patients with stage IV Hodgkin's disease who received ABVD as salvage treatment. The Stanford experience with the B-CAVe regimen (Porzig et al., 1978) is clearly more favorable than that with ABVD and appears to be comparable to that of the Harvard group with B-DOPA (Lokich et al., 1976). Among the patients who entered complete remission after treatment with B-DOPA, the median duration of complete

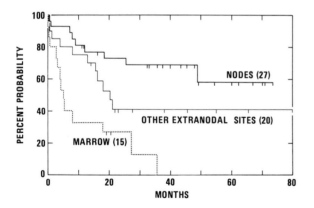

Figure 11.53 Influence of site of first relapse on the probability and time course of a second relapse in patients treated with various types of salvage therapy for initial relapses developing after radiotherapy or combined modality therapy. (Reprinted, by permission of the authors and the Editor of *Blood,* from the paper by Portlock et al., 1978.)

Table 11.7 Efficacy of Cross-over Combination Chemotherapy Regimens in Patients Relapsing after MOPP Chemotherapy

Cross-over Regimen	No. of Patients Treated	No. of Patients Evaluable	Remissions (%)		Reference
			Complete	Partial	
ABVD	15	15	9 (60)	1 (7)	Bonadonna et al., 1977
ABVD	27	27	6 (22)	4 (15)	Krikorian et al., 1978
B-CAVe	25	22	11 (50)	6 (27)	Porzig et al., 1978
B-DOPA	20	15	9 (60)	3 (20)	Lokich et al., 1976
SCAB	17	17	6 (35)	4 (24)	Levi et al., 1977

remission was 14 + months, and six of nine patients remained in remission at 21 months. Although these complete remission data provide some degree of encouragement, the followup intervals in these studies have been relatively short, and data on much larger numbers of patients followed for much longer intervals of time will be required before it can be ascertained whether any of these cross-over regimens can offer more than a small chance of long-term salvage in patients who relapse following MOPP chemotherapy.

General Treatment Recommendations

This section presents a distillation of my current views, slightly modified from those set forth by Kaplan and Rosenberg (1975), concerning the optimal management of Hodgkin's disease in relation to site(s) and stage of disease, constitutional symptoms, histopathology, and prior treatment, based on experience with a series of controlled clinical trials under way at Stanford University Medical Center since 1962 and on selected data from other institutions. The fact that certain aspects of treatment are in a state of flux implies that some of the recommendations offered here represent merely my best clinical judgment at this time. It is also to be anticipated that in the years ahead these recommendations will be altered by the results emerging from the randomized clinical trials currently in progress at major medical centers. Continuing refinements in combined modality therapy during the next several years will undoubtedly again make obsolete some of the recommendations which appear in this chapter. It is to be hoped that readers will therefore use these recommendations judiciously and will be prepared to modify them as indicated, after taking into account the skill and experience of the oncologic specialists with whom they collaborate.

Treatment Recommendations for Previously Untreated Patients. Treatment recommendations for patients with previously untreated Hodgkin's disease are set forth in Table 11.8 as a graded sequence of options related to stage, symptoms, histopathology, and presenting site. Local, involved field radiotherapy still has a valid place in the management of certain stage IA and IIA presentations (examples 1a, 2, 3a), and subtotal lymphoid radiotherapy in others (examples 4a, 4b, and 5a). For more extensive or symptomatic stage II disease, or in cases with unfavorable histologic patterns, however, total lymphoid radiotherapy must now be regarded as the treatment of choice, either alone (examples 1, 3, 4c, 5b) or supplemented by six cycles of combination chemotherapy, omitting prednisone (examples 7, 8). In stage III_SA with documented involvement of the spleen, total lymphoid radiotherapy should be supplemented with hepatic irradiation (2,200 rads/four weeks); when massive involvement of lymph nodes and/or spleen is present, adjuvant combination chemotherapy is indicated (Hoppe et al., 1979a). In the presence of constitutional symptoms (stage IIIB, III_SB), both hepatic irradiation and combination chemotherapy are added to total lymphoid radiotherapy. Patients with stage IV disease usually require combination chemotherapy as the mainstay of their management, but those treated with chemotherapy alone have a relatively high rate of relapse in sites of initially bulky lymphadenopathy. Hence strategies which incorporate moderate dose radiotherapy in a split course or alternating approach are recommended in many stage IV situations (examples 11–13). Such combined chemotherapy-radiotherapy programs are formidable and should be used selectively in relatively young patients who are in good general health, reserving chemotherapy alone for elderly patients and those in frail condition.

Table 11.8   Treatment Recommendations for Previously Untreated Patients

Stage	Histologic Type	Description	Recommended treatment
1.(a) PSIA	LP or NS	Limited to *one upper cervical region;* negative lymphangiogram and laparotomy	Local cervical-supraclavicular (involved field) or mini-mantle and Waldeyer field radiotherapy only
(b) PSIA	MC or LD	Same as 1(a)	Total lymphoid radiotherapy
2. CSIA	NS	Limited to *mediastinal* nodes; clinically negative cervical-supraclavicular nodes, negative lymphangiogram	Mantle field radiotherapy only
3.(a) PSIA	LP or NS	Limited to one *inguinal-femoral region;* negative lymphangiogram and laparotomy	Inverted-Y (pelvis, para-aortic, and splenic pedicle) field radiotherapy only
(b) PSIA	MC or LD	Same as 3(a)	Total lymphoid radiotherapy
4.(a) PSIA	LP or NS	Limited to *one lower cervical-supraclavicular region;* negative lymphangiogram and laparotomy	Subtotal lymphoid radiotherapy only (mantle and spade fields; Waldeyer field also when upper cervical nodes involved)
(b) PSIIA	LP or NS	Involvement of *two or more lymph node regions above the diaphragm;* negative lymphangiogram and laparotomy	Same as 4(a)
(c) PSIA	MC or LD	Same as 4(a) or (b)	Total lymphoid radiotherapy
5.(a) PSIIA	LP	Involvement of *two or more lymph node regions below the diaphragm;* negative spleen, liver and bone marrow	Subtotal lymphoid radiotherapy only (full inverted-Y and mini-mantle fields)
(b) PSIIA	NS, MC, or LD	Same as 5(a)	Total lymphoid radiotherapy (including mediastinal and hilar nodes)
6. PSIB	LP or NS	As in 1–5, but with *constitutional symptoms*	Total lymphoid radiotherapy (mantle and full inverted-Y fields; Waldeyer field also when upper cervical nodes involved)
7. PSII$_E$A, II$_E$B	LP or NS	As in 4, 5, or 6, but with *one or two localized extralymphatic site(s)* of involvement	Total lymphoid radiotherapy plus local irradiation of the extralymphatic lesion(s); if lymphadenopathy is massive, this may be followed (after a 6–8 week rest period) by 6 cycles of combination chemotherapy (omitting prednisone)
8. PSIB, IIB,	MC or LD	As in 6 or 7	Combined modality therapy: total lymphoid radiotherapy (mantle and full inverted-Y fields; Waldeyer field also when upper cervical nodes involved) and combination chemotherapy in an alternating sequence, starting with radiotherapy to the involved region

	Stage	Histologic Type	Description	Recommended treatment
9.	PSIIA, III$_S$A, III$_E$A, III$_{ES}$A	Any	Involvement of *nodes above and below diaphragm,* with or without *spleen;* no marrow or liver involvement; *constitutional symptoms absent*	Total lymphoid radiotherapy (plus local irradiation of "E" lesion(s), if present); when spleen is involved, hepatic field irradiation in addition; with massive spleen or nodal involvement, adjuvant combination chemotherapy is indicated
10.	PSIIIB, III$_S$B, III$_E$B, III$_{ES}$B	Any	As in 9, but *with constitutional symptoms*	Combined modality therapy: total lymphoid radiotherapy (mantle, para-aortic/hepatic, and pelvic fields) and combination chemotherapy in a split course or alternating sequence, beginning with 2 cycles of chemotherapy
11.	PSIV$_{H+}$A, IV$_{H+}$B	Any	*Biopsy-proven liver involvement* with spleen and node involvement	Alternating combined modality therapy: 2–3 cycles of combination chemotherapy, then para-aortic/hepatic field radiotherapy; 2 more cycles of chemotherapy, then mantle field radiotherapy followed by 2 more cycles of chemotherapy (omitting prednisone) and ending with pelvic field radiotherapy
12(a)	CS or PSIV$_{L,P}$	Any	Multiple bilateral pulmonary lesions, or pulmonary and biopsy-proven pleural lesions	Combination chemotherapy (3–6 cycles), followed by low to moderate dose (2,000–3,000 rads) radiotherapy to regions of initially bulky lymph node involvement, and 3–6 consolidation cycles of chemotherapy; no maintenance chemotherapy
(b)	CS or PSIV$_o$	Any	Multiple disseminated lesions of bone	
(c)	PSIV$_{M+}$	Any	Biopsy-proven bone marrow involvement	
(d)	CS or PSIV	Any	Stage IV lesions other than the above	

Treatment Recommendations for Previously Treated Patients in Relapse. The nature and extent of previous treatment are the major new variables which influence, and often severely limit, the treatment of relapsing disease. Nonetheless, modern treatment modalities make possible a very gratifying rate of salvage, especially of first relapses. When the full extent of disease is not apparent at the time of first relapse, a complete diagnostic workup should be performed, including a repeat lymphangiogram, and if necessary, laparotomy with splenectomy and biopsies of para-aortic nodes, liver, and marrow. The proper course of action cannot be arrived at without objective knowledge of the distribution of relapsing sites of disease. Relapses in lymph nodes, spleen, or localized osseous or subcutaneous sites in patients previously treated with radiotherapy only (Table 11.9, examples 1–5, 10) call for treatment with at least six cycles of MOP (or other combination) chemotherapy, supplemented in most instances by additional radiotherapy to the site(s) of relapse and to previously untreated lymphoid regions. Relapses in liver, lung, bone marrow, or multiple, disseminated sites in patients previously treated with radiotherapy only are best treated with MOP or other combination chemotherapy regimens (six or more cycles), supplemented in some instances with low to moderate dose radiotherapy to the site(s) of relapse, as in examples 6, 8, and 9. Patients who relapse following single-drug chemotherapy may be moderately to severely cytopenic and have limited

Table 11.9   Recommended Treatment of Previously Treated Patients in First Relapse

Description of disease	Recommended treatment
1 *Recurrence in treated lymph node chain* in patients previously treated *with radiotherapy only*	6 (or more) cycles of MOP combination chemotherapy followed by low-dose (1,500–2,000 rads, 2–2½ weeks) local radiotherapy
2 *Recurrence at margin of treated lymph node chain* in patients previously treated *with radiotherapy*	MOP chemotherapy followed by local radiotherapy, with dose limited to 1,500–2,000 rads to previously irradiated area but carried to 4,000 rads/4 weeks to marginal recurrence
3 *Extension* to previously *untreated lymph node chain* on *same* side of diaphragm	High-dose radiotherapy (4,000 rads/4 weeks) to newly involved chain and to all other previously unirradiated lymphoid regions on *both* sides of diaphragm, plus MOP chemotherapy using split course or alternating sequence

4 *Extension* to previously *untreated lymph node chains* on *opposite* side of diaphragm.
  a Extension from *below* diaphragm to *cervical-supraclavicular* nodes;
  b Extension from *above* diaphragm to *para-aortic* nodes
	a High-dose radiotherapy as in 3, above.
	b Laparotomy, if not previously done; if *spleen* or *liver* found to be involved, then as per 5 or 6, respectively; if nodes alone are involved and spleen removed, high-dose radiotherapy to full inverted-Y field, plus MOP chemotherapy using split course or alternating sequence

5 *Extension to spleen,* usually associated with para-aortic node involvement, in patients previously treated *with radiotherapy above diaphragm*	*Splenectomy* with *liver and bone marrow biopsies;* if biopsies positive, then as per 6 or 7, respectively; if negative, MOP chemotherapy, using split course or alternating sequence, plus high-dose radiotherapy to para-aortic/hepatic field (4,400 rads/2,200 rads/4 weeks), then to other previously unirradiated fields (4,400 rads/4 weeks)
6 *Biopsy-proven extension* to *liver,* with or without evident lymph node disease, in patients previously treated *with radiotherapy only*	Split course MOP chemotherapy (usually 2–4 cycles initially), then low dose radiotherapy (2,000 rads/3–4 weeks) to the liver and regions of bulky lymphadenopathy, then 3–6 more cycles of MOP
7 *Biopsy-proven extension* to *bone marrow,* with or without concurrent involvement of spleen and lymph nodes, in patients previously treated *with radiotherapy only*	MOP chemotherapy (6-9 cycles), followed by low-dose (1,500–2,000 rads/2 weeks) radiotherapy to areas of bulky lymphadenopathy and 2–4 consolidation cycles of MOP chemotherapy in patients attaining documented complete remission
8 *Solitary* lesion in *one lung* in patients previously treated *with radiotherapy only*	MOP chemotherapy (usually 6 cycles), supplemented by ipsilateral whole-lung irradiation (1,500 rads/3–4 weeks)
9 *Multiple* lesions in *both lungs* in patients previously treated *with radiotherapy only*	MOP chemotherapy (6 or more cycles) and optional low-dose radiotherapy to both lung fields (1,200–1,500 rads/4 weeks)
10 *Apparently solitary extension to bone* or *subcutaneous* tissues in patients previously treated *with radiotherapy only*	Local radiotherapy (4,000 rads/4 weeks) if region previously unirradiated; MOP chemotherapy, 6 cycles, optionally supplemented by 1,500 rads/2 weeks if region previously irradiated to dose not exceeding 4,500 rads and not in proximity to vital tissues or organs
11 *Multiple* scattered *osseous* or *subcutaneous* lesions in patients previously treated *with radiotherapy only*	MOP chemotherapy (6–9 cycles); supplemental low-dose radiotherapy to sites of incomplete response
12 In *lymph node(s)* in patients previously treated *with single drug chemotherapy only*	Careful diagnostic evaluation and restaging, then high-dose, total lymphoid radiotherapy if no extranodal disease is detected and hematologic tolerance is good; high-dose local radiotherapy to involved areas plus 6 cycles of MOP chemotherapy is acceptable alternative

Description of disease	Recommended treatment
13 In *extranodal site(s)* (bone marrow, liver, lungs, etc.) in patients previously treated *with single-drug chemotherapy only*	MOPP, ABVD, B-CAVe, B-DOPA, or other combination chemotherapy, selecting combination with agents to which resistance has not yet been demonstrated
14 In patients previously treated *with MOPP (or other combination) chemotherapy*	MOPP chemotherapy may be tried again when first relapse occurs more than 12 months after end of first course of MOPP; for earlier relapses, crossover to other drug combinations, such as ABVD, B-CAVe, B-DOPA when hematologic tolerance is good; high-dose radiotherapy may be the treatment of choice in selected patients with nodal relapses following MOPP or other combination chemotherapy who have had no prior irradiation in the region of relapse; palliative single-drug chemotherapy and/or local radiotherapy (for localized relapses) when hematologic tolerance is too poor to permit intensive chemotherapy

tolerance for combination chemotherapy; if so, the regimen selected for them should comprise agents with little or no myelotoxicity and, when possible, those agents to which their tumor has not yet established resistance. Patients who develop "late" relapses following MOPP chemotherapy (more than 12 months after completion of the last MOPP cycle) occasionally do well again on MOPP; those relapsing earlier are best regarded as MOPP failures and treated with one of the "cross-over" combinations (ABVD, B-CAVe, B-DOPA, SCAB). Treatment options inevitably become more and more severely restricted in patients with multiple, sequential relapses (Table 11.10), both because of the limitations on tissue tolerance imposed by prior therapy and because of the dwindling list of agents to which tumor resistance has not yet developed. Nonetheless, skillful use of the available options can provide months and even years of useful and productive life, despite the fact that such patients are ultimately destined to die of Hodgkin's disease.

Typical Responses to the Initial and Subsequent Courses of Treatment

It is important to distinguish objective responses—the diminution in size and disappearance of enlarged lymph nodes, radiographic evidence of regression of lymphadenopathy in para-aortic or iliac lymph nodes opacified during prior lymphangiography, radiographic clearing of pulmonary infiltrates, defervescence, progressive improvement in hemoglobin or hematocrit levels, or other laboratory indices of response—from purely subjective responses such as an improvement in general well-being, disappearance of malaise or fatigue, or increased appetite. In the chemotherapy of Hodgkin's disease, not only the completeness but also the duration of response is considered in scoring objective remissions as complete or partial. It is generally accepted practice to score remissions as complete only when all manifestations of disease disappear and remain inapparent for a period of at least two to three months after completion of an

Table 11.10   Recommended Treatment of Previously Treated Patients with Second and Later Relapses

Description	Recommended treatment
Relapse involving *multiple* or *extralymphatic* or *heavily irradiated* sites; hematologic tolerance good to adequate	MOP(P) chemotherapy, omitting prednisone if mantle region previously irradiated
Relapse involving *local nodal* or *osseous* sites; hematologic tolerance poor or marginal	Local radiotherapy if local tissue tolerance permits
Relapse in *multiple* or *extralymphatic* sites after attempted MOPP salvage therapy of initial relapse; hematologic tolerance adequate	B-CAVe, ABVD, B-DOPA, or other crossover regimen of combination chemotherapy
Relapse involving *multiple* or *extralymphatic* or *heavily irradiated* sites; hematologic tolerance poor	Single-drug, palliative chemotherapy

inducing course of chemotherapy. The higher doses of modern megavoltage radiotherapy that are now employed yield complete remissions in almost 100 percent of instances, and most relapses tend to occur in previously unirradiated sites. However, radiotherapists do not ordinarily score responses in terms of remissions, which connote a temporary response, often followed by relapse.

That spontaneous remissions may occur prior to the initiation of specific therapy in patients with Hodgkin's disease was documented many years ago by Obrecht and Caspers (1960). With the advent of modern, highly effective methods of treatment, few if any patients with Hodgkin's disease are left untreated; thus, the opportunity for the observation of spontaneous remissions seldom occurs. For the same reason, there are no modern data on survival in untreated patients with Hodgkin's disease. Valid estimates on the frequency with which spontaneous remissions might be expected to occur are not possible with the limited data available.

Objective regression of palpable or radiographically demonstrable lymphadenopathy usually begins within the first one to two weeks after the initiation of radiotherapy and is not infrequently complete by the time a course of radiotherapy is finished. However, the response rate is also a function of the histopathologic type of Hodgkin's disease being treated. In the lymphocyte predominance form of the disease, responses are often dramatic; large, conglomerate masses of lymph nodes may virtually "melt away" within a few days. In contrast, lesions containing relatively large amounts of collagen, as is common in the nodular sclerosing form of the disease, not infrequently appear to respond slowly or not at all for long periods of time, owing to the fact that collagenous bands comprise such a large proportion of the total tumor volume. We have observed instances in which firm lymph nodes in the neck remained palpable after the completion of treatment; subsequent surgical excision revealed only dense masses of collagen, with no viable lymphoid or abnormal reticulum cells.

Since large mediastinal masses, particularly in young female patients, are usually of the nodular sclerosing type, slower regression should be anticipated in a significant proportion of such cases. An example of such delayed response in the nodular sclerosing form of Hodgkin's disease is illustrated in Figure 5.6, Chapter 5. Persistent enlargement of the mediastinal silhouette does not necessarily indicate relapsing disease. In three such cases submitted to exploratory thoracotomy, cystic lesions were discovered, and no evidence of residual Hodgkin's disease was present (Katz et al., 1977). In most instances, the split course technique of radiotherapy described in Chapter 9 can be used successfully to eradicate large mediastinal masses while preserving pulmonary ventilatory function. However, when regression of the mediastinal mass is slow, it may sometimes be necessary to interrupt the radiotherapy and to give two or more cycles of MOPP chemotherapy to reduce the size of the mediastinal mass sufficiently to permit completion of mantle irradiation (Figs. 11.54, 11.55). Some investigators (Mauch, Goodman, and Hellman, 1978) have argued for the routine use of combined modality therapy in patients with very large mediastinal masses to decrease the risk of local recurrence and/or relapse. However, we have preferred to use split course radiotherapy alone in those cases in which rapid regression is observed and to hold combination chemotherapy in reserve for the infrequent instances in which relapses later develop. In patients with Hodgkin's disease of the lymphocytic depletion subtype, responses are also likely to be relatively slow and are often incomplete at a time when the full course of initially planned treatment has been delivered, necessitating supplementary radiation, usually through reduced fields, to the areas of persistent disease.

Constitutional symptoms usually disappear within the first two to three weeks after the initiation of radiotherapy. However, in patients with stage IIIB disease, symptoms may persist, sometimes with diminished intensity, during the initial part of the course, while radiotherapy is directed to the supradiaphragmatic manifestations of disease, and disappear only when the infradiaphragmatic areas of involvement have also been irradiated. When symptoms persist throughout a course of radiotherapy in patients with disease initially staged as IIB or IIIB, the presence of occult disease in an extralymphatic site, such as the bone marrow or liver, should be strongly suspected and renewed diagnostic investigation of such sites undertaken. Some authorities have recommended the use of single-drug chemotherapy prior to radiotherapy in patients with constitutional symptoms. Although profoundly debilitating high fever or drenching sweats may occasionally provide an adequate indication for such preliminary chemotherapy, it is unnecessary in the great majority of symptomatic cases and should, in our opinion, be avoided whenever possible, since the hematopoietic insult produced by the chemotherapy may jeop-

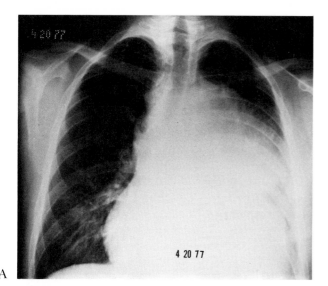

A

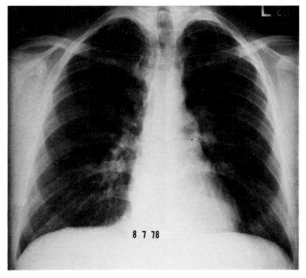

C

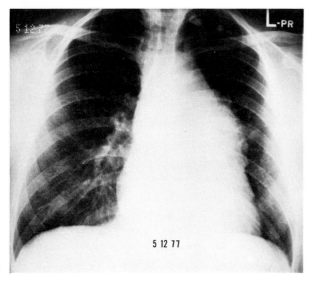

B

Figure 11.54 Combined modality therapy in the management of massive mediastinal and intrathoracic involvement. *A,* initial chest film revealing an enormous mediastinal and left hilar mass with pericardial and left pulmonary invasion. The patient was treated to 1,650 rads with a mantle field, omitting the left lung shield, with modest regression *(B).* A lymphangiogram was then performed and was negative. The patient then received six cycles of MOP chemotherapy from May through October 1977, with marked further regression of his intrathoracic disease. Mantle field irradiation was resumed in January 1978, and an additional 3,400 rads was delivered to the mediastinum, followed by treatment of a paraaortic-splenic field to 3,500 rads, with the liver receiving 1,500 rads through a 50 percent transmission block. *C,* a repeat chest roentgenogram in August 1978 was essentially normal.

ardize the delivery of full tumor-sterilizing doses of radiotherapy.

In patients treated with chemotherapeutic agents, objective regressions are noted earlier with some agents than with others, even though the objective remission rate may be similar. Examples include the alkylating agents such as nitrogen mustard, the response to which is likely to be rapid, and the vinca alkaloids, to which the response is typically slow. Response rates with MOPP or other multiple drug combinations are usually rapid, since most such regimens include an alkylating agent. Disappearance of fever may be noted within a few days, and objective regression of lymph node masses within one to three weeks after a single intravenous injection of nitrogen mustard or a single cycle of MOPP (cf. Figs. 4.3 and 10.1). Indeed, the persistence of disease four to six weeks later usually indicates that only a partial and short-lived remission can be anticipated (Fig. 11.56).

The response to subsequent courses of treatment depends a good deal on circumstances. In the case of radiotherapy, the response to a second course of treatment is likely to be just as prompt and complete as the initial response if a new area of involvement, not encompassed within the previous radiotherapeutic fields, is being treated. However, disease developing within a previously irradiated area commonly responds more sluggishly to a second course of treatment. Moreover, re-irradiation is associated with a distinctly higher rate of recurrence and, when relatively high doses have accumulated, of radiation-induced injury to the normal tissues in the treated volume. The radiotherapist today seldom sees patients whose Hodgkin's disease has become completely refrac-

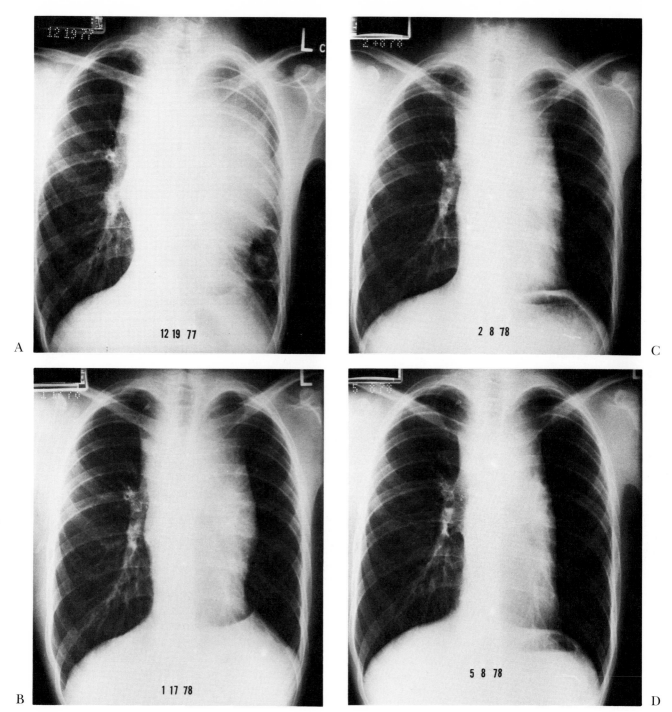

Figure 11.55 Slow regression of a mediastinal mass during combined modality therapy. *A,* massive mediastinal and subcarinal adenopathy is evident on the initial chest film; tomograms also revealed bilateral hilar adenopathy and a left lung nodule. The patient received 1,500 rads to the mantle field, with the left lung unshielded, from 12/20/77 to 1/4/78, with good but obviously incomplete regression evident on repeat chest films taken 1/17/78 and 2/8/78 (*B, C*). He was then treated with two cycles of MOP in February and March 1978 and showed further, but still incomplete, regression on another film taken 5/8/78 (*D*), at which time mantle field irradiation was resumed and carried to a combined total dose of 5,000 rads. He then received MOP cycles 3 and 4, para-aortic–splenic pedicle irradiation, MOP cycles 5 and 6, and pelvic irradiation. Later chest films in July and September 1978 remained essentially unchanged.

tory to radiation, as was commonly observed during the era of palliative radiotherapy and multiple successive courses of retreatment of the same involved lymph nodes, largely because patients in whom relapses occur after one or two courses of radiotherapy usually become candidates for chemotherapy.

Evidence suggesting that Hodgkin's disease recurring in lymph nodes after prior chemotherapy may also be more resistant to subsequent radiotherapy has been presented by Johnson and Brace (1966). They noted eight recurrences in a total of twenty-one radiation treatment fields in eight patients previously treated with one or more courses of chemotherapy; during the same interval, there were no recurrences in ten treatment fields in four previously untreated patients.

The development of refractoriness to any given chemotherapeutic agent is the rule in all cases of Hodgkin's disease managed with a single agent, though the rapidity with which the refractory state appears may vary widely. Disease that has become refractory to one drug in a given category is likely to be refractory to all other drugs in the same category. For example, patients who are no longer responsive to nitrogen mustard or Chlorambucil are not likely to respond to another alkylating agent such as Cytoxan. However, the same patient may respond well if a new class of agent, such as a *Vinca* alkaloid, is employed at this stage. This provided the rationale for several of the "cross-over" combination chemotherapy regimens developed for the treatment of MOPP-resistant disease. After several relapses, progressive erosion of hematopoietic reserves and increasing hematologic, neurologic, or other manifestations of toxicity occur. As responsiveness to one category of drug after another becomes exhausted, a preterminal state will ultimately ensue in which the remaining choice of chemotherapeutic agents becomes severely restricted, drugs may be employed only at reduced dose levels, and responses become increasingly feeble, transient, or negligible.

Therapeutic Errors in Management

Hodgkin's disease is usually a cruel and ruthless adversary, which seldom permits the physician to commit an error in judgment without serious consequences to his patient. Although the long-term salvage afforded by retreatment of cases in which relapse has developed after primary treatment has improved greatly, the chance for cure which it offers is undoubtedly far less than that afforded by primary treatment. Data from several treatment centers (Lauwers and Dancot, 1966; Papillon et al., 1966b; Kaplan, 1968b; Spittle et al., 1973; Weller et al., 1976) convincingly document the fact that patients who have had a relapse during any given interval of time after primary treatment are much more likely to die of Hodgkin's disease than those patients who have not. Musshoff and Boutis (1968, 1969) noted that virtually all of their surviving patients at fourteen to twenty years were those who entered complete remission during the first course of treatment and remained relapse-free for nine or more years thereafter. Errors in clinical judgment unquestionably contribute to the probability of relapse and may thus contribute directly to the impairment of a patient's chance for survival.

We have observed several categories of error (both our own and those of others):

1. *Errors in diagnosis.* This category includes not only errors in histopathologic interpretation, with ensuing delay in the diagnosis of Hodgkin's disease, but also undue procrastination in obtaining a biopsy of enlarged lymph nodes, sometimes with prolonged antibiotic treatment for supposed inflammatory disease, and poor surgical judgment or bad luck in the selection of lymph nodes for excisional biopsy.

2. *Errors in the diagnostic evaluation of the extent of disease.* Prior to the advent of lymphangiography, this was probably the single most frequent type of error. Lymph node involvement below the diaphragm was formerly likely to remain undetected and thus untreated until it reached massive proportions. In our opinion, lymphangiography remains an indispensable part of the routine diagnostic evaluation of patients with Hodgkin's disease, except for those presenting specific contraindications to the procedure. Moreover, as the data presented in Chapters 4, 7, and 8 attest, the staging laparotomy with splenectomy is the only reliable way to detect the all-too-frequent presence of spleen involvement. The omission of a bone marrow biopsy or reliance on a negative marrow aspirate in patients subjected to radical radiotherapy for apparent stage IIB or stage IIIB disease is most unwise. Perhaps the most indefensible error of all is the discouragingly prevalent practice of proceeding with local radiotherapy or with chemotherapy for clinically obvious disease without any serious attempt to conduct a thorough diagnostic search for other possible sites of involvement.

3. *Errors in the selection of primary treatment with curative versus palliative intent.* As recently as a decade ago, a frequent and serious error was the use

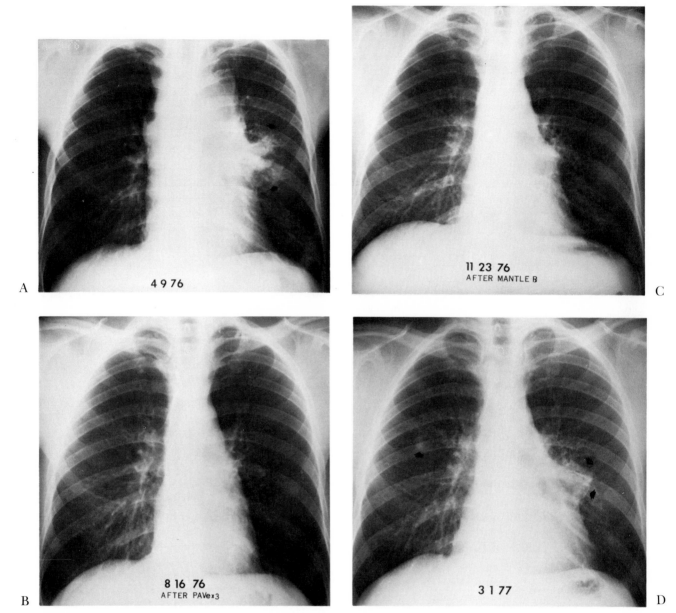

Figure 11.56 Incomplete regression followed by recrudescence of intrathoracic disease. *A,* initial chest film revealing massive mediastinal, left hilar, and left pulmonary involvement (arrows) in a 35-year-old male patient with fever and night sweats. After diagnostic evaluation, he was staged as having PS III_EB nodular sclerosing Hodgkin's disease and randomized to split course PAVe chemotherapy and total lymphoid irradiation in the S-5 protocol. After three cycles of PAVe (*B*), marked regression was evident, but there was still infiltration into the left lung from the hilum, and his disease began to grow again during mantle field irradiation (*C*). He was then treated with a succession of other drug regimens, but new pulmonary lesions continued to appear (*D, E, F*) and enlarged to massive size (*G, H*) before his death in November 1977.

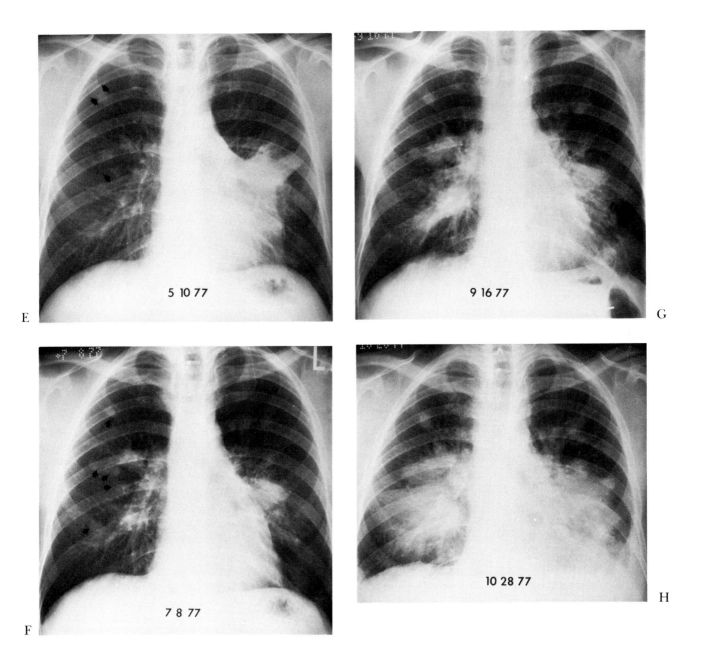

E   G

F   H

of palliative treatment in the mistaken belief that a previously untreated patient with Hodgkin's disease had no significant chance for cure. The problem is well illustrated by a patient seen by us in consultation several years ago after prior diagnosis and treatment elsewhere. The patient, a ten-year-old female, had a relatively favorable diagnosis of stage IIA Hodgkin's disease of the nodular sclerosing type. Her parents stated that nine consecutive physicians whom they consulted after the initial biopsy diagnosis was made, including pediatricians, surgeons, and hematologists, had informed them that their daughter's case was hopeless and that only palliative therapy was indicated. Fortunately, they were stubborn enough to seek a tenth opinion, that of a qualified radiotherapist, who told them that their daughter had a relatively good chance for cure (a statement which by that time they found almost difficult to believe) and who administered intensive megavoltage radiotherapy, achieving a complete remission which has been maintained to date. Even those physicians who do accept the possibility of cure of Hodgkin's disease may believe that cures are attainable only in the relatively limited group of stage I cases. It is important for physicians to recognize that modern diagnostic and therapeutic advances have indeed extended the potential for cure to include essentially all cases, irrespective of stage, unless intensive therapy is contraindicated by old age or some coexistent life-threatening medical condition.

4. *Errors in the selection of the modality for treatment with curative intent.* Intensive radiotherapy is clearly the treatment of choice in patients with stage I, II, and IIIA Hodgkin's disease. Since megavoltage radiotherapy carried to tumoricidal doses can eradicate localized disease with a significantly smaller probability of local recurrence and an essentially perfect cosmetic result, it no longer seems justifiable to subject patients to a needlessly disfiguring procedure such as radical surgical node dissection. The selection of single-drug chemotherapy as the modality for treatment with curative intent is an equally serious error. A careful search of the literature fails to reveal a single instance of relapse-free survival for intervals long enough to suggest probable cure in patients with Hodgkin's disease treated with single-drug chemotherapy alone. Moreover, there have been some indications that when relapses develop after chemotherapy, the tumor may have been rendered relatively more radioresistant (Johnson and Brace, 1966). Multiple-drug combination chemotherapy has now been shown to have curative potential in patients with advanced disease (De Vita et al., 1976), and is the treatment of choice, alone or combined with radiotherapy, in all those who present no specific contraindication to its use.

5. *Errors in the diagnosis of relapsing disease.* It is essential that patients be seen for followup examination at relatively frequent intervals during the first two years after completion of primary therapy. The patient who is not brought back for followup examination for six months or more after initial treatment may well have far-advanced, incurable disease when finally examined. The character of the followup examination, presented in Chapter 4, is likewise of importance. Although relatively brief, it must be thoughtfully oriented to the detection of all of the reasonably probable manifestations of relapsing disease. Leaving aside patients who have never had a lymphangiogram, who are obviously subject to the risk of missed diagnosis of retroperitoneal node disease not only initially but also during the followup period, we have observed occasional instances in which patients who had had an apparently negative lymphangiogram prior to treatment later developed far-advanced abdominal disease, either because abdominal roentgenograms were not routinely obtained as part of their followup examination, or because the significance of changes in the size, contour, and consistency of opacified retroperitoneal nodes seen on such followup films was not appreciated (cf. Fig. 5.65).

Conversely, as Craver (1964, p. 1048) has emphasized, "One must guard against assuming that every new symptom or sign is caused by Hodgkin's disease." Biopsy confirmation of recurrence or extension of Hodgkin's disease is highly desirable in all instances, particularly those in which re-irradiation of a previously irradiated field might be required. A related problem is the misinterpretation of transient effects of treatment, such as postirradiation paramediastinal pneumonitis and fibrosis, as uncontrolled, recurrent mediastinal adenopathy, with the initiation of a potentially very hazardous second course of radiotherapy or of chemotherapy for nonexistent disease.

6. *Errors in the selection of treatment for relapsing disease.* In general, patients with relapsing disease should be given the benefit of the doubt and treated with intensive radiotherapy and/or combination chemotherapy for whatever chance of cure they may still have, rather than being prematurely relegated to palliative therapy. However, the phy-

sician must take into consideration the age and general clinical condition of the patient in arriving at this decision.

7. *Errors in the technique of treatment.* Technical considerations are of the greatest importance to the efficacy and safety of both radiotherapy and chemotherapy. Although the details of technique have been presented in previous chapters, it is important to stress here that the skill and experience of the radiotherapist or chemotherapist is a vitally important factor in the optimal management of patients with Hodgkin's disease. The advanced techniques utilized in modern megavoltage radiotherapy and multiple-drug chemotherapy are often available only in major medical centers, to which patients with previously untreated Hodgkin's disease should be referred for expert primary care. The converse policy of treating such patients with whatever methods are readily available in the local community, and deferring referral to a major medical center until relapse supervenes, leads almost inevitably to disaster.

Special Topics

Elderly Patients. It is perhaps fortunate that patients over sixty-five years of age are encountered relatively infrequently in most large series of cases of Hodgkin's disease, at least in North America and western Europe. Elderly patients may pose difficult problems for either the radiotherapist or the chemotherapist, in part because they are more likely to have other serious coexistent medical conditions and in part because the hematopoietic capacity of the bone marrow decreases significantly in old age, with the consequence that bone marrow suppression is much more often a serious limiting factor in the delivery of a complete course of treatment.

The general clinical condition and physiologic status of every patient over sixty years of age with Hodgkin's disease should be evaluated with particular care. A patient who is a "young" sixty-five years of age (i.e., whose physiologic age appears to be substantially younger than his chronologic age) is likely to tolerate quite well the same intensive radiotherapy and/or combination chemotherapy indicated in younger adults. Conversely, a frail or senile patient in this age range is likely to tolerate such treatment very poorly and is therefore an appropriate candidate for a more limited, perhaps even palliative, treatment regimen. Old age may also influence the technique of treatment. For ex-

ample, radiotherapists who would ordinarily use subtotal or total lymphoid irradiation in adolescent or young adult patients with stage I or stage II Hodgkin's disease might elect to encompass only the clinically involved regions in elderly patients with similarly localized disease. Finally, the risk associated with treatment with curative intent may not be warranted in elderly patients with stage IIIB or stage IV disease, particularly if they are not otherwise in good general health; in such patients, it may be the better part of valor to elect treatment with palliative intent, either with single-drug chemotherapy or with localized-field radiotherapy limited to moderate dose levels.

Children. It was once widely believed that young children with Hodgkin's disease tolerate treatment poorly and have a relatively poor prognosis. We have been at a loss to discover the evidence on which this widely prevailing view was based. Even in the prelymphangiography era of low-dose, essentially palliative radiotherapy, five-year survival in the Memorial Hospital series of 40 patients was 50 percent; after the introduction of lymphangiography and high-dose radiotherapy (1960–1969), an additional 69 patients were treated, with a five-year survival of 62 percent; and with the advent of staging laparotomy and combination chemotherapy, 45 patients treated during 1970–1974 experienced a five-year survival rate of 82 percent (Tan et al., 1975). Indeed, many studies during the past decade testify that children do about as well as (or somewhat better than) young adults (Teillet and Schweisguth, 1969; K. L. Smith et al., 1974; Jenkin et al., 1975; Tan et al., 1975; Donaldson et al., 1976b; I. E. Smith et al., 1977).

Donaldson et al. (1976a,b) have presented a detailed analysis of the Stanford experience during the ten-year period 1962–1972 with the treatment of 79 previously untreated children, aged 15 years or less, with Hodgkin's disease of all stages. Staging laparotomy was performed in 41 children, yielding diagnostic information which resulted in a change of stage in 12 instances (29 percent). Seven patients (8.8 percent) had localized extralymphatic (E) sites of disease at presentation. High-dose radiotherapy alone was used in stages I–III during most of this period; stage IV patients were treated with single-drug chemotherapy until late 1968, after which MOPP combination chemotherapy was used, with or without supplemental irradiation. Only 5 of these patients were part of the pediatric protocol described earlier in this chapter in the section on modification of dose in combined modality therapy (page 511) in which low-dose radiotherapy was combined with six cycles of MOPP chemotherapy. For the entire series of 79 patients, actuarial survival was 89 percent at 5 years and 70 percent at 9.5 years. Moreover, 66 percent were relapse-free at 5 years (Fig. 11.57). Although relapse rates were significantly higher among children who were staged clinically (45 percent at 5 years) than among those submitted to staging laparotomy (18 percent at 5 years), survival in these two groups at 5 years was only slightly, and not significantly, better among the surgically staged patients (Fig. 11.58).

It was entirely possible to deliver intensive megavoltage radiotherapy to all of the major lymph node chains and the spleen in children as young as five years of age. However, treatment fields must be delineated with particular care (cf. Fig. 9.18, Chapter 9) and every effort made to shield the lungs, kidneys, and other vital organs and tissues during the irradiation of such patients (Donaldson, Glatstein, and Kaplan, 1976a). Despite these precautions, there was one death due to severe radiation pneumonitis in our series, and impairment of bone growth and development was observed in several of the smaller children treated with high-dose radiotherapy (Probert, Parker, and Kaplan, 1973; Probert and Parker, 1975). Due to the penumbra and scatter of kilovoltage X-ray beams, effective protection of vital organs, even in small children, requires the use of megavoltage energies. Accordingly, a particularly strong case can be made for the referral of young children with Hodgkin's disease to major medical centers, where they can be treated by radiotherapists highly expe-

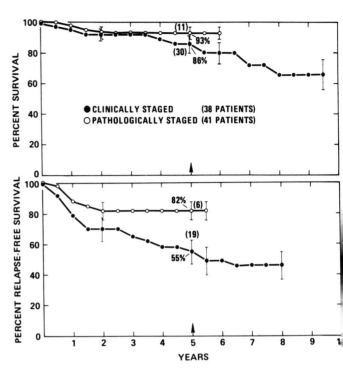

Figure 11.58 Comparative analysis of survival (upper panel) and freedom from relapse (lower panel) among 38 pediatric patients who were clinically staged and 41 who were pathologically staged. (Reprinted, by permission of the authors and the Editor of *Cancer,* from the paper by Donaldson et al., 1976b.)

rienced in these techniques, employing optimal modern megavoltage equipment. Combination chemotherapy may also be attended by serious complications in the pediatric age group. There were three deaths due to infection in our series in children receiving chemotherapy; one other fatal infection occurred in a child who had completed low-dose irradiation plus six cycles of MOPP. Azoospermia apparently occurs in essentially all male children treated with MOPP, though some may later manifest partial recovery of spermatogenesis. No secondary leukemias have been observed in this series of children. However, one adolescent boy with Ollier's syndrome who had been treated with multiple courses of radiotherapy, MOPP, and various single drugs for relapsing Hodgkin's disease developed an inoperable chondrosarcoma in a region of high-dose irradiation.

Pregnancy. Two quite different situations are represented by the patient who becomes pregnant during the course of treatment for a previously established diagnosis of Hodgkin's disease and the patient in whom a diagnosis of Hodgkin's disease is

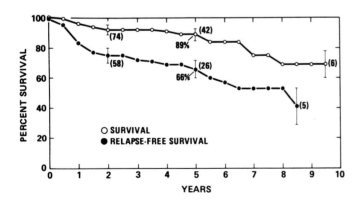

Figure 11.57 Actuarial analysis of survival and freedom from relapse in a series of 79 children with Hodgkin's disease of all stages treated at Stanford University Medical Center, 1962–1972. (Reprinted, by permission of the authors and the Editor of *Cancer,* from the paper by Donaldson et al., 1976b.)

made during the course of an established pregnancy. In the former instance, it may be assumed that all of the diagnostic procedures required for proper staging, including lymphangiography and staging laparotomy with splenectomy, have already been completed. Several clinical possibilities deserve consideration. In the case of clinical stage IA disease apparently limited to the neck or axilla, particularly disease of a favorable histopathologic type, an acceptable compromise from the standpoint of both the mother and the fetus would be to irradiate only the involved chain of lymph nodes to a "holding" dose (about 2,000 rads in 2 weeks) and then to observe the patient carefully at serial intervals, hoping that the pregnancy can be carried to full term before any new clinical manifestations of disease appear. The treatment regimen indicated by the initial pathologic stage of disease can then be carried to completion.

Obviously, this plan would not be appropriate for stage I disease presenting in the groin, since the amount of scattered irradiation reaching the fetus would be prohibitively great. Similarly, more extensive stage II disease, confined either to the upper abdominal lymph node chains or to supradiaphragmatic sites, would very likely require such large treatment fields as to entail at least a significant probability of damage to the fetus by scattered radiation, despite careful beam collimation (Covington and Baker, 1969). In all of these situations, we would recommend therapeutic abortion, after which the treatment plan that would have been employed in a nonpregnant patient with disease of similar distribution may be carried to completion. When it is possible during such a course of treatment to preserve ovarian function, it is entirely possible for such patients to become pregnant again at a later date and to deliver normal, full-term offspring.

Finally, we may consider the patient with advanced, disseminated disease in whom pregnancy supervenes. Despite earlier fears that the major chemotherapeutic agents utilized in Hodgkin's disease would be likely to have teratogenic effects on the fetus, a number of case reports (Deuschle and Wiggins, 1953; Sokal and Lessmann, 1960; Armstrong et al., 1964; Lacher, 1964; Lacher and Durant, 1966) have appeared suggesting that normal, full-term children may be born to mothers who are receiving chemotherapy for advanced Hodgkin's disease. However, the teratogenic effects of chlorambucil, vinblastine, and vincristine have been documented in rats and hamsters (Monie, 1961; Ferm, 1963), and there have been

isolated reports of congenital anomalies in human fetuses born to mothers treated with alkylating agents during pregnancy (Shotton and Monie, 1963; Greenberg and Tanaka, 1964; Chauvergne, 1971; Garrett, 1974). Accordingly, the most prudent policy is that stated by Lacher and Geller (1966): "Because of the meager experience with chemotherapeutic agents during pregnancy, . . . it is desirable to avoid treatment in all trimesters in all cases whenever possible. The late effects of chemotherapy are still unknown and complacency concerning the use of these potentially teratogenic agents should be avoided."

Let us consider now the converse situation of the patient who has a biopsy diagnosis of Hodgkin's disease made during the course of an established pregnancy. Here, not only the pathologic type of the Hodgkin's disease but also the duration of the pregnancy at the time of diagnosis must be taken into consideration. When the disease is localized and histologically favorable and the pregnancy is at or beyond the seventh month, it is obviously desirable to minimize therapeutic intervention in order to avoid injury to the nearly mature fetus. When the lymphadenopathy is truly of minimal extent and apparently indolent, it is probably best simply to observe the patient carefully, deferring both the diagnostic evaluation and the treatment until after delivery, unless an abrupt acceleration of growth rate or the appearance of new manifestations of disease elsewhere provide a more pressing indication for treatment. Under the latter circumstance, the early induction of labor or even a caesarian section for the delivery of a viable premature infant may gain precious time for the initiation of definitive diagnostic and therapeutic measures.

The patient in whom relatively far-advanced Hodgkin's disease is first discovered too late in the course of a pregnancy to permit therapeutic abortion is probably best treated conservatively with single-drug chemotherapy. It may be possible to carry the pregnancy to term in this way and then to reassess the patient carefully prior to the initiation of combination chemotherapy or combined modality therapy with curative intent.

In many respects, the most difficult situation is that in which a biopsy diagnosis of Hodgkin's disease is made during the first or early in the second trimester of pregnancy. It is unlikely that the disease will remain quiescent long enough for the fetus to mature to extrauterine viability. In very exceptional cases of apparently localized, indolent disease of favorable histopathologic type, a policy of watchful waiting may indeed permit a full-term fetus to be obtained without significant progression of the disease. However, in the great majority of instances, the disease will progress during this interval of several months, and the extent of progression is likely to threaten the prognosis of the mother. Accordingly, it has been our policy in pregnancies that have not passed the first half of the second trimester to recommend therapeutic abortion followed by diagnostic evaluation of the extent of disease and the initiation of appropriate treatment. When the extent of disease has been sufficiently limited to make possible the preservation of ovarian function, some patients have been able to conceive and bear normal, full-term children at a later date.

Although unsubstantiated claims have long circulated that pregnancy may rekindle persistent but dormant Hodgkin's disease to renewed activity (Craver, 1964), there is little or no documentation for this view in the published literature. On the contrary, the reported studies suggest that pregnancy has little or no adverse effect on prognosis (Smith et al., 1958; Barry et al., 1962).

The Role of Surgery. It hardly needs to be restated that the diagnosis of Hodgkin's disease cannot be made without biopsy and microscopic examination of affected tissue. Where lymphadenopathy is present, excisional biopsy of one or more lymph nodes is the procedure of choice. Incisional biopsy is strongly contraindicated, since it may promote local invasion and spread of the disease and provide an inadequate tissue sample. Aspiration biopsy of lymph nodes does not provide enough tissue to permit reliable pathologic diagnosis and classification. The practice of treating patients for presumptive Hodgkin's disease without biopsy verification is strongly condemned. In patients with mediastinal lymphadenopathy who present no palpably enlarged peripheral nodes, blind scalene node biopsy should be considered. Although a negative scalene node biopsy is not helpful, a positive biopsy obviates the need for thoracotomy.

Slaughter, Economou, and Southwick (1958) documented the fact that only a fraction of the lymph nodes in a radical node dissection specimen are likely to contain Hodgkin's disease and that other nodes immediately adjacent to them may be uninvolved. Accordingly, the surgeon must exercise careful judgment in deciding which lymph node to excise for biopsy. Often, the most accessible and freely movable node is one that is least likely to be involved and thus may yield a potentially misleading pathologic diagnosis. The characteristically firm, "rubbery" consistency of lymph nodes extensively involved by Hodgkin's disease is often helpful to the surgeon in deciding which node to remove.

Surgery now has an additional role in the diagnostic evaluation of patients with Hodgkin's disease (Enright et al., 1970). Laparotomy with splenectomy and biopsy of the para-aortic nodes and liver has yielded such a high incidence of positive results in patients with no other clinical or radiographic evidence of infradiaphragmatic involvement as to indicate the desirability of incorporating these surgical measures routinely into the diagnostic workup (cf. Chapters 4,8). The procedure is particularly valuable for the detection of Hodgkin's disease in the spleen. Obviously, when Hodgkin's disease is shown to be present in the spleen, it becomes a semantic question whether the splenectomy should be regarded as diagnostic or therapeutic.

Evidence presented in Chapters 4 and 7 indicates that the probability of liver involvement is high, even in the face of negative wedge or needle liver biopsies, whenever splenic involvement preexists. Conversely, the liver is unlikely to be involved when the splenectomy specimen reveals no evidence of Hodgkin's disease. Accordingly, the gross and histologic findings revealed by splenectomy have extremely important implications for treatment planning, particularly with respect to the liver. When performed by experienced surgeons in previously untreated patients with Hodgkin's disease, routine laparotomy, splenectomy, para-aortic node biopsy, and liver biopsy are remarkably free of morbidity and mortality (Glatstein et al., 1969; Enright et al., 1970; Ferguson et al., 1973; Cannon et al., 1975; Poulsen et al., 1977). These results stand in striking contrast to the reported surgical experience with splenectomy in patients with advanced Hodgkin's disease complicated by hemolytic anemia or pancytopenia attributable to hypersplenism (Strawitz et al., 1961; Rousselot et al., 1962; Schultz, Denny, and Ross, 1964). Moreover, the staging laparotomy affords an opportunity to perform oophoropexies, thus permitting shielding of the ovaries and preservation of ovarian function in young female patients who require subsequent irradiation of the pelvic lymph nodes (Ray et al., 1970; Trueblood et al., 1970). Nonetheless, a note of caution is in order: staging laparotomy and splenectomy should not be attempted by surgeons who are likely to perform them sporadically and infrequently, since the experience essential to maintaining a low level of morbidity and mortality cannot be acquired under these circumstances.

Mediastinal exploration may be necessary for diagnostic purposes in patients with roentgenographic evidence of mediastinal adenopathy who lack biopsy-accessible enlargement of peripheral nodes. In such instances, it is highly desirable to limit the procedure to the excision of one or two lymph nodes when possible. However, the surgeon not infrequently encounters a large fused conglomerate mass of nodes, with invasion of other mediastinal tissues, and then must make a decision whether simply to take an incisional biopsy and close the chest again or to attempt complete or incomplete resection of the mass. When frozen-section histopathologic diagnosis is attempted, erroneous diagnoses are not infrequently arrived at initially in patients with malignant lymphomas and particularly in Hodgkin's disease. Such erroneous diagnoses may encourage the surgeon to attempt an extirpative resection, which is usually incomplete, after which permanent sections reveal Hodgkin's disease in the resected specimen. This is a most unfortunate situation, since such patients will, in any case, require postoperative radiotherapy.

Careful exploration by the surgeon may reveal direct invasion of the pericardium or the lung. Tissue samples taken from such sites are helpful in staging, and the placement of silver clips at the biopsied sites assists the radiotherapist in delineating treatment fields of adequate size. Thoracotomy may sometimes be necessary for biopsy of suspicious pulmonary nodules or infiltrates or for biopsy of pleural nodules under direct vision. When pleural disease is suspected, however, it is sometimes possible to obtain biopsy confirmation with the Cope needle, thus obviating the need for thoracotomy. Thoracentesis may document the presence of fluid in the pleural and/or pericardial cavities and provide information concerning the protein content and specific gravity of such effusions, but such evidence should not be relied on too heavily in assessing whether the pleura or pericardium is actually invaded by Hodgkin's disease.

Unlike the situation in the leukemias and lymphocytic lymphomas where bone marrow aspiration is likely to be diagnostic, involvement of the bone marrow by Hodgkin's disease is usually focal in distribution, rendering simple aspiration virtually worthless. Instead, actual tissue biopsy samples must be obtained, usually from the marrow of the iliac crest, either by open surgical removal of a substantial core of bone and bone marrow with the Stryker saw, or by the use of a trephine type of needle, such as the Jamshidi needle, which cuts a core of tissue.

Patients with Hodgkin's disease are by no means immune to a host of other illnesses that afflict mankind. The usual surgical indications are likely to prevail in such patients if they should develop bleeding ulcers, cholelithiasis, gastrointestinal perforations, empyema, lung abscess, appendicitis, or strangulated hernia, to mention only a few examples. In some of these situations, as also those instances in which other primary malignant tumors become manifest, the scope of the surgical procedure should take into account the status of the patient's Hodgkin's disease. When the extent of the Hodgkin's disease is relatively limited and it has responded or is likely to respond well to treatment, major surgery may be indicated for the intercurrent disease; otherwise, and especially in far-advanced cases, more limited surgical procedures may be preferable.

Hemolytic anemia or pancytopenia is a not-uncommon complication in patients with advanced Hodgkin's disease. The presence of palpable splenomegaly in such patients suggests that peripheral blood elements may be undergoing sequestration and destruction in the spleen. Direct confirmation of this possibility is sometimes feasible with the aid of red blood cells tagged with radioactive ^{51}Cr. Although the presence of an autoimmune disorder is usually thought to be the underlying mechanism, direct evidence of circulating red blood cell antibodies, as indicated by a positive Coombs' test, is seldom obtainable. Beneficial responses to steroid therapy are sometimes obtained, but are seldom of long duration. Radiotherapy of the spleen for hypersplenism has in most instances yielded equivocal or disappointing results (Comas et al., 1968). Surgical splenectomy is followed by a prompt and sometimes dramatic restoration of peripheral blood elements to or toward normal levels. However, the procedure is associated with an appreciable operative mortality, in part related to the fact that surgery is often postponed until steroid therapy and other conservative measures have been exhausted, by which time the clinical condition of the patient may have deteriorated to a degree that greatly increases the operative risk (Strawitz et al., 1961; Rousselot et al., 1962; Duckett, 1963; Schultz et al., 1964; Grace and Mittelman, 1966).

One of the complications of radiotherapy that may require surgical intervention is radiation pericarditis (Stewart et al., 1967). Although the great majority of cases are manifested as simple pericardial effusions with few or no cardiac symptoms, clearing spontaneously with bed rest and diuretics, occasional cases progress to tamponade, which may require pericardiocentesis, and some of these, representing an even smaller fraction of the total, go on to chronic constrictive pericarditis. In this small group of cases with irreversible fibrotic and constrictive changes in the pericardium, surgical pericardiectomy is likely to be required and, in our experience to date, has been curative in all but one of the six cases in which it has been attempted.

Radical surgical lymph node dissection alone or in association with postoperative radiotherapy was used for many years for the treatment of selected cases of Hodgkin's disease or other malignant lymphomas presenting as an apparently solitary primary focus. As early as 1922, Yates, in a general discusson of surgical treatment of malignant disease involving lymph nodes, mentions a case with six-and-one-half-year survival after a bilateral groin dissection. Baker and Mann (1939) cited two patients with apparently cured Hodgkin's disease, one surviving without relapse for twelve years after left cervical lymph node dissection in 1926, the other surviving free of disease ten years after right axillary node dissection in 1928. However, both had received modest doses of postoperative X-ray therapy.

Stimulated by these early reports and aware of the limitations of the kilovoltage radiotherapy techniques available in that era, an increasing number of surgeons began to report favorable experiences in selected, apparently localized cases of Hodgkin's disease (Slaughter and Craver, 1942; Slaughter et al., 1958; Holloway, 1965; Schamaun, 1966; Pack and Molander, 1966; Catlin, 1966). By 1947, Hellwig was able to report that 25 percent of his series of 130 patients had survived for five years or more and that of 21 patients with a single primary focus in which radical surgery alone was employed, 12 had survived without recurrence of disease for periods of five to twenty years.

However, Lacher (1963) analyzed in detail the 11 cases among a total of 544 seen at Memorial Hospital in New York in which radical surgery for apparently primary Stage I Hodgkin's disease had been performed. Surgical dissection had been used alone, without supplementary X-ray therapy, in only three of these patients, two of whom survived more than five years, one with active disease to which he later succumbed. The remaining eight patients had also received postoperative X-ray therapy; five of these survived more than five

years, one later dying of Hodgkin's disease. Thus, in the entire group, seven of eleven (64 percent) had survived five years. Lacher noted, however, that the five-year survival of the entire group of ninety-three Stage I patients treated with X-ray therapy alone in the interval between 1949 and 1955 was 66 percent. He concluded that radical surgery had been used in a negligibly small fraction of highly favorable stage I cases, that at least a part of the credit for long survival in some of these cases may have been due to the postoperative X-ray therapy employed, and that the survival rates in this selected group were not superior to those achieved with kilovoltage X-ray therapy alone in a much larger (and presumably less favorable) group of stage I cases.

Today, with the advent of megavoltage radiotherapy, few surgeons still advocate radical lymph node dissection as definitive treatment for localized Hodgkin's disease. Slaughter (1965) made the incomprehensible statement that radical surgery is to be preferred to radiotherapy because its cosmetic results are better! Even in the hands of the most experienced and skilled of surgeons, radical lymph node dissection is, of necessity, a cosmetically disfiguring procedure which may also be associated with significant functional disability, whereas it is now commonplace knowledge that tumoricidal doses of megavoltage radiotherapy may be delivered to entire chains of superficial or deep lymph nodes with little or no skin reaction and, in most instances, no later cosmetic evidence that the area had ever been treated.

Moreover, even the best surgical results, in highly selected cases, are no longer competitive with those obtainable by megavoltage radiotherapy. This is clearly revealed in data from various published series tabulated by Afkham et al. (1969). It is known that the true recurrence rate in involved lymph node chains treated with megavoltage radiotherapy to doses of 4,000 rads or more is only 1 to 4 percent (Kaplan, 1966,1970). In contrast, Afkham et al. observed local recurrences in five of twenty cases (25 percent) treated with radical surgery at Freiburg. Confirming the earlier report of Lacher (1963), they found that the five-year survival in a series of twenty-six patients with stage I disease treated with X-ray therapy alone was 66.8 percent, whereas that in a series of twenty patients treated with surgical resection followed by postoperative X-ray therapy was 57.8 percent; the proportion of patients who remained relapse-free for five years was 43.5 percent versus 20 percent, respectively. They concluded that there is no valid indication for surgery, either alone or in combination with postoperative X-ray therapy, in stage I cases and that the curative method of choice is early wide-field radiotherapy carried to tumoricidal doses. We concur with this view, with two minor exceptions: (1) the rare cases of apparently primary extranodal Hodgkin's disease arising in organs such as the stomach, small intestine, or thyroid, in which surgical resection followed by radiotherapy appears to be the treatment of choice; and (2) isolated instances of local recurrence after high-dose radiotherapy which, in our experience, may sometimes be controlled by limited excisional surgery.

Finally, it should be mentioned that limited excisional surgery also has a useful, though limited, place in the palliative management of some cases of Hodgkin's disease. There are occasional patients among those who develop generalized disseminated disease in whom, despite otherwise satisfactory chemotherapeutic palliation, localized lymph node enlargement may cause pressure or obstructive symptoms. When such lymph node areas have previously received one or more courses of high-dose radiotherapy, limited surgical excision of the enlarging lymph node or nodes may afford prompt and effective palliation without the need of subjecting the patient to the serious hazard of additional radiotherapy in an area where normal tissue tolerance for additional radiation has been significantly depleted.

Nonspecific Supportive Care. Transfusion of whole blood is often required for the relief of anemia in patients with advanced Hodgkin's disease and should be considered when hemoglobin levels fall below 8 to 10 gm. percent. Decisions concerning blood transfusion should be individualized for each patient rather than tied automatically to any arbitrarily selected hemoglobin level. The potential hazards of serum hepatitis, transfusion reactions, and, after large numbers of transfusions, of hemochromatosis must be weighed against the severity of the symptoms attributable to the anemia and the anticipated benefits of transfusion.

Severe thrombocytopenia due to radiotherapy or chemotherapy may be temporarily alleviated and the patient tided over until the marrow can recover sufficiently to produce platelets again in adequate numbers by transfusion of fresh whole blood or of platelet packs. In instances of autoimmune thrombocytopenia or pancytopenia with hypersplenism, transfusion of fresh whole blood or

platelet packs immediately prior to and during surgical splenectomy is indicated to reduce the hazard of hemorrhagic complications, which are not infrequently fatal in such cases. Cryopreserved platelets have also been used in such situations (Schiffer, Aisner, and Wiernik, 1976).

Most infections in Hodgkin's disease occur when the disease is far advanced and becoming increasingly refractory to chemotherapy. As Casazza et al. (1966) have stated: "Successful management of these infections requires effective antineoplastic chemotherapy, accurate diagnosis, and specific therapy of the infectious complication. If the disseminated neoplastic disease cannot be controlled, the patient usually will either die with the initial infection, or with a subsequent episode occurring shortly thereafter." Every effort should be made to identify a specific bacterial or other infectious agent. Careful auscultatory and radiographic examination of the lungs and urinalysis with urine culture are indicated in all cases; less often the locus of infection will be in the skin, gastrointestinal tract, or central nervous system, in which case localizing symptoms or signs are likely to be present. Serial blood, sputum, urine, throat, or stool cultures, as indicated, should be carried out to identify specific organisms and to ascertain their specific antibiotic sensitivity whenever possible. Where the severity of infection requires the initiation of treatment in the absence of an identified specific organism, the high incidence of staphylococcal and gram-negative bacillary infection suggests the desirability of using one of the broad-spectrum agents. Tuberculous infection usually responds well to streptomycin and isonicotinic acid hydrazide.

Fungal infections are likely to be much more insidious, and their antemortem diagnosis often depends on the alertness of the physician to an otherwise unexplained deterioration in the condition of a patient with far-advanced disease. Amphotericin B is generally considered the most effective agent in the treatment of cryptococcosis, histoplasmosis, candidiasis, and aspergillosis, but its use in individual cases must be carefully weighed against the hazard of its considerable nephrotoxicity (Duvall and Carbone, 1966; Littman and Walter, 1968). Sulfonamides are indicated in the treatment of infections due to *Nocardia* and *Toxoplasma*. Pentamidine isethionate, pyrimethamine-sulfadiazine, and trimethoprim-sulfamethoxazole have all been reported to be effective in the treatment of *Pneumocystis carinii* infection (Ivády and Páldy, 1958; Ruskin and Remington,

1968; Minielly et al., 1969; Hughes, Feldman, and Sanyal, 1975; Lau and Young, 1976; Hughes, 1976; Young and De Vita, 1976). To date, no specific therapy is available for disseminated cytomegalic inclusion disease. Localized herpes zoster resolves spontaneously and requires no specific therapy. Recent evidence indicates that life-threatening dissemination may be prevented by prompt administration of human leukocyte interferon (Merigan et al., 1978a).

Pain and tenderness due to bone erosion or pressure on nerves is most effectively treated with radiotherapy when local and with chemotherapy when diffuse. However, when such specific therapy is no longer possible, as in patients with far-advanced, preterminal Hodgkin's disease, the use of analgesic and narcotic drugs of increasing potency may be required for the control of pain. The milder analgesics should always be tried first and for as long as they remain effective before recourse is had to the more powerful narcotics.

Fever and night sweats occurring relatively early in the course of the disease are seldom a therapeutic problem, since they almost invariably respond to the radiotherapeutic or chemotherapeutic measures undertaken for control of other disease manifestations. Recurring in the patient with far-advanced, relatively refractory disease, however, they may be severely debilitating and uncomfortable. Symptomatic treatment with acetylsalicylic acid or indomethacin (Silberman, McGinn, and Kremer, 1965) may then afford effective relief, though these drugs have no effect on the course of the disease. One of our patients with severe fever and night sweats, whose disease had become refractory to certain chemotherapeutic agents but who could not be safely treated with others because of severe leukopenia, was maintained essentially fever-free and in relative comfort with indomethacin alone for slightly more than one month, by which time the white blood cell count had recovered sufficiently to permit the initiation of a new chemotherapeutic agent. Cycloheximide has also been reported to be of value as an antipyretic in Hodgkin's disease (Young and Dowling, 1975).

Generalized pruritus responds well to treatment of the underlying Hodgkin's disease with irradiation or chemical agents. When specific therapy is no longer effective in patients with far-advanced disease, itching may become a profoundly distressing symptom, and the excoriations produced by scratching become an important site of entry for infection. Starch baths and other topical dermatologic measures may then afford some degree of relief. A variety of drugs, such as para-aminobenzoic acid, have also been advocated but appear to have only sporadic effectiveness.

Coexistent Illnesses. Particularly in the older age group, patients with Hodgkin's disease may present one or more coexistent medical conditions that are either immediately or potentially life-threatening. The list includes heart disease, hypertension, severe diabetes, nephritis, extensive tuberculosis, or other malignant tumors. Each such instance must be evaluated individually to assess the severity of the coexistent condition. Not infrequently the grave prognosis of uncontrolled cardiac failure or diabetes or of an independent primary malignant tumor may preempt the physician's therapeutic attention and relegate the Hodgkin's disease to secondary status. Where the situation created by the other illness is less immediately life-threatening, it may nonetheless carry significant implications with respect to the patient's probable tolerance for intensive treatment and thus temper the physician's judgment in the direction of more limited forms of curative therapy or toward treatment with palliative rather than curative intent.

Miscellaneous Other Factors. Patients of certain religious sects are not permitted by their religious convictions to accept blood transfusions. Those with localized disease are readily treated with local radiotherapy, with essentially no significant hematopoietic risk. When the disease is more extensive, however, and would ordinarily entail the intensive irradiation of virtually all major lymph node regions or the use of combination chemotherapy, during which hematopoietic depression is occasionally severe enough to require transfusion, the appropriateness of such treatment must be weighed with particular care. Sometimes, it may be possible to proceed with only slight modifications of the treatment plan, such as the utilization of longer rest intervals between the irradiation of successive lymphoid regions to ensure more complete hematopoietic recovery. When combination chemotherapy is employed, it is desirable to watch the peripheral blood cell counts with particular care and to be prepared to reduce drug dose levels, particularly in the later cycles of the course of treatment, somewhat more readily than would ordinarily be the case. Despite the potential added risk which the prohibition of blood transfusions introduces into their care, we have encountered no really serious difficulty in the treatment of several such patients in recent years, some with intensive radiotherapy and others with chemotherapy.

Patients with Hodgkin's disease who live in remote areas with relatively poor access to medical care and who may have to travel long distances to the nearest major medical center often represent very difficult problems of management. Complications of radiotherapy such as radiation pneumonitis or pericarditis are unlikely to come to medical attention early and thus constitute a serious hazard. Patients requiring prolonged maintenance chemotherapy cannot travel to the major medical center at frequent intervals and may not even be able to visit their personal physicians as often as would be desired for serial blood cell counts and adjustment of chemotherapeutic doses. A final category includes patients with psychoses or mental retardation who are unable to comprehend or cooperate in more complex forms of treatment. These patients, as well as those coming from remote rural areas, are sometimes best treated with limited measures, such as local radiotherapy or single-drug chemotherapy, employing agents of relatively low toxicity whenever possible.

Chapter 12

Prognosis

Survival as Related to Treatment

Historical Aspects. It has been recognized since the turn of the century that survival times in Hodgkin's disease may display an almost bewildering variability (Ziegler, 1911). Some patients are first seen with generalized disease and severe constitutional symptoms; the disease runs a fulminating course, and the patient dies within a few weeks or months. In others, asymptomatic peripheral lymphadenopathy may progress indolently, sometimes almost imperceptibly, over a period of several years, sometimes punctuated by episodes of spontaneous regression before finally becoming generalized and going on to a fatal termination many years after its first manifestation. As the number of such anecdotal reports proliferated, it was not surprising that clinicians came to regard the course of the disease as notoriously unpredictable, with the exception of one seeming certainty, its eventually fatal outcome. It was not until survival data on several large series of consecutive cases became available that the powerful methods of modern statistical analysis could be applied to bring order and predictability out of seeming chaos.

In important papers which have not received the attention they deserved, Osgood (1958) and Rigat (1958) independently discovered that the survival of patients dying of Hodgkin's disease follows a logarithmic probability distribution, as had previously been shown to be true for many types of cancer and leukemia (Boag, 1949). When a logarithmic scale is used to plot survival time, measured either from the time of apparent onset of the disease or from the time of diagnosis or first treatment, and the proportion of patients surviving at various intervals of time is plotted on a probability unit (probit) scale, the resulting survival curve is seen to be approximately linear. Osgood emphasized the importance of observing certain criteria in the selection of data from the literature for such statistical analyses: "The series should

show evidence that all ages and both sexes were included, that all patients whose biopsies revealed Dorothy Reed cells and who were referred for treatment were included, and that at least five and preferably more points for plotting the survival curves were given."

By pooling 650 cases of Hodgkin's disease from the series reported by Nathanson and Welch (1937), Shimkin et al. (1955), and Stout (1949), which he considered a representative sample of cases reflecting the standards of treatment prevailing at major centers in the 1930's and 1940's, Osgood obtained a linear reference curve for the duration of the disease, *measured from the time of onset of symptoms.* This curve indicated a median survival time of 33.3 months with a log standard deviation (SD) of 0.412, yielding estimates that 15.9 percent of patients die within 12.9 months and that 84.1 percent die within 86 months. The cases reported by Nice and Stenstrom (1954) and by Bethell et al. (1950) were similarly combined to yield a second series of 343 cases in which the duration of the disease *measured from the time of diagnosis or first treatment* could be estimated from the linear reference curve obtained on a logarithmic-probability plot. This curve was characterized by a median survival of 20.8 months, with log SD = 0.612, corresponding to 15.9 percent mortality by five months and 84.1 percent mortality at 85 months.

Osgood discussed a number of alternative methods for valid statistical comparison of other series of cases with the survival pattern described by these two reference curves: "For large series, individual points of the series may be compared with these reference curves using two standard errors for binomial probability determined as described by Mosteller and Tukey (1949). By connecting a series of such points, a confidence band at any desired level for any number of cases may be drawn on either side of the reference curve." As an example, he plotted the data of Hall and Olson (1956) on thirty-one patients treated with nitrogen mustard with or without X-ray therapy and on thirty-one other patients treated with X-ray therapy only and showed that both series of points lay within the 95 percent confidence intervals for the reference curve for survival plotted from the time of onset of the disease. In smaller series, Osgood advocated the use of the random number sign test, described by Dixon and Massey (1957), as a simple and convenient method which can also be utilized for comparisons of specific factors within a series under investigation, such as age, sex, and other variables. The maximum likelihood method of logarithmic probability analysis (Lea, 1945) is available for more rigorous evaluations. The considerably greater mathematical complexity of this method was formerly a deterrent to its use, but this problem has been largely eliminated by the increasing availability of modern digital computers.

A longstanding misconception about Hodgkin's disease is that treatment does not significantly influence survival. This view dates back to 1926, when Minot and Isaacs analyzed the survival of 401 patients known to have died of malignant lymphomas, of whom 238 had received some form of radiotherapy. Although the remaining 163 had not received any irradiation, 33 are stated to have had surgery "with removal of a considerable amount of disease tissue." From this study, Minot and Isaacs reached the following conclusion: "These data suggest that this therapy (irradiation) had lengthened particularly the life of patients destined by nature to have their disease less than two and a half years, and has not influenced the course of those living long." It is ironic that this paper came to be regarded as a classic, whereas that of Osgood remained largely unheralded and unappreciated, particularly since the ill-founded conclusion reached by Minot and Isaacs immediately withers under critical scrutiny. Indeed, the pitfalls in their study are almost too numerous to mention. They considered the various histologic types of malignant lymphomas not separately but rather as an indiscriminate mixture of 477 cases, of which only 173 were stated to have been instances of Hodgkin's disease. They made no attempt to analyze the quality or scope of the radiotherapy given to their treated series; presumably even the patients with disease so far advanced that they were able to receive only a few palliative X-ray treatments before death are also included in the "treated" series. Finally, they excluded living patients from their analysis, and thus the small group of long-term survivors who might have provided the first indication of the curative potential of radiotherapy were effectively eliminated from

consideration. Yet, their conclusion continued to be handed down almost as an article of faith from decade to decade for more than forty years! As recently as 1964, in an otherwise excellent review of the subject, a leading authority again reiterated this view (Aisenberg, 1964): "Although statistical proof that therapy alters prognosis is not yet available, there can be no question of the marked improvement in morbidity that can be achieved by judicious treatment."

It is undoubtedly true that serious pitfalls beset any attempt to evaluate the influence of treatment on survival solely on the basis of retrospective analysis of published series of cases. Some of the difficulties have been clearly stated by Shimkin (1964): "It is still impossible, however, to determine what proportion of the survival results can be attributed to specific therapy when we consider the actual data. None of these retrospective analyses includes acceptable controls, or concurrent groups of similar patients treated by different modalities. Moreover, it is difficult to establish comparative reports because the data are too widespread and varied to be conclusive. Such variations as characteristics of patients, extent of the disease at diagnosis, diagnostic criteria, medical procedures that have been introduced or discarded, and reasons for selection of patients for admission and for treatment, all invalidate sound comparison . . . In order to replace clinical opinions with scientific quantitation, we must use the biometrically designed clinical trial, in which we compare treatments on patients by randomization . . . These clinical trials would not only define the best available procedures, but they would also create a foundation for further progress in the therapy of Hodgkin's disease."

Influence of Treatment on Survival. Though undoubtedly aware of these pitfalls, Osgood (1958) nonetheless attempted to assess whether any of the larger series of reported cases treated by radiotherapy showed a significantly better survival than that characterized by his reference curves, taking pains to consider only those published reports that met his stringent criteria quoted above. He was able to find only three series of patients whose survival differed significantly from the reference curves. Of these, the data from the 1950 report of Dr. Vera Peters were the most impressive, yielding a best fit log-probability curve with an observed median of 50 months, extrapolating to 14 percent survival at 25 years. The survival data reported by Medinger and Craver (1942) were also stated to be significantly better than Osgood's reference curve, though scrutiny of the data points plotted by Osgood suggests that this superiority is valid only for the first four years after treatment, after which the survival in the Medinger-Craver series becomes equal to and then inferior to that of the reference curve. The third reported series is that of Smetana and Cohen (1956), which is open to the criticism that it represents a highly selected military population.

Curiously, Osgood made no attempt to ascertain whether the survival of his reference curve cases, representing the composite data of Nice and Stenstrom (1954) and of Bethell et al. (1950) on patients treated predominantly by low-dose kilovoltage radiotherapy, was significantly better than that of patients receiving no specific therapy at all. Since few physicians today would withhold therapy from patients with biopsy-proved Hodgkin's disease, data on survival of essentially untreated patients must necessarily be derived from studies published many years ago, when certain forms of supportive therapy such as antibiotics and blood transfusions, as well as specific chemotherapy, were unavailable. However, Osgood pointed out that survival of the first 102 patients treated by Nice and Stenstrom in the preantibiotic era before 1935 did not differ significantly from that of their 122 patients treated subsequently. Similarly, Gellhorn and Collins (1951), Osgood (1958), and Shimkin et al. (1955) observed no significant difference in survival of patients treated before and after the introduction of alkylating agents. Accordingly, it seems permissible to use the data from the older published reports to construct a composite baseline reference curve for the anticipated survival of essentially untreated cases of Hodgkin's disease.

In the analysis that follows, a great many reported series of cases in the literature have been reviewed, and those have been selected which either met the criteria of Osgood, stated above, or were otherwise deemed essential for the purposes of this analysis, despite certain drawbacks. These series have been grouped into four categories according to the major form of treatment employed: (a) essentially untreated patients; (b) patients treated with low-dose kilovoltage radiotherapy, without "prophylactic" treatment to apparently uninvolved lymph node regions; (c) patients treated with high-dose kilovoltage radiotherapy, usually with "prophylactic" or "segmental" treatment of apparently uninvolved lymph node regions; and (d) patients treated to high doses with megavoltage radiotherapy, using the extended-field or "total lymphoid" techniques described in Chapter 9. It should be recognized that, although all stages of disease are included in each of these series, they are not necessarily represented in equal proportions. Even in those series in which the stage distribution is stated, progress in the methods of diagnostic evaluation and staging make valid comparisons within stages impossible. It should also be noted that some of the reported data refer to observed survival at different time intervals, whereas survival in other series has been analyzed by the actuarial methods of Boag (1949), Berkson and Gage (1950), or Haybittle (1959).

The series selected for analysis and the actual data are set forth in Tables 12.1, 12.2, and 12.3. A conventional linear plot of percentage survival versus time has been constructed by plotting data points from representative series of each of the four therapeutic categories, as shown in Figure 12.1. After the first year, there is no overlap between the survival data on patients receiving no specific therapy and those receiving low-dose kilovoltage radiotherapy without "prophylactic" treatment. Further improvement in results is seen in the group treated with high-dose kilovoltage radiotherapy, and another increment of improvement has resulted from the introduction of extended-field megavoltage radiotherapy techniques.

In an effort to provide a more rigorous comparison, the data of seven series of essentially untreated cases summarized in Table 12.1 have been pooled to construct a composite reference curve in an Osgood-type logarithmic-probability plot. This curve is compared in Figure 12.2 with Osgood's reference curve for survival measured from the time of apparent onset of disease, which was constructed from the 650 pooled patients of Shimkin et al. (1955), Stout (1949), and Nathanson and Welch (1937), most of whom were probably treated with low-dose kilovoltage radiotherapy. Consistent with this surmise, it may be seen that the data of Merner and Stenstrom (1947) for survival from the time of apparent onset in a series of 185 patients treated with low-dose kilovoltage radiotherapy without "prophylactic" therapy, and the data of Videbaek (1950) on similarly treated patients, conform very closely to Osgood's reference curve (Fig. 12.3). In contrast, the composite reference curve for essentially untreated patients shows a significantly poorer survival than that of patients receiving low-dose kilovoltage radiotherapy. It is important to recognize that these "essentially untreated" patients constitute a motley collection. As stated, some of the patients of Minot and

Table 12.1 Survival as Related to Treatment in Hodgkin's Disease (All Stages)

A. No Specific Therapy; Untreated Cases

Author and year	No. of cases	Survival (years)[a]																		
		1		2		3		4		5		6		7		8		9		10
		No.	%	No.	%	No.	%	No.	%	No.	%	No.	%	No.	%	No.	%	No.	%	No.	%
1. Craft, 1940	52	18	34.6	11	21.2	8	15.4	3	5.8	3	5.8	2	3.8	2	3.8	2	3.8	2	3.8	0	—
2. Minot & Isaacs, 1926	163[b]	106	65.0	64	39.0	39	24.0	29	18.0	18	11.0	13	8.0	9	5.5	6	3.5	4	—	3	1.4
3. Desjardins and Ford, 1923	135[c]	—	—	—	—	—	—	—	—	10	7.4	—	—	—	—	—	—	—	—	—	—
4. Uddströmer, 1934	494[d]	331	67.0	203	41.0	109	22.0	55	11.2	30	6.1	11	2.3	7	1.5	3	0.7	0	0	—	—
5. Shimkin et al., 1955	13	7		4		2		2		2	16.0										
6. Stout, 1949	32[e]	7	47	2	32	1	11	1		1		1		1		1		1		1	
7. Greco et al., 1974	80	20	25	17	21	11	14	9	11	8	10	8	10	8	10	8	10	6	8	6	8
Composite totals	834	$\frac{489}{834} = 58.6$		$\frac{301}{812} = 37.1$		$\frac{170}{807} = 21.1$		$\frac{99}{803} = 12.3$		$\frac{72}{938} = 7.7$		$\frac{35}{803} = 4.4$		$\frac{27}{803} = 3.4$		$\frac{20}{803} = 2.5$		$\frac{13}{803} = 1.6$		$\frac{9}{802} = 1.1$	

[a] From onset of disease.

[b] All types of malignant lymphomas; only 36% had Hodgkin's disease; 33/163 had incomplete surgical resections.

[c] Only 92 available for analysis.

[d] Minority of patients received small doses of radiotherapy.

[e] Thirty-one died within three years, last in ninth year. Actuarial analysis of survival derived from raw data.

Table 12.2   Survival as Related to Treatment in Hodgkin's Disease (All Stages)
B. *Low-dose Radiotherapy: No "Prophylactic" Irradiation; Prechemotherapy Era*

Author and year	No. of cases	Survival (years)[a]																			
		1		2		3		4		5		6		7		8		9		10	
		No.	%	No.	%	No.	%	No.	%	No.	%	No.	%	No.	%	No.	%	No.	%	No.	%
1. Craft, 1940	179	131	73.2		58	65/149	43.6		29	30/128	23.4	14/100	17		14.0		10.5		9	5/45	11.1
2. Westling, 1965	31[b]	21	68			14	45			9	29										
3. Videbaek, 1950	172		89[d]		72		52		38		28		20		16		9		4		3
4. Lampe and Fayos, 1968	69									14	20.3										
5.a Merner and Stenstrom, 1947	185	111	60[e]	85	46	67	36	53/170	31	33/160	21	21/147	14	19/134	14	16/122	13	12/107	11	8/102	8
5.b Merner and Stenstrom, 1947			85[f]		62				44		34		29				18				10
6. Peters, 1966	49[c]										12										2
7. Rigat, 1958	140									30	21.4							7/86	8.1		
8. Appel, Jaeschke, and Vermund, 1961	121	72	59	55	45	43	35	39	32	32	26	12/87	14		14	8/64	12			1/25	4

[a] After first treatment unless otherwise stated.
[b] Patients admitted 1926–1935 (his tables 26, 27, and 28).
[c] Low-dose group; no prophylactic treatment.
[d] Survival calculated from date of onset.
[e] Survival computed from date of first treatment.
[f] Survival computed from date of onset of disease.

Table 12.3 Survival as Related to Treatment in Hodgkin's Disease (All Stages)

C. *High-dose (Kilovoltage) Radiotherapy*

Author and year	No. of cases	Survival (years)[a]																				Comment
		1		2		3		4		5		6		7		8		9		10		
		No.	%	No.	%	No.	%	No.	%	No.	%	No.	%	No.	%	No.	%	No.	%	No.	%	
1. Gilbert, 1939	46									13	34.2											21 patients not treated by "segmental" technique were excluded
2. Gilbert, 1951	94									32	34									17/67	25	10.6% at 15 yrs.; 8.5% at 20 yrs.
3. Hynes, 1955	31									16	52									4/19	21	"Segmental" technique
4. Peters, 1950	113		77		62		57		54	58	51		43		39		34		34	19/54	35	31% at 15 yrs.
5. Peters & Middlemiss, 1958	221									95	43									40/139	29	16/64 (25%) at 15 yrs.; 6/23 (26%) at 20 yrs.
6. Peters, 1966	319									127	40									82	26	43/215 (20%) at 15 yrs.; 23/127 (18%) at 20 yrs.
7. Easson, 1966	1064									342	32.1									148/686	21.6	67/319 (21.0%) at 15 yrs.
8. Healy, Amory & Friedman, 1955	216									82	37									15	6	"Prophylactic" treatment in stages I and II
9. Lampe & Fayos, 1968	106							55		43	40.6											No "prophylactic" treatment
10. Hynes, 1969	64		94		67		61			32	50				38					18/57	32	"Sequential" technique
11. Jelliffe & Thomson, 1955	171									50	29											
12. Papillon et al, 1966	231			148	64	123	53			89	39									20/113	18	6/47 (13%) at 15 yrs.
13. Musshoff & Boutis, 1968	340		87.5				63.4			127/264	48.0									39/136	23.7	27 treated with ^{60}Co, 1964–66; 20 treated with chemotherapy only
13a. Musshoff, Boutis, Laszlo & Laszlo, 1966	287	248	87.1	202/284	71.1	157/268	58.6	120/254	47.2	91/224	40.6	73/197	37	55/162	34	44/148	30	34/121	28	20/79	20.2	
14. Westling, 1965	112	89	79	54	48					42	37											
15. Glinska et al, 1969	617									163	26											Patients admitted 1946–55 (from his tables 27 & 28)

[a] After diagnosis or start of treatment.

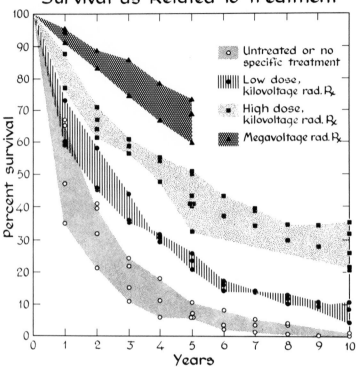

Figure 12.1 The progressive and dramatic change in survival of patients with Hodgkin's disease of all stages from (1) the era in which no specific therapy was utilized (open circles, dark stippling) to (2) the era of relatively low-dose kilovoltage radiotherapy (solid circles, vertical stripes) to (3) the era of high-dose kilovoltage radiotherapy, usually accompanied by "prophylactic" treatment of apparently uninvolved regions (closed squares, pale stippling) to (4) the era of intensive extended-field or total-lymphoid megavoltage radiotherapy (closed triangles, cross-hatching). The data points are those of the references cited in Tables 12.1, 12.2, and 12.3.

Isaacs (1926) did not have Hodgkin's disease but had other malignant lymphomas, and some were treated by incomplete surgical resection. An unstated number of the patients reported by Uddströmer (1934) probably received small doses of X-rays, and an unstated number of patients in several of the series, particularly those treated in the earliest decades represented by these reports, received arsenicals and various sera and vaccines. Nonethless, for all their limitations, these are the only—and therefore the best—data we have, and any prolongation of survival resulting from any of the nonspecific treatments mentioned would only have had the effect of minimizing rather than ex-

aggerating any differences in survival which this analysis has disclosed.

The other Osgood reference curve refers to survival after diagnosis or first treatment and is based on the pooled data of Nice and Stenstrom (1954) and of Bethell et al. (1950), which may be considered representative of survival from the time of diagnosis or first treatment in patients treated with low-dose kilovoltage radiotherapy without "prophylactic" treatment. Confirming this impression, the data of Merner and Stenstrom (1947), computed from the time of first treatment for patients treated with low-dose kilovoltage radiotherapy, are again shown to conform closely to Osgood's reference curve. The median survival times from diagnosis in a series of 33 patients with advanced Hodgkin's disease treated with sequential single-agent chemotherapy (25 months in 14 patients with stage IIIB, 16 months in 19 patients with stage IV disease; Brook and Gocka, 1972) also fall

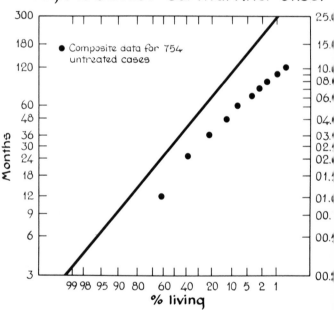

Figure 12.2 Logarithm of survival after the time of onset of Hodgkin's disease plotted against the proportion of cases (in probability units, or probits) surviving for various intervals (log-probit plot). The heavy solid line is the reference curve of Osgood (1958), constructed from 650 cases pooled from the series of Nathanson and Welch (1937), Stout (1949), and Shimkin et al. (1955). The solid circles are the composite data on 754 essentially untreated patients from the six published series of Table 12.1. The survival of the untreated patients appears significantly poorer than that of patients included in Osgood's reference curve.

Hodgkin's Disease: Survival After Onset

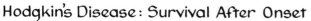

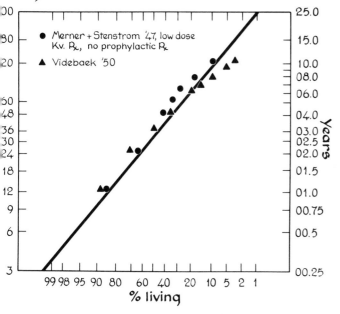

Figure 12.3 Log probit plot showing the survival data (from time of onset) of Merner and Stenstrom (1947) and of Videbaek (1950) for patients with Hodgkin's disease of all stages treated with low-dose kilovoltage radiotherapy. The excellent fit to Osgood's reference curve strongly suggests that the latter was comprised predominantly of cases treated in the same way.

in close proximity to the reference curve. In striking contrast are two other sets of data also presented in Figure 12.4: the survival data reported by Dr. Vera Peters in 1950, predominantly but not exclusively composed of patients treated with high-dose kilovoltage radiotherapy with "prophylactic" treatment to apparently uninvolved regions; and an early analysis (Kaplan, 1970) of our own survival experience with a homogeneous series of patients treated with high-dose megavoltage radiotherapy, most of whom also received "prophylactic" high-dose treatment to apparently uninvolved lymphoid structures. Dr. Peters' data, as was earlier established by Osgood, are significantly better than those of Osgood's reference curve, and our megavoltage data are significantly better than both the reference curve and Peters' (1950) data. To further illustrate the historical change in prognosis, five-year survival data for patients with all stages of disease from the untreated series of Craft (1940), the high-dose kilovoltage X-ray-treated series of Peters (1961), and our current treatment results (Kaplan, 1978) are compared in Figure 12.5.

Moreover, there has been a significant and progressive improvement in prognosis during the past two decades. This is evident from the curves for survival and freedom from relapse in previously untreated patients with disease of all stages admitted to Stanford University Medical Center during three successive five-year accession periods (Fig. 12.6), as well as in a comparison of data on survival and freedom from relapse in all of the early Stanford clinical trials (1962–1968), as contrasted with the most recent series of protocols initiated in 1974 (Fig. 12.7). Similarly, Aisenberg and Qazi (1976) noted that five-year survival, which was only 34 percent in a series of patients seen at the Massachusetts General Hospital between 1948 and 1964, improved to 65 percent in the group admitted between July 1965 and November 1968, with a further improvement to 87 percent among patients admitted between November 1968 and

Hodgkin's Disease: Survival After 1ST Treatment or Diagnosis

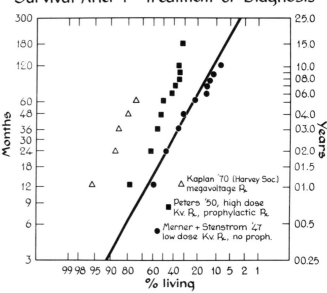

Figure 12.4 Log probit plot of Osgood's reference curve for survival from the time of diagnosis or start of treatment (solid line), together with data for three other comparable series of cases: those of Merner and Stenstrom (1947), treated with low-dose kilovoltage radiotherapy; those of Peters (1950), treated with high-dose kilovoltage radiotherapy, including prophylactic treatment of apparently uninvolved regions; and those of Kaplan (1970), treated with intensive megavoltage radiotherapy. Whereas the data of Merner and Stenstrom lie on the reference curve, those of Peters are significantly more favorable; and the megavoltage data are shifted still further toward greater longevity.

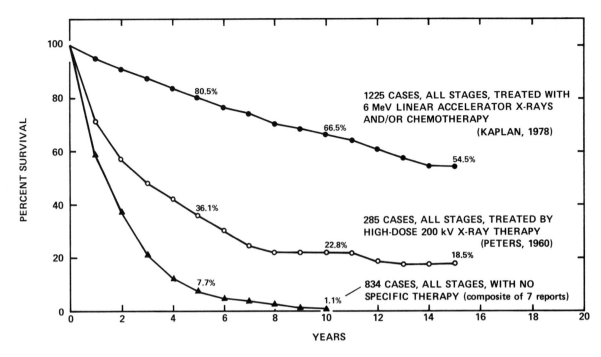

Figure 12.5 Comparison of representative five-year survival data from three different eras for patients with Hodgkin's disease of all stages: the series of untreated cases summarized in Table 12.1; the series reported by Peters (1960), treated with high-dose kilovoltage radiotherapy; and the Stanford University Medical Center series, treated with intensive megavoltage radiotherapy and/or (since 1968) combination chemotherapy.

July 1973. Thus, contrary to the discredited dictum of Minot and Isaacs (1926), it is clear that treatment does indeed significantly prolong survival of patients with Hodgkin's disease and that survival has progressively improved with advances in staging, radiotherapy, and chemotherapy.

Clinical Factors Correlated with Prognosis of Previously Untreated Patients

A number of clinical factors have been reported to relate to the prognosis of Hodgkin's disease. Of these, undoubtedly the most important are the

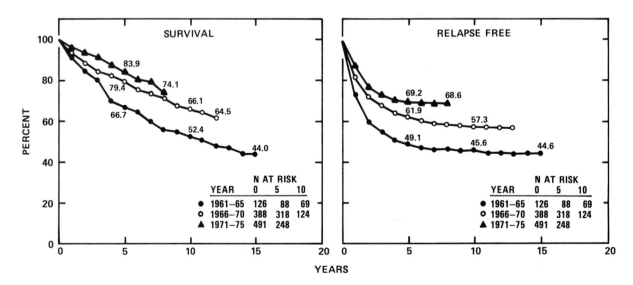

Figure 12.6 Actuarial analysis of survival and freedom from relapse of patients with Hodgkin's disease of all stages admitted and treated at Stanford University Medical Center during three successive five-year accession periods.

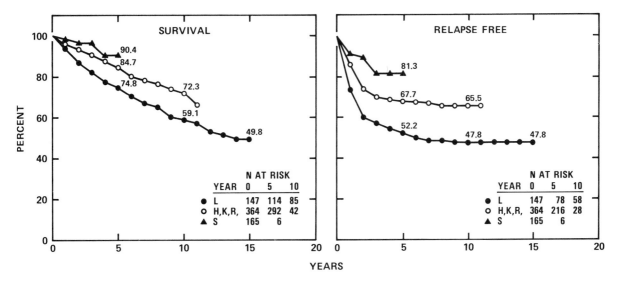

Figure 12.7 Actuarial analysis of survival and freedom from relapse of patients admitted to randomized clinical trials at Stanford University Medical Center during three different periods: 1962–1967, the L-1 and L-2 protocols, dealing with stages I–III; 1967–1974, the H-1 through H-7, R-1, and K-1 protocols (stages I–IV); and 1974 to 1979, the S-1 through S-8 protocols (stages I–IV). The design of each of these clinical trials is described in Chapter 11.

clinical stage of the disease at the time of diagnosis, the presence or absence of constitutional symptoms, and the histopathologic form of the disease. The influence of such other factors as age and sex is more difficult to evaluate, since these are not independent variables but are, in themselves, related to the clinical extent of disease, to histopathologic type, and to the probability of occurrence of certain constitutional symptoms. Axtell et al. (1972) have applied adjustment procedures developed by Hankey and Myers (1971) to separate out the individual contributions to prognosis of multiple interacting factors.

During the interval from 1961 through 1977, 1,225 previously untreated patients with Hodgkin's disease were admitted and treated at Stanford University Medical Center. Essentially all patients were staged with the aid of lymphangiography, and since July 1968 all but overt stage IV cases have been staged with the aid of laparotomy and splenectomy. All cases have been staged prospectively or retrospectively in accordance with the Ann Arbor classification. Retrospective restaging was of course subject to significant error in patients admitted between 1961 and July 1968. Treatment policies have also undergone evolution during this interval. For example, virtually all patients with stage III and stage IV disease were treated palliatively prior to 1962, and the "total lymphoid" radiotherapy technique did not come into use until that year. MOPP combination chemotherapy for

advanced and for relapsing disease was adopted at Stanford in August 1968. Despite these limitations, the data have the merit of being relatively homogeneous in two respects: the patients were nearly all evaluated by one group of clinical investigators; and they represent the first large series in which primary treatment of all but the most advanced, disseminated cases was with megavoltage radiotherapy techniques, employing dose levels which are acceptable by current standards.

This series of 1,225 cases has been submitted to actuarial analysis of survival and freedom from relapse (Fig. 12.8) by the method of Berkson and Gage (1950, 1952). Survival and freedom from relapse curves for the more homogeneous subset of 923 patients admitted since 1968 and staged prospectively after laparotomy are presented in Figure 12.9. In the section that follows, the Stanford data are further analyzed with respect to such factors as the anatomic extent of disease (clinical stage), presence or absence of constitutional symptoms, and histopathologic type.

Anatomic Extent of Disease. Peters (1950) was the first to call attention to the fact that the anatomic extent of involvement at the time of admission determines survival of patients with Hodgkin's disease. Indeed, the three-stage clinical classification which she introduced evolved out of a retrospective analysis of factors correlated with survival. She observed that in patients with disease of stage I ex-

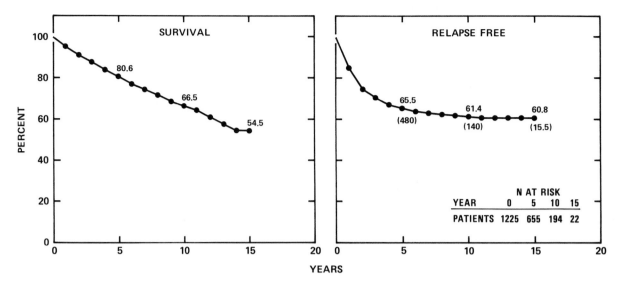

Figure 12.8   Actuarial analysis of survival and freedom from relapse of 1,225 patients with Hodgkin's disease of all stages admitted and treated at Stanford University Medical Center from 1961 through 1977. The numbers of patients at risk at 5, 10, and 15 years are indicated in the insert.

tent, defined as involvement of a single lymph node region or a single lesion elsewhere in the body, the survival rate was consistently high at both the five- (88 percent) and the ten-year mark (79 percent). In stage II, defined as involvement of two or more "proximal" lymph node regions of either the upper or the lower trunk, the five-year survival was high (72 percent), but there was a tremendous drop by ten years (21 percent), suggesting that stage II cases have an intermediate prognosis. Finally, the stage III group, defined as having in-

volvement of two or more lymph node regions of both the upper and lower trunk, showed a consistently poor prognosis, with a five-year survival of only 9 percent and no survivors at the end of ten years.

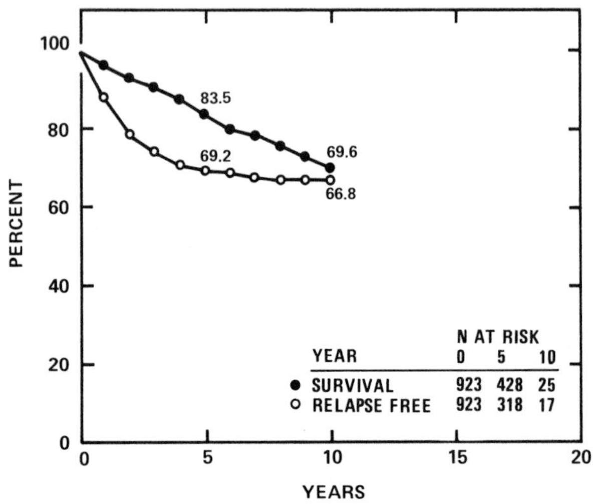

Although the staging definitions and the survival figures have both undergone modification in the course of time (Chapter 8), the basic observation of Peters, that the anatomic extent of disease is the single most important factor influencing survival of patients with Hodgkin's disease, still holds true today. Virtually all publications on the subject since 1950 and particularly those involving relatively large numbers of cases (Jelliffe and Thomson, 1955; Easson and Russell, 1963; Westling, 1965; Easson, 1966; Kaplan, 1966, 1970, 1973; Musshoff and Boutis, 1968; Aisenberg and Qazi, 1976; Björkholm et al., 1977b) have provided additional documentation of this conclusion.

Survival and freedom from relapse of the entire 1961–1977 Stanford series of 1,225 patients have been analyzed with respect to Ann Arbor clinical stage in Figure 12.10 and Table 12.4. A similar analysis has been made of the more homogeneous subset of 923 patients admitted since 1968 and staged with the aid of lymphangiography, marrow biopsy, and laparotomy with splenectomy (Fig. 12.11). It is again evident in these curves that survival and freedom from relapse are related to the anatomic extent of disease at the time of admission. Analysis of survival and freedom from relapse in three successive five-year accession periods (Kaplan, 1977) reveals that improvement in prognosis,

Figure 12.9   Actuarial analysis of the more homogeneous subset of 923 patients admitted to Stanford University Medical Center since 1968 and staged prospectively with the aid of laparotomy and splenectomy.

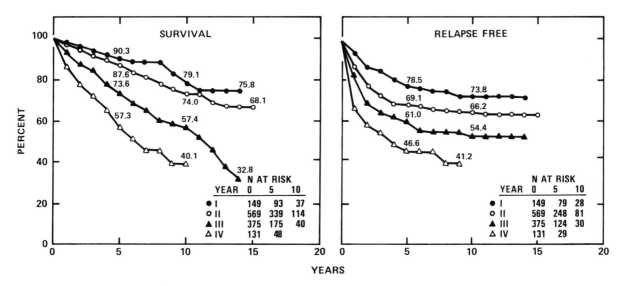

Figure 12.10   Actuarial analysis of survival and freedom from relapse of the entire Stanford series of 1,225 patients, subclassified with respect to Ann Arbor clinical stage.

as expected, has been most dramatic in stages III and IV, a conclusion also supported by the data of Aisenberg and Qazi (1976).

There is also some evidence that prognosis may depend upon the anatomic extent of disease within a single stage. At the Royal Marsden Hospital, Peckham et al. (1975) found that relapse-free survival in patients with stage IIA disease was a function of the number of lymph node sites involved. Among patients with only two or three involved lymph node chains, relapse rate by three to four

years was only about 40 percent, whereas among those with more than three lymph node chains involved, it was in excess of 90 percent at two years. Carmel and Kaplan (1976) found an approximately linear relationship between the number of supradiaphragmatic sites initially involved and the probability of supradiaphragmatic relapse (Fig. 12.12). In an analysis of patients with pathologic stage IIIA disease, Hoppe et al. (1979a) also found that those with more than four sites (lymph node regions and/or spleen) involved had a significantly

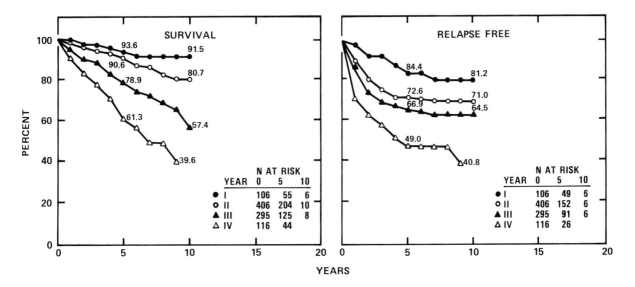

Figure 12.11   Influence on prognosis of anatomical extent of disease. Actuarial analysis of survival and freedom from relapse of the more homogeneous subset of 923 laparotomy-staged patients admitted since 1968, subclassified with respect to Ann Arbor clinical stage.

Table 12.4 Actuarial Survival of 1,225 Previously Untreated Patients with Hodgkin's Disease Staged According to the Ann Arbor (1971) Clinical Staging Classification and Treated at Stanford University Medical Center, 1961–1977

Years at risk	No. cases at risk[b]	Actuarial survival[a] (%) by clinical stage										
		IA, I_EA (n = 140)	IIA, II_SA (n = 355)	IB, I_EB + IIB, II_SB (n = 127)	II_EA, II_{ES}A + II_EB, II_{ES}B (n = 97)	IIIA (n = 217)	IIIB (n = 158)	IVA (n = 40)	IVB (n = 91)	All A's (n = 814)	All B's (n = 411)	All cases (n = 1,225)
0–1	1,200.0	98.6	98.8	96.7	95.8	96.7	87.7	87.5	85.6	97.4	90.8	95.2
1–2	1,062.5	97.0	97.0	88.1	95.8	93.0	79.6	82.0	76.3	95.1	82.9	91.0
2–3	909.0	95.2	95.3	83.7	86.9	91.2	75.9	78.7	69.6	92.9	77.5	87.7
3–4	781.0	93.2	93.0	82.8	84.1	86.2	66.9	78.7	60.0	90.0	71.8	83.7
4–5	654.5	91.1	91.7	78.4	84.1	83.7	60.4	78.7	48.4	88.4	65.6	80.5
5–6	536.5	89.9	86.7	75.9	84.1	77.5	57.2	71.5	43.4	84.2	62.6	76.8
6–7	433.5	89.9	83.8	73.1	84.1	75.1	53.5	71.5	37.2	82.3	59.2	74.3
7–8	349.0	89.9	81.8	68.1	81.2	69.1	50.4	—	37.2	79.7	56.2	71.5
8–9	268.0	84.1	79.4	63.7	81.2	65.1	50.4	—	37.2	76.1	54.5	68.6
9–10	195.5	79.4	76.5	63.7	81.2	65.1	47.6	—	37.2	73.5	53.4	66.5
10–11	134.5	76.1	76.5	63.7	81.2	60.3	43.8	—	—	72.1	50.2	64.5
11–12	88.5	76.1	70.7	63.7	81.2	54.2	37.9	—	—	67.8	47.8	60.9
12–13	57.0	76.1	70.7	54.6	81.2	47.0	28.4	—	—	66.2	41.2	57.7
13–14	36.5	76.1	70.7	54.6	—	37.6	—	—	—	63.8	36.4	54.5
14–15	21.5	—	70.7	—	—	—	—	—	—	63.8	36.4	54.5

[a] Method of Berkson and Gage (1950).

[b] Number of cases at risk at the middle of each year, before adjustment for patients dying of intercurrent disease or no longer at risk. Tabulation stopped when fewer than 5 cases remained at risk in any group.

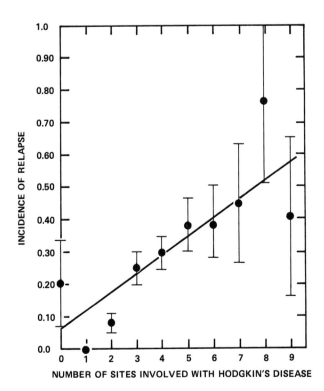

Figure 12.12 Supradiaphragmatic relapse rate as a function of the number of supradiaphragmatic sites initially involved. (Reprinted, by permission of the Editor of *Cancer,* from the paper by Carmel and Kaplan, 1976.)

greater risk of relapse than those with fewer stage III sites involved; in the subgroup of patients admitted to the H-5 and S-4 clinical trials, this was also reflected in a significant difference in survival.

Desser et al. (1977) subdivided patients with stage III disease into two substages, III_1 and III_2, on the basis of the anatomic sites of lymph node involvement documented at staging laparotomy. Stage III_1 included patients with involvement limited to those lymphatic structures related to the celiac axis vessels: the spleen, splenic hilar nodes, celiac nodes, and/or porta hepatis nodes. Stage III_2 included patients with involvement in the lower abdominal and pelvic lymph node chains (para-aortic, iliac, and/or mesenteric nodes) with or without involvement of the spleen or the splenic hilar, celiac, or porta hepatis nodes. In their series of 23 patients with stage III_1 disease, five-year survival was 93 percent, whereas that among the 29 patients with stage III_2 disease was only 57 percent, a difference which was significant at the 5 percent level. Parallel differences were also observed for dissemination-free and relapse-free survival (Fig. 12.13). Similar findings have been reported by

Stein et al. (1978). A slightly different approach to the subclassification of stage IIIA disease was used by Levi and Wiernik (1977b). They subclassified such patients into two categories: III_{S+} (disease limited to the spleen with or without splenic hilar node involvement) and III_{S+N+} (spleen involvement with more extensive intra-abdominal involvement). This is similar to the substaging employed by Desser et al. except for the fact that the celiac and porta hepatis nodes are not specifically included in the III_{S+} category. Again, overall survival and relapse-free survival were significantly better in their III_{S+} group than in their III_{S+N+} group, and relapses in the III_{S+N+} group were primarily in extralymphatic sites.

We have attempted to verify these findings in the much larger series of pathologic stage IIIA patients available for analysis at Stanford University Medical Center (Hoppe et al., 1979a). Since the celiac, porta hepatis, and splenic hilar lymph nodes are not visualized by lower extremity lymphangiography, patients with stage III_1 disease would be expected to have negative lymphangiograms, whereas most of those with stage III_2 disease would be expected to have positive lymphangiograms. In an analysis which attempted to correlate lymphangiographic findings with anatomic substage, Desser et al. (1977) had previously reported that the lymphangiogram correctly predicted the anatomic substage in 28 of 38 patients. Thus, a reasonable approximation of the substages described by Desser et al. can be achieved by comparing patients with clinical stage IA or IIA supradiaphragmatic disease (and negative lymphangiograms) who are found at laparotomy to have spleen involvement, with or without involvement of the splenic hilar, celiac, or porta hepatis nodes (CS I–IIA/PS III_SA), and patients with clinical stage III disease (positive lymphangiograms) in whom involvement of the spleen and other subdiaphragmatic sites was documented at staging laparotomy (CS IIIA/PS IIIA). Survival and freedom from relapse have been analyzed separately in these two subsets of patients in relation to treatment, since some received total lymphoid radiotherapy alone (supplemented by hepatic irradiation in those with positive spleens) whereas others received both total lymphoid irradiation and adjuvant combination chemotherapy. The results of this analysis are presented in Figure 12.14. In contrast to the findings of Desser et al. (1977), Levi and Wiernik (1977b) and Stein et al. (1978), the Stanford data reveal no significant difference in survival or relapse-free survival in these

A

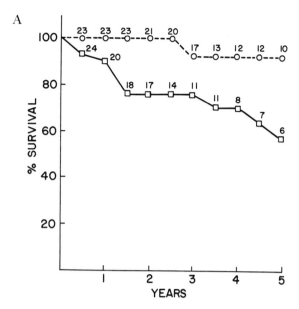

B

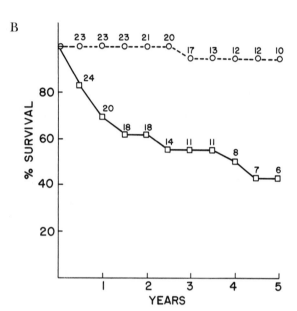

C

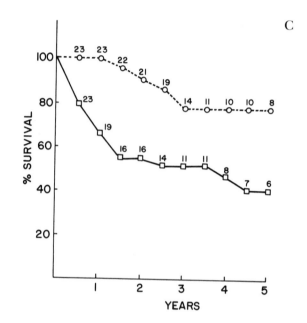

Figure 12.13 Influence on prognosis of substage III₁ versus III₂ (as defined by Desser et al., 1977). Stage III₁, o—o; stage III₂, □—□. *A*, survival; *B*, dissemination-free survival; *C*, relapse-free survival. (Reprinted, by permission of the authors and the Editor of *Blood*, from the paper by Desser et al., 1977.)

two anatomic substages when compared within their respective treatment groups: radiotherapy alone or combined modality therapy.

Constitutional Symptoms. It has long been recognized that patients with Hodgkin's disease who experience severe constitutional symptoms tend to show a more rapidly progressive course. A great many published reports attest to the adverse influence of constitutional symptoms on survival (Finkbeiner et al., 1954; Peters and Middlemiss, 1958; Westling, 1965; Keller et al., 1968; Musshoff and Boutis, 1968; and Smithers, 1969).

In the course of time, two clinical forms of disease have been distinguished; an essentially asymp-

tomatic A form and a symptomatic B form. However, there has been a good deal of controversy as to the criteria by which these clinical forms of the disease are defined. Although Peters and Middlemiss presented evidence indicating the prognostic significance of constitutional symptoms, they did not clearly define which symptoms had been considered in their analysis. Musshoff et al. (1968) have used a relatively complex schema, whereby any of the following manifestations or any combination thereof sufficed to classify a patient in clinical form B: bad general condition; erythrocyte sedimentation rate exceeding 50 mm. per hour; body temperature exceeding 37.6 C; loss of appetite; loss of weight; sweating, itching, pains, or ma-

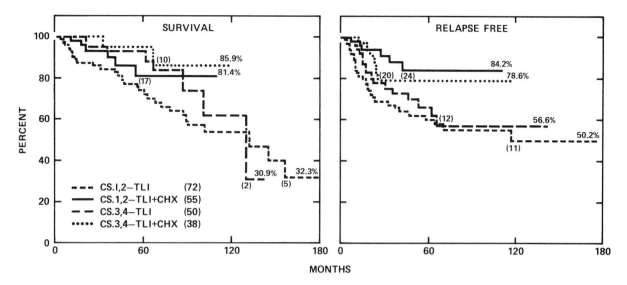

Figure 12.14   Actuarial analysis of survival and freedom from relapse of Stanford patients with CS I or II/PS IIIA versus lymphangiogram-positive, CS III (or IV)/PS IIIA disease. Some patients in each group had been treated with total lymphoid radiotherapy (TLI) alone, others with total lymphoid radiotherapy plus combination chemotherapy (TLI + CHX); the numbers of patients are given in parenthesis.

laise; severe anemia with dyspnea; thrombocytopenia with hemorrhagic diathesis; and leukocytosis with a strong shift to the left. At the Rye conference in 1965, the prevailing view was that only those constitutional symptoms regarded as relatively specific for Hodgkin's disease should be utilized in defining the B category. Accordingly, such relatively nonspecific symptoms as fatigue, malaise, weight loss, and anemia were discarded, leaving only night sweats, otherwise unexplained fever, and/or generalized pruritus as the constitutional symptoms considered significant for the purposes of clinical staging (Rosenberg, 1966). These symptoms were further revised at the Ann Arbor conference (Carbone et al., 1971), where generalized pruritis was deleted from the list and weight loss exceeding 10 percent of normal body weight was added (Chapter 8). Thus, the data presented by Musshoff and Boutis (1968) on the relationship between the clinical form of the disease and survival are not directly comparable with data on series of cases classified in strict accordance with either the Rye criteria, as in the study of Keller et al. (1968), or the Ann Arbor criteria (Kaplan, 1976, 1977). The adverse influence of constitutional symptoms on prognosis is again evident in the updated actuarial analysis of survival presented in Table 12.4.

Our experience in attempting to adhere as closely as possible to the Ann Arbor criteria during the past several years has brought to light a number of problems with this classification. Although

the patient with drenching night sweats and classical Pel-Ebstein cyclic fever is easy to classify, many patients give a much more equivocal history (a modest increase in perspiration noted for only a few nights or a single, relatively brief episode of moderate fever), which is much more difficult to evaluate. Patients also differ considerably in their awareness of these symptoms and in the reliability with which they respond to questioning about them. Accordingly, it would be quite advantageous if general agreement could be reached in future revisions of the Ann Arbor staging classification on objective laboratory criteria which have prognostic implications similar to those of the constitutional symptoms and which could thus be taken into consideration, together with subjective symptoms, in evaluating whether a given patient belongs in clinical form A or B. Some of the possible laboratory criteria which might be relevant to such a proposal have been discussed in Chapter 4.

A second difficulty with the existing data on the prognostic significance of constitutional symptoms in Hodgkin's disease is that many of the published analyses do not take into consideration the fact that the anatomic extent of disease and the presence of constitutional symptoms are not independent variables. It is well established that constitutional symptoms are relatively infrequent in stage I cases, whereas the great majority of stage III and stage IV cases are symptomatic (cf. Table 8.7). Thus, the observation that survival is less favorable in symptomatic than in asymptomatic patients might be

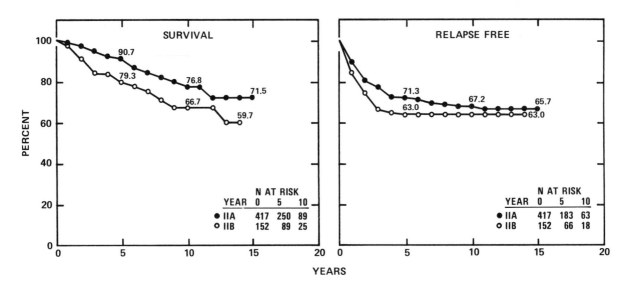

Figure 12.15 Influence of constitutional symptoms on prognosis. Actuarial analysis of survival and freedom from relapse of Stanford patients with stage II disease without (IIA) and with (IIB) constitutional symptoms, as defined by the Ann Arbor classification. The numbers of patients at risk at 0, 5, and 10 years are indicated in the insert.

due simply to the greater proportion of anatomically advanced cases in the symptomatic group.

In order to assess whether such constitutional symptoms as night sweats, fever, and weight loss have an impact on prognosis independent of the anatomic extent of the disease, an actuarial analysis has been made of survival and freedom from relapse in previously untreated patients with and without these symptoms within Ann Arbor stage II, and similarly within stage III (Figs. 12.15 and 12.16). It will be seen that the occurrence of these constitutional symptoms exerts only a small, though significant, adverse influence on survival, and no significant long-term influence on relapse rate, in patients with stage II Hodgkin's disease, whereas their impact on survival and relapse rate in stage III is much more serious (Fig. 12.16).

Confirming the conclusion previously reached by Justin-Besançon et al. (1958), Musshoff et al. (1966), Ennuyer et al. (1966), and Chawla et al.

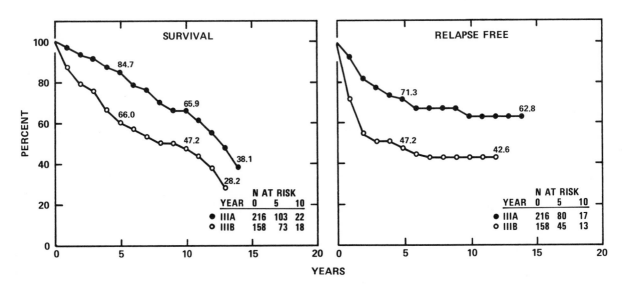

Figure 12.16 Influence of constitutional symptoms on prognosis. Actuarial analysis of survival and freedom from relapse of Stanford patients with stage III disease without (IIIA) and with (IIIB) constitutional symptoms, as defined by the Ann Arbor classification. The numbers of patients at risk at 0, 5, and 10 years are indicated in the insert.

(1970), generalized pruritus did not appear to exert any adverse influence whatever on survival in either the regionally localized or the more advanced stages of the disease (Kaplan, 1972). Accordingly, this symptom was deleted from the list of constitutional symptoms in the Ann Arbor clinical staging classification. It is, however, of some interest that pruritus tended to be relatively more abundant in females than in males, whereas the occurrence of constitutional symptoms, defined according to the Ann Arbor classification, was distinctly more prevalent in males than in females (Table 8.7). Inasmuch as the nodular sclerosing histologic form of Hodgkin's disease is also known to be more prevalent in females, it would be of interest to analyze whether nodular sclerosing disease and generalized itching are correlated, possibly reflecting the existence of a constitutional and local tissue host defense reaction to the Hodgkin's disease process.

Histopathologic Type. This subject has already been considered in Chapter 3. Jackson and Parker (1947) clearly established many years ago the existence of a correlation between the histopathologic morphology of Hodgkin's disease and its prognosis. They reported a 55 percent five-year survival in the paragranuloma group, compared with 14 percent among the granulomas, and no survivor beyond the third year among the sarcoma category. Confirmatory evidence of a correlation with prognosis was reported by a number of other authors (Peters, 1950; Lennert and Hippchen, 1954; Jelliffe and Thomson, 1955; Smetana and Cohen, 1956; Wright, 1956; and others), using the Jackson-Parker or similar histopathologic classifications. However, the existence of such a correlation was disputed by a number of other investigators (Craver, 1934; Finkbeiner et al., 1954; Videbaek, 1950; Winterhalter, 1961; and others). Moreover, as has been discussed in Chapter 3, the Jackson-Parker classification suffered from the disadvantage that between 80 and 90 percent of all cases fell in the heterogeneous granuloma group, leaving only some 5 to 10 percent in the relatively benign paragranuloma group and from 1 to 8 percent in the sarcoma category at the other extreme. Accordingly, the prognostic information revealed by the Jackson-Parker classification was not really clinically useful. Both the prognostic gradient from paragranuloma through granuloma to sarcoma and the concentration of cases in the granuloma category are clearly revealed in an analysis by Westling (1965).

Lukes and his colleagues (1963, 1966a,b) provided the basis for a fresh approach. Using survival data on cases submitted to the Armed Forces Institute of Pathology, they reported an excellent correlation between survival and their proposed new six-category histopathologic classification. At the Rye conference in 1965, this histopathologic classification was simplified to four categories: lymphocyte predominance, nodular sclerosis, mixed cellularity, and lymphocyte depletion. The Rye classification (Lukes et al., 1966c) has been applied to the retrospective analysis of survival in several relatively large series of cases (Franssila et al., 1967; Keller et al., 1968; Landberg and Larsson, 1969; Gough, 1970). Data on 179 previously untreated patients with Hodgkin's disease admitted to Stanford University Medical Center between 1956 and 1966 were reviewed by Keller et al. They observed a distinct difference in survival, computed by the actuarial method, among the various histologic types (cf. Fig. 3.42), and these differences were sustained when only cases of limited anatomic extent (stages I and II) were considered (Fig. 3.43). Thus, it was concluded that anatomic extent of disease and histopathologic type each exert a significant impact on prognosis.

That they are not truly independent variables, however, was indicated by an analysis of our data, which indicated that lymphocyte predominance and nodular sclerosis tend to be concentrated among the relatively localized (stage I and II) cases, whereas mixed cellularity and lymphocyte depletion tend to predominate in the clinically more advanced cases and among those with constitutional symptoms. Similar observations have also been reported by Berard et al. (1971). Moreover, data from the Stanford series of over 800 consecutive staging laparotomies clearly indicate that histology influences the probability of spleen (and thus also of liver and bone marrow) involvement. The spleen was involved in 85 (59.9 percent) of 142 laparotomized patients with mixed cellularity or lymphocyte depletion, and in only 226 (33.7 percent) of 670 patients with lymphocyte predominance, nodular sclerosis, or interfollicular and other unclassified types (cf. Chapter 7). Confirming the previous reports of Hanson (1964) and of Lukes, Butler, and Hicks (1966b), nodular sclerosis was found to involve the mediastinum and the cervical-supraclavicular nodes significantly more often than the mixed cellularity or lymphocyte predominance types; contrary to expectation, however, it involved the infradiaphragmatic lymph nodes only slightly less frequently (Kadin, Glatstein, and Dorfman, 1971; Dorfman, 1971). Nodular sclerosis also tended to occur in a somewhat younger age group and to occur preponderantly among female patients, reversing the usual sex ratio in Hodgkin's disease, as initially reported by Lukes et al. (1963, 1966b).

The influence of the four Rye histopathologic types on survival and on freedom from relapse of patients with previously untreated Hodgkin's disease admitted and treated at Stanford University Medical Center from 1961 through 1977 is graphically displayed in Figure 12.17. Lymphocyte predominance disease again had the best prognosis, with 5- and 10-year survival rates of 95.9 and 79.9 percent, respectively, and a 10-year relapse-free survival of 72.9 percent. Nodular sclerosis was also prognostically favorable; 5-year survival was 84.3 percent, 10-year survival 70.6 percent, and 15-year survival 60.9 percent. Moreover, 63.3 percent of patients with nodular sclerosing disease remained relapse-free, and there were no relapses beyond the eighth year. Mixed cellularity, which once had a prognosis almost as poor as that of lymphocyte depletion, has shown marked improvement; 69.8 percent of such patients survived five years, and 54.3 percent were alive at ten years, with a relapse-free survival which flattened out at 50.2 percent at about ten years. When the analysis was further subdivided according to stage, there was no longer any significant difference in either survival or freedom from relapse between mixed cellularity and nodular sclerosing disease in patients with stage I,

II, and IIIA disease (Fig. 12.18); a difference in survival persisted, in favor of nodular sclerosing disease, in patients with stage IIIB and IV disease, although the difference in relapse-free survival was not statistically significant (Fig. 12.19). Fuller et al. (1977) also noted that mixed cellularity was not prognostically unfavorable in patients with stage I and II disease. However, prognosis in lymphocyte depletion disease remains grim. Only 26.3 percent of such patients survived five years, and only 17.4 percent were relapse-free at three years. In a series of 39 patients studied by Bearman et al. (1978) median survival time in the reticular form of lymphocyte depletion disease was 25.1 months; in the diffuse fibrosis subtype, 22.4 months.

Vascular invasion, which is also seen more often in lymphocyte depletion disease (Rappaport and Strum, 1970; Naeim, Waisman, and Coulson, 1974), is also a prognostically unfavorable histopathologic manifestation. In an analysis of tissues from 71 patients, Naeim, Waisman, and Coulson reported that the median survival time in those with vascular invasion was only 21.8 months, compared with 65.8 months in those without vascular invasion. Kirschner et al. (1974) noted vascular invasion in 7 of 44 spleens involved with Hodgkin's disease, and found that these patients were at greater risk of spread to the liver and bone marrow, early relapse, and decreased survival.

The prognostic significance of differences in relative abundance of specific cell types has been ana-

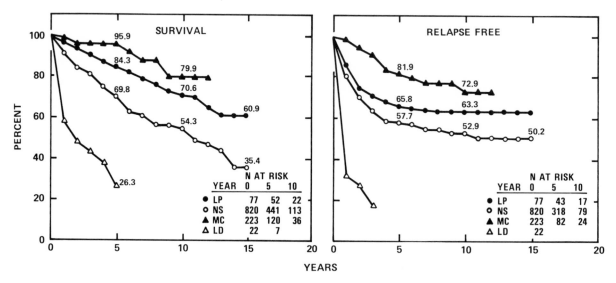

Figure 12.17   Influence of histopathologic type on prognosis. Actuarial analysis of survival and freedom from relapse of the Stanford 1961–1977 series of 1,225 patients, subclassified with respect to the Rye histopathologic scheme. LP, lymphocyte predominance; NS, nodular sclerosis; MC, mixed cellularity; LD, lymphocyte depletion.

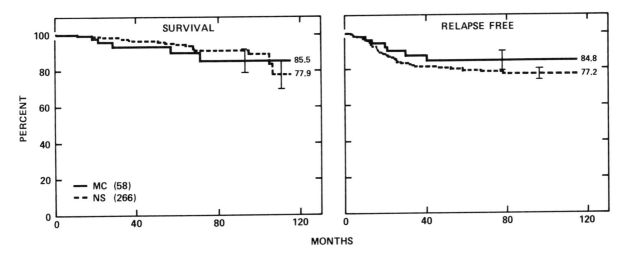

Figure 12.18 Actuarial analysis (by the method of Kaplan and Meier, 1958) of survival and freedom from relapse of patients in the Stanford 1961–1977 series who had stage I, II, or IIIA disease of mixed cellularity (MC) versus nodular sclerosing (NS) type.

lyzed by Coppleson et al. (1973). They found that a stroma rich in lymphocytes was associated with a distinctly more favorable prognosis in either the nodular sclerosis or mixed cellularity forms of the disease. Conversely, an abundance of either benign or malignant histiocytes was an unfavorable prognostic indicator. Curiously, the numbers of Sternberg-Reed cells showed no significant correlation with prognosis, despite the fact that they were highly correlated with numbers of malignant histiocytes. Plasma cells and eosinophils had no evident prognostic significance in this study. However, in an analysis of 327 biopsy specimens from patients with Hodgkin's disease, Tóth,

Dworák, and Sugár (1977) encountered 10 cases with dense eosinophilic infiltration, principally in association with fibrotic changes. The survival time of these 10 patients with "eosinophilic predominance" was significantly shorter than that of comparable controls.

Age. Survival is best in the pediatric and young adult (twenty- to forty-year-old) age groups. There is a good deal of evidence to suggest that prognosis is appreciably less favorable in elderly patients, in whom Jackson and Parker reported the sarcoma form of the disease to be most prevalent. Lokich, Pinkus, and Moloney (1974) compared the histo-

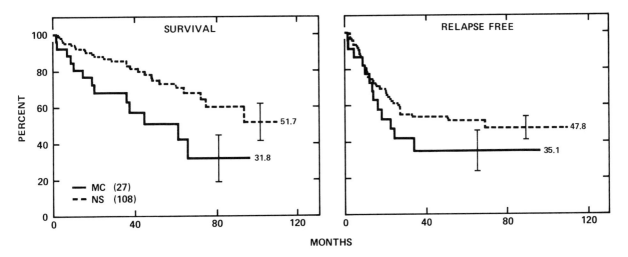

Figure 12.19 Actuarial analysis (by the method of Kaplan and Meier, 1958) of survival and freedom from relapse of patients in the Stanford 1961–1977 series who had stage IIIB or IV disease of mixed cellularity (MC) versus nodular sclerosing (NS) type.

pathologic findings, clinical presentation, distribution of disease, and survival in a series of 47 patients with onset of Hodgkin's disease after age 60 with those of a younger adult control group. Adenopathy was the presenting manifestation in only 24 of the elderly group, as compared with 37 of the younger adults, whereas constitutional symptoms were present at presentation in 12 of the elderly patients and only 1 of the younger group. In 8 of the 12 elderly patients with constitutional symptoms, fever of unknown origin was present. There was a significantly greater frequency of inguinal lymphadenopathy and a decreased frequency of mediastinal involvement in the elderly group. Spleen involvement was clinically evident in 17 of the elderly group, as compared with only 6 of the younger group; however, few patients in either group had staging laparotomies. Clinical evidence of liver involvement was detected in 12 of the elderly and none of the younger adult group, and intestinal involvement was reported to be present in 8 of the elderly group and none of the controls.

Stage distribution was also strikingly different. Only 9 of the elderly patients were in clinical stages I or II; 16 were in clinical stage III; and 22 in clinical stage IV. In contrast, the younger controls included 7 stage I, 17 stage II, 18 stage III, and only 4 stage IV cases. Of 37 patients in the elderly group whose initial biopsies were classified according to the Rye histopathologic classification, mixed cellularity and lymphocyte depletion were present in 31 (83 percent) and nodular sclerosis was observed in only 4 patients (10 percent). In contrast, lymphocyte predominance or nodular sclerosis were present in 15 (47 percent) of 32 patients in the younger age group, and lymphocyte depletion in only 6 percent.

Median survival among the elderly patients with stage I and II disease was only 27 months, that in patients with stage III disease was 15 months, and in stage IV patients, only 3 months. Survival in the elderly group was compared with a second control group matched for symptoms and histopathologic type. The median survival for the elderly group was only 5 months, that for the control group 40 months, a highly significant difference. In considerable measure, however, these differences in survival may have been related to differences in aggressiveness of treatment rather than to an intrinsically more rapid course of the disease in elderly patients. Five of the 47 elderly patients received only supportive therapy, and 8 others received local palliative therapy supplemented with a single course of nitrogen mustard. Single-agent chemotherapy was used in 19 patients. Only 9 patients with stage IIA or IIIA disease were treated with curative intent using intensive radiotherapy, and 6 other patients, all with stage IV disease, received MOPP combination chemotherapy. In contrast, 42 of 47 patients in the younger age group received intensive radiotherapy with or without adjuvant combination chemotherapy, and 3 other patients were treated with combination chemotherapy alone. Thus, the differences in survival reflect differences in intensity of treatment, and perhaps also decreased tolerance for intensive treatment among elderly patients.

The prognosis in the pediatric age group was once much more controversial. Ziegler reported in 1911 that children with Hodgkin's disease have a particularly adverse prognosis, and this view was echoed by a number of other authors (Smith, 1934; Charache, 1946; Vogelgesang and Többen, 1956), with the result that it became widely accepted. However, there was no evidence indicating a particulary unfavorable prognosis in children in the large series of Swedish cases reviewed by Uddströmer in 1934 or in the smaller series of cases studied by Pitcock et al. (1959). Westling (1965) observed a 50 percent five- and ten-year survival among a small group of patients in the zero- to fourteen-year age range, as compared with a five-year survival of 43.8 percent and a ten-year survival of 26.7 percent in the fifteen- to forty-nine-year age bracket. In contrast, patients in his series who were over fifty years of age at the time of admission had a significantly poorer survival at both five and ten years (16.7 and 11.4 percent, respectively).

One difficulty in evaluating the published reports just cited is that clinical staging data are either unavailable or antedate lymphangiography and staging laparotomy and are thus subject to serious error. An analysis of the previously untreated patients with Hodgkin's disease admitted to Stanford University Medical Center between 1961 and 1977 confirms the existence of a relationship between age at the time of admission and clinical extent of disease (Table 8.8). It may be seen that there is a significantly greater fraction of cases in the one- to sixteen-year age range in the regionally localized group (64 percent in stages I and II), and a significantly greater proportion of cases fifty years of age or older (49 percent) in stages III and IV. It is therefore clear that many of the earlier analyses which purported to show a more unfavorable prognosis among older patients were, at least in part, reflecting the greater abundance of far-advanced clinical stages, rather than an influence of age per se.

The Stanford cases have been subjected to actuarial analysis of survival as a function of age, clinical stage, and the presence or absence of constitutional symptoms. The survival curves and numbers at risk in each group are presented in Figures 12.20 and 12.21. Overall survival was only 54.8 percent at five years and 30 percent at ten years among patients who were 50 years of age or older at the time of admission. In contrast, 82.5 percent of the patients 17 to 49 years of age at the time of admission and 91.6 percent of the pediatric age group were alive at five years; the corresponding figures at ten years were 69.3 and 81.1 percent, respectively. The survival figures have not been corrected for attrition due to intercurrent deaths, and this is likely to be a significant factor in the apparently poorer survival of the older age group. This is also reflected in the fact that the relapse-free survival curves for the older age group, though again less favorable than those of the young adult and pediatric age groups, are less dramatically different. The prognostic influence of age is clearly stage-dependent. There is little difference between the pediatric and young adult patients with stage IA and IIA disease; however, survival among the older patients is distinctly less favorable even with such regionally localized disease. The very poor survival of symptomatic patients with regionally localized disease (stages IB and IIB) in the older age group is based on too few

cases to permit statistically valid comparison. Survival in the young adult age group was comparable to that of the pediatric age group with stage IIIA or IVA disease, but significantly worse in stages IIIB and IVB. Survival among the older group with stage III or IV disease was significantly worse than that of children or young adults, whether constitutional symptoms were present or not at the time of admission (Fig. 12.21).

Prognosis in the pediatric age group is slightly better than that in the young adult age group in both the asymptomatic and symptomatic stage I and II cases and very much better in stages IIIB and IVB. Thus, there is no longer any justification for the outdated view that prognosis among patients in the pediatric age group is unfavorable. On the contrary, it would appear that overall survival in the pediatric age group is slightly superior to that of young adults. Similar conclusions emerge from the data of several other groups who have analyzed survival and freedom from relapse in children with Hodgkin's disease staged and treated by modern techniques (Jenkin et al., 1975; Tan et al., 1975; Donaldson et al., 1976a,b; I. E. Smith et al., 1977). Although the course of Hodgkin's disease is generally similar in children and adolescents (Smith and Rivera, 1976), 83 percent of the children 10 years of age or less studied by Donaldson et al. (1976a) were relapse-free, as compared with 61 percent of adolescents 11 years of age or more. The same authors noted a marked difference in relapse-free survival of clinically versus pathologi-

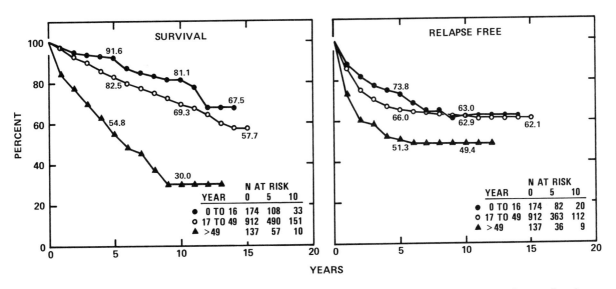

Figure 12.20   Influence of age on prognosis. Actuarial analysis of survival and freedom from relapse of patients in the Stanford 1961–1977 series who were ≤16 years of age, 17 to 49 years of age, or ≥50 years of age at the time of admission. Numbers of patients at risk at 0, 5, and 10 years are indicated in the insert.

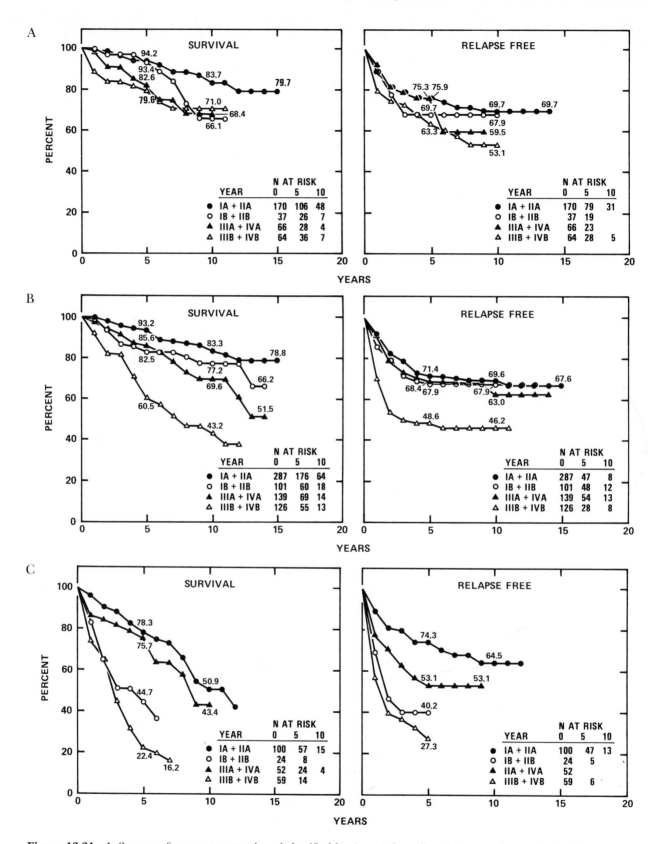

Figure 12.21 Influence of age on prognosis, subclassified by Ann Arbor clinical stage and constitutional symptoms. *A*, ≤20 years of age; *B*, 21–40 years of age; *C*, ≥41 years of age at the time of admission. Numbers of patients at risk at 0, 5, and 10 years are indicated in the insert.

cally staged patients at five years; only 55 percent of the clinically staged patients were relapse-free, as compared to 82 percent of those staged with the aid of laparotomy, and there were no relapses after two years in patients staged with the aid of laparotomy. The prognostic influence of histopathologic type was again evident in the pediatric age group. Survival was 100 percent at eight years in children and adolescents with lymphocyte predominance histology, 88 percent at five years in those with nodular sclerosis, and 81 percent at five years among those with mixed cellularity disease (Donaldson et al., 1976a).

Sex. The possible influence of sex on the prognosis of patients with Hodgkin's disease was first reported by Epstein (1939), who compared the longevity of 204 cases in females with that of 180 cases among males, all collated from the medical literature. His conclusion was that females have a better prognosis than males. Though founded on evidence that is clearly unacceptable by current standards, this view has nonetheless been supported by a plethora of subsequent studies (Peters, 1950; Jelliffe and Thomson, 1955; Heilmeyer et al., 1957; Croizat et al., 1958; Meighan and Ramsay, 1963; and others). The magnitude of the difference in prognosis appears to be statistically significant in the data collected by Hohl et al. (1951); Shimkin et al. (1955); Peters and Middlemiss (1958); Musshoff et al. (1964 and 1966); Westling (1965); Peters et al. (1966); and Gross et al. (1966).

However, it is known that sex and histopathologic type are not independent variables. The nodular sclerosing type is significantly more abundant among females, and this alone might contribute to the apparently better survival among female patients with Hodgkin's disease. The observed difference in survival may also be attributable in part to differences in the distribution of the various clinical stages among the two sexes. Musshoff and Boutis (1968) have suggested that the greater preponderance of stage III and IV cases among males may account for the observed difference. A similar inference can be drawn from the data of Peters et al. (1966).

An actuarial analysis of survival and freedom from relapse in the Stanford cases as related to sex, clinical stage, and the presence or absence of constitutional symptoms reveals the data summarized in Figures 12.22 and 12.23. It is clear that there is no appreciable difference attributable to sex in the regionally localized, asymptomatic cases (stages IA and IIA) and only a modest difference among the stage IB and IIB or IIIA and IVA cases. However, the most dramatic difference in prognosis is observed in patients with stage III and IV disease with constitutional symptoms; whereas survival among the females with such far-advanced disease is only moderately less than that among females with regionally localized disease, survival among the males is sharply decreased. This difference between males and females with stage IIIB and IVB disease accounts for most of the net (10–12

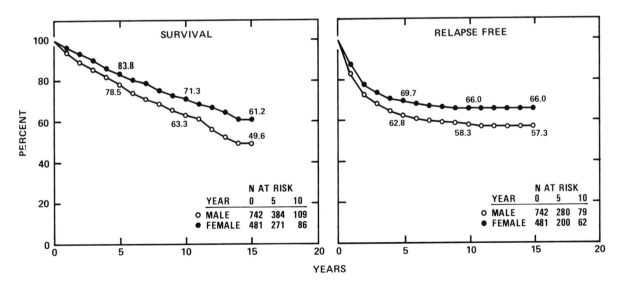

Figure 12.22 Influence of sex on prognosis. Actuarial analysis of survival and freedom from relapse of male versus female patients in the Stanford 1961–1977 series. The numbers of patients at risk at 0, 5, and 10 years are indicated in the insert.

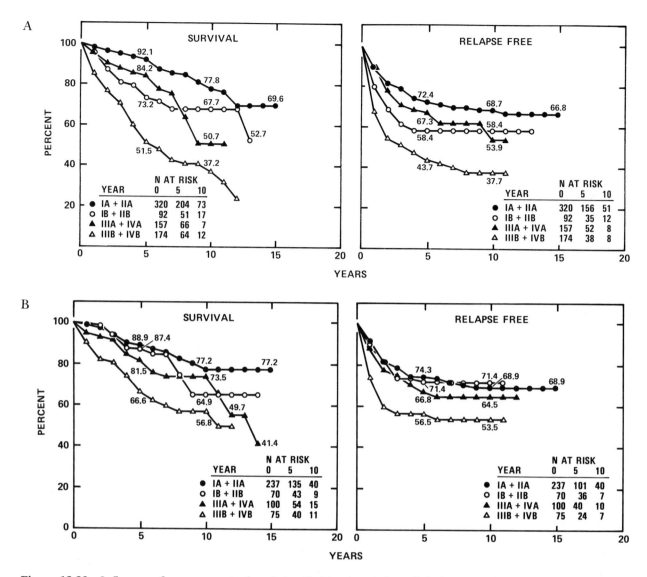

Figure 12.23   Influence of sex on prognosis, subclassified by Ann Arbor clinical stage and constitutional symptoms. *A*, males; *B*, females.

percent) sex-related difference in overall survival and freedom from relapse (Fig. 12.22). Differences in the distribution of the various histopathologic types may well account in part for these striking differences in prognosis of males and females with far-advanced stages of disease. It is conceivable that differences in host resistance to the disease may also be involved; if so, it is curious that they remain inapparent while the disease is still regionally localized and become manifest only when the disease has spread widely through the lymphatic system or beyond and has elicited constitutional symptoms.

Pregnancy. Data on the influence of pregnancy on prognosis in Hodgkin's disease have been pub-

lished by many authors (Hultberg, 1954; Hartvigsen, 1955; Smith et al., 1958; Peters and Middlemiss, 1958; Braun and Rummel, 1965; Morgenfeld et al., 1965). There is fairly general agreement that pregnancies occurring subsequent to the first course of treatment of female patients with Hodgkin's disease do not significantly alter prognosis. The same general conclusion has been reached in most, but not in all, studies to date of patients who were pregnant at the time when the diagnosis was established. It seems likely that, in part, the isolated reports of an adverse influence of pregnancy on prognosis of Hodgkin's disease may be due to the fact that pregnant patients are not usually subjected to lymphangiography or to laparotomy with splenectomy and liver biopsy and thus that the full extent of their disease is less likely to be appreciated.

Initial Localization of Involvement. There has been general agreement that Hodgkin's disease presenting with intra-abdominal and especially with retroperitoneal lymph node involvement has a particularly poor prognosis. This point has been documented by Westling (1965), who found a five-year survival of only 4.9 percent and ten-year survival of 2.4 percent in a series of forty-one cases with retroperitoneal onset, as compared with five-year survival of approximately 42 percent and ten-year survival of 25 to 31 percent in groups with presenting localization in the mediastinal and in the superficial lymph nodes, respectively. However, it must be remembered that these data are derived from an era in which lymphangiography was not employed. It is reasonable to assume that cases with a predominantly abdominal localization were those in which the disease had grown to such massive size as to become clinically evident. The excellent survival observed in the stage IIIA cases in the Stanford series (Fig. 12.11), in which retroperitoneal involvement was often detected at a relatively early stage by lymphangiography and/or laparotomy with biopsy, strongly suggests that it was the massive size that intra-abdominal involvement was formerly permitted to attain, rather than intra-abdominal node involvement per se, that may have been responsible for the poor prognosis of this type of localization. The possible prognostic influence of different sites of lymph node involvement within the abdomen has already been discussed in the section on the influence of clinical stage. The data of two groups (Desser et al., 1977; Stein et al., 1978) suggest that patients with stage III$_1$ disease whose subdiaphragmatic involvement is limited to the spleen and/or celiac, splenic hilar, or porta hepatis nodes have a better prognosis than patients with para-aortic, mesenteric, and/or pelvic lymphadenopathy (stage III$_2$).

Whether involvement of the spleen per se adversely affects prognosis has been more difficult to ascertain. Shipley, Piro, and Hellman (1974) attempted to evaluate this question by matched pair analysis in a retrospective study. Their data indicate that relapse-free survival at three years was 85–95 percent among the spleen-negative matched controls, as compared to approximately 60 percent among the spleen-positive group. There were 8 relapses (28 percent) among 29 patients with involved spleens; 4 of these occurred within two to nine months and were extralymphatic in location, whereas the 8 relapses among 54 spleen-negative patients (15 percent) tended to occur somewhat later and only 1 was extralymphatic in location. Three of the four extranodal relapses in the spleen-positive patients occurred in the liver; it is of interest that one of these patients had only microscopic involvement in the spleen. These observations provide support for the policy of using supplementary external beam radiotherapy to the liver in patients with documented involvement of the spleen, as described by Schultz, Glatstein, and Kaplan (1975). The data of Levi and Wiernik (1977b) tend to suggest that the unfavorable prognosis in patients with stage III disease is associated to a greater extent with involvement of lower abdominal lymph nodes in addition to the spleen, rather than with splenic involvement alone. The Stanford experience in patients with pathologic stage III disease with spleen involvement as the only site of subdiaphragmatic disease (S+N−), as contrasted with a group of patients with pathologic stage III disease in whom lymph node involvement was documented but the spleen was uninvolved (S−N+), is presented in Figure 12.24. It is evident that the differences in prognosis are minor, although the slight differences observed both among PS IIIA and among PS IIIB cases are in favor of those with spleen involvement in the absence of subdiaphragmatic node involvement. However, a recent analysis of our PS IIIA data (Hoppe et al., 1979a) suggests that the extent of spleen involvement, rather than the mere presence or absence of any disease in the spleen, may be prognostically important. Patients with diffuse involvement throughout the spleen had a significantly worse prognosis with respect to both survival and freedom from relapse than did those with only one or a few small nodules in the spleen.

Krikorian et al. (1979b) analyzed the course of 19 patients with pathologic stage I or II disease presenting below the diaphragm (usually in the groin), and found that their prognosis did not differ significantly from that of 223 similarly staged patients with supradiaphragmatic disease. Those with subdiaphragmatic disease included a preponderance of males (74 versus 53 percent), tended to be somewhat older (mean age 40 versus 27, respectively), and were often of mixed cellularity subtype. At eight to ten years, 76.6 percent of the subdiaphragmatic group and 78.0 percent of the supradiaphragmatic group were relapse-free, and survival in the former group was 92.3 percent at eight years.

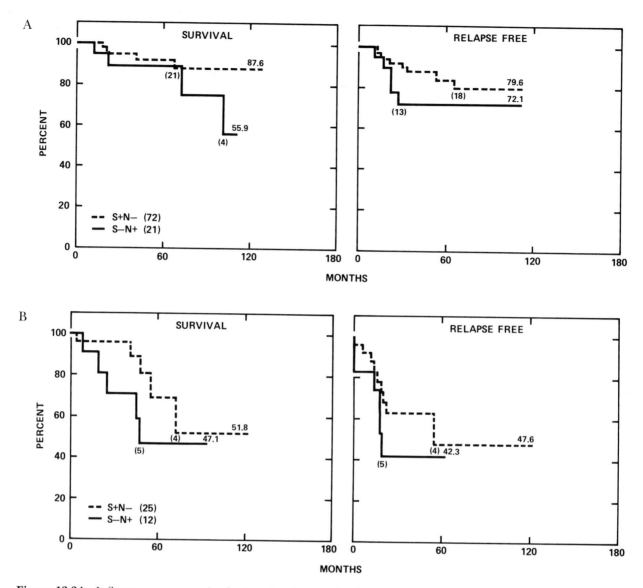

Figure 12.24   Influence on prognosis of spleen involvement in the absence of subdiaphragmatic node involvement (S + N −) versus node involvement without spleen involvement (S − N +) among laparotomy-staged patients in the Stanford series. *A*, PS IIIA; *B*, PS IIIB.

As is readily apparent from the data of three successive five-year accession periods (Fig. 12.25), the prognosis of patients with pathologically documented stage IV disease has improved dramatically. Nonetheless, there remain some differences in prognosis which depend on the specific stage IV site involved. Involvement of the liver, once inevitably fatal, now appears to be curable in a surprisingly high proportion of all patients treated with either radiotherapy alone (Fig. 11.11), MOPP combination chemotherapy alone (Fig. 11.28), or combined modality therapy (Fig. 11.28; Chapter 11). Indeed, the prognosis of patients with stage IV_HA or B disease is probably not significantly different

from that of patients with stage III_SA or B disease, respectively.

The bone marrow has long been considered the least favorable of all stage IV sites. Weiss, Brunning, and Kennedy (1975) reported a median survival of only nine months among patients in whom bone marrow involvement was detected at the time of presentation, and of only five months among those in whom bone marrow involvement developed later in the course of the disease. In an analysis of the first 81 Stanford patients treated with MOPP combination chemotherapy, Moore et al. (1973) reported that complete remissions were induced in 13 of 17 patients with bone marrow in-

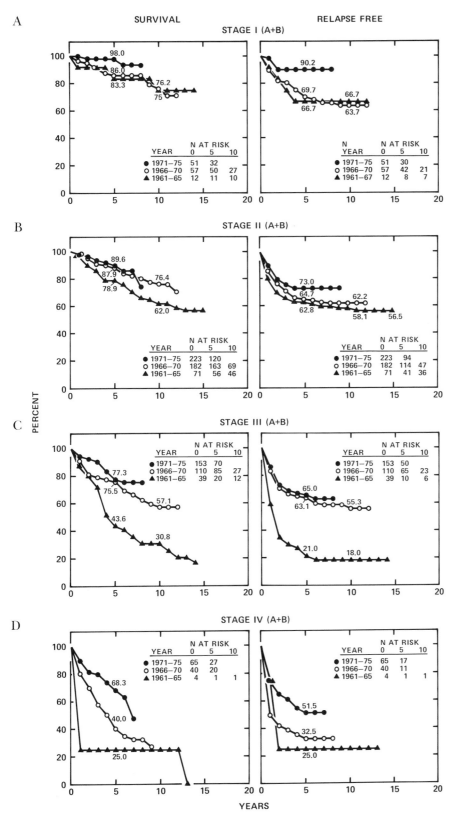

Figure 12.25 Actuarial analysis of survival and freedom from relapse of patients admitted to Stanford University Medical Center during three successive five-year accession periods, subdivided by Ann Arbor clinical stage. *A*, stage I; *B*, stage II; *C*, stage III; *D*, stage IV.

volvement (76 percent), approximately the same proportion as for all other extralymphatic sites of involvement, but relapses occurred in 8 of the 13 patients with bone marrow involvement who entered complete remission, a relapse rate of 62 percent, whereas the relapse rate among patients with other extralymphatic sites of stage IV involvement who entered complete remission was only about 20 percent. However, the experience of the National Cancer Institute group with MOPP chemotherapy in patients with bone marrow involvement has been appreciably more favorable. Myers et al. (1974) reported that 13 (72 percent) of 18 such patients treated with MOPP entered complete remission. The median duration of remission was over 25 months, and 49 percent of these patients were still in complete remission after more than three years, two for more than six years. Overall, the four-year survival in the marrow-positive group was about 70 percent, slightly higher than in the entire stage IV group. The more recent Stanford experience in patients with bone marrow involvement in the H-7 and S-8 protocols (Figs. 11.29 and 11.33) is also encouraging, though not as good as that among stage IV patients with liver involvement.

The influence of localized extralymphatic lesions, formerly designated as stage IV sites in the Rye clinical staging classification, but now designated as "E" lesions in the Ann Arbor classification (Carbone et al., 1971), is currently somewhat controversial. The earlier data of Musshoff et al. (1968) and of Peters, Hasselback, and Brown (1968) had indicated that the prognosis of patients with such localized extralymphatic lesions was not significantly worse than that of patients with the corresponding extent of lymph node disease who were devoid of extralymphatic lesions. Indeed, their data provided much of the impetus for the change from the Rye to the Ann Arbor staging classification. However, Levi and Wiernik (1977a), in an analysis of 84 patients with PS IIA and IIIA disease, and of 18 patients with PS II$_E$A and III$_E$A disease, noted a relapse rate after irradiation alone of 29 percent among the former and of 82 percent among the latter. Most of the relapses among the patients with "E" lesions were recurrences within the lung parenchyma. However, it is noteworthy that the radiotherapy technique used in these patients did not include ipsilateral or bilateral low-dose lung irradiation in patients with hilar and mediastinal disease. Carmel and Kaplan (1976) have presented evidence that patients with hilar or bulky mediastinal adenopathy are at increased risk

of extension to the lungs, and that pulmonary irradiation by the thin lung block technique (Palos, Kaplan, and Karzmark, 1971) can reduce the frequency of such intrapulmonary relapses. Only 1 ipsilateral pulmonary relapse occurred among 30 lungs treated with the thin lung block technique. Moreover, in patients with "E" lesions in the lung in association with mediastinal and/or hilar adenopathy, they found that the combination of full-dose irradiation to the "E" lesion and prophylactic low-dose ipsilateral whole lung irradiation was capable of controlling pulmonary Hodgkin's disease. Of 27 patients with pulmonary lesions, 17 remained free of relapse after treatment with radiation alone. Of 11 patients with lung lesions who eventually relapsed, only 4 developed their initial relapses in the lung.

Torti et al. (1978) have undertaken a more extensive analysis of the Stanford experience in 63 patients with "E" lesions in a total series of 406 patients with stage I, II, or III (A + B) Hodgkin's disease who had been entered in randomized clinical trials comparing radiation therapy alone versus radiation therapy plus adjuvant combination chemotherapy. Of the 63 patients with "E" lesions, 36 were asymptomatic and 27 had constitutional symptoms. Relapse-free survival at five years for the "E" patients treated with radiotherapy alone was 50 percent, whereas that in the patients of similar stage distribution without "E" lesions was 71 percent ($p = 0.09$); that among patients treated with both radiotherapy and combination chemotherapy was 81 percent in the "E" group and 85 percent in the non-"E" group. However, actuarial survival at five years for patients treated with radiotherapy alone was 89 percent in the group with "E" lesions and 91 percent in the group without "E" lesions. Among those treated with radiotherapy plus chemotherapy, survival at five years was 81 percent in the "E" group and 89 percent in the non-"E" group. It was concluded that patients with "E" lesions treated with radiotherapy alone have rates of survival and freedom from relapse comparable to those of patients without "E" lesions. It seems likely that the much lower relapse rate in the Stanford patients with "E" lesions treated with radiotherapy alone is attributable to such refinements of radiotherapeutic technique as prophylactic low-dose whole lung irradiation in patients with hilar and/or bulky mediastinal lymphadenopathy, and prophylactic whole liver irradiation among those with spleen involvement. The Stanford data suggest that although supplementation of radiotherapy with adjuvant chemotherapy decreases relapse rates among patients with "E" lesions, adjuvant chemotherapy has no significant influence on their survival.

A number of reports suggest that mediastinal involvement is not a prognostically unfavorable localization. Indeed, the data of Kurohara et al. (1967), Fuller et al. (1973), and Papillon (1974) suggest that mediastinal involvement may be associated with a significantly more favorable prognosis, particularly when relatively localized. However, it must be remembered that histopathologic type influences anatomic distribution and that the prognostically favorable nodular sclerosing form is well known to exhibit a strong predilection for involvement of the mediastinum. Thus, histopathology rather than anatomic locus per se may account for the good survival in most cases with a mediastinal presentation. There is some evidence that bulky or massive mediastinal lymphadenopathy may be associated with an increased relapse rate, perhaps due in part to the fact that such massive lesions must often be treated by split course or low-dose radiation techniques. Carmel and Kaplan (1976) reported that relapses occurred in 18 (29.5 percent) of 61 patients with bulky mediastinal adenopathy in whom total mantle treatment time exceeded 34 days, as compared with only 7 relapses (15.6 percent) among 45 patients whose treatment time was 34 days or less. The corresponding relapse rates among patients with minimal mediastinal adenopathy were 9.7 percent and 5.5 percent, respectively. Mauch, Goodman, and Hellman (1978) have also reported an increased relapse rate among patients with mediastinal lymphadenopathy that exceeds one-third of the transverse thoracic diameter in width, and Thar et al. (1979) found that the risk of lung or pleural involvement was strongly dependent on size of mediastinal/hilar adenopathy. Only 2 (5 percent) of 43 patients with a mediastinal diameter less than 6 cm had lung or pleural involvement, as contrasted with 10 (71 percent) of 14 patients with a diameter greater than 6 cm.

Mauch, Goodman, and Hellman (1978) have suggested that adjuvant combination chemotherapy is routinely indicated in patients with bulky or massive mediastinal adenopathy. However, the Stanford experience with those patients whose mediastinal disease responds rapidly to treatment, and in whom mantle treatment can therefore be carried to completion in 34 days or less, indicates that relapse rate is not sufficiently high to warrant the routine use of adjuvant combination chemotherapy with its attendant increased complication

rate and risk of late secondary hematologic neoplasia. We have therefore preferred to observe the initial response of massive mediastinal lymphadenopathy when the first phase of split course mantle treatment has been completed, at a dose of about 1,500 to 2,000 rads. If response is rapid, the mantle treatment is carried to completion using new lung shielding blocks shaped to the reduced contours of the mediastinum (cf. Figs. 5.1 and 9.63), and adjuvant chemotherapy is not employed. Conversely, when there is little or no evidence of regression after the first 1,500 to 2,000 rads of mantle irradiation has been delivered, we proceed with two or more cycles of MOPP combination chemotherapy and then complete the mantle treatment, usually with a "boost" to approximately 5,000 rads total dose (cf. Figs. 11.54 and 11.55, Chapter 11). Excellent results with respect to mediastinal regression, preservation of pulmonary function, and long-term relapse-free survival have been obtained with both techniques, suggesting that this selective policy, linked to the initial rate of mediastinal regression, is an appropriate one.

Craver (1964) suggested that lymphadenopathy localized to the upper cervical region may have a more favorable outlook than disease in the lower cervical and supraclavicular region. This relationship, which has been confirmed in our own experience to date, as well as that of Fuller et al. (1971), is perhaps attributable to the fact that the upper cervical nodes, unlike those in the lower cervical and supraclavicular chains, do not communicate directly with the thoracic duct. They would therefore not be expected to exhibit as frequent an association with involvement of the upper lumbar para-aortic nodes (cf. Chapter 7). It is also known that lymphocyte predominance disease tends to present in the high cervical nodes, and this may also contribute to the more favorable prognosis of such localizations.

Duration of Disease prior to Diagnosis or Treatment. Peters and Middlemiss (1958) reported that among patients with regionally localized disease (stages I or II), survival was directly related to the duration of the disease. Five-year survival in stage I was 59 percent for those with a duration of disease prior to treatment of less than six months; 82 percent for those with a duration of six to twenty-four months; and 87 percent for those with a duration exceeding twenty-four months. The five-year survival figures for the corresponding groups with stage II disease were 46 percent, 53 percent, and 83 percent, respectively. In contrast, there was no significant difference in patients found to have stage III disease at the time of admission. The data are probably best interpreted as reflecting the selection of slowly evolving cases.

Westling (1965) found that patients with a duration of disease before admission of less than six months had a significantly smaller proportion of stage III cases, as well as a lower incidence of fever, elevated sedimentation rate, and anemia, than those with longer preadmission histories and that they also had a somewhat better survival. He concluded that the earlier the diagnosis and treatment, the better the survival rate after admission. Musshoff and Boutis (1969) found that the duration of the history had no significant relationship to prognosis in their series. Since dating of the onset of symptoms or signs of the disease is highly subjective and thus subject to appreciable error, it seems undesirable to place undue emphasis on this factor in attempting to assess prognosis in individual cases.

Hematologic Indicators. Many investigators have reported the unfavorable prognostic significance of anemia, as measured by the erythrocyte count, hemoglobin, and packed red blood cell volume (Bethell et al., 1950; Levinson et al., 1957; Justin-Besançon et al., 1958; Westling, 1965; Musshoff, Boutis, Laszlo, and Laszlo, 1966; Tubiana et al., 1971). However, anemia is not an independent variable but is linked to generalized disease. It is therefore likely that the poor prognosis of these patients is primarily a reflection of the anatomic extent of their disease. There is, to our knowledge, no documentary evidence of the prognostic influence of anemia per se within a given clinical stage.

Marked leukocytosis has been reported to be a grave sign by some investigators (Bethell et al., 1950; Levinson et al., 1957), whereas others have reported that leukopenia is an unfavorable prognostic manifestation (Levinson et al., 1957; Croizat et al., 1958). In a more recent analysis, Westling (1965) found that patients with leukopenia (fewer than 4,000 white blood cells per cubic millimeter) had a five-year survival of only 11.1 percent, versus 38.3 percent for those with either a normal white blood cell count or leukocytosis at the time of admission. There was no significant relationship to the eosinophil count, but those patients with an absolute lymphocyte count of fewer than 800 per cubic millimeter had a five-year survival of 13.2 percent and a ten-year survival of 0 percent, as compared with five- and ten-year survivals of 41.0 and 28.9 percent, respectively, in those with

lymphocyte counts in the normal range. Eight of nine patients in whom the lymphocyte count was less than 500 per cubic millimeter were dead within one year; it is of interest that only three of these were leukopenic, suggesting that the absolute lymphocyte count is a more sensitive indicator of prognosis than the total white blood cell count. Swan and Knowelden (1971) and Tubiana et al. (1971) also reported that survival was significantly decreased in patients with lymphocyte counts below 900–1,000 per cubic millimeter. However, Musshoff, Boutis, Laszlo, and Laszlo (1966) failed to observe a significant correlation between survival and absolute lymphocyte count, although they did note such a relationship with the absolute monocyte count.

Westling (1965) observed thrombocytopenia (less than 100,000 platelets per cubic millimeter) at the time of admission in three patients, all with relatively advanced disease, none of whom survived as long as three months after admission. However, four other patients had platelet counts exceeding 400,000 per cubic millimeter, and none of these survived more than seven months. In a study of fifty-six cases of Hodgkin's disease, Barry et al. (1966) noted that a sudden, pronounced elevation of platelet levels was often correlated with the spread of disease to new lymph node chains. In cases in which peripheral lymphadenopathy was not available as a clinical indicator, they suggested that thrombocytosis, together with elevation of the erythrocyte sedimentation rate, may represent a useful index of incipient relapse and that a return to normal platelet values may anticipate a remission of the disease.

As early as 1934, Uddströmer called attention to the prognostic significance of an elevated erythrocyte sedimentation rate. His observation was soon confirmed by Wise (1942) and more recently by Westling (1965), Musshoff et al. (1966), and Tubiana et al. (1971). For example, when the ESR was greater than 25 mm. in one hour, Westling observed a five-year survival of only 27.5 percent and a ten-year survival of 17.5 percent, as compared with 54.7 and 36.3 percent, respectively, for ESR values in the 0 to 25 mm. range. Tubiana et al. (1971) reported a 49 percent five-year survival among 57 patients whose initial ESR was <30 mm/hr, as compared with only 27 percent among 67 patients whose initial ESR level exceeded 30 mm/hr. There was no correlation between ESR and histologic type or clinical stage. Although ESR was strongly correlated with constitutional symptoms such as weight loss and fever, an elevation of ESR had an unfavorable prognostic significance even in afebrile patients.

Several authors have suggested that the ESR may also be a useful indicator of prognosis later in the course of the disease and that an otherwise unexplained elevation of ESR may herald an impending relapse. For example, Le Bourgeois and Tubiana (1977), in a followup study of 68 patients with clinical stage I or II Hodgkin's disease, reported that relapses which occurred in 28 patients were preceded or accompanied by an increase in ESR levels; the average interval from the elevation of ESR to the detection of relapse was 4.5 months. However, the ESR level remained normal in 7 other relapsing patients, increased to abnormal levels in 8 patients who remained relapse-free, and failed to return to normal levels following treatment in 12 other patients who apparently entered complete remission. It is of course important to remember that the ESR is a relatively nonspecific indicator, which may respond to a host of infectious and nonspecific inflammatory conditions. This is particularly true in children, in whom Wilimas, Thompson, and Smith (1978) observed false positive ESR elevations in 62 of 109 cases. Accordingly, although an otherwise unexplained elevation of a previously normal ESR in a patient with Hodgkin's disease in remission should alert the physician to search with particular care for signs of relapse, it would be quite unwarranted to accept the elevated ESR alone as evidence of a relapse and to institute treatment solely on the basis of this manifestation.

Biochemical Indicators. Serum copper levels were reported to be elevated in patients with active Hodgkin's disease by Koch et al. (1957), Pagliardi and his associates (1960, 1963), and Jensen et al. (1964). Using a modification of Jensen's method, Hrgovcic et al. (1968) reported data on 153 normal subjects, as well as on 28 patients with Hodgkin's disease and a number of others with other types of malignant lymphoma and with acute leukemias. They found that the normal range was 69 to 133, with an average of 101 μg $\pm$ 16 μg percent; in children up to five years of age the upper limit of normal was somewhat higher, approximately 180 μg percent. In five cases of Hodgkin's disease in apparently complete remission, the serum copper values were all within the normal range (71 to 130 μg percent), whereas in four other patients with active disease, serum copper values were 170, 195, 275, and 280 μg percent, respectively. Similar observations on varying numbers of patients have been reported by several other groups (Mortazavi

et al., 1972; Ray, Wolf, and Kaplan, 1973; Cappelaere et al., 1975; Thorling and Thorling, 1976). Tessmer, Hrgovcic, and Wilbur (1973) presented serum copper data on 37 children with Hodgkin's disease. In those with previously untreated disease, the mean serum copper level was 185 μg percent, falling to about 120 among those who had entered complete remission after treatment, whereas patients with uncontrolled or relapsing disease had a mean of 188 μg percent. Thorling and Thorling (1976) reported that serum copper levels fell to less than 145 μg percent in 55 of 56 males and 34 of 39 females who entered complete remission; 27 of 63 males and 10 of 40 females who entered partial remission; and only 1 of 14 males and 1 of 5 females who had little or no response to treatment.

Hrgovcic et al. (1968) also studied cases in which serial determinations of the serum copper level were available. Seven of their patients had active disease which had been treated with chemotherapy. Of these, three showed a good to excellent clinical response, with a concomitant decrease of their serum copper levels from pretreatment values in the 210 to 260 μg percent range down to 80 to 100 μg percent after treatment. In contrast, four other patients responded poorly and failed to enter remission, and the serum copper values remained elevated in three instances and actually increased further in one. Similarly, four of nine patients treated with radiation therapy who entered complete remission all had elevated pretreatment serum copper levels which fell to the normal range after treatment. Five other patients, who experienced a partial remission after radiotherapy, showed a slight to moderate decrease in their serum copper levels, but these remained significantly elevated. These studies were later extended by Hrgovcic et al. (1975) to a series of 39 adult patients who had a total of 318 serum copper determinations on two or more occasions. Sequential serum copper values remained relatively stable and within the normal range among two groups of patients in remission: 12 who were on maintenance chemotherapy (Fig. 12.26) and 20 who were no longer receiving treatment (Fig. 12.27). Conversely, there appeared to be a good correlation between renewed elevation of serum copper levels and the development of relapsing disease. Thus, all but 4 of 63 serum copper determinations in 44 patients studied during relapse by Hrgovcic et al. (1975) were elevated (Fig. 12.28). Warren et al. (1969) analyzed serial serum copper determinations in relation to the course of the disease in a series of sixty-four cases. They concluded that there

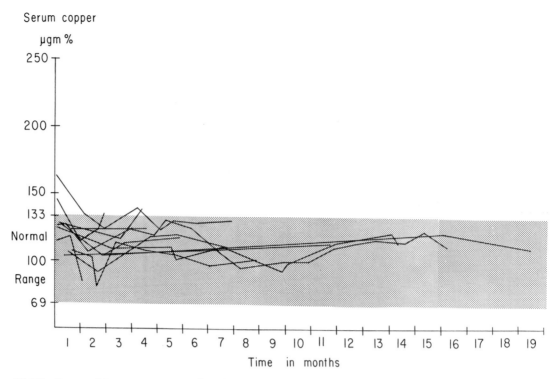

Figure 12.26   Sequential serum copper values in 12 patients with two or more serum copper levels during a period of two months or longer while remaining in remission with maintenance therapy. No significant variations in serum copper levels occur, with time or maintenance therapy, in any one individual. (Reprinted, by permission of the authors and *Texas Medicine,* from the paper by Hrgovcic et al., 1975.)

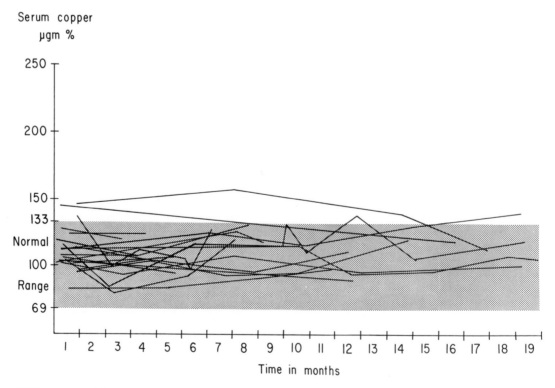

Figure 12.27   Sequential serum copper levels in 20 patients with two or more serum copper levels during a period of two months or longer while remaining in remission without maintenance therapy. No significant variations in serum copper levels occur with time in any one individual. (Reprinted, by permission of the authors and *Texas Medicine,* from the paper by Hrgovcic et al., 1975.)

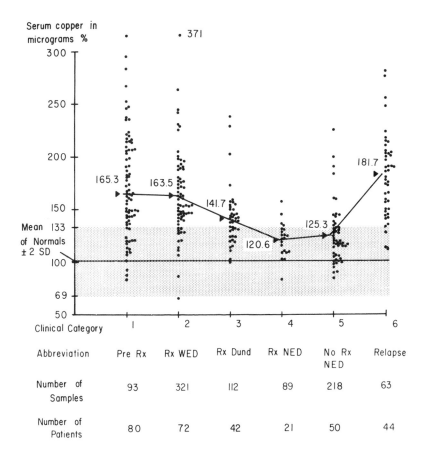

Figure 12.28 Serum copper levels in relation to disease activity. The stippled area indicates the normal range (mean ± 2 S.D.). Each point is the mean of all serum copper values for a single patient in any given clinical category. The data are grouped in six clinical categories: 1) pretreatment (Pre R); 2) under treatment with evidence of disease (R WED); 3) under treatment, activity of disease undetermined (R Dund); 4) under treatment, no evidence of disease (R NED); 5) no current treatment, no evidence of disease (No R NED); and 6) relapse, or recurrent disease, with or without maintenance treatment (Relapse). (Reprinted, by permission of the authors and the Editor of *Cancer,* from the paper by Hrgovcic et al., 1973.)

	Pre Rx	Rx WED	Rx Dund	Rx NED	No Rx NED	Relapse
Clinical Category	1	2	3	4	5	6
Number of Samples	93	321	112	89	218	63
Number of Patients	80	72	42	21	50	44

is a close correlation between the pattern of fluctuation of the serum copper level and prognosis and that the persistence of a level of 150 μg percent or higher strongly suggests the presence of active disease. A typical example in our own experience of an increase in serum copper level as a premonitory indicator of relapse is presented in Figure 12.29.

However, serum copper levels may be elevated for reasons that have nothing to do with disease activity. Wilimas, Thompson, and Smith (1978) observed false positive elevations of serum copper levels in 8 of 19 children with Hodgkin's disease, in whom upper respiratory infection and inflammatory disease are common, and observed increases in consecutive values of the serum copper in nearly 20 percent of patients in remission which exceeded those among patients who relapsed. Hrgovcic et al. (1975) have also stressed that the serum copper is nonspecific and that false positive levels may be observed secondary to infection or inflammation, in pregnancy, and in patients taking certain medications, notably contraceptive pills containing estrogen, or certain dyes, such as phenazopyridine hydrochloride (Pyridium). In the series of 50 patients studied at Stanford University Medical Center

(Chapter 4), serial determinations again indicate the importance of interpreting elevated levels with caution. Serum copper levels returned to normal following treatment in 83 percent of the patients in whom levels were elevated prior to treatment. There was a general correlation between subsequent renewed elevation of serum copper levels and the development of relapses. However, it is noteworthy that on one or more followup visits 43 (86 percent) of the patients had an inflammatory condition which could well have caused an elevation of the serum copper level. For this and other reasons, a much more detailed analysis of these longitudinal data will be required before any estimate can be offered of the reliability of an elevated serum copper level as an indicator of impending relapse.

Significantly reduced zinc contents in the plasma, whole blood, and erythrocytes of patients with Hodgkin's disease have been reported by Koch et al. (1957), Auerbach (1965), and Valberg, Holt, and Card (1966). Bucher and Jones (1977) stated that the copper/zinc ratio (CZR) correlated well with disease activity in a series of patients with Hodgkin's disease. Previously untreated and relapsing patients had mean CZR values of 2.1 and

A

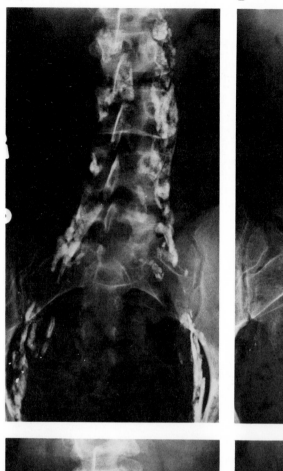

B

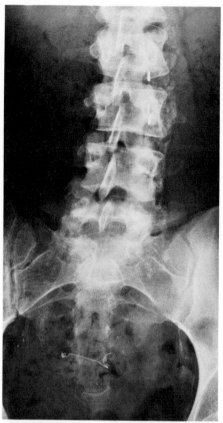

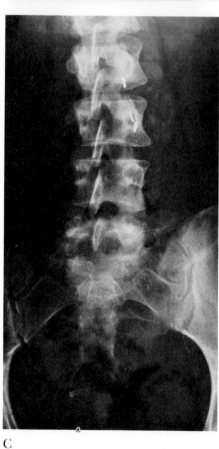

C

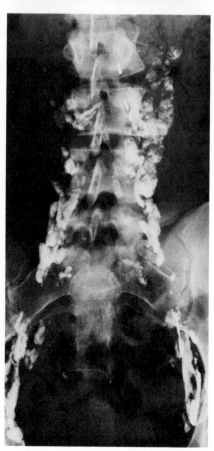

D

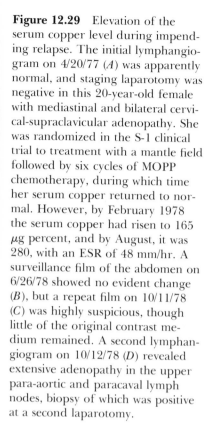

Figure 12.29 Elevation of the serum copper level during impending relapse. The initial lymphangiogram on 4/20/77 (*A*) was apparently normal, and staging laparotomy was negative in this 20-year-old female with mediastinal and bilateral cervical-supraclavicular adenopathy. She was randomized in the S-1 clinical trial to treatment with a mantle field followed by six cycles of MOPP chemotherapy, during which time her serum copper returned to normal. However, by February 1978 the serum copper had risen to 165 μg percent, and by August, it was 280, with an ESR of 48 mm/hr. A surveillance film of the abdomen on 6/26/78 showed no evident change (*B*), but a repeat film on 10/11/78 (*C*) was highly suspicious, though little of the original contrast medium remained. A second lymphangiogram on 10/12/78 (*D*) revealed extensive adenopathy in the upper para-aortic and paracaval lymph nodes, biopsy of which was positive at a second laparotomy.

2.2, respectively, whereas those with partial and complete remissions had mean ratios of 1.7 and 1.5, respectively. Decreased levels of serum iron have also been thought to mirror the extent and activity of Hodgkin's disease. Indeed, it has been stated by Teillet, Boiron, and Bernard (1971) that hyposideremia is the most reliable of a constellation of biological signs indicative of a "systemic syndrome" in Hodgkin's disease; the other relevant biological signs include: ESR $\geq$ 40 mm/hr, serum fibrin $\geq$ 0.5 g/100 ml, serum α-2-globulin $\geq$ 1 g/100 ml, and granulocytosis $\geq$ 9,000/mm³. One or more of these biological signs was present in 20 of 22 patients with splenic relapses in the series studied by Teillet, Boiron, and Bernard. However, there is little or no evidence that decreased serum iron levels have prognostic significance independently of other laboratory indicators or of constitutional symptoms. For a limited time, we routinely determined serum iron levels and total iron binding capacity in consecutive, previously untreated patients, but discontinued both tests when we found that they were frequently normal in patients whose ESR and/or serum copper levels were distinctly elevated.

Leukocyte alkaline phosphatase, which is known to be elevated in the presence of infection and in polycythemia (Martinez-Maldonado et al., 1964), has also been reported to fluctuate in parallel with disease activity in patients with Hodgkin's disease. Flury and Wegmann (1964) observed a mean value of 149 in 51 cases of Hodgkin's disease, as compared with a mean of 44.8 in 25 normal individuals (range 20 to 76). Patients whose Hodgkin's disease was clinically active had a mean of 194, whereas the mean level in those in remission was 95. In a series of sixteen patients treated with intensive radiotherapy, the mean level prior to treatment was 192 and after treatment 88; in contrast, fourteen other patients treated with palliative radiotherapy showed a slight increase from the pretreatment level of 191 to a post-treatment level of 205. Seven others treated palliatively with chemotherapy similarly showed no decrease of the leukocyte alkaline phosphatase into the normal range. Bennett et al. (1968) reported that leukocyte alkaline phosphatase levels were significantly elevated in twenty-two of twenty-three patients with active Hodgkin's disease and were normal in fifteen of nineteen with clinically inactive disease. Similar data have been reported by Lille-Szyskowicz et al. (1966) and Simmons, Spiers, and Fayers (1973).

Eilam et al. (1968) reported that the mean level of bradykininogen in a series of seventeen patients with active Hodgkin's disease was 4.2 ± 0.32 μg per ml., as compared with a mean of 6.08 ± 0.28 μg per ml. in twenty-three normal subjects and 6.79 ± 0.41 μg per ml. in twenty-eight patients with clinically inactive Hodgkin's disease. LeRoy et al. (1966) observed elevated plasma levels of a hydroxyproline-containing protein in thirteen patients with active Hodgkin's disease. Eight of these patients responded well to therapy, with a concomitant return of the hydroxyproline-containing protein to normal levels, whereas two others failed to enter remission, and their elevated hydroxyproline-containing protein levels persisted. Similar observations have been reported for serum haptoglobin (Krauss et al., 1966a), C-reactive protein (Wood et al., 1958; Pecori et al., 1959), acid glycoprotein (Schmid et al., 1964), serum hexosamine (Spiers and Malone, 1966), serum protein-bound hexose (Goulian and Fahey, 1961; Abdou et al., 1966), and serum transcobalamin-II levels (Rachmilewitz and Rachmilewitz, 1976) in patients with Hodgkin's disease, though the relationship to disease activity has been less extensively studied. Child et al. (1978) noted that the levels of several acute phase reactant proteins tended to fluctuate in relation to disease activity.

A general difficulty in the interpretation of all of these reported abnormalities is that many, and perhaps all, of the biochemical indicators studied are known to respond nonspecifically to a variety of febrile and inflammatory disorders. Accordingly, as in the case of the ESR, it would be hazardous to place excessive reliance on alterations in any one indicator alone. Moreover, most of the reported biochemical studies to date have not been carried out on series of cases in which complete diagnostic evaluation of the extent of the disease, reliable clinical staging, and definitive therapy have also been utilized. It seems desirable to acquire additional data on several of these biochemical parameters in a series of patients who are properly staged, treated in accordance with a well-defined policy, and subsequently carefully followed for the detection and timing of relapses in relation to fluctuations in levels of one or more biochemical parameters. It is to be hoped that, when such careful correlative studies have been carried out, the utilization of one or more of these biochemical indicators as additional prognostic aids can be more confidently recommended.

Immunologic Responses. The available evidence concerning the existence and nature of an immunologic defect and its correlation with clinical stage and prognosis in patients with Hodgkin's disease has been detailed in Chapter 6. Few published studies have been specifically directed at the question whether disease activity is reliably mirrored in immunologic responsiveness. Ciampelli and Pèlu (1963) reported that the course of the disease was favorable in twelve of sixteen patients who were tuberculin-positive both initially and after radiotherapy and in six of eight initially tuberculin-negative patients who converted to positive reactions after treatment, whereas an unfavorable course was observed in seven of eight initially tuberculin-positive patients who became unresponsive after irradiation, and in nine of fifteen who were initially, and subsequently remained, tuberculin negative. They also noted suggestive evidence of a correlation between survival and the post-irradiation tuberculin response. Sokal and Primikirios (1961) also noted conversion of initially tuberculin-negative responses to normal reactivity in patients with Hodgkin's disease who remained in long-sustained remission after treatment.

Sokal and Aungst (1969) studied thirty-two patients with advanced Hodgkin's disease and negative cutaneous reactions to second-strength purified protein derivative who were vaccinated with the bacillus of Calmette and Guérin (BCG) during a period of quiescent or mildly active disease. They reported that seven of eight whose tuberculin reaction failed to convert were dead within one year, as compared with only one such death among twenty-four patients who were successfully converted, suggesting that BCG vaccination may be a prognostically useful procedure in tuberculin-negative patients (cf. Fig. 6.12).

Aisenberg (1962), studying the capacity of patients to respond to active sensitization with dinitrochlorobenzene (DNCB), noted that those whose disease had been clinically inactive for two years or longer tended to have normal cutaneous reactions and that occasional initially unresponsive patients became DNCB-positive one to two years after radiotherapy. We have noted such "reversals" to DNCB reactivity in a high proportion of our apparently successfully irradiated patients (Fuks et al., 1976b; cf. Chapter 6); however, reversals are not always a reliable indicator of persistent remission or cure, since we have also observed them in occasional patients with well-documented activity or progression of disease.

The correlation between immune responses and disease activity may be masked, at least for some time, by the effects of treatment on immunity. Jackson, Garrett, and Craig (1970) studied the phytohemagglutinin-induced blastoid transformation response in vitro of lymphocytes from forty-one patients at serial intervals during the course of the disease. They noted some correlation with clinical stage, a depressed response for about six months after radiotherapy, and a return to normal in patients whose disease entered remission thereafter. Kun and Johnson (1975), in a followup study of 69 patients treated with intensive radiotherapy, observed apparently complete recovery of delayed hypersensitivity responses and serum immunoglobulin levels within five years.

However, it is clear that some immunologic responses are profoundly impaired by intensive total lymphoid radiotherapy and that such impairment may persist for many years thereafter in patients who remain in complete remission. Fuks et al. (1976b) studied several immunologic parameters before and at various intervals up to ten years after intensive radiotherapy in a series of 227 patients with Hodgkin's disease treated at Stanford University Medical Center between 1965 and 1975. They observed a striking absolute T-lymphocytopenia immediately after radiotherapy which persisted in patients who had been treated as long as ten years previously. In contrast, the profound fall in absolute B-lymphocyte count immediately following radiotherapy was transient and gave way to an absolute B-lymphocytosis in over 60 percent of patients which was sustained for up to ten years. Stimulation of peripheral blood lymphocytes by phytohemagglutinin (PHA) was profoundly depressed over a wide range of PHA concentrations immediately following radiotherapy and remained at approximately the same low levels in patients who had been in continuous remission for as long as ten years after treatment. Similar impairment of the stimulation response to concanavalin A was observed. In contrast, the mixed lymphocyte reaction, though decreased immediately following treatment, gradually recovered between two and five years thereafter.

Depressed lymphocyte responses to PHA in vitro were also observed by Case et al. (1977a) in patients with Hodgkin's disease in long-sustained continuous remission. Björkholm et al. (1977a) reported similar observations with respect to T-lymphocytopenia and impaired lymphocyte stimulation responses to concanavalin A and to tuberculin in patients remaining in complete remission for 15–18 months after completion of radiotherapy, and Weitzman et al. (1977b) also observed impairment of humoral immunity in treated patients in remission. Thus, it appears that in most patients the profound and long-sustained effects of treatment on the immune response preclude the use of the immune response as a guide to prognosis in treated patients. Although it is probably generally true that restoration of cell-mediated immune responses is an indication of a favorable prognosis, the converse is by no means true. Many patients who remain anergic for years following treatment may nonetheless remain relapse-free indefinitely.

It has long been recognized that noncaseating epithelioid granulomas (Fig. 3.51) occur in a small but significant proportion of patients with Hodgkin's disease (Kadin, Donaldson, and Dorfman, 1970). Some observers formerly considered these lesions an atypical expression of the disease process itself, whereas others have speculated that they may reflect an immunologic response of the body to the disease. In an attempt to assess the significance of these granulomas, Sacks et al. (1978a) examined the records of 608 consecutive patients with biopsy-proven Hodgkin's disease who were surgically staged and treated at Stanford University Medical Center between July 1968 and January 1974. They found a total of 55 patients who had histologically verified noncaseating epithelioid granulomas. The course of the disease in this study group was compared with that in 553 concurrently treated patients in whom granulomas were not found at staging laparotomy. There were no significant differences in stage distribution, histopathologic type, or proportion with constitutional symptoms between the two groups. After a minimum followup interval of two years, and a median followup time of 60 months, the actuarial probability of survival and of freedom from relapse was calculated, yielding the curves seen in Figure 12.30. A separate analysis of survival among patients with stage I and II versus stage III and IV disease (Fig. 12.31) again shows significant differences in survival in favor of patients who had noncaseating epithelioid granulomas. The five-year survival rate for patients with granulomas was 94.7 percent, that for the group without granulomas, 81.2 percent. O'Connell et al. (1975a) also observed improved survival among 17 patients with granulomas among a series of 91 patients with Hodgkin's disease. Both groups were unable to detect any correlation between the presence or absence of such granulomas and the immune responsiveness of patients. Indeed, an inverse relationship was suggested by the Stanford data, in which a difference in delayed hypersensitivity responsiveness to DNCB was observed in favor of the nongranuloma group which was nearly significant at the 5 percent

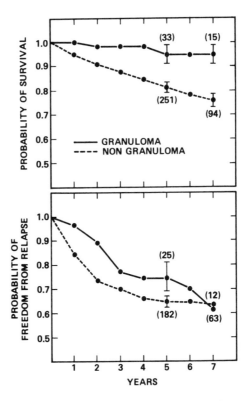

Figure 12.30 Actuarial survival and relapse-free survival in patients with and without epithelioid granulomas, showing significant differences in both survival curves ($p = 0.005$) and relapse-free survival curves ($p = 0.03$) in favor of those patients with granulomas. (Reprinted, by permission of the authors and the Editor of *Cancer,* from the paper by Sacks et al., 1978a.)

level (Sacks et al., 1978a). Although the mechanism underlying their prognostic influence remains obscure, it appears that the presence of noncaseating epithelioid granulomas in association with Hodgkin's disease is correlated with an increased probability of survival in all stages of disease.

The Concept of a Composite Prognostic Index. The concept that a more effective prognostic index could be constructed by taking multiple prognostic indicators simultaneously into consideration has been considered by a number of investigators. As early as 1953, Gilbert alluded to this idea when he stated that the experienced clinician could learn to evaluate the duration and type of symptoms prior to admission, the clinical picture and extent of disease at the time of diagnosis, and the response to therapy and early post-treatment course of the disease in estimating the *Entwicklungspotential,* i.e., the potential of the disease to develop and progress.

Perhaps the first specific attempt to utilize a combination of prognostic factors was the modification

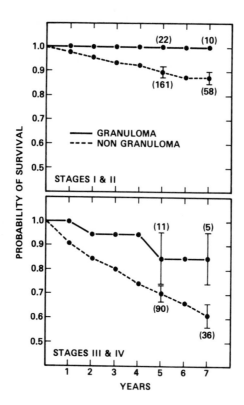

Figure 12.31 Actuarial survival curves for "early" (stages I and II) and "advanced" (stages III and IV) Hodgkin's disease, comparing survival of patients with and without granulomas. Both sets of curves show significant differences in favor of those patients with granulomas. (Reprinted, by permission of the authors and the Editor of *Cancer,* from the paper by Sacks et al., 1978a.)

of the original Peters' (1950) staging classification by Peters and Middlemiss (1958), in which a subdivision of anatomic stage II into subgroups with and without constitutional symptoms was proposed. This concept was extended to all four anatomic stages in the Rye staging classification and has since been adopted in other proposed classifications (Musshoff et al., 1968; Rosenberg and Kaplan, 1970; Carbone et al., 1971).

Westling (1965), after a detailed analysis of his case material, identified six factors as the major prognostic indicators in Hodgkin's disease. Since each of these influenced survival by about 15 to 25 percent, he constructed a "forecaster index" simply by adding the number of these factors that were present in any given case. Accordingly, his index ranged between 0 and 6. He also suggested the substitution of certain auxiliary factors in instances in which no data were available on the major prognostic criteria. As might have been expected, survival of his cases, when reanalyzed on the basis of index points, showed an excellent correlation with this composite index. However, relatively few cases were available for consideration in the highest index point groups 5 and 6 and in the lowest category 0. Accordingly, he proposed a simplified version of the index, which grouped together cases with either 0 or 1 point, considered cases with 2 points as a separate category, and grouped together those with 3 or more points. Survival curves for this modified forecaster index again revealed an excellent correlation. The six prognostic factors that were utilized in constructing his index were: stage III disease, fever (or "subfebrility"), leukopenia, ESR greater than 25, age greater than fifty years, and signs of abdominal disease. Westling recognized that certain of his prognostic factors were interrelated rather than independent and that they did not all carry equal prognostic weight. Accordingly, he attempted to estimate weighting factors for each of the various criteria; the most significant were fever, abdominal signs, and stage III disease, each of which was apparently associated with an influence on survival of between 20 and 30 percent.

Papillon et al. (1966c) divided unfavorable prognostic signs in their series of 231 cases into two categories. Their particularly unfavorable group (series A) included: generalized superficial adenopathy; visceral involvement; the Peters and Middlemiss subcategory B for symptoms of generalized disease; alteration of the general condition of the patient; the presence of numerous small, hard lymph nodes; the presence of interbronchial lymph nodes; and the diffuse fibrosis histopathologic type of Lukes. Their series B included prognostic indicators which were also unfavorable, but less so in their opinion than those of series A. The factors associated with series B included age of less than fifteen years or more than forty years, male sex, lymphangiographic evidence of stage III disease, bilateral inguinal or spinal adenopathy, and delayed diagnosis. On the basis of these groupings, they suggested that three types of Hodgkin's disease could be prognostically defined. Their group I, comprising patients presenting at least two signs from series A, was the most unfavorable, with particularly rapid evolution of the disease and survival in general not exceeding two years. Their group II, which included those with a single sign from series A or two signs from series B, was also relatively unfavorable, the duration of first remission frequently being relatively short, but survival of appreciable duration was considered possible. Finally, group III included patients who presented no signs from either series A or series B. Papillon et al. suggest that it is in this "privileged" group that virtually all of the long remissions and long survivals occur. The most typical member of this group would be a female patient between twenty and forty years of age, with supraclavicular and mediastinal adenopathy without fever or other systemic signs. They noted that among their twelve clinically cured patients in remission for ten to twenty-five years, nine were female, the age range at time of diagnosis was sixteen to thirty-one years, nine had supraclavicular and anterior mediastinal adenopathy, two had generalized pruritus, and two were pregnant.

Another type of composite prognostic index (CPI) was suggested by Keller, Kaplan, Lukes, and Rappaport (1968). This index takes into consideration the anatomic extent of disease, the presence or absence of constitutional symptoms, and the histopathologic type of Hodgkin's disease present, using the Rye modification of the Lukes classification:

> To a baseline score of 0, the index for any given case is obtained by adding the following arbitrarily assigned values: one each for systemic symptoms (unexplained fever, night sweats, and/or significant weight loss), mixed cellularity, and stage III; two each for lymphocyte depletion and stage IV. Thus, for example, a stage IA case of the lymphocyte predominance type would have an index of 0, a stage IIB case of nodular sclerosis would have an index of $0 + 1 + 0 = 1$; a stage IIIA case of mixed cellularity type an index of $1 + 0 + 1 = 2$; and a stage IVB case of lymphocyte depletion type, an index of $2 + 1 + 2 = 5$.

Retrospective analysis of survival in the Stanford series indicated that patients with a CPI of 0 had a significantly better five-year survival than those with a CPI of 1 or 2, and these in turn had a significantly better survival at three years than patients with a CPI of 3 or more (Fig. 12.32). An advantage of this prognostic index is that relatively large groups of patients fell into the most favorable and least favorable groups, rather than clustering in the intermediate range. It was suggested that, as further data are accumulated, more accurate weighting factors can be substituted for the arbitrarily assigned values of 1 or 2 for the various categories to further refine the index.

To date, there has been no general agreement on the adoption of any of these composite prognostic indices, though the need for such an index is widely recognized (Schilling, 1978). The funda-

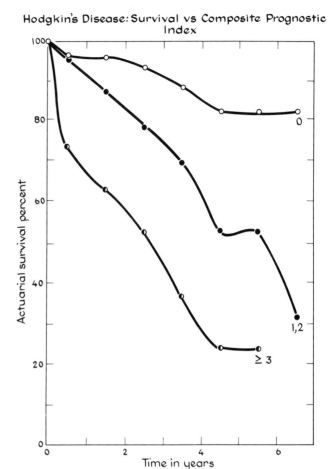

Figure 12.32 Actuarial survival versus composite prognostic index (see text for details). (Reprinted, by permission, from the paper by Keller et al., 1968.)

mental idea of combining multiple factors into an index with greater prognostic discriminatory power seems eminently sound, and the effectiveness of such indices in sharpening estimates of prognosis has been convincingly demonstrated. The specific indices proposed to date are relatively crude and somewhat arbitrary, however. What seems needed at this point is a computer-assisted analysis of the relative significance and mutual interdependence of the various prognostic factors from which valid estimates of appropriate prognostic weighting factors could be obtained. Methods for the statistical analysis of such multiple factor interactions and for the application of adjustment factors to take account of their influence on survival have been proposed and discussed by Hankey and Myers (1971), Axtell et al. (1972), and Myers and Axtell (1973). It is to be hoped that an internationally acceptable composite prognostic index of this type can be developed and widely introduced during the next several years.

The Curability of Hodgkin's Disease

Historical Aspects. There are few diseases in which the word "cure" arouses as much emotion and controversy as in Hodgkin's disease. It is not difficult to understand some of the reasons why controversy continues to rage about a question that should be as amenable to rational definition and solution as the curability of any other malignant tumor. A dominant factor is the "image" of Hodgkin's disease, dating back to the turn of the century, as having a remarkable quality of inexorability in its fatal course, despite occasional unpredictable remissions. The concept of Hodgkin's disease as inevitably fatal has continued to be handed down in medical teaching, almost to the present decade, with the consequence that some older physicians still hold firmly to this conviction.

The introduction of radiotherapy in the first decade of the century did little to alter the situation; when the initial, almost magical regressions of lymphadenopathy were followed by recurrence and progression of the disease, the first wave of enthusiasm and hope was succeeded by a pessimistic attitude more deeply entrenched than ever. Thus, when a slowly increasing number of long-term, disease-free survivors began to be recorded in the 1920's and 1930's, the stage was set for their being explained away as anything but the cures that they may well have represented. The dilemma of the era was well expressed by Minot and Isaacs in 1926; "It does remain true and noteworthy that there is a high frequency among the cases of long duration of those treated early by surgery and irradiation, the latter being continued in a suitable manner. It becomes difficult not to believe that therapy does, at least sometimes, influence the duration of the disease. Even so, the facts might not be reconciled in this way; for it is true that similar cases, either with or without any irradiation or surgery, or such treatment very late in the course of the disease, are alike in duration, and that among the cases of all types are some with long intervals, even years between irradiation treatments."

Gilbert (1939) clearly believed that individual foci of disease in lymph nodes could be eradicated by appropriate doses of radiotherapy; yet he could not bring himself to use the word "cure." The ambivalence of his attitude is clearly reflected in his statement: "The aim should always be to obtain *prolonged remission equivalent to clinical cures,* remis-

sions that can be renewed without risk on the appearance of the *inevitable recurrences*" [my italics]. In 1949, the distinguished pathologist Arthur Purdy Stout pondered the same question: "Is it possible to suppose that any of the long survival symptom-free patients are cures? It would be hazardous to affirm it when it is noted that so many have survived an equally long time with the disease still persisting." Certainly, the persistence of Hodgkin's disease among long-term survivors has been well documented (Henry, 1970; Strum and Rappaport, 1971b; Wright, 1975). However, it should be noted that most, if not all, of the long-term survivors in these studies had been clinically staged prior to the advent of lymphangiography or staging laparotomy, and many had been treated with low-dose, involved field radiotherapy alone. Moreover, most of the individuals who were ultimately found to have persistent Hodgkin's disease at autopsy had had one or more clinically overt relapses at some time after their initial course of treatment.

One of the first investigators to appreciate clearly the important distinction between disease-free survival and survival with periodically relapsing disease was Hynes (1955). In an article boldly entitled "Radiocurability of Malignant Lymphoma," he stated: "The malignant lymphomas differ from other cancers in that they include an appreciable number of cases which evolve slowly and are amenable to palliative treatment long after most cancers would prove fatal. We must therefore be extremely conservative in the estimation of probable cures when we report upon malignant lymphomas. Those patients who remain well with periodic therapy must be considered as 'survivors'; but those who remain well for many years after a single course of treatment should be considered as possible 'cures.'"

Other skeptics have discounted long-term, disease-free survivors as instances of erroneous diagnosis or of the relatively "benign" paragranuloma or lymphocyte predominance histopathologic types, which are well known to run a remarkably indolent course with or without specific therapy. It must be admitted that erroneous histopathologic diagnosis unquestionably accounts for some of the long survivals, but it can no longer be seriously proposed as a valid explanation for the great majority of them (Kaplan, 1966c).

Lukes, Gompel, and Nezelof (1966d) reviewed the original biopsy slides on a large number of cases of Hodgkin's disease in which disease-free survival for over ten years had been documented. They were able to reconfirm the diagnosis of

Hodgkin's disease in all but a small proportion of these cases. Moreover, they established that the frequency of the paragranuloma form among the ten-year survivors was not significantly greater than what might have been expected at the time of original diagnosis. Thus, there is no longer any reason to doubt that many patients who had unequivocally confirmed histopathologic evidence of Hodgkin's disease initially have survived relapse-free for ten years or more after intensive radiotherapy. Once this is accepted as established fact, the next question is whether such patients can appropriately be considered cured, and this in turn brings us to the difficult problem of providing acceptable definitions of cure.

Definitions of "Cure." Many physicians insist that the word "cure" be used only in an absolute sense to refer to patients in whom all manifestations of a disease have been completely and permanently eradicated, never to recur during the remainder of their normal life span. They reject as unacceptable definitions of cure based on statistical analysis, since statistics by its nature deals with probabilities rather than with certainties. This attitude is clearly reflected in the criticism, expressed by Craver and Miller (1965), of the important article entitled "The Cure of Hodgkin's Disease," which was published by Easson and Russell in 1963: "Their use of the word 'cure' seems an exercise in semantics, inasmuch as they mean only that between ten and fifteen years after treatment the death-rate curve of disease-free survivors runs parallel to that of the general population of the same age and sex." Yet, as we shall discuss later, this is an eminently practical and meaningful definition of the word "cure."

It has been possible to prove conclusively by sacrifice, careful postmortem examination, and microscopic examination of serial sections that mice appropriately treated for autochthonous malignant lymphomas may indeed be cured in an absolute sense (Kaplan and Nagareda, 1961). Of course, such a procedure is clearly untenable for human patients afflicted with Hodgkin's disease or other malignant lymphomas. There are, however, increasing numbers of cases on record of patients who died of intercurrent disease at relatively long intervals after definitive treatment for a confirmed diagnosis of Hodgkin's disease, in whom careful postmortem examination failed to reveal gross or histopathologic evidence of residual disease. The principal drawback of such autopsy evidence is that it is essentially anecdotal in character. The au-

topsy-negative cases who die in automobile accidents or of intercurrent disease will inevitably comprise too small a sample to provide any valid estimate of the proportion of long-term survivors who are really cured in an absolute sense. Thus, any practical definition of cure, if it is to be applicable to large populations of patients with Hodgkin's disease rather than merely to isolated, anecdotal cases, must necessarily be predicated on statistical considerations.

The article by Hynes (1955), cited above, which was probably the first to claim that Hodgkin's disease and other malignant lymphomas can be cured by radiotherapy, was unfortunately published in a relatively obscure journal and received little attention. It was not until 1963, when Easson and Russell published their article with the deliberatively provocative title, "The Cure of Hodgkin's Disease," that this possibility began to receive widespread attention. Of equal importance was the pragmatic definition of "cure" which they offered: "Cure of a disease is taken to connote that in time . . . probably a decade or two after treatment . . . there remains a group of disease-free survivors whose annual death rate from all causes is similar to that of a normal population group of the same sex and age distribution." Analyzing the survival of a large series of patients with Hodgkin's disease treated at Manchester, they found that the survival curve became progressively less steep with time until, about twelve years after treatment, it paralleled that of an age- and sex-matched normal population. For regionally localized cases, their curve flattened at about 40 percent survival; for "generalized" cases, at between 10 and 15 percent.

Schwartz (1966), acknowledging that the Easson-Russell definition of cure is a valid one, nonetheless listed four objections to it: (1) the choice of the control population may be arbitrary; (2) proof that the survival curve has indeed become parallel to that of the age- and sex-matched normal population is difficult and not very sensitive; (3) parallelism attained at any given time interval may not persist because of later deaths; and (4) not all cases in the parallel segment of the curve need be true cures. He called attention to the existence of more powerful methods for the statistical analysis of such data, involving the separation of observed survival into two distributions: (*a*) that of the cured patients, which should simulate that of the normal population, and (*b*) that of non-cured patients.

Such an analysis requires a model or an a priori hypothesis regarding the form of these two distributions. A suitable model for the distribution of survivals among the cured patients is the known distribution of survival times for the normal control population. For the non-cured patients, any one of three mathematical models which have been proposed to fit the survival curves of patients with cancer may be selected: the Berkson and Gage (1950, 1952) model, based on exponentially decreasing survival; Boag's model (1949), based on a log-normal distribution of survival; or the extrapolated actuarial model proposed by Haybittle (1959). It is then possible to evaluate the proportion of cases in the apparently cured group and its confidence interval and to calculate the probability that this proportion differs significantly from zero. These methods are appreciably more rigorous than the original Easson-Russell concept of parallelism and are not subject to objections (2) and (4) cited above.

Haybittle (1963) carried out such an analysis on the original data of Easson and Russell, applying both the Berkson-Gage and his own (Haybittle, 1959) models of the survival distribution in patients dying of the disease to obtain an estimate of c, the fraction cured, together with its standard error. He also tested both models for their goodness of fit to the data, and established that both were acceptable. The average of the estimates provided by the two models indicates that 34 ± 5 percent of the localized cases and 13 ± 3 percent of the generalized cases of Easson and Russell can properly be considered true cures, since both values of c differ from zero by more than twice their standard error.

Frei and Gehan (1971) used the *relative* survival rate to analyze national data on Hodgkin's disease collected by the National Cancer Institute. The relative survival rate is defined as the ratio of the observed percentage of survival to the percentage of survival expected on the basis of general population experience adjusted for age, sex, race, and calendar year. By this definition, a population of patients that was cured after a given period of time would yield a horizontal straight line in a plot of relative survival rate against time following treatment. The excess mortality due to Hodgkin's disease was found to decrease from 15 percent to 10 percent and then to 5 percent in successive five-year intervals after the sixth year. After the twentieth year, there were no deaths from Hodgkin's disease among the 87 patients who were at risk at the start of that interval. Thus, although there is a decreasing risk of death from Hodgkin's disease with time, cure, by this definition, does not occur until after the twentieth year.

The Relapse-Free Interval and Cure. A serious disadvantage of any method of analysis which uses survival as its sole endpoint is that appreciable numbers of late deaths occur beyond the tenth year. Such long intervals are particularly vexing to investigators exploring the efficacy of new modes of treatment and therefore desirous of valid answers at the earliest possible date. Accordingly, attention has turned to other criteria of response that might serve as earlier indicators of potential survival. That the duration of remission after the first course of treatment might constitute such an early criterion of potential survival was perhaps first suggested by Hynes (1955), who stated: "When remission of signs and symptoms persists for ten or more years, without the need of continued treatment, it is proper to describe such remission as apparent cure."

Hall and Olson (1956) provided the first documentary evidence indicating that the length of the first remission is correlated with ultimate survival time in Hodgkin's disease. They found that nineteen patients whose first remission lasted for one year or more had a five-year survival of 53 percent, whereas twenty-eight other patients with a first remission shorter than one year had only a 7.1 percent five-year survival. The existence of a relationship between the duration of first remission and survival has since been amply confirmed by other investigators (Gnatyshek and Kuznetsova, 1960; Croizat et al., 1962; Roxin et al., 1962; Musshoff et al., 1966; Papillon et al., 1966c).

In 1962, I compiled a summary of my own data and the relatively sparse published information in the literature to obtain an estimate of the temporal distribution of relapses after the first course of radiotherapy. I found that twenty-nine of thirty-five documented initial relapses (83 percent) occurred within twenty-four months after the start of the first course of treatment. Moreover, the average interval to relapse in a series of 117 cases reported by Heilmeyer et al. (1957) was twelve months, in good agreement with estimates based on individual case reports. I therefore proposed that freedom from relapse at two years might be a reasonably stringent test of the efficacy of any method of treatment. Since several of the patients treated with radical megavoltage radiotherapy in my series had survived free of disease for several multiples of the average time interval to first relapse, I suggested that at least some of these patients may have been cured (Kaplan, 1962).

In successive analyses of Stanford University Medical Center experience, a much more voluminous mass of evidence has now been gathered in support of this approach. I have presented data on the relapse-free interval in a series of 145 patients with stage I and II Hodgkin's disease and of 76 patients with stage III and IV disease (Kaplan, 1968b). The annual relapse rates after radiotherapy were high during the first two to three years after treatment and rapidly diminished to approach the zero baseline by the fourth or fifth year. In this analysis, about 85 percent of the observed relapses had occurred by the end of three years.

Spittle et al. (1973) analyzed a series of 114 primary relapses occurring among a total of 462 previously untreated patients with Hodgkin's disease of stages I–III admitted between 1961 and 1971. There was surprisingly little variation of relapse rate with clinical stage. Relapses occurred in 14 (21.9 percent) of 66 patients with stage IA or IB disease; 64 (24.9 percent) of 257 patients with stage IIA or IIB disease; and 36 (25.9 percent) of 139 patients with stage IIIA or IIIB disease. However, there appeared to be a relationship between relapse rate and histopathologic type. There were only 6 relapses among the 49 patients with LP histology (12 percent); 68 among the 277 patients with NS (25 percent); 33 among 121 with MC (27 percent); and 7 of 15 with LD histopathology (47 percent). The cumulative relapse curve indicated that nearly 50 percent of all of the recorded relapses occurred within the first year, and 82 percent had occurred by the end of the second year, in excellent agreement with the data of the 1962 and 1968 studies. There were no recorded relapses beyond the fifth year following radiotherapy. Fifty-seven patients were available for analysis of the relationship between the time interval to first relapse and the interval to a second relapse. The data are plotted in a scattergram (Fig. 12.33). Despite considerable variability, second relapses tended to occur at intervals consistent with the tempo of the initial relapse. For 29 patients whose first relapse occurred within less than one year and who had a second relapse, 19 (66 percent) of the second relapses were again within one year. Conversely, for 28 patients whose first interval to relapse was greater than one year and who had a second relapse, 17 (61 percent) of the second relapses again occurred after an interval exceeding one year. Actuarial analysis of survival, calculated from the time of first admission of these 114 patients with relapsing disease, was only 53 percent at five years. There was some indication that the interval to relapse may influence postrelapse prognosis. Among 59 patients whose primary relapse

Relationships Between Intervals to Relapse

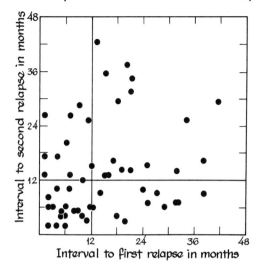

Figure 12.33 Scattergram of the interval to second relapse in relation to the interval to first relapse in a series of 57 patients with Hodgkin's disease. (Reprinted by permission from the paper by Spittle et al., 1973.)

occurred within the first 12 months, 61 percent were dead with disease and only 25 percent remained apparently relapse-free. Among 35 patients whose initial relapses occurred during the second year, 51 percent were dead with disease and 23 percent were apparently disease-free. Finally, of 20 patients whose primary relapses occurred beyond two years, only 40 percent were dead with disease and 30 percent remained disease-free.

The next Stanford studies were those of Weller et al. (1976, 1977), who analyzed 243 relapses occurring among 701 consecutive patients treated between 1961 and 1973. They found that 87 percent of all primary relapses occurred within the first three years, and 96 percent within five years after the initial course of treatment, again in good agreement with previously published data. However, in a subset of 40 patients whose initial relapses were retrograde transdiaphragmatic extensions from initially supradiaphragmatic stage I or stage II disease, 5 relapses (12.5 percent) occurred after five years (Weller et al., 1977). Relapse rates were essentially identical for both males and females. As may be seen in Table 12.5, there was an increasing risk of relapse in patients with unfavorable (MC and LD) histopathologic types of disease. The data of Table 12.6 indicate that the risk of relapse increased with advancing clinical stage, from 17 percent in patients with stage I to 55 percent in patients with stage IV disease.

Table 12.5 Initial Relapse Rates versus Histopathologic Type

Histologic type	No. of patients	Initial relapses	
		No.	%
Lymphocyte predominance	51	9	18
Nodular sclerosis	433	154	36
Mixed cellularity	151	60	40
Lymphocyte depletion	19	16	84
Unclassified	47	4	

Source: Stanford University Medical Center data, from the paper by Weller et al., 1976.

Musshoff and Boutis (1968) have published data on the relapse rates in a series of 340 cases of Hodgkin's disease. Their data indicate that 67 percent of the relapses occurred in the first year and that the cumulative relapse curve increased to 87 percent by the end of three years and to 96 percent by the end of five years. Between the fifth and tenth year, the proportion of cases remaining in complete remission decreased by only 3.5 percent, and there were no relapses at all between the ninth and the fifteenth year after treatment. Thus, the curve for cumulative relapses rises rapidly in the first two years but tends to flatten out progressively thereafter, reaching a plateau by about the fifth year (Fig. 12.34). This is again clearly evident in the curves published by Prosnitz et al. (1969) and Musshoff et al. (1976) and in the data reviewed by Frei and Gehan (1971).

The probability of a primary relapse after the fifth year is small, almost certainly less than 5 percent. Analysis of the Stanford 1961–1977 series of 1,225 consecutive, previously untreated patients (Kaplan, unpublished) reveals an ultimate relapse rate of 39.1 percent, with the last recorded relapse occurring during the eleventh year (Fig. 12.33). Relapses occurred earlier and cumulative relapse rates rose to higher levels, as expected, among patients with stage III and IV disease than among those in stages I and II (Fig. 12.35). Similar differences were evident in relation to the presence or absence of constitutional symptoms (Fig. 12.36). Only 6 (3.3 percent) of 184 patients who remained relapse-free for the first five years developed primary relapses thereafter. It follows, therefore, that at least 95 percent of patients who remain relapse-free for five years or more are in fact cured.

Additional evidence of the prognostic significance of the relapse-free interval is to be found in data on the after-survival of persons with Hodgkin's disease who have experienced one or more relapses during a given time interval, as compared

Table 12.6 Initial Relapse Rates versus Ann Arbor Clinical Stage

Stage	No. of patients	Initial relapses	
		No.	%
I	98	17 (6)[a]	17
IIA	240	70 (28)	29
IIB	97	30 (15)	31
IIIA	105	34 (19)	32
IIIB	96	47 (27)	49
IV	65	36 (5)	55
Exclusions		9	
Totals	701	243 (100)	35

Source: Stanford University Medical Center data, from the paper by Weller et al., 1976.

[a] (—) Numbers in parentheses represent number of patients pathologically staged at presentation.

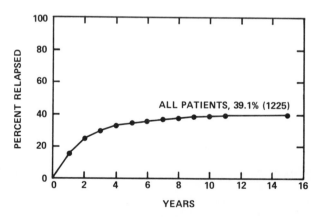

Figure 12.34 Cumulative relapse curve to 15 years in the Stanford 1961–1977 series of 1,225 consecutive, previously untreated patients with Hodgkin's disease of all stages. The final relapse rate was 39.1 percent. The last recorded relapse occurred during the eleventh year, though the curve is nearly flat after the fifth year.

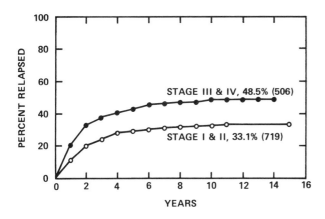

Figure 12.35 Cumulative relapse curves of the Stanford series plotted separately for patients with Ann Arbor stage III and IV versus stage I and II disease. It is evident that relapse rates rise earlier among the patients with advanced disease. Total numbers of patients in each group are indicated in parentheses.

with those who have remained relapse-free during the same interval. Papillon et al. (1966b) analyzed a series of ninety-nine cases of Hodgkin's disease treated at Lyon during the years 1935 to 1954, who had been at risk for more than ten years after treatment. They found that nineteen patients had survived more than ten years. Seven of these had developed one or more relapses before ten years, two having developed their initial relapse at about 9.5 years; of these, three subsequently died of Hodgkin's disease in the eleventh to the thirteenth year, and the remaining four all had active disease under treatment with chemotherapeutic agents. In contrast, the remaining twelve patients had all sur-

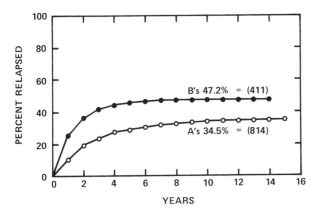

Figure 12.36 Cumulative relapse curves of the Stanford series plotted separately with respect to the presence (B's) or absence (A's) of constitutional symptoms. It is evident that relapse rates rise earlier among the patients with symptoms. Total numbers of patients in each group are indicated in parentheses.

vived for more than ten years with no interval relapse before the tenth year. All of these twelve continued free of Hodgkin's disease for periods of eleven to twenty-five years at the time of the report. The authors stated: "After a complete remission for ten years, we have never seen a relapse in the eleventh or twelfth year, and in the literature there is not to our knowledge any observation of an initial recurrence so late." These conclusions remained valid in a subsequent update of the data by Papillon (1974).

Lauwers and Dancot (1966) analyzed in detail 69 biopsy-proved five-year survivors out of a total series of 320 patients with Hodgkin's disease treated at the Institut Jules Bordet in Brussels from 1926 to 1950. Of the sixty-nine five-year survivors, forty-seven had had a primary relapse before the fifth year, and twenty-two had not. They found that forty of the forty-seven (85 percent) with interval relapses before the fifth year later died with active Hodgkin's disease. In contrast, only three of the twenty-two who were relapse-free at five years later developed a primary relapse (after six, seven, and twelve years). All three of these were successfully treated and alive, but two other patients died of unknown causes. Thus, the ultimate survival in the former group was only seven of forty-seven (15 percent), compared with seventeen (including four who died of intercurrent disease) of the twenty-two patients relapse-free at five years (77 percent).

Seydel, Bloedorn, and Wizenberg (1969) analyzed the course of thirty-nine patients with stage I and IIA Hodgkin's disease, of whom twenty-three had recurrence or extension of disease for which they received adequate radiotherapy. Whereas the eight-year survival after the initial course of radiotherapy, computed by the actuarial method, was 69 percent for the sixteen patients without extension or recurrence, it was only 24 percent for the thirteen patients with "localized extension," defined as involvement of lymph nodes on one side of the diaphragm without systemic symptoms, and 0 percent for ten patients with "generalized extension," defined as the development of lymph node disease on both sides of the diaphragm or with systemic symptoms or extralymphatic involvement. They concluded that extension of disease is associated with a poor prognosis, even within a given stage of the disease and despite adequate retreatment.

Musshoff and Boutis (1968) have published curves for survival and for the percentage of cases remaining in primary remission in a series of 340 cases of Hodgkin's disease. Their data (Fig. 12.37) clearly indicate that survival for the entire series

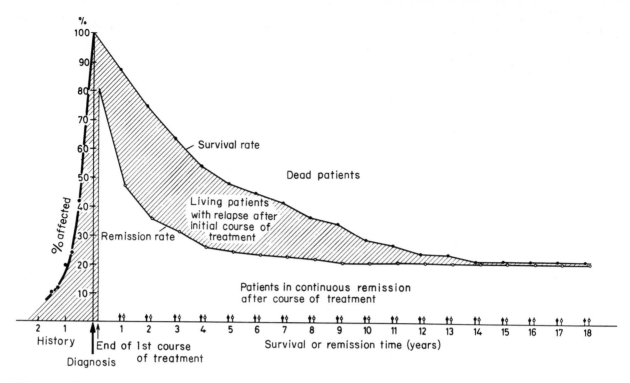

Figure 12.37 Natural history of previously untreated patients with Hodgkin's disease treated at Freiburg i. Br. from 1945 to 1966, n = 340. "History" = percentage of patients with signs or symptoms of disease for the indicated time interval (in years) prior to the time of diagnosis. "Survival rate" = survival curve of entire series; "Remission rate" = survival curve of relapse-free patients; shaded area between curves = surviving patients with relapse after first treatment; lower open area = patients in continuous remission. It is evident that the curve for long-surviving patients approaches that for the proportion of patients still in primary remission. (Reprinted, with translations inserted, by permission from the paper by Musshoff and Boutis, 1968.)

approaches and becomes essentially identical with the survival curve for patients remaining in primary remission at about the fourteenth year, at which time 20.9 percent of their patients remained in primary remission and 21.2 percent survived. This difference of 0.3 percent represents a single individual, who was the only relapsing patient in their entire series to survive longer than fourteen years.

A previous analysis of Stanford data on after-survival of patients with and without interval relapse during the first one and two years following intensive megavoltage radiotherapy again revealed a striking difference in the prognosis of those who remained relapse-free, compared with those with an interval relapse (Kaplan, 1968b). An updated analysis of 512 patients with pathological stage I or II Hodgkin's disease, admitted after July 1, 1968 and all staged with the aid of laparotomy and splenectomy, is presented in Figure 12.38. There were 467 patients who were at risk for at least one year. Of these, 33 had developed an initial relapse within the first year; their after-survival rate of

55.9 percent at about seven years is clearly far worse than that of the 434 patients who had no interval relapse during the first year (86.8 percent at eight years). The pairs of curves for 403 patients at risk for two years or more who did or did not develop relapses during the first two years are virtually identical to those in the first-year panel. Finally, the after-survival of 226 patients at risk for five years or more again shows a similar, though slightly lesser difference in prognosis of the 42 patients who relapsed during but were still alive at five years, and those who were relapse-free for the first five years. Collectively, these data provide compelling evidence to support the view that there is a prognostically vital distinction between survival with periodic relapsing disease and relapse-free survival for five years or more after the initial course of radiotherapy of Hodgkin's disease. The long-term survival data of Papillon et al. and of Lauwers and Dancot, as well as the thirty-year survival curves published by Hynes (1969; Fig. 12.39) and isolated cases of 40-year survival recorded by Peters (1973) and by Niblett (1975), clearly support

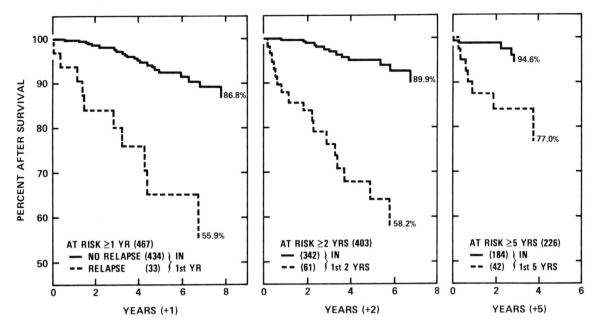

Figure 12.38 Actuarial analysis (by the method of Kaplan and Meier, 1958) of after-survival as a function of interval relapse in a series of 512 patients with PS I or II Hodgkin's disease. There were 467 patients at risk for at least one year (left panel), of whom 33 had suffered a relapse during the first year. Of the 403 patients at risk for at least two years (middle panel), 61 had suffered a relapse during that interval but were still alive at the start of the third year. Similarly, the 226 patients at risk for five years or more (right panel) included 42 who had relapsed during that interval and were still alive at the start of the sixth year. Note that the time scale is staggered: time 0 is one year after admission in the left panel, two years in the middle panel, and five years in the right panel. The strongly unfavorable influence of an interval relapse on after-survival is evident at all three time intervals.

the conclusion that patients who remain relapse-free for five to ten years after treatment are likely to be permanently cured.

At one time, the occurrence of a relapse consti-

tuted virtually a sentence of death in Hodgkin's disease. This is evident in the data of Musshoff and Boutis (1968), reproduced in Figure 12.37, in which only a single patient who developed an in-

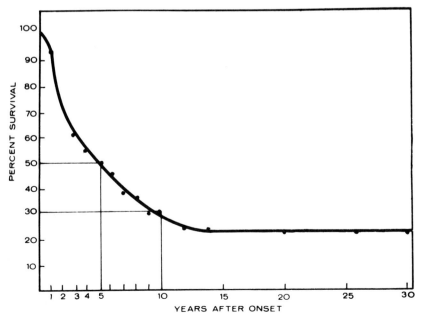

Figure 12.39 Hodgkin's disease (1935–1967). Actuarial survival from onset. (Reprinted, by permission, from the paper by Hynes, 1969.)

terval relapse survived beyond the fourteenth year. However, the prognosis of patients with relapsing Hodgkin's disease has undergone a very gratifying improvement, and it is now clear that a very appreciable long-term salvage of these cases can be achieved. In some cases, particularly those in which relapses occur in previously unirradiated lymph node chains, salvage can be accomplished with a second course of radiotherapy alone. Crosbie (1962) reported that six of ten patients with initial stage I disease and eleven of twenty-five with initial stage II disease, reirradiated for relapsing disease, survived five years from the date of their *initial* radiotherapy. In a study of twenty-six recurrences of mediastinal Hodgkin's disease after prior radiotherapy, Vaeth (1962) reported that six patients were again treated with radiotherapy and that two of these survived five years. Musshoff et al. (1976) reported that 27 (41 percent) of 66 patients who relapsed after initial radiotherapy were restored to complete remission by a second course of radiotherapy. The outlook was particularly favorable for patients whose primary relapses followed a period of complete remission after the first course of radiotherapy; 86 percent of such patients again entered complete remission, and 57 percent survived relapse-free for five years or more. In contrast, only 24 percent of patients whose primary relapses occurred after an initial partial remission entered complete remission after re-irradiation, but all of these remained relapse-free for five years. Relapses in previously nonirradiated lymph node regions had the best prognosis for retreatment by radiotherapy alone. Similar observations have been reported by Tubiana et al. (1973).

As had been noted in Chapter 11, sequential analyses of our Stanford University Medical Center data on the prognosis of patients with relapsing Hodgkin's disease indicate a dramatically improving situation. Spittle et al. (1973) found that of 87 patients with initial stage I or stage II disease who were treated primarily with radiotherapy for their primary relapses, survival was only about 20 percent at six years after retreatment (Fig. 11.47, Chapter 11). Weller et al. (1976) carried out a historical comparison of survival and freedom from second relapse in patients treated for relapsing disease during two different time intervals. In 83 patients treated between 1961 and August 1978, primary reliance was placed on radiotherapy, with single-agent chemotherapy reserved for patients with extralymphatic relapses. MOPP combination chemotherapy was introduced at Stanford in August 1968. Among a second group of 126 relapsing

patients treated between August 1968 and January 1973, 88 received MOPP chemotherapy alone or in combination with supplemental radiotherapy. As may be seen in Figure 11.48, Chapter 11, there was a very appreciable improvement in relapse-free survival, which was only 14 percent at five years in the earlier group as compared to 39 percent in the more recent group. Survival was also improved during the first four years, but the difference was largely abolished by interval deaths during the fifth year. The outlook was best for patients whose primary relapses occurred in lymph nodes, either within or outside of previous radiation treatment fields, and in the lung and other sites such as bone, whereas those whose primary relapses occurred in the liver and bone marrow had a distinctly less favorable prognosis with retreatment (Fig. 11.51). There was some indication that survival was particularly favorable among the patients treated with both radiotherapy and MOPP (Fig. 11.50), and that there was little or no difference between those treated with MOPP alone or with radiotherapy alone. However, this is in part due to the fact that patients with bone marrow relapses, who had the least favorable prognosis, were treated with MOPP alone, whereas a high proportion of those treated with both radiotherapy and MOPP had relapses in previously irradiated lymph node chains.

In an analysis confined to 244 previously untreated patients with stage I–III Hodgkin's disease who had participated in randomized clinical trials in which they received radiotherapy (RT) alone versus radiotherapy plus adjuvant MOPP chemotherapy (RT + CT), Portlock et al. (1978) studied the survival and freedom from disease progression after retreatment of 64 evaluable patients who developed primary relapses, 46 after RT and 18 after RT + CT (Fig. 12.40). After retreatment, 29 of these patients appeared to have been salvaged; this group included 23 of the 46 patients (50 percent) previously treated with RT alone, who were retreated with MOPP and/or additional RT, and 6 (33 percent) of the 18 patients with relapsing disease after initial treatment with RT + CT, who were retreated with either chemotherapy or RT (Fig. 11.52). The actuarial probability of remaining free of second relapse was not significantly different for the two groups. However, the median survival of those relapsing after RT + CT was only 33 months, as compared to 58 percent survival at five years for those relapsing after RT alone, a difference which was nearly significant at the five percent level. In this group of patients, the occurrence of a primary relapse within less than 12 months

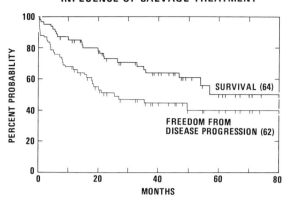

RELAPSING HODGKIN'S DISEASE: INFLUENCE OF SALVAGE TREATMENT

Figure 12.40 Actuarial analysis, by the method of Kaplan and Meier (1958), of survival and freedom from second relapse, from the date of initial relapse, in 64 patients with relapsing Hodgkin's disease. (Reprinted by permission, from the paper by Portlock et al., 1978.)

after RT alone was not associated with a significantly poorer chance of salvage than that of patients whose first relapse after RT alone occurred beyond the first year; at three years after retreatment, 40.8 percent of the former and 51.1 percent of the latter group were free of second relapses, a difference which is not statistically different. Actuarial survival of these two groups was also similar and in excess of 60 percent at three years in both groups. However, for patients who relapsed after RT + CT, early relapses occurring within the first 12 months were associated with a significantly shorter interval to second relapse and significantly impaired survival. All 5 of the patients treated with RT + CT who relapsed during the first 12 months developed progressive disease again within 6 months of the initiation of salvage therapy, with an actuarial survival at three years of only 20 percent,

whereas 44 percent of those whose relapses developed later than 12 months remained free of second relapse at three years, and 54 percent were alive.

Sites of relapse were related to initial stage, and had a strong influence on prognosis after retreatment. Only 1 of 24 patients with initial stage I or II disease relapsed in the bone marrow, as compared to 14 of 40 with initial stage III disease ($p < 0.05$). Relapses confined to lymph nodes occurred in 16 of 24 patients with initial stage I or II disease, as contrasted with only 13 of 40 patients with initial stage III disease ($p < 0.05$). Salvage treatment was significantly less effective in patients whose primary relapses occurred in bone marrow (Fig. 11.53). Only 2 of 15 such patients were salvaged, and the median interval to second relapse was only 5 months, as compared to 20 months among patients with relapses in other extranodal sites. Of patients whose initial relapse occurred in lymph nodes, 58 percent remained free of progressive disease at five years, and 78 percent were alive, as compared to less than 20 percent of patients with bone marrow relapses.

In summary, there is no longer any justification for the view that Hodgkin's disease is an inexorably fatal condition. An impressive mass of evidence, derived from autopsy studies on long-term survivors dying of intercurrent disease, as well as from rigorous statistical analyses of both survival and relapse-time data, leaves little doubt that a very significant proportion of all patients with Hodgkin's disease can indeed be permanently cured. Moreover, the data cited in Chapter 11 and in this chapter strongly suggest that a dramatic improvement in survival, and thus in the numbers of cured patients, has been achieved in the past two decades as a consequence of the introduction of intensive, total lymphoid megavoltage radiotherapy, combination chemotherapy, and combined modality treatment programs.

Chapter 13

Summary and Outlook for the Future

It seems appropriate to summarize here some of the major new advances in our concepts of the nature of Hodgkin's disease and of its diagnostic evaluation, staging, and treatment, for which detailed evidence has been marshaled in earlier chapters of this book. I have selected only those points which seemed of greatest importance for such special emphasis. This summary also provides a convenient introduction to the final section of the chapter, in which I have attempted to look into the future and to delineate the areas of greatest promise for ongoing investigation in this fascinating disease.

Nature of Hodgkin's Disease

Chromosomal studies clearly indicate that a significant fraction of the mitotic cells in lymph nodes involved by Hodgkin's disease are aneuploid and that some of them contain distinctive abnormal marker chromosomes which, in some instances, are present in multiple cells from the lymph nodes of one individual. These observations thus satisfy the most stringent biological definition of neoplasia currently available, namely, that of clonal proliferation of aneuploid cells, and thus provide irrefutable evidence that Hodgkin's disease is fundamentally neoplastic in character. Studies using labeled DNA precursors have revealed that both the abnormal mononuclear Hodgkin cells and the Sternberg-Reed cells are capable of DNA synthesis, and binucleate mitotic figures have been demonstrated in long-term cultures of such cells. Chromosome numbers of mitotic cells in culture have consistently been aneuploid and often hyper-tetraploid; functional and surface marker studies have demonstrated that such cultured cells are phagocytic, secrete lysozyme, and bear Fc and complement receptors. Taken together, these findings clearly identify Sternberg-Reed and Hodgkin cells as malignant neoplastic cells of macrophage-monocyte lineage.

Etiology and Epidemiology

It is now well established that C-type RNA viruses are the causative agents of most of the leukemias and lymphomas developing in chickens, mice, cats, cattle, and subhuman primates. Moreover, such viruses have now been isolated from leukemias and embryonic cell strains of human origin, as well as from cultures of non-Hodgkin's lymphoma cell lines. DNA viruses of the herpesvirus class have also been incriminated in the genesis of certain lymphomas of chickens, rabbits, and monkeys, and a human virus of this class, the Epstein-Barr virus, is consistently found in the tumor cells of African Burkitt's lymphomas. Although much circumstantial evidence suggests that Hodgkin's disease may also be of viral etiology, no firm evidence to substantiate this view is yet available, either in the laboratory or at the clinical level. The observation of a bimodal age-specific incidence curve for both sexes in the United States and western Europe has suggested that the disease may be comprised of two or more different entities or subtypes, perhaps with differing specific etiologies. However, the preponderance of evidence favors the view that such differences result from the interplay of environmental and host factors influencing the natural history of a single disease. Although there have been a number of reports of time-space clustering, virtually all such observations have been open to serious methodological criticisms. Studies purporting to demonstrate direct case-case or indirect case-contact-case transmission of Hodgkin's disease have also been beset with methodological flaws and have not yet been confirmed by more rigorously designed investigations. Preliminary evidence suggests that individuals with a prior history of infectious mononucleosis may be at an increased risk of developing Hodgkin's disease, but the fact that the genome of the etiologic agent of infectious mononucleosis, the Epstein-Barr virus, is absent in Sternberg-Reed and Hodgkin's giant cells in culture apparently rules out any etiologic role for this virus in Hodgkin's disease.

Histopathology

The importance of biopsy diagnosis in all cases and the many serious pitfalls which beset histopathologic interpretation in this complex field are stressed. Although identification of one or more morphologically acceptable Sternberg-Reed cells is an essential precondition for the diagnosis of Hodgkin's disease, it is not alone a sufficient condition, since morphologically similar or indistinguishable cells have now been seen in a variety of other neoplastic and non-neoplastic conditions, notably infectious mononucleosis. The histopathologic classification adopted at Rye, New York, encompassing four categories designated as lymphocyte predominance, nodular sclerosis, mixed cellularity, and lymphocyte depletion, appears to be the best classification thus far devised and correlates well with prognosis in clinical use. The preponderance of evidence indicates that the same histologic type is likely to be observed in the original biopsy and in other concurrently involved sites, and that progression from one type to another is a relatively slow process which is usually unidirectional from favorable to unfavorable type. Vascular invasion occurs in about 10 percent of all cases and may significantly alter the patterns of dissemination and progress of the disease.

Diagnostic Evaluation

Experience with lymphangiography and with laparotomy and splenectomy has firmly documented the fact that silent, sometimes microscopic foci of Hodgkin's disease often exist well beyond the sites of clinically apparent presenting manifestations of the disease. Clinically unsuspected disease may be found in the retroperitoneal lymph nodes, the spleen, and sometimes even in extralymphatic organs and tissues. Newer noninvasive procedures such as computed tomography and grey-scale ultrasonography have also been useful in detecting such intra-abdominal lesions. The detection of all involved sites is essential for the rational selection and execution of optimal treatment. A thorough, meticulous diagnostic investigation of each patient must be carried out prior to the institution of treatment, utilizing an integrated combination of clinical, roentgenologic, radioisotopic, laboratory, and surgical diagnostic procedures, including, in most instances, lymphangiography and laparotomy with

splenectomy. Laboratory indicators of disease activity, such as sustained elevation of the erythrocyte sedimentation rate or the serum copper in treated patients in otherwise complete clinical remission, may be helpful in the detection of impending relapse, but must be used with great caution because they are nonspecific.

Clinical Staging Classification

The four-stage clinical classification adopted at Rye has been found to suffer from certain significant drawbacks. In particular, the assignment of localized, as well as disseminated, forms of extralymphatic organ or tissue involvement to Rye stage IV has been shown to be inappropriate, since such localized extralymphatic disease has a far more favorable prognosis than the stage IV designation would imply. The newer Ann Arbor classification proposed to circumvent these difficulties has the added virtue of distinguishing between the clinical stage, based solely on the original tissue biopsy, history, physical examination, and radiographic findings, and the pathologic stage, based in addition on histologic findings in tissues obtained at laparotomy or supplementary biopsies. The Ann Arbor classification has now been field-tested for several years and has proven to be eminently satisfactory.

Immunology

There is now ample evidence that patients with Hodgkin's disease suffer from an immunologic deficiency which is specific in the sense that it selectively affects immune responses of the cell-mediated type, such as delayed hypersensitivity and homograft rejection. Humoral antibody formation appears to be little if at all impaired until the advanced stages of the disease. The pathophysiologic mechanisms underlying this selective immunologic deficiency state have been extensively investigated. Current evidence implicates an E-rosette inhibitor in the serum and spleens of patients with Hodgkin's disease, which reversibly binds to and interferes with the function of a subpopulation of T-lymphocytes. Binding of ferritin to the lymphocyte membrane and suppressor activity by monocytes are among the alternative reported mechanisms. Patients in long-sustained complete remission following total lymphoid irradiation continue to exhibit impaired cell-mediated immunity, associated with a T-lymphocytopenia and a B-lymphocytosis.

Radiotherapy

The cardinal features of successful radiotherapy for Hodgkin's disease are the use of sufficiently high total doses; of large fields, carefully shaped to encompass multiple lymph node chains in continuity; and of megavoltage beam energies. Sophisticated beam alignment and dosimetric procedures have been developed to permit the irradiation of essentially all lymphoid structures in the body to tumoricidal dose levels. Though potentially hazardous, total-lymphoid radiotherapy, when carried out with meticulous attention to detail by qualified, experienced radiotherapists, has in fact proved to be remarkably well tolerated. Specialized techniques have been developed to permit concurrent irradiation of one or both lungs, the entire liver, and the mesenteric lymph nodes. Refinements in technique have eliminated several potential complications and reduced the frequency of others to acceptably low levels.

Chemotherapy

A widening spectrum of highly effective drugs has become available for the palliative treatment of advanced Hodgkin's disease. However, a careful search of the literature fails to reveal a single, well-documented instance of apparent cure of a patient with biopsy-proved Hodgkin's disease treated with a single chemotherapeutic agent alone. The fact that the toxic manifestations of these drugs are in some instances directed at nonoverlapping systems within the body has opened the possibility of using combinations of multiple chemotherapeutic agents simultaneously to achieve additive effects on the disease within acceptable limits of overall toxicity. The MOPP quadruple combination chemotherapy program has yielded significantly improved rates of induction of complete remission and significantly prolonged duration of unmaintained remissions. The fact that some patients with advanced disease have now remained relapse-free for more than ten years strongly suggests that this regimen has curative potential. Several other multiple drug combinations have been clinically tested, but none to date have shown any clear superiority over MOPP. Some of these combinations appear, however, to offer promise as "cross-over" regimens in MOPP-resistant patients. Combination chemotherapy has also greatly improved the salvage of patients who develop relapses after prior radiotherapy or, to a lesser extent, chemotherapy. Azoospermia, usually sustained, is an almost invariable complication of MOPP therapy. There is also evidence of an increased risk of acute myeloblastic leukemia and possibly also of other secondary malignant neoplasms.

Combined Modality Therapy

Clinical trials utilizing total lymphoid radiotherapy followed by or alternating with multiple cycles of combination chemotherapy have demonstrated that this formidable program of treatment is surprisingly well tolerated in most previously untreated patients with far-advanced Hodgkin's disease. Such combined modality therapy has significantly decreased relapse rates and appears also to have significantly improved survival in patients with stage IIIB, and perhaps also in those with CS IIIA/PS IIIA disease. It has also been demonstrated in patients with stage I or stage II disease that localized radiotherapy plus adjuvant combination chemotherapy yields long-term results comparable to those of total or subtotal radiotherapy alone, suggesting that combination chemotherapy can effectively eradicate microscopic disease in unirradiated lymph node chains. Finally, low-dose radiotherapy plus adjuvant combination chemotherapy has yielded unexcelled survival and freedom from relapse in children with Hodgkin's disease, while permitting essentially normal growth and development. However, the risk of secondary acute leukemias or non-Hodgkin's lymphomas following combined modality therapy greatly exceeds the risks associated with either radiotherapy or combination chemotherapy alone. Accordingly, combined modality therapy should not be used indiscriminately; its use is indicated only in those clinical situations in which the improved long-term survival which it offers clearly exceeds potential mortality attributable to late hematologic or other neoplasia.

Management Recommendations

In my opinion, radiotherapy alone remains the treatment of choice for essentially all patients with stage I and stage II Hodgkin's disease. Laparotomy-staged patients with disease confined to one upper cervical region or to the mediastinum may appropriately be treated with localized, involved-field radiotherapy, whereas those with low cervical-supraclavicular adenopathy on one or both sides, with or without associated axillary or mediastinal involvement, require treatment of both the mantle and para-aortic–splenic pedicle regions, sparing the pelvis (subtotal lymphoid irradiation). Finally, total lymphoid irradiation is indicated in all patients with stage IB or IIB disease. In stage IIIA, total lymphoid radiotherapy appears to yield significantly better results than MOPP combination chemotherapy alone. However, randomized clinical trials have not yet established whether combined modality therapy is significantly better than total lymphoid irradiation alone. Pending further clarification of this question, it seems reasonable to recommend total lymphoid radiotherapy alone for those patients with PS IIIA or III$_S$A disease who have minimal or no spleen involvement and limited lymphadenopathy, and combined modality therapy for those patients who have extensive, diffuse spleen involvement and/or generalized or massive lymphadenopathy. Combined modality therapy is clearly the treatment of choice for all patients with stage IIIB or stage III$_S$B disease. In patients with stage IVA or IVB disease, combination chemotherapy is the treatment of choice, supplemented in selected patients with low-dose irradiation to sites of initially bulky or massive lymphadenopathy. Low-dose radiotherapy to all initially involved sites supplemented by adjuvant combination chemotherapy is also the treatment of choice for children with all stages of Hodgkin's disease.

Prognosis

There is now ample evidence to disprove the old notion that treatment does not significantly prolong survival of patients with Hodgkin's disease. On the contrary, it is clear that significant prolongation of survival has occurred in each of the major eras of advance in the field of radiotherapy, including the modern megavoltage era, and that survival has continued to improve with the advent of staging laparotomy and of combination chemotherapy. Of the many factors that have been shown to correlate closely with prognosis, those which appear to be of greatest significance are the anatomic extent of disease, the presence or absence of constitutional symptoms, the histopathologic type, and the age of the patient. The long-standing, deeply rooted conviction that Hodgkin's disease is incurable and inevitably fatal is no longer tenable. Data from extensive series of cases from many major medical centers throughout the world clearly satisfy several different definitions of "cure": absence of histologic evidence of persistent disease at autopsy in previously treated patients dying of intercurrent or accidental causes; flattening of survival curves to parallel the slope of the survival curve for

a cohort from the general population; various statistical tests of the significance of the difference of observed survival from that expected in mathematical models of the projected survival of patients destined to die of Hodgkin's disease; and freedom from relapse for five years or more.

Outlook for the Future

Despite the tremendous advances of the past two decades in our knowledge concerning the fundamental nature, clinical manifestations, and therapeutic management of Hodgkin's disease, many mysteries remain to be unraveled by further research. In this section, I have attempted to set forth a number of the more important unresolved problems which deserve emphasis in the years ahead.

At the fundamental level, what are the immunobiologic implications of the identification of Sternberg-Reed cells as neoplastic macrophages? The tight apposition of T-cells around Sternberg-Reed cells in electron micrographs of biopsy specimens has long suggested that the T-lymphocytes might be attempting to mount an immunological attack against the neoplastic cells. Yet the natural history of Hodgkin's disease tells us that the Sternberg-Reed cells, in untreated patients, inevitably win this battle, and that a profound depletion of lymphocytes occurs in the lymphoid tissues of the host. The newly available Sternberg-Reed and Hodgkin's cell lines may make it possible to study the interaction between these cells and T-lymphocytes in vitro, using autologous T-cells frozen at the time of initiation of the Hodgkin's cell cultures. The availability of pure cultures of these giant cells should also permit studies of their surface membranes to ascertain whether they bear distinctive differentiation antigens capable of eliciting a response by T-lymphocytes. Sophisticated new techniques for the production of monospecific antibodies by the "hybridoma" technique will greatly facilitate such studies and render them far more reliable and meaningful than has been possible with heterologous antibody preparations in the past.

Similar considerations apply to ongoing studies of the mechanism of impairment of cell-mediated immunity in patients with Hodgkin's disease. Several possible mechanisms have now been elucidated, but it has not yet been established which of these is in fact the relevant mechanism in the induction of the immune defect. The evidence suggesting a possible role for suppressor cells suffers from an apparent lack of specificity, whereas the E-rosette inhibitor detected in the sera and spleens of patients with Hodgkin's disease appears to act selectively on the T-lymphocytes of patients with the disease and not on those of normal individuals. It will be of interest to ascertain whether this E-rosette inhibitor is secreted by the Sternberg-Reed and Hodgkin's giant cells in culture and whether it binds specifically to the surface membrane of T-lymphocytes from patients with Hodgkin's disease. If so, a highly plausible immunobiologic mechanism whereby the Sternberg-Reed and Hodgkin's giant cells paralyze the immune system will have emerged. However, this mechanism also carries the implication that some subtle change, the nature of which remains unknown, must have occurred in the surface membranes of a major subpopulation of T-lymphocytes in these patients.

If it should become possible to identify the relevant immunosuppressive mechanism with reasonable certainty, can it be reversed, and immunity restored to normal in vivo? Recent studies by various groups suggest that levamisole may be able to reverse the defect in cell-mediated immunity, at least temporarily. Further studies are needed to ascertain whether the use of levamisole as an adjuvant would significantly improve prognosis in those patients shown initially to have overt impairment of their immune responses. Other approaches to the restoration of immune responsiveness also deserve exploration.

The availability of permanently established cell cultures of Sternberg-Reed and Hodgkin's giant cells will now make it possible to apply the sophisticated techniques of modern molecular virology in a search for the presence of the "fingerprints" of possible RNA or DNA tumor viruses in these cells. Such studies have been greatly hampered in the past by the fact that in tissue samples Hodgkin's cells are so greatly outnumbered by normal stromal cells. Moreover, tumor viruses, if indeed they do exist, might well be masked by antibody both in vivo and in fresh tissue samples and would be expected to emerge only after cells had been in culture long enough for preexisting antibody to disappear. Although recent evidence strongly suggests that the Epstein-Barr virus is not directly implicated in the genesis of Hodgkin's disease, an etiologic role for C-type RNA viruses, or for as-yet-unidentified DNA tumor viruses, remains a distinct possibility.

Will staging laparotomy with splenectomy continue to have an important role in the diagnostic assessment of patients with Hodgkin's disease? This seems likely to depend in part on the development of new or improved methods for minimizing the hazard of late bacterial sepsis, thus encouraging continued recourse to splenectomy. On the other hand, the development of new drug combinations which can be shown to be safe and effective when used as adjuvants in conjunction with radiotherapy would, by extending the indications for routine combined modality therapy, greatly diminish the importance of documenting the presence and extent of involvement of the spleen and would thus tend to render splenectomy obsolete. At present, studies are in progress of the antibody response to immunization with polyvalent pneumococcal vaccine prior to splenectomy. If these studies yield encouraging results with respect to antibody titers, immunization prior to laparotomy of all pediatric patients, and perhaps also of adult patients, should confer substantial protection and would become highly desirable.

Alternatively, it is known that implantation of autologous splenic tissue (splenosis) may occur following trauma or during surgical removal of the spleen (Brewster, 1973). In such instances, islands of functional splenic tissue may be detected by the uptake of ^{99m}Tc sulfur colloid; the "pitted" erythrocytes which appear in the peripheral blood of splenectomized individuals again diminish or disappear; and selected indices of immune function return toward normal levels, indicating that the spleen has been functionally "born again" (Pearson et al., 1978). It is thus conceivable that spleen tissue, after having been sliced and carefully examined under sterile conditions and found not to contain any macroscopic nodules of Hodgkin's disease, could be returned to the peritoneal cavity for the deliberate induction of splenosis in selected patients, and in particular, young children. Finally, specific replacement therapy may become a possibility in the future. Tuftsin, a tetrapeptide extracted from the spleen (Najjar and Nishioka, 1970; Nishioka et al., 1972), has been shown to restore opsonizing antibody production and other immune functions (Tzehoval et al., 1978). Although native tuftsin in vivo decays too rapidly to make its use practical, synthetic derivatives have been prepared, some of which may prove to have a sufficiently long half-life to be clinically useful in this setting.

At present, staging laparotomy with splenectomy remains a highly important diagnostic procedure. For example, there is no present evidence that adjuvant chemotherapy significantly improves survival in patients with pathologic stage I or stage II (A or B) disease, whereas combined modality therapy is clearly essential in pathological stage IIIB disease and also in those patients with IIIA disease in whom massive lymphadenopathy or spleen involvement has been demostrated. To make a reliable distinction between these two groups of patients usually requires laparotomy with splenectomy. Accordingly, unless new drug combinations are developed which can be shown to be at least as efficacious as the MOPP combination and which are devoid of the leukemogenic, teratogenic, and sterilizing hazards associated with MOPP chemotherapy, staging laparotomy with splenectomy will probably retain its present important role in the diagnostic assessment and therapeutic management of patients with Hodgkin's disease.

Much remains to be learned about the mode of spread of the neoplastic cells in Hodgkin's disease. Since they have now been identified as neoplastic macrophages or closely related cells of the mononuclear phagocyte system, arguments based on the "homing" properties of the lymphocyte no longer seem entirely relevant. Unfortunately, we lack detailed information about the patterns of migration of normal macrophages within the body, though it is clear that they do not exhibit a dynamic recirculation comparable to that of lymphocytes (Roser, 1970). The hypothesis of contiguous spread via lymphatic channels from one lymph node to another appears to be well supported by the available evidence for limited degrees of involvement confined to a few lymph node chains. However, we do not at present have a good explanation for the frequent occurrence of Hodgkin's disease in the spleen as the apparently sole site of subdiaphragmatic involvement in patients with cervical and supraclavicular lymphadenopathy, with or without concomitant mediastinal or axillary involvement. If the tumor cells travel in the retrograde direction via the thoracic duct, why do they not routinely produce macroscopic disease in the upper para-aortic lymph nodes as a prerequisite for migration to the hilum of the spleen and thence into the splenic substance? Conversely, if the tumor cells reach the spleen by the hematogenous route, why do they lodge in the spleen alone and not in other organs and tissues such as the liver, lungs, and bone marrow, which are at least as well endowed with a vascular supply? Since many patients with documented stage III_SA disease may be permanently cured with total lymphoid irradiation alone, it does not seem likely that they could have had microscopic disease in bone marrow, liver, and/or other visceral organs. The fact that spleen involve-

ment is the common denominator for either concomitant or subsequent involvement of the liver and the bone marrow continues to suggest that the pathway for spread of the disease is from lymph nodes to other lymph nodes, then secondarily from lymph nodes to spleen, and finally from spleen to liver and/or bone marrow. There is no good reason to doubt that the first phase of this sequence, spread from node to node, occurs via lymphatic channels, nor is there reason to doubt that the third phase, spread from spleen to liver and bone marrow, is blood-borne, but the pathway of spread from the lymph nodes to the spleen remains obscure.

The treatment of Hodgkin's disease is now entering a phase in which increasing attention must be paid to refinements of both radiotherapy and chemotherapy that preserve current gains with respect to survival and freedom from relapse while diminishing late complications and the hazard of secondary neoplasia. Carefully designed clinical trials will be needed to assess the extent to which radiation dose can be decreased, in conjunction with adjuvant chemotherapy, without diminution of ultimate tumor cell kill. Conversely, the reduction of drug toxicity is an equally important goal. Recent studies (Bristow, Billingham, and Daniels, 1979) indicate that increased levels of histamine and catecholamines are responsible for the cardiotoxicity of adriamycin and that effective protection can be conferred by combined histaminergic and adrenergic blockade. Such studies are needed with respect to the toxic effects of several of the other currently available compounds. We also need to know urgently whether two- or three-drug regimens that omit procarbazine and alkylating agents can be devised which are as effective as present combinations when used in the adjuvant setting. It will of course be essential to document that low-dose irradiation followed by new adjuvant chemotherapy combinations is attended by a significantly lower risk of secondary hematologic neoplasms than has been the experience with present high-dose total lymphoid irradiation and MOPP chemotherapy.

Another important direction for future investigation is the use of relatively nontoxic adjuvant agents such as levamisole or interferon in patients in whom complete remissions have been induced by prior radiotherapy, combination chemotherapy, or combined modality therapy. Recent preliminary studies suggest that interferon has a modest degree of antitumor activity in patients with stage IV follicular lymphomas (Merigan et al.,

1978b). If this substance can be more extensively purified and perhaps produced at substantially reduced cost, it would clearly be of interest as a possible adjuvant in patients with Hodgkin's disease.

Finally, a particularly intensive effort is needed to develop improved treatment regimens for patients with Hodgkin's disease who present one or more of the unfavorable prognostic indicators: stage IV extent, constitutional symptoms, lymphocyte depletion histopathologic type, age over 50 years, and documented initial relapses. Why do Sternberg-Reed and Hodgkin's cells become so refractory to eradication in the relapsing patient, especially following MOPP combination chemotherapy? This is an intriguing problem which may now become susceptible of investigation at the laboratory level by adapting permanently established cell lines to clonal culture in semisolid agar or methyl cellulose, thus making possible quantitative studies of the efficacy of graded doses of radiation, various drugs and combinations of drugs, and possible immunotherapeutic interactions in killing the tumor giant cells. Biochemical studies after exposure of such cells to sublethal drugs or radiation may permit detection of the activation of alternative biosynthetic pathways, of gene amplification mechanisms, and of other adaptations which have the net effect of rendering the surviving cells significantly more resistant to the same or related therapeutic agents. Perhaps such laboratory investigations will generate new therapeutic strategies for the treatment of relapses and thus bring us even closer to the total therapeutic conquest of this once inexorably fatal neoplasm.

Appendix

This section contains diagrammatic representations of the clinical course in a series of cases selected to reflect a cross-section of the natural history of Hodgkin's disease, with emphasis on patterns of extension to the abdomen. Patient identification data, age, sex, histology, and clinical stage are given in the caption. The small manikin at the far left indicates the sites of involvement documented during the initial hospital admission, and the adjacent manikin indicates the radiotherapeutic fields and doses employed in the first course of treatment. The essential diagnostic data of the first admission are summarized below these manikins, together with the lowest white blood cell (WBC) and platelet counts recorded during the first course of radiotherapy. The time scale along the lower edge is expanded in some sections to accommodate additional detail and contracted during periods of routine followup observation; the letters N, F, M, and A refer to November, February, May, and August, respectively, with the years indicated above. Other abbreviations include: LAG = lymphangiogram; IVC = inferior vena cavagram; IVP = intravenous pyelogram; BSP = bromsulphalein retention; Hgb = hemoglobin; PCV = packed red blood cell volume; Alk. phos. = serum alkaline phosphatase; LATS = long-acting thyroid stimulator; BEI = butanol-extractable iodide; T_3 = triiodothyronine; and NED = no evidence of disease. Sites of relapse of disease, when observed, have been indicated on additional manikins in the mid- or right-hand sections of each figure, together with the radiotherapy and/or chemotherapy employed in each such instance.

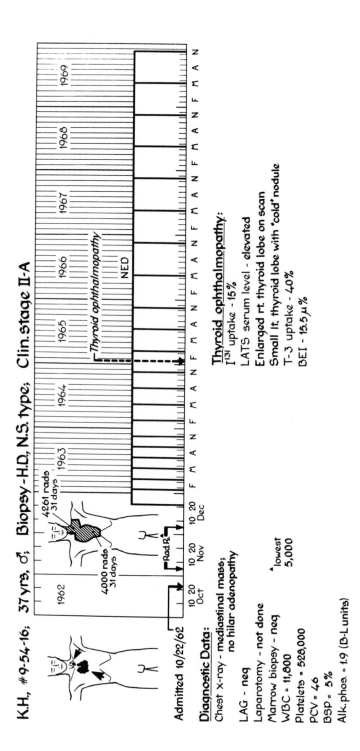

Case 1   K. H. Successful primary radiotherapy. This case is illustrative of the course of the majority of patients treated with intensive megavoltage radiotherapy at Stanford during the past 25 years. Despite the limited fields employed, there has been no relapse to date (nearly 18 years at the time of publication), and the patient is considered probably cured. An incidental complication of interest was the thyroid dysfunction and ophthalmopathy which became evident about two years after treatment.

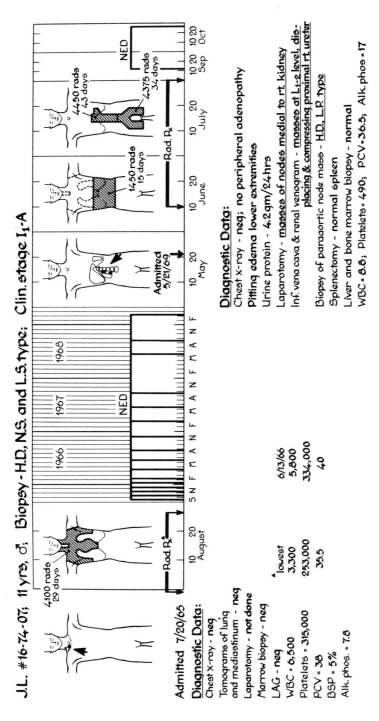

J.L. #16-74-07; 11 yrs, ♂; Biopsy - H.D., N.S. and L.S. type;   Clin. stage I₁-A

Admitted 7/20/65

Diagnostic Data:
Chest x-ray - neg
Tomograms of lung
and mediastinum - neg
Laparotomy - not done
Marrow biopsy - neg

		6/13/66
LAG - neg		
WBC = 6,500	lowest 3,300	5,800
Platelets = 315,000	253,000	334,000
PCV = 38	35.5	40
BSP = 5%		
Alk. phos. = 7.8		

4,100 rads 29 days

1966   1967   1968

NED

4,450 rads 15 days

4,450 rads 43 days

4,375 rads 34 days

NED

Admitted 5/21/69

Diagnostic Data:
Chest x-ray - neg; no peripheral adenopathy
Pitting edema lower extremities
Urine protein - 4.2 gm/24 hrs
Laparotomy - masses of nodes medial to rt. kidney
Inf. vena cava & renal venogram - masses at L₁-2 level, displacing & compressing proximal rt. ureter
Biopsy of paraaortic node mass - H.D., L.P. type
Splenectomy - normal spleen
Liver and bone marrow biopsy - normal
WBC = 8.8; Platelets = 490; PCV = 36.5, Alk. phos = 17

Case 2   J. L. Apparent salvage of a late intra-abdominal relapse with supplementary radiotherapy. Despite treatment to a full mantle field for disease apparently localized to the right neck, this patient developed a nephrotic syndrome nearly four years later due to massive enlargement of the upper lumbar para-aortic nodes, with compression and displacement of the left renal vein and the right upper ureter. Additional radiotherapy to the upper abdomen and the para-aortic and pelvic nodes afforded prompt and dramatic relief of his edema, and he remained well at the time of his last followup visit in January, 1979.

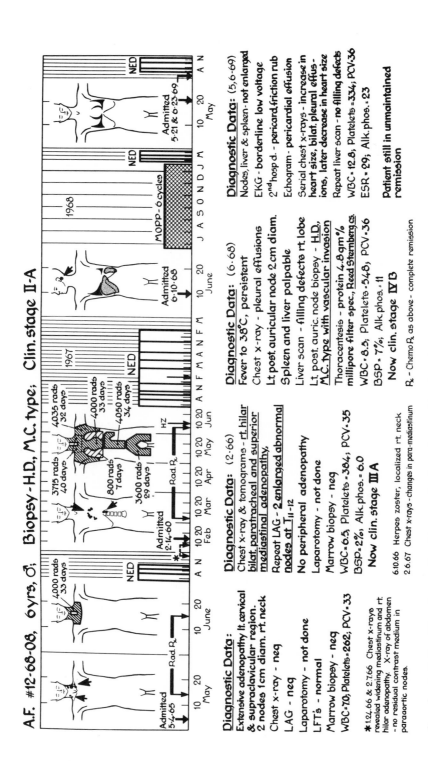

A.F. #12-68-08, 6 yrs, ♂;   Biopsy-H.D., M.C. type;   Clin. stage II-A

Admitted 5·4·65   4000 rads 33 days   NED   Rad R̯x   Admitted 2·14·60   3715 rads 40 days   4035 rads 32 days   4000 rads 33 days   800 rads 7 days   3600 rads 29 days   4050 rads 34 days   Rad R̯x   HZ   NED   1967   1968   Admitted 6·10·68   MOPP-6 cycles   NED   NED   Admitted 5·21 & 6·23·69   NED

10 20 June   A N   10 20 Feb   10 20 Mar   10 20 Apr   10 20 May   10 20 Jun   A N F M A N F M   10 20 June   A N F M A N F M   J A S O N D J M   10 20 May

Diagnostic Data:
Extensive adenopathy lt. cervical & supraclavicular region. 2 nodes 1 cm diam. rt. neck

Chest x-ray - neg

LAG - neg

Laparotomy - not done

LFT's - normal

Marrow biopsy - neg

WBC=7.0, Platelets=262, PCV=33

*1·24·66 & 2·7·66 Chest x-rays revealed widening mediastinum and rt. hilar adenopathy. X-ray of abdomen - no residual contrast medium in paraaortic nodes.

Diagnostic Data: (2·66)
Chest x-ray & tomograms - rt. hilar bilat. paratracheal and superior mediastinal adenopathy.

Repeat LAG - 2 enlarged abnormal nodes at T₁₁-₁₂

No peripheral adenopathy

Laparotomy - not done

Marrow biopsy - neg

WBC=6.5, Platelets=384, PCV-35

BSP=2%, Alk.phos.= 6.0

Now clin. stage IIIA

6.10.66 Herpes zoster, localized rt. neck

2.6.67 Chest x-rays - changes in para-mediastinum

Diagnostic Data: (6·68)
Fever to 38°C, persistent

Chest x-ray - pleural effusions

Lt post. auricular node 2 cm diam.

Spleen and liver palpable

Liver scan - filling defects rt. lobe

Lt. post. auric. node biopsy - H.D., M.C. type with vascular invasion

Thoracentesis - protein 4.8 gm% millipore filter spec., Read-Sternberg cs.

WBC-8.5, Platelets-548, PCV-36

BSP- 7%, Alk.phos.-11

Now clin. stage IVB

R̯x - Chemo R̯x as above - complete remission

Diagnostic Data: (5,6-69)
Nodes, liver & spleen - not enlarged

EKG - borderline low voltage

2ⁿᵈ hosp d. - pericard.friction rub

Echogram- pericardial effusion

Serial chest x-rays - increase in heart size, bilat. pleural effusions, later decrease in heart size

Repeat liver scan - no filling defects

WBC-12.8, Platelets-334, PCV-36

ESR - 29, Alk.phos. - 23

Patient still in unmaintained remission

Case 3   A. F. Possible salvage of a widespread relapse by combination chemotherapy. Localized irradiation of adenopathy apparently confined to both cervical-supraclavicular regions in this young boy was followed within a few months by the development of mediastinal and right hilar adenopathy and para-aortic involvement demonstrated on a repeat lymphangiogram. Despite his youth, he tolerated total lymphoid radiotherapy well, except for localized herpes zoster. However, in June 1968, clinical and biopsy evidence of Hodgkin's disease involving the pleura, liver, spleen, and a left postauricular node became manifest. He was treated with six cycles of MOPP quadruple chemotherapy, which he tolerated surprisingly well despite the prior radiotherapy. He remained relapse free thereafter, but developed a slowly growing chondrosarcoma in the heavily irradiated left supraclavicular region which was refractory to all attempts at treatment, and died in May, 1977 without evidence of persistent Hodgkin's disease.

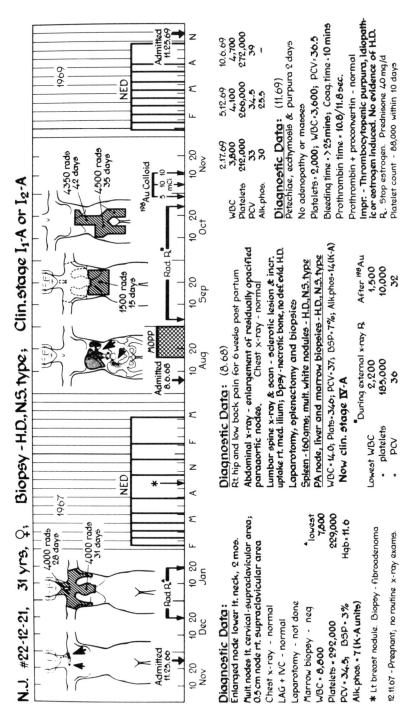

N.J. #22-12-21, 31 yrs, ♀; Biopsy - H.D., N.S. type; Clin. stage I₁-A or I₂-A

Diagnostic Data:
Enlarged node lower lt. neck, 2 mos.
Mult. nodes lt. cervical-supraclavicular area; 0.5 cm node rt. supraclavicular area
Chest x-ray - normal
LAG + IVC - normal
Laparotomy - not done
Marrow biopsy - neg
                                        lowest
WBC - 8,600   7,600
Platelets - 292,000   229,000
PCV - 34.5, BSP - 3%   Hgb - 11.6
Alk. phos. - 7 (K-A units)

* Lt. breast nodule. Biopsy - fibroadenoma
12.11.67 - Pregnant, no routine x-ray exams.

Diagnostic Data: (8.68)
Rt. hip and low back pain for 6 weeks post partum
Abdominal x-ray - enlargement of residually opacified paraaortic nodes.   Chest x-ray - normal
Lumbar spine x-ray & scan - sclerotic lesion & incr. uptake rt. med. ilium; Bpsy-necrotic bone, no def. evid. H.D.
Laparotomy, splenectomy and biopsies
Spleen -160 gms: mult. white nodules - H.D., N.S. type
PA node, liver and marrow biopsies - H.D., N.S. type
WBC=4.0; Plats=340; PCV=37; BSP=7%; Alk.phos=14(K-A)
Now clin. stage IV-A

	During external x-ray Rx	After ¹⁹⁸Au
Lowest WBC	2,200	1,500
platelets	185,000	10,000
PCV	36	32

	2.17.69	5.12.69	10.6.69
WBC	3,800	4,100	4,700
Platelets	212,000	266,000	272,000
PCV	33	34.5	39
Alk. phos.	30	25.5	-

Diagnostic Data: (11.69)
Petechiae, ecchymosis & purpura 2 days
No adenopathy or masses
Platelets - 2,000; WBC - 3,600; PCV - 36.5
Bleeding time - > 25 mins; Coag. time - 10 mins
Prothrombin time - 10.8/11.8 sec.
Prothrombin + proconvertin - normal
Impr. - Thrombocytopenic purpura, idiopathic or estrogen induced. No evidence of H.D.
Rx. Stop estrogen. Prednisone 40 mg/d
Platelet count - 88,000 within 10 days

Case 4 N. J. Possible salvage of a widespread relapse by combined quadruple chemotherapy, external radiotherapy, and colloidal radioactive gold (¹⁹⁸Au). Detection of this patient's intra-abdominal extension was undoubtedly delayed several months by a pregnancy which forced discontinuation of surveillance X-ray films. By the time it was detected, her disease had spread to involve not only the para-aortic and iliac nodes but also the spleen, liver, right iliac bone, and the adjacent bone marrow. She was treated with one cycle of MOPP chemotherapy, external radiotherapy to the liver, splenic pedicle, para-aortic nodes, and pelvis, and a total of 25 mCi of colloidal ¹⁹⁸Au in fractionated intravenous injections. She remained free of disease nearly 10 years later, at the time of her last followup visit in October, 1978, although her course was punctuated by idiopathic or estrogen-induced thrombocytopenic purpura which responded to prednisone and discontinuation of estrogen.

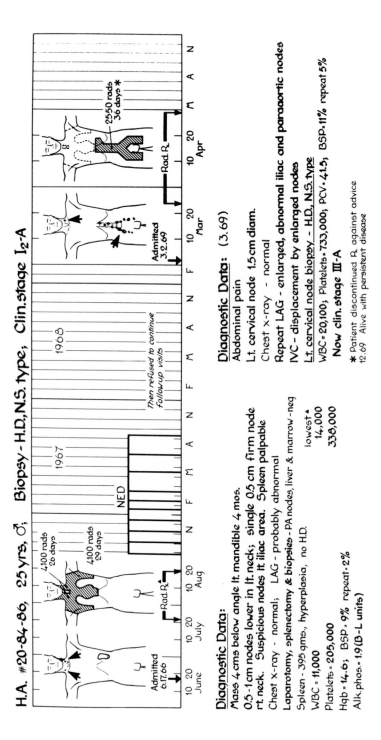

H.A. #20-84-86, 25 yrs, ♂;   Biopsy - H.D., N.S. type,   Clin. stage I₂-A

1967   1968

NED

Then refused to continue
follow-up visits

Admitted
6.17.66

10 20 | 10 20 | 10 20
June | July | Aug

4100 rads
26 days

4100 rads
29 days

Rad. Rx

Admitted
3.2.69

Rad. Rx

2550 rads
36 days *

10 20 | 10 20 | 10 20
F | Mar | Apr
N | M | A | N

Diagnostic Data:

Mass 4 cms below angle lt. mandible 4 mos.
0.5-1 cm nodes lower in lt. neck; single 0.5 cm firm node
rt. neck.   Suspicious nodes lt. iliac area.   Spleen palpable
Chest x-ray - normal;   LAG - probably abnormal
Laparotomy, splenectomy & biopsies - PA nodes, liver & marrow-neg
Spleen - 395 gms., hyperplasia, no H.D.
WBC = 11,000   lowest ↑
                                                        14,000
Platelets = 205,000   338,000
Hgb = 14.6;   BSP = 9% repeat = 2%
Alk. phos = 1.9 (B-L units)

Diagnostic Data: (3.69)
Abdominal pain
Lt. cervical node 1.5cm diam.
Chest x-ray - normal
Repeat LAG - enlarged, abnormal iliac and paraaortic nodes
IVC - displacement by enlarged nodes
Lt. cervical node biopsy - H.D., N.S. type
WBC = 20,100; Platelets=733,000; PCV= 41.5;   BSP=11% repeat 5%
Now clin. stage III-A

* Patient discontinued Rx against advice
12.69 Alive with persistent disease

Case 5   H. A. Intra-abdominal relapse, despite a negative initial staging laparotomy. This patient was noted to have a palpable spleen and a probably abnormal lymphangiogram, but none of the surgical tissue specimens revealed Hodgkin's disease. He remained well for nearly 3 years after his first course of radiotherapy to a mantle field, then was seen with a biopsy-proved recurrence in the left neck. Repeat lymphangiography and inferior vena cavography revealed marked para-aortic and iliac adenopathy, and reirradiation was started but discontinued by the patient against advice. He subsequently also started and discontinued MOPP chemotherapy, and is alive with persistent, slowly progressive disease 10 years later.

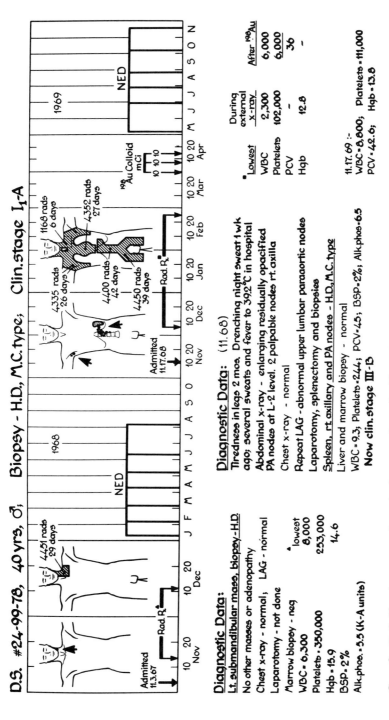

D.S. #24-99-78, 40 yrs, ♂;   Biopsy - H.D., M.C. type;   Clin. stage I₁-A

Diagnostic Data:
Lt. submandibular mass, biopsy - H.D.
No other masses or adenopathy
Chest x-ray - normal;   LAG - normal
Laparotomy - not done

	▲lowest
WBC - 6,300	8,000
Platelets - 350,000	253,000
Hgb - 15.9	14.6
BSP - 2%	
Alk. phos. - 5.5 (K-A units)	

Diagnostic Data: (11.68)
Tiredness in legs 2 mos. Drenching night sweat 1 wk ago; several sweats and fever to 39.2°C in hospital
Abdominal x-ray - enlarging residually opacified PA nodes at L-2 level. 2 palpable nodes rt. axilla
Chest x-ray - normal
Repeat LAG - abnormal upper lumbar paraaortic nodes
Laparotomy, splenectomy and biopsies
Spleen, rt. axillary and PA nodes - H.D., M.C. type
Liver and marrow biopsy - normal
WBC - 9.3; Platelets - 244; PCV - 45; BSP - 2%; Alk. phos - 6.5
Now clin. stage III-B

	During external x-ray	After ¹⁹⁸Au
•Lowest		
WBC	2,300	6,000
Platelets	102,000	6,000
PCV	-	36
Hgb	12.8	-

11.17.69 :-
WBC - 8,800;   Platelets - 111,000
PCV - 42.6;   Hgb - 13.8

Case 6 D. S. Simultaneous relapse in the contralateral axilla and upper abdomen after local radiotherapy to left upper cervical adenopathy. Although this patient was initially asymptomatic, the onset of his abdominal relapse was signaled by the development of night sweats and fever, which recurred again in 1970, about 18 months after total lymphoid radiotherapy supplemented with colloidal radiogold. He was unsuccessfully treated with MOPP quadruple chemotherapy but was maintained in remission for several years on single-drug chemotherapy. During the summer of 1978, he developed a rapidly progressive upper abdominal non-Hodgkin's lymphoma of undifferentiated type. This tumor proved refractory to chemotherapy, and he died in August, 1978.

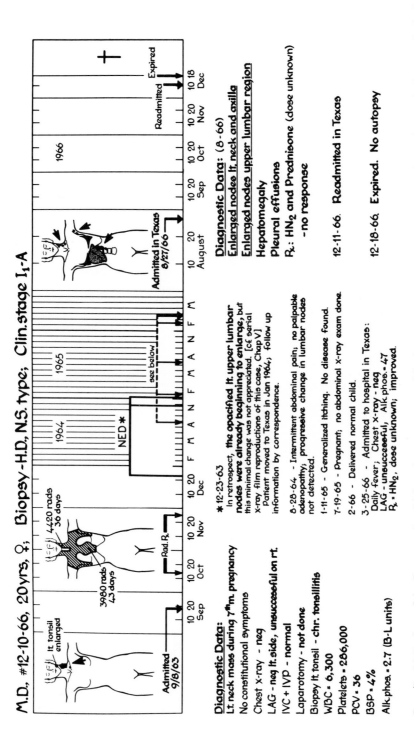

M.D., #12-10-66, 20yrs, ♀; Biopsy-H.D., N.S. type; Clin. stage I₁-A

Diagnostic Data:
Lt. neck mass during 7ᵗʰm. pregnancy
No constitutional symptoms
Chest x-ray - neg
LAG - neg lt. side, unsuccessful on rt.
IVC + IVP - normal
Laparotomy - not done
Biopsy lt. tonsil - chr. tonsillitis
WBC = 6,300
Platelets = 286,000
PCV = 36
BSP = 4%
Alk. phos. = 2.7 (B-L units)

* 12-23-63
In retrospect, the opacified lt. upper lumbar nodes were already beginning to enlarge, but this minimal change was not appreciated. [cf. serial x-ray film reproductions of this case, Chap V] Patient moved to Texas in Jan 1964; follow up information by correspondence.

8-28-64 - Intermittent abdominal pain; no palpable adenopathy; progressive change in lumbar nodes not detected.

1-11-65 - Generalized itching. No disease found.
7-19-65 - Pregnant; no abdominal x-ray exam done.
2-66 - Delivered normal child.
3-25-66 - Admitted to hospital in Texas:
Daily fever; Chest x-ray - neg
LAG - unsuccessful, Alk. phos. = 47
Rx - HN₂, dose unknown; improved.

Diagnostic Data: (8-66)
Enlarged nodes lt. neck and axilla
Enlarged nodes upper lumbar region
Hepatomegaly
Pleural effusions
Rx: HN₂ and Prednisone (dose unknown)
        - no response

12-11-66. Readmitted in Texas

12-18-66. Expired. No autopsy.

Case 7 M. D. One of the first cases in which we became aware of the hazard of transthoracic extension from the cervical-supraclavicular region to the upper abdomen. Unfortunately, this case antedates our use of elective staging laparotomy, which might have been particularly helpful inasmuch as the lymphangiogram was incomplete. Disease was believed to be confined to the left neck, and the mantle field employed seemed to go well beyond the involved nodes in all directions. Soon thereafter, changes in size and configuration of the opacified upper lumbar para-aortic nodes became visible on serial surveillance films, but were not appreciated until several months later, after the patient had moved to Texas and become temporarily lost to followup. Her subsequent downhill course was only transiently altered by single-drug chemotherapy.

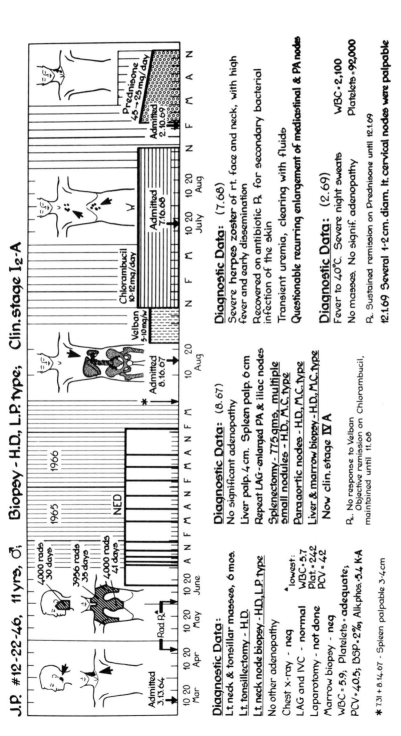

J.P. #12-22-46, 11 yrs, ♂;   Biopsy - H.D, L.P. type;   Clin. stage I₂-A

Diagnostic Data:
Lt. neck & tonsillar masses, 6 mos.
Lt. tonsillectomy - H.D.
Lt. neck node biopsy - H.D, L.P. type
No other adenopathy

Chest x-ray - neg   lowest:
LAG and IVC - normal   WBC = 5.7
Laparotomy - not done   Plat. = 242
Marrow biopsy - neg   PCV = 42
WBC = 5.9, Platelets = adequate,
PCV = 40.5; BSP = 2%, Alk phos.= 5.4 KA

* 7.31 + 8.14.67 - Spleen palpable 3-4 cm

Diagnostic Data: (8.67)
No significant adenopathy
Liver palp. 4 cm. Spleen palp. 6 cm
Repeat LAG - enlarged PA & iliac nodes
Splenectomy - 775 gms, multiple
small nodules - H.D, M.C. type
Paraaortic nodes - H.D, M.C. type
Liver & marrow biopsy - H.D, M.C. type
Now clin. stage Ⅳ A

R₂. No response to Velban
      Objective remission on Chlorambucil,
      maintained until 11.68

Diagnostic Data: (7.68)
Severe herpes zoster of rt. face and neck, with high
fever and early dissemination
Recovered on antibiotic R₂ for secondary bacterial
infection of the skin
Transient uremia, clearing with fluids
Questionable recurring enlargement of mediastinal & PA nodes

Diagnostic Data: (2.69)
Fever to 40°C. Severe night sweats   WBC = 2,100
No masses. No signif. adenopathy   Platelets = 92,000

R₂. Sustained remission on Prednisone until 12.1.69

12.1.69 Several 1-2 cm. diam. lt. cervical nodes were palpable

Case 8   J. P. Another early case with clinically silent spread to the para-aortic nodes, liver, spleen, and bone marrow from the left neck. This young boy was entirely well for more than three years after mantle and Waldeyer field irradiation of his left tonsillar and cervical-supraclavicular disease. In retrospect, it would have been helpful to have performed a repeat lymphangiogram in early 1966, by which time all of the contrast material in his para-aortic nodes had disappeared. By July 1967, when his spleen was first palpated, stage IV disease had already developed in his liver and bone marrow. His course thereafter, with successive response and failure on a series of drugs, was typical of single-drug chemotherapy, and he died on October 11, 1970.

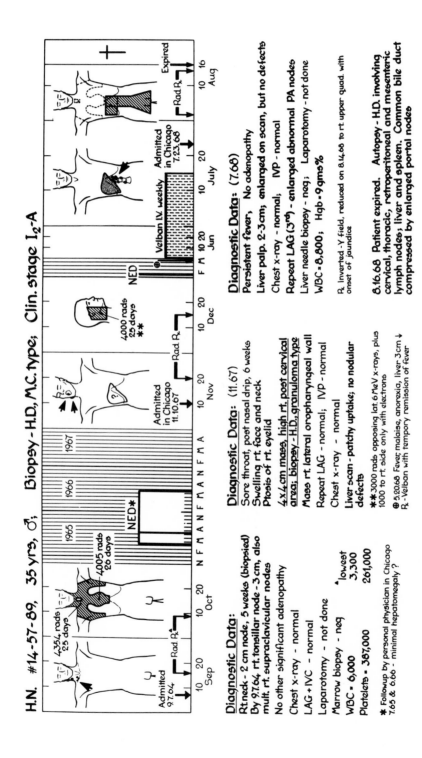

Case 9 H. N. Extension to Waldeyer's ring and later to the para-aortic nodes, spleen, and liver from disease apparently localized to the right neck and supraclavicular region. The patient remained well for more than 3 years following mantle-field radiotherapy. It is noteworthy that a second lymphangiogram late in 1967, at the time of the oropharyngeal and right cervical relapse, was still normal. Within a few months, however, constitutional symptoms and hepatomegaly appeared, and a third lymphangiogram shortly before death revealed para-aortic adenopathy, which was confirmed at autopsy. This was one of the cases that led to our present practice of irradiating the Waldeyer ring region whenever cervical nodes are involved in the upper half of the neck on either side.

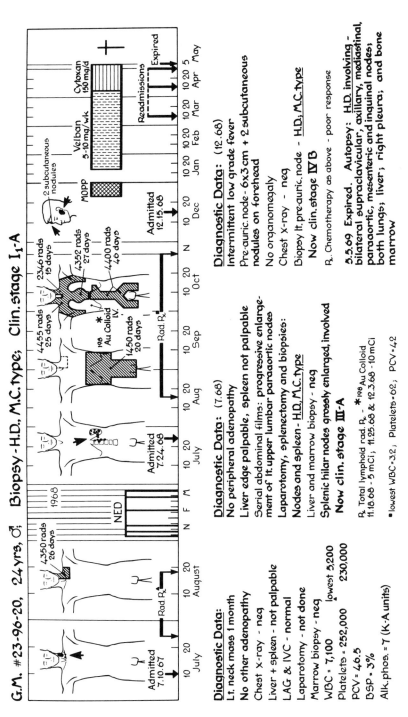

Case 10 G. M. Extension to the para-aortic nodes, and later dissemination and death, after local radiotherapy for disease apparently confined to the left neck. Once the disease had spread, it appeared to gain momentum and responded poorly to total lymphoid radiotherapy supplemented with ¹⁹⁸Au colloid, and later to MOPP and single-drug chemotherapy. This case was one of the last of a series of cases with transthoracic extension to the para-aortic nodes which, together with the startling results of our selective laparotomies, led to our initiation of routine staging laparotomy with splenectomy in the summer of 1968.

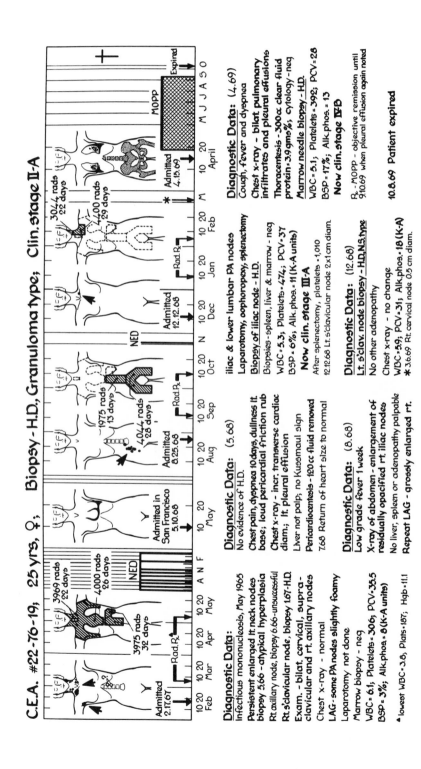

C.E.A. #22-76-19; 25 yrs, ♀; Biopsy - H.D., Granuloma type; Clin. stage II-A

Admitted 2.17.67 — 3969 rads 22 days — 4000 rads 26 days — 3975 rads 32 days — NED — Rad Rx

Admitted in San Francisco 5.10.68 — 4044 rads 28 days — 1975 rads 13 days — Admitted 8.25.68 — NED — Admitted 12.12.68 — 4400 rads 29 days

3044 rads 22 days — Rad Rx — Admitted 4.15.69 — MOPP — Expired

10 20 Feb Mar Apr May A N F 10 20 May 10 20 Aug Sep Oct N Dec 10 20 Jan Feb M April M J J A S O

Diagnostic Data:
Infectious mononucleosis, May 1965
Persistent enlarged lt. neck nodes biopsy 5.66 - atypical hyperplasia
Rt. axillary node, biopsy 6.66-unsuccessful
Rt. s'clavicular node, biopsy 1.67-H.D.
Exam. - bilat. cervical, supra-clavicular and rt. axillary nodes
Chest x-ray - normal
LAG - some PA nodes slightly foamy
Laparotomy not done
Marrow biopsy - neg
WBC = 6.1; Platelets = 306; PCV=35.5
BSP = 3%; Alk.phos.= 8 (K-A units)
▲ lowest WBC=3.6, Plats=187; Hgb=11.1

Diagnostic Data: (5.68)
No evidence of H.D.
Chest pain, dyspnea 10 days, dullness lt. base; loud pericardial friction rub
Chest x-ray - incr. transverse cardiac diam.; lt. pleural effusion
Liver not palp; no Kussmaul sign
Pericardiocentesis - 120 cc fluid removed
7.68 Return of heart size to normal

Diagnostic Data: (8.68)
Low grade fever 1 week
X-ray of abdomen - enlargement of residually opacified rt. iliac nodes
No liver, spleen or adenopathy palpable
Repeat LAG - grossly enlarged rt.

iliac & lower lumbar PA nodes
Laparotomy, oophoropexy, splenectomy
Biopsy of iliac node - H.D.
Biopsies-spleen, liver & marrow - neg
WBC=5.3; Platelets=474; PCV=37
BSP=6%; Alk.phos.=11(K-A units)
Now clin. stage III-A
After splenectomy, platelets = 1,010
12.12.68 Lt. s'clavicular node 2x1 cm diam.

Diagnostic Data: (12.68)
Lt. s'clav. node biopsy - H.D.N.S.type
No other adenopathy
Chest x-ray - no change
WBC=59; PCV=31; Alk.phos.=18 (K-A)
* 3.6.69 Rt. cervical node 0.5 cm diam.

Diagnostic Data: (4.69)
Cough, fever and dyspnea
Chest x-ray - bilat. pulmonary infiltrates and pleural effusions
Thoracentesis - 300cc clear fluid protein-3.9 gm%, cytology - neg
Marrow needle biopsy - H.D.
WBC=5.1; Platelets=392; PCV=28
BSP=17%; Alk.phos.= 13
Now clin. stage IV-B

Rx - MOPP - objective remission until 9.10.69 when pleural effusion again noted

10.8.69 Patient expired

Case 11   C. E. A. Retrograde spread to the iliac nodes, with later dissemination and death, after radiotherapy to mantle and para-aortic-spleen fields. In retrospect, laparotomy would have been helpful, since the original lymphangiogram revealed a few suspicious para-arotic nodes which, if they had been confirmed by biopsy, would have led us to treat the pelvic nodes as well, instead of attempting to preserve ovarian function, with fatal consequences, in this young female patient. Note the occurrence of radiation pericarditis in May 1 1968, with prompt and permanent clearing after pericardiocentesis and treatment with bed rest and diuretics.

References

Abdou, M. S., Salem, E. and el-Mahdy, H. M. (1966). Mucoprotein and protein bound hexose in reticulosis. *J. Egypt. Med. Assoc.* 49:619–625.

Abe, T., Morita, M., Misawa, S. and Masuda, M. (1976). Banding analysis of human leukemic and malignant lymphoma cell chromosomes. *Japan J. Hum. Genet.* 20:250–251 (abst.).

Abel, C. A. and Good, T. A. (1966). Isolation of an acid α_1-glycoprotein from the urine of a patient with Hodgkin's disease. *Clin. Chim. Acta* 14:802–806.

Abele, R., Alberto, P., Germano, G., Obrecht, J. P. and Wagenknecht, L. (1976). Simultaneous combination of adriamycin, bleomycin, cyclohexyl-chloroethyl nitrosourea with dimethyl-triazeno imidazole carboxamide in the treatment of Hodgkin's lymphoma. *Schweiz. Med. Wchnschr.* 106:961–963.

Aboul Nasr, A. L., Tawfik, H. N. and El-Einen, M. A. (1973). Lymphoreticular tumors and leukemias in Egypt. *J. Nat. Cancer Inst.* 50:1619–1621.

Abramson, J. H. (1973). Infective agents in the causation of Hodgkin's disease. A review of the epidemiological evidence. *Israel J. Med. Sci.* 9:932–953.

Abt, A. B., Kirschner, R. H., Belliveau, R. E., O'Connell, M. J., Sklansky, B. D., Greene, W. H. and Wiernik, P. H. (1974). Hepatic pathology associated with Hodgkin's disease. *Cancer* 33:1564–1571.

Acheson, E. D. (1967). Hodgkin's disease in woodworkers. *Lancet* 2:988–989.

Ackerman, G. A., Knouff, R. A. and Hoster, H. A. (1951). Cytochemistry and morphology of neoplastic and non-neoplastic human lymph nodes with special reference to Hodgkin's disease. *J. Nat. Cancer Inst.* 12:465–489.

Afkham, I. K., Musshoff, K., Boutis, L. and Lenz, H. (1969). Die operative Behandlung der malignen Lymphogranulomatose. *Sonderband 69 zur Strahlenther.*, pp. 105–112.

Agliozzo, C. M. and Reingold, I. M. (1971). Infectious mononucleosis simulating Hodgkin's disease. *Am. J. Clin. Path.* 56:730–735.

Aisenberg, A. C. (1962). Studies on delayed hypersensitivity in Hodgkin's disease. *J. Clin. Invest.* 41:1964–1970.

Aisenberg, A. C. (1964a). Immunologic aspects of Hodgkin's disease. *Medicine* 43:189–193.

Aisenberg, A. C. (1964b). Hodgkin's disease: prognosis, treatment and etiologic and immunologic considerations. *New Engl. J. Med.* 270:508–514; 565–570; 617–622.

Aisenberg, A. C. (1965a). Studies of lymphocyte transfer reactions in Hodgkin's disease. *J. Clin. Invest.* 44:555–564.

Aisenberg, A. C. (1965b). Lymphocytopenia in Hodgkin's disease. *Blood* 25:1037–1042.

Aisenberg, A. C. (1965c). Quantitative estimation of the reactivity of normal and Hodgkin's disease lymphocytes with thymidine-2-C^{14}. *Nature* 205:1233–1234.

Aisenberg, A. C. (1966). Immunologic status of Hodgkin's disease. *Cancer* 19:385–394.

Aisenberg, A. C. (1972). Hematogenous dissemination of Hodgkin's disease. *Ann. Int. Med.* 77:810–811.

Aisenberg, A. C., Kaplan, M. M., Rieder, S. V. and Goldman, J. M. (1970). Serum alkaline phosphatase at the onset of Hodgkin's disease. *Cancer* 26:318–326.

Aisenberg, A. C. and Leskowitz, S. (1963). Antibody formation in Hodgkin's disease. *New Engl. J. Med.* 268:1269–1272.

Aisenberg, A. C. and Qazi, R. (1974). Abdominal involvement at the onset of Hodgkin's disease. *Am. J. Med.* 57:870–874.

Aisenberg, A. C. and Qazi, R. (1976). Improved survival in Hodgkin's disease. *Cancer* 37:2423–2429.

Aisenberg, A. C., Weitzman, S. and Wilkes, B. (1978). Lymphocyte receptors for concanavalin A in Hodgkin disease. *Blood* 51:439–443.

Aiuti, F., Schirrmacher, V., Ammirati, P. and Fiorilli, M. (1975). Effect of thymus factor on human precursor T lymphocytes. *Clin. Exper. Immunol.* 20:499–503.

Aiuti, F. and Wigzell, H. (1973). Function and distribution pattern of human T lymphocytes. II. Presence of T lymphocytes in normal humans and in humans with various immunodeficiency disorders. *Clin. Exper. Immunol.* 13:183–189.

Akazaki, K. and Wakasa, H. (1974). Frequency of lymphoreticular tumors and leukemias in Japan. *J. Nat. Cancer Inst.* 52:339–343.

Alderson, M. R. and Nayak, R. (1971). A study of space-time clustering in Hodgkin's disease in the Manchester region. *Brit. J. Prev. Soc. Med.* 25:168–173.

Alderson, M. R. and Nayak, R. (1972). Epidemiology of Hodgkin's disease. *J. Chronic Dis.* 25:253–259.

Ali, M. K., Khalil, K. G., Fuller, L. M., Leachman, R. D., Sullivan, M. P., Loh, K. K., Gamble, J. F. and Shullenberger, C. C. (1976). Radiation-related myocardial injury. Management of two cases. *Cancer* 38:1941–1946.

Allen, L. W., Ultmann, J. E., Ferguson, D. R. and Rappaport, H. (1969). Laparotomy and splenectomy in the staging of Hodgkin's disease. *J. Lab. Clin. Med.* 74:845 (abst.).

Alslev, J. (1956). Klinischer Beitrag zur isolierten Lymphogranulomatose der Milz. *Arztl. Wchnschr.* 11:163–164.

Amadini, S. and Novi, C. (1975). Considerazioni su un caso di morbo di Hodgkin esclusivamente splenico, con riconoscimento solo istologico. *Minerva med.* 66:405–407.

Amblard, P., Schaerer, R., Sotto, J.-J., Martel, J., Bensa, J.-C. and Fillon, J.-P. (1973). Les manifestations cutanées de la maladie de Hodgkin. A propos de l'étude systématique de 94 sujets porteurs de cette affection. *Sem. Hôp. Paris* 49:3073–3078.

Amiel, J. L. (1967). Study of the leucocyte phenotypes in Hodgkin's disease. *In* Histocompatibility Testing 1967, Copenhagen: Munksgaard; Baltimore: Williams and Wilkins, pp. 79–81.

Amlot, P. L. and Green, L. A. (1978). Atopy and immunoglobulin E concentration in Hodgkin's disease and other lymphomas. *Brit. Med. J.* 1:327–329.

Amlot, P. L., Slaney, J. M. and Williams, B. D. (1976). Circulating immune complexes and symptoms in Hodgkin's disease. *Lancet* 1:449–451.

Ammann, A. J., Addiego, J., Wara, D. W., Lyman, B., Smith, W. B. and Mentzer, W. C. (1977). Polyvalent pneumococcal-polysaccharide immunization of patients with sickle-cell anemia and patients with splenectomy. *New Engl. J. Med.* 297:897–900.

Anagnostou, D., Parker, J. W., Taylor, C. R., Tindle, B. H. and Lukes, R. J. (1977). Lacunar cells of nodular sclerosing Hodgkin's disease. *Cancer* 39:1032–1043.

Andersen, R. E., D'Angio, G. J. and Khan, F. M. (1969). Dosimetry of irregularly shaped radiation therapy fields. II. Isodose contours obtained utilizing a simulated human thorax. *Radiology* 92:1097–1100.

Anderson, E. (1974). Depletion of thymus dependent lymphocytes in Hodgkin's disease. *Scand. J. Haemat.* 12:263–269.

André, R., Dreyfus, B. and Bessis, M. (1955). La ponction ganglionnaire dans la maladie de Hodgkin, examinée au microscope électronique. *Presse méd.* 63:967–970.

Antonio, J. and Sherwood, P. M. (1976). Idiopathic thrombocytopenic purpura in Hodgkin's disease after splenectomy. *Am. J. Hematol.* 1:115–120.

Appel, L., Jaeschke, H. and Vermund, H. (1961). Follow-up study on patients with Hodgkin's disease seen at the University of Wisconsin between 1948 and 1954. *Wisconsin Med. J.* 60:435–440.

Archibald, R. B. and Frenster, J. F. (1973). Quantitative ultrastructural analysis of *in vivo* lymphocyte–Reed-Sternberg cell interactions in Hodgkin's disease. *Nat. Cancer Inst. Monograph* 36:239–245.

Arends, T., Coonrad, E. V. and Rundles, R. W. (1954). Serum proteins in Hodgkin's disease and malignant lymphomas. *Am. J. Med.* 16:833–841.

Arkin, A. (1926). Familial mediastinal lymphogranuloma. *Am. J. Med. Sci.* 171:669–682.

Armenta, D., Pretty, H. M., Long, L. A., Neemeh, J. A. and Gosselin, G. (1975). Maladie de Hodgkin évoluant en leucémie aiguë. Présentation de deux cas. *Union Med. Canad.* 104:744–748.

Armstrong, D. I. and Tait, J. J. (1973). The matching of adjacent fields in radiotherapy. *Radiology* 108:419–422.

Armstrong, J. G., Dyke, R. W., Fouts, P. J., Hawthorne, J. J., Jansen, C. J., Jr. and Peabody, A. M. (1967). The initial clinical experience with vinglycinate sulfate, a molecular modification of vinblastine. *Cancer Res.* 27:221–227.

Armstrong, J. G., Dyke, R. W., Fouts, P. J. and Jansen, C. J. (1964). Delivery of a normal infant during the course of oral vinblastine sulfate therapy for Hodgkin's disease. *Ann. Int. Med.* 61:106–107.

Armstrong, M. Y. K., Ruddle, N. H., Lipman, M. B. and Richards, F. F. (1973). Tumor induction by immunologically activated murine leukemia virus. *J. Exper. Med.* 137:1163–1179.

Arseneau, J. C., Canellos, G. P., De Vita, V. T., Jr. and Sherins, R. J. (1974). Recently recognized complications of cancer chemotherapy. *Ann. N.Y. Acad. Sci.* 230:481–488.

Arseneau, J. C., Canellos, G. P., Johnson, R. and De Vita, V. T., Jr. (1977). Risk of new cancers in patients with Hodgkin's disease. *Cancer* 40:1912–1916.

Arseneau, J. C., Sponzo, R. W., Levin, D. L., Schnipper, L. E., Bonner, H., Young, R. C., Canellos, G. P., Johnson, R. E. and De Vita, V. T. (1972). Nonlymphomatous malignant tumors complicating Hodgkin's disease; possible association with intensive therapy. *New Engl. J. Med.* 287:1119–1122.

Arundell, F. D., Wilkinson, R. D. and Haserick, J. R. (1960). Dermatomyositis and malignant neoplasms in adults: a survey of 20 years' experience. *Arch. Dermatol.* 82:772–775.

Asbjørnsen, G., Molne, K., Klepp, O. and Aakvaag, A. (1976a). Testicular function after radiotherapy to inverted 'Y' field for malignant lymphoma. *Scand. J. Haematol.* 17:96–100.

Asbjørnsen, G., Molne, K., Klepp, O. and Aakvaag, A. (1976b). Testicular function after combination chemotherapy for Hodgkin's disease. *Scand. J. Haematol.* 16:66–69.

Asher, M. W. and Freimanis, A. K. (1969). Echographic diagnosis of retroperitoneal lymph node enlargement—ultrasonic scanning technique and diagnostic findings. *Am. J. Roentgenol.* 105:438–445.

Åström, K. -E., Mancall, E. L. and Richardson, E. P., Jr. (1958). Progressive multifocal leukoencephalopathy: a hitherto unrecognized complication of chronic lymphatic leukemia and Hodgkin's disease. *Brain* 81:93–111.

Atkinson, M. K., Austin, D. E., McElwain, T. J. and Peckham, M. J. (1976a). Alcohol pain in Hodgkin's disease. *Cancer* 37:895–899.

Atkinson, M. K., McElwain, T. J., Peckham, M. J. and Thomas, P. R. (1976b). Hypertrophic pulmonary osteoarthropathy in Hodgkin's disease: reversal with chemotherapy. *Cancer* 38:1729–1734.

Auerbach, S. (1965). Zinc content of plasma, blood, and erythrocytes in normal subjects and in patients with Hodgkin's disease and various hematologic disorders. *J. Lab. Clin. Med.* 65:628–637.

Aulakh, G. S. and Gallo, R. C. (1977). Rauscher-leukemia-virus-related sequences in human DNA: presence in some tissues of some patients with hematopoietic neoplasias and absence in DNA from other tissues. *Proc. Nat. Acad. Sci. U.S.* 74:353–357.

Axtell, L. M., Myers, M. H., Thomas, L. H., Berard, C. W., Kagan, A. R. and Newell, G. R. (1972). Prognostic indicators in Hodgkin's disease. *Cancer* 29:1481–1488.

Azzam, S. A. (1966). High incidence of Hodgkin's disease in children in Lebanon. *Cancer Res.* 26:1202–1203.

Bacci, G., Bianchi, F. B. and Ferramosca, B. (1969). Morbo di Hodgkin ad esclusiva localizzazione splenica. Descrizione di due casi e revisione della letteratura. (con particolare riguardo al problema della splenectomia). *Arch. Patol. Clin. Med.* 45:268–288.

Bagley, C. M., Roth, J. A., Thomas, L. B. and De Vita, V. T. (1972). Liver biopsy in Hodgkin's disease. Clinicopathologic correlations in 127 patients. *Ann. Int. Med.* 76:219–225.

Bagley, C. M., Jr., Thomas, L. B., Johnson, R. E., Chretien, P. B. and De Vita, V. T., Jr. (1973). Diagnosis of liver involvement by lymphoma: results in 96 consecutive peritoneoscopies. *Cancer* 31:840–847.

Bajoghli, M. (1961). Generalized lymphadenopathy and hepatosplenomegaly induced by diphenylhydantoin. *Pediatrics* 28:943–945.

Baker, C. and Mann, W. N. (1939). Hodgkin's disease; a study of sixty-five cases. *Guy's Hosp. Rep.* 89:83–107.

Baker, J. W., Morgan, R. L., Peckham, M. J. and Smithers, D. W. (1972). Preservation of ovarian function in patients requiring radiotherapy for para-aortic and pelvic Hodgkin's disease. *Lancet* 1:1307–1308.

Baker, M. C. and Atkin, N. B. (1965). Chromosomes in short-term cultures of lymphoid tissue from patients with reticulosis. *Brit. Med. J.* 1:770–771.

Baldetorp, L., Landberg, T. and Svahn-Tapper, G. (1976). Clinical course after mantle treatment of non-laparotomized patients with Hodgkin's disease. *Acta Radiol. Ther. Phys. Biol.* 15:193–200.

Ball, J. K. and McCarter, T. A. (1971). Repeated demonstration of a mouse leukemia virus after treatment with chemical carcinogens. *J. Nat. Cancer Inst.* 46:751–762.

Ballas, S. K., Saidi, P. and Coccia, P. (1975). Infectious mononucleosis in asymptomatic Hodgkin disease. *J.A.M.A.* 234:1162–1163.

Baltimore, D. (1970). RNA-dependent DNA polymerase in virions of RNA tumor viruses. *Nature* 226:1209–1211.

Balzola, F., Berruti, C. and Segre, E. (1964). II comportamento del complemento e delle sue frazioni nelle emopatie sistemiche. *Cancro* 17:520–530.

Bandt, P. D., Blank, N. and Castellino, R. A. (1972). Needle diagnosis of pneumonitis. Value in high-risk patients. *J.A.M.A.* 220:1578–1580.

Banfi, A., Bonadonna, G., Buraggi, G., Chiappa, S., Di Pietro, S., Dragoni, G., Pizzetti, F., Uslenghi, C. and Veronesi, U. (1965). Proposta di classificazione e terapia della malattia de Hodgkin. *Tumori* 51:97–112.

Banfi, A., Bonadonna, G., Carnevali, G. and Fossati-Bellani, F. (1969). Malignant lymphomas: further studies on their preferential sites of involvement and possible mode of spread. *Lymphology* 2:130–138.

Banfi, A., Bonadonna, G., Carnevali, G., Oldini, C. and Salvini, E. (1968). Preferential sites of involvement and spread in malignant lymphomas. *Europ. J. Cancer* 4:319–324.

Barge, J. and Potet, F. (1971). Étude anatomopathologique du foie dans la maladie de Hodgkin. *Presse Méd.* 79:565–568.

Barnes, D. W. H., Ford, C. E., Ilbery, P. L. T., Jones, K. W. and Loutit, J. F. (1959). Murine leukaemia. *Acta Unio Internat. Contra Cancrum* 15:544–548.

Barr, M. and Fairley, G. H. (1961). Circulating antibodies in reticuloses. *Lancet* 1:1305–1310.

Barry, A., Laroche, A. and Delâge, J. M. (1966). Les plaquettes sanguines dans la maladie de Hodgkin. *Laval Méd.* 37:784–787.

Barry, R. M., Diamond, H. D. and Craver, L. F. (1962). Influence of pregnancy on course of Hodgkin's disease. *Am. J. Obst. Gynec.* 84:445–454.

Baum, S., Bron, K. M., Wexler, L. and Abrams, H. L. (1963). Lymphangiography, cavography, and urography: Comparative accuracy in diagnosis of pelvic and abdominal metastases. *Radiology* 81:207–218.

Beachley, M. D., Lau, B. P. and King, E. R. (1972). Bone involvement in Hodgkin's disease. *Am. J. Roentgenol.* 114:559–563.

Beamish, M. R., Jones, P. A., Trevett, D., Evans, L. H. and Jacobs, A. (1972). Iron metabolism in Hodgkin's disease. *Brit. J. Cancer* 26:444–452.

Bearman, R. M., Pangalis, G. A. and Rappaport, H. (1978). Hodgkin's disease, lymphocyte depletion type: a clinicopathologic study of 39 patients. *Cancer* 41:293–302.

Begent, R. H. J. and Wiltshaw, E. (1974). The effect of splenectomy on the haematological response to radiotherapy in Hodgkin's disease. *Brit. J. Haematol.* 27:331–336.

Bell, E. G., McAfee, J. G. and Constable, W. C. (1969). Local radiation damage to bone and marrow demonstrated by radioisotopic imaging. *Radiology* 92:1083–1088.

Bell, T. M., Massie, A., Ross, M. G. R., Simpson, D. I. H. and Griffin, E. (1966). Further isolations of Reovirus type 3 from cases of Burkitt's lymphoma. *Brit. Med. J.* 1:1514–1517.

Belliveau, R. E., Wiernik, P. H. and Abt, A. B. (1974). Liver enzymes and pathology in Hodgkin's disease. *Cancer* 34:300–305.

Benassi, M., Paoluzi, R., LePera, V., Guadagni, A., Arcangeli, G. and Nervi, C. (1974). A computer method of shield construction for extended field irradiation of Hodgkin's disease. *Brit. J. Radiol.* 47:732–736.

Ben-Bassat, H. and Goldblum, N. (1975). Concanavalin A receptors on the surface membrane of lymphocytes from patients with Hodgkin's disease and other malignant lymphomas. *Proc. Nat. Acad. Sci. U.S.* 72:1046–1049.

Benda, C. (1904). Zur Histologie der pseudoleukämischen Geschwülste. *Verhandl. deut. patholog. Gesell.* 7:123–131.

Bendixen, H. J. (1965). Studies of bovine leucosis in Denmark. II. Pathogenic and enzootic aspects of infectious bovine leucosis. *Deut. tierärztl. Wchnschr.* 67:57–63.

Benjamin, S., McCormack, L., Effler, D. and Groves, L. (1972). Primary lymphatic tumors of the mediastinum. *Cancer* 30:708–712.

Bennett, J. H. (1845). Case of hypertrophy of the spleen and liver, in which death took place from suppuration of the blood. *Edinburgh Med. Surg. J.* 64:413–423.

Bennett, J. M., Nathanson, L. and Rutenburg, A. M. (1968). Significance of leukocyte alkaline phosphatase in Hodgkin's disease. *Arch. Int. Med.* 121:338–341.

Bennett, J. S., Bond, J., Singer, I. and Gottlieb, A. J. (1972). Hypouricemia in Hodgkin's disease. *Ann. Int. Med.* 76:751–756.

Benninghoff, D. L., Medina, A., Alexander, L. L. and Camiel, M. R. (1970). The mode of spread of Hodgkin's disease to the skin. *Cancer* 26:1135–1140.

Bentwich, Z., Cohen, R. and Brautbar, C. (1976). T and

B blocking factors in Hodgkin's disease. *Adv. Exper. Med. Biol.* 66:685–690.

Berard, C. W., Thomas, L. B., Axtell, L. M., Kruse, M., Newell, G. and Kagan, R. (1971). The relationship of histopathological subtype to clinical stage of Hodgkin's disease at diagnosis. *Cancer Res.* 31:1776–1785.

Beretta, G., Spinelli, P., Rilke, F., Tancini, G., Canetta, R., Gennari, L., and Bonadonna, G. (1976). Sequential laparoscopy and laparotomy combined with bone marrow biopsy in staging Hodgkin's disease. *Cancer Treat. Rep.* 60:1231–1237.

Bergevin, P. R. and Blom, J. (1972). Hodgkin's disease terminating in acute erythromyeloblastic leukemia with diabetes insipidus. A case report and review. *Med. Ann. D.C.* 41:625–629.

Bergh, N. P., Gatzinsky, P., Larsson, S., Lundin, P. and Ridell, B. (1978). Tumors of the thymus and thymic region: II. Clinicopathological studies on Hodgkin's disease of the thymus. *Ann. Thor. Surg.* 25:99–106.

Berkson, J. and Gage, P. (1950). Calculation of survival rates for cancer. *Proc. Staff Meet. Mayo Clin.* 25:270–286.

Berkson, J. and Gage, P. (1952). Survival curve for cancer patients following treatment. *J. Am. Stat. Assoc.* 47:501–515.

Berliner, A. D. and Distenfeld, A. (1972). Hodgkin's disease in a married couple. *J.A.M.A.* 221:703–704.

Bernhard, W. and Leplus, R. (1964). The Fine Structure of the Normal and Malignant Human Lymph Node. Oxford: Pergamon Press.

Bernier, J. J., Christol, D., Vic-DuPont, D., Geffroy, Y., Rambaud, J. C., Bognel, C. and Prost, A. (1967). Maladie de Hodgkin de l'intestin grêle, à forme diarrhéique. *Presse méd.* 75:2255–2259.

Bernuth, G. von, Minielly, J. A., Logan, G. B. and Gleich, G. J. (1970). Hodgkin's disease and thymic alymphoplasia in a 5-month-old infant. *Pediatrics* 45:792–799.

Bertrams, J., Kuwert, E., Böhme, U., Reis, H. E., Gallmeier, W. M., Wetter, O. and Schmidt, C. G. (1972). HL-A antigens in Hodgkin's disease and multiple myeloma. Increased frequency of W18 in both diseases. *Tissue Antigens* 2:41–46.

Besuschio, S. and Ghinelli, C. (1973). Lymphoreticular tumors in Argentina. *J. Nat. Cancer Inst.* 50:1639–1643.

Bethell, F. H., Andrews, G. A., Neligh, R. B. and Meyers, M. C. (1950). Treatment of Hodgkin's disease with roentgen irradiation and nitrogen mustard. *Am. J. Roentgenol.* 64:61–73.

Bichel, J. (1959). The alcohol-intolerance syndrome in Hodgkin's disease. *Acta Med. Scand.* 164:105–112.

Bichel, J. (1972). Is the alcohol-intolerance syndrome in Hodgkin's disease disappearing? *Lancet* 1:1069.

Bichel, J. (1976). Postvaccinial lymphadenitis developing into Hodgkin's disease. *Acta Med. Scand.* 199:523–525.

Bickel, G. S. (1971). Die lymphogranulomatose Hodgkin des spinalkanals. *Schweiz. Arch. Neurol. Neurochir. Psychiatr.* 108:193–208.

Bickel, P. G. and Rutishauser, E. (1942). Syndrome de sprue symptomatique d'une lymphogranulomatose de l'intestin et des ganglions mésentériques. *Helvet. Med. Acta* 9:697–719.

Bieber, C. P. and Bieber, M. M. (1973). Detection of ferritin as a circulating tumor-associated antigen in Hodgkin's disease. *Nat. Cancer Inst. Monogr.* 36:147–157.

Bieber, M. M., Fuks, Z. and Kaplan, H. S. (1977). E-rosette inhibiting substance in Hodgkin's disease spleen extracts. *Clin. Exper. Immunol.* 29:369–375.

Bieber, M. M., King, D. P., Strober, S. and Kaplan, H. S. (1979). Characterization of an E-rosette inhibitor (ERI) in the serum of patients with Hodgkin's disease as a glycolipid. *Clin. Res.* 27:81A (abst.).

Bierman, H. R. (1968). Human appendix and neoplasia. *Cancer* 21:109–118.

Bignotti, G., Tognella, S., and Grifoni, V. (1970). Caso di malattia di Hodgkin con quadro terminale di leucemia acuta. *Haematologica* 55:699–710.

Bilgutay, A. M., Jensen, M. K., Schmidt, W. R., Garanella, J. J., Lynch, M. F. and Kelly, W. D. (1969). Mediastinoscopy. *J. Thor. Cardiovasc. Surg.* 57:841–847.

Billingham, M. E., Bristow, M. R., Glatstein, E., Mason, J. W., Masek, M. A. and Daniels, J. R. (1977). Adriamycin cardiotoxicity: endomyocardial biopsy evidence of enhancement by irradiation. *Am. J. Surg. Path.* 1:17–23.

Billingham, M. E., Rawlinson, D. G., Berry, P. F. and Kempson, R. L. (1975). The cytodiagnosis of malignant lymphomas and Hodgkin's disease in cerebrospinal, pleural, and ascitic fluids. *Acta Cytol.* 19:547–556.

Billingsley, J. G. and Fukunaga, F. F. (1963). An unusual case of Hodgkin's disease presenting the x-ray appearance of lung abscess. *New Eng. J. Med.* 269:1025–1026.

Biniaminov, M. and Ramot, B. (1974). Possible T-lymphocyte origin of Reed-Sternberg cells. *Lancet* 1:368.

Bizzozero, O. J., Jr., Johnson, K. G. and Ciocco, A. (1966). Radiation-related leukemia in Hiroshima and Nagasaki, 1946–1964. I. Distribution, incidence and appearance time. *New Engl. J. Med.* 274:1095–1101.

Bjelke, E. (1969). Hodgkin's disease in Norway. Mortality trends, incidence, and survival. *Acta Med. Scand.* 185:73–81.

Björkholm, M., Holm, G., Johansson, B., Mellstedt, H. and Moller, E. (1975a). A prospective study of HL-A antigen phenotypes and lymphocyte abnormalities in Hodgkin's disease. *Tissue Antigens* 6:247–256.

Björkholm, M., Holm, G. and Mellstedt, H. (1977a). Persisting lymphocyte deficiencies during remission in Hodgkin's disease. *Clin. Exper. Immunol.* 28:389–393.

Björkholm, M., Holm, G., Mellstedt, H. and Johansson, B. (1975b). Immunodeficiency and prognosis in Hodgkin's disease. *Acta Med. Scand.* 198:275–279.

Björkholm, M., Holm, G., Mellstedt, H., Johansson, B., Askergren, J. and Söderberg, G. (1977b). Prognostic factors in Hodgkin's disease. I. Analysis of histopathology, stage distribution and results of therapy. *Scand. J. Haematol.* 19:487–495.

Björkholm, M., Holm, G., Mellstedt, H., Johansson, B., Killander, D., Sundblad, R. and Söderberg, G. (1978). Prognostic factors in Hodgkin's disease. II. Role of the lymphocyte defect. *Scand. J. Haematol.* 20:306–318.

Björkholm, M., Holm, G., Mellstedt, H. and Pettersson, D. (1975c). Immunological capacity of lymphocytes from untreated patients with Hodgkin's disease evaluated in mixed lymphocyte culture. *Clin. Exper. Immunol.* 22:373–377.

Björklund, A., Cavallin-Stahl, E., Landberg, T., Lindberg, L. G. and Akerman, M. (1975). Biopsy of nasopharynx as staging procedure in Hodgkin's disease. *Brit. Med. J.* 4:517–518.

Blaese, R. M., Oppenheim, J. J., Seeger, R. C. and Waldmann, T. A. (1972). Lymphocyte-macrophage interaction in antigen induced *in vitro* lymphocyte transformation in patients with the Wiskott-Aldrich syndrome and other diseases with anergy. *Cell. Immunol.* 4:228–242.

Blank, N. and Castellino, R. A. (1972). Patterns of pleural reflections of the left superior mediastinum. Normal anatomy and distortions produced by adenopathy. *Radiology* 102:585–589.

Bloch, C. (1967). Roentgen features of Hodgkin's disease of the stomach. *Am. J. Roentgenol.* 99:175–181.

Blomgren, H., Cantell, K., Johansson, B., Lagergren, C., Ringborg, U. and Strander, H. (1976). Interferon therapy in Hodgkin's disease. A case report. *Acta Med. Scand.* 199:527–532.

Bloomfield, C. D., Weiss, R. B., Fortuny, I., Vosika, G. and Kennedy, B. J. (1976). Combined chemotherapy with cyclophosphamide, vinblastine, procarbazine, and prednisone (CVPP) for patients with advanced Hodgkin's disease—an alternative program to MOPP. *Cancer* 38:42–48.

Bluefarb, S. M. (1959). Cutaneous Manifestations of the Malignant Lymphomas. Springfield, Ill.: Charles C Thomas.

Bluefarb, S. M. (1967). Cutaneous manifestations of the leukemia-lymphoma group. *Postgrad. Med.* 41:476–485.

Blum, R. H. and Carter, S. K. (1974). Adriamycin, a new anticancer drug with significant clinical activity. *Ann. Int. Med.* 80:249–259.

Blum, R. H., Carter, S. K. and Agre, K. (1973). A clinical review of bleomycin: a new antineoplastic agent. *Cancer* 31:903–913.

Boag, J. W. (1949). Maximum likelihood estimates of the proportion of patients cured by cancer therapy. *J. Roy. Stat. Soc., B.* 11:15–53.

Bobrove, A. M., Fuks, Z., Strober, S. and Kaplan, H. S. (1975). Quantitation of T and B lymphocytes and cellular immune function in Hodgkin's disease. *Cancer* 36:169–179.

Bobrove, A. M., Strober, S., Herzenberg, L. A. and DePamphilis, J. D. (1974). Identification and quantitation of thymus-derived lymphocytes in human peripheral blood. *J. Immunol.* 112:520–527.

Bodel, P. (1974). Pyrogen release *in vitro* by lymphoid tissues from patients with Hodgkin's disease. *Yale J. Biol. Med.* 47:101–112.

Bodmer, W. F. (1973). Genetic factors in Hodgkin's disease: association with disease-susceptibility locus (DSA) in the HL-A region. *Nat. Cancer Inst. Monograph* 36:127–134.

Boecker, W. R., Hossfeld, D. K., Gallmeier, W. M. and Schmidt, C. G. (1975). Clonal growth of Hodgkin cells. *Nature* 258:235–236.

Bohunický, L., Poliaková, L., Krizan, Z., Cerný, V. and Halko, J. (1971) The incidence of lymphogranulomatosis in single-ovum twins. *Neoplasma* 18:283–288.

Bonadonna, G., Chiappa, S., Di Pietro, S., Marano, P., Molinari, R. and Uslenghi, C. (1967). L'association de la radiothérapie endolymphatique et des agents alkylants dans le traitement des hématosarcomes rétropéritonéaux. *Nouv. rev. franç. hématol.* 7:381–392.

Bonadonna, G., DeLena, M., Banfi, A. and Lattuada, A. (1973). Secondary neoplasms in malignant lymphomas after intensive therapy. *New. Engl. J. Med.* 88:1242–1243.

Bonadonna, G., DeLena, M., Monfardini, S., Bajetta, E. and Tancini, G. (1972a). Intensive treatment with chemotherapy and radiotherapy for Hodgkin's disease. *In* Thyroid Tumours, Lymphoma, Granulocytic Leukemia, M. Fiorentino, R. Vangelista, and E. Grigoletto (eds.), Padova: Piccin Med. Books, pp. 155–175.

Bonadonna, G., DeLena, M., Monfardini, S., Bartoli, C., Bajetta, E., Beretta, G. and Fossati-Bellani, F. (1972b). Clinical trials with bleomycin in lymphomas and in solid tumors. *Europ. J. Cancer* 8:205–215.

Bonadonna, G., Fossati, V. and DeLena, M. (1978). MOPP vs. MOPP plus ABVD in stage IV Hodgkin's disease. *Proc. Am. Assoc. Cancer Res.* 19:363 (abst.).

Bonadonna, G., Zucali, R., DeLena, M. and Valagussa, P. (1977). Combined chemotherapy (MOPP or ABVD)-radiotherapy approach in advanced Hodgkin's disease. *Cancer Treat. Rep.* 61:769–777.

Bonadonna, G., Zucali, R., Monfardini, S., DeLena, M. and Uslenghi, C. (1975). Combination chemotherapy of Hodgkin's disease with adriamycin, bleomycin, vinblastine, and imidazole carboxamide versus MOPP. *Cancer* 36:252–259.

Bostick, W. L. (1948). The serial passage of Hodgkin's disease tissue extract in chicken eggs. *J. Immunol.* 59:189–193.

Bostick, W. L. (1950). Virus interference by serially passed Hodgkin's disease extracts in chicken eggs. *Proc. Soc. Exper. Biol. Med.* 74:519–521.

Bostick, W. L. and Hanna, L. (1955). Characteristics of a virus isolated from Hodgkin's disease lymph nodes. *Cancer Res.* 15:650–656.

Bourdon, R., Desprez-Curely, J. P., Bismuth, V., Dana, M. and Markovits, P. (1966). Incidences de la lymphographie sur la classification clinique de la maladie de Hodgkin. *Nouv. rev. franç. hématol.* 6:32–46.

Bouroncle, B. A. (1966). Sternberg-Reed cells in the peripheral blood of patients with Hodgkin's disease. *Blood* 27:544–556.

Bouroncle, B. A., Old, J. W., Jr. and Vazques, A. G. (1962). Pathogenesis of jaundice in Hodgkin's disease. *Arch. Int. Med.* 110:872–883.

Boutis, L., Hoffmann, P. and Musshoff, K. (1967). Veränderungen im peripheren Blutbild während und nach einer systematischen Bestrahlung bei der Lymphogranulomatose. *Strahlenther.* 133:539–548.

Bowdler, A. J. and Glick, I. W. (1966). Autoimmune hemolytic anemia as the herald state of Hodgkin's disease. *Ann. Int. Med.* 65:761–767.

Brace, K., Serpick, A. A., Block, J. B. and Wiernick, P. H. (1973). Combination radiotherapy and chemotherapy in the treatment of early Hodgkin's disease. *Oncology* 27:484–492.

Branch, A. (1931). Avian tubercle bacillus infection with special reference to mammals and to man; its reported association with Hodgkin's disease. *Am. J. Path.* 12:253–274.

Branco, F. and Gander, G. (1964). Lymphadenopathies

et disprotéinémie d'origine médicamenteuse simulant une maladie maligne. *Arq. pat.* 36:107–115.

Brandt, K., Cathcart, E. S. and Cohen, A. S. (1968). A clinical analysis of the course and prognosis of 42 patients with amyloidosis. *Am. J. Med.* 44:955–969.

Brant-Zawadzki, M. and Enzmann, D. R. (1978). Computed tomographic brain scanning in patients with lymphoma. *Radiology* 129:67–71.

Brascho, D. J., Durant, J. R. and Green, L. E. (1977). The accuracy of retroperitoneal ultrasonography in Hodgkin's disease and non-Hodgkin's lymphoma. *Radiology* 125:485–487.

Braun, E., Manley, C., Liao, K. and Boyarsky, S. (1972). Intrinsic Hodgkin's disease of the ureter. *J. Urol.* 107:952–954.

Braun, H. and Rummel, A. (1965). Schwangerschaft bei Hämoblastosen. *Zbl. Gynaek.* 87:1713–1723.

Braylan, R. C., Jaffe, E. S. and Berard, C. W. (1974). Surface characteristics of Hodgkin's lymphoma cells. *Lancet* 2:1328–1329.

Brazinsky, J. H. (1973). Metastatic intracerebral and intracerebellar Hodgkin's disease. Case report. *J. Neurosurg.* 38:635–637.

Bredesgaard, P. (1966). Lymfogranulomatoselignende sygdomsbillede fremkaldt af fenytoin (Difhydan). *Ugeskr. Laeg.* 128:1019–1021.

Brehmer-Andersson, E. (1976). Mycosis fungoides and its relation to Sézary's syndrome, lymphomatoid papulosis, and primary cutaneous Hodgkin's disease. A clinical, histopathologic and cytologic study of fourteen cases and a critical review of the literature. *Acta Dermato-Venereol.* 56:3–142.

Breiman, R. S., Castellino, R. A., Harell, G. S., Marshall, W. H., Glatstein, E. and Kaplan, H. S. (1978). CT-pathologic correlations in Hodgkin's disease and non-Hodgkin's lymphoma. *Radiology* 126:159–166.

Brennan, M. J. (1956). Case cited by Devore and Doan (1957).

Brent, L. and Medawar, P. B. (1964). Nature of the normal lymphocyte transfer reaction. *Nature* 204:90–91.

Brewin, T. B. (1966). Alcohol intolerance in neoplastic disease. *Brit. Med. J.* 2:437–441.

Brewster, D. C. (1973). Splenosis—report of two cases and review of the literature. *Am. J. Surg.* 126:14–19.

Brieux de Salum, S., Pavlovsky, S., Bachmann, A. E. and Pavlovsky, A. (1973) Estudio morfológico, ultraestructural y citoquímico de células cultivadas in vitro provenientes de nos linfomas de Hodgkin. *Sangre* 18:341–348.

Bright, R. (1838). Observations on abdominal tumours and intumescence. *Guy's Hosp. Rep.* 3:401–460.

Brill, N. E., Baehr, G. and Rosenthal, N. (1925). Generalized giant lymph follicle hyperplasia of lymph nodes and spleen. A hitherto undescribed type. *J.A.M.A.* 84:668–671.

Brincker, H. (1970). Epithelioid-cell granulomas in Hodgkin's disease. *Acta Path. Microbiol. Scand.* 78:19–32.

Bristow, M. R., Mason, J. W., Billingham, M. E. and Daniels, J. R. (1978). Doxorubicin cardiomyopathy: evaluation by phonocardiography, endomyocardial biopsy, and cardiac catheterization. *Ann. Int. Med.* 88:168–175.

Bristow, M. R., Billingham, M. E. and Daniels, J. R. (1979). Histamine and catecholamines mediate adria-mycin cardiotoxicity. *Proc. Am. Assoc. Cancer Res.* 20:(abst. in press).

Bristowe, J. S. and Pick, T. P. (1870). Report of the committee on morbid growth on Dr. Tuckwell's case. *Trans. Path. Soc. London* 21:365–368.

British National Lymphoma Investigation (1975). The value of laparotomy and splenectomy in the management of early Hodgkin's disease. *Clin. Radiol.* 26:151–157.

British National Lymphoma Investigation (1976). Initial treatment of stage IIIA Hodgkin's disease. Comparison of radiotherapy with combined chemotherapy. *Lancet* 2:991–995.

Britten, R. J. and Kohne, D. E. (1968). Repeated sequences in DNA. *Science* 161:529–540.

Brodovsky, H. S., Samuels, M. L., Migliore, P. J. and Howe, C. D. (1968). Chronic lymphocytic leukemia, Hodgkin's disease, and the nephrotic syndrome. *Arch. Int. Med.* 121:71–75.

Brody, R. S., Schottenfeld, D. and Reid, A. (1977). Multiple primary cancer risk after therapy for Hodgkin's disease. *Cancer* 40:1917–1926.

Brook, J. and Gocka, E. E. (1972). Prediction and analysis of survival in advanced Hodgkin's disease. *Comput. Biomed. Res.* 5:659–672.

Brookes, P. and Lawley, P. D. (1961). The reaction of mono- and di-functional alkylating agents with nucleic acids. *Biochem. J.* 80:496–503.

Brooks, R. E. and Siegel, B. V. (1967). Nuclear bodies of normal and pathological human lymph node cells: an electron microscopic study. *Blood* 29:269–275.

Brooks, W. H., Netsky, M. G., Normansell, D. E. and Horwitz, D. A. (1972). Depressed cell-mediated immunity in patients with primary intracranial tumors. Characterization of a humoral immunosuppressive factor. *J. Exper. Med.* 136:1631–1647.

Brown, C. A., Hall, C. L., Long, J. C., Carey, K., Weitzman, S. A. and Aisenberg, A. C. (1978). Circulating immune complexes in Hodgkin's disease. *Am. J. Med.* 64:289–294.

Brown, D. V. and Thorson, T. A. (1956). Reticulum-cell sarcoma of rats. Experimental production with trypan blue. *J. Nat. Cancer Inst.* 16:1181–1195.

Brown, F. A. and Kaplan, H. S. (1957). Hodgkin's disease: a revised clinical classification and an approach to the treatment of its localized form. *Stanford Med. Bull.* 15:183–190.

Brown, J. M. (1971). Drug-associated lymphadenopathies with special reference to the Reed-Sternberg cell. *Med. J. Australia* 1:375–378.

Brown, R. S., Haynes, H. A., Foley, H. T., Godwin, H. A., Berard, C. W. and Carbone, P. P. (1967). Hodgkin's disease. Immunologic, clinical and histologic features of 50 untreated patients. *Ann. Int. Med.* 67:291–302.

Browse, N. L., Lord, R. S. A. and Taylor, A. (1971). Pressure waves and gradients in the canine thoracic duct. *J. Physiol.* 213:507–524.

Bruce, W. R., Meeker, B. E., Powers, W. E. and Valeriote, F. A. (1969). Comparison of the dose and time-survival curves for normal hematopoietic and lymphoma colony-forming cells exposed to vinblastine, vincristine, arabinosyl cytosine, and amethopterin. *J. Nat. Cancer Inst.* 42:1015–1023.

Bruce, W. R., Meeker, B. E. and Valeriote, F. A. (1966).

Comparison of the sensitivity of normal hematopoietic and transplanted lymphoma colony-forming cells to chemotherapeutic agents administered *in vivo*. *J. Nat. Cancer Inst.* 37:233–245.

Bruce, W. R., Valeriote, F. A. and Meeker, B. E. (1967). Survival of mice bearing a transplanted syngeneic lymphoma following treatment with cyclophosphamide, 5-fluorouracil, or 1,3-bis(2-chloroethyl)-1-nitrosourea. *J. Nat. Cancer Inst.* 39:257–266.

Brunner, K. W. and Young, C. W. (1965). A methylhydrazine derivative in Hodgkin's disease and other malignant neoplasms. *Ann. Int. Med.* 62:69–86.

Bruun, S. and Engeset, A. (1956). Lymphadenography. A new method for the visualization of enlarged lymph nodes and lymphatic vessels. (Preliminary report.) *Acta Radiol.* 45:389–395.

Bucher, W. C. and Jones, S. E. (1977). Serum copper-zinc ratio (CZR) in patients with malignant lymphoma. *Am. J. Clin. Path.* 68:104–105 (abst.).

Buehler, S. K., Firme, F., Fodor, G., Fraser, G. R., Marshall, W. H. and Vaze, P. (1975). Common variable immunodeficiency, Hodgkin's disease, and other malignancies in a Newfoundland family. *Lancet* 1:195.

Buge, A., Escourolle, R., Poisson, M. and Gray, F. (1977). Diffuse nongranulomatous reticular cerebral infiltration in a patient treated for Hodgkin's disease. *Ann. Méd. Int. (Paris)* 128:969–972.

Bull, J. M., De Kiewiet, J. W. C., Rosenberg, S. A. and Kaplan, H. S. (1970). Cyclic chemotherapy (MOPP) combined with extended field radiotherapy for Hodgkin's disease. *Clin. Res.* 18:189 (abst.)

Bunting, C. H. (1914a). The blood picture in Hodgkin's disease. *Bull. Johns Hopkins Hosp.* 25:173–177.

Bunting, C. H. (1914b). Hodgkin's disease. *Bull. Johns Hopkins Hosp.* 25:177–180.

Bunting, C. H. and Yates, J. L. (1915). Bacteriologic results in chronic leukemia and pseudoleukemia. *Bull. Johns Hopkins Hosp.* 26:376–377.

Burgers, J. M. V., Tierie, A. H., Somers, R. and van Unnik, J. A. M. (1976). Hodgkin, EORTC trial no. 1 (H-1). Annual Report, Netherlands Cancer Institute, Amsterdam, pp. 95–96.

Burkitt, D. (1958). A sarcoma involving the jaws in African children. *Brit. J. Surg.* 46:218–223.

Burkitt, D. P. (1969). Etiology of Burkitt's lymphoma—an alternative hypothesis to a vectored virus. *J. Nat. Cancer Inst.* 42:19–28.

Burkitt, D. and Wright, D. (1966). Geographical and tribal distribution of African lymphoma in Uganda. *Brit. Med. J.* 1:569–573.

Burmester, B. R. (1952). Studies on fowl lymphomatosis. *Ann. New York Acad. Sci.* 54:992–1003.

Burn, C., Davies, J. N. P., Dodge, O. G. and Nias, B. C. (1971). Hodgkin's disease in English and African children. *J. Nat. Cancer Inst.* 46:37–41.

Burns, C. P., Stjernholm, R. L. and Kellermeyer, R. W. (1971). Hodgkin's disease terminating in acute lymphosarcoma cell leukemia. A metabolic study. *Cancer* 27:806–811.

Butler, J. J. (1969). Non-neoplastic lesions of lymph nodes of man to be differentiated from lymphomas. *Nat. Cancer Inst. Monograph* 32:233–255.

Byhardt, R., Brace, K., Ruckdeschel, J., Chang, P., Martin, R. and Wiernik, P. (1975). Dose and treatment factors in radiation-related pericardial effusion associated with the mantle technique for Hodgkin's disease. *Cancer* 35:795–802.

Cadman, E. C., Capizzi, R. L. and Bertino, J. R. (1977). Acute nonlymphocytic leukemia. A delayed complication of Hodgkin's disease therapy: analysis of 109 cases. *Cancer* 40:1280–1296.

Cambier, J., Boivin, P., Girauld, A., Lechevalier, B., Weiss, A.-M. and Lhuillier, M. (1973). Les déterminations cérébrales de la maladie de Hodgkin. *Ann. Med. Int.* 124:65–74.

Cameron, H. C. (1954). Mr. Guy's Hospital. London: Longmans Green.

Cammarata, R. J., Rodnan, G. P. and Jensen, W. N. (1963). Systemic rheumatic disease and malignant lymphoma. *Arch. Int. Med.* 111:330–337.

Canellos, G. P., Arseneau, J. C., De Vita, V. T., Whang-Peng, J. and Johnson, R. E. (1975). Second malignancies complicating Hodgkin's disease in remission. *Lancet* 1:947–949.

Cannon, W. B., Kaplan, H. S., Dorfman, R. F. and Nelsen, T. S. (1975). Staging laparotomy with splenectomy in Hodgkin's disease. *In* Surgery Annual 1975, L. M. Nyhus (ed.). New York: Appleton-Century-Crofts, pp. 103–114.

Cannon, W. B. and Nelsen, T. S. (1976). Staging of Hodgkin's disease: a surgical perspective. *Am. J. Surg.* 132:224–230.

Cappelaere, P., Sulman, Ch., Chechan, Ch. and Gosselin-Dulaquais, P. (1975). Les concentrations plasmatiques du cuivre et du zinc au cours de la maladie de Hodgkin. *Lille méd.* 20:904–913.

Capron, P. and Menne, M. (1969). Découverte de cellules de Sternberg dans le sang d'un sujet atteint de maladie de Hodgkin à forme disséminée. *Lille méd.* 14:1196–1197.

Carbone, P. P. (1967). The role of chemotherapy in the management of patients with Hodgkin's disease. *Ann. Int. Med.* 67:433–437.

Carbone, P. P., Kaplan, H. S., Musshoff, K., Smithers, D. W. and Tubiana, M. (1971). Report of the committee on Hodgkin's disease staging. *Cancer Res.* 31:1860–1861.

Carbone, P. P. and Spurr, C. (1968). Management of patients with malignant lymphoma: a comparative study with cyclophosphamide and Vinca alkaloids. *Cancer Res.* 28:811–822.

Carmel, R. J. and Kaplan, H. S. (1976). Mantle irradiation in Hodgkin's disease. An analysis of technique, tumor eradication, and complications. *Cancer* 37:2813–2825.

Carnes, W. H., Lieberman, M., Marchildon, M. and Kaplan, H. S. (1968). Replication of type C virus particles in thymus grafts of C57BL mice inoculated with radiation leukemia virus. *Cancer Res.* 28:98–103.

Carpenter, J. L. and Blom, J. (1976). *Corynebacterium equi* pneumonia in a patient with Hodgkin's disease. *Am. Rev. Respir. Dis.* 114:235–239.

Carr, I. (1975). The ultrastructure of the abnormal reticulum cells in Hodgkin's disease. *J. Path.* 115:45–50.

Carson, P., Hendee, W. and Ahluwalia, B. (1973). Target-skin distance for x-ray films used as templates for styrofoam molds in large-field radiation therapy. *Radiology* 107:447–448.

Carter, S. K. and Livingston, R. B. (1973). Single-agent

therapy for Hodgkin's disease. *Arch. Int. Med.* 131: 377–387.

Carvalho, A. R. L. de. (1973). Malignant lymphomas in northeastern Brazil. *J. Nat. Cancer Inst.* 50:1645–1650.

Carvalho, R. P. S., Evans, A. S., Frost, P., Dalldorf, G., Camargo, M. E. and Jamra, M. (1973). EBV infections in Brazil. I. Occurrence in normal persons, in lymphomas and in leukemias. *Internat. J. Cancer* 11:191–201.

Casazza, A. R., Duvall, C. P. and Carbone, P. P. (1966). Summary of infectious complications occurring in patients with Hodgkin's disease. *Cancer Res.* 26:1290–1296.

Case, D. C., Jr., Hansen, J. A., Corrales, E., Young, C. W., DuPont, B., Pinsky, C. M. and Good, R. A. (1976a). Comparison of multiple in vivo and in vitro parameters in untreated patients with Hodgkin's disease. *Cancer* 38:1807–1815.

Case, D. C., Hansen, J. A., Corrales, E., Young, C. W., Dupont, B., Pinsky, C. M. and Good, R. A. (1977a). Depressed in vitro lymphocyte responses to PHA in patients with Hodgkin's disease in continuous long remissions. *Blood* 49:771–778.

Case, D. C., Young, C. W. and Lee, B. J. (1977b). Combination chemotherapy of MOPP-resistant Hodgkin's disease with adriamycin, bleomycin, dacarbazine and vinblastine (ABDV). *Cancer* 39:1382–1386.

Case, D. C., Jr., Young, C. W., Nisce, L., Lee, B. J., III and Clarkson, B. D. (1976b). Eight-drug combination chemotherapy (MOPP and ABDV) and local radiotherapy for advanced Hodgkin's disease. *Cancer Treat. Rep.* 60:1217–1223.

Casirola, G., Ippoliti, G. and Marini, G. (1973). Laparoscopy in Hodgkin's disease. *Acta Haematol.* 49:1–5.

Cassady, J. R., Richter, M. P., Piro, A. J. and Jaffe, N. (1975). Radiation-adriamycin interactions: preliminary clinical observations. *Cancer* 36:946–949.

Cassileth, P. A. and Trotman, B. W. (1973). Inappropriate antidiuretic hormone in Hodgkin's disease. *Am. J. Med. Sci.* 265:233–235.

Castaigne, P., Buge, A., Escourolle, R. and Masson, M. (1964). L'atrophie cérébelleuse paranéoplasique. A propos d'une observation. *Presse méd.* 72:2639–2644.

Castaigne, P., Cambier, J., Escourolle, R., Lechevalier, B., Tanzer, J. and Lhuillier, M. (1970). Les myélopathies post-radiothérapiques au cours de la maladie de Hodgkin. A propos de 4 observations. *Rev. Neurol.* 123:369–386.

Castellino, R. A., Billingham, M. and Dorfman, R. F. (1974a). Lymphographic accuracy in Hodgkin's disease and malignant lymphoma with a note on the "reactive" lymph node as a cause of most false-positive lymphograms. *Invest. Radiol.* 9:155–165.

Castellino, R. A. and Blank, N. (1972). Adenopathy of the cardiophrenic angle (diaphragmatic) lymph nodes. *Am. J. Roentgenol.* 114:509–515.

Castellino, R. A., Blank, N., Cassady, J. R. and Kaplan, H. S. (1973a). Roentgenologic aspects of Hodgkin's disease. II. Role of routine radiographs in detecting initial relapse. *Cancer* 31:316–323.

Castellino, R. A., Filly, R. and Blank, N. (1976). Routine full-lung tomography in the initial staging and treatment planning of patients with Hodgkin's disease and non-Hodgkin's lymphoma. *Cancer* 38:1130–1136.

Castellino, R. A., Fuks, Z., Blank, N. and Kaplan, H. S. (1973b). Roentgenologic aspects of Hodgkin's disease: repeat lymphangiography. *Radiology* 109:53–58.

Castellino, R. A., Glatstein, E., Turbow, M. M., Rosenberg, S. and Kaplan, H. S. (1974b). Latent radiation injury of lungs or heart activated by steroid withdrawal. *Ann. Int. Med.* 80:593–599.

Castellino, R. A., Silverman, J. F., Glatstein, E., Blank, N. and Wexler, L. (1972). Splenic arteriography in Hodgkin's disease. A roentgenologic-pathologic study of 33 consecutive untreated patients. *Am. J. Roentgenol.* 114:574–582.

Castleman, B. (1955). Tumors of the Thymus Gland. Atlas of Tumor Pathology, Sect. 5, Fascicle 19, Washington, D.C.: Armed Forces Institute of Pathology.

Castoldi, G. (1973). La citogenetica nel morbo di Hodgkin. *Recenti Prog. Med.* 55:278–287.

Castro, G. A. M., Church, A., Pechet, L. and Snyder, L. M. (1973). Leukemia after chemotherapy of Hodgkin's disease. *New Engl. J. Med.* 289:103–104.

Catalano, L. W., Jr. and Goldman, J. M. (1972). Antibody to *Herpesvirus hominis* types 1 and 2 in patients with Hodgkin's disease and carcinoma of the nasopharynx. *Cancer* 29:597–602.

Catlin, D. (1966). Surgery for head and neck lymphomas. *Surgery* 60:1160–1166.

Cavallero, P., Sartoris, S., Vergano, F., Pegoraro, L. and Fazio, M. (1966). Anergie lymphocytaire à la phytohémagglutinine (PHA) dans la maladie de Hodgkin. *Presse méd.* 74:11–12.

Cavalli, F., Garber, A., Mosimann, W., Sonntag, R. W. and Tschopp, L. (1977). Acute myeloid leukemia in the course of Hodgkin's disease. *Deut. Med. Wchnschr.* 102:1019–1024.

Cavallin-Ståhl, E., Landberg, T., Ottow, Z. and Mitelman, F. (1977). Hodgkin's disease and acute leukaemia. A clinical and cytogenetic study. *Scand. J. Haematol.* 19:273–280.

Cavdar, A. O., Gozdasoglu, S., Arcasoy, A., Topuz, U. and Babacan, E. (1974). High frequency of Hodgkin's disease in Turkish children. *New Istanbul Contrib. Clin. Sci.* 11:31–38.

Cazenave, J.-P., Gagnon, J. A. E., Girouard, E. and Bastarache, A. (1973). Autoimmune hemolytic anemia terminating seven years later in Hodgkin's disease. *Canad. Med. Assoc. J.* 109:748–749.

Cerilli, J., Rynasiewicz, J. J., Lemas, L. B. and Rothermel, W. S., Jr. (1977). Hodgkin's disease in human renal transplantation. *Am. J. Surg.* 133:182–184.

Chabner, B. A., De Vita, V. T., Livingston, D. M. and Oliverio, V. T. (1970). Abnormalities of trytophan metabolism and plasma pyridoxal phosphate in Hodgkin's disease. *New Engl. J. Med.* 282:838–843.

Chabner, B. A., Myers, C. E., Coleman, C. N. and Johns, D. G. (1975). The clinical pharmacology of antineoplastic agents. *New Engl. J. Med.* 292:1107–1113, 1159–1168.

Chaiken, B. H., Goldberg, B. I. and Segal, J. P. (1950). Dilantin sensitivity; report of a case of hepatitis with jaundice, pyrexia and exfoliative dermatitis. *New Engl. J. Med.* 242:897–898.

Champion, A. E., Coup, A. J. and Hancock, B. W. (1976). Hodgkin's disease and chronic renal failure. *Cancer* 38:1867–1868.

Chan, B. W. B. and McBride, J. A. (1972). Hodgkin's disease and leukemia. *Canad. Med. Assoc. J.* 106:558–561.

Chang, T. C., Stutzman, L. and Sokal, J. E. (1975). Correlation of delayed hypersensitivity responses with chemotherapeutic results in advanced Hodgkin's disease. *Cancer* 36:950–955.

Chaoul, H. and Lange, K. (1923). Die Röntgenbestrahlung bei der Lymphogranulomatose. *Strahlenther.* 15:620–623.

Charache, H. (1941). Tumors in one of homologous twins. Hodgkin's disease: osteogenic sarcoma. *Am. J. Roentgenol.* 46:69–74.

Charache, H. (1946). Hodgkin's disease in children. *New York State J. Med.* 46:507–509.

Chase, M. W. (1966). Delayed-type hypersensitivity and the immunology of Hodgkin's disease, with a parallel examination of sarcoidosis. *Cancer Res.* 26:1097–1120.

Chaudhuri, T. K., Chaudhuri, T. K., Suzuki, Y., Go, R. T. and Christie, J. H. (1972). Splenic accumulation of ^{87m}Sr in a patient with Hodgkin's disease. *Radiology* 105:617–618.

Chauvergne, J. (1971). Les risques gynécologiques et obstétricaux de la chimiothérapie anticancéreuse. *Bordeaux méd.* 4:1559–1574.

Chauvergne, J., Cappelaere, P., Carton, M., Gary-Bobo, J. and Klein, T. (1978). Rubidazone (22 050 RP): clinical study. Phase II trial in solid tumors and lymphomas. *Bull. Cancer* 65:19–24.

Chawla, P. L., Stutzman. L., DuBois, R. E., Kim, U. and Sokal, J. E. (1970). Long survival in Hodgkin's disease. *Am. J. Med.* 48:85–92.

Chebat, J., Uzzan, D., Gilbert, J., Lechien, J., Seigneur, F. and Israel-Asselain, R. (1977). Complications of mediastinal cobalt therapy for Hodgkin's disease. Report of 15 cases. *Rev. fr. mal. respir.* 5:189–200.

Check, J. H., Damsker, J. I., Brady, L. W. and O'Neill, E. A. (1973). Effect of radiation therapy on mumps-delayed type hypersensitivity reaction in lymphoma and carcinoma patients. *Cancer* 32:580–584.

Cheever, A. W., Valsamis, M. P. and Rabson, A. S. (1965). Necrotizing toxoplasmic encephalitis and herpetic pneumonia complicating treated Hodgkin's disease. *New Engl. J. Med.* 272:26–29.

Chelloul, N., Burke, J., Motteram, R., LeCapon, J. and Rappaport, H. (1972). HL-A antigens and Hodgkin's disease. Report on the histological analysis. *In* Histocompatibility Testing, 1972, Copenhagen: Munksgaard, pp. 769–771.

Chen, K. T. K., Bloomfield, C. D., McKenna, R. W. and Brunning, R. D. (1977). Double bilateral bone marrow biopsies in staging patients with lymphoma. *Proc. Am. Assoc. Cancer Res.* 18:179 (abst.).

Cheson, B. D. (1978). Hodgkin's disease, alcohol, and vena caval obstruction. *J.A.M.A.* 239:23–24.

Chevalier, P. and Bernard, J. (1932). La Maladie de Hodgkin. Paris: Masson.

Chezzi, C., Dettori, G., Manzari, V., Agliano, A. M. and Sanne, A. (1976). Simultaneous detection of reverse transcriptase and high molecular weight RNA in tissue of patients with Hodgkin's disease and patients with leukemia. *Proc. Nat. Acad. Sci. U.S.* 73:4649–4652.

Chiappa, S., Bonadonna, G., Uslenghi, C., Marano, P. and Milinari, R. (1966). The role of endolymphatic radiotherapy in the treatment of chronic lymphatic leukemia. *Brit. J. Cancer* 20:480–484.

Chiari, H. (1951). Ueber das feingewebliche Bild der bei Mesantoinbehandlung zu beobachtenden Lymphknotenschwellung. *Wien. Klin. Wchnschr.* 63:77–81.

Chilcote, R. R., Baehner, R. L., Hammond, D. and Children's Cancer Study Group (1976). Septicemia and meningitis in children splenectomized for Hodgkin's disease. *New Engl. J. Med.* 295:798–800.

Child, J. A., Cooper, E. H., Illingworth, S. and Worthy, T. S. (1978). Biochemical markers in Hodgkin's disease and non-Hodgkin's lymphoma. *In* Recent Results in Cancer Research, G. Mathé, M. Seligmann, and M. Tubiana (eds.), Berlin, Heidelberg: Springer-Verlag. Vol. 64, pp. 180–189.

Chin, A. H., Saiki, J. H., Trujillo, J. M. and Williams, R. C., Jr. (1973). Peripheral blood T- and B-lymphocytes in patients with lymphoma and acute leukemia. *Clin. Immunol. Immunopathol.* 1:499–510.

Chisari, F. V. and Edgington, T. S. (1975). Lymphocyte E rosette inhibitory factor: a regulatory serum lipoprotein. *J. Exper. Med.* 142:1092–1107.

Chisesi, T., Capnist, G. and Barbui, T. (1976). Two serum IgG-M components of different light-chain types in a case of Hodgkin's disease. *Acta Haematol.* 55:250–255.

Ciampelli, E. and Pèlu, G. (1963). Comportamento della intradermoreazione alla tubercolina nei pazienti affetti da morbo di Hodgkin trattati radiologicamente. *Radiol. Med.* 49:683–690.

Cionini, L. (1973). Bone marrow damage following total nodal irradiation in Hodgkin's disease. *Brit. J. Radiol.* 46:67–68.

Clamon, G. H. and Corder, M. P. (1978). ABVD treatment of MOPP failures in Hodgkin's disease: a re-examination of goals of salvage therapy. *Cancer Treat. Rep.* 62:363–367.

Clarke, E. A., Anderson, T. W. and Davidson, J. W. (1974). Hodgkin's disease among Japanese Americans. *Lancet* 1:745.

Clarke, J. M. (1901). Discussion on lymphadenoma. *Brit. Med. J.* 2:701–709.

Clemmesen, J. (1965). Statistical studies in malignant neoplasms. I. Review and results. Copenhagen: Munksgaard, pp. 453–455.

Clemmesen, J. and Sorensen, J. (1958). Malignant neoplasms of haemopoietic and connective tissues in various countries. *Danish Med. Bull.* 5:73–123.

Cline, M. J. and Berlin, N. I. (1963). Anemia in Hodgkin's disease. *Cancer* 16:526–532.

Cohen, A. B. and Cline, M. J. (1971). The human alveolar macrophage: isolation, cultivation *in vitro*, and studies of morphologic and functional characteristics. *J. Clin. Invest.* 50:1390–1398.

Cohen, B. M., Smetana, H. F. and Miller, R. W. (1964). Hodgkin's disease: long survival in a study of 388 World War II Army cases. *Cancer* 17:856–866.

Cohen, J. R. (1978). Idiopathic thrombocytopenic purpura in Hodgkin's disease. A rare occurrence of no prognostic significance. *Cancer* 41:743–746.

Cohen, N. and Canter, J. W. (1959). Hodgkin's disease of the small intestine. Report of six cases. *Am. J. Digest. Dis.* 4:361–377.

Cohn, K. E., Stewart, J. R., Fajardo, L. F. and Hancock,

E. W. (1967). Heart disease following radiation. *Medicine* 46:281–298.

Cohn, Z. A. and Wiener, E. (1963). The particulate hydrolases of macrophages. I. Comparative enzymology, isolation, and properties. *J. Exper. Med.* 118:991–1008.

Cohnen, G., Augener, W., Brittinger, J. and Douglas, S. D. (1973a). Rosette-forming lymphocytes in Hodgkin's disease. *New Engl. J. Med.* 289:863.

Cohnen, G., Augener, W., König, E. and Brittinger, G. (1973b). B lymphocytes in Hodgkin's disease. *New Engl. J. Med.* 288:161–162.

Cohnen, G., Douglas, S. D., König, E. and Brittinger, G. (1973c). *In vitro* lymphocyte response to phytohemagglutinin and pokeweed mitogen in Hodgkin's disease. An electron microscopic and functional study. *Cancer* 31:1346–1353.

Cole, L. J. and Nowell, P. C. (1970). Parental-F$_1$ hybrid bone marrow chimeras: high incidence of donor-type lymphomas. *Proc. Soc. Exper. Biol. Med.* 134:653–657.

Cole, P. (1972). Epidemiology of Hodgkin's disease. *J.A.M.A.* 222:1636–1639.

Cole, P., Mack, T., Rothman, K., Henderson, B. and Newell, G. (1973). Tonsillectomy and Hodgkin's disease. *New Engl. J. Med.* 288:634.

Cole, P., MacMahon, B. and Aisenberg, A. (1968). Mortality from Hodgkin's disease in the United States. Evidence for the multiple aetiology hypothesis. *Lancet* 2:1371–1376.

Coleman, C. N., Williams, C. J., Flint, A., Glatstein, E. J., Rosenberg, S. A. and Kaplan, H. S. (1977). Hematologic neoplasia in patients treated for Hodgkin's disease. *New Engl. J. Med.* 297:1249–1252.

Collaborative Study. (1976). Survival and complications of radiotherapy following involved and extended field therapy of Hodgkin's disease, stages I and II—a collaborative study. *Cancer* 38:288–305.

Colomb, D., Plauchu, M., and Piante, M. (1969). Nouveau cas d'ichthyose paranéoplasique révélatrice d'une maladie de Hodgkin totalement méconnue. Guérison après traitement de l'affection causale. *Bull. soc. franç. derm. syph.* 76:64–67.

Colombani, J., Colombani, M. and Dausset, J. (1964). Leucocyte antigens and skin homograft in man demonstrating humoral antibodies after homografting by the antiglobulin consumption test. *Ann. New York Acad. Sci.* 120:307–321.

Coltman, C. A., Jr., Frei, E., III and Moon, T. E. (1976). MOPP maintenance versus unmaintained remission for MOPP induced complete remission of advanced Hodgkin's disease: 7.2 year followup. *Proc. Am. Soc. Clin. Oncol.* 17:289 (abst.).

Coltman, C. A., Jr. and Jones, S. E. (1978). MOPP plus low dose bleomycin (MOPP+LDB) for advanced Hodgkin's disease (HD)—a five year followup. *Proc. Am. Soc. Clin. Oncol.* 19:329 (abst.).

Coltman, C. A., Jr., Montague, E. and Moon, T. E. (1977). Chemotherapy and total nodal radiotherapy in pathological stage IIB, IIIA, and IIIB Hodgkin's disease. *In* Adjuvant Therapy of Cancer, S. E. Salmon and S. E. Jones (eds.), Amsterdam: North-Holland Press, pp. 529–536.

Comas, F. D., Andrews, G. A. and Nelson, B. (1968). Spleen irradiation in secondary hypersplenism. *Am. J. Roentgenol.* 104:668–673.

Comstock, G. W., Livesay, V. T. and Webster, R. G. (1971). Leukaemia and B. C. G. A controlled trial. *Lancet* 2:1062–1063.

Connelly, R. R. and Christine, B. W. (1974). A cohort study of cancer following infectious mononucleosis. *Cancer Res.* 34:1172–1178.

Connolly, E. (1975). Hodgkin's disease complicated by acute leukaemia. *Irish Med. J.* 68:6–8.

Cook, J. C., Krabbenhoft, K. L. and Leucutia, T. (1959). Combined radiation and nitrogen mustard therapy in Hodgkin's disease as compared with radiation therapy alone. *Am. J. Roentgenol.* 82:651–657.

Cook, P. L., Jelliffe, A. M., Kendall, B. and McLoughlin, M. J. (1966). The role of lymphography in the diagnosis and management of malignant reticuloses. *Brit. J. Radiol.* 39:561–574.

Cooper, E. H., Peckham, M. J., Millard, R. E., Hamlin, I. M. E. and Gérard-Marchant, R. (1968). Cell proliferation in human malignant lymphomas. Analysis of labeling index and DNA content in cell populations obtained by biopsy. *Europ. J. Cancer* 4:287–296.

Cooper, I. A., Rana, C., Madigan, J. P., Motteram, R., Maritz, J. S. and Turner, C. N. (1972). Combination chemotherapy (MOPP) in the management of advanced Hodgkin's disease. A progress report on 55 patients. *Med. J. Australia* 1:41–49.

Cooray, G. H. and Perera, R. (1966). The pattern of neoplastic disease in Ceylonese infants and children. An analysis of 600 tumours. *Brit. J. Cancer* 20:1–11.

Coppleson, L. W., Factor, R. M., Strum, S. B., Graff, P. W. and Rappaport, H. (1970). Observer disagreement in the classification and histology in Hodgkin's disease. *J. Nat. Cancer Inst.* 45:731–740.

Coppleson, L. W., Rappaport, H., Strum, S. B. and Rose, J. (1973). Analysis of the Rye classification of Hodgkin's disease. The prognostic significance of cellular composition. *J. Nat. Cancer Inst.* 51:379–390.

Corder, M. P., Young, R. C., Brown, R. S. and De Vita, V. T. (1972). Phytohemagglutinin-induced lymphocyte transformation: the relationship to prognosis of Hodgkin's disease. *Blood* 39:595–601.

Correa, P. (1973). Hodgkin's disease in Latin America. *Nat. Cancer Inst. Monograph* 36:9–14.

Correa, P. (1977). Hodgkin's disease. International mortality patterns and time trends. *World Health Stat. Rep.* 30:146–154.

Correa, P. and O'Conor, G. T. (1971). Epidemiologic patterns of Hodgkin's disease. *Internat. J. Cancer* 8:192–201.

Correa, P. and O'Conor, G. T. (1973). Geographic pathology of lymphoreticular tumors: summary of survey from the Geographic Pathology Committee of the International Union Against Cancer. *J. Nat. Cancer Inst.* 50:1609–1617.

Correa, P., O'Conor, G. T., Berard, C. W., Axtell, L. M. and Myers, M. H. (1973). International comparability and reproducibility in histologic subclassification of Hodgkin's disease. *J. Nat. Cancer Inst.* 50:1429–1435.

Cossman, J., Deegan, M. J. and Schnitzer, B. (1977). Complement receptor B lymphocytes in nodular sclerosing Hodgkin's disease. *Cancer* 39:2166–2173.

Court Brown, W. M. (1958). Radiation-induced leukemia in man, with particular reference to the dose-response relationship. *J. Chron. Dis.* 8:113–122.

Court Brown, W. M. and Doll, R. (1957). Leukaemia and aplastic anaemia in patients irradiated for ankylosing spondylitis. Med. Res. Council Special Report Series 295, London.

Coutinho, V., Bottura, C. and Falcao, R. P. (1971). Cytogenetic studies in malignant lymphomas: a study of 28 cases. *Brit. J. Cancer* 25:789–801.

Covington, E. E. and Baker, A. S. (1969). Dosimetry of scattered radiation to the fetus. *J.A.M.A.* 209:414–415.

Cowley, J. G. (1978). *In vitro* cell proliferation studies in Hodgkin's disease. *Neoplasma* 25:83–90.

Cox, F. and Hughes, W. T. (1975). Contagious and other aspects of nocardiosis in the compromised host. *Pediatrics* 55:135–138.

Craft, C. B. (1940). Results with roentgen ray therapy in Hodgkin's disease. *Bull. Staff Meet. Univ. Minn. Hosp.* 11:391–409.

Craigie, D. (1828). Elements of General and Pathological Anatomy. Edinburgh: Adam Black.

Craigie, D. (1845). Case of disease of the spleen, in which death took place in consequence of the presence of purulent matter in the blood. *Edinburgh Med. Surg. J.* 64:400–413.

Craver, L. F. (1934). Five-year survival in Hodgkin's disease. *Am. J. Med. Sci.* 188:609–612.

Craver, L. F. (1951). Hodgkin's disease. *In* Practice of Medicine, F. Tice (ed.), Hagerstown, Md.: W. F. Prior. Vol. 5, pp. 107–152.

Craver, L. F. (1964). Hodgkin's disease. *In* Practice of Medicine, F. Tice and E. M. Harvey (eds.). Hagerstown, Md.: W. F. Prior. Vol. 6. pp. 1017–1063.

Craver, L. F. (1968). Etiology and pathogenesis. *In* Hodgkin's Disease, D. W. Molander and G. T. Pack (eds.). Springfield, Ill.: Charles C. Thomas, p. 3.

Craver, L. F. and Miller, D. G. (1965). Treatment and prognosis of Hodgkin's disease. *Ca* 15:246–251.

Creagan, E. T. and Fraumeni, J. F., Jr. (1972). Familial Hodgkin's disease. *Lancet* 2:547.

Crepaldi, G. and Parpajola, A. (1964). Excretion of tryptophan metabolites in different forms of haemoblastosis. *Clin. Chim. Acta* 9:106–117.

Cridland, M. D. (1961). Seasonal incidence of clinical onset of Hodgkin's disease. *Brit. Med. J.* 1:621–623.

Croft, W. A., Jr., Skibba, J. L. and Bryan, G. T. (1975). Carcinogenicity of the antineoplastic agent 4(5)-(3,3-dimethyl-1-triazeno)imidazole-5(4)-carboxamide (NSC-45388, *DTIC*) in germfree rats. *Fed. Proc.* 34:229 (abst.).

Croizat, P., Galy, P., Papillon, J., Revol, L., Chassard, J. L., Contamin, A. and Bretagnolle, G. (1962). Les formes médiastinales de début de la maladie de Hodgkin. (A propos de 41 observations.) *J. radiol. électrol.* 43:1–11.

Croizat, P., Ponthus, P., Papillon, J., Revol, L., Dargent, M., Pinet, F., Kuentz, M. and Lenoble, E. (1958). Le pronostic de la maladie de Hodgkin. *Presse méd.* 66:1135–1138.

Crosbie, J. (1962). A clinical study of Hodgkin's disease. *In* Progress in Radiation Therapy, F. Buschke (ed.). New York: Grune and Stratton. Vol. 2, pp. 153–163.

Cross, R. M. (1968). A clinicopathologic study of nodular sclerosing Hodgkin's disease. *J. Clin. Path.* 21:303–310.

Cross, R. M. (1969). Hodgkin's disease: histological classification and diagnosis. *J. Clin. Path.* 22:165–182.

Crowe, J. E. (1975). Cardiophrenic adenopathy in Hodgkin disease. *Am. J. Dis. Child.* 129:116–117.

Crowther, D. (1973). Some aspects of the immunology of Hodgkin's disease. *Tumori* 59:351–362.

Crowther, D., Fairley, G. H. and Sewell, R. L. (1967a). Lymphoid cells in Hodgkin's disease. *Nature* 215:1086–1088.

Crowther, D., Fairley, G. H. and Sewell, R. L. (1967b). Desoxyribonucleic acid synthesis in the lymphocytes of patients with malignant disease. *Europ. J. Cancer* 3:417–421.

Cruickshank, W. (1786). The Anatomy of the Absorbing Vessels of the Human Body. London: G. Nicol.

Cundiff, J. H., Cunningham, J. R., Golden, R., Lanzl, L. H., Meurk, M. L., Ovadia, J., Last, V. P., Pope, R. A., Sampierre, V. A., Saylor, W. L., Shalek, R. J., and Suntharalingam, N. (1973). A method for the calculation of dose in the radiation treatment of Hodgkin's disease. *Am. J. Roentgenol.* 117:30–44.

Cuny, G., Penin, F., Guerci, O. and Peroz, F. (1973). Hodgkin's disease associated with acute leukemia. *Ann. méd. Nancy* 12:1103–1110.

Curran, R. C. and Jones, E. L. (1977). Dendritic cells and B lymphocytes in Hodgkin's disease. *Lancet* 2:349.

Custer, R. P. and Bernhard, W. G. (1948). The interrelationship of Hodgkin's disease and other lymphatic tumors. *Am. J. Med. Sci.* 216:625–642.

Cuttner, J., Meyer, R. and Huang, Y. P. (1979). Intracerebral involvement in Hodgkin's disease. A report of 6 cases and review of the literature. *Cancer* 43:1497–1506.

Dalla Pria, A. F. (1967). La prognosi nel rapporto tri i caratteri istologici e l'evoluzione clinica della malattia de Hodgkin. Studio eseguito su 110 casi. *Minerva med.* 58:2910–2914.

Dalldorf, G., Bergamini, F. and Frost, P. (1966). Further observations of the lymphomas of African children. *Proc. Nat. Acad. Sci.* 55:297–302.

Damascelli, B., Bonadonna, G., Musumeci, R. and Uslengli, C. (1969). Two-dimensional pulsed echo detection of para-aortic lymph nodes. *Surg. Gynec. Obst.* 128:772–776.

Dameshek, W., Weisfuse, L. and Stein, T. (1949). Nitrogen mustard therapy in Hodgkin's disease. Analysis of 50 consecutive cases. *Blood* 4:338–379.

Damon, H. F. (1964). Leucocythemia. Boston: DeVries, Ibarra.

Dana, M., Weisgerber, C., Teillet, F., Desprez-Curely, J. P., Goguel, A., Chotin, G. and Bernard, J. (1976). Problèmes de stérilité chez l'homme et la femme après irradiation par grand champ sous-diaphragmatique. *J. radiol. électrol. méd. nucl.* 57:405–408.

Danforth, D. N., Jr. and Javadpour, N. (1975). Total unilateral renal destruction caused by irradiation for Hodgkin's disease. *Urology* 5:790–793.

Davidson, J. W. (1969). Malignant lymphoma. *In* Fuchs, W. A., Davidson, J. W. and Fischer, H. W., Lymphography and Cancer. Berlin: Springer-Verlag. Chap. 8, pp. 176–237.

Davidson, J. W. and Clarke, E. A. (1968). Influence of modern radiological techniques on clinical staging of malignant lymphomas. *Canad. Med. Assoc. J.* 99:1196–1204.

Dawson, P. J. (1968). The original illustrations of Hodgkin's disease. *Arch. Int. Med.* 121:288–290.

Dawson, P. J., Cooper, R. A. and Rambo, O. N. (1964). Diagnosis of malignant lymphoma. A clinical pathological analysis of 158 difficult lymph node biopsies. *Cancer* 17:1405–1413.

Declève, A., Niwa, O., Hilgers, J. and Kaplan, H. S. (1974). An improved murine leukemia virus immunofluorescence assay. *Virology* 57:491–502.

De Gast, G. C., Halie, M. R. and Nieweg, H. O. (1975). Immunological responsiveness against two primary antigens in untreated patients with Hodgkin's disease. *Europ. J. Cancer* 11:217–224.

DeGowin, R. L., Chandhuri, T. K., Christie, J. H., Callis, M. N. and Mueller, A. L. (1974). Marrow scanning in evaluation of hemopoiesis after radiotherapy. *Arch. Int. Med.* 134:297–303.

DeLena, M., Guzzon, A., Monfardini, S. and Bonadonna, G. (1972). Clinical, radiologic and histopathologic studies on pulmonary toxicity induced by treatment with bleomycin. *Cancer Chemother. Rep.* 56:343–356.

De Marval, L. (1940). Los pacientes afectados de limfogranulomatosis maligna son insensibles a dosis masivas de tuberculina bruta inyectida por via subcutanea. *Prensa méd. Argent.* 27:2310–2312.

Demin, A. A., Radzhabli, S. I., Loseva, M. I. and Metelkina, N. V. (1972). Cytogenetic studies in Hodgkin's disease and some other reticuloses. *Sov. Genet.* 8:126–141.

Denton, P. M. and Field, E. O. (1973). Immunofluorescent studies of lymphoid tissue in Hodgkin's disease. *Tumori* 59:375–382.

Deresinski, S. C. and Stevens, D. A. (1975). Coccidioidomycosis in compromised hosts. Experience at Stanford University Hospital. *Medicine* 54:377–395.

Desjardins, A. U. (1945). Salient factors in the treatment of Hodgkin's disease and lymphosarcoma with roentgen rays. *Am. J. Roentgenol.* 54:707–722.

Desjardins, A. U. and Ford, F. A. (1923). Hodgkin's disease and lymphosarcoma; clinical and statistical study. *J.A.M.A.* 81:925–927.

DeSousa, M., Tan, C., Tan, R., Dupont, B. and Good, R. A. (1977). Immunological parameters of prognosis in childhood Hodgkin's disease (HD). *Proc. Am. Soc. Clin. Oncol.* 18:333 (abst.).

Desser, R. K., Golomb, H. M., Ultmann, J. E., Ferguson, D. J., Moran, E. M., Griem, M. L., Vardiman, J., Miller, B., Oetzel, N., Sweet, D., Kinzie, J. J. and Blough, R. (1977). Prognostic classification of Hodgkin disease in pathologic stage III, based on anatomic considerations. *Blood* 49:883–893.

Desser, R. K., Moran, E. M. and Ultmann, J. E. (1973). Staging of Hodgkin's disease and lymphoma. Diagnostic procedures including staging laparotomy and splenectomy. *Med. Clin. North Amer.* 57:479–498.

Desser, R. K. and Ultmann, J. E. (1972). Risk of severe infection in patients with Hodgkin's disease or lymphoma after diagnostic laparotomy and splenectomy. *Ann. Int. Med.* 77:143–146.

Desser, R. K. and Ultmann, J. E. (1973). The sensitivity of Hodgkin's disease to chemotherapeutic agents administered singly. *Ser. Haematol.* 6:152–181.

Deuschle, K. W. and Wiggins, W. S. (1953). The use of nitrogen mustard in the management of two pregnant lymphoma patients. *Blood* 8:576–579.

De Vita, V. T. (1973). Lymphocyte reactivity in Hodgkin's disease: a lymphocyte civil war. *New Engl. J. Med.* 289:801–802.

De Vita, V. T., Jr., Bagley, C. M., Jr., Goodell, D., O'Kieffe, D. A. and Trujillo, N. P. (1971a). Peritoneoscopy in the staging of Hodgkin's disease. *Cancer Res.* 31:1746–1750.

De Vita, V., Canellos, G., Hubbard, S., Chabner, B. and Young, R. (1976). Chemotherapy of Hodgkin's disease (HD) with MOPP: a 10 year progress report. *Proc. Am. Soc. Clin. Oncol.* 17:269 (abst.).

De Vita, V. T., Chabner, B. A., Livingston, D. M. and Oliverio, V. T. (1971b). Anergy and tryptophan metabolism in Hodgkin's disease. *Am. J. Clin. Nutr.* 24:835–840.

De Vita, V. T., Jr., Denham, C., Davidson, J. D. and Oliverio, V. T. (1967). The physiological deposition of the carcinostatic 1,3-bis(2-chloroethyl)-1-nitrosourea (BCNU) in man and animals. *Clin. Pharmacol. Ther.* 8:566–577.

De Vita, V. T., Jr., Serpick, A. and Carbone, P. P. (1970). Combination chemotherapy in the treatment of advanced Hodgkin's disease. *Ann. Int. Med.* 73:881–895.

De Vita, V. T., Jr., Young, R. C. and Canellos, G. P. (1975). Combination versus single agent chemotherapy: a review of the basis for selection of drug treatment of cancer. *Cancer* 35:98–110.

DeVore, J. and Doan, C. (1957). Studies in Hodgkin's syndrome. XII. Hereditary and epidemiologic aspects. *Ann. Int. Med.* 47:300–316.

Dhingra, H. K. and Flance, I. J. (1970). Cavitary primary pulmonary Hodgkin's disease presenting as pruritus. *Chest* 58:71–73.

Dhru, R. and Templeton, A. C. (1972). Postmortem findings in Ugandans with Hodgkin's disease. *Brit. J. Cancer* 26:331–334.

Di Bella, N. J., Blom, J. and Slawson, R. G. (1973). Splenectomy and hematologic tolerance to irradiation in Hodgkin's disease. *Radiology* 107:195–200.

Dickler, H. B. and Kunkel, H. G. (1972). Interaction of aggregated γ-globulin with B lymphocytes. *J. Exper. Med.* 136:191–196.

Diggs, C. H., Wiernik, P. H. and Aisner, J. (1978). SCAB (streptozotocin, CCNU, adriamycin, bleomycin) for advanced untreated Hodgkin's disease. *Proc. Am. Soc. Clin. Oncol.* 19:370 (abst.).

Diggs, C. H., Wiernik, P. H., Levi, J. A. and Kvols, L. K. (1977). Cyclophosphamide, vinblastine, procarbazine and prednisone with CCNU and vinblastine maintenance for advanced Hodgkin's disease. *Cancer* 39:1949–1954.

Dixon, F. J., Talmage, D. W. and Maurer, P. H. (1952). Radiosensitive and radioresistant phases in the antibody response. *J. Immunol.* 68:693–700.

Dixon, W. J. and Massey, F. J., Jr. (1957). Introduction to Statistical Analysis. New York: McGraw-Hill.

Dmochowski, L. (1968). Viral studies in human leukemia and lymphoma. *In* International Conference on Leukemia-Lymphoma, C. J. D. Zarafonetis (ed.). Philadelphia: Lea and Febiger, pp. 97–113.

Doan, C. A., Bouroncle, B. A. and Wiseman, B. (1960). Idiopathic and secondary thrombocytopenic purpura: clinical study and evaluation of 381 cases over a period of 28 years. *Ann. Int. Med.* 53:861–876.

Dörken, H. (1960). Über die Altersverteilung der Lymphogranulomatose. *Klin. Wchnschr.* 38:944–947.

Dörken, H. (1975). M. Hodgkin: Eine epidemiologische

Studie über 140 Kinder; Stadt/Land-Relation, Berufe der Eltern, Kontakte mit Haustieren. *Arch. Geschwulstforsch.* 45:283–298.

Dollinger, M. R., Lavine, D. M. and Foye, L. V., Jr. (1966). Myocardial infarction due to post-irradiation fibrosis of the coronary arteries. *J.A.M.A.* 195:316–319.

Dominok, G. W. (1964). Die histologischen veränderungen menschlicher Lymphknoten nach Lymphographien. *Virchow's Arch. f. path. Anat.* 338:143–149.

Donaldson, S. S., Glatstein, E. and Kaplan, H. S. (1976a). Radiotherapy of childhood lymphoma. *In* Trends in Childhood Cancer, M. M. Donaldson and H. G. Seydel (eds.), John Wiley and Sons, pp. 38–66.

Donaldson, S. S., Glatstein, E., Rosenberg, S. A. and Kaplan, H. S. (1976b). Pediatric Hodgkin's disease. II. Results of therapy. *Cancer* 37:2436–2447.

Donaldson, S. S., Glatstein, E. and Vosti, K. L. (1978). Bacterial infections in pediatric Hodgkin's disease: relationship to radiotherapy, chemotherapy, and splenectomy. *Cancer* 41:1949–1958.

Dorfman, R. F. (1961). Enzyme histochemistry of the cells in Hodgkin's disease and allied disorders. *Nature* 190:925–926.

Dorfman, R. F. (1964). Enzyme histochemistry of normal, hyperplastic, and neoplastic lymphoreticular tissues. *In* Symposium on Lymphatic Tumours in Africa. Paris, 1963. Basel: S. Karger. pp. 304–326.

Dorfman, R. F. (1971). Relationship of histology to site in Hodgkin's disease. *Cancer Res.* 31:1786–1793.

Dorfman, R. F., Rice, D. F., Mitchell, A. D., Kempson, R. L. and Levine, G. (1973). Ultrastructural studies of Hodgkin's disease. *Nat. Cancer Inst. Monograph* 36:221–238.

Dougherty, T. F. and White, A. (1943). Effect of pituitary adrenotrophic hormone on lymphoid tissue. *Proc. Soc. Exper. Biol. Med.* 53:132–133.

Doyle, A. P. and Hellstrom, H. R. (1963). Mesantoin lymphadenopathy morphologically simulating Hodgkin's disease. *Ann. Int. Med.* 59:363–368.

Dreschfeld, J. (1892). Clinical lecture on acute Hodgkin's (or pseudoleucocythemia). *Brit. Med. J.* 1:893–896.

Dubin, I. N. (1947). The poverty of the immunological mechanism in patients with Hodgkin's disease. *Ann. Int. Med.* 27:898–913.

Duckett, J. W. (1963). Splenectomy in the treatment of secondary hypersplenism. *Ann. Surg.* 157:737–746.

Duhamel, G., Najman, A. and André, R. (1971). Les localisations à la moelle osseuse de la maladie de Hodgkin. Leur place dans l'évolution de la maladie. Etude par biopsie médullaire de 100 observations. *Presse méd.* 79:2305–2308.

Dumont, A. E. and Martelli, A. B. (1973). Experimental studies bearing on the question of retrograde spread of Hodgkin's disease via the thoracic duct. *Cancer Res.* 33:3195–3202.

Dunn, T. B. (1954). Normal and pathologic anatomy of the reticular tissue in laboratory mice, with a classification and discussion of neoplasms. *J. Nat. Cancer Inst.* 14:1281–1433.

Dunn, T. B. and Deringer, M. K. (1968). Reticulum cell neoplasm, type B, or the "Hodgkin's-like" lesion of the mouse. *J. Nat. Cancer Inst.* 40:771–821.

Durant, J. R. and Tassoni, E. M. (1967). Coexistent Di

Guglielmo's leukemia and Hodgkin's disease. A case report with cytogenetic studies. *Amer. J. Med. Sci.* 254:824–830.

Ďurkovský, J. and Krajči, M. (1972). Complications after radiation treatment in Hodgkin's disease. *Neoplasma* 19:227–233.

Dutton, R. W. (1975). Suppressor T cells. *Transplant. Rev.* 26:39–55.

Duvall, C. P. and Carbone, P. P. (1966). *Cryptococcus* and *neoformans* pericarditis associated with Hodgkin's disease. *Ann. Int. Med.* 64:850–856.

Dworsky, R. L. and Henderson, B. E. (1974). Hodgkin's disease clustering in families and communities. *Cancer Res.* 34:1161–1163.

Earle, J. D. and Bagshaw, M. A. (1967). A rapid optical method for preparation of complex field shapes. *Radiology* 88:1162–1165.

Easson, E. C. (1966). Possibilities for the cure of Hodgkin's disease. *Cancer* 19:345–350.

Easson, E. C. and Russell, M. H. (1963). The cure of Hodgkin's disease. *Brit. Med. J.* 1:1704–1707.

Ebstein, W. von (1887). Das chronische Rückfallsfieber, eine neu Infectionskrankheit. *Berlin Klin. Wchnschr.* 24:565–568.

Ecker, M. D., Jay, B. and Keshane, M. F. (1978). Procarbazine lung. *Am. J. Roentgenol.* 131:527–528.

Eckhardt, S., Döbrentey, E. and Bodrogi, I. (1975). Results obtained with combination therapy of VM-26, natulan and prednisolone in generalized Hodgkin's disease. *Chemotherapy* 21:248–254.

Eden, A., Miller, G. W. and Nussenzweig, V. (1973). Human lymphocytes bear membrane receptors for C_{3b} and C_{3d}. *J. Clin. Invest.* 52:3239–3242.

Ederer, F., Myers, M. H., Eisenberg, H. and Campbell, P. C. (1965). Temporal-spatial distribution of leukemia and lymphoma in Connecticut. *J. Nat. Cancer Inst.* 35:625–629.

Edington, G. M. and Hendrickse, M. (1973). Incidence and frequency of lymphoreticular tumors in Ibadan and the western state of Nigeria. *J. Nat. Cancer Inst.* 50:1623–1631.

Edington, G. M., Osunkoya, B. O. and Hendrickse, M. (1973). Histologic classification of Hodgkin's disease in the western state of Nigeria. *J. Nat. Cancer Inst.* 50:1633–1637.

Edland, R. W. and Hansen, H. (1969). Irregular field-shaping for ^{60}Co teletherapy. *Radiology* 92:1567–1569.

Edward, D. G. F. (1938). Observations on the nature of Gordon's encephalitogenic agent. *J. Path. Bact.* 47:481–487.

Edwards, C. L. and Hayes, R. L. (1969). Tumor scanning with ^{67}Ga citrate. *J. Nucl. Med.* 10:103–105.

Edwards, J. M., Gimlette, T. M. D., Clapham, W. F., Rutt, D. L. and Kinmonth, J. B. (1966). Endolymphatic therapy of tumours with particular reference to the VX_2 tumour in *Lepus cuniculus*. *Brit. J. Surg.* 53:969–978.

Edwards, J. M., Lloyd-Davies, R. W. and Kinmonth, J. B. (1967). Selective lymphopenia in man after intralymphatic injection of radioactive ^{131}I Lipiodol. *Brit. Med. J.* 1:331–335.

Edwards, R. T., III. (1969). Hodgkin's sarcoma of the small bowel. *Virginia Med. Monthly* 96:521–525.

Eggleston, J. C. and Hartmann, W. H. (1968). Hodgkin's

disease involving the spinal epidural space. *Johns Hopkins Med. J.* 123:265–270.

Eidelman, S., Parkins, R. A. and Rubin, C. E. (1966). Abdominal lymphoma presenting as malabsorption. *Medicine* 45:111–138.

Eilam, N., Johnson, P. K., Johnson, N. L. and Creger, W. P. (1968). Bradykininogen levels in Hodgkin's disease. *Cancer* 22:631–634.

Eisinger, M., Fox, S. M., de Harven, E., Biedler, J. L. and Sanders, F. K. (1971). Virus-like agents from patients with Hodgkin's disease. *Nature* 233:104–108.

Eisner, E., Ley, A. D. and Mayer, K. (1967). Coombs'-positive hemolytic anemia in Hodgkin's disease. *Ann. Int. Med.* 66:258–273.

Ellermann, V. and Bang, O. (1908). Experimentelle Leukämie bei Hühnern. Vorlaufige mitteilung. *Zentr. Bakteriol. Parasitenk, Abt.* I Orig. 46:4–5.

Eltringham, J. R., Fajardo, L. F. and Stewart, J. R. (1975). Adriamycin cardiomyopathy: enhanced cardiac damage in rabbits with combined drug and cardiac irradiation. *Radiology* 115:471–472.

Eltringham, J. R. and Kaplan, H. S. (1973). Impaired delayed hypersensitivity responses in 154 patients with untreated Hodgkin's disease. *Nat. Cancer Inst. Monograph* 36:107–115.

Eltringham, J. R., and Weissman, I. (1970). Regional lymph node irradiation: effect on immune responses. *Radiology* 94:438–441.

Elves, M. W., Roath, S. and Israëls, M. C. G. (1963). The response of lymphocytes to antigen challenge *in vitro*. *Lancet* 1:806–807.

Emmerson, R. W. (1969). Follicular mucinosis: a study of 47 patients. *Brit. J. Dermatol.* 81:395–413.

Engeset, A., Abrahamsen, A. F., Bremer. K., Brennhovd, I. O., Christensen, I., Fröland, S. S., Hager, B., Høeg, K., Høst, H. and Nesheim, A. (1973). Peripheral and central lymph in Hodgkin's disease: preliminary report. *Nat. Cancer Inst. Monograph* 36:247–252.

Engeset, A., Brennhovd, I. O., Christensen, I., Hagen, S., Høeg, K., Høst, H., Liverud, K. and Nesheim, A. (1968). Sternberg-Reed cells in the thoracic duct lymph of patients with Hodgkin's disease. A preliminary report. Cytologic studies in connection with lymphography. *Blood* 31:99–103.

Engeset, A., Fröland, S. S., Bremer, K. and Høst, H. (1973). Blood lymphocytes in Hodgkin's disease. Increase of B-lymphocytes following extended field irradiation. *Scand. J. Haematol.* 11:195–200.

Engeset, A., Høeg, K., Høst, H., Liverud, K. and Nesheim, A. (1969). Thoracic duct lymph cytology in Hodgkin's disease. *Internat. J. Cancer* 4:735–742.

Engleman, E. G., Hoppe, R.. Kaplan, H. S., Comminskey, J. and McDevitt, H. O. (1978). Suppressor cells of the mixed lymphocyte reaction in healthy subjects and patients with Hodgkin's disease and sarcoidosis. *Clin. Res.* 26:513A (abst.).

English, J. M. III (1970). Infectious mononucleosis followed by Hodgkin's disease. *Lancet* 1:948.

English, R. S., Hurley, H. J., Witkowski, J. A. and Sanders, J. (1963). Generalized anhidrosis associated with Hodgkin's disease and acquired ichthyosis. *Ann. Int. Med.* 58:676–681.

Ennuyer, A., Bataini, P. and Franiatte, J. (1966). Résultats lointains obtenus par radiothérapie dans la maladie de Hodgkin. *Nouv. rev. franç. hématol.* 6:76–79.

Ennuyer, A., Bataini, P. and Hélary, J. (1961). Maladie de Hodgkin des voies aero-digestives supérieures. Porte d'entrée éventuelle de l'agent causal de la lymphogranulomatose maligne. *Annales oto-laryngol.* 78:474–509.

Enright, L. P., Trueblood, H. W. and Nelsen, T. S. (1970). The surgical diagnosis of abdominal Hodgkin's disease. *Surg. Gynec. Obst.* 130:853–858.

E.O.R.T.C. Radiotherapy-Chemotherapy Cooperative Group. (1972). A randomized study of irradiation and vinblastine in stages I and II of Hodgkin's disease. *Europ. J. Cancer* 8:353–362.

Epstein, A. L., Henle, W., Henle, G., Hewetson, J. F. and Kaplan, H. S. (1976). Surface marker characteristics and Epstein-Barr virus studies of two established North American Burkitt's lymphoma cell lines. *Proc. Nat. Acad. Sci. U.S.* 73:228–232.

Epstein, A. L. and Kaplan, H. S. (1974). Biology of the human malignant lymphomas. I. Establishment in continuous cell culture and heterotransplantation of diffuse histiocytic lymphomas. *Cancer* 34:1851–1872.

Epstein, E. (1939). Sex as a factor in the prognosis of Hodgkin's disease. *Am. J. Cancer* 35:230–233.

Epstein, M. A. and Achong, B. G. (1968). A specific immunofluorescence test for the herpes-type EB virus of Burkitt lymphoblasts, authenticated by electron microscopy. *J. Nat. Cancer Inst.* 40:593–607.

Epstein, M. A., Achong, B. G. and Barr, Y. M. (1964). Virus particles in cultured lymphoblasts from Burkitt's lymphoma. *Lancet* 1:702–703.

Epstein, M. A. and Barr, Y. M. (1964). Cultivation *in vitro* of human lymphoblasts from Burkitt's malignant lymphoma. *Lancet* 1:252–253.

Epstein, W. L. (1958). Induction of allergic contact dermatitis in patients with the lymphoma-leukemia complex. *J. Invest. Derm.* 30:39–40.

Ertel, I. J., Boles, E. T., Jr. and Newton, W. A., Jr. (1977). Infection after splenectomy. *New Engl. J. Med.* 296:1174.

Eshhar, Z., Order, S. E. and Katz, D. H. (1974). Ferritin, a Hodgkin's disease associated antigen. *Proc. Nat. Acad. Sci. U.S.* 71:3956–3960.

Evans, A. R., Hancock. B. W., Brown, M. J. and Richmond, J. (1977). A small cluster of Hodgkin's disease. *Brit. Med. J.* 1:1056–1057.

Evans, A. S. (1960). Infectious mononucleosis in University of Wisconsin students. *Am. J. Hyg.* 71:342–362.

Evans, A. S., Niederman, J. C. and McCollum, R. W. (1968). Seroepidemiologic studies of infectious mononucleosis with EB virus. *New Engl. J. Med.* 279:1121–1127.

Evans, H. E. and Nyhan, W. L. (1964). Hodgkin's disease in children. *Bull. Johns Hopkins Hosp.* 114:237–248.

Evans, R. F., Sagerman, R. H., Ringrose, T. L., Auchincloss, J. H. and Bowman, J. (1974). Pulmonary function following mantle-field irradiation for Hodgkin's disease. *Radiology* 111:729–731.

Ewing, J. (1928). Neoplastic Diseases. Philadelphia: W. B. Saunders.

Ezdinli, E. Z., Sokal, J. E., Aungst, C. W., Kim, U. and Sandberg, A. A. (1969). Myeloid leukemia in Hodgkin's disease: chromosomal abnormalities. *Ann. Int. Med.* 71:1097–1104.

Ezdinli, E. Z. and Stutzman, L. (1968). Vinblastine vs. nitrogen mustard therapy of Hodgkin's disease. *Cancer* 22:473–479.

Fabian, C. E., Nudelman, E. J. and Abrams, H. L. (1966).

Postlymphangiogram film as an indicator of tumor activity in lymphoma. *Invest. Radiol.* 1:386–393.

Fadem, R. S., Berson, S. S., Jacobson, A. S., and Straus, B. (1951). The effects of cortisone on the bone marrow in Hodgkin's disease. *Am. J. Clin. Path.* 21:799–813.

Faerberg, E., Yárre, H., Pastor Mengide, J. and Casareto, R. C. M. (1965). Linfogranulomatosis maligna del apendice ileocecal (enfermedad de Hodgkin-Paltauf-Sternberg). *Prensa med. Argent.* 52:2175–2176.

Faguet, G. B. (1975). Quantitation of immunocompetence in Hodgkin's disease. *J. Clin. Invest.* 56:951–957.

Fairbanks, V. F., Tauxe, W. N.. Kiely, J. M. and Miller, W. E. (1972). Scintigraphic visualization of abdominal lymph nodes with ^{99m}Tc-pertechnetate-labeled sulfur colloid. *J. Nucl. Med.* 13:185–190.

Fairley, G. H., and Akers, R. J. (1962). Antibodies to blood group A and B substances in reticuloses. *Brit. J. Haemat.* 8:375–391.

Fajardo, L. F., Stewart, J. R. and Cohn, K. E. (1968). Morphology of radiation-induced heart disease. *Arch. Path.* 86:512–519.

Falk, J. and Osoba, D. (1971). HL-A antigens and survival in Hodgkin's disease. *Lancet* 2:1118–1120.

Falkson, H. C., Portugal, M. A. and Falkson, G. (1976). Leukemia in Hodgkin's disease. *S. Afr. Med. J.* 50:1429–1431.

Falletta, J. M., Ramanujam, N., Starling, K. A. and Fernbach, D. J. (1973). Ig-positive lymphocytes in Hodgkin's disease. *New Engl. J. Med.* 288:581–582.

Farber, L. R., Prosnitz, L. R., Bertino, J. R., Cadman, E. C., Fischer, D. S., Lutes, R. A. and Pezzimenti, J. F. (1978). Long term results of combined modality therapy for advanced Hodgkin's disease. *Proc. Am. Assoc. Cancer Res.* 19:385 (abst.).

Farber, S. (1949). Some observations on the effect of folic acid antagonists on acute leukemia and other forms of incurable cancer. *Blood* 4:160–167.

Farber, S., Diamond, L. K., Mercer, R. D., Silvester, R. F., Jr. and Wolfe, J. A. (1948). Temporary remissions in acute leukemia in children produced by folic acid antagonist 4-aminopteroylglutamic acid (Aminopterin). *New Engl. J. Med.* 238:787–793.

Farney, R. J., Morris, A. H., Armstrong, J. D., Jr. and Hammer, S. (1977). Diffuse pulmonary disease after therapy with nitrogen mustard, vincristine, procarbazine, and prednisone. *Am. Rev. Respir. Dis.* 115:135–145.

Farrer-Brown, G., Bennett, M. H., Harrison, C. V., Millett, Y. and Jelliffe, A. M. (1971). The pathological findings following laparotomy in Hodgkin's disease. *Brit. J. Cancer* 25:449–457.

Favre, R., Carcassonne, Y. and Meyer, G. (1977). A surface antigen associated with Hodgkin's disease. *J. Nat. Cancer Inst.* 59:1727–1730.

Faw, F. L., Johnson, R. E., Warren, C. A. and Glenn, D. W. (1971). A standard set of "individualized" compensating filters for mantle field radiotherapy of Hodgkin's disease. *Am. J. Roentgenol.* 111:376–381.

Fayos, J. V. and Lampe, I. (1971). Cardiac apical mass in Hodgkin's disease. *Radiology* 99:15–18.

Fazekas, J., Greenberg, C. and Rambo, O. N. (1974). Primary thymic Hodgkin's disease. A clinicopathologic study of 27 cases. *Radiol. Clin. Biol.* 43:456–464.

Fazio, M. and Bachi, C. (1967). Combined action of phytohaemagglutinin and RNA in lymphocytes from patients with Hodgkin's disease. *Nature* 215:629–630.

Fazio, M. and Calciati, A. (1962). An attempt to transfer tuberculin hypersensitivity in Hodgkin's disease. *Panminerva Med.* 4:164–167.

Fazio, M., Calciati, A. and De Paoli, M. (1962). Dermatite allergica de contatto nel linfogranuloma maligno. *Minerva derm.* 37:259–261.

Fechner, R. E. (1969). Hodgkin's disease of the thymus. *Cancer* 23:16–23.

Fellows, K. E., Jr., Abell, M. R. and Martel, W. (1969). Intrapulmonary lymph node detected roentgenologically; case report. *Am. J. Roentgenol.* 106:601–603.

Felsburg, P. J. and Edelman, R. (1977). The active E-rosette test: a sensitive *in vitro* correlate for human delayed-type hypersensitivity. *J. Immunol.* 118:62–66.

Fenelly, J. J. and McBride, A. (1974). Immunological depletion contributing to familial Hodgkin's disease. *Brit. J. Cancer* 30:182 (abst.).

Ferguson, D. J., Allen, L. W., Griem, M. L., Moran, M. E., Rappaport, H. and Ultmann, J. (1973). Surgical experience with staging laparotomy in 125 patients with lymphoma. *Arch. Int. Med.* 131:356–361.

Ferm, V. H. (1963). Congenital malformations in hamster embryos after treatment with vinblastine and vincristine. *Science* 141:426.

Ferrant, A., Rodhain, J., Michaux, J. L., Piret, L., Maldague, B. and Sokal, G. (1975). Detection of skeletal involvement in Hodgkin's disease: a comparison of radiography, bone scanning, and bone marrow biopsy in 38 patients. *Cancer* 35:1346–1353.

Ferrer, J. F. and Kaplan, H. S. (1968). Antigenic characteristics of lymphomas induced by radiation leukemia virus (RadLV) in mice and rats. *Cancer Res.* 28:2522–2528.

Filly, R., Blank, N. and Castellino, R. A. (1976a). Radiographic distribution of intrathoracic disease in previously untreated patients with Hodgkin's disease and non-Hodgkin's lymphoma. *Radiology* 120:277–281.

Filly, R. A., Marglin, S. and Castellino, R. A. (1976b). The ultrasonographic spectrum of abdominal and pelvic Hodgkin's disease and non-Hodgkin's lymphoma. *Cancer* 38:2143–2148.

Finkbeiner, J. A., Craver, L. F. and Diamond, H. D. (1954). Prognostic signs in Hodgkin's disease. *J.A.M.A.* 156:472–477.

Fischer, H. W. (1969). Complications of lymphography. *In* W. A. Fuchs, J. W. Davidson and H. W. Fischer, Lymphography in Cancer. Berlin and Heidelberg: Springer-Verlag. Chap. 4, pp. 24–41.

Fisher, A. M. H., Kendall, B. and Van Leuven, B. D. (1962). Hodgkin's disease: a radiological survey. *Clin. Radiol.* 13:115–127.

Fisher, R. I., De Vita, V. T., Hubbard, S. M. and Young, R. C. (1977). Prolonged disease free survival in Hodgkin's disease following reinduction with MOPP. *Proc. Am. Soc. Clin. Oncol.* 18:318 (abst.).

Fleischman, E. V., Prigogina, E. L., Platonova, G. M., Chudina, A. P., Kruglova, G. V. and Kaverzneva, M. M. (1974). Comparative chromosome characteristics of reticulosarcomas and Hodgkin's disease. *Neoplasma* 21:51–61.

Fleischmann, T., Hakanson, C. H., and Levan, A. (1971). Fluorescent marker chromosomes in malignant lymphomas. *Hereditas* 69:311–314.

Fleischmann, T. and Krizsa, F. (1976). Chromosomák malignus lymphomákban. *Orv. Hetil.* 117:1263–1266.

Flury, R. and Wegmann, T. (1964). The behavior of leukocytic alkaline phosphatase in Hodgkin's disease. *Schweiz. Med. Wchnschr.* 94:958–961.

Focan, C., Brictieux, N., Lemaire, M. and Hugues, J. (1974). Néoplasies secondaires compliquant une maladie de Hodgkin. *Nouv. presse méd.* 3:1385.

Forbes, J. F. and Morris, P. J. (1972). Analysis of HL-A antigens in patients with Hodgkin's disease and their families. *J. Clin. Invest.* 51:1156–1163.

Forbus, W. D. (1942). Studies on Hodgkin's disease and its relation to infection by Brucella. *Am. J. Path.* 18: 745–748.

Fordham, E. W., Hibbs, G. G. and Hendrickson, F. R. (1969). Shield construction for extended field therapy of Hodgkin's disease. *Radiology* 92:1374–1376.

Forteza Bover, G., Báguena Candela, J., Forteza Vila, J., Barbera Guillem, E. and Báguena Candela, R. (1968). Estudio de la ultrastructura de la célula gigante de Sternberg y de sus relaciones con otras células immunocompetentes. *Medicina española* 59:430–435.

Forteza Bover, G., Báguena Candela, R., Marco Orts, F. and Esquerdo Mañez, J. (1965). Analisis cromosomico mediante puncion ganglion en un caso de enfermedad de Hodgkin. *Medicina española* 54:263–268.

Fox, H. (1926). Remarks on microscopical preparations made from some of the original tissue described by Thomas Hodgkin, 1832. *Ann. Med. History* 8:370–374.

Foxon, G. E. H. (1966). Thomas Hodgkin, 1798–1866; a biographical note. *Guy's Hosp. Rep.* 115:243–254.

Frajola, W. J., Greider, M. A. and Bouroncle, B. A. (1958). Cytology of the Sternberg-Reed cell as revealed by the electron microscope. *Ann. New York Acad. Sci.* 73:221–236.

Franssila, K. O., Heiskala, M. K. and Heiskala, H. J. (1977). Epidemiology and histopathology of Hodgkin's disease in Finland. *Cancer* 39:1280–1288.

Franssila, K. O., Kalima, T. V. and Voutilainen, A. (1967). Histologic classification of Hodgkin's disease. *Cancer* 20:1594–1601.

Fraumeni, J. F., Jr. (1969). Constitutional disorders of man predisposing to leukemia and lymphoma. *Nat. Cancer Inst. Monograph* 32:221–232.

Fraumeni, J. F., Jr. (1971). Infectious mononucleosis and acute leukemia. *J.A.M.A.* 215:1159.

Fraumeni, J. F., Jr. (1974). Family studies in Hodgkin's disease. *Cancer Res.* 34:1164–1165.

Fraumeni, J. F., Jr. and Li, F. P. (1969). Hodgkin's disease in childhood: an epidemiologic study. *J. Nat. Cancer Inst.* 42:681–691.

Frei, E., III and Gamble, J. F. (1966). Progress in the chemotherapy of Hodgkin's disease. *Cancer* 19:378–384.

Frei, E., III and Gehan, E. A. (1971). Definition of cure for Hodgkin's disease. *Cancer Res.* 31:1828–1833.

Frei, E., III, Luce, J. K., Gamble, J. F., Coltman, C. A., Jr., Constanzi, J. J., Talley, R. W., Monto, R. W., Wilson, H. E., Hewlett, J. S., Delaney, F. C. and Gehan, E. A. (1973). Combination chemotherapy in advanced Hodgkin's disease. Induction and maintenance of remission. *Ann. Int. Med.* 79:376–382.

Frei, E., III, Luce, J. K., Talley, R. W., Vaitkevicius, V. K. and Wilson, H. E. (1972). 5-(3,3-dimethyl-1-triazeno)imidazole-4-carboxamide (NSC-45388) in the treatment of lymphoma. *Cancer Chemother. Rep.* 56: 667–670.

Friedman, M., Kim, T. H. and Panahon, A. M. (1976). Spinal cord compression in malignant lymphoma. Treatment and results. *Cancer* 37:1485–1491.

Friedman, M., Pearlman, A. W. and Turgeon, L. (1967). Hodgkin's disease: tumor lethal dose and iso-effect recovery curve. *Am. J. Roentgenol.* 99:843–850.

Friend, C. (1957). Cell-free transmission in adult Swiss mice of a disease having the character of a leukemia. *J. Exper. Med.* 105:307–318.

Froissart, M., Mizon, J.-P., Morcamp, D. and Demay, J.-P. (1976). Atrophie cérébelleuse subaiguë paranéoplasique au cours d'une maladie de Hodgkin. *Nouv. presse méd.* 5:2549–2550.

Fröland, S. S. (1972). Binding of sheep erythrocytes to human lymphocytes: a probable marker of T lymphocytes. *Scand. J. Immunol.* 1:269–280.

Fuchs, W. A. (1969). Normal anatomy. *In* W. A. Fuchs, J. W. Davidson and H. W. Fischer, Lymphography in Cancer. Berlin: Springer-Verlag. Chap. 5, pp. 42–86.

Fuchs, W. A., Davidson, J. W., and Fischer, H. W. (1969). Lymphography in Cancer. Berlin: Springer-Verlag.

Fuks, Z., Glatstein, E., Marsa, G. W., Bagshaw, M. A. and Kaplan, H. S. (1976a). Long-term effects of external radiation on the pituitary and thyroid glands. *Cancer* 37:1152–1161.

Fuks, Z., Strober, S., Bobrove, A. M., Sasazuki, T., McMichael, A. and Kaplan, H. S. (1976b). Long term effects of radiation on T and B lymphocytes in peripheral blood of patients with Hodgkin's disease. *J. Clin. Invest.* 58:803–814.

Fuks, Z., Strober, S. and Kaplan, H. S. (1976c). Interaction between serum factors and T lymphocytes in Hodgkin's disease. *New Engl. J. Med.* 295:1273–1278.

Fuks, Z., Strober, S., King, D. P. and Kaplan, H. S. (1976d). Reversal of cell surface abnormalities of T lymphocytes in Hodgkin's disease after *in vitro* incubation in fetal sera. *J. Immunol.* 117:1331–1335.

Fukuhara, S. and Rowley, J. D. (1978). Chromosome 14 translocations in non-Burkitt lymphomas. *Internat. J. Cancer* 22:14–21.

Fuller, L. M. (1967). Results of intensive regional radiation therapy in the treatment of Hodgkin's disease and the malignant lymphomas of the head and neck. *Am. J. Roentgenol.* 99:340–351.

Fuller, L. M., Gamble, J. F., Ibrahim, E., Jing, B.-S., Butler, J. J. and Shullenberger, C. C. (1973). Stage II Hodgkin's disease. Significance of mediastinal and non-mediastinal presentations. *Radiology* 109:429–435.

Fuller, L. M., Gamble, J. F., Shullenberger, C. C., Butler, J. J. and Gehan, E. A. (1971). Prognostic factors in localized Hodgkin's disease treated with regional radiation. Clinical presentation and specific histology. *Radiology* 98:641–654.

Fuller, L. M., Madoc-Jones, H., Gamble, J. F., Butler, J. J., Sullivan, M. P., Fernandez, C. H. and Gehan, E. A. (1977). New assessment of the prognostic significance of histopathology in Hodgkin's disease for laparotomy-negative stage I and stage II patients. *Cancer* 39:2174–2182.

Furth, J. and Furth, O. B. (1936). Neoplastic disease produced in mice by general irradiation with X-rays. Incidence and types of neoplasms. *Am. J. Cancer* 28:54–65.

Gailani, S., Ezdinli, E., Nussbaum, A., Silvernail, P. and Elias, E. G. (1974). Studies on tryptophan metabolism in patients with lymphoma. *Cancer Res.* 34:1664–1667.

Gaines, J. D., Gilmer, M. A. and Remington, J. S. (1973). Deficiency of lymphocyte antigen recognition in Hodgkin's disease. *Nat. Cancer Inst. Monograph* 36:117–121.

Gajl-Peczalska, K. J., Hansen, J. A., Bloomfield, C. D. and Good, R. A. (1973). B lymphocytes in untreated patients with malignant lymphoma and Hodgkin's disease. *J. Clin. Invest.* 52:3064–3073.

Galan, H. M., Lida, E. J. and Kleisner, E. H. (1963). Chromosomes of Sternberg-Reed cells. *Lancet* 1:335.

Gall, E. A. and Mallory, T. B. (1942). Malignant lymphoma. A clinical-pathologic survey of 618 cases. *Am. J. Path.* 18:381–429.

Gallagher, R. E. and Gallo, R. C. (1975). Type C RNA tumor virus isolated from cultured human acute myelogenous leukemia cells. *Science* 187:350–353.

Gallmeier, W. M., Boecker, W. R., Bruntsch, U., Hossfeld, D. K. and Schmidt, C. G. (1977). Characterization of a human Hodgkin cell line and a lymphoblastic EBNA-negative cell line derived from a non-Hodgkin's lymphoma patient. *Haematol. Blood Transfus.* 20:277–281.

Gallmeier, W. M., Bruntsch, U., Pfeiffer, R., Bestek, U. and Schmidt, C. G. (1973). T and B lymphocytes in Hodgkin's disease. *Z. Krebsforsch.* 80:247–254.

Gallo, R. C., Gallagher, R. E., Wong-Staal, F., Aoki, T., Markham, P. D., Schetters, H., Ruscetti, F., Valerio, M., Walling, M. J., O'Keeffe, R. T. O., Saxinger, W. C., Smith, R. G., Gillespie, D. H. and Reitz, M. S., Jr. (1978). Isolation and tissue distribution of type-C virus and viral components from a gibbon ape (*Hylobates lar*) with lymphocytic leukemia. *Virology* 84:359–373.

Gamble, J. F., Fuller, L. M., Martin, R. G., Sullivan, M. P., Jing, B.-S., Butler, J. J. and Shullenberger, C. C. (1975). Influence of staging celiotomy in localized presentations of Hodgkin's disease. *Cancer* 35:817–825.

Gams, R. A., Neal, J. A. and Conrad, F. G. (1968). Hydantoin-induced pseudo-lymphoma. *Ann. Int. Med.* 69:557–568.

Gardner, W. U. (1937). Influence of estrogenic hormones on abnormal growths. *In* Occasional Publications of the American Association for the Advancement of Science. Vol. IV, pp. 67–75. Lancaster, Pa.: Science Press.

Garrett, M. J. (1974). Teratogenic effects of combination chemotherapy. *Ann. Int. Med.* 80:667.

Garrett, M. J., Das, S., Smith, J. D. and Freeman, L. S. (1977). Long term experience with combination chemotherapy in advanced Hodgkin's disease. *Clin. Oncol.* 3:145–154.

Garvin, A. J., Spicer, S. S., Parmley, R. T. and Munster, A. M. (1974). Immunohistochemical demonstration of IgG in Reed-Sternberg and other cells in Hodgkin's disease. *J. Exper. Med.* 139:1077–1083.

Gastearena, J., Martinez, J., Lizaur, J., Arcas, D. and Chacón, J. (1969). Estudio de una anomalia cromosomica en la enfermedad de Hodgkin. *Rev. clin. española* 113:453–454.

Gates, G. F. and Dore, E. K. (1978). Streamline flow in the human portal vein. *J. Nucl. Med.* 14:79–83.

Gazet, J. C. (1973). Laparotomy and splenectomy. *In* Hodgkin's Disease, D. W. Smithers (ed.). Edinburgh: Churchill Livingstone, pp. 190–200.

Gearhart, P. J., Sigal, N. H. and Klinman, N. R. (1975). Production of antibodies of identical idiotype but diverse immunoglobulin classes by cells derived from a single stimulated B cell. *Proc. Nat. Acad. Sci. U.S.* 72:1707–1711.

Geering, G., Old, L. J. and Boyse, E. A. (1966). Antigens of leukemias induced by naturally occurring murine leukemia virus: their relation to the antigens of Gross virus and other murine leukemia viruses. *J. Exper. Med.* 124:753–772.

Gehan, E. A. (1965). A generalized Wilcoxon test for comparing arbitrarily singly-censored samples. *Biometrika* 52:203–233.

Geller, S. A. and Stimmel, B. (1973). Diagnostic confusion from lymphatic lesions in heroin addicts. *Ann. Int. Med.* 78:703–705.

Geller, W. (1953). A study of antibody formation in patients with malignant lymphomas. *J. Lab. Clin. Med.* 42:232–237.

Gellhorn, A. and Collins, V. P. (1951). A quantitative evaluation of the contribution of nitrogen mustard to the therapeutic management of Hodgkin's disease. *Ann. Int. Med.* 35:1250–1259.

Geslin, P., Fraboulet, J. Y., Delhumeau, A., Victor, J., Larra, F., and Tadei, A. (1977). Pericarditis after mediastinal irradiation for Hodgkin's disease. *Rev. fr. mal. respir.* 5:219–226.

Ghatak, N. R. (1975). Unusual infections of the nervous system in malignant lymphomas. *Acta Neuropathol.* 6:261–265.

Ghosh, L. and Muehrcke, R. C. (1970). The nephrotic syndrome: a prodrome to lymphoma. *Ann. Int. Med.* 72:379–382.

Giannopoulos, P. P. and Bergsagel, D. E. (1959). The mechanism of the anemia associated with Hodgkin's disease. *Blood* 14:856–869.

Gilbert, E. H., Earle, J. D., Glatstein, E., Goris, M. L., Kaplan, H. S. and Kriss, J. P. (1976a). [111]Indium bone marrow scintigraphy as an aid in selecting marrow biopsy sites for the evaluation of marrow elements in patients with lymphoma. *Cancer* 38:1560–1567.

Gilbert, E. H., Earle, J. D., Goris, M. L., Kaplan, H. S. and Kriss, J. P. (1976b). The accuracy of ^{111}In Cl$_3$ as a bone marrow scanning agent. *Radiology* 119:167–168.

Gilbert, R. (1925). La roentgenthérapie de la granulomatose maligne. *J. radiol. électrol.* 9:509–514.

Gilbert, R. (1939). Radiotherapy in Hodgkin's disease (malignant granulomatosis): anatomic and clinical foundations; governing principles; results. *Am. J. Roentgenol.* 41:198–241.

Gilbert, R. (1951). Lymphogranulome, lymphosarcome, réticulosarcome, radiothérapie. *Radiol. Clin.* 20:313–336.

Gilbert, R. and Babaïantz, L. (1931). Notre méthode de roentgenthérapie de la lymphogranulomatose (Hodgkin); résultats éloignés. *Acta Radiol.* 12:523–529.

Gillman, J., Gillman, T., Gilbert, C. and Spence, I. (1952). The pathogenesis of experimentally produced lymphomata in rats (including Hodgkin's-like sarcoma). *Cancer* 5:792–846.

Gillman, T., Kinns, M. and Cross, R. M. (1969). Hodgkin's disease: a possible experimental model in rats. *Lancet* 2:1421–1422.

Gillman, T., Kinns, A. M., Hallowes, R. C. and Lloyd, J. B. (1973). Malignant lymphoreticular tumors induced by trypan blue and transplanted in inbred rats. *J. Nat. Cancer Inst.* 50:1179–1193.

Gilmore, H. R., Jr. and Zelesnick, G. (1962). Environmental Hodgkin's disease and leukemia. *Penn Med. J.* 65:1047–1049.

Ginzton, E. L., Mallory, K. B. and Kaplan, H. S. (1957). The Stanford medical linear accelerator. I. Design and development. *Stanford Med. Bull.* 15:123–140.

Givler, R. L., Brunk, S. F., Hass, C. A. and Gulesserian, H. E. (1971). Problems of interpretation of liver biopsy in Hodgkin's disease. *Cancer* 28:1335–1342.

Glatstein, E. (1974). Hodgkin's disease and non-Hodgkin's lymphomas: how important is histology? *Front. Radiation Ther. Oncol.* 9:203–216.

Glatstein, E. (1977). Radiotherapy in Hodgkin's disease. Past achievements and future progress. *Cancer* 39:834–842.

Glatstein, E., Guernsey, J. M., Rosenberg, S. A. and Kaplan, H. S. (1969). The value of laparotomy and splenectomy in the staging of Hodgkin's disease. *Cancer* 24:709–718.

Glatstein, E., Trueblood, H. W., Enright, L. P., Rosenberg, S. A. and Kaplan, H. S. (1970). Surgical staging of abdominal involvement in unselected patients with Hodgkin's disease. *Radiology* 97:425–432.

Glatstein, E., McHardy-Young, S., Brast, N., Eltringham, J. R. and Kriss, J. P. (1971). Alterations in serum thyrotropin (TSH) and thyroid function following radiotherapy in patients with malignant lymphoma. *J. Clin. Endocrinol. Metab.* 32:833–841.

Glees, J. P., Gazet, J.-C., Macdonald, J. S. and Peckham, M. J. (1974). The accuracy of lymphography in Hodgkin's disease. *Clin. Radiol.* 25:5–11.

Glees, J., Taylor, K., Gazet, J.-C., Peckham, M. and McCready, V. (1977). Accuracy of grey-scale ultrasonography of liver and spleen in Hodgkin's disease and the other lymphomas compared with isotope scans. *Clin. Radiol.* 28:233–238.

Glenn, D. W., Faw, F. L., Kagan, A. R. and Johnson, R. E. (1968). Field separation in multiple portal radiation therapy. *Am. J. Roentgenol.* 102:199–206.

Glenn, D. W. and Johnson, R. E. (1972). Male gonadal shielding during cobalt teletherapy. *Radiology* 104:214.

Glick, A. D., Leech, J. H., Flexner, J. M. and Collins, R. D. (1976). Ultrastructural study of Reed-Sternberg cells. Comparison with transformed lymphocytes and histiocytes. *Am. J. Pathol.* 85:195–208.

Glick, J. H. (1978). The treatment of stage IIIA Hodgkin's disease: what is the role of combined modality therapy? *Internat. J. Radiation Oncol. Biol. Phys.* 4:909–911.

Glicksman, A. S. and Nickson, J. J. (1973). Acute and late reactions to irradiation in the treatment of Hodgkin's disease. *Arch. Int. Med.* 131:369–373.

Glinska, H., Slomska, J. and Madejczyk, A. (1969). Le pronostic dans la maladie de Hodgkin et dans les autres lymphomes malins—A propos de 1239 cas traités et suivis dans 3 instituts d'oncologie en Pologne, 1951–1960. *Bull. assoc. méd. étrangers Inst. Gustave Roussy* 8:74–83.

Gnatyshek, A. I. and Kuznetsova, L. I. (1960). Results of treatment of patients with Hodgkin's disease. *Vrach. Delo* 12:77–79.

Godeau, P., Guillevin, L., de Saxce, H. and Le Porrier, M. (1975). Purpura thrombopénique révélateur de la maladie de Hodgkin. *Sem. hôp. Paris* 51:2401–2405.

Goffinet, D. R., Glatstein, E., Fuks, Z. and Kaplan, H. S. (1976). Abdominal irradiation in non-Hodgkin's lymphomas. *Cancer* 37:2797–2805.

Goffinet, D. R., Glatstein, E. J. and Merigan, T. C. (1972). Herpes zoster-varicella infections and lymphoma. *Ann. Int. Med.* 76:235–240.

Goldberg, I. H. and Rabinowitz, M. (1962). Actinomycin D inhibition of deoxyribonucleic acid-dependent synthesis of ribonucleic acid. *Science* 136:315–316.

Goldberg, I. H. and Reich, E. (1964). Actinomycin inhibition of RNA synthesis directed by DNA. *Fed. Proc.* 23:958–964.

Goldin, A., Venditti, J. M., Humphreys, S. R. and Mantel, N. (1956). Influence of the concentration of leukemic inoculum on the effectiveness of treatment. *Science* 123:840.

Goldin, A., Venditti, J. M., Humphreys, S. R. and Mantel, N. (1958). Quantitative evaluation of chemotherapeutic agents against advanced leukemia in mice. *J. Nat. Cancer Inst.* 21:495–511.

Golding, B., Golding, H., Lomnitzer, R., Jacobson, R., Koornhof, H. J. and Rabson, A. R. (1977). Production of leukocyte inhibitory factor (LIF) in Hodgkin's disease: spontaneous production of an inhibitor of normal lymphocyte transformation. *Clin. Immunol. Immunopathol.* 7:114–122.

Goldman, J. M. (1971). Parasternal chest wall involvement in Hodgkin's disease. *Chest* 59:133–137.

Goldman, J. M. and Aisenberg, A. C. (1970). Incidence of antibody to EB virus, herpes simplex and cytomegalovirus in Hodgkin's disease. *Cancer* 26:327–331.

Goldman, J. M. and Dawson, A. A. (1975). Combination therapy for advanced resistant Hodgkin's disease. *Lancet* 2:1224–1227.

Goldman, J. M. and Hobbs, J. R. (1967). The immunoglobulins in Hodgkin's disease. *Immunology* 13:421–431.

Goldman, R., Fishkin, B. G. and Peterson, E. T. (1950). The value of the heterophile antibody reaction in the lymphomatous diseases. *J. Lab. Clin. Med.* 35:681–687.

Goldman, R. L. (1970). Granulomas in Hodgkin's disease. *New Engl. J. Med.* 283:1410.

Goldmann, E. E. (1892). Beitrag zu der Lehre von dem "malignen Lymphom". *Centr. Allg. Path. Anat.* 3:665–690.

Good, R. A. and Finstad, J. (1968). The association of lymphoid malignancy and immunologic functions. *In* Proceedings of the International Conference on Leukemia-Lymphoma, C. J. D. Zarafonetis (ed.). Philadelphia: Lea & Febiger. pp. 175–197.

Good, R. A., Kelly, W. D., Rotstein, J. and Varco, R. L. (1962). Hodgkin's disease and other lymphomas. *Prog. Allergy* 6:275–291.

Goodman, L. S., Wintrobe, M. M., Dameshek, W., Goodman, M. J., Gilman, A. Z. and McLennan, M. T. (1946). Nitrogen mustard therapy. Use of methyl-bis-(β-chloroethyl)amine hydrochloride and tris-(β-chloroethyl) amine hydrochloride for Hodgkin's disease, lymphosarcoma, leukemia and certain allied and miscellaneous disorders. *J.A.M.A.* 132:126–132.

Goodman, R., Jaffe, N., Filler, R. and Cassady, J. R. (1976a). Herpes zoster in children with stage I–III Hodgkin's disease. *Radiology* 118:429–431.

Goodman, R. L., Piro, A. J. and Hellman, S. (1976b). Can

pelvic irradiation be omitted in patients with pathologic stages IA and IIA Hodgkin's disease? *Cancer* 37:2834–2839.

Goodwin, J. S., Messner, R. P., Bankhurst, A. D., Peake, G. T., Saiki, J. H. and Williams, R. C., Jr. (1977). Prostaglandin-producing suppressor cells in Hodgkin's disease. *New Engl. J. Med.* 297:963–968.

Gordon, I., Stoker, D. J. and Macdonald, J. S. (1976). The lymphographic pattern in Hodgkin's disease: a correlation with the Rye histological classification. *Clin. Radiol.* 27:57–64.

Gordon, M. H. (1932). Studies on Aetiology of Lymphadenoma. Rose Research on Lymphadenoma. Bristol, England: John Wright & Sons. pp. 7–76.

Gordon, M. H. (1936). Aetiology of lymphadenoma. Synthetized vaccine of elementary bodies. *Lancet* 231:65–68.

Gordon, M. H., Gow, A. E., Levitt, W. M. and Weber, F. P. (1934). Recent advances in pathology and treatment of lymphadenoma. *Proc. Roy. Soc. Med.* 27:1035–1050.

Gotoff, S. P., Lolekha, S., Lopata, M., Kopp, J., Kopp, R. L. and Malecki, T. J. (1973). The macrophage aggregation assay for cell-mediated immunity in man. Studies of patients with Hodgkin's disease and sarcoidosis. *J. Lab. Clin. Med.* 82:682–691.

Gough, J. (1970) Hodgkin's disease; a correlation of histopathology with survival. *Internat. J. Cancer* 5:273–281.

Goulian, M. and Fahey, J. L. (1961). Abnormalities in serum protein-bound hexose in Hodgkin's disease. *J. Lab. Clin. Med.* 57:408–419.

Gowans, J. L. and Knight, E. J. (1964). The route of recirculation of lymphocytes in the rat. *Proc. Roy. Soc., B* 159:257–282.

Gowers, W. R. (1879). Hodgkin's disease. *In* A System of Medicine, J. R. Reynolds (ed.). London: Macmillan, pp. 306–352.

Grace, J. T., Jr. and Mittelman, A. (1966). Surgery in the management of Hodgkin's disease. *Cancer* 19:351–355.

Graff, K. S., Simon, R. M., Yankee, R. A., De Vita, V. T. and Rogentine, G. N. (1974). HL-A antigens in Hodgkin's disease: histopathologic and clinical correlations. *J. Nat. Cancer Inst.* 52:1087–1090.

Grand, C. G. (1944). Tissue culture studies of cytoplasmic inclusion bodies in lymph nodes of Hodgkin's disease. *Proc. Soc. Exper. Biol. Med.* 56:229–230.

Grand, C. G. (1949). Cytoplasmic inclusions and the characteristics of Hodgkin's disease lymph node in tissue culture. *Cancer Res.* 9:183–192.

Granger, W. and Whitaker, R. (1967). Hodgkin's disease in bone, with special reference to periosteal reaction. *Brit. J. Radiol.* 40:939–948.

Grann, V., Pool, J. L. and Mayer, K. (1966). Comparative study of bone marrow aspiration and biopsy in patients with neoplastic disease. *Cancer* 19:1898–1900.

Gravell, M., Levine, P. H., McIntyre, R. F., Land, V. J. and Pagano, J. S. (1976). Epstein-Barr virus in an American patient with Burkitt's lymphoma: detection of viral genome in tumor tissue and establishment of a tumor-derived cell line (NAB). *J. Nat. Cancer Inst.* 56:701–704.

Graves, D. and Ferrer, J. (1976). *In vitro* transmission and propagation of the bovine leukemia virus in monolayer cell cultures. *Cancer Res.* 36:4152–4159.

Gray, J. G. and Russell, P. S. (1963). Donor selection in human organ transplantation. *Lancet* 2:863–865.

Gray, L. and Prosnitz, L. R. (1975). Dosimetry of Hodgkin's disease therapy using a 4 MV linear accelerator. *Radiology* 116:423–428.

Greco, F., Kolins, J., Rajjoub, R. and Brereton, H. (1976). Hodgkin's disease and granulomatous angitis of the central nervous system. *Cancer* 38:2027–2032.

Greco, R. S., Acheson, R. M. and Foote, F. M. (1974). Hodgkin disease in Connecticut from 1935 to 1962. The bimodal incidence curve in the general population and survival in untreated patients. *Arch. Int. Med.* 134:1039–1042.

Green, I. and Corso, P. (1958). Experiences with skin homografting in patients with lymphoma. *Transp. Bull.* 5:427–428.

Green, I., Inkelas, M. and Allen, L. B. (1960). Hodgkin's disease: a maternal-to-foetal lymphocyte chimaera? *Lancet* 1:30–32.

Greenberg, L. H. and Cohen, M. (1962). Histiomonocytic leukemia occurring in patient with Hodgkin's disease. *N.Y. State J. Med.* 62:3817–3821.

Greenberg, L. H. and Tanaka, K. R. (1964). Congenital anomalies probably produced by cyclophosphamide. *J.A.M.A.* 188:423–426.

Greenfield, W. S. (1878). Specimens illustrative of the pathology of lymphadenoma and leucocythemia. *Trans. Path. Soc. London* 29:272–304.

Greenwood, R., Smellie, H., Barr, M. and Cunliffe, A. C. (1958). Circulating antibodies in sarcoidosis. *Brit. Med. J.* 1:1388–1391.

Griesshaber, W. von (1964). Beitrag zur chronischen Mesantoinvergiftung. *Med. Klin.* 59:932–934.

Griffin, F. M., Jr., Bianco, C. and Silverstein, S. C. (1975). Characterization of the macrophage receptor for complement and demonstration of its functional independence from the receptor for the Fc portion of immunoglobulin G. *J. Exper. Med.* 141:1269–1277.

Griffin, J. W., Thompson, R. W., Mitchinson, M. J., De Kiewiet, J. C. and Welland, F. H. (1971). Lymphomatous leptomeningitis. *Am. J. Med.* 51:200–208.

Grifoni, V. (1973). Recent immunological findings in Hodgkin's disease. *Tumori* 59:363–374.

Grifoni, V., Del Giacco, G. S., Tognella, S., Manconi, P. E. and Mantovani, G. (1970). Lymphocytotoxins in Hodgkin's disease. *Ital. J. Immunol. Immunopathol.* 1:21–31.

Grifoni, V., Del Giacco, G. S., Tognella, S., Spano, G., Manconi, P. E. and Rugarli, C. (1968a). Anticorpi antilinfonodo nella malattia di Hodgkin. *Boll. soc. ital. biol. sper.* 44:2137–2140.

Grifoni, V., Del Giacco, G. S., Tognella, S., Spano, G., Manconi, P. E. and Rugarli, C. (1969). Ulteriori osservazioni sulla presenza di anticorpi antilinfonodo nella malattia di Hodgkin. *Boll. soc. ital. biol. sper.* 45:1283–1286.

Grifoni, V., Rugarli, C., Tossi, B., Besana, C. and Scorza, R. (1968b). Effetti di estratti linfonodali autologhi su culture di linfociti di soggetti con malattia di Hodgkin. *Haematologica* 53:958–968.

Gross, L. (1951). "Spontaneous" leukemia developing in C3H mice following inoculation, in infancy, with AKleukemia extracts, or AK-embryos. *Proc. Soc. Exper. Biol. Med.* 76:27–32.

Gross, L. (1958). Attempt to recover filterable agents from X-ray-induced leukemia. *Acta Haematol.* 19:353–361.

Gross, L. (1961). "Vertical" transmission of passage A virus from inoculated C3H mice through their untreated offspring. *Proc. Soc. Exper. Biol. Med.* 107:90–93.

Gross, N. J. (1977). Pulmonary effects of radiation therapy. *Ann. Int. Med.* 86:81–92.

Gross, R., Zach, J. and Schulten, H. K. (1966). Die Lymphogranulomatose. Diagnostisch-prognostische Hinweise anhand von 700 Fällen. *Deut. Med. Wchnschr.* 91:521–529.

Groth, C. G., Hellström, K., Hofvendahl, S., Nordenstam, H. and Wengle, B. (1972). Diagnosis of malignant lymphoma at laparotomy disclosing intrahepatic cholestasis. *Acta Chir. Scand.* 138:186–189.

Grover, S. and Hardas, U. D. (1972). Childhood malignancies in central India. *J. Nat. Cancer Inst.* 49:953–958.

Grufferman, S. (1977). Clustering and aggregation of exposures in Hodgkin's disease. *Cancer* 39:1829–1833.

Grufferman, S. G., Cole, P., Smith, P. G. and Lukes, R. J. (1977). Hodgkin's disease in sibs. *New Engl. J. Med.* 296:248–250.

Grufferman, S., Duong, T. and Cole, P. (1976). Occupation and Hodgkin's disease. *J. Nat. Cancer Inst.* 57:1193–1195.

Gutensohn, N. and Cole, P. (1977). Epidemiology of Hodgkin's disease in the young. *Internat. J. Cancer* 19:595–604.

Gutensohn, N., Cole, P. and Li, F. P. (1975a). Sibship size and Hodgkin's disease. *New Engl. J. Med.* 292:1025–1028.

Gutensohn, N., Li, F. P., Johnson, R. E. and Cole, P. (1975b). Hodgkin's disease, tonsillectomy and family size. *New Engl. J. Med.* 292:22–25.

Gutjahr, P., Greinbacher, I. and Kutzner, J. (1976). Late effects of tumor treatment. Structural changes in the spinal column seen on x-ray. *Deut. Med. Wchnschr.* 101:988–992.

Haas, E. (1953). Beitrag zum Morbus Hodgkin und seiner Stadieneinteilung. *Klin. Wchnschr.* 31:694–697.

Habeshaw, J. A., Stuart, A. E., Dewar, A. E. and Young, G. (1976). IgM receptors on cells in Hodgkin's disease. *Lancet* 1:916.

Haddow, A. J. (1963). An improved map for the study of Burkitt's lymphoma syndrome in Africa. *E. Afr. Med. J.* 40:429–432.

Hagans, J. A. (1950). Hodgkin's granuloma with pericardial effusion. *Am. Heart J.* 40:624–629.

Hahn, E. W., Feingold, S. M. and Nisce, L. (1976). Aspermia and recovery of spermatogenesis in cancer patients following incidental gonadal irradiation during treatment: a progress report. *Radiology* 119:223–225.

Halazun, J. F., Kerr, S. E. and Lukens, J. N. (1972). Hodgkin's disease in three children from an Amish kindred. *J. Pediatr.* 80:289–291.

Hale White, Sir W. (1924). Thomas Hodgkin. *Guy's Hosp. Rep.* 74:117–136.

Halie, M. R., Eibergen, R. and Nieweg, H. O. (1972a). Observations on abnormal cells in the peripheral blood and spleen in Hodgkin's disease. *Brit. Med. J.* 2:609–611.

Halie, M. R., Huiges, W. and Nieweg, H. O. (1974a). Abnormal cells in the peripheral blood of patients with Hodgkin's disease. I. Observations with light microscopy. *Brit. J. Haematol.* 28:317–322.

Halie, M. R., Seldenrath, J. J., Stam, H. C. and Nieweg, H. O. (1972b). Curative radiotherapy in Hodgkin's disease: significance of haematogenous dissemination established by examination of peripheral blood and spleen. *Brit. Med. J.* 2:611–613.

Halie, M. R., Splett-Romascano, M., Molenaar, I. and Nieweg, H. O. (1974b). Abnormal cells in the peripheral blood of patients with Hodgkin's disease. II. Ultrastructural studies. *Brit. J. Haematol.* 28:323–328.

Hall, C. A. and Olson, K. B. (1955). Alcohol-induced pain in Hodgkin's disease. *New Engl. J. Med.* 253:608–609.

Hall, C. A. and Olson, K. B. (1956). Prognosis of the malignant lymphomas. *Ann. Int. Med.* 44:687–706.

Hall, T. C. (1966). New chemotherapeutic agents in Hodgkin's disease. *Cancer Res.* 26:1297–1302.

Hall, T. C., Choi, E. S., Abadi, A. and Krant, M. J. (1967). High-dose corticoid therapy in Hodgkin's disease and other lymphomas. *Ann. Int. Med.* 66:1144–1153.

Hambly, C. K. and Blundell, J. E. (1968). Hodgkin's disease of the oesophagus. *Australasian Radiol.* 12:43–48.

Hamilton, P. J. and Dawson, A. A. (1973). Thrombocytopenic purpura as the sole manifestation of a recurrence of Hodgkin's disease. *J. Clin. Path.* 26:70–72.

Han, T. (1972). Effect of sera from patients with Hodgkin's disease on normal lymphocyte response to phytohemagglutinin. *Cancer* 29:1626–1631.

Han, T. (1973). Immune RNA-mediated transfer of delayed skin reactivity in patients with Hodgkin's disease. *Clin. Exper. Immunol.* 14:213–217.

Han, T. (1974). Transfer of cell-mediated skin reactivity with "immune" RNA in Hodgkin's disease and other neoplastic diseases. *Cancer* 33:497–502.

Han, T. and Sokal, J. E. (1970). Lymphocyte response to phytohemagglutinin in Hodgkin's disease. *Am. J. Med.* 48:728–734.

Han, T. and Stutzman, L. (1967). Mode of spread in patients with localized malignant lymphomas. *Arch. Int. Med.* 120:1–7.

Han, T., Stutzman, L. and Roque, A. L. (1971). Bone marrow biopsy in Hodgkin's disease and other neoplastic diseases. *J.A.M.A.* 217:1239–1241.

Hancock, B. W., Bruce, L., Dunsmore, I. R., Ward, A. M. and Richmond, J. (1977a). Follow-up studies on the immune status of patients with Hodgkin's disease after splenectomy and treatment, in relapse and remission. *Brit. J. Cancer* 36:347–354.

Hancock, B. W., Bruce, L. and Richmond, J. (1976a). Neutrophil function in lymphoreticular malignancy. *Brit. J. Cancer* 33:496–500.

Hancock, B. W., Bruce, L. and Richmond, J. (1976b). Sensitization to Hodgkin's disease spleen tissue in patients with malignant lymphoma: follow-up study. *Brit. Med. J.* 2:351–352.

Hancock, B. W., Bruce, L., Ward, A. M. and Richmond, J. (1977b). The immediate effects of splenectomy, radiotherapy and intensive chemotherapy on the immune status of patients with malignant lymphoma. *Clin. Oncol.* 3:137–144.

Hancock, B. W. and Henry, L. (1977). Renal papillary necrosis associated with renal candidiasis in a patient with Hodgkin's disease. *Cancer* 40:2309–2311.

Hankey, B. F. and Myers, M. H. (1971). Evaluating differences in survival between two groups of patients. *J. Chron. Dis.* 24:523–532.

Hanks, G. E., Newsome, J. F. and Lewis, N. T. (1971). The value of laparotomy in staging lymphomas. *South. Med. J.* 64:585–588.

Hansen, H. E., Skov, P. E., Askjaer, S. A. and Albertsen, K. (1972). Hodgkin's disease associated with the nephrotic syndrome without kidney lesion. *Acta Med. Scand.* 191:307–313.

Hansen, J. A., Young, C. W., Whitsett, C., Case, D. C., Jr., Jersild, C., Good, R. A. and Dupont, B. (1977). HLA and MLC typing in patients with Hodgkin's disease. *Prog. Clin. Biol. Res.* 16:217–227.

Hanson, T. A. S. (1964). Histological classification and survival in Hodgkin's disease. A study of 251 cases with special reference to nodular sclerosing Hodgkin's disease. *Cancer* 17:1595–1603.

Haran-Ghera, N. (1967). A leukemogenic filtrable agent from chemically-induced lymphoid leukemia in C57BL mice. *Proc. Soc. Exper. Biol. Med.* 124:697–699.

Haran-Ghera, N., Kotler, M. and Meshorer, A. (1967). Studies on leukemia development in the SJL/J strain of mice. *J. Nat. Cancer Inst.* 39:653–662.

Harbert, J. C. and Ashburn, W. L. (1968). Radiostrontium bone scanning in Hodgkin's disease. *Cancer* 22:58–63.

Hardin, V. M. and Johnston, G. S. (1971). Liver and spleen scintigraphy in staging Hodgkin's disease. *J. Surg. Oncol.* 3:109–115.

Hardmeier, T. H. and Rellstab, H. (1975). Family studies in cases with malignant lymphomas. *Acta Neuropathol.* 6:205–208.

Harlan, J. M., Fennessy, J. J. and Gross, N. J. (1974). Bronchial brush biopsy in Hodgkin's disease. *Chest* 66:136–138.

Harned, R. K. and Sorrell, M. F. (1976). Hodgkin's disease of the rectum. *Radiology* 120:319–320.

Harris, V. J. and Seeler, R. A. (1973). Ataxia-telangiectasia and Hodgkin's disease. *Cancer* 32:1415–1420.

Harrison, C. V. (1952). Benign Hodgkin's disease (Hodgkin's paragranuloma). *J. Path. Bact.* 64:513–518.

Harrison, D. T. and Neiman, P. E. (1977). Primary treatment of disseminated Hodgkin's disease with BCNU alone and in combination with vincristine, procarbazine, and prednisone. *Cancer Treat. Rep.* 61:789–795.

Hartley, J. W., Rowe, W. P., Capps, W. I. and Huebner, R. J. (1965). Complement fixation and tissue culture assays for mouse leukemia viruses. *Proc. Nat. Acad. Sci. U.S.* 53:931–938.

Hartsock, R. J. (1968). Postvaccinial lymphadenitis. Hyperplasia of lymphoid tissue that simulates malignant lymphomas. *Cancer* 21:632–649.

Hartvigsen, B. (1955). Hodgkin's disease and pregnancy. *Acta Radiol.* 44:317–324.

Hartwich, G. and Schlabeck, H. (1970). Lymphogranulo-matose: Jahreszeitliche Verteilung der Erstmanifestation. *Deut. Med. Wchnschr.* 95:1387–1389.

Hashimoto, M. and Hanazato, D. (1961). Study on bone marrow of autopsy cases in Hodgkin's disease. *J. Kyushu Hemat. Soc.* 11:193–208.

Hass, A. C., Brunk, S. F., Gulesserian, H. P. and Givler, R. L. (1971). The value of exploratory laparotomy in malignant lymphoma. *Radiology* 101:157–165.

Haybittle, J. L. (1959). The estimation of the proportion of patients cured after treatment for breast cancer. *Brit. J. Radiol.* 32:725–733.

Haybittle, J. L. (1963). Cure of Hodgkin's disease. *Brit. Med. J.* 2:933–934.

Hayhoe, F. G., Burns, F., Cawley, J. C. and Stewart, J. W. (1978). Cytochemical, ultrastructural, and immunological studies of circulating Reed-Sternberg cells. *Brit. J. Haematol.* 38:485–490.

Healy, R. J., Amory, H. I. and Friedman, M. (1955). Hodgkin's disease—a review of two hundred and sixteen cases. *Radiology* 64:51–55.

Heath, C. W., Jr., Everett, J. R., II, Stewart, J. R., Daines, J. and Daines, P. H. (1973). Clustering in Hodgkin's disease. *Lancet* 1:669–670.

Hehlmann, R., Kufe, D. and Spiegelman, S. (1972). Viral-related RNA in Hodgkin's disease and other human lymphomas. *Proc. Nat. Acad. Sci. U.S.* 69:1727–1731.

Heidenberg, W. J., Lupovitch, A. and Tarr, N. (1966). "Pulseless disease" complicating Hodgkin's disease; a case apparently caused by radiotherapy. *J.A.M.A.* 195:488–491.

Heier, H. E. and Normann, T. (1974). Blood lymphocytes in Hodgkin's disease. Lymphocytopenia related to stages and histological groups. *Scand. J. Haematol.* 13:199–202.

Heilman, F. R. and Kendall, E. D. (1944). The influence of 11-dehydro-17-hydroxycorticosterone (compound E) on the growth of a malignant tumor in the mouse. *Endocrinology* 34:416–420.

Heilmeyer, L., Mössner, G. and Hunstein, W. (1957). Hodgkin's disease (lymphogranulomatosis): symptomatology and results of treatment in 200 cases. *Deut. Med. Wchnschr.* 82:1046–1050.

Heine, K. M. and Stobbe, H. (1967). Tests of immunological competence in lymphogranulomatosis with different antigens in lymphocyte culture. *Helv. Med. Acta* 34:36–43.

Hellman, S. and Fink, M. E. (1965). Granulocyte reserve following radiation therapy as studied by the response to a bacterial endotoxin. *Blood* 25:310–324.

Hellman, S., Mauch, P., Goodman, R. L., Rosenthal, D. S. and Moloney, W. C. (1978). The place of radiation therapy in the treatment of Hodgkin's disease. *Cancer* 42:971–978.

Hellwig, C. A. (1947). Malignant lymphoma; the value of radical surgery in selected cases. *Surg. Gynec. Obst.* 84:950–958.

Henderson, B. E., Dworsky, R., Menek, H., Alena, B., Henle, W., Henle, G., Terasaki, P., Newell, G. R., Rawlings, W. and Kinnear, B. K. (1973). Case-control study of Hodgkin's disease. II. Herpesvirus group antibody titers and HL-A type. *J. Nat. Cancer Inst.* 51:1437–1441.

Henle, G. and Henle, W. (1966a). Studies on cell lines

derived from Burkitt's lymphoma. *Trans. New York Acad. Sci.* 29:71–79.

Henle, G. and Henle, W. (1966b). Immunofluorescence in cells derived from Burkitt's lymphoma. *J. Bact.* 91:1248–1256.

Henle, W. and Henle, G. (1973). Epstein-Barr virus-related serology in Hodgkin's disease. *Nat. Cancer Inst. Monograph* 36:79–84.

Henle, G., Henle, W. and Diehl, V. (1968). Relation of Burkitt's tumor-associated herpes-type virus to infectious mononucleosis. *Proc. Nat. Acad. Sci. U.S.* 59:94–101.

Hennig, K., Franke, W. G., Woller, P. and Platzbecker, H. (1971). Ergebnisse der endolymphatischen Therapie bei malignen Lymphomen. *Radiobiol. Radiother.* 12:607–610.

Henry, L. (1970). Long survival in Hodgkin's disease. *Clin. Radiol.* 21:203–210.

Henry, L. (1971). Partial involvement of the lymph node in Hodgkin's disease. *Clin. Radiol.* 22:405–410.

Herman, T. S. and Jones, S. E. (1977). Systematic restaging in Hodgkin's disease. *Proc. Am. Assoc. Cancer Res.* 18:97 (abst.).

Herrera, N. E., Gonzalez, R., Schwarz, R. D., Diggs, A. M. and Belsky, J. (1965). ^{75}Se-methionine as a diagnostic agent in malignant lymphoma. *J. Nucl. Med.* 6:792–804.

Hersh, E. M. (1973). Kinetic approach to the study of cell-mediated immunity in Hodgkin's disease. *Nat. Cancer Inst. Monograph* 36:123–124.

Hersh, E. M. and Oppenheim, J. J. (1965a). Inhibition of *in vitro* lymphocyte transformation during chemotherapy in man. *Proc. Am. Assoc. Cancer Res.* 6:27 (abst.).

Hersh, E. M. and Oppenheim, J. J. (1965b). Impaired *in vitro* lymphocyte transformation in Hodgkin's disease. *New Engl. J. Med.* 273:1006–1012.

Hesse, J., Andersen, E., Levine, P. H., Ebbesen, P., Halberg, P. and Reisher, J. I. (1973). Antibodies to Epstein-Barr virus and cellular immunity in Hodgkin's disease and chronic lymphatic leukemia. *Internat. J. Cancer* 11:237–243.

Hesse, J., Levine, P. H., Ebbesen, P., Connelly, R. R. and Mordhorst, C. H. (1977). A case control study on immunity to two Epstein-Barr virus-associated antigens, and to herpes simplex virus and adenovirus in a population-based group of patients with Hodgkin's disease in Denmark, 1971-1973. *Internat. J. Cancer* 19:49–58.

Hilgers, J., Nowinski, R. C., Geering, G. and Hardy, W. (1972). Detection of avian and mammalian oncogenic RNA viruses (oncornaviruses) by immunofluorescence. *Cancer Res.* 32:98–106.

Hill, J. M., Marshall, G. J. and Falco, D. J. (1956). Massive prednisone and prednisolone therapy in leukemia and lymphomas in the adult. *J. Am. Geriat. Soc.* 4:627–640.

Hill, W. (1966). Thomas Hodgkin—A bibliography. *Guy's Hosp. Rep.* 115:281–303.

Hilleman, M. R., McLean, A. A., Vella, P. P., Weibel, R. E. and Woodhour, A. F. (1978). Polyvalent pneumococcal polysaccharide vaccines. *Bull. World Health Org.* 56:371–375.

Hillinger, S. M. and Herzig, G. P. (1978). Impaired cell-mediated immunity in Hodgkin's disease mediated by suppressor lymphocytes and monocytes. *J. Clin. Invest.* 61:1620–1627.

Hirsch, M. S., Phillips, S. M., Solnik, C., Black, P. H.,

Schwartz, R. S. and Carpenter, C. B. (1972). Activation of leukemia viruses by graft-versus-host and mixed lymphocyte reactions *in vitro*. *Proc. Nat. Acad. Sci. U.S.* 69:1069–1072.

Hirschhorn, K., Bach, F., Kolodny, R. L., Firschein, I. I. and Hashem, N. (1963). Immune response and mitosis of human peripheral blood lymphocytes *in vitro*. *Science* 142:1185–1187.

Hirshaut, Y., Reagan, R. L., Perry, S., De Vita, V. and Barile, M . F. (1974). The search for a viral agent in Hodgkin's disease. *Cancer* 34:1080–1089.

Hodgkin, T. (1832). On some morbid appearances of the absorbent glands and spleen. *Med.-Chir. Trans.* 17:68–114.

Hoerni, B., Chauvergne, J., Hoerni-Simon, G., Durand, M. and Lagarde, C. (1971). BCG-nonspecific immunotherapy of Hodgkin's disease. Preliminary results from a controlled investigation. *Acta Haematol.* 52:214–219.

Hoerni, B., Chauvergne, J. and Parsi, M. (1970). La fièvre de la maladie de Hodgkin. Hypothèse pathogénique. *Presse méd.* 78:1317–1319.

Hövelborn, C. (1932). Die isolierte Lymphogranulomatose der Haut. *Arch. Derm. Syph.* 166:136–151.

Hoffbrand, B. I. (1964). Hodgkin's disease and hypogammaglobulinemia—a rare association. *Brit. Med. J.* 1:1156–1158.

Hoffbrand, B. I. (1965). Hodgkin's disease, autoimmunity, and the thymus. *Brit. Med. J.* 1:1592–1594.

Hoffer, P. B., Turner, D., Gottschalk, A., Harper, P. V. and Ultmann, J. E. (1973). Whole-body radiogallium scanning for staging of Hodgkin's disease and other lymphomas. *Nat. Cancer Inst. Monograph* 36:277–285.

Hoffmann, G. T. and Rottino, A. (1950a). Phase microscopy studies of Hodgkin's disease lymph nodes in relation to histogenesis of the Sternberg-Reed cell. *Blood* 5:74–78.

Hoffmann, G. T. and Rottino, A. (1950b). Studies of immunologic reactions of patients with Hodgkin's disease. Antibody reaction to typhoid immunization. *Arch. Int. Med.* 86:872–876.

Hohl, K., Sarasin, P. and Bessler, W. (1951). Therapie und Prognose der Lymphogranulomatose. Zürcher Erfahrungen von 1922-1950. *Oncologia* 4:1–20.

Holloway, J. B., Jr. (1965). Definitive surgery for malignant lymphomas. *Am. Surg.* 31:349–353.

Holm, G., Björkholm, M., Mellstedt, H. and Johansson, B. (1975). Cytotoxic activity of lymphocytes from patients with Hodgkin's disease. *Clin. Exper. Immunol.* 21:376–383.

Holm, G., Mellstedt, H., Björkholm, M., Johansson, B., Killander, D., Sundblad, R. and Söderberg, G. (1976). Lymphocyte abnormalities in untreated patients with Hodgkin's disease. *Cancer* 37:751–762.

Holm, G., Perlmann, P. and Johansson, B. (1967). Impaired phytohaemagglutinin-induced cytotoxicity *in vitro* of lymphocytes from patients with Hodgkin's disease or chronic lymphatic leukaemia. *Clin. Exper. Immunol.* 2:351–360.

Hoogstraten, B., Gottlieb, J. A., Caoili, E., Tucker, W. G., Talley, R. W. and Haut, A. (1973). CCNU (1-(2-chloroethyl)-3-cyclohexyl-1-nitrosourea, NSC-79037) in the treatment of cancer. Phase II study. *Cancer* 32:38–43.

Hoover, R. (1974). Hodgkin's disease in schoolteachers. *New Engl. J. Med.* 291:473.

Hopfan, S., Reid, A., Simpson, L. and Ager, P. J. (1977). Clinical complications arising from overlapping of adjacent radiation fields—physical and technical considerations. *Internat. J. Rad. Oncol. Biol. Phys.* 2: 801–808.

Hoppe, R. T., Cox, R. S., Rosenberg, S. A. and Kaplan, H. S. (1979a). Prognostic factors in pathologic stage (PS) IIIA Hodgkin's disease. *Proc. Am. Soc. Clin. Oncol.* 20:429 (abst.).

Hoppe, R. T., Portlock, C. S., Glatstein, E., Rosenberg, S. A. and Kaplan, H. S. (1979b). Alternating chemotherapy and irradiation in the treatment of advanced Hodgkin's disease. *Cancer* 43:472–481.

Horan, F. T. (1969). Bone involvement in Hodgkin's disease. A survey of 201 cases. *Brit. J. Surg.* 56:277–281.

Horn, N. L., Ray, G. R. and Kriss, J. P. (1976). Gallium-67 citrate scanning in Hodgkin's disease and non-Hodgkin's lymphoma. *Cancer* 37:250–257.

Horwich, L., Buxton, P. H. and Ryan, G. M. S. (1966). Cerebellar degeneration with Hodgkin's disease. *J. Neurol. Neurosurg. Psychiat.* 29:45–51.

Hossfeld, D. K. and Schmidt, C. G. (1978). Chromosome findings in effusions from patient with Hodgkin's disease. *Internat. J. Cancer* 21:147–156.

Høst, H. and Vale, J. R. (1973). Lung function after mantle field irradiation in Hodgkin's disease. *Cancer* 32:328–332.

Hoster, H. A., Doan, C. A. and Schumacher, M. (1944). Studies in Hodgkin's syndrome; search for Brucella in Hodgkin's syndrome. *Proc. Soc. Exper. Biol. Med.* 57:86–88.

Hoster, H. A., Dratman, M. V., Craver, L. F. and Rolnick, H. A. (1948). Hodgkin's disease—1832-1947. *Cancer Res.* 8:1–48; 49–78.

Hoster, H. A. and Reiman, M. S. (1950). Studies in Hodgkin's syndrome. X. The morphology and growth patterns of explant cells cultivated *in vitro. Cancer Res.* 10:423–430.

Howard, A. and Pelc, S. R. (1953). Synthesis of desoxyribonucleic acid in normal and irradiated cells and its relation to chromosome breakage. *Heredity* (Supp.) 6: 261–273.

Hreshchyshyn, M. M., Sheehan, F. R. and Holland, J. F. (1961). Visualization of retroperitoneal lymph nodes. Lymphangiography as an aid in the measurement of tumor growth. *Cancer* 14:205–209.

Hrgovcic, M., Tessmer, C. F., Minckler, T. M., Mosier, B. and Taylor, G. H. (1968). Serum copper levels in lymphoma and leukemia. Special reference to Hodgkin's disease. *Cancer* 21:743–755.

Hrgovcic, M. J., Tessmer, C. F., Mumford, D. M., Ong, P. S., Gamble, J. F. and Shullenberger, C. C. (1975). Interpreting serum copper levels in Hodgkin's disease. *Texas Med.* 71:53–63.

Hrgovcic, M., Tessmer, C. F., Thomas, F. B., Fuller, L. M., Gamble, J. F. and Shullenberger, C. C. (1973). Significance of serum copper levels in adult patients with Hodgkin's disease. *Cancer* 31:1337–1345.

Huber, C., Huber, H., Schmalzl, F., Lederer, B., Bütterich, D. and Braunsteiner, H. (1970). DNS-synthese in Blut-lymphozyten beim malignen Lymphogranulom. *Acta Haematol.* 44:222–232.

Huber, C., Michlmayr, G., Falkensamer, M., Fink, U., Nedden, G. Z., Braunsteiner, H. and Huber, H. (1975). Increased proliferation of T lymphocytes in the blood of patients with Hodgkin's disease. *Clin. Exper. Immunol.* 21:47–53.

Huber, H., Polley, M. J., Linscott, W. D., Fudenberg, H. H. and Muller-Eberhard, H. J. (1968). Human monocytes: distinct receptor sites for the third component of complement and for immunoglobulin G. *Science* 162:1281–1283.

Huber, S. C., Webb, W. R., Kuykendall, J. D. and Meier, W. L. (1978). Abnormal cardiac silhouette in a patient with Hodgkin's disease. *J.A.M.A.* 239:2785–2786.

Hughes, W. T. (1976). Treatment of *Pneumocystis carinii* pneumonitis; editorial. *New Engl. J. Med.* 295:726–727.

Hughes, W. T., Feldman, S. and Sanyal, S. K. (1975). Treatment of *Pneumocystis carinii* pneumonitis with trimethoprim-sulfamethoxazole. *Canad. Med. Assoc. J.* 112:47S–50S.

Huguley, C. M., Durant, J. R., Moores, R. R., Chan, Y.-K., Dorfman, R. F. and Johnson, L. (1975). A comparison of nitrogen mustard, vincristine, procarbazine, and prednisone (MOPP) vs. nitrogen mustard in advanced Hodgkin's disease. *Cancer* 36:1227–1240.

Hultberg, S. (1954). Pregnancy in Hodgkin's disease. *Acta Radiol.* 41:277–289.

Hunter, C. P., Pinkus, G., Woodward, L., Moloney, W. C. and Churchill, W. H. (1977). Increased T lymphocytes and IgMEA-receptor lymphocytes in Hodgkin's disease spleens. *Cell Immunol.* 31:193–198.

Hutchison, G. B. (1972). Anatomic patterns by histologic type of localized Hodgkin's disease of the upper torso. *Lymphology* 5:1–14.

Hutchison, G. B. (1973). Progress report. Hodgkin's clinical trial, 1972. *Nat. Cancer Inst. Monograph* 36:387–393.

Hyams, L. and Wynder, E. L. (1968). Appendectomy and cancer risk. An epidemiological evaluation. *J. Chronic Dis.* 21:319–415.

Hyman, G. and Sommers, S. (1966). The development of Hodgkin's disease and other lymphomas during anticonvulsant therapy. *Blood* 28:416–427.

Hynes, J. F. (1955). Radiocurability of malignant lymphoma. *Acta Unio Internat. Contra Cancrum* 11:514–525.

Hynes, J. F. (1969). Curative treatment of Hodgkin's disease. *Am. J. Roentgenol.* 105:629–635.

Hynes, J. F. and Frelick, R. W. (1953). Roentgen therapy of malignant lymphoma with special reference to segmental radiation therapy. *Am. J. Roentgenol.* 70:247–257.

Iacovino, J. R., Leitner, J., Abbas, A. K., Lokich, J. J. and Snider, G. L. (1976). Fatal pulmonary reaction from low doses of bleomycin. An idiosyncratic tissue response. *J.A.M.A.* 235:1253–1255.

Igel, H. J., Huebner, R. J., Turner, H. C., Kotin, P. and Falk, H. L. (1969). Mouse leukemia virus activation by chemical carcinogens. *Science* 166:1624–1626.

Ihde, D. C. and De Vita, V. T. (1975). Osteonecrosis of the femoral head in patients with lymphoma treated with intermittent combination chemotherapy (including corticosteroids). *Cancer* 36:1585–1588.

Ingold, J. A., Reed, G. B., Kaplan, H. S. and Bagshaw, M. A. (1965). Radiation hepatitis. *Am. J. Roentgenol.* 93:200–208.

Innes, J. and Newall, J. (1961). Seasonal incidence in clinical onset of Hodgkin's disease. *Brit. Med. J.* 2:765.

Ioachim, H. L., Schmidt, E. C. and Keller, S. E. (1976). Morphologic studies of cell receptors of lymphocytes and lymphomas. *Bibl. Haematol.* 43:29–33.

Irino, S., Ota, Z., Sezaki, T. and Suzaki, K. (1963). Cell-free transmission of 20-methylcholanthrene-induced Rf mouse leukemia and electron microscopic demonstration of virus particles in its leukemic tissue. *Gann* 54:225–237.

Irunberry, J. and Colonna, P. (1970). Intérêt de l'immunoélectrophorèse des protéines sériques au cours de la maladie de Hodgkin. *Presse méd.* 78:187–188.

Irving, M. (1975). The role of surgery in the management of Hodgkin's disease. *Brit. J. Surg.* 62:853–862.

Isard, H. J. and Sklaroff, D. M. (1967). Thermography in Hodgkin's disease of the breast. *J.A.M.A.* 202:552.

Ito, Y., Shiratori, O., Kurita, S., Takahashi, T., Kurita, Y. and Ota, K. (1968). Some characteristics of a human cell line (AICHI-4) established from tumorous lymphatic tissue of Hodgkin's disease. *J. Nat. Cancer Inst.* 41:1367–1375.

Ivády, G. and Páldy, L. (1958). Ein neues Behandlungsverfahren der interstitiellen plasmazelligen Pneumonie frühgeborener mit fünfwertigem Stibium und aromatischen Diamidinen. *Monatschr. Kinderheilk.* 106:10–14.

Iyer, B. N. and Szybalski, W. (1963). A molecular mechanism of mitomycin action: linking of complementary DNA strands. *Proc. Nat. Acad. Sci. U.S.* 50:355–362.

Jackson, F. C., Ney, E. C. and Fisher, E. R. (1959). Surgical implantation of Hodgkin's disease of the stomach to the skin of the abdominal wall. *Ann. Surg.* 150:1000–1006.

Jackson, H., Jr. (1937). Classification and prognosis of Hodgkin's disease and allied disorders. *Surg. Gynec. Obst.* 64:465–467.

Jackson, H., Jr. (1939). Hodgkin's disease and allied disorders. *New Engl. J. Med.* 220:26–30.

Jackson, H., Jr. and Parker, F., Jr. (1944a). Hodgkin's disease. I. General considerations. *New Engl. J. Med.* 230:1–8.

Jackson, H., Jr. and Parker, F., Jr. (1944b). Hodgkin's disease. II. Pathology. *New Engl. J. Med.* 231:35–44.

Jackson, H., Jr. and Parker, F., Jr. (1947). Hodgkin's Disease and Allied Disorders. New York: Oxford University Press.

Jackson, H. L., Hass, A. C., Sooby, D. and Marschke, C. H. (1970). The gonadal exposure of boys and young men treated with inverted "Y" fields: its reduction and genetic significance. *Radiology* 96:181–186.

Jackson, S. M., Garrett, J. D. and Craig, A. W. (1970). Lymphocyte transformation changes during the clinical course of Hodgkin's disease. *Cancer* 25:843–850.

Jacobs, A., Slater, A., Whittaker, J. A., Canellos, G. and Wiernik, P. H. (1976). Serum ferritin concentration in untreated Hodgkin's disease. *Brit. J. Cancer* 34:162–166.

Jacobs, C., Portlock, C. S. and Rosenberg, S. A. (1976). Prednisone in MOPP chemotherapy for Hodgkin's disease. *Brit. Med. J.* 2:1469–1471.

Jacobs, E. M., Peters, F. C., Luce, J. K., Zoppin, C. and Wood, D. A. (1968). Mechlorethamine HCl and cyclophosphamide in the treatment of Hodgkin's disease and the lymphomas. *J.A.M.A.* 203:104–110.

Jacobson, L. O., Spurr, C. L., Guzman Barron, E. S., Smith, T., Lushbaugh, C. and Dick, G. F. (1946). Nitrogen mustard therapy; studies on the effect of methylbis-(β-chloroethyl) amine hydrochloride on neoplastic disorders and allied disorders of the hemopoietic system. *J.A.M.A.* 132:263–271.

Jacobson, R. J., Sagel, J., Distiller, L. A. and Morley, J. E. (1978). Leydig cell dysfunction in male patients with Hodgkin's disease receiving chemotherapy. *Clin. Res.* 26:437 (abst.).

Jacquillat, C., Belpomme, D., Weil, M., Auclerc, G., Teillet, F., Weisgerber, C., Tanzer, J., Boiron, M. and Bernard, J. (1973). Les néoplasies simultanées et successives. A propos de 18 observations d'affections malignes compliquant l'évolution de la maladie de Hodgkin. *Nouv. presse méd.* 2:3089–3092.

Jaffe, E. S., Shevach, E. M., Sussman, E. H., Frank, M., Green, I. and Berard, C. W. (1975). Membrane receptor sites for the identification of lymphoreticular cells in benign and malignant conditions. *Brit. J. Cancer* 31:107–120.

Jaffe, N. and Bishop, Y. M. M. (1970). The serum iron level, hematocrit, sedimentation rate, and leukocyte alkaline phosphatase level in pediatric patients with Hodgkin's disease. *Cancer* 26:332–337.

James, A. H. (1960). Hodgkin's disease with and without alcohol-induced pain. A clinical and histological comparison. *Quart. J. Med.* 29:47–66.

Jamshidi, K. and Swaim, W. R. (1971). Bone marrow biopsy with unaltered architecture. A new biopsy device. *J. Lab. Clin. Med.* 77:335–342.

Janossy, G. and Greaves, M. F. (1972). Lymphocyte activation. II. Discriminating stimulation of lymphocyte subpopulations by phytomitogens and heterologous antilymphocyte sera. *Clin. Exper. Immunol.* 10:525–536.

Jantet, G. H. (1962). Direct intralymphatic injections of radioactive colloidal gold in the treatment of malignant disease. *Brit. J. Radiol.* 35:692–697.

Jarrett, W. F. H., Crawford, E. M., Martin, W. B. and Davie, F. (1964). Leukemia in the cat. A virus-like particle associated with leukemia (lymphosarcoma). *Nature* 202:567–569.

Jarvis, J. E., Ball, G., Rickinson, A. B. and Epstein, M. A. (1974). Cytogenetic studies on human lymphoblastoid cell lines from Burkitt's lymphomas and other sources. *Internat. J. Cancer* 14:716–721.

Jelliffe, A. M., Millett, Y. L., Marston, J. A. P., Bennett, M. H., Farrer-Brown, G., Kendall, B. and Keeling, D. H. (1970). Laparotomy and splenectomy as routine investigations in the staging of Hodgkin's disease before treatment. *Clin. Radiol.* 21:439–445.

Jelliffe, A. M. and Thomson, A. D. (1955). The prognosis in Hodgkin's disease. *Brit. J. Cancer* 9:21–36.

Jenkin, R. D. T., Brown, T. C., Peters, M. V. and Sonley, M. J. (1975). Hodgkin's disease in children. A retrospective analysis: 1958-73. *Cancer* 35:979–990.

Jenkin, R. D. T., Peters, M. V. and Darte, J. M. M. (1967). Hodgkin's disease in children. *Am. J. Roentgenol.* 100:222–226.

Jennings, F. L. and Arden, A. (1962). Development of radiation pneumonitis. Time and dose factors. *Arch. Path.* 74:351–360.

Jensen, F. C., Gwatkin, R. B. L. and Biggers, J. D. (1964). A simple organ culture method which allows simultaneous isolation of specific types of cells. *Exper. Cell Res.* 34:440–447.

Jensen, K. D., Thorling, E. B. and Andersen, C. J. (1964). Serum copper in Hodgkin's disease. *Scand. J. Haemat.* 1:63–74.

Johansson, B., Klein, G., Henle, W. and Henle, G. (1970). Epstein-Barr virus (EBV)-associated antibody patterns in malignant lymphoma and leukemia. I. Hodgkin's disease. *Internat. J. Cancer* 6:450–462.

Johnson, R. E. and Brace, K. C. (1966). Radiation response of Hodgkin's disease recurrent after chemotherapy. *Cancer* 19:368–370.

Johnson, R. E., Kagan, A. R., Hafermann, M. D. and Keyes, J. W., Jr. (1969). Patient tolerance to extended irradiation in Hodgkin's disease. *Ann. Int. Med.* 70:1–6.

Johnson, R. E., Ruhl, R., Johnson, S. K. and Glover, M. (1976). Split-course radiotherapy of Hodgkin's disease. Local tumor control and normal tissue reactions. *Cancer* 37:1713–1717.

Johnson, R. E., Thomas, L. B. and Chretien, P. (1970). Correlation between clinicohistologic staging and extranodal relapse in Hodgkin's disease. *Cancer* 25:1071–1075.

Johnson, R. E., Thomas, L. B., Schneiderman, M., Glenn, D. W., Faw, F. and Hafermann, M. D. (1970). Preliminary experience with total nodal irradiation in Hodgkin's disease. *Radiology* 96:603–608.

Johnson, S. K. and Johnson, R. E. (1972). Tonsillectomy history in Hodgkin's disease. *New Engl. J. Med.* 287:1122–1125.

Johnston, G. S., Go, M. F., Benua, R. S., Larson, S. M., Andrews, G. A. and Hubner, K. F. (1977). Gallium-67 citrate imaging in Hodgkin's disease: final report of cooperative group. *J. Nucl. Med.* 18:692–698.

Jondal, M., Holm, G. and Wigzell, H. (1972). Surface markers on human T and B lymphocytes. I. A large population of lymphocytes forming nonimmune rosettes with sheep red blood cells. *J. Exper. Med.* 136:207–215.

Jondal, M. and Klein, G. (1973). Surface markers on human B and T lymphocytes. II. Presence of Epstein-Barr virus receptors on B lymphocytes. *J. Exper. Med.* 138:1365–1378.

Jondal, M., Klein, G., Oldstone, M. B. A., Bokish, V. and Yefenof, E. (1976). Surface markers on human B and T lymphocytes. VIII. Association between complement and Epstein-Barr virus receptors on human lymphoid cells. *Scand. J. Immunol.* 5:401–410.

Jones, A. (1964). Transient radiation myelopathy (with reference to Lhermitte's sign of electrical paraesthesia). *Brit. J. Radiol.* 37:727–744.

Jones, J. V., Peacock, D. B., Greenham, L. W. and Bullimore, J. A. (1976). Antibody production in preclinical Hodgkin's disease. *Lancet* 1:92–93.

Jones, P. A. E., Miller, F. M., Worwood, M. and Jacobs, A. (1973). Ferritinaemia in leukaemia and Hodgkin's disease. *Brit. J. Cancer* 27:212–217.

Jones, S. E. (1973). Autoimmune disorders and malignant lymphoma. *Cancer* 31:1092–1098.

Jones, S. E., Moore, M., Blank, N. and Castellino, R. A. (1972). Hypersensitivity to procarbazine (Matulane) manifested by fever and pleuropulmonary reaction. *Cancer* 29:498–500.

Jones, S. E., Tucker, W. G., Haut, A., Tranum, B. T., Vaughn, C., Chase, E. M. and Durie, B. G. M. (1977). Phase II trial of piperazinedione in Hodgkin's disease, non-Hodgkin's lymphoma, and multiple myeloma: a Southwest Oncology Group study. *Cancer Treat. Rep.* 61:1619–1621.

Jonsson, K. and Lunderquist, A. (1974). Angiography of the liver and spleen in Hodgkin's disease. *Am. J. Roentgenol.* 121:789–792.

Justin-Besançon, L., Lamotte-Barrillon, S. and Lubetzki, D. (1958). Éléments du pronostic dans la maladie de Hodgkin. *Sem. hôp. Paris* 34:1697–1703.

Kademian, M. T. and Wirtanen, G. W. (1977). Accuracy of bipedal lymphography in Hodgkin's disease. *Am. J. Roentgenol.* 129:1041–1042.

Kadin, M. E. (1973). *In vitro* study of multinucleated cells in Hodgkin's disease. *Nat. Cancer Inst. Monograph* 36:211–217.

Kadin, M. E. and Asbury, A. K. (1973). Long term cultures of Hodgkin's tissue. A morphologic and radioautographic study. *Lab. Investigation* 28:181–184.

Kadin, M. E., Donaldson, S. S. and Dorfman, R. F. (1970). Isolated granulomas in Hodgkin's disease. *New Engl. J. Med.* 283:859–861.

Kadin, M. E., Glatstein, E. and Dorfman, R. F. (1971). Clinical-pathologic studies of 117 untreated patients subjected to laparotomy for the staging of Hodgkin's disease. *Cancer* 27:1277–1294.

Kadin, M. E., Newcom, S. R., Gold, S. B. and Stites, D. P. (1974). Origin of Hodgkin's cell. *Lancet* 2:167–168.

Kadin, M. E., Stites, D. P., Levy, R. and Warnke, R. (1978). Exogenous origin of immunoglobulin in Reed-Sternberg cells of Hodgkin's disease. *New Engl. J. Med.* 299:1208–1214.

Kaiser-McCaw, B., Epstein, A. L., Kaplan, H. S. and Hecht, F. (1977). Chromosome 14 translocations in African and North American Burkitt's lymphoma. *Internat. J. Cancer* 19:482–486.

Kahn, L. B., Selzer, G. and Kaschula, R. O. C. (1972). Primary gastrointestinal lymphoma. A clinicopathologic study of fifty-seven cases. *Am. J. Dig. Dis.* 17:219–232.

Kaplan, E. S. and Meier, P. (1958). Non-parametric estimation from incomplete observation. *Am. Stat. Assoc. J.* 53:457–480.

Kaplan, H. S. (1948). Comparative susceptibility of lymphoid tissues of strain C57 Black mice to induction of lymphoid tumors by irradiation. *J. Nat. Cancer Inst.* 8:191–197.

Kaplan, H. S. (1949). Preliminary studies of the effectiveness of local irradiation in the induction of lymphoid tumors in mice. *J. Nat. Cancer Inst.* 10:267–270.

Kaplan, H. S. (1957). The pathogenesis of experimental lymphoid tumors in mice. *In* Proc. Second Canadian Cancer Conference, R. W. Begg (ed.). Vol. II, pp. 127–141. New York: Academic Press.

Kaplan, H. S. (1962). The radical radiotherapy of regionally localized Hodgkin's disease. *Radiology* 78:553–561.

Kaplan, H. S. (1965). Radiotherapeutic management of the malignant lymphomas. *Med. Rec. Ann.* 58:43–46.

Kaplan, H. S. (1966a). Evidence for a tumoricidal dose level in the radiotherapy of Hodgkin's disease. *Cancer Res.* 26:1221–1224.

Kaplan, H. S. (1966b). Long-term results of palliative and radical radiotherapy of Hodgkin's disease. *Cancer Res.* 26:1250–1252.

Kaplan, H. S. (1966c). Role of intensive radiotherapy in

the management of Hodgkin's disease. *Cancer* 19:356–367.

Kaplan, H. S. (1967). On the natural history of the murine leukemias: presidential address. *Cancer Res.* 27:1325–1340.

Kaplan, H. S. (1968a). Clinical evaluation and radiotherapeutic management of Hodgkin's disease and the malignant lymphomas. *New Engl. J. Med.* 278:892–899.

Kaplan, H. S. (1968b). Prognostic significance of the relapse-free interval after radiotherapy in Hodgkin's disease. *Cancer* 22:1131–1136.

Kaplan H. S. (1970). On the natural history, treatment, and prognosis of Hodgkin's disease. Harvey Lectures, 1968–1969. New York: Academic Press. pp. 215–259.

Kaplan, H. S. (1971). Role of immunological disturbance in human oncogenesis: some facts and fancies. *Brit. J. Cancer* 25:620–634.

Kaplan, H. S. (1973). Survival and relapse rates in Hodgkin's disease: Stanford experience, 1961–71. *Nat. Cancer Inst. Monograph* 36:487–496.

Kaplan, H. S. (1974). Leukemia and lymphoma in experimental and domestic animals. *Ser. Haematol.* 7:94–163.

Kaplan, H. S. (1976). Hodgkin's disease and other human malignant lymphomas: advances and prospects. G. H. A. Clowes Memorial Lecture. *Cancer Res.* 36:3863–3878.

Kaplan, H. S. (1977). Hodgkin's disease: multidisciplinary contributions to the conquest of a neoplasm. Erskine Memorial Lecture, 1976. *Radiology* 123:551–558.

Kaplan H. S. (1978a). Lymphomas. *In* Cancer in China, H. S. Kaplan and P. J. Tsuchitani (eds.). New York: Alan Liss, pp. 153–158.

Kaplan, H. S. (1978b). Etiology of lymphomas and leukemias: role of C-type RNA viruses. *Leukaemia Res.* 2:253–271.

Kaplan, H. S. and Bagshaw, M. A. (1968). Radiation hepatitis: possible prevention by combined isotopic and external radiation therapy. *Radiology* 91:1214–1220.

Kaplan, H. S., Bagshaw, M. A. and Rosenberg, S. A. (1964). Présentation du protocole d'essai radiothérapique des lymphomes malins de l'Université de Stanford. *Nouv. rev. franç. hématol.* 4:95–100.

Kaplan, H. S. and Brown, M. B. (1951). Further observations on inhibition of lymphoid tumor development by shielding and partial body irradiation of mice. *J. Nat. Cancer Inst.* 12:427–436.

Kaplan, H. S. and Brown, M. B. (1952). A quantitative dose-response study of lymphoid tumor development in irradiated C57 Black mice. *J. Nat. Cancer Inst.* 13:185–208.

Kaplan, H. S. and Brown, M. B. (1954). Development of lymphoid tumors in nonirradiated thymic grafts in thymectomized irradiated mice. *Science* 119:439–446.

Kaplan, H. S., Brown, M. B. and Paull, J. (1953). Influence of bone marrow injections on involution and neoplasia of mouse thymus after systemic irradiation. *J. Nat. Cancer Inst.* 14:303–316.

Kaplan, H. S., Carnes, W. H., Brown, M. B. and Hirsch, B. B. (1956). Indirect induction of lymphomas in irradiated mice. I. Tumor incidence and morphology in mice bearing nonirradiated thymic grafts. *Cancer Res.* 16:422–425.

Kaplan, H. S., Dorfman, R. F., Nelsen, T. S. and Rosen-

berg, S. A. (1973). Staging laparotomy and splenectomy in Hodgkin's disease: analysis of indications and patterns of involvement in 285 consecutive, unselected patients. *Nat. Cancer Inst. Monograph* 36:291–301.

Kaplan, H. S. and Gartner, S. (1977). "Sternberg-Reed" giant cells of Hodgkin's disease: cultivation *in vitro,* heterotransplantation, and characterization as neoplastic macrophages. *Internat. J. Cancer* 19:511–525.

Kaplan, H. S., Gartner, S., Goodenow, R. S. and Bieber, M. M. (1979). Biology and virology of the human malignant lymphomas. *Cancer* 43:1–24.

Kaplan, H. S., Goodenow, R. S., Epstein, A. L., Gartner, S., Declève, A. and Rosenthal, P. N. (1977). Isolation of a type C RNA virus from an established human histiocytic lymphoma cell line. *Proc. Nat. Acad. Sci. U.S.* 74:2564–2568.

Kaplan, H. S., Hirsch, B. B. and Brown, M. B. (1956). Indirect induction of lymphomas in irradiated mice. IV. Genetic evidence of the origin of the tumor cells from the thymic grafts. *Cancer Res.* 16:434–436.

Kaplan, H. S. and Nagareda, C. S. (1961). On the possibility of cure of malignant lymphoid tumors. I. Treatment of autochthonous lymphoid tumors in C57BL mice with massive doses of lymphocytolytic agents. *Blood* 18:166–175.

Kaplan, H. S. and Rosenberg, S. A. (1966a). La radiothérapie segmentaire de la maladie de Hodgkin. Premiers résultats de deux essais thérapeutiques contrôlés. *Nouv. rev. franç. hématol.* 6:121–133.

Kaplan, H. S. and Rosenberg, S. A. (1966b). Extended-field radical radiotherapy in advanced Hodgkin's disease: Short-term results of 2 randomized clinical trials. *Cancer Res.* 26:1268–1276.

Kaplan, H. S. and Rosenberg, S. A. (1966c). The treatment of Hodgkin's disease. *Med. Clin. North Amer.* 50:1591–1610.

Kaplan, H. S. and Rosenberg, S. A. (1968). The cure of malignant lymphomas. *Hosp. Practice* 3:28–33.

Kaplan, H. S. and Rosenberg, S. A. (1973). Current status of clinical trials: Stanford experience, 1962–72. *Nat. Cancer Inst. Monograph* 36:363–371.

Kaplan, H. S. and Rosenberg, S. A. (1975). The management of Hodgkin's disease. *Cancer* 36:796–803.

Kaplan, H. S. and Smithers, D. W. (1959). Autoimmunity in man and homologous disease in mice in relation to the malignant lymphomas. *Lancet* 2:1–4.

Kaplan, H. S. and Stewart, J. R. (1973). Complications of intensive megavoltage radiotherapy for Hodgkin's disease. *Nat. Cancer Inst. Monograph* 36:439–444.

Kardinal, C. G., Barnes, A. and Pugh, R. P. (1974). Acute leukemia: a disease of medical progress? Case reports. *Missouri Med.* 71:683–684.

Karnofsky, D. A. (1966a). The staging of Hodgkin's disease. *Cancer Res.* 26:1090–1094.

Karnofsky, D. A. (1966b). Chemotherapy of Hodgkin's disease. *Cancer* 19:371–377.

Karnofsky, D. A. (1968). Chemotherapy of the lymphomas. *In* Proceedings of the International Conference on Leukemia-Lymphoma, C. J. D. Zarafonetis (ed.). Philadelphia: Lea & Febiger. pp. 409–422.

Karnofsky, D. A. and Clarkson, B. D. (1963). Cellular effects of anti-cancer drugs. *Ann. Rev. Pharmacol.* 3:357–428.

Karnofsky, D. A., Craver, L. F., Rhoads, C. P. and Abels, J. C. (1947). An evaluation of methyl-bis-(β-chloroethyl) amine hydrochloride and tris-(β-chloroethyl) amine hydrochloride (nitrogen mustards) in the treatment of lymphomas, leukemia and allied diseases. *In* Approaches to Tumor Chemotherapy. Washington, D. C.: American Association for the Advancement of Science. pp. 319–337.

Karnofsky, D. A., Miller, D. G. and Phillips, R. F. (1963). Role of chemotherapy in the management of early Hodgkin's disease. *Am. J. Roentgenol.* 90:968–977.

Karnofsky, D. A., Parisette, L. M., Patterson, P. A. and Jacquez, J. A. (1948). The behavior and growth of homologous and heterologous normal and neoplastic tissues on the chick embryo; and the influence of various agents on tumor growth. *Acta Unio Internal. Contra Cancrum.* 6:642–651.

Karpas, A., Wreghitt, T. G. and Nagington, J. (1978). Transformation of normal bone-marrow cells by a leukaemic cell line associated with a presumptive new human virus. *Lancet* 2:1016–1019.

Kass, L. and Schnitzer, B. (1972). Ammoniacal silver staining of Reed-Sternberg cells in Hodgkin's disease. *Acta Haematol.* 48:288–291.

Katin, M. J. (1977). Reasons for familial aggregation in Hodgkin's disease. *New Engl. J. Med.* 296:940.

Katz, A. and Lattes, R. (1969). Granulomatous thymoma or Hodgkin's disease of thymus? A clinical and histologic study and a re-evaluation. *Cancer* 23:1–15.

Katz, D. H., Order, S. E., Graves, M. and Benacerraf, B. (1973). Purification of Hodgkin's disease tumor-associated antigens. *Proc. Nat. Acad. Sci. U.S.* 70:396–400.

Katz, M., Piekarski, J. D., Bayle-Weisgerber, Ch., Laval-Jeantet, M., and Teillet, F. (1977). Residual mediastinal masses after radiotherapy for Hodgkin's disease. *Ann. Radiol.* 20:667–672.

Kauffman, C. A., Israel, K. S., Smith, J. W., White, A. C., Schwarz, J. and Brooks, G. F. (1978). Histoplasmosis in immunosuppressed patients. *Am. J. Med.* 64:923–932.

Kaur, J., Spiers, A. S. D., Catovsky, D. and Galton, D. A. G. (1974). Increase of T lymphocytes in the spleen in Hodgkin's disease. *Lancet* 2:800–802.

Kávai, M., Berényi, E., Pálkovi, E. and Szegedi, G. (1976). Immune complexes in Hodgkin's disease. *Lancet* 1:1249.

Kawakami, T. G., Huff, S. D., Buckley, P. M., Dungworth, D. S. and Snyder, S. P. (1972). C-type virus associated with gibbon lymphosarcoma. *Nature New Biol.* 235:170–171.

Kawakami, T. G., Theilen, G. H., Dungworth, D. L., Munn, R. J. and Beall, S. G. (1967). "C"-type viral particles in plasma of cats with feline leukemia. *Science* 158:1049–1050.

Kay, D. N. and McCready, V. R. (1972). Clinical isotope scanning using ^{67}Ga citrate in the management of Hodgkin's disease. *Brit. J. Radiol.* 45:437–443.

Kay, M. M. B. (1976). Hodgkin's disease: a war between T-lymphocytes and transformed macrophages? *In* Lymphocytes, Macrophages, and Cancer, G. Mathé, I. Florentin, and M. C. Simmler (eds). Berlin: Springer-Verlag. *Recent Results Cancer Res.* 56:111–121.

Kay, M. M. B. and Kadin, M. (1975). Surface characteristics of Hodgkin's cells. *Lancet* 1:748–749.

Kay, N. E. and Gottlieb, A. J. (1973). Hypouricemia in Hodgkin's disease. Report of an additional case. *Cancer* 32:1508–1511.

Keelan, M. H. and Rudders, R. A. (1974). Successful treatment of radiation pericarditis with corticosteroids. *Arch. Int. Med.* 134:145–147.

Keller, A. R. and Castleman, B. (1974). Hodgkin's disease of the thymus gland. *Cancer* 33:1615–1623.

Keller, A. R., Kaplan, H. S., Lukes, R. J. and Rappaport, H. (1968). Correlation of histopathology with other prognostic indicators in Hodgkin's disease. *Cancer* 22:487–499.

Kelley, M. L., Jr. (1968). Intraluminal manometry in the evaluation of malignant disease of the esophagus. *Cancer* 21:1011–1018.

Kellum, J. M., Jr., Jaffe, B. M., Calhoun, T. R. and Ballinger, W. F. (1977). Gastric complications after radiotherapy for Hodgkin's disease and other lymphomas. *Am. J. Surg.* 134:314–317.

Kelly, F. (1965). Hodgkin's disease in children. *Am. J. Roentgenol.* 95:48–51.

Kelly, W. D., Good, R. A., Varco, R. L. and Levitt, M. (1958). The altered response to skin homografts and to delayed allergens in Hodgkin's disease. *Surg. Forum* 9:785–789.

Kelly, W. D., Lamb, D. L., Varco, R. L. and Good, R. A. (1960). An investigation of Hodgkin's disease with respect to the problem of homotransplantation. *Ann. New York Acad. Sci.* 87:187–202.

Kenis, Y., Dustin, P., Jr. and Peltzer, T. (1958). Un cas de maladie de Hodgkin avec syndrome hématologique et sérologique de mononucléose infectieuse. *Acta Haematol.* 20:329–336.

Kern, W. H., Crepeau, A. G. and Jones, J. C. (1961). Primary Hodgkin's disease of the lung: report of 4 cases and review of the literature. *Cancer* 14:1151–1165.

Kesselman, M., Sasyniuk, A. and Hryniuk, W. (1973). Buffy-coat leucocytes in Hodgkin's disease. *Lancet* 2:977.

Khan, A., Hill, J. M., MacLellan, A., Loeb, E., Hill, N. O. and Thaxton, S. (1975). Improvement in delayed hypersensitivity in Hodgkin's disease with transfer factor: lymphapheresis and cellular immune reactions of normal donors. *Cancer* 36:86–89.

Khan, A., Thometz, D., Garrison, O. and Hill, J. M. (1976). Increase in E-rosettes after transfer factor (TF) treatment: fractionation of TF. *Ann. Allergy* 36:330–336.

Kiely, T. M., Wagoner, R. D. and Holley, K. E. (1969). Renal complications of lymphoma. *Ann. Int. Med.* 71:1159–1175.

Killander, D., Lindblom, D. and Lundell, G. (1977). ^{75}Se-selenite scintigraphy in the clinical staging of malignant lymphomas. *Acta Radiol.* 16:81–85.

Kim, I. and Harley, J. B. (1972). Hodgkin's disease terminating in acute leukemia. *W. Va. Med. J.* 68:23–26.

Kinmonth, J. D. (1952). Lymphangiography in man. Method of outlining lymphatic trunks and operation. *Clin. Sc.* 11:13–20.

Kirschbaum, A. and Mixer, H. W. (1947). Induction of leukemia in eight inbred stocks of mice varying in susceptibility to the spontaneous disease. *J. Lab. Clin. Med.* 32:720–731.

Kirschner, R. H., Abt, A. B., O'Connell, M. J., Sklansky, B. D., Greene, W. H. and Wiernik, P. H. (1974). Vascular invasion and hematogenous dissemination of Hodgkin's disease. *Cancer* 34:1159–1162.

Kissmeyer-Nielsen, F., Kjerbye, K. E. and Lamm, L. U.

(1975). HL-A in Hodgkin's disease. III. A prospective study. *Transplant. Rev.* 22:168–174.

Klein, G. (1975a). Studies on the Epstein-Barr virus (EBV)-genome and the EBV-determined nuclear antigen in human malignant disease. *Cold Spring Harbor Symp. Quant. Biol.* 39:783–790.

Klein, G. (1975b). The Epstein-Barr virus and neoplasia. *New Engl. J. Med.* 293:1353–1357.

Klein, G., Clifford, P., Klein, E. and Stjernswärd, J. (1966). Search for tumor-specific immune reactions in Burkitt lymphoma patients by the membrane immunofluorescence reaction. *Proc. Nat. Acad. Sci. U.S.* 55:1628–1635.

Klinger, R. J. and Minton, J. P. (1973). Case clustering of Hodgkin's disease in a small rural community, with associations among cases. *Lancet* 1:168–171.

Knospe, W. H., Rayudu, V. M. S., Cardello, M., Friedman, A. M. and Fordham, E. W. (1976). Bone marrow scanning with ^{52}iron (^{52}Fe). Regeneration and extension of marrow after ablative doses of radiotherapy. *Cancer* 37:1432–1442.

Koch, H. J., Jr., Smith, E. R. and McNeely, J. (1957). Analysis of trace elements in human tissues. II. The lymphomatous diseases. *Cancer* 10:151–160.

Krakoff, I. (1974). Bleomycin activity in lymphomas and solid tumors. *In* New Drug Seminar on Bleomycin, W. T. Soper and A. B. Gott (eds.). Bethesda, Md.: National Cancer Institute, pp. 82–96.

Krasznai, G. (1966). Hydantoin lymphadenopathia. *Magy. Onkol.* 10:105–112.

Krauss, S., Schrott, M. and Sarcione, E. J. (1966). Haptoglobin metabolism in Hodgkin's disease. *Am. J. Med. Sci.* 252:184–191.

Krauss, S. and Sokal, J. E. (1966). Paraproteinemia in the lymphomas. *Am. J. Med.* 40:400–413.

Kraut, J. W., Kaplan, H. S. and Bagshaw, M. A. (1972). Combined fractionated isotopic and external irradiation of the liver in Hodgkin's disease. A study of 21 patients. *Cancer* 30:39–46.

Krick, J. A. and Remington, J. S. (1976). Opportunistic invasive fungal infections in patients with leukaemia and lymphoma. *Clin. Haematol.* 5:249–310.

Krikorian, J. G., Burke, J. S., Rosenberg, S. A. and Kaplan, H. S. (1979a). The occurrence of non-Hodgkin's lymphoma following therapy for Hodgkin's disease. *New Engl. J. Med.* 300:452–458.

Krikorian, J. G., Portlock, C. S. and Rosenberg, S. A. (1978). Treatment of advanced Hodgkin's disease with adriamycin, bleomycin, vinblastine, and imidazole carboxamide (ABVD) after failure of MOPP therapy. *Cancer* 41:2107–2111.

Krikorian, J. G., Portlock, C. S., Rosenberg, S. A. and Kaplan, H. S. (1979b). Hodgkin's disease, stages I and II, occurring below the diaphragm. *Cancer* 43:1866–1871.

Kriss, J. P. (1969). Diagnosis of pericardial effusion by radioisotopic angiocardiography. *J. Nucl. Med.* 10:233–241.

Kruchen, C. (1929). Beitrag zur Röntgentherapie der Lymphogranulomatose mit besonderer Berücksichtigung der neueren klinischen Ergebnisse. *Strahlenther.* 31:623–670.

Kryscio, R. J., Myers, M. H., Prusiner, S. T., Heise, H. W. and Christine, B. W. (1973). The space time distribution of Hodgkin's disease in Connecticut, 1940–69. *J. Nat. Cancer Inst.* 50:1107–1110.

Kufe, D. W., Peters, W. P. and Spiegelman, S. (1973). Unique nuclear DNA sequences in the involved tissues of Hodgkin's and Burkitt's lymphomas. *Proc. Nat. Acad. Sci. U.S.* 70:3810–3814.

Kuiper, D. H. and Papp, J. T. (1969). Supraclavicular adenopathy demonstrated by the Valsalva maneuver. *New Engl. J. Med.* 280:1007–1008.

Kuisk, H. (1973). New methods to facilitate radiotherapy planning and treatment, including a method for fast production of solid lead blocks with diverging walls for cobalt 60 beam. *Am. J. Roentgenol.* 117:161–167.

Kun, L. E., De Vita, V. T., Young, R. C. and Johnson, R. E. (1976). Treatment of Hodgkin's disease using intensive chemotherapy followed by irradiation. *Internat. J. Radiat. Oncol. Biol. Phys.* 1:619–626.

Kun, L. E. and Johnson, R. E. (1975). Hematologic and immunologic status in Hodgkin's disease 5 years after radical radiotherapy. *Cancer* 36:1912–1916.

Kundrat, H. (1893). Über Lympho-sarkomatosis. *Wien. Klin. Wchnschr.* 6:211–234.

Kunii, A., Takemoto, H. and Furth, J. (1965). Leukemogenic filterable agent from estrogen-induced thymic lymphoma in Rf mice. *Proc. Soc. Exper. Biol. Med.* 119:1211–1215.

Kuper, S. W. A. and Bignall, J. R. (1964). Tritiated-thymidine uptake by tumour cells in blood. *Lancet* 1:1412–1414.

Kurnick, J. E., White, M., Ware, D. E. and Robinson, W. A. (1975). Bleomycin (NSC-125066) and CCNU (NSC-79037) in the combination chemotherapy of MOPP-resistant Hodgkin's disease. *Cancer Chemother. Rep.* 59:1147–1150.

Kurohara, S. S., George, F. W. III, Levitt, S. H. and Rubin, P. (1967). The influence of certain clinical factors on survival in Hodgkin's disease. *Radiol. Clin.* 36:41–52.

Kushner, L. N. (1969). Hodgkin's disease simulating inflammatory breast carcinoma on mammography. A case report. *Radiology* 92:350.

Kyaw, M. and Koehler, P. R. (1969). Renal and perirenal lymphoma: arteriographic findings. *Radiology* 93:1055–1058.

Lacassagne, A. (1937). Sarcomes lymphoïdes apparus chez des souris longuement traités par des hormones oestrogènes. *Compt. rend. soc. biol.* 126:193–195.

Lacher, M. J. (1963). Role of surgery in Hodgkin's disease. *New Engl. J. Med.* 268:289–292.

Lacher, M. J. (1964). Use of vinblastine sulfate to treat Hodgkin's disease during pregnancy. *Ann. Int. Med.* 61:113–115.

Lacher, M. J. and Durant, J. R. (1965). Combined vinblastine and chlorambucil therapy of Hodgkin's disease. *Ann. Int. Med.* 62:468–476.

Lacher, M. J. and Geller, W. (1966). Cyclophosphamide and vinblastine sulfate in Hodgkin's disease during pregnancy. *J.A.M.A.* 195:486–488.

Lacher, M. J. and Sussman, L. N. (1963). Leukemia and Hodgkin's disease. *Ann. Int. Med.* 59:369–378.

Lagarde, C., Chauvergne, J., Hoerni, B., Touchard, J., Durand, M., Hoerni-Simon, G. and Brunet, R. (1976). Traitement des stades cliniques I et II de maladie de Hodgkin. Résultats obtenus chez 100 malades par l'association à la radiothérapie d'un ou deux cycles de chimiothérapie. *Acta Haematol.* 55:257–264.

Laird, H. M., Jarrett, O., Crighton, G. W. and Jarrett, W. F. H. (1968). An electron microscopic study of virus particles in spontaneous leukemia in the cat. *J. Nat. Cancer Inst.* 41:867–878.

Lamb, D., Pilney, F., Kelly, W. D. and Good, R. A. (1962). A comparative study of the incidence of anergy in patients with carcinoma, leukemia, Hodgkin's disease and other lymphomas. *J. Immunol.* 89:555–558.

Lamoureux, K. B., Jaffe, E. S., Berard, C. W. and Johnson, R. E. (1973). Lack of identifiable vascular invasion in patients with extranodal dissemination of Hodgkin's disease. *Cancer* 31:824–825.

Lampe, I. and Fayos, J. V. (1968). Hodgkin's disease: radiotherapeutic experience. *In* Proceedings of the International Conference on Leukemia-Lymphoma, C. J. D. Zarafonetis (ed). Philadelphia: Lea & Febiger. pp. 393–401.

Lanaro, A. E., Bosch, A. and Frías, Z. (1971). Red blood cell survival in patients with Hodgkin's disease. *Cancer* 28:658–661.

Lancaster, H. O. (1955). The mortality in Australia from leukaemia. *Med. J. Australia* 2:1064–1065.

Landaas, T. O., Godal, T. and Halvorsen, T. B. (1977). Characterization of immunoglobulins in Hodgkin cells. *Internat. J. Cancer* 20:717–722.

Landberg, T. and Larsson, L.-E. (1968). Studium des klinischen Verlaufs bei Sternbergscher Erkrankung. *Radiol. Austriaca* 18:197–210.

Landberg, T. and Larsson, L.-E. (1969). Hodgkin's disease—retrospective clinico-pathologic study in 149 patients. *Acta radiol.* 8:390–414.

Landberg, T., Lidén, K. and Forslo, H. (1973). Split-course radiation therapy of mediastinal Hodgkin's disease. TSD and CRE concepts. *Acta Radiol.* 12:33–39.

Lang, J. M., Bigel, P., Oberling, F. and Mayer, S. (1977). Normal active rosette-forming cells in untreated patients with Hodgkin's disease. *Biomedicine* 27:322–324.

Lang, J. M., Bigel, P., Oberling, F. and Mayer, S. (1978). Decreased "active" rosette-forming cells during remission in Hodgkin's disease. *Biomedicine* 29:83–84.

Lang, J. M., Oberling, F., Bigel, P., Mayer, S. and Waitz, R. (1974). Lymphocyte reactivity to phytohaemagglutinin and allogeneic lymphocytes in 32 untreated patients with Hodgkin's disease. *Biomedicine* 21:372–377.

Lang, J. M., Oberling, F., Tongio, M., Mayer, S. and Waitz, R. (1972). Mixed lymphocyte reaction as assay for immunological competence of lymphocytes from patients with Hodgkin's disease. *Lancet* 1:1261–1263.

Langenhuysen, M. M. A. C., Cazemier, T., Houwen, B., Brouwers, T. M., Halie, M. R., The, T. H. and Nieweg, H. O. (1974). Antibodies to Epstein-Barr virus, cytomegalovirus and Australia antigen in Hodgkin's disease. *Cancer* 34:262–267.

Langhans, T. (1872). Das Maligne Lymphosarkom (Pseudoleukämie). *Virchow's Arch f. path. Anat.* 54:509–537.

Langlands, A. O., MacLean, N., Pearson, J. G. and Williamson, E. R. D. (1967). Lymphadenopathy and megaloblastic anemia in patient receiving primidone. *Brit. Med. J.* 1:215–217.

Lantorp, K., Wahren, B. and Hanngren, A. (1972). Infectious mononucleosis and depression of cellular immunity. *Brit. Med. J.* 4:668–669.

Larsen, J. and Brincker, H. (1977). The incidence and characteristics of acute myeloid leukemia arising in Hodgkin's disease. *Scand. J. Haematol.* 18:197–206.

Lassvik, C., Rosengren, B. and Wranne, B. (1977). Pulmonary gas exchange following irradiation of cervical,

mediastinal, hilar and axillary nodes. *Acta Radiol.* 16:27–31.

Latarjet, R., and Ennuyer, A. (1969). Un traitement complémentaire de la maladie de Hodgkin par extrait tumoral irradié. (Expérimentation et essais cliniques). *Bull. Cancer* 56:221–230.

Lattes, R. (1962). Thymoma and other tumors of the thymus. An analysis of 107 cases. *Cancer* 15:1224–1260.

Lau, W. K. and Young, L. S. (1976). Trimethoprim-sulfamethoxazole treatment of *Pneumocystis carinii* pneumonia in adults. *New Engl. J. Med.* 295:716–718.

Lauwers, L. and Dancot, H. (1966). Rélation entre le degré d'activité de la maladie de Hodgkin au cours des cinq prémières années et le devenir des malades survivants à cinq ans. *Nouv. rev. franç. hématol.* 6:98–101.

Law, L. W. and Potter, M. (1956). The behavior in transplant of lymphocytic neoplasms arising from parental thymic grafts in irradiated, thymectomized hybrid mice. *Proc. Nat. Acad. Sci. U. S.* 42:160–167.

Lawler, M. R., Jr. and Riddell, D. H. (1966). Hodgkin's disease of the breast. *Arch. Surg.* 93:331–334.

Lawler, S. D., Pentycross, C. R. and Reeves, B. R. (1967). Lymphocyte transformation and chromosome studies in Hodgkin's disease. *Brit. Med. J.* 2:704–708.

Lawrence H. S. (1949). The cellular transfer of cutaneous hypersensitivity to tuberculin in man. *Proc. Soc. Exper. Biol. Med.* 71:516–522.

Lawrence, H. S. (1956). The delayed type of allergic inflammatory response. *Am. J. Med.* 20:428–447.

Lea, D. E. (1945). Biological assay of carcinogens. *Cancer Res.* 5:633–640.

Leb, L. and Merritt, J. A. (1978). Decreased monocyte function in patients with Hodgkin's disease. *Cancer* 41:1794–1803.

Le Bourgeois, J. P. and Bouhnik, H. (1976). The importance of fractionation in radiotherapy for Hodgkin's disease. *J. radiol. électrol. méd. nucl.* 57:828–830.

Le Bourgeois, J. P. and Tubiana, M. (1977). The erythrocyte sedimentation rate as a monitor for relapse in patients with previously treated Hodgkin's disease. *Internat. J. Radiat. Oncol. Biol. Phys.* 2:241–247.

Lecanet, D., Bernageau, J., Basch, A., Goguel, A. and Bismuth, V. (1971). Les localisations osseuses de la maladie de Hodgkin. *Ann. Radiol.* 14:845–861.

Lee, B. J., Nelson, J. H. and Schwarz, G. (1964). Evaluation of lymphangiography, inferior venacavography and intravenous pyelography in the clinical staging and management of Hodgkin's disease and lymphosarcoma. *New Engl. J. Med.* 271:327–337.

Lee, J. K. T., Stanley, R. J., Sagel, S. S. and Levitt, R. G. (1978). Accuracy of computed tomography in detecting intraabdominal and pelvic adenopathy in lymphoma. *Am. J. Roentgenol.* 131:311–315.

Leech, J. (1973). Immunoglobulin-positive Reed Sternberg cells in Hodgkin's disease. *Lancet* 1:265–266.

LeFloch, O., Donaldson, S. S. and Kaplan, H. S. (1976). Pregnancy following oophoropexy and total nodal irradiation in women with Hodgkin's disease. *Cancer* 38:2263–2268.

Lefrak, E. A., Pitha, J., Rosenheim, S. and Gottlieb, J. (1973). A clinicopathologic analysis of adriamycin cardiotoxicity. *Cancer* 32:302–314.

Leighton, P., Smith, P. G., Draper, G. J. and Pike, M. C. (1974). Malignant disease in the parents of children dying of Hodgkin's disease. *Brit. J. Cancer* 30:373–375.

Lenaz, L. and Page, J. A. (1976). Cardiotoxicity of adriamycin and related anthracyclines. *Cancer Treatment Rev.* 3:111–120

Lennert, K (1958). Die Frühveränderungen der Lymphogranulomatose. *Frankfurt. Z. Path.* 69:103–122.

Lennert, K. and Hippchen, A. M. (1954). Zur Prognose der Lymphogranulomatose. Abhängigkeit von histologischen Bild, Alter and Geschlecht. *Frankfurt. Z. Path.* 65:378–389.

Lennert, K. and Mestdagh, J. (1968). Lymphogranulomatosen mit konstant hohem Epithelioidzellgehalt. *Virchow's Arch. f. path. Anat.* 344:1–20.

Le Roy, E. C., Carbone, P. P. and Sjoerdsma, A. (1966). Elevated plasma levels of a hydroxyproline-containing protein in Hodgkin's disease and their relation to disease activity. *J. Lab. Clin. Med.* 67:891–897.

Leshan, L., Marvin S. and Lyerly, O. (1959). Some evidence of relationship between Hodgkin's disease and intelligence. *Arch. Gen. Psychiat.* 1:477–479.

L'Esperance, E. S. (1929). Experimental inoculation of chickens with Hodgkin's nodes. *J. Immunol.* 16:37–60.

L'Esperance, E. S. (1931). Studies in Hodgkin's disease. *Ann. Surg.* 93:162–168.

Lessner, H. E. (1969). BCNU (1,3,bis(β-chloroethyl)-1-nitrosourea). Effects on advanced Hodgkin's disease and other neoplasia. *Cancer* 22:451–456.

Le Van, P. and Bierman, S. (1962). Idiosyncratic drug eruption to Dilantin and trimethadione. *Arch. Derm.* 86:254–256.

Levi, J. A. and Wiernik, P. H. (1977a). Limited extranodal Hodgkin's disease. Unfavorable prognosis and therapeutic implications. *Am. J. Med.* 63:365–372.

Levi, J. A. and Wiernik, P. H. (1977b). The therapeutic implications of splenic involvement in stage IIIA Hodgkin's disease. *Cancer* 39:2158–2165.

Levi, J. A., Wiernik, P. H. and Diggs, C. H. (1977). Combination chemotherapy of advanced previously treated Hodgkin's disease with streptozotocin, CCNU, adriamycin and bleomycin. *Med. Pediatr. Oncol.* 3:33–40.

Levin, A. G, McDonough, E. F., Jr., Miller, D. G. and Southam, C. M. (1964). Delayed hypersensitivity response to DNFB in sick and healthy persons. *Ann. New York Acad. Sci.* 120:400–409.

Levine, P. H. (1974). The etiology of Hodgkin's disease. *Pathobiology Annual* 4:143–170.

Levine, P. H., Ablashi, D. V., Berard, C. W., Carbone, P. P., Waggoner, D. E. and Malan, L. (1971). Elevated antibody titers to Epstein-Barr virus in Hodgkin's disease. *Cancer* 27:416–421.

Levinson, B., Walter, B. A., Wintrobe, M. M. and Cartwright, G. E. (1957). A clinical study in Hodgkin's disease. *Arch. Int. Med.* 99:519–535.

Levitan, R. (1966). Unrelated gastro-intestinal disorders in patients with generalized Hodgkin's disease. *Am. J. Digest. Dis.* 11:307–313.

Levitan, R., Diamond, H. D. and Craver, L. F. (1961). Liver in Hodgkin's disease. *Gut* 2:60–71.

Levitt, M., DeConti, R. C., Pearson, H. A., March, J. C., Zanes, R. P., Mitchell, M. S., Kaetz, H. W. and Bertino, J. R. (1970). The Yale combination chemotherapy program for advanced Hodgkin's disease: a preliminary report. *Connecticut Med.* 34:862–866.

Levo, Y., Rotter, V. and Ramot, B. (1975). Restoration of cellular immune response by levamisole in patients with Hodgkin's disease. *Biomedicine* 23:198–200.

Levy, R. A. and Kaplan, H. S. (1974). Impaired lympho-cyte function in untreated Hodgkin's disease. *New Engl. J. Med.* 290:181–186.

Levy, R., Warnke, R., Dorfman, R. F. and Haimovich, J. (1977). The monoclonality of human B cell lymphomas. *J. Exper. Med.* 145:1014–1028.

Lewis, M. R. (1941). The behavior of Dorothy Reed cells in tissue cultures. *Am. J. Med. Sci.* 201:467 (abst.).

Li, F. P., Willard, D. R., Goodman, R. and Vawter, G. (1975). Malignant lymphoma after diphenylhydantoin (Dilantin) therapy. *Cancer* 36:1359–1362.

Liao, K. T. (1971). The superiority of histologic sections of aspirated bone marrow in malignant lymphomas. A review of 1,124 examinations. *Cancer* 27:618–628.

Libánský, J., Lukášová, M. and Piňosová, I. (1973). Blastogenic transformation of lymphocytes following phytohaemagglutinin treatment *in vitro* in malignant lymphomas. I. Hodgkin's disease. (Correlation with immunity response of the cellular type and with the clinical status). *Neoplasma* 20:51–60.

Libshitz, H. I., Brosof, A. B. and Southard, M. E. (1973). Radiographic appearance of the chest following extended field radiation therapy for Hodgkin's disease. A consideration of time-dose relationships. *Cancer* 32:206–215.

Lichtenfeld, J. L., Wiernik, P. H., Mardiney, M. R., Jr., and Zarco, R. M. (1976). Abnormalities of complement and its components in patients with acute leukemia, Hodgkin's disease, and sarcoma. *Cancer Res.* 36:3678–3680.

Lieberman, M. and Kaplan, H. S. (1959). Leukemogenic activity of filtrates from radiation-induced lymphoid tumors of mice. *Science* 130:387–388.

Lieberman, M. and Kaplan, H. S. (1966). Lymphoid tumor induction by mouse thymocytes infected *in vitro* with radiation leukemia virus. *Nat. Cancer Inst. Monograph* 22:549–554.

Liebow, A. A., Carrington, C. R. B. and Friedman, P. J. (1972). Lymphomatoid granulomatosis. *Human Path.* 3:457–558.

Lilien, D. L., Berger, H. G., Anderson, D. P. and Bennett, L. R. (1973). ^{111}In-chloride: a new agent for bone marrow imaging. *J. Nucl. Med.* 14:184–186.

Lilien, D. L., Jones, S. E., O'Mara, R. E., Salmon, S. E. and Durie, B. G. M. (1975). A clinical evaluation of indium-111 bleomycin as a tumor-imaging agent. *Cancer* 35:1036–1049.

Lille-Szyszkowicz, I., Gabay, P., Saracino, R. T. and Bourdin, J. S. (1966). La phosphatase alcaline leucocytaire chez les malades atteints de tumeurs ou d'hémopathies malignes. *Nouv. rev. franç. hématol.* 6:187–194.

Lillicrap, S. C. (1973). Modes of spread of Hodgkin's disease. *Brit. J. Radiol.* 46:18–23.

Lilly, F. and Pincus, T. (1973). Genetic control of murine viral leukemogenesis. *In* Advances in Cancer Research, G. Klein and S. Weinhouse (eds.), New York: Academic Press. Vol. 17, pp. 231–277.

Lindqvist, T. (1957). Lupus erythematosus disseminatus after administration of Mesantoin. Report of two cases. *Acta Med. Scand.* 158:131–138.

Lingeman, C. H. (1969). Epidemiologic pathology of leukemias and lymphomas of man. *Nat. Cancer Inst. Monograph* 32:177–209.

Linke, A. (1960). Die Behandlung der Hämoblastosen und malignen Tumoren mit Trisaethyleniminobenzochinon. *Deut. Med. Wchnscher.* 85:1928–1933.

Linke. A. (1965). Hypercalcämie bei Lymphogranulomatose. *Verh. Deut. Ges. Inn. Med.* 71:896–898.

Lipsky, P. E. and Rosenthal, A. S. (1973). Macrophage-lymphocyte interaction. I. Characteristics of the antigen-independent binding of guinea pig thymocytes and lymphocytes to syngeneic macrophages. *J. Exper. Med.* 138:900–924.

Lipton, M. J., DeNardo, G. L., Silverman, S. and Glatstein, E. (1972). Evaluation of the liver and spleen in Hodgkin's disease. I. The value of hepatic scintigraphy. *Am. J. Med.* 52:356–361.

Lisak, R. P., Mitchell, M., Zweiman, B., Orrechio, E. and Asbury, A. K. (1977). Guillain-Barré syndrome and Hodgkin's disease: three cases with immunological studies. *Ann. Neurol.* 1:72–78.

Littman, M. L. and Walter, J. E. (1968). Cryptococcosis: Current status. *Am. J. Med.* 45:922–932.

Loh, K. K., Gamble, J. F., Shullenberger, C. C. and Fuller, L. M. (1977). Combination chemotherapy in MOPP resistant Hodgkin's disease. *Proc. Am. Soc. Clin. Oncol.* 18:267 (abst.).

Lohmann, H. I. (1965). Prognostic significance of histopathology in Hodgkin's granuloma. *Acta path. microbiol. Scand.* 64:16–30.

Lokich, J. J., Bass, H., Eberly, F. E., Rosenthal, D. S. and Moloney, W. C. (1973). The pulmonary effect of mantle irradiation in patients with Hodgkin's disease. *Radiology* 108:397–402.

Lokich, J. J., Frei, E., III, Jaffe, N. and Tullis, J. (1976). New multiple-agent chemotherapy (B-DOPA) for advanced Hodgkin's disease. *Cancer* 38:667–671.

Lokich, J. J., Galvanek, E. G. and Moloney, W. C. (1973). Nephrosis of Hodgkin disease. An immune complex-induced lesion. *Arch. Int. Med.* 132:597–600.

Lokich, J. J., Pinkus, G. S. and Moloney, W. C. (1974). Hodgkin's disease in the elderly. *Oncology* 19:484–500.

Long, J. C., Aisenberg, A. C., Zamecnik, M. V. and Zamecnik, P. C. (1973). A tumor antigen in tissue cultures derived from patients with Hodgkin's disease. *Proc. Nat. Acad. Sci. U.S.* 70:1540–1544.

Long, J. C., Aisenberg, A. C. and Zamecnik, P. C. (1974a). An antigen in Hodgkin's disease tissue cultures: fluorescent antibody studies. *Proc. Nat. Acad. Sci. U.S.* 71:2285–2289.

Long, J. C., Aisenberg, A. C. and Zamecnik, P. C. (1974b). An antigen in Hodgkin's disease tissue cultures: radioiodine-labeled antibody studies. *Proc. Nat. Acad. Sci. U.S.* 71:2605–2609.

Long, J. C., Aisenberg, A. C. and Zamecnik, P. C. (1977a). Chromatographic and electrophoretic analysis of an antigen in Hodgkin's disease tissue cultures. *J. Nat. Cancer Inst.* 58:223–227.

Long, J. C., Hall, C. L., Brown, C. A., Stamatos, C., Weitzman, S. S. and Carey, K. (1977b). Binding of soluble immune complexes in sera of patients with Hodgkin's disease to tissue cultures derived from the tumor. *New Engl. J. Med.* 297:295–299.

Long, J. C., Zamecnik, P. C., Aisenberg, A. C. and Atkins, L. (1977c). Tissue culture studies in Hodgkin's disease. Morphologic, cytogenetic, cell surface, and enzymatic properties of cultures derived from splenic tumors. *J. Exper. Med.* 145:1484–1500.

Long, J. P. and Patchefsky, A. S. (1971). Primary Hodgkin's disease of the ovary. A case report. *Obstet. Gynecol.* 38:680–682.

Longcope, W. T. (1903). On the pathological histology of Hodgkin's disease, with a report of a series of cases. *Bull. Ayer Clin. Lab., Pennsylvania Hosp.* 1:1–76.

Longcope, W. T. (1907). Notes on the experimental inoculation of monkeys with glands from cases of Hodgkin's disease. *Bull. Ayer Clin. Lab., Pennsylvania Hosp.* 4:18–21.

Longcope, W. T. and McAlpin, K. R. (1920). Hodgkin's disease. *Oxford Medicine* Vol. 4, part 1, pp. 1–43.

Longmire, R. L., McMillan, R., Yelenosky, R., Armstrong, S., Lang, J. E. and Craddock, C. G. (1973). *In vitro* splenic IgG synthesis in Hodgkin's disease. *New Engl. J. Med.* 289:763–767.

Lorenz, E., Congdon, C. C. and Uphoff, D. (1953). Prevention of irradiation-induced lymphoid tumors in C57BL mice by spleen protection. *J. Nat. Cancer Inst.* 14:291–301.

Lowenbraun, S., Ramsey, H., Sutherland, J. and Serpick, A. A. (1970). Diagnostic laparotomy and splenectomy for staging Hodgkin's disease. *Ann. Int. Med.* 72:655–663.

Lowenhaupt, E. and Brown, R. (1951). Carcinoma of the thymus of granulomatous type; clinical and pathological studies. *Cancer* 4:1193–1209.

Lowy, D. R., Rowe, W. P., Teich, N. and Hartley, J. W. (1971). Murine leukemia virus: high frequency activation *in vitro* by 5-iododeoxyuridine and 5-bromodeoxyuridine. *Science* 174:155–156.

Lucas, P. F. (1955). Lymph node smears in the diagnosis of lymphadenopathy: A review. *Blood* 10:1030–1054.

Luce, J. K., Frei, E., III, Gehan, E. A., Coltman, C. A., Jr., Talley, R. and Monto, R. W. (1973). Chemotherapy of Hodgkin's disease. Maintenance therapy vs. no maintenance after remission induction with combination chemotherapy. *Arch. Int. Med.* 131:391–395.

Luk, K. H., Castro, J. R., Meyler, T. S., Potter, L. and Purser, P. R. (1977). Individualized low-melting alloy shielding blocks for external-beam radiation therapy. *Applied Radiology* 6:115.

Lukes, R. J. (1963). Relationship of histologic features to clinical stages in Hodgkin's disease. *Am. J. Roentgenol.* 90:944–955.

Lukes, R. J. (1971). Criteria for involvement of lymph node, bone marrow, spleen, and liver in Hodgkin's disease. *Cancer Res.* 31:1755–1767.

Lukes, R. J. and Butler, J. J. (1966a). The pathology and nomenclature of Hodgkin's disease. *Cancer Res.* 26:1063–1081.

Lukes, R. J., Butler, J. J. and Hicks, E. B. (1966b). Natural history of Hodgkin's disease as related to its pathologic picture. *Cancer* 19:317–344.

Lukes, R. J. and Collins, R. D. (1974). Immunologic characterization of human malignant lymphomas. *Cancer* 34:1488–1503.

Lukes, R. J., Craver, L. F., Hall, T. C., Rappaport, H. and Rubin, P. (1966c). Report of the nomenclature committee. *Cancer Res.* 26:1311.

Lukes, R. J., Gompel, C. and Nezelof, C. (1966d). Le diagnostic histopathologique de la maladie de Hodgkin. Analyse préliminaire d'une étude conduite à l'aveugle sur 395 observations, par trois pathologistes de nationalité différente. *Nouv. rev. franç. hématol.* 6:11–14.

Lukes, R. J. and Tindle, B. H. (1975). Immunoblastic

lymphadenopathy. A hyperimmune entity resembling Hodgkin's disease. *New Engl. J. Med.* 292:1–8.

Lukes, R. J., Tindle, B. H. and Parker, J. W. (1969). Reed-Sternberg-like cells in infectious mononucleosis. *Lancet* 2:1003–1004.

Lumb, G. (1954). Tumours of Lymphoid Tissue. Edinburgh and London: E & S Livingstone. Chap. 8, pp. 71–99.

Lundh, B., Mitelman, F., Nilsson, P. G., Stenstam, M. and Söderström, N. (1975). Chromosome abnormalities identified by banding technique in a patient with acute myeloid leukaemia complicating Hodgkin's disease. *Scand. J. Haematol.* 14:303–307.

Lundin, F. E., Jr., Fraumeni, J. F., Jr., Lloyd, J. W. and Smith, E. M. (1966). Temporal relationships of leukemia and lymphoma deaths in neighborhoods. *J. Nat. Cancer Inst.* 37:123–133.

Luxton, R. (1953). Radiation nephritis. *Quart. J. Med.* 22:215–242.

Lycette, R. R. and Pearmain, G. E. (1963). Further observations on antigen-induced mitosis. *Lancet* 2:386.

Lynch, H. T., Saldivar, V. A., Guirgis, H. A., Terasaki, P. I., Bardawil, W. A., Harris, R. E., Lynch, J. F. and Thomas, R. (1976). Familial Hodgkin's disease and associated cancer. A clinical-pathological study. *Cancer* 38:2033–2041.

Macaulay, W. L. (1968). Lymphomatoid papulosis: a continuing self-healing eruption, clinically benign, histologically malignant. *Arch. Derm.* 97:23–30.

MacDonald, C. A., Jr. and Lacher, M. J. (1966). Oral vinblastine sulfate in Hodgkin's disease. *Clin. Pharmacol. Ther.* 7:534–541.

MacDonald, D. M. and Sarkany, I. (1976). Lymphomatoid granulomatosis. *Clin. Exper. Dermatol.* 1:163–173.

MacDonald, J. S., Laugier, A. and Schlienger, M. (1968). Observations on the growth of tumours in lymph nodes changing from normal to abnormal while remaining opacified after lymphography. *Clin. Radiol.* 19:120–127.

Machado, J. C., Jamra, M., Okuyama, M. H. and Marigo, C. (1973). Lymphoreticular tumors in São Paulo, Brazil. *J. Nat. Cancer Inst.* 50:1651–1655.

Mack, T. (1974). Role of the case-control design in the study of Hodgkin's disease. *Cancer Res.* 34:1166–1169.

MacMahon, B. (1957). Epidemiological evidence on the nature of Hodgkin's disease. *Cancer* 10:1045–1054.

MacMahon, B. (1966). Epidemiology of Hodgkin's disease. *Cancer Res.* 26:1189–1200.

MacMahon, B., Cole, P. and Newell, G. R. (1971). Hodgkin's disease: one entity or two? *Lancet* 1:240–241.

MacMahon, B. and Koller, E. K. (1957). Ethnic differences in the incidence of leukemia. *Blood* 12:1–10.

Madsen, B. and Davidsen, D. (1973). Splenic angiography in Hodgkin's disease. *Danish Med. Bull.* 20:42–46.

Maldonado, J. E., Taswell, H. F. and Kiely, J. M. (1972). Familial Hodgkin's disease. *Lancet* 2:1259.

Mallory, F. B. (1914). Principles of Pathologic Histology. Philadelphia: W. B. Saunders.

Malpas, J. S. and Fairley, G. H. (1964). Changes in γ-2 globulins in reticuloses. *J. Clin. Path.* 17:651–654.

Maneche, H. C. (1966). Blood pyruvate in malignant neoplastic disorders. *Clin. Chem.* 12:158–164.

Mankin, Z. W. (1936). Experimentell-histologische Untersuchungen über normale und pathologisch veränderte Lymphknoten des Menschen. *Beitr. path. Anat.* 96:248–308.

Manners, J. S. (1977). The radiology of the neurological complications of the reticuloses. *Clin. Radiol.* 28:221–227.

Manolov, G. and Manolova, Y. (1972). Marker band in one chromosome 14 from Burkitt lymphomas. *Nature* 237:33–34.

Mantel, N. and Blot, W. J. (1976). Is Hodgkin's disease infectious? Discussion of an epidemiologic method used to impute that it is. *J. Nat. Cancer Inst.* 56:413–414.

Marigo, C., Muller, H. and Davies, J. N. P. (1969). Survey of cancer in children admitted to a Brazilian charity hospital. *J. Nat. Cancer Inst.* 43:1231–1240.

Marinello, M., Tkachenko, G., Gavilondo, J. and Baeza, B. (1975). *In vitro* incorporation of tritiated thymidine by the Sternberg-Reed cells in Hodgkin disease. *Neoplasma* 22:185–193.

Marinone, G., Colle, R. and Mombelloni, P. (1978). Long-term evaluation of the effect of combined chemotherapy with vincristine, adriamycin, procarbazine, and prednisone (VAPP) on advanced Hodgkin's disease. *Minerva med.* 69:1255–1261.

Markiewicz, W., Glatstein, E., London, E. J. and Popp, R. L. (1977). Echocardiographic detection of pericardial effusion and pericardial thickening in malignant lymphoma. *Radiology* 123:161–164.

Markovits, P., Gasquet, C., and Parmentier, C. (1968). La rate Hodgkinienne. Étude par artériographie coeliaque sélective. (A propos d'une observation.) *J. radiol. électrol.* 49:297–299.

Markowitz, M. and Tringali, M. (1962). Hodgkin's disease and exfoliative dermatitis. *New York State J. Med.* 62:3970–3973.

Marks, J. E., Haus, A. G., Sutton, H. G. and Griem, M. L. (1974a). Localization error in the radiotherapy of Hodgkin's disease and malignant lymphoma with extended mantle fields. *Cancer* 34:83–90.

Marks, J. E., Moran, E. M., Griem, M. L. and Ultmann, J. E. (1974b). Extended mantle radiotherapy in Hodgkin's disease and malignant lymphoma. *Am. J. Roentgenol.* 121:772–788.

Marks, J. E., Pinsky, S. M. and Griem, J. L. (1971). The extended mantle field in the radiotherapeutic treatment of malignant lymphoma. *Radiology* 100:423–425.

Marks, R. D., Jr., Agarwal, S. K. and Constable, W. C. (1973). Increased rate of complications as a result of treating only one prescribed field daily. *Radiology* 107:615–619.

Marmont, A. M. and Damasio, E. E. (1967). The effects of two alkaloids derived from *Vinca Rosea* on the malignant cells in Hodgkin's disease, lymphosarcoma and acute leukemia *in vivo*. *Blood* 29:1–21.

Marquardt, H. and Marquardt, H. (1977). Induction of malignant transformation and mutagenesis in cell cultures by cancer chemotherapeutic agents. *Cancer* 40:1930–1934.

Marsh, J. C., DeConti, R. C. and Hubbard, S. P. (1971). Treatment of Hodgkin's disease and other cancers with 1,3-Bis(2-chloroethyl)-1-nitrosourea (BCNU; NSC-409962). *Cancer Chemother. Rep.* 55:599–606.

Marshall, A. H. E. (1953). The production of tumours of the reticular tissue by di-azo vital dyes. *Acta microbiol. Scand.* 33:1–9.

Marshall, A. H. E. (1956). An Outline of the Cytology and Pathology of the Reticular Tissue. Edinburgh: Oliver and Boyd. pp. 203–211.

Marshall, A. H. E. and Wood, C. (1957). The involvement of the thymus in Hodgkin's disease. *J. Path. Bact.* 73:163–166.

Marshall, G., Roessmann, U. and Van Den Noort, S. (1968). Invasive Hodgkin's disease of the brain. Report of two new cases and review of American and European literature with clinical-pathologic correlations. *Cancer* 22:621–630.

Marshall, W. H., Jr., Breiman, R. S., Harell, G. S., Glatstein, E. and Kaplan, H. S. (1977). Computed tomography of abdominal paraaortic lymph node disease: preliminary observations with a 6 second scanner. *Am. J. Roentgenol.* 128:759–764.

Martin, R., Sureau, B., Véron, M. and Barme, M. (1954). Accidents cutanés et ganglionnaires au cours d'un traitement par la diphényl-hydantoïne et la phénacety-lurée. *Arch. franç. pediat.* 11:979–982.

Martinez-Maldonado, M., Menéndez-Corrada, R. and Rivera De Sala, A. (1964). Diagnostic value of alkaline phosphatase in leukocytes. *Am. J. Med. Sci.* 248:175–183.

Martinez-Maldonado, M. and Ramírez De Arrelano, G. A. (1966). Renal involvement in malignant lymphomas: a survey of 49 cases. *J. Urol.* 95:485–488.

Martire, J. R. (1974). Histologic correlation of lymphangiograms in Hodgkin's disease: an evaluation of diagnostic criteria. *South. Med. J.* 67:1317–1321.

Maruyama, Y., Moore, V. C., Burns, D. and Hilger, N. T. J. (1969). Individualized lung shields constructed from lead shot imbedded in plastic. *Radiology* 92:634–635.

Masland, D. S., Rotz, C. T. and Harris, J. H. (1968). Postradiation pericarditis with chronic pericardial effusion. *Ann. Int. Med.* 69:97–102.

Mason, T. J. and Fraumeni, J. F., Jr. (1974). Hodgkin's disease among Japanese Americans. *Lancet* 1:215.

Massey, F. C., Lane, L. L. and Imbriglia, J. E. (1953). Acute infectious mononucleosis and Hodgkin's disease occurring simultaneously in the same patient. *J.A.M.A.* 151:994–995.

Matanoski, G. M., Sartwell, P. E. and Elliott, E. A. (1975). Hodgkin's disease mortality among physicians. *Lancet* 1:926–927.

Matchett, K. M., Huang, A. T. and Kremer, W. B. (1973). Impaired lymphocyte transformation in Hodgkin's disease. Evidence for depletion of circulating T-lymphocytes. *J. Clin. Invest.* 52:1908–1917.

Mathé, G. (1969). Approaches to the immunological treatment of cancer in man. *Brit. Med. J.* 4:7–10.

Mathé, G., Amiel, J. L., Schwarzenberg, L., Schneider, M., Cattan, A., Schlumberger, J. R., Hayat, M. and de Vassal, F. (1969). Active immunotherapy for acute lymphoblastic leukaemia. *Lancet* 1:697–699.

Mathé, G., Schweisguth, O., Schneider, M., Amiel, J. L., Berumen, L., Brule, G., Cattan, A. and Schwarzenberg, L. (1963). Methylhydrazine in the treatment of Hodgkin's disease. *Lancet* 2:1077–1080.

Mauch, P., Goodman, R. L. and Hellman, S. (1978). The significance of mediastinal involvement in early stage Hodgkin's disease. *Cancer* 42:1039–1045.

Mauri, C. and Quaglino, D. (1974). Hodgkin's disease terminating in acute myeloid leukaemia. *Haematologica* 59:86–90.

Mavor, W. O. and Adams, P. (1967). Hodgkin's disease: an unusual termination. *Postgrad. Med. J.* 43:490–491.

May, K. and Hancock, B. W. (1977). Plasma ferritin levels in untreated patients with malignant lymphoma. *Clin. Sci. Mol. Med.* 53:14 (abst.).

Mazar, S. A. and Straus, B. (1951). Marital Hodgkin's disease. *Arch. Int. Med.* 88:819–830.

McCord, D. L., Million, R. R., Northrop, M. and Kavanaugh, H. V. Z. (1973). Daily reproducibility of lung blocks in the mantle technique. *Radiology* 109:735–736.

McCormick, D. P., Meyer, W. J. and Nesbit, M. E. (1971). Coexistence of Hodgkin's disease and Down's syndrome. *Am. J. Dis. Child.* 122:71–73.

McDougall, I. R., Saunders, W., Coleman, C. N. and Kaplan, H. S. (1979). Thyroid carcinoma after high dose external radiotherapy for Hodgkin's disease—report of 3 cases. *Cancer* (in press).

McElwain, T. J., Toy, J., Smith, E., Peckham, M. J. and Austin, D. E. (1977). A combination of chlorambucil, vinblastine, procarbazine and prednisolone for treatment of Hodgkin's disease. *Brit. J. Cancer* 36:276–280.

McElwain, T. J., Wrigley, P. F. M., Hunter, A., Crowther, D., Malpas, J. S., Peckham, M. J., Smithers, D. W. and Fairley, G. H. (1973). Combination chemotherapy in advanced and recurrent Hodgkin's disease. *Nat. Cancer Inst. Monograph* 36:395–402.

McGregor, J. K. (1960). Hodgkin's disease of the breast. *Am. J. Surg.* 99:348–351.

McHeffey, G. and Peterson, R. (1934). Hodgkin's disease occurring simultaneously in two brothers. *J.A.M.A.* 102:521–522.

McIntire, K. R. (1969). Reticular neoplasms of SJL/J mice. *Nat. Cancer Inst. Monograph* 32:49–58.

McIntire, K. R. and Law, L. W. (1967). Abnormal serum immunoglobulins occurring with reticular neoplasms in an inbred strain of mouse. *J. Nat. Cancer Inst.* 39:1197–1211.

McNaught, J. B. (1938). The Gordon test for Hodgkin's disease. A reaction to eosinophils. *J.A.M.A.* 111:1280–1284.

McMahon, N. J., Gordon, H. W. and Rosen, R. B. (1970). Reed-Sternberg cells in infectious mononucleosis. *Am. J. Dis. Child.* 120:148–150.

McReynolds, R. A., Gold, G. L. and Roberts, W. C. (1976). Coronary heart disease after mediastinal irradiation for Hodgkin's disease. *Am. J. Med.* 60:39–45.

Meadows, R. (1965). Hodgkin's disease of the colon presenting as disseminated sclerosis with associated ulcerative colitis. *Aust. New Zeal. J. Surg.* 35:80–82.

Medinger, F. G. and Craver, L. F. (1942). Total body irradiation, with review of cases. *Am. J. Roentgenol.* 48:651–671.

Meier, R., Posern, E. and Weitzmann, G. (1937). Das Wachstum menschlichen Lymphogranulomes *in vitro*. *Virchow's Arch. f. path. Anat.* 299:329–338.

Meighan, S. S. and Ramsay, J. D. (1963). Survival in Hodgkin's disease. *Brit. J. Cancer* 17:24–36.

Meistrich, M. L., Hunter, N. R., Suzuki, N., Trostle, P. K. and Withers, H. R. (1978). Gradual regeneration of mouse testicular stem cells after exposure to ionizing radiation. *Radiat. Res.* 74:349–362.

Melamed, M. R. (1963). The cytological presentation of malignant lymphomas and related diseases in effusions. *Cancer* 16:413–431.

Meller, R. L. and Resch, J. A. (1949). Convulsive disorders in adults. *Postgrad. Med.* 6:452–458.

Mennuti, M. T., Shepard, T. H. and Mellman, W. J. (1975). Fetal renal malformation following treatment of Hodgkin's disease during pregnancy. *Obstet. Gynecol.* 46:194–196.

Merigan, T. C., Rand, K. H., Pollard, R. B., Abdallah, P. S., Jordan, G. W. and Fried, R. P. (1978a). Human leukocyte interferon for the treatment of herpes zoster in patients with cancer. *New Engl. J. Med.* 298:981–987.

Merigan, T. C., Sikora, K., Breeden, J. H., Levy, R. and Rosenberg, S. A. (1978b). Preliminary observations of the effect of human leukocyte interferon in non-Hodgkin's lymphoma. *New Engl. J. Med.* 299:1449–1453.

Merner, T. B. and Stenstrom, K. W. (1947). Roentgen therapy in Hodgkin's disease. *Radiology* 48:355–368.

Messinetti, S., Zelli, G. P., Marcellino, L. R. and Alcini, E. (1966). Le indagini citogenetiche nel morbo di Hodgkin. Analisi cromosomica diretta in un caso di paragranuloma. *Ann. ital. chir.* 42:909–919.

Meurk, M. L., Green, J. T., Nussbaum, H. and Vaeth, J. M. (1968). Phantom dosimetry study of shaped cobalt-60 fields in the treatment of Hodgkin's disease. *Radiology* 91:554–558.

Meyer, H. A. (1967). Der diagnostische Wert der supraclaviculären Lymphknotenbiopsie nach Daniels. *Schweiz. Med. Wchnschr.* 97:1023–1027.

Meytes, D. and Modan, B. (1969). Selected aspects of Hodgkin's disease in a whole community. *Blood* 34:91–95.

Michaels, L. and Todd, G. B. (1976). Biopsy of nasopharynx as a staging procedure in Hodgkin's disease. *Brit. Med. J.* 1:41–42.

Michel, J., Ardichvili, D., Somerhausen, M., Kenis, Y. and Heuson, J. C. (1973). Hodgkin's disease with massive hepatic involvement and uninvolved spleen. *Europ. J. Cancer* 9:701–702.

Milder, M. S., Larson, S. M., Bagley, C. M., Jr., De Vita, V. T., Jr., Johnson, R. E. and Johnston, G. S. (1973). Liver-spleen scan in Hodgkin's disease. *Cancer* 31:826–834.

Miles, C. P., Geller, W. and O'Neill, F. (1966). Chromosomes in Hodgkin's disease and other malignant lymphomas. *Cancer* 19:1103–1116.

Milham, S., Jr. (1974). Hodgkin's disease as an occupational disease of schoolteachers. *New Engl. J. Med.* 290:1329.

Milham, S., Jr. and Hesser, J. (1967). Hodgkin's disease in woodworkers. *Lancet* 2:136–137.

Millard, R. E. (1968). Chromosome abnormalities in malignant lymphomas. *Europ. J. Cancer* 4:97–105.

Miller, D. G. (1962). Patterns of immunological deficiency in lymphomas and leukemias. *Ann. Int. Med.* 57:703–716.

Miller, D. G., Lizardo, J. G. and Snyderman, R. K. (1961). Homologous and heterologous skin transplantation in patients with lymphomatous disease. *J. Nat. Cancer Inst.* 26:569–583.

Miller, N. R. and Iliff, W. J. (1975). Visual loss as the initial symptom in Hodgkin disease. *Arch. Ophthalmol.* 93:1158–1161.

Miller, R. A., Gartner, S. and Kaplan, H. S. (1978). Stimulation of mitogenic responses in human peripheral blood lymphocytes by lipopolysaccharide: serum and T helper cell requirements. *J. Immunol.* 121:2160–2164.

Miller, R. W. (1966). Mortality in childhood; Hodgkin's disease. An etiologic clue. *J.A.M.A.* 198:1216–1217.

Miller, R. W. and Beebe, G. W. (1973). Infectious mononucleosis and the empirical risk of cancer. *J. Nat. Cancer Inst.* 50:315–321.

Minielly, J. A., Mills, S. D. and Holley, K. E. (1969). *Pneumocystis carinii* pneumonia. *Canad. Med. Assoc. J.* 100:846–854.

Minot, G. R. and Isaacs, R. (1926). Lymphoblastoma (malignant lymphoma); age and sex incidence, duration of disease, and the effect of roentgen-ray and radium irradiation and surgery. *J.A.M.A.* 86:1185–1189; 1265–1270.

Minow, R. A., Benjamin, R. S. and Gottlieb, J. A. (1975). Adriamycin (NSC-123127) cardiomyopathy—an overview with determination of risk factors. *Cancer Chemother. Rep.* 6:195–201.

Mintz, U. and Sachs, L. (1975). Membrane differences in peripheral blood lymphocytes from patients with chronic lymphocytic leukemia and Hodgkin's disease. *Proc. Nat. Acad. Sci. U.S.* 72:2428–2432.

Misad, O., Brandon, J. G. and Albujar, P. (1973). Lymphoreticular tumors in Peru. *J. Nat. Cancer Inst.* 50:1663–1668.

Mitchell, R. K., Peters, M. V. Brown, T. C. and Rideout, D. (1972). Laparotomy for Hodgkin's disease: some surgical observations. *Surgery* 71:694–703.

Modan, B., Goldman, B., Shani, M., Meytes, D. and Mitchell, B. S. (1969). Epidemiological aspects of neoplastic disorders in Israeli migrant population. V. The lymphomas. *J. Nat. Cancer Inst.* 42:375–381.

Mody, A. E. Mascarenhas, A. F. A., Vora, N. K. and Dalal, K. A. (1965). Hodgkin's disease of the stomach; a case report. *J. Postgrad. Med.* 11:137–140.

Moloney, W. C., Davis, S. and Hieber, R. D. (1961). The use of steroid hormones in the management of hematologic disorders. *G.P.* 24:101–106.

Moloney, W. C. and Long, J. C. (1974). Anemia and thrombocytopenia after therapy for Hodgkin's disease. *New Engl. J. Med.* 290:1012–1017.

Molyneux, M. E. (1973). Mediastinal reticulosis with hypertrophic pulmonary osteoarthropathy. *Brit. J. Dis. Chest* 67:66–70.

Monfardini, S., Bajetta, E., Arnold, C. A., Kenda, R. and Bonadonna, G. (1975). Herpes zoster-varicella infection in malignant lymphomas. Influence of splenectomy and intensive treatment. *Europ. J. Cancer* 11:51–57.

Monie, I. W. (1961). Chlorambucil-induced abnormalities of urogenital system of rat fetuses. *Anat. Rec.* 139:145–153.

Moolten, S. E. (1934). Hodgkin's disease of the lung. *Am. J. Cancer* 21:253–294.

Moore, D. F., Migliore, P. J., Shullenberger, C. C. and Alexanian, R. (1970). Monoclonal macroglobulinemia in malignant lymphoma. *Ann. Int. Med.* 72:43–47.

Moore, M. R., Bull, J. M., Jones, S. E., Rosenberg, S. A. and Kaplan, H. S. (1972). Sequential radiotherapy and chemotherapy in the treatment of Hodgkin's disease: a progress report. *Ann. Int. Med.* 77:1–9.

Moore, M. R., Jones, S. E., Bull, J. M., William, L. A. and

Rosenberg, S. A. (1973). MOPP chemotherapy for advanced Hodgkin's disease. Prognostic factors in 81 patients. *Cancer* 32:52–60.

Moorthy, A. V., Zimmerman, S. W. and Burkholder, P. M. (1976). Nephrotic syndrome in Hodgkin's disease. Evidence for pathogenesis alternative to immune complex deposition. *Am. J. Med.* 61:471–477.

Morano, E. and Orecchia, C. (1965). Su un caso di linfogranuloma primitivo del stomaco. *Cancro* 18:86–93.

Morardet, N., Parmentier, C. and Flamant, R. (1973). Étude par le fer⁵⁹ des effets de la radiothérapie étendue des hématosarcomes sur l'érythropoïèse. *Biomedicine* 18:228–234.

Morgenfeld, M. C., De Piterbarg, S. M. and De Bonaparte, Y. P. (1965). Enfermedad de Hodgkin y embarazo. *Rev. asoc. med. Argent.* 79:341–342.

Morgenfeld, M. C., Goldberg, V., Parisier, H., Bugnard, S. C. and Bur, G. E. (1972). Ovarian lesions due to cytostatic agents during the treatment of Hodgkin's disease. *Surg. Gynec. Obst.* 134:826–828.

Mori, Y. and Lennert, K. (1969). Electron Microscopic Atlas of Lymph Node Cytology and Pathology. Berlin and Heidelberg: Springer-Verlag.

Moroz, C., Giler, S., Kupfer, B. and Urea, I. (1977a). Lymphocytes bearing surface ferritin in patients with Hodgkin's disease and breast cancer. *New Engl. J. Med.* 296:1172–1173.

Moroz, C., Lahat, N., Biniaminov, M. and Ramot, B. (1977b). Ferritin on the surface of lymphocytes in Hodgkin's disease patients. A possible blocking substance removed by levamisole. *Clin. Exper. Immunol.* 29:30–35.

Morris, L. L., Cassady, J. R. and Jaffe, N. (1975). Sternal changes following irradiation for childhood Hodgkin's disease. *Radiology* 115:701–705.

Morris, P. J., Lawler, S. and Oliver, R. T. (1972). HL-A and Hodgkin's disease. *In* Histocompatibility Testing, 1972. Copenhagen: Munksgaard, pp. 669–677.

Mortazavi, S. H., Bani-Hashemi, A., Mozafari, M. and Raffi, A. (1972). Value of serum copper measurement in lymphomas and several other malignancies. *Cancer* 29:1193–1198.

Mortensen, R. F., Osmand, A. P. and Gewurz, H. (1975). Effects of C-reactive protein on the lymphoid system. I. Binding to thymus-dependent lymphocytes and alteration of their functions. *J. Exper. Med.* 141:821–839.

Morton, J. J., and Mider, G. B. (1938). The production of lymphomatosis in mice of known genetic constitution. *Science* 87:327–328.

Moses, A. M. and Spencer, H. (1963). Hypercalcemia in patients with malignant lymphoma. *Ann. Int. Med.* 59:531–536.

Moss, W. T., Haddy, F. J. and Sweany, S. K. (1960). Some factors altering the severity of acute radiation pneumonitis: variation with cortisone, heparin, and antibiotics. *Radiology* 75:50–54.

Moulton, J. D. and Bostick, W. L. (1958). Canine malignant lymphoma simulating Hodgkin's disease in man. *J. Am. Vet. Med. Assoc.* 132:204–210.

Moxley, J. H. III, De Vita, V. T., Jr., Brace, K. and Frei, E. III. (1967). Intensive combination chemotherapy and x-irradiation in Hodgkin's disease. *Cancer Res.* 27:1258–1263.

Müftüöglu, A. U. and Balkuv, S. (1967). Passive transfer of tuberculin sensitivity to patients with Hodgkin's disease. *New Engl. J. Med.* 277:126–129.

Muggeo, M., DeAntoni, A., Allegri, G., Costa, C. and Crepaldi, G. (1970). The influence of nicotinamide on the urinary excretion of tryptophan metabolites in Hodgkin's disease. *Clin. Chim. Acta* 30:779–785.

Mundkur, B. and Greenwood, H. (1968). Amido black 10B as a nucleolar stain for lymph nodes in Hodgkin's disease. *Acta Cytologica* 12:218–226.

Mundkur, B. and Stibitz, M. (1969). Selective effects of a new metal-complex azo dye on proteins of the Reed-Sternberg cell. *Cancer Res.* 29:1485–1497.

Munoz, N., Davidson, R. J., Witthoff, B., Ericsson, J. E. and De-The, G. (1978). Infectious mononucleosis and Hodgkin's disease. *Internat. J. Cancer* 22:10–13.

Murphy, E. D. (1963). SJL/J, a new inbred strain of mouse with a high, early incidence of reticulum-cell neoplasms. *Proc. Am. Assoc. Cancer Res.* 4:46 (abst.).

Murphy, W. T. and Bilge, N. (1964). Compression of the spinal cord in patients with malignant lymphoma. *Radiology* 82:495–501.

Musshoff, K. (1970). Therapy and prognosis of two different forms of organ involvement in cases of malignant lymphoma (Hodgkin's disease, reticulum cell sarcoma, lymphosarcoma) as well as a report about stage division in these diseases. *Klin. Wchnschr.* 48:673–678.

Musshoff, K. and Boutis, L. (1968). Therapy results in Hodgkin's disease, Freiburg i. Br., 1948-1966. *Cancer* 21:1100–1113.

Musshoff, K. and Boutis, L. (1969) Beurteilung Behandlungsgrundsätze und -ergebnisse bei der Lymphogranulomatose. *Sonderband 69 zur Strahlenther.*, pp. 59–74.

Musshoff, K., Boutis, L., Laszlo, A. M. and Laszlo, I. (1966). Prognostische Krankheitssymptome und -zeichen bei Morbus Hodgkin und ihre Bedeutung für die Therapie der Erkrankung. *Strahlenther.* 131:482–504.

Musshoff, K., Busch, M. and Kaminski, H. (1964). Lymphogranulomatose (Morbus Hodgkin) mit Knochenbefall. Symptomatologie mit besonderer Berücksichtigung des Röntgenbildes, Therapie und Prognose. Ein Bericht über 66 Fälle (Freiburger Krankengut 1948-1961). *Fortschr. Geb. Röntgenstr.* 101:117–137.

Musshoff, K., Hartmann, Chr., Niklaus, B. and Rössner, R. (1976). The prognostic significance of first and second remission after first and second relapse radiotherapy in Hodgkin's disease. *Z. Krebsforsch* 85:243–270.

Musshoff, K., Renemann, H., Boutis, L. and Afkham, J. (1968). Die extranoduläre Lymphogranulomatose. Diagnose, Therapie und Prognose bei zwei unterschiedlichen Formen des Organbefalls. Ein Beitrag zur Stadieneinteilung des Morbus Hodgkin. *Fortschr. Geb. Röntgenstr.* 109:776–786.

Musshoff, K., Stamm, H., Lummel, G., and Gössel, K. (1964). Zur Prognose der Lymphogranulomatose. Klinisches Bild und Strahlentherapie. Freiburger Krankengut 1938-1958. *Beitrag Inn. Med.* Stuttgart: F. K. Schattauer-Verlag. pp. 549–561.

Myers, C. E., Chabner, B. A., De Vita, V. T. and Gralnick, H. R. (1974). Bone marrow involvement in Hodgkin's disease: pathology and response to MOPP chemotherapy. *Blood* 44:197–204.

Myers, M. H. and Axtell, L. M. (1973). Statistical procedures for evaluating survival in Hodgkin's disease. *Nat. Cancer Inst. Monograph* 36:555–559.

Naeim, F., Waisman, J. and Coulson, W. F. (1974). Hodgkin's disease: the significance of vascular invasion. *Cancer* 34:655–662.

Nagata, Y., Hayakawa, T. and Ariyama, Y. (1966). Autopsy case of Hodgkin's disease originating in the appendix. *Jap. J. Clin. Med.* 24:791–795.

Nahhas, W. A., Nisce, L. Z., D'Angio, G. J. and Lewis, J. L., Jr. (1971). Lateral ovarian transposition. Ovarian relocation in patients with Hodgkin's disease. *Obstet. Gynecol.* 38:785–788.

Najjar, V. A. and Nishioka, K. (1970). "Tuftsin": a natural phagocytosis stimulating peptide. *Nature* 228:672–673.

Nanba, K., Itagaki, T. and Iijima, S. (1975). Enzyme histochemical investigations of human malignant lymphomas. *Beitr. Path.* 154:233–242.

Nathanson, I. T. and Welch, C. E. (1937). Life expectancy and incidence of malignant disease. V. Malignant lymphoma, fibrosarcoma, malignant melanoma, and osteogenic sarcoma. *Am. J. Cancer* 31:598–608.

Navone, R., Palestro, G. and Resegotti, L. (1975). Quantitative studies of macrophages in blood cultures in Hodgkin's disease. *Acta Haematol.* 53:25–29.

Naysmith, A. and Hancock, B. W. (1976). Hodgkin's disease and pemphigus. *Brit. J. Dermatol.* 94:695–696.

Neely, R. A. and Neill, D. W. (1956). Electrophoretic studies on the serum proteins in neoplastic disease involving the haemopoietic and reticuloendothelial systems. *Brit. J. Haematol.* 2:32–40.

Neiman, R. S., Rosen, P. J. and Lukes, R. J. (1973). Lymphocyte-depletion Hodgkin's disease. A clinicopathologic entity. *New Engl. J. Med.* 288:751–755.

Neufeld, H., Weinerman, B. H. and Kemel, S. (1978). Secondary malignant neoplasms in patients with Hodgkin's disease. *J.A.M.A.* 239:2470–2471.

Newberry, W. M. and Sanford, J. P. (1971). Defective cellular immunity in renal failure: depression of reactivity of lymphocytes to phytohemagglutinin by renal failure serum. *J. Clin. Invest.* 50:1262–1271.

Newberry, W. M., Shorey, J. W., J. P. Sanford, and Combes, B. (1973). Depression of lymphocyte reactivity to phytohemagglutinin by serum from patients with liver disease. *Cell Immunol.* 6:87–97.

Newbold, P. C. H. (1970). Skin markers of malignancy. *Arch. Dermatol.* 102:680–692.

Newell, G. R. (1972). Seasonal occurrence of Hodgkin's disease. *Lancet* 1:1024–1025.

Newell, G. R., Cole, S. R., Miettinen, O. S. and MacMahon, B. (1970). Age differences in the histology of Hodgkin's disease. *J. Nat. Cancer Inst.* 45:311–317.

Newell, G. R., Harris, W. W., Bowman, K. O., Boone, C. W. and Anderson, N. G. (1968). Evaluation of "virus-like" particles in the plasmas of 255 patients with leukemia and related diseases. *New Engl. J. Med.* 278:1185–1191.

Newell, G. R. and Rawlings, W. (1972). Evidence for environmental factors in the etiology of Hodgkin's disease. *J. Chronic Dis.* 25:261–267.

Newell, G. R., Rawlings, W., Kinnear, B. K., Correa, P., Henderson, B. E., Dworsky, R., Menck, H., Thompson, R. and Sheehan, W. W. (1973). Case-control study of Hodgkin's disease. I. Results of the interview questionnaire. *J. Nat. Cancer Inst.* 51:1437–1441.

Newman, D. R., Maldonado, J. E., Harrison, E. G., Jr., Kiely, J. M. and Linman, J. W. (1970). Myelomonocytic leukemia in Hodgkin's disease. *Cancer* 25:128–134.

Neyazaki, T., Kupic, E. A., Marshall, W. H. and Abrams, H. L. (1965). Collateral lymphatico-venous communication after experimental obstruction of the thoracic duct. *Radiology* 85:423–431.

Niblett, J. S. (1975). Forty-year survival in Hodgkin's disease with calcified lymph nodes. *Brit. J. Radiol.* 48:396–400.

Nice, C. M. and Stenstrom, K. W. (1954). Irradiation therapy in Hodgkin's disease. *Radiology* 62:641–653.

Nicholson, W. M., Beard, M. E. J., Crowther, D., Stansfeld, A. G., Vartan, C. T., Malpas, J. S., Fairley, G. H. and Bodley Scott, R. (1970). Combination chemotherapy in generalized Hodgkin's disease. *Brit. Med. J.* 3:7–10.

Nickels, J., Franssila, K. and Hjelt, L. (1973). Thymoma and Hodgkin's disease of the thymus. *Acta Path. Microbiol. Scand.* 81:1–5.

Nickson, J. J. (1966). Hodgkin's disease clinical trial. *Cancer Res.* 26:1279–1283.

Nickson, J. J. and Hutchison, G. B. (1972). Extensions of disease, complications of therapy, and deaths in localized Hodgkin's disease: preliminary report of a clinical trial. *Am. J. Roentgenol.* 114:564–573.

Niederman, J. C., McCollum, R. W., Henle, G. and Henle, W. (1968). Infectious mononucleosis: clinical manifestations in relation to EB virus antibodies. *J.A.M.A.* 203:205–209.

Nilsen, L. B., Missal, M. E. and Condemi, J. J. (1967). Appearance of Hodgkin's disease in a patient with systemic lupus erythematosus. *Cancer* 20:1930–1933.

Nilsson, K. and Pontén, J. (1975). Classification and biological nature of established human hematopoietic cell lines. *Internat. J. Cancer* 15:321–341.

Nisce, L. Z. and D'Angio, G. J. (1973). A new technique for the irradiation of large fields in patients with lymphoma. *Radiology* 106:641–644.

Nishioka, K., Constantopoulos, A., Satoh, P. S. and Najjar, V. A. (1972). The characteristics, isolation and synthesis of the phagocytosis stimulating peptide tuftsin. *Biochem. Biophys. Res. Commun.* 47:172–179.

Nishiyama, H. and Inoue, T. (1970). Some epidemiological features of Hodgkin's disease in Japan. *Gann* 61:197–205.

Nissen, N. I., Pajak, T. F., Glidewell, O., Pedersen-Bjergaard, J., Stutzman, L., Falkson, G., Cuttner, J., Blom, J., Leone, L., Sawitsky, A., Coleman, M., Haurani, F., Spurr, C. L., Jones, B., Seligman, B., Cornell, C., Jr., Henry, P., Senn, H., Brunner, K., Martz, G., Maurice, P. and Holland, J. F. (1979). A comparative study of a BCNU containing 4-drug program versus MOPP versus 3-drug combinations in advanced Hodgkin's disease. A cooperative study by the Cancer and Leukemia Group B. *Cancer* 43:31–40.

Nixon, D. W. and Aisenberg, A. C. (1974). Combination chemotherapy of Hodgkin's disease. *Cancer* 33:1499–1504.

Noble, R. L., Beer, C. T. and Cutts, J. H. (1958a) Role of chance observations in chemotherapy: *Vinca rosea*. *Ann. New York Acad. Sci.* 76:882–894.

Noble, R. L., Beer, C. T. and Cutts, J. H. (1958b). Further biological activities of vincaleukoblastine—an alkaloid isolated from *Vinca rosea* (L). *Biochem. Pharmacol.* 1:347–348.

Nobrega, F. T., Kyle, R. A. and Harrison, E. G., Jr. (1973). Malignant lymphoma including Hodgkin's disease occurring in the vicinity of a large medical center (Olmsted County, Minn., 1945 through 1969). *Cancer* 31:295–302.

Noetzli, M. and Sheline, G. E. (1962). Local recurrence in lymph nodes irradiated for Hodgkin's disease. *In* Progress in Radiation Therapy, F. Buschke (ed.). New York: Grune and Stratton. Vol. 2, pp. 188–194.

Nonoyama, M., Kawai, Y., Huang, C. H., Pagano, J. S., Hirshaut, Y. and Levine, P. H. (1974). Epstein-Barr virus DNA in Hodgkin's disease, American Burkitt's lymphoma, and other human tumors. *Cancer Res.* 34:1228–1231.

Nonoyama, M. and Pagano, J. S. (1973). Homology between Epstein-Barr virus DNA and viral DNA from Burkitt's lymphoma and nasopharyngeal carcinoma determined by DNA-DNA reassociation kinetics. *Nature* 242:44–47.

Nooter, K., Aarssen, A. M., Bentvelzen, P., de Groot, F. G., and van Pelt, F. G. (1975). Isolation of infectious C-type oncornavirus from human leukaemic bone marrow cells. *Nature* 256:595–597.

Nordentoft, A. M., Jensen, K. B., Andersen, E., Videbaek, A., Nielsen, H. M., Hansen, L. K., Hastrup, J. and Madsen, B. (1973). Diagnostic laparotomy in Hodgkin's disease. *Danish Med. Bull.* 20:33–41.

Nordman, E. (1977). Complications after megavoltage therapy of Hodgkin's disease. *Ann. Clin. Res.* 9:35–38.

Nováková, I. (1978). Diagnosis, treatment and prognosis in 20 patients with 24 cases of spinal cord compression caused by epidural localization of malignant lymphomas. *Nederl. Tijdschr. Geneesk.* 122:184–187.

Nowell, P. C. (1960). Phytohemagglutinin: an initiator of mitosis in cultures of normal human lymphocytes. *Cancer Res.* 20:462–466.

Oberling, C. (1928). Les réticulosarcomes et les réticuloendothéliosarcomes de la moelle osseuse (sarcomes d'Ewing). *Bull. assoc. franç. étude du cancer* 17:259–296.

Obrecht, P. and Caspers, I. (1960). Zur Frage des Therapieeinflusses bei Lymphogranulomatose. *Schweiz. Med. Wchnschr.* 90:1202–1205.

O'Carroll, D. L., McKenna, R. W. and Brunning, R. D. (1976). Bone marrow manifestations of Hodgkin's disease. *Cancer* 38:1717–1728.

O'Connell, M. J., Schimpff, S. F., Kirschner, R. H., Abt, A. B. and Wiernik, P. H. (1975a). Epithelioid granulomas in Hodgkin's disease—a favorable prognostic sign? *J.A.M.A.* 233:886–889.

O'Connell, M. J., Wiernik, P. H., Brace, K. C., Byhardt, R. W. and Greene, W. H. (1975b). A combined modality approach to the treatment of Hodgkin's disease. Preliminary results of a prospectively randomized clinical trial. *Cancer* 35:1055–1065.

O'Connell, M. J., Wiernik, P. H., Sklansky, B. D., Greene, W. H., Abt, A. B., Kirschner, R. H., Ramsey, H. E. and Murphy, W. L. (1974). Staging laparotomy in Hodgkin's disease. Further evidence in support of its clinical utility. *Am. J. Med.* 57:86–91.

O'Gara, R. W., Adamson, R. H., Kelly, M. G. and Dalgard, D. W. (1971). Neoplasms of the hematopoietic system in non-human primates—report of one spontaneous tumor and two leukemias induced by Procarbazine. *J. Nat. Cancer Inst.* 46:1121–1130.

Okada, H. and Nishioka, K. (1973). Complement receptors on cell membranes. I. Evidence for two complement receptors. *J. Immunol.* 111:1444–1449.

Olinici, C. D. (1972). Cytogenetic observations on different cell lines in Hodgkin's disease. *Acta Haematol.* 48:283–287.

Olisa, E. G., Kovi, J., Kennedy, J., Kish, M. H., Lanava, T. S. and Williams, A. O. (1976). Hodgkin's disease in American Negroes. Histologic classification of the disease in 143 untreated patients, and age distribution. *Am. J. Clin. Path.* 66:537–544.

Ollivier, A. and Ranvier, L. (1867). Observation pour servir a l'histoire de l'adénie. *In* Mémoires lus à le société de biologie, pp. 99–112.

Olmer, J., Paillas, J., Roger, J., Muratore, R. and Badier, M. (1952). Manifestations ganglionnaires au cours de traitements par la methyl-3-phenyl-ethyl 5-5 hydantoine. *Presse méd.* 60:1748–1750.

Olweny, C. L., Katongole-Mbidde, E., Kiire, C., Lwanga, S. K., Magrath, I. and Ziegler, J. L. (1978). Childhood Hodgkin's disease in Uganda: a ten year experience. *Cancer* 42:787–792.

Olweny, C. L., Ziegler, J. L., Bernard, C. and Templeton, A. C. (1971). Adult Hodgkin's disease in Uganda. *Cancer* 27:1295–1301.

Oort, J. and Turk, J. L. (1965). A histologic and autoradiographic study of lymph nodes during the development of contact sensitivity in the guinea pig. *Brit. J. Exper. Path.* 46:147–154.

Opler, S. R. (1967). Animal model of viral oncogenesis. *Nature* 215:184.

Order, S. E., Bloomer, W. D., Jones, A. G., Kaplan, W. D., Davis, M. A., Adelstein, S. J. and Hellman, S. (1975). Radionuclide immunoglobulin lymphangiography: a case report. *Cancer* 35:1487–1492.

Order, S. E., Colgan, J. and Hellman, S. (1974). Distribution of fast-and slow-migrating Hodgkin's tumor-associated antigens. *Cancer Res.* 34:1182–1186.

Order, S. E. and Hellman, S. (1972). Pathogenesis of Hodgkin's disease. *Lancet* 1:571–573.

Order, S. E., Porter, M., and Hellman, S. (1971). Hodgkin's disease: evidence for a tumor associated antigen. *New Engl. J. Med.* 285:471–474.

Osgood, E. E. (1958). Methods for analyzing survival data, illustrated by Hodgkin's disease. *Am. J. Med.* 24:40–47.

Osserman, E. F. and Lawlor, D. P. (1966). Serum and urinary lysozyme (muramidase) in monocytic and monomyelocytic leukemia. *J. Exper. Med.* 124:921–952.

Osta, S., Wells, M., Viamonte, M. and Harkness, D. (1970). Hodgkin's disease terminating in acute leukemia. *Cancer* 26:795–799.

Ouyang, A., Chao, C. H., Chao, C. T., Hsi, Y. J. and Liu, C. M. (1966). Reed-Sternberg cell leukemia. Report of a case. *Chin. Med. J.* 85:124–129.

Pack, G. T. and Molander, D. W. (1966). The surgical treatment of Hodgkin's disease. *Cancer Res.* 26:1254–1263.

Paffenbarger, R. S., Jr., Wing, A. L. and Hyde, R. T. (1977). Characteristics in youth indicative of adult-onset Hodgkin's disease. *J. Nat. Cancer Inst.* 58:1489–1491.

Pagano, J. S., Huang, C. H. and Levine, P. (1973). Absence of Epstein-Barr viral DNA in American Burkitt's lymphoma. *New Engl. J. Med.* 289:1395–1399.

Page, A. R., Hansen, A. E. and Good, R. A. (1963). Occurrence of leukemia and lymphoma in patients with agammaglobulinemia. *Blood* 21:197–206.

Page, V., Gardner, A. and Karzmark, C. J. (1970a). Physical and dosimetric aspects of the radiotherapy of malignant lymphomas. I. The mantle technique. *Radiology* 96:609–618.

Page, V., Gardner, A. and Karzmark, C. J. (1970b). Physical and dosimetric aspects of the radiotherapy of malignant lymphomas. II. The inverted-Y technique. *Radiology* 96:619–626.

Paglia, M. A., Lacher, M. J., Hertz, R. E. L., Geller, W., Watson, R. C., Lewis, J. L., Nisce, L. Z. and Lieberman, P. H. (1973). Surgical aspects and results of laparotomy and splenectomy in Hodgkin's disease. *Am. J. Roentgenol.* 117:12–18.

Pagliardi, E., Cravario, A., Brusa, L., Cantino, D. and Giangrandi, E. (1963). Indigene sul metabolismo del rame nel morbo di Hodgkin. *Haematol.* 48:209–228.

Pagliardi, E. and Giangrandi, E. (1960). Clinical significance of the blood copper in Hodgkin's disease. *Acta Haemat.* 24:201–212.

Palmer, C. G., Livengood, D., Warren, A. K., Simpson, P. J. and Johnson, I. S. (1960). The action of vincaleukoblastine on mitosis *in vitro*. *Exper. Cell Res.* 20:198–201.

Palos, B., Kaplan, H. S. and Karzmark, C. J. (1971). The use of "thin" lead lung shields to deliver limited whole lung irradiation during mantle field treatment of Hodgkin's disease. *Radiology* 101:441–442.

Papatestas, H. E., Genkins, G. and Kark, A. E. (1973). Thymus transplantation in leukemia and malignant lymphogranulomatosis. *Lancet* 2:795.

Papillon, J. (1974). The curability of Hodgkin's disease. *In* Diagnosis and Therapy of Malignant Lymphoma, K. Musshoff (ed.). Berlin: Springer-Verlag, pp. 195–200.

Papillon, J., Chassard, J. L. and Contamin, A. (1966a). Problème de la dose optimale dans l'irradiation de la maladie de Hodgkin. *Nouv. rev. franç. hématol.* 6:161–163.

Papillon, J., Croizat, P., Revol, L., Chassard, J. L., Feroldi, J., Contamin, A. and Dutou, L. (1966b). Les survies de plus de 10 ans dans la maladie de Hodgkin. *Nouv. rev. franç. hématol.* 6:79–83.

Papillon, J., Croizat, P., Revol, L., Chassard, J. L., Chassard, E. and Contamin, A. (1966c). Le pronostic de la maladie de Hodgkin. *J. de radiol. et d'électrol.* 47:381–390.

Pappas, A., Pees, H. and Girmann, G. (1977). A micromethod for PHA-induced stimulation of human lymphocytes. II. Communication: effect of splenectomy on the inhibitory activity of serum in patients with Hodgkin's disease. *Z. Immun.-Forsch.* 153:1–10.

Parker, B. R., Blank, N. and Castellino, R. A. (1974). Lymphographic appearance of benign conditions simulating lymphoma. *Radiology* 111:267–274.

Parker, F., Jr., Jackson, H., Jr., Fitzhugh, G. and Spies, T. D. (1932). Studies of diseases of the lymphoid and myeloid tissues. IV. Skin reactions to human and avian tuberculin. *J. Immunol.* 22:277–282.

Parker, J. C., Jr. (1972). Intramedullary spinal cord involvement in Hodgkin's disease with an atypical systemic distribution. *Cancer* 30:545–552.

Parks, W. P. and Scolnick, E. M. (1972). Radioimmunoassay of mammalian type-C viral proteins: interspecies antigenic reactivities of the major internal polypeptide. *Proc. Nat. Acad. Sci. U.S.* 69:1766–1770.

Parks, W. P., Scolnick, E. M., Ross, J., Todaro, G. J. and Aaronson, S. A. (1972). Immunologic relationships of reverse transcriptases from ribonucleic acid tumor viruses. *J. Virol.* 9:110–115.

Parmentier, C., Askienazy, S., Gérard-Marchant, R., Lacour, J., Amiel, J.-L., Lemerle, J. and Tubiana, M. (1969). Confrontations entre les données de la scintigraphie splénique et les constatations anatomiques dans la maladie de Hodgkin. (A propos de 20 observations.) *Ann. Radiol.* 12:43–56.

Parmley, R. T., Spicer, S. S. and Garvin, A. J. (1976). Multilaminar endoplasmic reticulum and abnormal mitosis in Hodgkin's disease. *Cancer Res.* 36:1717–1724.

Parmley, R., Spicer, S., Morgan, S. and Grash, O. (1975). Ultrastructural and immunochemical studies in a patient with Hodgkin's disease and acute monomyelogenous leukemia. *Blood* 46:1013 (abst.).

Parsons, P. B. and Poston, M. A. (1939). Pathology of human brucellosis; a report of 4 cases with one autopsy. *South. Med. J.* 32:7–13.

Patchefsky, A. S., Brodovsky, H., Southard, M., Menduke, H., Gray, S. and Hoch, W. S. (1973). Hodgkin's disease. A clinical and pathologic study of 235 cases. *Cancer* 32:150–161.

Paterson, E. (1958). The evaluation of chemotherapeutic compounds in the reticuloses. *Brit. J. Cancer* 12:332–341.

Paterson, R. and Tod, M. (1953). Reticulo-endothelial system. *In* The Treatment of Malignant Disease by Radium and X-ray, R. Paterson (ed.). London: Edw. Arnold. pp. 414–437.

Patey, D. H. (1963). A contribution to the study of Hodgkin's disease. *Brit. J. Surg.* 50:389–392.

Payne, S. V., Jones, D. B., Haegert, D. G., Smith, J. L. and Wright, D. H. (1976). T and B lymphocytes and Reed-Sternberg cells in Hodgkin's disease lymph nodes and spleens. *Clin. Exper. Immunol.* 24:280–286.

Pearmain, G., Lycette, R. R. and Fitzgerald, P. H. (1963). Tuberculin induced mitosis in peripheral blood lymphocytes. *Lancet* 1:637–638.

Pearson, H. A., Johnston, D., Smith, K. A. and Touloukian, R. J. (1978). The born-again spleen. Return of splenic function after splenectomy for trauma. *New Engl. J. Med.* 298:1389–1392.

Peck, B. (1976). Hypertrophic osteoarthropathy with Hodgkin's disease in the mediastinum. *J.A.M.A.* 238:1400–1401.

Peckham, M. J. (1973). Quantitative cytology and cytochemistry of Hodgkin's tissue labelled *in vivo* with tritiated thymidine. *Brit. J. Cancer* 28:332–339.

Peckham, M. J. and Cooper, E. H. (1969). Proliferation characteristics of the various classes of cells in Hodgkin's disease. *Cancer* 24:135–146.

Peckham, M. J. and Cooper, E. H. (1973). Cell proliferation in Hodgkin's disease. *Nat. Cancer Inst. Monograph* 36:179–189.

Peckham, M. J., Ford, H. T., McElwain, T. J., Harmer, C. L., Atkinson, K. and Austin, D. E. (1975). The results of radiotherapy for Hodgkin's disease. *Brit. J. Cancer* 32:391–400.

Pecori, V., Turrisi, E., Altucci, P. and Buonanno, G. (1959). Behavior of C-reactive protein in malignant blood diseases, with special regard to Hodgkin's lymphogranuloma. *Riforma med.* 73:1–3.

Pel, P. K. (1887). Zur Symptomatologie der sogenannten Pseudoleukämie. II. Pseudoleukämie oder chronisches Rückfallsfieber? *Berlin Klin. Wchnschr.* 24:644–646.

Penn, I. (1976). Second malignant neoplasms associated with immunosuppressive medications. *Cancer* 37: 1024–1032.

Perera, D. R., Greene, M. L. and Fenster, L. F. (1974). Cholestasis associated with extrabiliary Hodgkin's disease. Report of three cases and review of four others. *Gastroenterology* 67:680–685.

Perez-Tamayo, R., Thornbury, J. R. and Atkinson, R. J. (1963). "Secondary-look" lymphangiography. *Am. J. Roentgenol.* 90:1078–1086.

Perlin, E., Levine, P. H., McCoy, J., Dean, J. and Herberman, R. (1976). Hodgkin's disease in siblings: a family study. *Oncology* 33:116–118.

Perlin, E., Ryan, T. F., Ebersole, J. H., Wilson, T. H. and Moquin, R. B. (1972). Diagnostic laparotomy and splenectomy in the clinical staging of Hodgkin's disease. *Military Med.* 137:97–102.

Perttala, Y. and Kijanen, I. (1965). Roentgenologic bone lesions in lymphogranulomatosis maligna. Analysis of 453 cases. *Ann. Chir. Gyn. Fenn.* 54:414–424.

Perttala, Y. and Svinhufvud, U. (1965). Cavity formation in the lung in Hodgkin's disease; analysis of 453 cases. *Ann. Med. Int. Fenn.* 54:19–24.

Peters, M. V. (1950). A study of survivals in Hodgkin's disease treated radiologically. *Am. J. Roentgenol.* 63: 299–311.

Peters, M. V. (1961). The place of irradiation in the control of Hodgkin's disease. *In* Proceedings of the 4th National Cancer Conference, 1960. Philadelphia: J. B. Lippincott Co. pp. 571–584.

Peters, M. V. (1966). Prophylactic treatment of adjacent areas in Hodgkin's disease. *Cancer Res.* 26:1232–1243.

Peters, M. V. (1973). The evolution of the radiotherapeutic concept in Hodgkin's disease. *Ser. Haemat.* 6:117–138.

Peters, M. V., Alison, R. E. and Bush, R. S. (1966). Natural history of Hodgkin's disease as related to staging. *Cancer* 19:308–316.

Peters, M. V., Hasselback, R. and Brown, T. C. (1968). The natural history of the lymphomas related to the clinical classification. *In* Proceedings of the International Conference on Leukemia-Lymphoma, C. J. D. Zarafonetis (ed.). Philadelphia: Lea and Febiger. pp. 357–370.

Peters, M. V. and Middlemiss, K. C. H. (1958). A study of Hodgkin's disease treated by irradiation. *Am. J. Roentgenol.* 79:114–121.

Petersen, G. R. and Milham, S., Jr. (1974). Hodgkin's disease mortality and occupational exposure to wood. *J. Nat. Cancer Inst.* 53:957–958.

Petrakis, N. L., Bostick, W. L. and Siegel, B. V. (1959). The deoxyribonucleic acid (DNA) content of Sternberg-Reed cells of Hodgkin's disease. *J. Nat. Cancer Inst.* 22:551–554.

Pezzimenti, J. F., Bruckner, H. W. and DeConti, R. C.

(1973). Paralytic brachial neuritis in Hodgkin's disease. *Cancer* 31:626–629.

Philips, F. S., Sternberg, S. S., Cronin, A. P. and Vidol, P. M. (1961). Cyclophosphamide and urinary bladder toxicity. *Cancer Res.* 21:1577–1589.

Phillips, T. L. and Fu, K. K. (1976). Quantification of combined radiation therapy and chemotherapy effects on critical normal tissues. *Cancer* 37:1186–1200.

Phillips, T. L. and Margolis, L. (1972). Radiation pathology and the clinical response of lung and esophagus. *Front. Rad. Ther. Oncol.* 6:254–273.

Pick, R. A., Castellino, R. A., and Seltzer, R. A. (1971). Arteriographic findings in renal lymphoma. *Am. J. Roentgenol.* 111:530–534.

Pierce, C. B., Jacox, H. W. and Hildreth, R. C. (1936). Roentgenologic considerations of lymphoblastoma. Roentgen pulmonary pathology of the Hodgkin's type. *Am. J. Roentgenol.* 36:145–164.

Pierce, R. H., Hafermann, M. D. and Kagan, A. R. (1969). Changes in the transverse cardiac diameter following mediastinal irradiation for Hodgkin's disease. *Radiology* 93:619–624.

Piessens, W. F. and Zeicher, M. (1970). Hodgkin's disease causing a reversible nephrotic syndrome by compression of the inferior vena cava. *Cancer* 25:880–884.

Pike, M. C. and Smith, P. G. (1973). Tonsillectomy and Hodgkin's disease. *Lancet* 1:434.

Pike, M . C. and Smith, P. G. (1974). Clustering of cases of Hodgkin's disease and leukemia. *Cancer* 34:1390–1394.

Pike, M. C., Thompson Hancock, P. E. and Ledlie, E. M. (1967). Treatment of early Hodgkin's disease. *Lancet* 2:1361.

Pilepich, M. V., Rene, J. B., Munzenrider, J. E. and Carter, B. L. (1978). Contribution of computed tomography to the treatment of lymphomas. *Am. J. Roentgenol.* 131:69–73.

Pilotti, S. and Rilke, F. (1972). La diagnosis citologica nella patologia linfonodale. *Tumori* 58:289–317.

Pinkard, K. J., Cooper, I. A., Motteram, R. and Turner, C. N. (1972). Purine and pyrimidine excretion in Hodgkin's disease. *J. Nat. Cancer Inst.* 49:27–38.

Pinkus, H. (1964). The relationship of alopecia mucinosa to malignant lymphoma. *Dermatologica* 129:266–270.

Piquet-Gauthier, G., Perrin, J., Vauzelle, J. L. and Revol, L. (1965). Maladie de Hodgkin avec envahissement vésical. A propos d'une observation récente. *Lyon méd.* 213:1869–1878.

Piringer-Kuchinka, A. (1953). Eigenartiger mikroskopischer befund an exzidierten Lymphknoten. *Verh. Deut. Ges. Path.* 36:352–362.

Piringer-Kuchinka, A., Martin, I. and Thalhammer, O. (1958). Über die vorzuglich cervico-nuchale Lymphadenitis mid kleinherdiger Epitheliodzellwucherung. *Virchow's Arch. f. Path. Anat.* 331:522–535.

Piro, A. J., Hellman, S. and Moloney, W. C. (1972). The influence of laparotomy on management decisions in Hodgkin's disease. *Arch. Int. Med.* 130:844–848.

Piro, A. J., Weiss, D. R. and Hellman, S. (1976). Mediastinal Hodgkin's disease: a possible danger for intubation anesthesia. *Internat. J. Radiat. Oncol. Biol. Phys.* 1:415–419.

Plager, J. and Stutzman, L. (1971). Acute nephrotic syndrome as a manifestation of active Hodgkin's disease.

Report of four cases and review of the literature. *Am. J. Med.* 50:56–66.

Pontén, J. (1967). Spontaneous lymphoblastoid transformation of long-term cell cultures from human malignant lymphoma. *Internat. J. Cancer* 2:311–325.

Pitcock, J. A., Bauer, W. A. and McGavran, M. H. (1959). Hodgkin's disease in children; a clinicopathologic study of 46 cases. *Cancer* 12:1043–1051.

Pope, J. H., Achong, B. G., Epstein, M. A. and Biddulph, J. (1967). Burkitt lymphoma in New Guinea: the establishment of a line of lymphoblasts *in vitro* and description of their fine structure. *J. Nat. Cancer Inst.* 39:933–945.

Portlock, C. S., Robertson, A., Turbow, M. M. and Rosenberg, S. A. (1976). MOPP chemotherapy for advanced Hodgkin's disease: prognostic factors in 242 patients. *Proc. Am. Soc. Clin. Oncol.* 17:248 (abst.).

Portlock, C. S., Rosenberg, S. A., Glatstein, E. and Kaplan, H. S. (1978). Impact of salvage treatment on initial relapses in patients with Hodgkin's disease, stages I–III. *Blood* 51:825–833.

Portmann, U. V., Dunne, E. F. and Hazard, J. B. (1954). Manifestations of Hodgkin's disease of the gastrointestinal tract. *Am. J. Roentgenol.* 72:772–787.

Porzig, K. J., Portlock, C. S., Robertson, A. and Rosenberg, S. A. (1978). Treatment of advanced Hodgkin's disease with B-CAVe following MOPP failure. *Cancer* 41:1670–1675.

Potolsky, A. I., Heath, C. W., Jr., Buckley, C. E., III and Rowlands, D. T., Jr. (1971). Lymphoreticular malignancies and immunologic abnormalities in a sibship. *Am. J. Med.* 50:42–48.

Poulsen, H., Bengmark, S., Borjesson, B., Flodgren, P., Kallum, B. and Landberg, T. (1977). Staging laparotomy with splenectomy in Hodgkin's disease. *Acta Chir. Scand.* 143:347–352.

Poussin-Rosillo, H., Nisce, L. Z. and D'Angio, G. J. (1976). Hepatic radiation tolerance in Hodgkin's disease patients. *Radiology* 121:461–464.

Poussin-Rosillo, H., Nisce, L. Z. and Lee, B. J. (1978). Complications of total nodal irradiation of Hodgkin's disease stages III and IV. *Cancer* 42:437–441.

Powers, W. E., Kinzie, J. J., Demidecki, A. J., Bradfield, J. J. and Feldman, A. (1973). A new system of field shaping for external-beam radiation therapy. *Radiology* 108:407–411.

Prager, D., Sembrot, J. T. and Southard, M. (1972). Cobalt-60 therapy of Hodgkin's disease and the subsequent development of hypothyroidism. *Cancer* 29:458–460.

Prandi, G., Alessi, E., Stefani, B. and Brugo, A. (1977). La papulose lymphomatoide. Role possible des IgA dans sa pathogénèse. *Ann. Dermatol. Venereol.* 104:165–166.

Prentice, R. T. W. (1965). Myocardial infarction following radiation. *Lancet* 2:388.

Press, B. O. and Shvetsova, F. V. (1975). Activity of non-specific esterase and acid phosphatase in Berezovsky-Sternberg's giant cells in patients with lymphogranulomatosis. *Probl. Gematol. Pereliv. Krovi.* 20:22–25.

Pretlow, T. G., II. (1978). Isolation of lymphocyte populations. *Nat. Cancer Inst. Monograph* 49:79–84.

Pretlow, T. G., II, Luberoff, D. E., Hamilton, L. J., Weinberger, P. C., Maddox, W. A. and Durant, J. R. (1973). Pathogenesis of Hodgkin's disease: separation and cul-

ture of different kinds of cells from Hodgkin's disease in a sterile isokinetic gradient of Ficoll in tissue culture medium. *Cancer* 31:1120–1126.

Price, P. J., Suk, W. A., Skeen, P. C., Chirigos, M. A. and Huebner, R. J. (1975). Transforming potential of the anticancer drug Adriamycin. *Science* 187:1200–1201.

Priesel, A. and Winkelbauer, A. (1926). Placentare Uebertragung des Lymphogranuloma. *Virchows Arch. path. Anat.* 262:749–765.

Primikirios, N., Stutzman, L. and Sandberg, A. A. (1961). Uric acid excretion in patients with malignant lymphomas. *Blood* 17:701–718.

Probert, J. C. and Parker, B. R. (1975). The effects of radiation therapy on bone growth. *Radiology* 114:155–162.

Probert, J. C., Parker, B. R. and Kaplan, H. S. (1973). Growth retardation in children after megavoltage irradiation of the spine. *Cancer* 32:634–639.

Prosnitz, L. R., Farber, L. R., Fischer, J. J. and Bertino, J. R. (1973). Low dose radiation therapy and combination chemotherapy in the treatment of advanced Hodgkin's disease. *Radiology* 107:187–193.

Prosnitz, L. R., Farber, L. R., Fischer, J. J., Bertino, J. R. and Fischer, D. B. (1976). Long term remissions with combined modality therapy for advanced Hodgkin's disease. *Cancer* 37:2826–2833.

Prosnitz, L. R., Hellman, S., Von Essen, C. F. and Kligerman, M. M. (1969). The clinical course of Hodgkin's disease and other malignant lymphomas treated with radical radiation therapy. *Am. J. Roentgenol.* 105:618–628.

Prosnitz, L. R., Montalvo, R. I., Fischer, D. B., Silverstein, A. B. and Berger, D. S. (1978). Treatment of stage IIIA Hodgkin's disease: is radiotherapy alone adequate? *Internat. J. Radiat. Oncol. Biol. Phys.* 4:781–789.

Prosnitz, L. R., Nuland, S. B. and Kligerman, M. M. (1972). Role of laparotomy and splenectomy in the management of Hodgkin's disease. *Cancer* 29:44–50.

Pusey, W. A. (1902). Cases of sarcoma and of Hodgkin's disease treated by exposures to X-rays: a preliminary report. *J.A.M.A.* 38:166–169.

Quaglino, D., Emilia, G., DiPrisco, A. U., DePasquale, A. and Zagni, G. (1975). Evoluzione terminale leucemica in un paziente con morbo di Hodgkin. *Minerva med.* 66:689–698.

Querleu, D., Vasseur, J. J., Triplet, I., Demaille, M. C., Crépin, G. and Demaille, A. (1977). Les métastases placentaires. *Rev. franç. gynéc.* 72:565–577.

Rabellino, E., Colon, S., Grey, H. M. and Unanue, E. R. (1971). Immunoglobulins on the surface of lymphocytes. I. Distribution and quantitation. *J. Exper. Med.* 133:156–167.

Rachmilewitz, B. and Rachmilewitz, M. (1976). Serum transcobalamin-II levels in acute leukemia and lymphoma. *Israel J. Med. Sci.* 12:583–586.

Raich, P. E., Carr, R. M., Meisner, L. F. and Korst, D. R. (1975). Acute granulocytic leukemia in Hodgkin's disease. *Am. J. Med. Sci.* 269:237–241.

Rall, D. T. and Zubrod, C. G. (1962). Mechanisms of drug absorption and excretion; passage of drugs in and out of the central nervous system. *Ann. Rev. Pharmacol.* 2:109–128.

Ramot, B., Biniaminov, M., Many, A. and Aghai, E. (1973). Thymus-derived lymphocyte (T-cell) depletion in Hodgkin's disease. *Israel J. Med. Sci.* 9:657–659.

Ramot, B., Biniaminov, M., Shoham, C. and Rosenthal, E. (1976). Effect of levamisole on E-rosette-forming cells *in vivo* and *in vitro* in Hodgkin's disease. *New Engl. J. Med.* 294:809–811.

Ramot, B., Shahin, M. and Bubis, J. J. (1965). Malabsorption syndrome in lymphoma of small intestine. *Israel J. Med. Sci.* 1:221–226.

Ramsey, N. M. (1975). Clustering of malignant lymphoma and Hodgkin's disease. *Med. J. Aust.* 2:779–780.

Ranlov, B. and Videbaek, A. (1963). Cyclic and haemolytic anaemia synchronous with Pel-Ebstein fever in a case of Hodgkin's disease. *Acta Med. Scand.* 174:583–588.

Ranney, H. M. and Gellhorn, A. (1957). The effect of massive prednisone and prednisolone therapy on acute leukemia and malignant lymphomas. *Am. J. Med.* 22:405–413.

Rao, G. U. V. and El-Mahdi, A. M. (1973). An optical minifier for shielding-block design in external-beam radiation therapy. *Radiology* 108:412.

Rappaport, H. (1966). Tumors of the Hematopoietic System. Atlas of Tumor Pathology, Section III, Fascicle 8, Armed Forces Institute of Pathology, Washington, D. C.

Rappaport, H., Berard, C. W., Butler, J. J., Dorfman, R. F., Lukes, R. J. and Thomas, L. B. (1971). Report of the committee on histopathological criteria contributing to staging of Hodgkin's disease. *Cancer Res.* 31:1864–1865.

Rappaport, H. and Strum, S. B. (1970). Vascular invasion in Hodgkin's disease: its incidence and relationship to the spread of the disease. *Cancer* 25:1304–1313.

Rappaport, H., Winter, W. J. and Hicks, E. B. (1956). Follicular lymphoma. A re-evaluation of its position in the scheme of malignant lymphoma, based on a survey of 253 cases. *Cancer* 9:792–821.

Rasker, J. J., van de Poll, M. A. P. C., Beekhuis, H., Woldring, M. G. and Nieweg, H. O. (1975). Some experience with ⁵⁷Co-labeled bleomycin as a tumor-seeking agent. *J. Nucl. Med.* 16:1058–1069.

Rassiga-Pidot, A. L. and McIntyre, O. R. (1974). *In vitro* leukocyte interferon production in patients with Hodgkin's disease. *Cancer Res.* 34:2995–3002.

Rather, L. J. (1972). Who discovered the pathognomonic giant cell of Hodgkin's disease? *Bull. New York Acad. Med.* 48:943–950.

Ratkóczy, N. (1936). Herdvernichtungsdosen in der Röntgentherapie der Lymphogranulomatose. *Strahlenther.* 56:325–336.

Ratti, A. (1962). La radioterapia endolinfatica con ¹³¹I: primi risultati, *Radiol. clin.* 31:220–228.

Ratti, A. and Chiappa, S. (1966). La lymphographie au Lipiodol radioactif dans la maladie de Hodgkin. *Nouv. rev. franç. hématol.* 6:155–156.

Rausing, A. and Trell, E. (1971). Malignant lymphogranulomatosis and anticonvulsant therapy. *Acta Med. Scand.* 189:131–136.

Ray, G. R., Trueblood, H. W., Enright, L. P., Kaplan, H. S. and Nelsen, T. S. (1970). Oophoropexy: a means of preserving ovarian function following pelvic megavoltage radiotherapy for Hodgkin's disease. *Radiology* 96:175–180.

Ray, G. R., Wolf, P. H. and Kaplan, H. S. (1973). Value of laboratory indicators in Hodgkin's disease: preliminary results. *Nat. Cancer Inst. Monograph* 36:315–323.

Razis, D., Diamond, H. and Craver, L. (1959a). Familial Hodgkin's disease: its significance and implications. *Ann. Int. Med.* 51:933–971.

Razis, D. V., Diamond, H. D. and Craver, L. F. (1959b). Hodgkin's disease associated with other malignant tumors and certain non-neoplastic diseases. *Am. J. Med. Sci.* 238:327–335.

Reagan, T. J. and Bennett, M. D. (1971). Intracerebral Hodgkin's disease. *Dis. Nerv. Syst.* 32:843–847.

Reboul, F., Donaldson, S. S. and Kaplan, H. S. (1978). Herpes zoster and varicella infections in children with Hodgkin's disease: an analysis of contributing factors. *Cancer* 41:95–99.

Redding, M. R., Anagnostopoulos, C. E. and Ultmann, J. E. (1971). The possible value of mediastinoscopy in staging Hodgkin's disease. *Cancer Res.* 31:1741–1745.

Redman, H. C., Glatstein, E., Castellino, R. A. and Federal, W. A. (1977). Computed tomography as an adjunct in the staging of Hodgkin's disease and non-Hodgkin's lymphomas. *Radiology* 124:381–385.

Reed, D. M. (1902). On the pathological changes in Hodgkin's disease, with especial reference to its relation to tuberculosis. *Johns Hopkins Hosp. Rep.* 10:133–196.

Reed, G. B., Jr. and Cox, A. J., Jr. (1966). The human liver after radiation injury: a form of veno-occlusive disease. *Am. J. Path.* 48:597–611.

Reedman, B. M. and Klein, G. (1973). Cellular localization of an Epstein-Barr virus (EBV)-associated complement-fixing antigen in producer and non-producer lymphoblastoid cell lines. *Internat. J. Cancer* 11:499–520.

Reeves, B. R. (1973). Cytogenetics of malignant lymphomas. *Humangenetik* 20:231–250.

Reiffers, J., Parsi, B., Hugues, A. and Hoerni, B. (1976). Hodgkin's disease localized in the thyroid gland. *Nouv. presse méd.* 5:1590.

Reiman, M. S., Stern, I. R., Ward, M. Z. and Hoster, H. A. (1950). Studies in Hodgkin's syndrome. XI. The influence of normal serum and Hodgkin's serum on cellular growth and morphology in tissue culture. *Cancer Res.* 10:467–473.

Reimann, H. A. (1977). Periodic (Pel-Ebstein) fever of lymphomas. *Ann. Clin. Lab. Sci.* 7:1–5.

Remington, J. S. (1972). The compromised host. *Hosp. Practice* 7:59–70.

Rewcastle, N. B. (1963). Subacute cerebellar degeneration with Hodgkin's disease. *Arch. Neurol.* 9:407–413.

Rewcastle, N. B. and Tom, M. I. (1962). Non-infectious granulomatous angiitis of the nervous system associated with Hodgkin's disease. *J. Neurol. Neurosurg. Psychiat.* 25:51–58.

Reynolds, H. Y., Atkinson, J. P., Newball, H. H. and Frank, M. M. (1975). Receptors for immunoglobulin and complement on human alveolar macrophages. *J. Immunol.* 114:1813–1819.

Ribacchi, R. and Giraldo, G. (1966). Leukemia virus release in chemically or physically induced lymphomas in BALB/c mice. *Nat. Cancer Inst. Monograph* 22:701–711.

Ricci, N., Punturieri, E., Bosi, L. and Castoldi, G. L. (1962). Chromosomes of Sternberg-Reed cells. *Lancet* 2:564.

Richmond, J., Sherman, R. S., Diamond, H. D. and

Craver, L. F. (1962). Renal lesions associated with malignant lymphomas. *Am. J. Med.* 32:184–207.

Rickard, C. G., Barr, L. M., Noronha, F., Dougherty, E. III and Post, J. E. (1967). C-type virus particles in spontaneous lymphocytic leukemia in a cat. *Cornell Vet.* 57:302–307.

Riederer, J. (1965). Ein Fall von primärer Lymphogranulomatose des Jejunums mit Dickdarmfistel. *Gastroenterologia* 104:302–308.

Rigat, L. (1958). Rendiconto clinico-statistico dei linofoblastomi maligni trattati dal 1928 al 1949. II. Illinofogranuloma maligno. *Radiol. Medica* 44:438–458.

Rigby, P., Pratt, P., Rosenlof, R. and Lemon, H. (1968). Genetic relationship in familial leukemia and lymphoma. *Arch. Int. Med.* 121:67–70.

Robb-Smith, A. H. G. (1947). The lymph node biopsy. In Recent Advances in Clinical Pathology, S. C. Dyke (ed.). London: J. and A. Churchill. Chap. 34, pp. 350–370.

Roberts, A. N., Smith, K. L., Dowell, B. L. and Hubbard, A. K. (1978). Cultural, morphological, cell membrane, enzymatic, and neoplastic properties of cell lines derived from a Hodgkin's disease lymph node. *Cancer Res.* 38:3033–3043.

Roberts, T. W. and Howard, R. G. (1963). Primary Hodgkin's disease of the thyroid: report of a case and review of the literature. *Ann. Surg.* 157:625–632.

Robinson, E. (1966). The occurrence of malignant lymphoma in Israel. *Harefuah* 71:339–340.

Robinson, T. J. (1976). Hodgkin's disease following infectious mononucleosis. *Postgrad. Med. J.* 52:239–240.

Rocchi, G., Hewetson, J. and Henle, W. (1973). Specific neutralizing antibodies in Epstein-Barr virus associated diseases. *Internat. J. Cancer* 11:637–647.

Rocchi, G., Tosato, G., Papa, G. and Ragona, G. (1975). Antibodies to Epstein-Barr virus-associated nuclear antigen and to other viral and nonviral antigens in Hodgkin's disease. *Internat. J. Cancer* 16:323–328.

Rodriguez Paradisi, E., De Bonaparte, Y. P. and Morgenfeld, M. C. (1969). Response in two groups of anergic patients to the transfer of leukocytes from sensitive donors. *New Engl. J. Med.* 280:859–861.

Roeser, H. P., Stocks, A. E. and Smith, A. J. (1978). Testicular damage due to cytotoxic drugs and recovery after cessation of therapy. *Aust. N.Z. J. Med.* 8:250–254.

Rogers, D. L. (1976). Precocious myocardial infarction after radiation treatment for Hodgkin's disease. *Chest* 70:675–677.

Rohmer, P. and Sacry, R. (1948). Un cas de nephrose lipoïdique au cours d'une maladie de Hodgkin. *Strasbourg méd.* 108:45–47.

Roozendaal, D. K. J. and Schreuder-Van Gelder, R. (1971). Ziekte van Hodgkin met terminale acute myelomonocyten leukemia. *Nederl. Tijdschr. Geneesk.* 115:1558–1562.

Rosdahl, N., Larsen, S. O. and Clemmesen, J. (1974). Hodgkin's disease in patients with previous infectious mononucleosis: 30 years' experience. *Brit. Med. J.* 2:253–256.

Rosenberg, N., Baltimore, D. and Scher, C. D. (1975). *In vitro* transformation of lymphoid cells by Abelson murine leukemia virus. *Proc. Nat. Acad. Sci. U.S.* 72:1932–1936.

Rosenberg, S. A. (1966). Report of the committee on the staging of Hodgkin's disease. *Cancer Res.* 26:1310.

Rosenberg, S. A. (1968). Contribution of lymphangiography to our understanding of lymphoma. *Cancer Chemother. Rep.* 52:213–228.

Rosenberg, S. A. (1970). The indication for chemotherapy in the lymphomas. *In* Proceedings of the Sixth National Cancer Conference, 1968. Philadelphia: J. B. Lippincott, pp. 83–89.

Rosenberg, S. A. (1971a). Hodgkin's disease of the bone marrow. *Cancer Res.* 31:1733–1736.

Rosenberg, S. A. (1971b). A critique of the value of laparotomy and splenectomy in the evaluation of patients with Hodgkin's disease. *Cancer Res.* 31:1737–1740.

Rosenberg, S. A. (1977). Personal comments on problems of interpretation of clinical trials presented at the conference on the adjuvant therapy of cancer. *In* Adjuvant Therapy of Cancer, S. E. Salmon and S. E. Jones (eds.). Amsterdam: North-Holland, pp. 609–611.

Rosenberg, S. A., Boiron, M., De Vita, V. T., Jr., Johnson, R. E., Lee, B. J., Ultmann, J. E. and Viamonte, M., Jr., (1971). Report of the committee on Hodgkin's disease staging procedures. *Cancer Res.* 31:1862–1863.

Rosenberg, S. A., Diamond, H. D., Jaslowitz, B. and Craver, L. F. (1961). Lymphosarcoma: a review of 1269 cases. *Medicine* 40:31–84.

Rosenberg, S. A. and Kaplan, H. S. (1966). Evidence for an orderly progression in the spread of Hodgkin's disease. *Cancer Res.* 26:1225–1231.

Rosenberg, S. A. and Kaplan, H. S. (1970). Hodgkin's disease and other malignant lymphomas. *Calif. Med.* 113:23–38.

Rosenberg, S. A. and Kaplan, H. S. (1975). The management of stages I, II, and III Hodgkin's disease with combined radiotherapy and chemotherapy. *Cancer* 35:55–63.

Rosenberg, S. A., Kaplan, H. S., Glatstein, E. and Portlock, C. S. (1977). The role of adjuvant MOPP in the radiation therapy of Hodgkin's disease: A progress report after eight years on the Stanford trials. *In* Adjuvant Therapy of Cancer, S. E. Salmon and S. E. Jones (eds.). Amsterdam: North-Holland, pp. 505–515.

Rosenberg, S. A., Kaplan, H. S., Glatstein, E. J. and Portlock, C. S. (1978). Combined modality therapy of Hodgkin's disease. A report on the Stanford trials. *Cancer* 42:991–1000.

Rosenberg, S. A., Moore, M. R., Bull, J. M., Jones, S. E. and Kaplan, H. S. (1972). Combination chemotherapy and radiotherapy for Hodgkin's disease. *Cancer* 30:1505–1510.

Rosenfeld, S., Swiller, A. I., Shenoy, Y. M. V. and Morrison, A. N. (1961). Syndrome simulating lymphosarcoma induced by diphenylhydantoin sodium. *J.A.M.A.* 176:491–493.

Rosenstock, J. G., D'Angio, G. J. and Kiesewetter, W. B. (1974). The incidence of complications following staging laparotomy for Hodgkin's disease in children. *Radiology* 120:531–535.

Rosenthal, S. R. (1936). Significance of tissue lymphocytes in the prognosis of lymphogranulomatosis. *Arch. Path.* 21:628–646.

Roser, B. (1970). The origins, kinetics, and fate of macrophage populations. *J. Reticuloendothelial Soc.* 8:139–161.

Rosner, F. and Grünwald, H. (1975). Hodgkin's disease and acute leukemia. Report of eight cases and review of the literature. *Am. J. Med.* 58:339–353.

Ross, G. D., Polley, M. J., Rabellino, E. M. and Grey, H. M. (1973). Two different complement receptors on human lymphocytes. One specific for C_3b and one specific for C_3b inactivator-cleaved C_3b. *J. Exper. Med.* 138:798–811.

Rostenberg, A., Jr., McCraney, H. C. and Bluefarb, S. M. (1956). Immunologic studies in the lymphoblastomas. II. The ability to develop an eczematous sensitization to a simple chemical and the ability to accept passive transfer antibody. *J. Invest. Derm.* 26:209–214.

Rottino, A. (1949). *In vitro* studies of lymph nodes involved in Hodgkin's disease. II. Tissue culture studies; formation, behavior and significance of the multinucleated giant cell. *Arch. Path.* 47:328–334.

Rottino, A. and Hoffmann, G. T. (1952). Cardiac involvement in Hodgkin's disease. *Am. Heart J.* 43:115–120.

Rottino, A. and Levy, A. L. (1959). Behavior of total serum complement in Hodgkin's disease and other malignant lymphomas. *Blood* 14:246–254.

Roulet, F. (1930). Das primäre Retothelsarkom der Lymphknoten. *Virchows Arch. path. Anat.* 277:15–47.

Rousselot, L. M., Rella, A. J. and Rottino, A. (1962). Splenectomy for hypersplenism in Hodgkin's disease. A reappraisal. *Am. J. Surg.* 103:769–774.

Routledge, R. C., Haun, I. M. and Morris Jones, P. H. (1976). Hodgkin's disease complicated by the nephrotic syndrome. *Cancer* 38:1735–1740.

Rouvière, H. (1932). Anatomie des lymphatiques de l'homme. Paris: Masson.

Rowe, W. P. (1973). Genetic factors in the natural history of murine leukemia virus infection. G. H. A. Clowes Memorial Lecture. *Cancer Res.* 33:3061–3068.

Rowe, W. P., Hartley, J. W., Lander, M. R., Pugh, W. E. and Teich, N. (1971). Noninfectious AKR mouse embryo cell lines in which each cell has the capacity to be activated to produce infectious murine leukemia virus. *Virology* 46:866–876.

Rowley, D. A., Fitch, F. W., Stuart, F. P., Kohler, H. and Cosenza, H. (1973). Specific suppression of immune responses. *Science* 181:1133–1141.

Rowley, J., Golomb, H. and Vardiman, J. (1977). Nonrandom chromosomal abnormalities in acute nonlymphocytic leukemia in patients treated for Hodgkin disease and non-Hodgkin lymphomas. *Blood* 50:759–770.

Roxin, T., Geib, R., Sighetea, E., Gociu, M., Bujar, H. and Grancea, A. (1962). Pozitia radioterapiei in tratamentul actual al limfogranulomatozei maligne. Studiu clinic şi radiologic pe 105 cazuri. *Stud. Cercetari Med. Int.* 3:631–640.

Royal, J. E. and Seller, R. A. (1978). Hemorrhagic cystitis with MOPP therapy. *Cancer* 41:1261–1264.

Rubin, P. and Casarett, G. W. (1968). Clinical Radiation Pathology. Philadelphia: W. B. Saunders. pp. 423–470.

Rubin, P. and Haluska, G. (1969). The basis for segmental sequential irradiation in Hodgkin's disease: extended vs. local fields in the radiocurability of the SJL/J

mouse Hodgkin's-like reticulum cell sarcoma. *Am. J. Roentgenol.* 105:806–813.

Rubin, P., Keys, H., Mayer, E. and Antemann, R. (1974). Nodal recurrences following radical radiation therapy in Hodgkin's disease. *Am. J. Roentgenol.* 120:536–548.

Rubin, P., Landman, S., Mayer, E., Keller, B. and Ciccio, S. (1973). Bone marrow regeneration and extension after extended field irradiation in Hodgkin's disease. *Cancer* 32:699–711.

Rubin, P. and Scarantino, C. W. (1978). The bone marrow organ: the critical structure in radiation-drug interaction. *Internat. J. Radiat. Oncol. Biol. Phys.* 4:3–23.

Rubio, M. and Sorensen, R. (1972). Enfermedad de Hodgkin en niños. Caracteristicas citoqumicas de las células de Sternberg. Adhesión de linfocitos a las células tumorales "in vivo". *Rev. Med. Chil.* 100:1071–1076.

Ruckdeschel, J. C., Chang, P., Martin, R. G., Byhardt, R. W., O'Connell, M. J., and Sutherland, J. C. (1975). Radiation-related pericardial effusions in patients with Hodgkin's disease. *Medicine* 54:245–259.

Rudders, R. A., Aisenberg, A. C. and Schiller, A. L. (1972). Hodgkin's disease presenting as "idiopathic" thrombocytopenic purpura. *Cancer* 30:220–230.

Rudolph, R., Stein, R. S. and Pattillo, R. A. (1976). Skin ulcers due to adriamycin. *Cancer* 38:1087–1094.

Rühl, H., Vogt, W., Bochert, G., Schmidt, S., Moelle, R. and Schaoua, H. (1975). Mixed lymphocyte culture stimulatory and responding capacity of lymphocytes from patients with lymphoproliferative diseases. *Clin. Exper. Immunol.* 19:55–65.

Rühl, H., Vogt, W., Bochert, G., Schmidt, S., Schaoua, H. and Moelle, R. (1974). Lymphocyte transformation and production of a human mononuclear leucocyte chemotactic factor in patients with Hodgkin's disease. *Clin. Exper. Immunol.* 17:407–415.

Rüttner, J. R. and Brunner, H. E. (1959). Zur Frage der experimentellen Induktion von Tumoren des lymphatischen Systems der Ratte mit den Diazo-Farbstoffen Trypanblau und Evans Blue. *Schweiz. z. Path. Bakt.* 22:519–535.

Rupp, J. J., Moran, J. J. and Griffith, J. R. (1962). Goiter as the initial manifestation of Hodgkin's disease. *Arch. Int. Med.* 110:386–388.

Ruskin, J. and Remington, J. S. (1967). *Pneumocystis carinii* infection in the immunosuppressed host. *Antimicrobial Agents Chemother.* 7:70–76.

Ruuskanen, O., Vanha-Perttula, T. and Kouvalainen, K. (1971). Tonsillectomy, appendicectomy, and Hodgkin's disease. *Lancet* 1:1127–1128.

Rzepecki, W. M., Lukasiewicz, M., Aleksandrowicz, J., Samigiel, Z., Skotnicki, A. and Lisiewicz, J. (1973). Thymus transplantation in leukemia and malignant lymphogranulomatosis. *Lancet* 2:508.

Sacks, E. L., Donaldson, S. S., Gordon, J. and Dorfman, R. F. (1978a). Epithelioid granulomas associated with Hodgkin's disease. Clinical correlations in 55 previously untreated patients. *Cancer* 41:562–567.

Sacks, E. L., Goris, M. L., Glatstein, E., Gilbert, E. and Kaplan, H. S. (1978b). Bone marrow regeneration following large field radiation: influence of volume, age, dose, and time. *Cancer* 42:1057–1065.

Sacks, M., Selzer, G. and Steinitz, R. (1973). Hodgkin's disease in Israel. *Nat. Cancer Inst. Monograph* 36:37–44.

Sahakian, G. J., Al-Mondhiry, H., Lacher, M. J. and Connolly, C. E. (1974). Acute leukemia in Hodgkin's disease. *Cancer* 33:1369–1375.

Sakai, H., Costanzi, J. J., Loukas, D. F., Jr., Gagliamo, R. G., Ritzmann, S. E. and Goldstein, A. L. (1975). Thymosin-induced increase in E-rosette-forming capacity of lymphocytes in patients with malignant neoplasms. *Cancer* 36:974–976.

Saksela, E. and Pontén, J. (1968). Chromosomal changes of immunoglobulin-producing cell lines from human lymph nodes with and without lymphoma. *J. Nat. Cancer Inst.* 41:359–372.

Salas, J. (1973). Lymphoreticular tumors in Costa Rica. *J. Nat. Cancer Inst.* 50:1657–1661.

Saltzstein, S. L. (1962). Lymphoma or drug reaction occurring during hydantoin therapy for epilepsy. *Am. J. Med.* 32:286–297.

Saltzstein, S. L. and Ackerman, L. V. (1959). Lymphadenopathy induced by anti-convulsant drugs and mimicking clinically and pathologically malignant lymphomas. *Cancer* 12:164–182.

Saltzstein, S. L., Jaudon, J. C., Luse, S. A. and Ackerman, L. V. (1958). Lymphadenopathy induced by Ethotoin (Peganone). Clinical and pathological mimicking of malignant lymphoma. *J.A.M.A.* 167:1618–1619.

Salvador, A. H., Harrison, E. G., Jr. and Kyle, R. A. (1971). Lymphadenopathy due to infectious mononucleosis: its confusion with malignant lymphoma. *Cancer* 5:1027–1041.

Salzman, J. R. and Kaplan, H. S. (1971). Effect of splenectomy on hematological tolerance during total lymphoid radiotherapy of patients with Hodgkin's disease. *Cancer* 27:471–478.

Sampson, D. and Lui, A. (1976). The effect of levamisole on cell-mediated immunity and suppressor cell function. *Cancer Res.* 36:952–955.

Sandusky, W. R., Jones, R. C., Horsley, J. S., Marsh, W. L., Tillack, T. W., Tegtmeyer, C. J. and Hess, C. E. (1978). Staging laparotomy in Hodgkin's disease. *Ann. Surg.* 187:485–489.

Sano, M. E. and Koprowska, I. (1965). Primary cytologic diagnosis of a malignant renal lymphoma. *Acta Cytol.* 9:194–196.

Santoro, A., Caillou, B. and Belpomme, D. (1977). T and B lymphocytes and monocytes in the spleen in Hodgkin's disease: the increase in T lymphocytes in involved spleens. *Europ. J. Cancer* 13:355–359.

Santos Silva, M. (1963). Experiences with thio-colciran in the chemotherapy of various types of cancer. *Rev. Brasil. Cancerol.* 19:55–74. (cf. *Cancer Chemother. Abst.* 5:648, 1964).

Santos Silva, M. (1965). Manifestações neurológicas dos linfomas. *J. Brasil. Med.* 9:256–277.

Sarcione, E. J., Smalley, J. R., Lema, M. J. and Stutzman, L. (1977). Increased ferritin synthesis and release by Hodgkin's disease peripheral blood lymphocytes. *Internat. J. Cancer* 20:339–346.

Sarcione, E. J., Stutzman, L. and Mittelman, A. (1975). Ferritin synthesis by splenic tumor tissue of Hodgkin's disease. *Experientia* 31:1334–1335.

Sarma, P. S., Turner, H. C. and Huebner, R. J. (1964). An avian leucosis group-specific complement fixation reaction. Application for the detection and assay of noncytopathogenic leucosis viruses. *Virology* 23:313–321.

Sartoris, S., Cavallero, P., Pegoraro, L., Vergnano, F. and Fazio, M. (1965). The absence of lymphocyte response *in vitro* to tuberculin challenge in Hodgkin's disease. *Panminerva Med.* 7:370–372.

Saslaw, S., Carlisle, H. D. and Bouroncle, B. A. (1961). Antibody response in hematologic patients. *Proc. Soc. Exper. Biol. Med.* 106:654–656.

Saxe, B. I. and Mandel, P. R. (1978). Hodgkin's disease. Radiotherapeutic management at a cancer oriented community hospital. *Cancer* 42:1046–1056.

Saxén, E. and Saxén, N. (1959). The histologic diagnosis of glandular toxoplasmosis. *Lab. Invest.* 8:386–394.

Sayoc, A. S. and Howland, W. J. (1974). Lymphangiographic findings of mesantoin-induced pseudolymphoma. *Radiology* 111:579–580.

Schabel, F. M., Jr., Skipper, H. E., Trader, M. W. and Wilcox, W. S. (1965). An experimental evaluation of potential anti-cancer agents. XIX. Sensitivity of nondividing leukemic cell populations to certain classes of drugs *in vivo*. *Cancer Chemother. Rep.* 48:17–30.

Schamaun, M. (1966). Chirurgische Behandlungsmöglichkeiten der Lymphogranulomatose. *Praxis* 55:754–758.

Schechter, G. P. and Soehnlen, F. (1978). Monocyte mediated inhibition of lymphocyte blastogenesis in Hodgkin's disease. *Blood* 52:261–271.

Schechter, J. P., Jones, S. E., Woolfenden, J. M., Lilien, D. L. and O'Mara, R. E. (1976). Bone scanning in lymphoma. *Cancer* 38:1142–1148.

Scheer, A. C. (1963). The course of stage I malignant lymphomas following local treatment. *Am. J. Roentgenol.* 90:939–943.

Scheerer, P. P., Pierre, R. V., Schwartz, D. L. and Linman, J. W. (1964). Reed-Sternberg-cell leukemia and lactic acidosis. Unusual manifestations of Hodgkin's disease. *New Engl. J. Med.* 270:274–278.

Schein, P. S., O'Connell, M. J., Blom, J., Hubbard, S., Bergevin, P., Wiernik, P. H., Ziegler, J. L. and De Vita, V. T. (1974). Clinical antitumor activity and toxicity of streptozotocin (NSC-85998). *Cancer* 34:993–1000.

Schellen, T.M.C.M. and Beek, J.J.H.M. (1974). The use of clomiphene treatment for male sterility. *Fertil. Steril.* 25:407–410.

Schellinger, D., Miller, W. E., Harrison, E. G., Jr. and Kiely, J. M. (1974). Lymphographic patterns of the subtypes of malignant lymphoma, including Hodgkin's disease. *Radiology* 111:257–266.

Scheurlen, P. G., Schneider, W. and Pappas, A. (1971). Inhibition of transformation of normal lymphocytes by plasma factor from patients with Hodgkin's disease and cancer. *Lancet* 2:1265.

Schick, P., Trepel, F. and Begemann, H. (1975). On the fate of DNA synthesizing lymphoid blood cells in Hodgkin's disease. *Scand. J. Haematol.* 14:17–23.

Schick, P., Trepel, F., Theml, H., Benedek, S., Trumpp, P., Kaboth, W., Begemann, H. and Fliedner, T. M. (1973). Kinetics of lymphocytes in Hodgkin's disease. *Blut* 27:223–235.

Schier, W. (1954). Familial Hodgkin's disease. *Blood* 9:236–240.

Schier, W. W., Roth, A., Ostroff, G. and Schrift, M. H. (1956). Hodgkin's disease and immunity. *Am. J. Med.* 20:94–99.

Schiffer, C. A., Aisner, J. and Wiernik, P. H. (1976). Clinical experience with transfusion of cryopreserved platelets. *Brit. J. Haematol.* 34:377–385.

Schiffer, C. A., Levi, J. A. and Wiernik, P. H. (1975). The significance of abnormal circulating cells in patients with Hodgkin's disease. *Brit. J. Haematol.* 31:177–183.

Schiffer, L. M. (1973). Proliferation of cells in Hodgkin's disease. *Nat. Cancer Inst. Monograph* 36:191–194.

Schilling, R. F. (1978). Complexities of classifying patients with Hodgkin's disease: a plea for a prognostic index. *Am. J. Hematol.* 4:93–95.

Schimpff, S. C., O'Connell, M. J., Greene, W. H. and Wiernik, P. H. (1975a). Infections in 92 splenectomized patients with Hodgkin's disease. A clinical review. *Am. J. Med.* 59:695–701.

Schimpff, S. C., Schimpff, C. R., Brager, D. M. and Wiernik, P. H. (1975b). Leukemia and lymphoma patients linked by prior social contact. *Lancet* 1:124–129.

Schimpff, S. C., Wiernik, P. H., Wiswell, J. and Salvatore, P. (1978). Radiation-related thyroid dysfunction in Hodgkin's disease. *Proc. Am. Soc. Clin. Oncol.* 19:376 (abst.).

Schlom, J. and Spiegelman, S. (1971). Simultaneous detection of reverse transcriptase and high molecular weight RNA unique to oncogenic RNA viruses. *Science* 174:840–843.

Schmid, K., Burke, J. F., Debray-Sachs, M. and Tokita, K. (1964). Sialic acid-deficient alpha-1-acid glycoprotein produced in certain pathological states. *Nature* 204:75–76.

Schmitt, D., Alario, A., Perrot, H. and Thivolet, J. (1977). Origin of Reed-Sternberg cell. *Lancet* 2:137.

Schnitzer, B. and Mead, M. L. (1975). Surface characteristics of Hodgkin's lymphoma cells. *Lancet* 1:223.

Scholten, J. B. (1968). Laparoscopie als hulpmiddel bij de dianostiek van de ziekte van Hodgkin. *Nederl. T. Geneesk.* 112:1685–1687.

Schreiber, M. and McGregor, J. (1968). Pseudolymphoma syndrome. A sensitivity to anticonvulsant drugs. *Arch. Derm.* 97:297–300.

Schreiner, B. F. and Mattick, W. L. (1924). Radiation therapy in 46 cases of lymphogranuloma (Hodgkin's disease). *Am. J. Roentgenol.* 12:133–137.

Schroeder, A. F., Scher, A. J. and Meurk, M. L. (1970). A rapid method of localization for the Hodgkin's mantle. *Radiology* 94:701–702.

Schuller, L., Cojolaru, I., Lörincz, J., Olariu, S. and Schapira, T. (1966). Primary malignant lymphogranulomatosis of the stomach associated with pregnancy. *Oncologia* 20:291–293.

Schultz, H. P., Glatstein, E. and Kaplan, H. S. (1975). Management of presumptive or proven Hodgkin's disease of the liver: a new radiotherapy technique. *Internat. J. Radiat. Oncol. Biol. Phys.* 1:1–8.

Schultz, J. C., Denny, W. F. and Ross, S. W. (1964). Splenectomy in leukemia and lymphoma. Report of twenty-four cases. *Am. J. Med. Sci.* 247:30–36.

Schultz, L. E. (1948). Heterophile antibody titer in diseases other than in infectious mononucleosis. *Arch. Int. Med.* 81:328–333.

Schwartz, D. (1966). Peut-on savoir si la maladie de Hodgkin est curable? Commentaire statistique. *Nouv. rev. franç. hématol.* 6:111–115.

Schwartz, R. S. and Beldotti, L. (1965). Malignant lymphomas following allogenic disease: transition from an immunological to a neoplastic disorder. *Science* 149:1511–1514.

Scott, J. L. (1963). The effect of nitrogen mustard and maintenance chlorambucil in the treatment of advanced Hodgkin's disease. *Cancer Chemother. Rep.* 27:27–32.

Scott, R. M. and Brizel, H. E. (1964). Time-dose relationships in Hodgkin's disease. *Radiology* 82:1043–1049.

Seabold, J. E., Votaw, M. L., Keyes, J. W., Jr., Foley, W. D., Balachandran, S. and Gill, S. P. (1976). Gallium citrate (Ga[67]) scanning. Clinical usefulness in lymphoma patients. *Arch. Int. Med.* 136:1370–1374.

Seif, G. S. F. and Spriggs, A. I. (1967). Chromosome changes in Hodgkin's disease. *J. Nat. Cancer Inst.* 39:557–570.

Seligmann, M., Preud'Homme, J. L. and Brouet, J. C. (1973). B and T cell markers in human proliferative blood diseases and primary immunodeficiencies, with special reference to membrane bound immunoglobulins. *Transplant Rev.* 16:85–113.

Seman, G. and Seman, C. (1968). Electron microscopic search for virus particles in patients with leukemia and lymphoma. *Cancer* 22:1033–1045.

Senn, N. (1903). Therapeutical value of röntgen ray in treatment of pseudoleukemia. *New York Med. J.* 77:665–668.

Seydel, H. G., Bloedorn, F. G. and Wizenberg, M. J. (1967). Time-dose-volume relationship in Hodgkin's disease. *Radiology* 89:919–922.

Seydel, H. G., Bloedorn, F. G. and Wizenberg, M. J. (1969). Results of radiotherapeutic treatment of relapsing Hodgkin's disease. *Cancer* 23:1033–1037.

Shalet, S. M., Rosenstock, J. D., Beardwell, C. G., Pearson, D. and Jones, P. H. M. (1977). Thyroid dysfunction following external irradiation to the neck for Hodgkin's disease in childhood. *Clin. Radiol.* 28:511–515.

Shapiro, H. A. (1961). Primary Hodgkin's disease of the rectum. *Arch. Int. Med.* 107:270–273.

Shapiro, R. F. and Zvaifler, N. J. (1973). Concurrent intrathoracic Hodgkin's disease and hypertrophic osteoarthropathy. *Chest* 63:912–916.

Sheagren, J. N., Block, J. B. and Wolff, S M. (1967). Reticuloendothelial system phagocytic function in patients with Hodgkin's disease. *J. Clin. Invest.* 46:855–862.

Sherins, R. T. and De Vita, V. T., Jr. (1973). Effect of drug treatment for lymphoma on male reproduction capacity. Studies on men in remission after therapy. *Ann. Int. Med.* 79:216–220.

Sherins, R. T., Olweny, C. L. M. and Ziegler, J. L. (1978). Gynecomastia and gonadal dysfunction in adolescent boys treated with combination chemotherapy for Hodgkin's disease. *New Engl. J. Med.* 299:12–16.

Sherman, M. J., Morales, J. B., Bayrd, E. D. and Schierman, W. D. (1955). Amyloid nephrosis secondary to Hodgkin's disease. *Arch. Int. Med.* 95:618–621.

Sherr, C. J., Fedele, L. A., Benveniste, R. E. and Todaro, G. J. (1975). Interspecies antigenic determinants of the reverse transcriptases and p30 proteins of mammalian type C virus. *J. Virol.* 15:1440–1448.

Shevach, E., Jaffe, E., Edelson, R. and Green, I. (1973). The immunological identification of malignant lymphoreticular cells. *Blood* 42:1025.

Shimaoka, K., Bross, I. D. and Tidings, J. (1973). Tonsillectomy and Hodgkin's disease. *New Engl. J. Med.* 288:634–635.

Shimkin, M. B. (1955). Hodgkin's disease. Mortality in the United States, 1921–1951; race, sex, and age distribution; comparison with leukemia. *Blood* 10:1214–1227.

Shimkin, M. B. (1964). Hodgkin's disease. Effectiveness of treatment in control. *J.A.M.A.* 190:916.

Shimkin, M. B., Oppermann, K. C., Bostick, W. L. and Low-Beer, B. V. A. (1955). Hodgkin's disease: an analysis of frequency distribution and mortality at the University of California Hospital, 1914–1951. *Ann. Int. Med.* 42:136–153.

Shipley, W. U., Piro, A. J. and Hellman, S. (1974). Radiation therapy of Hodgkin's disease: significance of splenic involvement. *Cancer* 34:223–229.

Shiratori, O., Ito, Y., Takahashi, T. and Imaeda, Y. (1969). Further studies on the established cell line (AICHI-4) derived from a patient with Hodgkin's disease. *Gann* 7:183–190.

Shotton, D. and Monie, I. W. (1963). Possible teratogenic effect of chlorambucil on a human fetus. *J.A.M.A.* 186:74–75.

Shreeve, D. R., Horrocks, P. and Mainwaring, A. R. (1968). Steatorrhoea and intra-abdominal lymphoma. *Scand. J. Gastroenterol.* 3:577–585.

Sibbitt, W. L, Bankhurst, A. D. and Williams, R. C. (1978). Studies of cell subpopulations mediating mitogen hyporesponsiveness in patients with Hodgkin's disease. *J. Clin. Invest.* 61:55–63.

Siber, G. R., Weitzman, S. A., Aisenberg, A. C., Weinstein, H. J. and Schiffman, G. (1978). Impaired antibody response to pneumococcal vaccine after treatment for Hodgkin's disease. *New Engl. J. Med.* 299:442–448.

Sieber, S. M. and Adamson, R. H. (1975). Toxicity of antineoplastic agents in man: chromosomal aberrations, antifertility effects, congenital malformations, and carcinogenic potential. *Adv. Cancer Res.* 22:57–155.

Sieber, S. M., Correa, P., Dalgard, D. W. and Adamson, R. H. (1978). Carcinogenic and other adverse effects of procarbazine in nonhuman primates. *Cancer Res.* 38:2125–2134.

Siegal, F. P. and Good, R. A. (1977). Human lymphocyte differentiation markers and their application to immune deficiency and lymphoproliferative diseases. *Clin. Haematol.* 6:355–422.

Siegel, B. V. (1961). Identification of a virus isolated from Hodgkin's disease lymph nodes serially passaged in mouse brain. *Virology* 14:378–379.

Siegel, B. V. and Smith, M. E. (1961). Tissue culture studies on the lymphomas with particular reference to Hodgkin's disease. *Path. Microbiol.* 24:1072–1079.

Silberman, H. R., McGinn, T. G. and Kremer, W. D. (1965). Control of fever in Hodgkin's disease by indomethacin. *J.A.M.A.* 194:597–600.

Silverman, H. (1969). Hodgkin's disease: Radical treatment by radiation therapy. *Radiol. Technol.* 41:1–14.

Silverman, L. and Rubinstein, L. J. (1965). Electron microscopic observations on a case of progressive multifocal leukoencephalopathy. *Acta Neuropathol.* 5:215–224.

Silverman, S., DeNardo, G. L., Glatstein, E. and Lipton, M. J. (1972). Evaluation of the liver and spleen in Hodgkin's disease. II. The value of splenic scintigraphy. *Am. J. Med.* 52:362–366.

Simmons, A. V., Spiers, A. S. D. and Fayers, P. M. (1973). Haematological and clinical parameters in assessing activity in Hodgkin's disease and other malignant lymphomas. *Quart. J. Med.* 42:111–124.

Simon, G. (1967). Intra-thoracic Hodgkin's disease. I.

Less common intra-thoracic manifestations of Hodgkin's disease. *Brit. J. Radiol.* 40:926–929.

Simon, N., Silverstone, S. M., Roach, L. C., Warner, R. R. P., Baron, M. G. and Rudavsky, A. Z. (1971). Intra-arterial irradiation of tumors, a safe procedure. *Am. J. Roentgenol.* 112:732–739.

Simons, P. J. and Ross, M. G. R. (1965). The isolation of herpes virus from Burkitt's tumours. *Europ. J. Cancer* 1:135–136.

Simpson, C. L. (1952). Trypan-blue induced tumours of rats. *Brit. J. Exper. Path.* 33:524–528.

Sinkovics, J. G. and Györkey, F. (1973). Hodgkin's disease: involvement of viral agents in the etiology. *J. Med.* 4:282–317.

Sinkovics, J. G., Shurato, E., Györkey, F., Cabiness, J. R. and Howe, C. D. (1969). Relationship between lymphoid neoplasms and immunologic functions. *In* Leukemia-Lymphoma. Chicago: Year-Book Publishers, pp. 53–92.

Sinks, L. F. and Clein, G. P. (1966). The cytogenetics and cell metabolism of circulating Reed-Sternberg cells. *Brit. J. Haemat.* 12:447–453.

Skegg, D. C. G. (1978). BCG vaccination and the incidence of lymphomas and leukemias. *Internat. J. Cancer* 21:18–21.

Skipper, H. E. (1968). Cellular kinetics associated with "curability" of experimental leukemias. *In* Perspectives in Leukemia, W. Dameshek and R. M. Dutcher (eds.). New York: Grune & Stratton. pp. 187–216.

Skipper, H. E. and Perry, S. (1970). Kinetics of normal and leukemic leukocyte populations and relevance to chemotherapy. *Cancer Res.* 30:1883–1897.

Skipper, H. E., Schabel, F. M., Jr. and Wilcox, W. S. (1964). Experimental evaluation of potential anticancer agents. XIII. On the criteria and kinetics associated with "curability" of experimental leukemia. *Cancer Chemother. Rep.* 35:3–111.

Slanina, J., Musshoff, K., Rahner, T. and Stiasny, R. (1977). Long-term side effects in irradiated patients with Hodgkin's disease. *Internat. J. Radiat. Oncol. Biol. Phys.* 2:1–19.

Slaughter, D. P. (1965). Radical surgery. *In* Symposium on Hodgkin's disease: curability of localized Hodgkin's disease by surgery, radiotherapy, and chemotherapy, P. Rubin (ed). *J.A.M.A.* 191:26–27.

Slaughter, D. P. and Craver, L. F. (1942). Hodgkin's disease; 5 year survival rate; value of early surgical treatment; notes on 4 cases of long duration. *Am. J. Roentgenol.* 47:596–606.

Slaughter, D. P., Economou, S. G., and Southwick, H. W. (1958). The surgical management of Hodgkin's disease. *Ann. Surg.* 148:705–710.

Slavin, R. and Nelsen, T. S. (1973). Complications from staging laparotomy for Hodgkin's disease. *Nat. Cancer Inst. Monograph* 36:457–459.

Sluys, F. (1931). La roentgenthérapie totale par champs séparés et la téléroentgenthérapie dans la lymphogranulomatose. *Ann. d'anat. path.* 8:926–929.

Smetana, H. F. and Cohen, B. M. (1956). Mortality in relation to histologic type in Hodgkin's disease. *Blood* 11:211–224.

Smith, C. A. (1934). Hodgkin's disease in childhood; clinical study with résumé of literature to date. *J. Pediat.* 4:12–38.

Smith, I. E., Peckham, M. J., McElwain, T. J., Gazet, J. C.

and Austin, D. E. (1977). Hodgkin's disease in children. *Brit. J. Cancer* 36:120–129.

Smith, K. L., Johnson, D., Hustu, O., Pratt, C. L., Fleming, I. and Holton, C. (1974). Concurrent chemotherapy and radiation therapy in the treatment of childhood and adolescent Hodgkin's disease. *Cancer* 33:38–46.

Smith, K. L. and Rivera, G. (1976). Comparison of the clinical course of Hodgkin's disease in children and adolescents. *Med. Pediatr. Oncol.* 2:361–370.

Smith, P. G., Kinlen, L. J. and Doll, R. (1974). Hodgkin's disease mortality among physicians. *Lancet* 2:525.

Smith, P. G. and Pike, M. C. (1974). Case clustering in Hodgkin's disease: a brief review of the present position and report of current work at Oxford. *Cancer Res.* 34:1156–1160.

Smith, P. G. and Pike, M. C. (1976). Current epidemiological evidence for transmission of Hodgkin's disease. *Cancer Res.* 36:660–662.

Smith, P. G., Pike, M. C., Kinlen, L. J., Jones, A. and Harris R. (1977). Contacts between young patients with Hodgkin's disease. A case-control study. *Lancet* 2:59–62.

Smith, R. A., Ezdinli, E., Bigley, N. J. and Han, T. (1973). Lawrence transfer factor and Hodgkin's disease. *Lancet* 1:434.

Smith, R. B. W., Sheehy, T. W. and Rothberg, H. (1958). Hodgkin's disease and pregnancy: case reports and discussion of treatment of Hodgkin's disease and leukemia during pregnancy. *Arch. Int. Med.* 102:777–789.

Smith, R. W., Terry, W. D., Buell, D. N. and Sell, K. W. (1973). An antigenic marker for human thymic lymphocytes. *J. Immunol.* 110:884–887.

Smithers, D. W. (1967). Hodgkin's disease. *Brit. Med. J.* 2:263–268; 337–341.

Smithers, D. W. (1969a). Clinical research in Hodgkin's disease. *In* The Scientific Basis of Medicine Annual Reviews, London: Athlone Press, pp. 95–111.

Smithers, D. W. (1969b). Factors influencing survival in patients with Hodgkin's disease. *Clin. Radiol.* 20:124–134.

Smithers, D. W. (1970a). Spread of Hodgkin's disease. *Lancet* 1:1262–1267.

Smithers, D. W. (1970b). Hodgkin's disease: one entity or two? *Lancet* 2:1285–1288.

Smithers, D. W. (1973). Modes of spread. *In* Hodgkin's Disease, D. W. Smithers (ed.). Edinburgh and London: Churchill-Livingstone, pp. 107–117.

Smithers, D. W., Lillicrap, S. C. and Barnes, A. (1974). Patterns of lymph node involvement in relation to hypotheses about the modes of spread of Hodgkin's disease. *Cancer* 34:1179–1786.

Snyder, E. M. (1977). The 3 and 2 technique for Hodgkin's disease at Memorial Hospital. *Radiol. Technol.* 49:293–300.

Søborg, M. and Bendixen, G. (1967). Human lymphocyte migration as a parameter of hypersensitivity. *Acta Med. Scand.* 181:247–256.

Sobrinho, L. G., Levine, R. A. and DeConti, R. C. (1971). Amenorrhea in patients with Hodgkin's disease treated with antineoplastic agents. *Am. J. Obstet. Gynecol.* 109:135–139.

Sokal, J. E. (1973). Immunologic deficiency in Hodgkin's disease. *Tumori* 59:343–350.

Sokal, J. E. and Aungst, C. W. (1969). Response to BCG vaccination and survival in advanced Hodgkin's disease. *Cancer* 24:128–134.

Sokal, J. E. and Lessmann, E. M. (1960). Effects of cancer chemotherapeutic agents on the human fetus. *J.A.M.A.* 172:1765–1771.

Sokal, J. E. and Primikirios, M. (1961). The delayed skin test response in Hodgkin's disease and lymphosarcoma. *Cancer* 14:597–607.

Sokal, J. E. and Shimaoka, A. (1967). Pyrogen in the urine of febrile patients with Hodgkin's disease. *Nature* 215:1183–1185.

Solidoro, A., Guzman, C. and Chang, A. (1966). Relative increased incidence of childhood Hodgkin's disease in Peru. *Cancer Res.* 26:1204–1208.

Somasundaram, M., Cho., E.-S. and Posner, J. B. (1975). Anterior horn cell degeneration as a "remote effect" of lymphoma. *Trans. Am. Neurol. Assoc.* 100:144–148.

Sonntag, R. W., Senn, H. J., Nagel, G., Giger, K. and Alberto, P. (1974). Experience with 4′-demethylepipodophyllotoxin 9-(4,6-o-2-thenylidene-beta-D-glucopyranoside); VM-26; NSC-122819 in the treatment of malignant lymphosis. *Europ. J. Cancer* 10:93–98.

Sørensen, N. E. (1973). Dose distribution in the treatment of Hodgkin's disease. *Danish Med. Bull.* 20:47–51.

Sorrell, T. C. and Forbes, I. J. (1975). Phenytoin sensitivity in a case of phenytoin-associated Hodgkin's disease. *Aust. N.Z. J. Med.* 5:144–147.

Sorrell, T. C., Forbes, I. J., Burness, F. R. and Rischbieth, R. H. C. (1971). Depression of immunological function in patients treated with phenytoin sodium (sodium diphenylhydantoin). *Lancet* 2:1233–1235.

Sparling, H. J., Jr., Adams, R. D. and Parker, F., Jr. (1947). Involvement of the nervous system by malignant lymphoma. *Medicine* 26:285–332.

Speiser, B., Rubin, P. and Casarett, G. (1973). Aspermia following lower truncal irradiation in Hodgkin's disease. *Cancer* 32:692–698.

Spencer, R. P., Montana, G., Scanlon, G. T. and Evans, O. R. (1967). Uptake of selenomethionine by mouse and in human lymphomas, with observations on selenite and selenate. *J. Nucl. Med.* 8:197–208.

Spiegelman, S., Kufe, D., Hehlmann, R. and Peters, W. P. (1973). Evidence for RNA tumor viruses in human lymphomas including Burkitt's disease. *Cancer Res.* 33:1515–1526.

Spiers, A. S. D. and Baikie, A. G. (1966). Cytogenetic studies in the malignant lymphomas. *Lancet* 1:506–510.

Spiers, A. S. D. and Malone, H. F. (1966). The significance of serum hexosamine levels in patients with cancer. *Brit. J. Cancer* 20:485–495.

Spiers, P. S. (1969). Hodgkin's disease in workers in the wood industry. *Public Health Rep.* 84:385–388.

Spittle, M. F. (1966). Inappropriate anti-diuretic hormone secretion in Hodgkin's disease. *Postgrad. Med. J.* 42:423–425.

Spittle, M. F., Harmer, C. L., Cassady, J. R. and Kaplan, H. S. (1973). Analysis of primary relapses after radiotherapy in Hodgkin's disease. *Nat. Cancer Inst. Monograph* 36:497–508.

Spriggs, A. I. and Boddington, M. M. (1962). Chromosomes of Sternberg-Reed cells. *Lancet* 2:153.

Squire, R. A. (1969). Spontaneous hematopoietic tumors of dogs. *Nat. Cancer Inst. Monograph* 32:97–116.

Stalsberg, H. (1973). Lymphoreticular tumors in Norway and in other European countries. *J. Nat. Cancer Inst.* 50:1685–1702.

Stanley, N. F., Walter, M. N. I., Leak, P. J. and Keast, D. (1966). The association of murine lymphoma with Reovirus type 3 infection. *Proc. Soc. Exper. Biol. Med.* 121:90–93.

Steigbigel, R. T., Lambert, L. H., Jr. and Remington, J. S. (1976). Polymorphonuclear leukocyte, monocyte, and macrophage bactericidal function in patients with Hodgkin's disease. *J. Lab. Clin. Med.* 88:54–62.

Stein, R. S., Hilborn, R. M., Flexner, J. M., Bolin, M., Stroup, S., Reynolds, V. and Krautz, S. (1978). Anatomical substages of stage III Hodgkin's disease. Implications for staging, therapy, and experimental design. *Cancer* 42:429–436.

Steinberg, M. H., Geary, C. G. and Crosby, W. H. (1970). Acute granulocytic leukemia complicating Hodgkin's disease. *Arch. Int. Med.* 125:496–498.

Steiner, P. E. (1934a). Etiology of Hodgkin's disease; skin reactions to avian and human tuberculin proteins in Hodgkin's disease. *Arch. Int. Med.* 54:11–17.

Steiner, P. E. (1934b). Hodgkin's disease; search for infective agent and attempts at experimental reproduction. *Arch. Path.* 17:749–763.

Steiner, P. E. (1943). Hodgkin's disease; the incidence, distribution, nature and possible significance of the lymphogranulomatous lesions in the bone marrow: a review with original data. *Arch. Path.* 36:627–637.

Steiner, R. M., Harell, G. S., Glatstein, E. and Wexler, L. (1970). Repeat lymphangiography in Hodgkin's disease. *Radiology* 97:613–618.

Stemmermann, G. N. (1970). Patterns of disease among Japanese living in Hawaii. *Arch. Environ. Health* 20:266–273.

Stenfert-Kroese, W. F., Sizoo, W. and Somers, R. (1976). Leukemia of the myeloid series in patients with Hodgkin's disease. *Neth. J. Med.* 19:234–238

Sterling, W. A., Wu, L. Y. F., Dowling, E. A. and Diethelm, A. G. (1974). Hodgkin's disease in a renal transplant recipient. *Transplantation* 17:315–317.

Sternberg, C. (1898). Über eine eigenartige unter dem Bilde der Pseudoleukämie verlaufende Tuberculose des lymphatischen Apparates. *Ztschr. Heilk.* 19:21–90.

Sternlieb, P., Mills, M. and Bellamy, J. (1961). Hodgkin's disease of the small bowel. *Am. J. Med.* 31:304–309.

Stewart, J. R., Cohn, K. E., Fajardo, L. F., Hancock, E. W. and Kaplan, H. S. (1967). Radiation-induced heart disease; a study of twenty-five patients. *Radiology* 89:302–310.

Stewart, S. E., Mitchel, E. Z., Whang, J. J., Dunlop, W. R., Ben, T. and Nomura, S. (1969). Viruses in human tumors. I. Hodgkin's disease. *J. Nat. Cancer Inst.* 43:1–14.

Stolberg, H. O., Patt, N. L., MacEwen, K. F., Warwick, O. H. and Brown, T. C. (1964). Hodgkin's disease of the lung. Roentgenologic-pathologic correlation. *Am. J. Roentgenol.* 62:96–115.

Stolinsky, D. C., Jacobs, E. M., Irwin, L. E., Pajak, Th.F. and Bateman, J. R. (1976a). Effect of trimethylcolchicinic acid methyl ether d-tartrate (TMCA) on Hodgkin's and non-Hodgkin's lymphoma. *Oncology* 33:151–153.

Stolinsky, D. C., Solomon, J., Weiner, J. M. and Bateman, J. R. (1976b). Results with CCNU in resistant Hodgkin's and non-Hodgkin's lymphoma. *Oncology* 33:271–273.

Stoopler, M. B., Caldwell, G. G., Zack, M. M., Housworth, W. J. and Heath, C. W., Jr. (1975). Sibship size and Hodgkin's disease. *New Engl. J. Med.* 292:1025.

Storgaard, L. and Karle, H. (1975). Fever and haemolysis in Hodgkin's disease. *Acta Med. Scand.* 197:311–316.

Stout, A. P. (1949). Lymphosarcoma and Hodgkin's disease. *Rhode Island Med. J.* 32:436–439.

Strand, M. and August, J. T. (1973). Structural proteins of oncogenic ribonucleic acid viruses. *J. Biol. Chem.* 248:5627–5633.

Strand, M. and August, J. T. (1974). Structural proteins of mammalian oncogenic RNA viruses: multiple antigenic determinants of the major internal protein and envelope glycoprotein. *J. Virol.* 13:171–180.

Straus, D., Young, C., Lee, B., Nisce, L., Case, D., Arlin, Z., Sykes, M. and Clarkson, B. (1978). Results at three years of 8-drug combination chemotherapy and local radiotherapy for advanced Hodgkin's disease. *Proc. Am. Assoc. Cancer Res.* 19:318 (abst.).

Strawitz, J. G., Sokal, J. E., Grace, J. T., Jr., Mukhtar, F. and Moore, G. E. (1961). Surgical aspects of hypersplenism in lymphoma and leukemia. *Surg. Gynec. Obst.* 112:89–95.

Strayer, D. R. and Bender, R. A. (1977). Eosinophilic meningitis complicating Hodgkin's disease. A report of a case and review of the literature. *Cancer* 40:406–409.

Strickland, B. (1967). Intra-thoracic Hodgkin's disease. II. Peripheral manifestations of Hodgkin's disease in the chest. *Brit. J. Radiol.* 40:930–938.

Strickstrock, K. H., Weissleder, H., Pfannenstiel, P., Afkham, I. K., Hoffmann, G. and Musshoff, K. (1968). Indikation und vorläufige ergebnisse der endolymphatischen Radio-Isotopen-Therapie bei malignen Erkrankungen des lymphatischen Systems. *Sonderband 69 zur Strahlenther.* pp. 197–210.

Strum, S. B. (1973). The natural history, histopathology, staging and mode of spread of Hodgkin's disease. *Ser. Haemat.* 6:20–115.

Strum, S. B., Allen, L. W. and Rappaport, H. (1971). Vascular invasion in Hodgkin's disease: its relationship to involvement of the spleen and other extranodal sites. *Cancer* 28:1329–1334.

Strum, S. B., Hutchison, G., Park, J. K. and Rappaport, H. (1971). Further observations on the biologic significance of vascular invasion in Hodgkin's disease. *Cancer* 27:1–6.

Strum, S. B., Park, J. K. and Rappaport, H. (1970). Observation of cells resembling Sternberg-Reed cells in conditions other than Hodgkin's disease. *Cancer* 26:176–190.

Strum, S. B. and Rappaport, H. (1970a). Significance of focal involvement of lymph nodes for the diagnosis and staging of Hodgkin's disease. *Cancer* 25:1314–1319.

Strum, S. B. and Rappaport, H. (1970b). Hodgkin's disease in the first decade of life. *Pediatrics* 46:748–759.

Strum, S. B. and Rappaport, H. (1971a). Interrelations of the histologic types of Hodgkin's disease. *Arch. Path.* 91:127–134.

Strum, S. B. and Rappaport, H. (1971b). The persistence of Hodgkin's disease in long-term survivors. *Am. J. Med.* 51:222–240.

Stuart, A. E., Williams, A. R. W. and Habeshaw, J. A. (1977). Rosetting and other reactions of the Reed-Sternberg cell. *J. Path.* 122:81–90.

Stuhlbarg, J. and Ellis, F. W. (1965). Hodgkin's disease of bone—favorable prognostic significance? *Am. J. Roentgenol.* 93:568–572.

Suprun, H. and Koss, L. G. (1964). The cytological study of sputum and bronchial washings in Hodgkin's disease with pulmonary involvement. *Cancer* 17:674–680.

Surks, M. I. and Guttman, A. B. (1966). Esophageal involvement in Hodgkin's disease. Report of a case. *Am. J. Dig. Dis.* 11:814–818.

Sutcliffe, S. B., Stansfeld, A. G., Wrigley, P. F. M., Katz, D., Shand, W. S. and Malpas, J. S. (1978). Post-treatment laparotomy in the management of Hodgkin's disease. *Lancet* 2:57–60.

Sutcliffe, S. B., Wrigley, P. F. M., Peto, J., Lister, T. A., Stansfeld, A. G., Whitehouse, J. M. A., Crowther, D. and Malpas, J. S. (1978). MVPP chemotherapy regimen for advanced Hodgkin's disease. *Brit. Med. J.* 1:679–683.

Sutcliffe, S. B. J., Wrigley, P. F. M., Smyth, J. F., Webb, J. A. W., Tucker, A. K., Beard, M. E. J., Irving, M., Stansfeld, A. G., Malpas, J. S., Crowther, D. and Whitehouse, J. M. A. (1976). Intensive investigation in management of Hodgkin's disease. *Brit. Med. J.* 2: 1343–1347.

Sutherland, J. C., Markham, R. V., Jr., Ramsey, H. E. and Mardiney, H. R., Jr. (1974). Subclinical immune complex nephritis in patients with Hodgkin's disease. *Cancer Res.* 34:1179–1181.

Sutherland, R. M., McCredie, J. A. and Inch, W. R. (1975). Effect of splenectomy and radiotherapy on lymphocytes in Hodgkin's disease. *Clin. Oncol.* 1:275–284.

Sutnick, A. I., London, W. T., Blumberg, B. S., Yankee, R. A., Gerstley, B. J. S. and Millman, I. (1970). Australia antigen (a hepatitis-associated antigen) in leukemia. *J. Nat. Cancer Inst.* 44:1241–1249.

Svahn-Tapper, G. and Landberg, T. (1971). Mantle treatment of Hodgkin's disease with cobalt 60. *Acta Radiol.* 10:33–55.

Svejgaard, A., Platz, P., Ryder, L. P., Nielsen, L. S. and Thomsen, M. (1975). HL-A and disease association—a survey. *Transplant. Rev.* 22:3–43.

Swain, A. and Trounce, J. R. (1974). Rosette formation in Hodgkin's disease. *Oncology* 30:449–457.

Swan, H. T. and Knowelden, J. (1971). Prognosis in Hodgkin's disease related to the lymphocyte count. *Brit. J. Haematol.* 21:343–349.

Sweet, D. L., Jr., Roth, D. G., Desser, R. K., Miller, J. B. and Ultmann, J. E. (1976). Avascular necrosis of the femoral head with combination therapy. *Ann. Int. Med.* 85:67–68.

Sybesma, J. P. H. B., Holtzer, J. D., Borst-Eilers, E., Moes, M. and Zegers, B. J. M. (1973). Antibody response in Hodgkin's disease and other lymphomas related to HL-A antigens, immunoglobulin levels and therapy. *Vox Sang* 25:254–262.

Sykes, J. A., Dmochowski, L., Shullenberger, C. C. and Howe, C. D. (1962). Tissue culture studies on human leukemia and malignant lymphoma. *Cancer Res.* 22: 21–26.

Sykes, M. D., Chu, F. C. H., Savel, H., Bonadonna, G. and Mathis, H. (1964). The effects of varying dosages

of irradiation upon sternal marrow regeneration. *Radiology* 83:1084–1087.

Symmers, D. (1927). Follicular lymphadenopathy with splenomegaly. A newly recognized disease of the lymphatic system. *Arch. Path. Lab. Med.* 3:816–820.

Symmers, W. St. C. (1968). Survey of the eventual diagnosis in 600 cases referred for a second histological opinion after an initial biopsy diagnosis of Hodgkin's disease. *J. Clin. Path.* 21:650–653.

Szur, L., Levene, G. M., Harrison, C. V., and Samman, P. D. (1970). Primary cutaneous Hodgkin's disease. *Lancet* 1:1016–1020.

Takahashi, M. and Abrams, H. L. (1967). The accuracy of lymphangiographic diagnosis in malignant lymphoma. *Radiology* 89:448–460.

Takashima, T. and Benninghoff, D. L. (1966). Effects of experimental thoracic duct obstruction in dogs. II. Chylous reflux. *Invest. Radiol.* 1:449–457.

Tan, C., D'Angio, G. J., Exelby, P. R., Lieberman, P. H., Watson, R. C., Cham, W. C. and Murphy, M. L. (1975). The changing management of childhood Hodgkin's disease. *Cancer* 35:808–816.

Tan, C., Etcubanas, E., Lieberman, P., Isenberg, H., King, O. and Murphy, M. L. (1971). Chediak-Higashi syndrome in a child with Hodgkin's disease. *Am J. Dis. Child.* 121:135–139.

Tan, K. K. and Shanmugaratnam, K. (1973). Incidence and histologic classification of malignant lymphomas in Singapore. *J. Nat. Cancer Inst.* 50:1681–1683.

Tannenbaum, A. (1947). Effects of varying caloric intake upon tumor incidence and tumor growth. *Ann. New York Acad. Sci.* 49:5–18.

Tauro, G. P. (1966). Hodgkin's disease associated with raised eosinophil counts. *Med. J. Aust.* 2:604–606.

Taylor, C. R. (1976). An immunohistological study of follicular lymphoma, reticulum cell sarcoma and Hodgkin's disease. *Europ. J. Cancer* 12:61–75.

Teillet, F., Boiron, M. and Bernard, J. (1971). A reappraisal of clinical and biological signs in staging of Hodgkin's disease. *Cancer Res.* 31:1723–1729.

Teillet, F. and Schweisguth, O. (1969). Hodgkin's disease in children; notes on diagnosis and prognosis based on experiences with 72 cases in children. *Clin. Pediatrics* 8:698–704.

Teillet, F., Weisgerber, C. and Feingold, N. (1973). Maladie de Hodgkin: essai d'évaluation de rôle joué par l'appendicectomie et l'amygdalectomie. *Nouv. Presse Méd.* 2:2097–2099.

Teitelman, S. L. and Brill, N. R. (1960). Localized Hodgkin's disease of the small intestine. *Am. J. Surg.* 99:247–248.

Temin, H. M. and Mizutani, S. (1970). RNA-dependent DNA polymerase in virions of Rous sarcoma virus. *Nature* 226:1211–1213.

Temine, P., Privat, Y. and Alerini, P. (1965). Localisation cutanée d'une maladie de Hodgkin. *Bull. soc. franç. derm. syph.* 72:750–752.

Terry, L. N., Jr. and Kligerman, M. M. (1970). Pericardial and myocardial involvement by lymphomas and leukemias. The role of radiotherapy. *Cancer* 25:1003–1008.

Teschendorf, W. (1927). Ueber Bestrahlung der ganzen menschlichen Körpers bei Blutkrankheiten. *Strahlenther.* 26:720–728.

Tessmer, C. F., Hrgovcic, M. and Wilbur, J. (1973).

Serum copper in Hodgkin's disease in children. *Cancer* 31:303–315.

Thar, T. L., Million, R. R., Hausner, R. J. and McKetty, M. H. B. (1979). Hodgkin's disease, stages I and II: relationship of recurrence to size of disease, radiation dose, and numbers of sites involved. *Cancer,*. 43:1101–1105.

Thomas, J. W., Boldt, W., Horrocks, G. and Low, B. (1967). Lymphocyte transformation by phytohemagglutinin. I. In Hodgkin's disease. *Canad. Med. Assoc. J.* 97:832–836.

Thomas, M. R., Steinberg, P., Votaw, M. L. and Bayne, N. K. (1976a). IgE levels in Hodgkin's disease. *Ann. Allergy* 37:416–419.

Thomas, P. R. M., Winstanly, D., Peckham, M. J., Austin, D. E., Murray, M. A. F. and Jacobs, H. S. (1976b). Reproductive and endocrine function in patients with Hodgkin's disease: effect of oophoropexy and irradiation. *Brit. J. Cancer* 33:226–231.

Thomson, A. D. (1955). The thymic origin of Hodgkin's disease. *Brit. J. Cancer* 9:37–50.

Thompson, R. W. and De Nardo, G. L. (1969). Intracranial Hodgkin's disease documented by brain scanning. *Cancer* 24:981–984.

Thompson Hancock, P. E. (1968). Thomas Hodgkin; The FitzPatrick Lecture. *J. Roy. Coll. Phys. London* 2:404–421.

Thompson Hancock, P. E., Austin, D. E. and Smith, P. G. (1973). Treatment of early Hodgkin's disease. *Lancet* 1:832–833.

Thompson Hancock, P. E. and Ledlie, E. M. (1967). Treatment of early Hodgkin's disease. *Lancet* 1:26–27.

Thorling, E. B. and Thorling, K. (1974). Serum-copper in Hodgkin's disease before and after herpes zoster. *Lancet* 2:1396–1397.

Thorling, E. B. and Thorling, K. (1976). The clinical usefulness of serum copper determinations in Hodgkin's disease—a retrospective study of 241 patients from 1963–1973. *Cancer* 38:225–231.

Thorling, K. (1973). Familial Hodgkin's disease. Occurrence in two brothers. *Danish Med. Bull.* 20:61–63.

Thuot, C., Gariépy, G., Monté, M. and Perron, L. (1973). Unusual symptomatology of Hodgkin's disease: massive invasion of the blood by abnormal cells. *Union Med. Can.* 102:1675–1678.

Timothy, A. R., Tucker, A. K., Malpas, J. S., Wrigley, P. F. M. and Sutcliffe, S. B. J. (1978). Osteonecrosis after intensive chemotherapy for Hodgkin's disease. *Lancet* 1:154.

Tindle, B. H., Parker, J. W. and Lukes, R. J. (1972). "Reed-Sternberg cells" in infectious mononucleosis? *Am. J. Clin. Path.* 58:607–617.

Tingelstad, J. B., McWilliams, N. B. and Thomas, C. E. (1976). Confirmation of a retrosternal mass by echocardiogram. *J. Clin. Ultrasound* 4:129–131.

Tittor, W., Drings, P. and Fritsch, H. (1975). Akute leukämie in der schlubphase eines morbus Hodgkin: folge der zellulären immunschwäche? *Med. Klin.* 70:607–612.

Todd, G. B. and Michaels, L. (1974). Hodgkin's disease involving Waldeyer's lymphoid ring. *Cancer* 34:1769–1778.

Tognella, S., Mantovani, G., Cengiarotti, L., Del Giacco, G. S., Manconi, P. E. and Grifoni, V. (1975a). Effetto del siero citotossico di pazienti con malattia di Hodgkin sulla mobilita elettroforetica di linfociti periferici normali e Hodgkiniani. *Tumori* 61:45–52.

Tognella, S., Mantovani, G., Floris, C. and Grifoni, V. (1975b). Herpes zoster and Hodgkin's disease. *Haematologica* 60:378.

Toland, D. M. and Coltman, C. A. (1975). Second malignancies complicating Hodgkin's disease. *Blood* 46:1013 (abst.).

Tonnesen, A. S. and Davis, F. G. (1976). Superior vena caval and bronchial obstruction during anesthesia. *Anesthesiology* 45:91–92.

Torti, F. M., Portlock, C. S., Rosenberg, S. A. and Kaplan, H. S. (1978). Extranodal (E) lesions in Hodgkin's disease (HD): prognosis and response to therapy. *Proc. Am. Soc. Clin. Oncol.* 19:367 (abst.).

Toth, B. (1963). Development of malignant lymphomas by cell-free filtrates prepared from a chemically induced mouse lymphoma. *Proc. Soc. Exper. Biol. Med.* 112:874–875.

Tóth, J., Dworák, O. and Sugár, J. (1977). Eosinophil predominance in Hodgkin's disease. *Z. Krebsforsch.* 89:107–111.

Tripodi, D., Parks, L. C. and Brugmans, J. (1973). Drug-induced restoration of cutaneous delayed hypersensitivity in anergic patients with cancer. *New Engl. J. Med.* 289:354–357.

Trotter, J. L., Hendin, B. A. and Osterland, C. K. (1976). Cerebellar degeneration with Hodgkin's disease. An immunological study. *Arch. Neurol.* 33:660–661.

Trousseau, A. (1965). De l'adénie. *Clin. méd. l'Hôtel-Dieu Paris* 3:555–581.

Trubowitz, S., Masek, B. and Del Rosario, A. (1966). Lymphocyte response to phytohemagglutinin in Hodgkin's disease, lymphatic leukemia and lymphosarcoma. *Cancer* 19:2019–2023.

Trueblood, H. W., Enright, L. P., Ray, G. R., Kaplan, H. S. and Nelsen, T. S. (1970). Preservation of ovarian function in pelvic radiation for Hodgkin's disease. *Arch. Surg.* 100:236–237.

Trujillo, J. M., Drewinko, B. and Athearn, M. A. (1972). The ability of tumor cells of the lymphoreticular system to grow *in vitro*. *Cancer Res.* 32:1057–1065.

Tsubota, T. (1972). Studies on lymphoblastoid cell lines derived from a patient with Hodgkin's disease. I. Comparative examination of lymphoblastoid cell lines established from lymph node and peripheral blood of a patient with Hodgkin's disease. *Acta Haematol. Jap.* 35:156–170.

Tubiana, M., Attié, E., Flamant, R., Gérard-Marchant, R. and Hayat, M. (1971). Prognostic factors in 454 cases of Hodgkin's disease. *Cancer Res.* 31:1801–1810.

Tubiana, M. and Mathé, G. (1973). Combined radiotherapy and chemotherapy in the treatment of Hodgkin's disease. *Ser. Haemat.* 6:202–243.

Tubiana, M., Mathé, G., Hayat, M., Le Bourgeois, J. P., Henry-Amar, M. and Laugier, A. (1977). Treatment of stage I and II Hodgkin's disease. *Nouv. rev. franç. hematol. Blood Cells* 18:463–472.

Tubiana, M., Rambert, P., Laugier, A. and Lalanne, C. M. (1966). Les irradiations étendues dans la maladie de Hodgkin. Réactions précoces. *Nouv. rev. franç. hématol.* 6:164–174.

Tubiana, M., Van der Werf-Messing, B., Laugier, A.,

Hayat, M., Henry-Amar, M., Attie, E. and Leroy, T. (1973). Survival after recurrence: prognostic factors and spread patterns in clinical stages I and II of Hodgkin's disease. *Nat. Cancer Inst. Monograph* 36:513–530.

Tucker, A. K., Pemberton, J. and Guyer, P. B. (1975). Pulmonary fungal infection complicating treated malignant disease. *Clin. Radiol.* 26:129–136.

Tuckwell, H. M. (1870). Enlargement of lymph glands in the abdomen, with formation of peculiar morbid growths in the spleen and peritoneum. *Trans. Path. Soc. London* 21:362–365.

Turk, J. L. (1967). Delayed Hypersensitivity. Amsterdam: North-Holland.

Turner, D. A., Pinsky, S. M., Gottschalk, A., Hoffer, P. B., Ultmann, J. E. and Harper, P. V. (1972). The use of ^{67}Ga scanning in the staging of Hodgkin's disease. *Radiology* 103:97–101.

Turner, J. C., Jackson, H., Jr. and Parker, F., Jr. (1938). Etiologic relation of eosinophils to Gordon phenomenon in Hodgkin's disease. *Am. J. Med. Sci.* 195:27–32.

Twomey, J. J., Laughter, A. H., Farrow, S. and Douglass, C. C. (1975). Hodgkin's disease. An immunodepleting and immunosuppressive disorder. *J. Clin. Invest.* 56:467–475.

Twomey, J. J., Laughter, A. H., Lazar, S. and Douglass, C. C. (1976). Reactivity of lymphocytes from primary neoplasms of lymphoid tissues. *Cancer* 38:740–747.

Twort, C. C. (1930). Etiology of lymphadenoma; summary of 6 years' researches. *J. Path. Bact.* 33:539–546.

Tyler, A. (1960). Clues to the etiology, pathology, and therapy of cancer provided by analogies with transplantation disease. *J. Nat. Cancer Inst.* 25:1197–1229.

Tzehoval, E., Segal, S., Stabinsky, Y., Fridkin, M., Spirer, Z. and Feldman, M. (1978). Tuftsin (an Ig-associated tetrapeptide) triggers the immunogenic function of macrophages: implications for activation of programmed cells. *Proc. Nat. Acad. Sci. U.S.* 75:3400–3404.

Uddströmer, M. (1934). On the occurrence of lymphogranulomatosis (Sternberg) in Sweden, 1915–1931 and some considerations as to its relation to tuberculosis. *Acta Tuberc. Scand. Supp.* 1:1–225.

Uhl, N. and Hunstein, W. (1969). Jahreszeitliche schwankungen im auftreten der lymphogranulomatose. *Arch. Klin. Med.* 216:355–370.

Uhr, J. W., and Scharff, M. (1960). Delayed hypersensitivity. V. The effect of X-irradiation on the development of delayed hypersensitivity and antibody formation. *J. Exper. Med.* 112:65–76.

Ultmann, J. E. (1966). Clinical features and diagnosis of Hodgkin's disease. *Cancer* 19:297–307.

Ultmann, J. E., Cunningham, J. K. and Gellhorn, A. (1966). The clinical picture of Hodgkin's disease. *Cancer Res.* 26:1047–1060.

Ultmann, J. E. and Moran, E. M. (1973). Clinical course and complications in Hodgkin's disease. *Arch. Int. Med.* 131:332–353.

Urbach, F., Sones, M. and Israel, H. L. (1952). Passive transfer of tuberculin sensitivity to patients with sarcoidosis. *New Engl. J. Med.* 247:794–797.

Urbanitz, D., Fechner, I., and Gross, R. (1975). Reduced monocyte phagocytosis in patients with advanced Hodgkin's disease and lymphosarcoma. *Klin. Wchnschr.* 53:437–440.

Vaeth, J. M. (1962). Retreatment of mediastinal Hodgkin's disease. *In* Progress in Radiation Therapy, F. Buschke (ed.). New York: Grune and Stratton. Vol. 2, pp. 164–187.

Valberg, L. S., Holt, M. M. and Card, R. T. (1966). Erythrocyte magnesium, copper and zinc in malignant diseases affecting the hemopoietic system. *Cancer* 19:1833–1841.

Valeriote, F. A., Bruce, W. R. and Meeker, B. E. (1968). Synergistic action of cyclophosphamides and 1,3-bis(2-chloroethyl)-1-nitrosourea on a transplanted murine lymphoma. *J. Nat. Cancer Inst.* 40:935–944.

Valeriote, F. and van Putten, L. (1975). Proliferation-dependent cytotoxicity of anticancer agents: a review. *Cancer Res.* 35:2619–2630.

Van der Maaten, M. J., Miller, J. M. and Boothe, A. D. (1974). Replicating type-C virus particles in monolayer cell cultures from cattle with lymphosarcoma. *J. Nat. Cancer Inst.* 52:491–497.

Van Der Meiren, L. (1948). Three cases of Hodgkin's disease with predominantly cutaneous localization. *Brit. J. Derm.* 60:181–184.

Van Dorssen, J. G., Mellink, J. H. and Thomas, P. (1970). Construction of auxiliary diaphragms for megavoltage irradiation of large, irregularly shaped fields. *Radiol. Clin. Biol.* 39:47–53.

van Furth, R. (1975). Mononuclear Phagocytes in Immunity, Infection, and Pathology, R. van Furth (ed.). Oxford: Blackwell Scientific Publ.

Van Rooyen, C. E. (1933). Etiology of Hodgkin's disease with special reference to B. Tuberculosis Avis. *Brit. Med. J.* 1:50–51.

Van Rooyen, C. E. (1934). Recent experimental work on the aetiology of Hodgkin's disease. *Brit. Med. J.* 2:519–524.

Van Wyk, J. J. and Hoffmann, C. R. (1948). Periarteritis nodosa. Case of fatal exfoliative dermatitis resulting from "dilantin sodium" sensitization. *Arch. Int. Med.* 81:605–611.

Varadi, S. (1960). Reed-Sternberg cells in peripheral blood and bone marrow in Hodgkin's disease. *Brit. Med. J.* 1:1239–1243.

Variakojis, D., Fennessy, J. J. and Rappaport, H. (1972). Diagnosis of Hodgkin's disease by bronchial brush biopsy. *Chest* 61:326–330.

Veenhof, C. H. N., van der Meer, J. and Doudsmit, R. (1973). Successfully treated priapism in acute myeloblastic leukemia complicating Hodgkin's disease. *Acta Med. Scand.* 194:349–352.

Verhaegen, H., De Cock, W., De Cree, J., Verbruggen, F., Verhaegen-Declercq, M. and Brugmans, J. (1975). *In vitro* restoration by levamisole of thymus-derived lymphocyte function in Hodgkin's disease. *Lancet* 1:978.

Veronesi, U., Bonadonna, G., Musumeci, R., Pizzetti, F. and Gennari, L. (1972). Diagnostic laparotomy with splenectomy in Hodgkin's disease and in the malignant lymphomas. *In* Thyroid Tumours, Lymphoma, Granulocytic Leukemia, M. Fiorentino, R. Vangelista, and E. Grigoletto (eds.) Padova: Piccin Medical Books, pp. 137–153.

Veronesi, U., Cascinelli, N. and Preda, F. (1966). Il linofogranuloma maligno primitivo della tiroide. *Tumori* 52:145–149.

Versé, M. (1931). Die Lymphogranulomatose der Lunge und des Brustfells. *In* Handbuch der speziellen pathologischen Anatomie und Histologie, F. Henke and O. Lubarsch (eds.). Berlin: Julius Springer. Vol III, part 3, pp. 280–343.

Vianna, N. J., Davies, J. N. P., Polan, A. K. and Wolfgang, P. (1974a). Familial Hodgkin's disease: an environmental and genetic disorder. *Lancet* 2:854–857.

Vianna, N. J., Greenwald, P., Brady, J., Polan, A. K., Dwork, A., Mauro, J. and Davies, J. N. P. (1972). Hodgkin's disease: cases with features of a community outbreak. *Ann. Int. Med.* 77:169–180.

Vianna, N. J., Greenwald, P. and Davies, J. N. P. (1971a). Extended epidemic of Hodgkin's disease in high-school students. *Lancet* 1:1209–1210.

Vianna, N. J., Greenwald and Davies, J. N. P. (1971b). Tonsillectomy and Hodgkin's disease: the lymphoid tissue barrier. *Lancet* 1:431–432.

Vianna, N. J., Keogh, M. D., Polan, A. K., and Greenwald, P. (1974b). Hodgkin's disease mortality among physicians. *Lancet* 2:131–133.

Vianna, N. J. and Polan, A. K. (1973). Epidemiological evidence for transmission of Hodgkin's disease. *New Engl. J. Med.* 289:499–502.

Vianna, N. J. and Polan, A. K. (1974). Infectious aspects of Hodgkin's disease. *New Engl. J. Med.* 290:342.

Vicente, J. and Cortés-Funes, H. (1976). ABVD for the treatment of advanced resistant lymphomas. *Proc. Am. Soc. Clin. Oncol.* 17:189 (abst.).

Videbaek, A. (1950). The course and prognosis of Hodgkin's disease. *Acta Med. Scand.* 136:203–208.

Videbaek, A. (1955). Familial Hodgkin's disease. *Acta Haemat.* 14:200–202.

Vieta, J. O. and Craver, L. F. (1941). Intrathoracic manifestations of the lymphomatoid diseases. *Radiology* 37:138–158.

Vinciguerra, V., Coleman, M., Jarowski, C. I., Degnan, T. J. and Silver, R. T. (1977). A new combination chemotherapy for resistant Hodgkin's disease. *J.A.M.A.* 239:33–35.

Virchow, R. (1845). Weisses blut. *Neue Notizen aus dem Geb. der Natur-und Heilkunde (Froriep's neue Notizen)* 36:151–156.

Vogel, J. M., Kimball, H. R., Foley, H. T., Wolff, S. M. and Perry, S. (1968). Effect of extensive radiotherapy on the marrow granulocyte reserves of patients wtih Hodgkin's disease. *Cancer* 21:798–804.

Vogelgesang, K. H., and Többen, A. (1956). Ein Beitrag zur Prognose und Therapie der Lymphogranulomatose. *Strahlenther.* 101:77–87.

Voorhoeve, N. (1925). La lymphogranulomatose maligne. *Acta Radiol.* 4:567–589.

Wagener, D. J. T., Geestman, E., Borgonjen, A. and Haanen, Cl. (1976). The influence of splenectomy on cellular immunologic parameters in Hodgkin's disease. *Cancer* 37:2212–2219.

Wagener, D. J. T. and Haanen, C. (1975). "Incubation period" in Hodgkin's disease. *Lancet* 2:747–748.

Wagener, D., Van Munster, P. and Haanen, C. (1976). The immunoglobulins in Hodgkin's disease. *Europ. J. Cancer* 12:683–688.

Wakasa, H. (1973). Hodgkin's disease in Asia, particularly in Japan. *Nat. Cancer Inst. Monograph* 36:15–22.

Wakem, C. J. and Bennett, J. M. (1972). Hodgkin's disease terminating as acute leukemia: case report and review of the literature. *New Zealand Med. J.* 76:187–194.

Walbom-Jorgensen, S., Cleemann, L., Nybo-Rasmussen, A. and Sorensen, P. B. (1972). Technical aids for the radiotherapy of Hodgkin's disease. *Brit. J. Radiol.* 45:949–953.

Waldmann, T., Trier, J. and Fallon, H. (1963). Albumin metabolism in patients with lymphoma. *J. Clin. Invest.* 42:171–178.

Wallace, S., Jackson, L., Schaeffer, B., Gould, J., Greening, R. R., Weiss, A. and Kramer, S. (1961). Lymphangiograms: their diagnostic and therapeutic potential. *Radiology* 76:179–199.

Wallhauser, A. (1933). Hodgkin's disease. *Arch. Path.* 16:522–562; 672–712.

Walsh, J. C. (1971). Neuropathy associated with lymphoma. *J. Neurol. Neurosurg. Psychiat.* 34:42–50.

Waltuch, G. and Sachs, F. (1968). Herpes zoster in a patient with Hodgkin's disease. Treatment with idoxuridine. *Arch. Int. Med.* 121:458–462.

Wara, W. M., Phillips, T. L., Margolis, L. W. and Smith, V. (1973). Radiation pneumonitis: a new approach to the determination of time-dose factors. *Cancer* 32:547–552.

Ward, P. A. and Berenberg, J. L. (1974). Defective regulation of inflammatory mediators in Hodgkin's disease. Supernormal levels of chemotactic factor activator. *New Engl. J. Med.* 290:76–80.

Warren, R. D., Bender, R. A., Norton, L. and Young, R. C. (1978). The treatment of combination chemotherapy-resistant Hodgkin disease with single-agent vinblastine. *Am. J. Hematol.* 4:47–55.

Warren, R. L., Jelliffe, A. M., Watson, J. V. and Hobbs, C. B. (1969). Prolonged observations on variations in the serum copper in Hodgkin's disease. *Clin. Radiol.* 20:247–256.

Warthin, A. S. (1931). Genetic neoplastic relationships of Hodgkin's disease, aleukemic and leukemic lymphoblastoma, and mycosis fungoides. *Ann. Surg.* 93:153–161.

Watkins, S. M. and Griffin, J. P. (1978). High incidence of vincristine-induced neuropathy in lymphomas. *Brit. Med. J.* 1:610–612.

Webb, D. I., Ubogy, G. and Silver, R. T. (1970). Importance of bone marrow biopsy in the clinical staging of Hodgkin's disease. *Cancer* 26:313–317.

Webb, D. R., Jr. and Jamieson, A. T. (1976). Control of mitogen induced transformation: characterization of a splenic suppressor cell and its mode of action. *Cell Immunol.* 24:45–57.

Weick, J. K., Kiely, J. M., Harrison, E. G., Jr., Carr, D. T. and Scanlon, P. W. (1973). Pleural effusion in lymphoma. *Cancer* 31:848–853.

Weiden, P. L., Lerner, K. G., Heywood, J. D., Fefer, A. and Thomas, E. D. (1973). Pancytopenia and leukemia in Hodgkin's disease: report of three cases. *Blood* 42:571–577.

Weinstein, P., Greenwald, E. S. and Grossman, J. (1976). Unusual cardiac reaction to chemotherapy following mediastinal irradiation in a patient with Hodgkin's disease. *Am. J. Med.* 60:152–156.

Weisenburger, T. H. and Juillard, G. J. F. (1977). Upper extremity lymphangiography in the radiation therapy of lymphomas and carcinoma of the breast. *Radiology* 122:227–230.

Weiss, R. B., Brunning, R. D. and Kennedy, B. J. (1975). Hodgkin's disease in the bone marrow. *Cancer* 36:2077–2083.

Weiss, R. B. and Jenkins, J. J., III. (1977). Hodgkin's disease presenting in epitrochlear lymph nodes. *South. Med. J.* 70:513–515.

Weitzman, S. and Aisenberg, A. C. (1977a). Fulminant sepsis after the successful treatment of Hodgkin's disease. *Am. J. Med.* 62:47–50.

Weitzman, S. A., Aisenberg, A. C., Siber, G. R. and Smith, D. H. (1977b). Impaired humoral immunity in treated Hodgkin's disease. *New Engl. J. Med.* 297:245–248.

Weitzman, S., Dvilansky, A. and Yanai, I. (1977c). Thrombocytopenic purpura as the sole manifestation of recurrence in Hodgkin's disease. *Acta Haemat.* 58:129–133.

Weller, S. A., Glatstein, E., Castellino, R. A., Kaplan, H. S. and Rosenberg, S. A. (1977). Initial relapse in previously treated Hodgkin's disease. II. Retrograde transdiaphragmatic extension. *Internat. J. Radiat. Oncol. Biol. Phys.* 2:863–872.

Weller, S. A., Glatstein, E., Kaplan, H. S. and Rosenberg, S. A. (1976). Initial relapses in previously treated Hodgkin's disease. I. Results of second treatment. *Cancer* 37:2840–2846.

Wernet, P. and Kunkel, H. G. (1973). Antibodies to a specific surface antigen of T cells in human sera inhibiting mixed leukocyte culture reactions. *J. Exper. Med.* 138:1021–1026.

Weshler, Z., Krasnokuki, D., Peshin, Y. and Biran, S. (1978). Thyroid carcinoma induced by irradiation for Hodgkin's disease. *Acta Radiol. Oncol.* 17:383–386.

Westling, P. (1965). Studies of the prognosis in Hodgkin's disease. *Acta Radiol.* (Supp.) 245:5–125.

Whitcomb, M. E., Schwarz, M. I., Keller, A. R., Flannery, E. P. and Blom, J. (1972). Hodgkin's disease of the lung. *Am. Rev. Resp. Dis.* 106:79–85.

White, A. A. and Palubinskas, A. J. (1970). Renal Hodgkin's disease; angiographic demonstration. *Radiology* 96:551–552.

Whitehead, R. H., Bolton, P. M., James, S. L. and Roberts, G. M. (1974). An *in vitro* method for assaying sensitivity to 2,4-dinitrochlorobenzene (DNCB) in man. *Europ. J. Cancer* 10:721–724.

Whitelaw, D. M. (1969). Chromosome complement of lymph node cells in Hodgkin's disease. *Canad. Med. Assoc. J.* 101:74–81.

Whiteside, J. D. and Begent, R. H. J. (1975). Toxoplasma encephalitis complicating Hodgkin's disease. *J. Clin. Path.* 28:443–445.

Wiernik, P. H. and Lichtenfeld, J. L. (1975). Combined modality therapy for localized Hodgkin's disease. A seven-year update of an early study. *Oncology* 32:208–213.

Wildner, G. P. and Eckert, H. (1965). Zur Morbiditätsstatistik der Lymphogranulomatose. Eine statistische Untersuchung von 1490 Fällen aus dem Krebskranken Register der Deutschen Demokratischen Republik. *Arch. Geschwulstforsch.* 26:216–222.

Wilimas, J., Thompson, E. and Smith, K. L. (1978). Value of serum copper levels and erythrocyte sedimentation rates as indicators of disease activity in children with Hodgkin's disease. *Cancer* 42:1929–1935.

Wiljasalo, S. (1969). Lymphographic polymorphism in Hodgkin's disease. Correlation of lymphography to histology and duration. *Acta Radiol.* (Supp.) 289:1–89.

Wilkey, I. S. (1973). Malignant lymphoma in Papua New Guinea: epidemiologic aspects. *J. Nat. Cancer Inst.* 50:1703–1711.

Wilks, Sir S. (1856). Cases of lardaceous disease and some allied affections, with remarks. *Guy's Hosp. Rep.* 17 (Ser. II, vol. 2):103–132.

Wilks, Sir S. (1865). Cases of enlargement of the lymphatic glands and spleen, (or, Hodgkin's Disease), with remarks. *Guy's Hosp. Rep.* 11:56–67.

Wilks, Sir S. (1909). A short account of the life and work of Thomas Hodgkin, M.D. *Guy's Hosp. Gaz.* 23:528–532.

Williams, L. H., Anastopulos, H. P. and Presant, C. A. (1969). Selective renal arteriography in Hodgkin's disease of the kidney. A case report. *Radiology* 93:1059–1060.

Williams, R. D., Andrews, M. C. and Zanes, R. P., Jr. (1951). Major surgery in Hodgkin's disease. *Surg. Gynec. Obst.* 93:636–640.

Williams, S. D. and Einhorn, L. H. (1977). Combination chemotherapy with doxorubicin and lomustine. Treatment of refractory Hodgkin's disease. *J.A.M.A.* 238:1659–1661.

Willson, J. K., Jr., Zaremba, J. L. and Pretlow, T. G., II. (1977). Functional characterization of cells separated from suspensions of Hodgkin's disease tumor cells in an isokinetic gradient. *Blood* 50:783–797.

Wilson, H. E. and Louis, J. (1967). The response of Hodgkin's disease to treatment with oral Vinblastine sulfate. *Ann. Int. Med.* 67:303–308.

Wilson, J. F., Marsa, G. W. and Johnson, R. E. (1972). Herpes zoster in Hodgkin's disease. Clinical, histologic, and immunologic correlations. *Cancer* 29:461–465.

Winawer, S. J. and Feldman, S. M. (1959). Amyloid nephrosis in Hodgkin's disease. *Arch. Int. Med.* 104:793–796.

Winchester, R. J., Fu, S. M., Hoffman, T. and Kunkel, H. G. (1975). IgG on lymphocyte surfaces: technical problems and the significance of a third cell population. *J. Immunol.* 114:1210–1212.

Winchester, R. J., Winfield, J. B., Siegal, F., Wernet, P., Bentwich, Z. and Kunkel, H. G. (1974). Analyses of lymphocytes from patients with rheumatoid arthritis and systemic lupus erythematosus. Occurrence of interfering cold-reactive antilymphocyte antibodies. *J. Clin. Invest.* 54:1082–1092.

Winkel, K. zum, Becker, J., Jahns, E., Scheurlen, H. and Herzfeld, U. (1967). Indikationsstellung und Dosimetrie bei der endolymphatischen Therapie mit J^{131}-Lipiodol. *Strahlenther.* 133:481–498.

Winkelstein, A., Mikulla, J. M., Sartiano, G. P. and Ellis, L. D. (1974). Cellular immunity in Hodgkin's disease: comparison of cutaneous reactivity and lymphoproliferative responses to phytohemagglutinin. *Cancer* 34:549–553.

Winterhalter, K. H. (1961). Verlauf und Prognose der Lymphogranulomatose anhand von 140 Fällen. Inaugural Dissertation. Zurich: Juris Verlag. (Cited by Westling, 1965.)

Wise, B. (1942). The sedimentation rate in Hodgkin's disease. *J. Lab. Clin. Med.* 27:1200–1206.

Wise, N. B. and Poston, M. A. (1940). Coexistence of brucella infection and Hodgkin's disease; clinical, bacteriologic and immunologic study. *J.A.M.A.* 115:1976–1984.

Wiseman, B. K. (1936). Blood picture in primary diseases

of lymphatic system; their character and significance. *J.A.M.A.* 107:2016–2022.

Witte, O. N., Weissman, I. L. and Kaplan, H. S. (1973). Structural characteristics of some murine RNA tumor viruses studied by lactoperoxidase iodination. *Proc. Nat. Acad. Sci. U.S.* 70:36–40.

Wolf, G. (1971). Verlaufskontrollen nach endolymphatischer radioisotopentherapie. *Strahlentherapie* 142:269–275.

Wolf, P., Dorfman, R., McClenahan, J. and Collins, F. (1970). False-positive infectious mononucleosis spot-test in lymphoma. *Cancer* 25:626–628.

Wood, H. F., Diamond, H. D., Craver, L. F., Pader, E. and Elster, S. K. (1958). Determination of C-reactive protein in the blood of patients with Hodgkin's disease. *Ann. Int. Med.* 48:823–833.

Woodall, J. P., Williams, M. C., Simpson, D. I. H. and Haddow, A. J. (1965). The isolation in mice of strains of herpes virus from Burkitt's tumours. *Europ. J. Cancer* 1:137–140.

World Health Organization. (1955). Mortality from Hodgkin's disease and from leukaemia and aleukaemia. *W.H.O. Epidemiol. and Vital Statist. Rep.* 8:81–114.

Wright, C. J. E. (1956). Hodgkin's paragranuloma. *Cancer* 9:773–777.

Wright, C. J. E. (1960). The "benign" form of Hodgkin's disease (Hodgkin's paragranuloma). *J. Path. Bact.* 80:157–171.

Wright, C. J. E. (1975). Death from Hodgkin's disease after 18 years' complete remission. *Cancer* 36:1132–1137.

Wright, D. (1967). The epidemiology of Burkitt's tumor. *Cancer Res.* 27:2424–2438.

Wright, D. H. (1973). Epidemiology and histology of Hodgkin's disease in Uganda. *Nat. Cancer Inst. Monograph* 36:25–30.

Wunderlich, C. A. (1858). Zwei Fälle von progressiven multiplen Lymphdrüsenhypertrophien. *Arch. physiol. Heilk.* 12:122–131.

Wybran, J., Carr, M. C. and Fudenberg, H. H. (1972). The human rosette-forming cell as a marker of a population of thymus-derived cells. *J. Clin. Invest.* 51:2537–2543.

Wychulis, A. R., Beahrs, O. H. and Woolner, L. B. (1966). Malignant lymphoma of the colon. A study of 69 cases. *Arch. Surg.* 93:215–225.

Yagoda, A., Mukherji, B., Young, C., Etcubanas, E., Lamonte, C., Smith, J. R., Tan, C. T. C. and Krakoff, I. H. (1972). Bleomycin, an antitumor antibiotic. *Ann. Int. Med.* 77:861–870.

Yam, L. T. and Li, C.-Y. (1976). Histogenesis of splenic lesions in Hodgkin's disease. *Am. J. Clin. Path.* 66:976–985.

Yang, Y. H. and Palmer, S. D. (1963). The morphology of Reed-Sternberg cells in bone marrow. *Am. J. Clin. Path.* 39:115–120.

Yates, J. L. (1922). Proper treatment of chronic malign diseases of the superficial lymph glands. *Arch. Surg.* 5:65–109.

Young, C. W. and Dowling, M. D., Jr. (1975). Antipyretic effect of cycloheximide, an inhibitor of protein synthesis, in patients with Hodgkin's disease or other malignant neoplasms. *Cancer Res.* 35:1218–1224.

Young, C., Eisinger, M. and Sanders, K. (1970). Growth of a cell line from a Hodgkin's disease node. *Proc. Am. Assoc. Cancer Res.* 11:86 (abst.).

Young, C. and Hodas, S. (1971a). Demonstration of a characteristic protein in plasma of febrile patients with Hodgkin's disease. *J. Clin. Invest.* 50:101A (abst.).

Young, C. W. and Hodas, S. (1971b). Excretion of a cationic protein in urine of febrile patients with Hodgkin's disease. *Proc. Am. Assoc. Cancer Res.* 12:37 (abst.).

Young, C. W., Hodas, S., Dessources, W. and Korngold, L. (1975). Observations on trace proteins in plasma of febrile patients by cationic disc electrophoresis in acrylamide gel at pH 3.8. *Cancer Res.* 35:1985–1990.

Young, C. W., MacDonald, R. N. and Karnofsky, D. A. (1964). Observations on effects of cycloheximide. *Proc. Am. Assoc. Cancer Res.* 5:263 (abst.).

Young, R. C., Canellos, G. P., Chabner, B. A., Hubbard, S. M. and De Vita, V. T., Jr. (1978). Patterns of relapse in advanced Hodgkin's disease treated with combination chemotherapy. *Cancer* 42:1001–1007.

Young, R. C., Canellos, G. P., Chabner, B. A., Schein, P. S. and De Vita, V. T. (1973a). Maintenance chemotherapy for advanced Hodgkin's disease in remission. *Lancet* 1:1339–1343.

Young, R. C., Corder, M. P., Berard, C. W. and De Vita, V. T. (1973b). Immune alterations in Hodgkin's disease. Effect of delayed hypersensitivity and lymphocyte transformation on course and survival. *Arch. Int. Med.* 131:446–454.

Young, R. C., Corder, M. P., Haynes, H. A. and De Vita, V. T. (1972). Delayed hypersensitivity in Hodgkin's disease. A study of 103 untreated patients. *Am. J. Med.* 52:63–72.

Young, R. C. and De Vita, V. T., Jr. (1976). Treatment of *Pneumocystis carinii* pneumonia: current status of the regimens of pentamidine isethionate and pyrimethamine-sulfadiazine. *Nat. Cancer Inst. Monogr.* 43:193–200.

Young, R. C., De Vita, V. T., Jr., Serpick, A. A. and Canellos, G. P. (1971). Treatment of advanced Hodgkin's disease with (1,3 bis(2-chloroethyl)-1-nitrosourea) BCNU. *New Engl. J. Med.* 285:475–479.

Yum, M. N., Edwards, J. L. and Kleit, S. (1975). Glomerular lesions in Hodgkin disease. *Arch. Path.* 99:645–649.

Zack, M. M., Jr., Heath, C. W., Jr., Andrews, M. D., Grivas, A. S., Jr. and Christine, B. W. (1977). High school contact among persons with leukemia and lymphoma. *J. Nat. Cancer Inst.* 59:1343–1349.

Zamecnik, P. C. and Long, J. C. (1977). Growth of cultured cells from patients with Hodgkin's disease and transplantation into *nude* mice. *Proc. Nat. Acad. Sci. U.S.* 74:754–758.

Zanes, R. P., Jr., Doan, C. A. and Hoster, H. A. (1948). Studies in Hodgkin's syndrome. VII. Nitrogen mustard therapy. *J. Lab. Clin. Med.* 33:1002–1018.

Zarembok, I. and Brace, K. C. (1972). Aorto-duodenal fistula following abdominal irradiation for Hodgkin's disease. A case report. *J. Canad. Assoc. Radiol.* 23:267–268.

Zarembok, I., Ramsey, H. E., Sutherland, J. and Serpick, A. A. (1972). Laparotomy and splenectomy in the staging of untreated patients with Hodgkin's disease. *Radiology* 102:673–678.

Zech, L., Haglund, U., Nilsson, K. and Klein, G. (1976). Characteristic chromosomal abnormalities in biopsies and lymphoid cell lines from patients with Burkitt and non-Burkitt lymphomas. *Internat. J. Cancer* 17:47–56.

Ziegler, J. B., Hansen, P. and Penny, R. (1975). Intrinsic lymphocyte defect in Hodgkin's disease: analysis of the phytohemagglutinin dose-response. *Cell. Immunol. Immunopath.* 3:451–460.

Ziegler, J. L., Bluming, A. Z., Fass, L., Magrath, I. T. and Templeton, A. C. (1972). Chemotherapy of childhood Hodgkin's disease in Uganda. *Lancet* 2:679–682.

Ziegler, K. (1911). Die Hodgkinsche Krankheit. Jena: Gustav Fischer.

Zorini, C. O., Neri, A., Comis, M., Mannella, E. and Paciucci, P. A. (1974). Influence of Hodgkin's serum on PHA stimulation of normal lymphocytes. *Lancet* 1: 745–746.

zur Hausen, H., Diehl, V., Wolf, H., Schulte-Holthausen, H. and Schneider, U. (1972). Occurrence of Epstein-Barr virus genomes in human lymphoblastoid cell lines. *Nature New Biol.* 237:189–190.

zur Hausen, H. and Schulte-Holthausen, H. (1970). Presence of EB virus nucleic acid homology in a "virus-free" line of Burkitt tumor cells. *Nature* 227:245–248.

ZuRhein, G. M. (1969). Association of papova-virions with a human demyelinating disease (progressive multifocal leukoencephalopathy). *Progr. Med. Virol.* 11: 185–247.

ZuRhein, G. M. and Chou, S. M. (1965). Particles resembling papova viruses in human cerebral demyelinating disease. *Science* 148:1477–1479.

Zwaan, F. E. and Speck, B. (1973). Acute myelomonocytic leukemia in a patient with Hodgkin's disease. *Acta Haematol.* 49:291–299.

Index